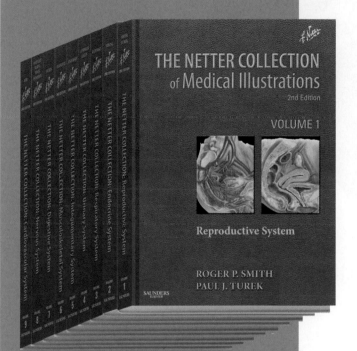

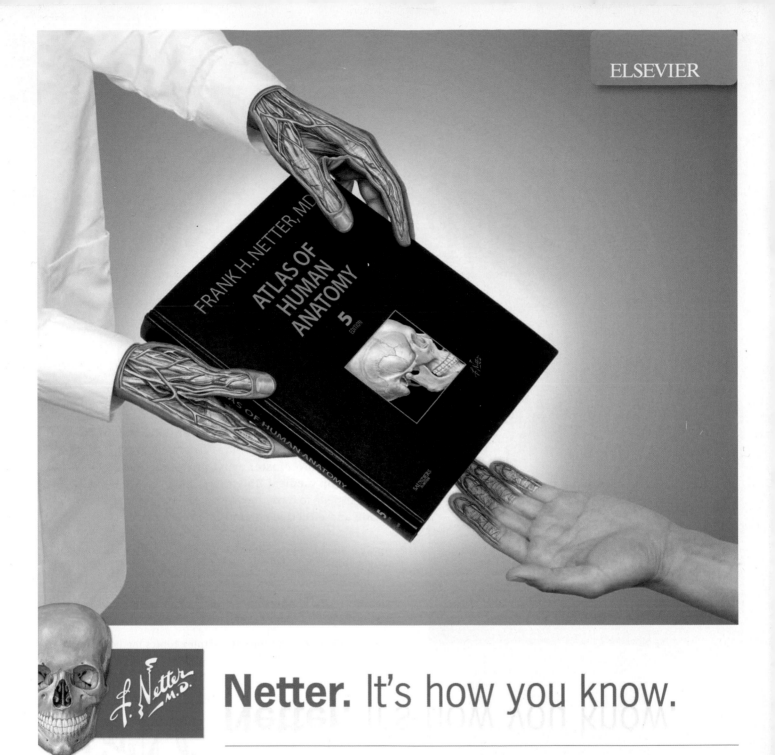

Netter's
Neurology
2nd edition

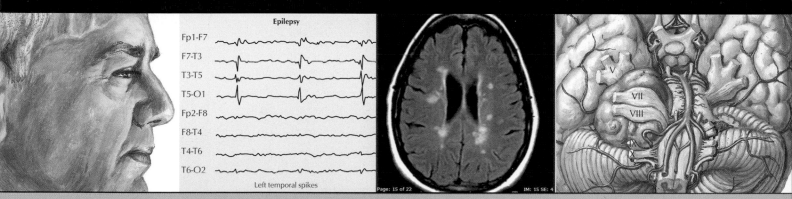

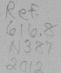
EDITOR-IN-CHIEF

H. ROYDEN JONES, JR., MD

Department of Neurology
Lahey Clinic
Burlington, Massachusetts;
Children's Hospital Boston
Boston, Massachusetts

EDITORS

JAYASHRI SRINIVASAN, MD, PhD

Department of Neurology
Lahey Clinic
Burlington, Massachusetts

GREGORY J. ALLAM, MD

Department of Neurology
Lahey Clinic
Burlington, Massachusetts

RICHARD A. BAKER, MD

Department of Radiology
Lahey Clinic
Burlington, Massachusetts

Illustrations by Frank H. Netter, MD

CONTRIBUTING ILLUSTRATORS

Carlos A. G. Machado, MD
John A. Craig, MD
James A. Perkins, MS, MFA
Anita Impagliazzo, MA, CMI

ELSEVIER
SAUNDERS

ELSEVIER
SAUNDERS

1600 John F. Kennedy Blvd.
Ste 1800
Philadelphia, PA 19103-2899

NETTER'S NEUROLOGY   ISBN: 978-1-4377-0273-6
Copyright © 2012 by Saunders, an imprint of Elsevier Inc.

Notices

ISBN: 978-1-4377-0273-6

Acquisitions Editor: Elyse O'Grady
Developmental Editor: Marybeth Thiel
Editorial Assistant: Chris Hazle-Cary
Publishing Services Manager: Patricia Tannian
Senior Project Manager: John Casey
Designer: Steven Stave

Printed in China

Last digit is the print number: 9 8 7 6 5 4 3 2 1

Dedication

To our dear patients and residents
*They taught us so much by providing unforgettable life
experiences in their own special way.
These special encounters continue to bring fond memories, very
poignantly motivating each of us.*

To our wonderful families:
*spouses, children, and grandchildren
with whom we each share a very extraordinary bond*

About the Artists

Frank H. Netter, MD

Frank Netter was born in 1906 in New York City. He studied art at the Art Student's League and the National Academy of Design before entering medical school at New York University, where he received his medical degree in 1931. During his student years, Dr. Netter's notebook sketches attracted the attention of the medical faculty and other physicians, allowing him to augment his income by illustrating articles and textbooks. He continued illustrating as a sideline after establishing a surgical practice in 1933, but he ultimately opted to give up his practice in favor of a full-time commitment to art. After service in the United States Army during World War II, Dr. Netter began his long collaboration with the CIBA Pharmaceutical Company (now Novartis Pharmaceuticals). This 45-year partnership resulted in the production of the extraordinary collection of medical art so familiar to physicians and other medical professionals worldwide.

In 2005 Elsevier, Inc., purchased the Netter Collection and all publications from Icon Learning Systems. There are now over 50 publications featuring the art of Dr. Netter available through Elsevier (in the US: www.us.elsevierhealth.com/Netter and outside the US: www.elsevierhealth.com).

Dr. Netter's works are among the finest examples of the use of illustration in the teaching of medical concepts. The 13-book *Netter Collection of Medical Illustrations*, which includes the greater part of the more than 20,000 paintings created by Dr. Netter, became and remains one of the most famous medical works ever published. *The Netter Atlas of Human Anatomy*, first published in 1989, presents the anatomical paintings from the Netter Collection. Now translated into 16 languages, it is the anatomy atlas of choice among medical and health professions students the world over.

The Netter illustrations are appreciated not only for their aesthetic qualities, but also, more important, for their intellectual content. As Dr. Netter wrote in 1949, "… clarification of a subject is the aim and goal of illustration. No matter how beautifully painted, how delicately and subtly rendered a subject may be, it is of little value as a *medical illustration* if it does not serve to make clear some medical point." Dr. Netter's planning, conception, point of view, and approach are what inform his paintings and what makes them so intellectually valuable.

Frank H. Netter, MD, physician and artist, died in 1991.

Learn more about the physician-artist whose work has inspired the Netter Reference collection: http://www.netterimages.com/artist/netter.htm.

Carlos A. G. Machado, MD

Carlos Machado was chosen by Novartis to be Dr. Netter's successor. He continues to be the main artist who contributes to the Netter collection of medical illustrations.

Self-taught in medical illustration, cardiologist Carlos Machado has contributed meticulous updates to some of Dr. Netter's original plates and has created many paintings of his own in the style of Netter as an extension of the Netter collection. Dr. Machado's photorealistic expertise and his keen insight into the physician-patient relationship informs his vivid and unforgettable visual style. His dedication to researching each topic and subject he paints places him among the premier medical illustrators at work today.

Learn more about his background and see more of his art at: http://www.netterimages.com/artist/machado.htm

About the Editors

H. Royden Jones, Jr., MD, was raised in semi-rural New Jersey but also frequently visited his grandmother, who lived a few blocks from the Atlantic Ocean. He graduated from Tufts College and Northwestern University Medical School, where during his first year he was intrigued by the introductory neuroanatomy course, which was particularly enhanced by his use of the first *Netter Nervous System* atlas and his teacher's presentation of active patients. Years later as Chair of the Alumni Advisory Board he received their Outstanding Service award.

After interning at the Philadelphia General Hospital, Royden began an internal medicine residency at the Mayo Clinic. He completed two years of internal medicine and took his last required rotation, neurology. This unexpectedly rekindled interests that began as a medical student, leading him to make a career shift from cardiology to neurology. One year later he volunteered for active duty, as a neurologist, with the United States Army Medical Corps, serving from 1966 to 1970 at the 5th General Hospital, Bad Cannstatt, Germany. Returning to Mayo, Royden completed his neurologic and clinical neurophysiology training.

In 1972 he joined the Lahey Clinic Neurology department, subsequently becoming their Chair and later the Chair of the Division of Medicine and Medical Specialties. Dr. Jones continues to practice at Lahey, where he holds the Jaime Ortiz-Patino chair in neurology. Currently his efforts are entirely dedicated to patient care and educational /clinical research pursuits. Royden is renowned for his astute clinical acumen and his compassionate care of patients. His wisdom is highly sought after by other physicians at Lahey, the surrounding community, as well as nationally. He is recognized as an exceptional teacher and has mentored numerous residents and fellows. His former students practice adult and pediatric neurology across the world. Dr. Jones developed the Lahey neurophysiology fellowship. A number of directors of EMG labs and several department chairs have been trained by Royden.

After having joined the Children's Hospital Boston neurology department, Royden was asked to develop their clinical electromyography laboratory in 1978. This presented an interesting challenge, since there was little written in the field of pediatric electromyography. Keeping careful prospective files of every patient studied there, Dr. Jones subsequently co-authored and edited three major texts of childhood clinical neurophysiology and neuromuscular disorders.

Dr. Jones is a Clinical Professor of Neurology at Harvard Medical School and a Lecturer at Tufts University School of Medicine. He served as a Director of the American Board of Psychiatry and Neurology from 1997 to 2004 and concomitantly was a member of the Residency Review Council of the Accreditation Council for Graduate Medical Education. He has served on the editorial boards of *Neurology Continuum* and *Muscle and Nerve* and is a reviewer for many neurologic journals. Dr. Jones was the recipient of the Distinguished Physician Award of the American Association of Neuromuscular and Electrodiagnostic Medicine in 2007 and the Frank Lahey award of the Lahey Clinic Staff Association of 2010.

In his free time Royden is a photographer and an amateur sea and landscape artist. He particularly enjoys opportunities to photograph his family, as well as record the magnificence of nature at the 40-mile long Moosehead Lake lying within the mountains of northwestern Maine. Here he spends part of his summer on remote Deer Island with his wife, four children, and five grandchildren. His daughter is a former prosecutor in Manhattan, and one of his sons is a college professor at the University of Rochester. His other two sons are physicians; one practices emergency medicine at a community hospital in suburban Boston, and his youngest son is the A. Bernard Ackerman Professor of the Culture of Medicine conjointly at Harvard College and Harvard Medical School. Their family particularly enjoys skiing, kayaking, and hiking together.

Jayashri Srinivasan, MD, PhD, grew up in Chennai, India, where she graduated from Stanley Medical College. She initially pursued her postgraduate training in Cardiff, Wales, where she received a doctorate in neurophysiology, as well as completing a residency in internal medicine and becoming a Fellow of the Royal College of Physicians (FRCP), United Kingdom. Jayashri moved to Boston to train at the Tufts neurology program; subsequently she completed a fellowship in neuromuscular disorders at Brigham & Women's Hospital and Harvard Medical School. She briefly returned to the Tufts faculty at Tufts Medical Center but soon thereafter moved to the Lahey Clinic in 2003. Jayashri is an associate professor of neurology at Tufts University School of Medicine.

At Lahey Dr. Srinivasan specializes in neuromuscular medicine, where she is a very skilful clinical neurophysiologist with particular interests in electromyography and autonomic disorders. She is director of the clinic's electromyography laboratory, the Lahey neuromuscular fellowship, as well as director of their Muscular Dystrophy Association clinic. Dr. Srinivasan has presented a number of papers at major North American neurologic societies and has written significantly within the neuromuscular field. When she is not practicing neurology, Jayashri devotes almost all of her free time to her family—her husband Bala, a nephrologist at Tufts, and their 2 children, a daughter in college at MIT, and a son in high school.

Gregory J. Allam, MD, has a dad and brother who are also physicians. Greg received his medical degree from the American University of Beirut before coming to Boston to pursue his neurology training though the Tufts University program, with additional training in EMG/neuromuscular disease and acute care neurology at the Saint Elizabeth's Medical Center in Boston. Greg joined the Lahey Clinic neurology department in 1997 as a member of the neurovascular team with interests in critical care neurology, as well as a skillful electromyographer. While at Lahey Greg was recognized as an astute and caring physician, especially by his many challenging patients whom he followed for their spasticity where his very careful Botox ministrations were often very successful.

Dr. Allam recently joined the Brigham and Woman's Hospital in Boston and is director of stroke care at the South Shore Hospital in South Weymouth, Massachusetts. He is a clinical instructor at the Harvard Medical School and lives in the Suburban Boston area with his wife Christina, an endocrinologist at Children's Hospital Boston, and their two young children.

Richard A. Baker, MD, was raised in rural Ohio and graduated from the College of Wooster and the Case Western Reserve Medical School in Cleveland. He interned at King County Hospital, Seattle, Washington, and began an internal medicine residency there. This was interrupted by service as a physician in the US Air Force. During his military tour Dick was stationed in Greenland, where in addition to his service responsibilities he also volunteered to care for the native Inuits. He then pursued a residency in radiology, initially at the University of Rochester, and then later at the Peter Bent Brigham Hospital in Boston for another year of radiology followed by a fellowship in neuroradiology there and at the Children's Hospital Boston. After completion of his training, Dr. Baker joined the staff of the Peter Bent Brigham Hospital and Harvard Medical School. The Lahey Clinic recruited him as their first neuroradiologist in 1978. Dick helped to develop this section and later became radiology department chairman, as well as president of the Lahey medical staff. He is currently an Associate Professor of Radiology at Tufts University School of Medicine.

His wisdom and clinical acumen are greatly appreciated and highly sought after at Lahey. Dick was a major force in the development of the first volume of *Netter's Nervous System, Part II, Neurologic and Neuromuscular Disorders* published in 1986 and the first edition of *Netter's Neurology*, published in 2005.

Dick has two children, one who followed in the footsteps of her mother as an infectious disease physician at Massachusetts General Hospital and Harvard, and a son who is working on his doctorate. Dr. Baker is a master gardener and a skilled woodworker, something he is pursuing with vigor now that he is working part time. He also enjoys a variety of outdoor activities with his wife, including skiing and hiking.

Acknowledgments

First and foremost I must thank Jaime Ortiz-Patino, my dear friend who underwrote the Jaime Ortiz-Patino Chair in Neurology at Lahey. This funding has provided me time to devote to this project. Equally important once again, my wonderful wife, Mary, has put up with my very frequent weekend and evening presence behind a laptop computer in our family room. Similarly, Jayashri, Greg, and Dick acknowledge the support and understanding of their families in bringing this project to completion. My many Lahey Clinic colleagues, in particular Paul T. Gross, MD, our department chairman, have been most gracious in their enthusiastic support of this project. The Elsevier team, including Marybeth Thiel, John Casey, Elyse O'Grady, and Carolyn Kruse, has always been very responsive and gracious in working with us. We are most appreciative of their expertise and support.

Foreword

Neurologic problems are among the most frequent encountered in medicine. The trainee in neurology, whether a medical student or resident, often has difficulty in fully grasping the subject, in part because of the complexities of the anatomy and physiology involved and in part also because of the mystery that still enshrouds the brain. The amazing advances made in the neurosciences over the past quarter century have, on the one hand, helped the clinician in the management of individual patients and, on the other hand, increased wonder about the elegance of cerebral function. The current edition is intended as a resource to aid students endeavoring to understand neurology and to keep up with advances in the field.

Netter's Neurology was first published in 2005 and met with immediate acceptance. Edited by H. Royden Jones, Jr., a clinical professor of neurology at Harvard Medical School, holder of the Jaime Ortiz-Patino chair in neurology at the Lahey Clinic, and one of the outstanding clinical neurologists of his generation, the book presented a concise account of the subject, illustrated by the renowned medical artwork of Frank Netter and others. Rapid advances in the field have underscored the need for a second edition of the book, however, and it is with especial pleasure that I welcome its publication.

The new edition is broader in scope than the earlier one, but improved design and an alteration in trim size have reduced the overall number of pages. Every chapter has been updated and many have been rewritten almost completely to incorporate the accumulated wisdom of recent years and provide more details on treatment. They contain numerous clinical vignettes exemplifying important points, such as clues to the site of the lesion, the features characterizing the typical course of a particular disorder, the investigative approach to clarify the likely diagnosis, and the optimal management plan. These vignettes focus the attention of readers on details that might otherwise be overlooked and help to make the volume clinically relevant, a feature that medical students will find particularly appealing. The artwork, too, has been updated, benefitting from the advances in neuroimaging in recent years. The illustrations, and particularly the rich color plates that made Frank Netter the premier medical artist of his time, help to convey to the reader an understanding of clinical neurology and its scientific underpinnings that it is hard to obtain with such facility elsewhere.

Dr. H. Royden Jones, the editor, is joined by three co-editors for this new edition. The authors of the individual chapters are drawn from the current or former staff of the Lahey Clinic, and many are former trainees of the senior editor. They are rich in clinical experience, and this is reflected in the text, where a practical approach to the evaluation and management of neurologic disorders is described with enviable clarity.

Readers will benefit greatly from this account of clinical neurology with its clear, flowing prose, amplified by the remarkably beautiful artwork contained within the volume. Together, the text and artwork will give students a firm grasp of the fundamentals of the subject. I congratulate the editors on their achievement in producing such an important addition to the medical literature.

Michael J. Aminoff, MD, DSc, FRCP
Distinguished Professor of Neurology
University of California, San Francisco

Preface

The second edition of *Netter's Neurology* speaks to the perpetuity of Frank Netter's incomparable artistic genius and educational vision. During my first year at Northwestern University Medical School we were forewarned as to how difficult the introductory neuroanatomy course was going to be, "the toughest one" that we would face. A few upperclassmen told me to purchase the *Netter Atlas of Neurosciences* and it would all fall into place. Indeed it did, and I became interested in a career in neurology. However, in 1960 when I discussed the possibility of a neurologic career with Northwestern's chairman of their combined psychiatry and neurology department, he told me that one could not make a living as a neurologist; instead I would need to eventually primarily practice Freudian psychiatry while just dabbling in neurology! That was not for me. A few years later my internal medicine residency at Mayo required 3 months of neurology; this was so interesting and intellectually challenging that I switched my career plans to neurology and gave up plans to become a cardiologist.

Having continued to be impressed with Dr. Netter's skillful renditions of many medical subjects, as presented in his semimonthly Ciba Symposia, some years later I enquired at an AMA meeting, where these were on display, as to whether he might have interest in illustrating the various mononeuropathies. Never did I think this suggestion would be transmitted directly to Dr. Netter. However, less than a year later, in 1982, I received a letter from him asking me to elaborate my ideas. I soon found myself visiting Dr. Netter at his new studio in Palm Beach. This was an undreamed of opportunity, especially as one of my hobbies includes rather amateur attempts at oil and water color painting. After a few visits with Frank, who was a very gracious and kind gentleman, he asked me to help him revise his *Neurologic and Neuromuscular Disorders* of his two-volume *Netter Nervous System* atlas, the very one that had so impressed me during my first-year neuroanatomy course. We spent many 3-day weekends together as he listened to my ideas as to how best illustrate each subject. The typical Netter day began in his studio at 7 AM … Frank always had a cigar going, and in self-defense I kept a pipe well stoked. With much help from some dear colleagues, this was published in 1986.

We planned to update this text every 6 to 8 years; however, with Frank's death in 1991 and Ciba Pharmaceutical's merging into Novartis, ongoing revisions seemed to be relegated to the publishing tundra. Much to my delight in 2000 Icon Publishers contacted me after they had purchased the rights to use the Netter paintings. Their vision led to the development of a number of more traditional, specialty oriented textbooks, and I had the honor of editing the first neurology edition in this more classic format.

Now 52 years after my introduction to Dr. Netter's artwork, we are finishing my third text utilizing his magnificent paintings and are already proceeding to a new edition of his *Neurosciences* atlas. On this occasion I have asked three colleagues to co-edit this volume with me. My dear friend, Richard Baker, a highly esteemed clinical neuroradiologist, has provided the neuroradiologic images for both of our earlier Netter texts. Concomitantly I recruited two outstanding younger Lahey colleagues, Jayashri Srinivasan and Gregory Allam, as our other co-editors. Both are master clinicians who are highly respected for their clinical acumen and teaching abilities. It has been an honor to work with both of them for more than a decade. As with the first edition of *Netter's Neurology* all of the authors have a Lahey Clinic heritage either as a current staff member, a former fellow, or former staff. This seemingly parochial approach has allowed us to minimize duplication and, more important, ensure the reader that what is discussed herein represents the latest approach to the patient with a clinical neurologic problem.

As Frank Netter often stated to me "a picture is worth a thousand words." Indeed they are, and his magnificent plates provide the foundation for this monograph. However, when conceiving the overall format for the first edition of *Netter's Neurology* it was very important for me not only to include an overview of a neurologic condition but also to use clinical case vignettes, particularly since these are my most effective means of teaching. Case-based methodologies are currently used at a number of medical schools; we have aimed this volume to complement such for both the undergraduate medical student as well as residents. My first neuroscience teachers at Northwestern very effectively used patient presentations to bring life to the complexities of basic neurologic anatomy and physiology. This didactic approach was very well received by the beginning student and resident alike in the first edition of *Netter's Neurology*. We also think that the practicing clinical neurologist will find this combination of basic anatomy and clinical neurology to be a refreshing alternative to the various forms of clinical review now available for our required recertification process. Concomitantly my co-editors and I hope that the internal medical resident and the general internist will find the blending of Netter paintings with clinical medicine to be similarly useful.

Every chapter in this second edition has been carefully reviewed and in most instances significantly rewritten. The total number of chapters was reduced, as we combined some subjects into one broader area. Many new vignettes have been added, and in a number of instances we replaced some of those in the first edition. The plates have a number of new MR images, and some are reedited in their entirety. New plates have also been added. Elsevier has changed the overall format to a standard text size that provides a slimmer volume. As in the first edition this is not a source for specific pharmacologic dosing, as such is an ever evolving standard. We are excited to be able to present this volume and are particularly pleased to be able to take advantage of the many publishing attributes that the Elsevier/Saunders staff brings to the table.

H. Royden Jones, Jr., MD
June 5, 2011

Contributors

Lloyd M. Alderson, MD
Department of Neurosurgery
Lahey Clinic
Burlington, Massachusetts

Timothy D. Anderson, MD
Department of Otolaryngology
Lahey Clinic
Burlington, Massachusetts

Diana Apetauerova, MD
Department of Neurology
Lahey Clinic
Burlington, Massachusetts

Jeffrey E. Arle, MD, PhD
Department of Neurosurgery
Lahey Clinic
Burlington, Massachusetts

Ritu Bagla
Department of Neurology
Lahey Clinic
Burlington, Massachusetts

Ted M. Burns, MD
University of Virginia Health Sciences
Department of Neurology
Charlottesville, Virginia

Ann Camac, MD
Department of Neurology
Lahey Clinic
Lexington, Massachusetts

Peter J. Catalano, MD
Department of Otolaryngology
Lahey Clinic
Burlington, Massachusetts

Claudia J. Chaves, MD
Department of Neurology
Lahey Clinic
Lexington, Massachusetts

Ellen Choi, MD
Attending Anesthesiologist
Santa Clara Valley Medical Center
San Jose, California

G. Rees Cosgrove, MD
Professor and Chairman
Department of Neurosurgery
Brown University Medical School
Providence, Rhode Island

Donald E. Craven, MD
Chairman, Department of Infectious Diseases
Lahey Clinic
Burlington, Massachusetts;
Professor of Medicine
Tufts University School of Medicine
Boston, Massachusetts

Carlos A. David, MD
Department of Neurosurgery
Lahey Clinic
Burlington, Massachusetts

Peter K. Dempsey, MD
Department of Neurosurgery
Lahey Clinic
Burlington, Massachusetts

Robert A. Duncan, MD
Department of Infectious Diseases
Lahey Clinic
Burlington, Massachusetts

Stephen R. Freidberg, MD
Department of Neurosurgery
Lahey Clinic
Burlington, Massachusetts

Paul T. Gross, MD
Chairman, Department of Neurology
Lahey Clinic
Burlington, Massachusetts

Jose A. Gutrecht
Department of Neurology
Lahey Clinic
Burlington, Massachusetts

Gisela Held, MD
Department of Neurology
Lahey Clinic Northshore
Peabody, Massachusetts

Doreen Ho
Department of Neurology
Lahey Clinic
Burlington, Massachusetts

Kinan K. Hreib, MD, PhD
Department of Neurology
Lahey Clinic
Burlington, Massachusetts

Allison Gudis Jackson, MS, CCC-SLP
Greenwich, Connecticut

Samuel E. Kalluvya, MD
Bugando Medical Centre
Mwanza, Tanzania

Johannes B. Kataraihya, MD
Bugando Medical Centre
Mwanza, Tanzania

Kenneth Lakritz, MD
Department of Psychiatry
Lahey Clinic
Burlington, Massachusetts

Julie Leegwater-Kim, MD, PhD
Department of Neurology
Lahey Clinic
Burlington, Massachusetts

Juliana Lockman
University of Virginia Health Sciences
Department of Neurology
Charlottesville, Virginia

Marie C. Lucey
Clinical Director
Gorden College Center for Balance, Mobility, and Wellness
Wenham, Massachusetts

Caitlin Macaulay, PhD
Department of Neurology
Lahey Clinic
Burlington, Massachusetts

Subu N. Magge, MD
Department of Neurosurgery
Lahey Clinic
Burlington, Massachusetts

John Markman, MD
Departments of Neurology and Anesthesiology
Lahey Clinic
Burlington, Massachusetts

Ippolit C. A. Matjucha, MD
Former Neuro-ophthalmologist
Lahey Clinic
Burlington, Massachusetts

Michelle Mauermann
Consultant in Neurology
Assistant Professor of Neurology
Mayo Clinic
Rochester, Minnesota

Daniel P. McQuillen, MD
Department of Infectious Diseases
Lahey Clinic
Burlington, Massachusetts

Eva M. Michalakis, MS
Department of Otolaryngology
Lahey Clinic
Burlington, Massachusetts

Carol Moheban, MD
Lahey Clinic Northshore

Mary Anne Muriello, MD
Department of Neurology
Lahey Clinic
Burlington, Massachusetts

Winnie W. Ooi
Department of Infectious Diseases
Lahey Clinic
Burlington, Massachusetts

Joel M. Oster, MD
Department of Neurology
Lahey Clinic
Burlington, Massachusetts

E. Prather Palmer, MD
Emeritus Staff
Department of Neurology
Lahey Clinic
Burlington, Massachusetts

Robert Peck, MD
Bugando Medical Centre
Mwanza, Tanzania

Dana Penney, MD
Department of Neurology
Lahey Clinic
Burlington, Massachusetts

James A. Russell, DO
Department of Neurology
Lahey Clinic
Burlington, Massachusetts

Monique M. Ryan, MB BS, M Med, FRACP
Royal Children's Hospital
Murdoch Children's Research Institute
Melbourne Australia

Clemens M. Schirmer
Director of Cerebrovascular and Endovascular Neurosurgery
Baystate Medical Center
Assistant Professor
Department of Neurosurgery
Tufts University School of Medicine
Boston, Massachusetts

Miruna Segarceanu, MD
Department of Neurology
Dartmouth-Hitchcock Clinic
Manchester, New Hampshire

Matthew Tilem, MD
Department of Neurology
Lahey Clinic
Burlington, Massachusetts

Michal Vytopil, MD
Department of Neurology
Lahey Clinic
Burlington, Massachusetts

Judith White, MD
Head, Section of Vestibular and Balance Disorders
Head and Neck Institute
Cleveland Clinic
Cleveland, Ohio

Yuval Zabar, MD
Department of Neurology
Lahey Clinic
Burlington, Massachusetts

Isabel A. Zacharias, MD
Transplant Department
Lahey Clinic
Burlington, Massachusetts

Contents

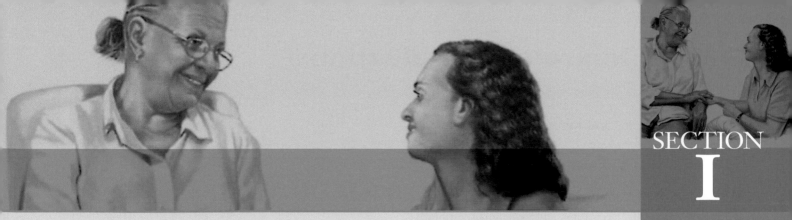

Initial Clinical Evaluation

Clinical Neurologic Evaluation

H. Royden Jones, Jr., and Kinan Hreib

*T*he neurologic sciences are the most intellectually challenging, unequivocally fascinating, and tremendously stimulating of the various clinical disciplines. Initially, the vast intricacies of basic neuroanatomy and neurophysiology often seem overwhelming to both medical student and neuroscience resident alike. However, eventually the various portions of this immense knowledge base come together in a discernible pattern, not unlike a Seurat canvas. Often one is expanding or revisiting our neurologic base as we are challenged by variations on the theme of our previous experiences. It is the keen observation and coding of these clinical experiences that leads the astute neurologic physician to solve new patient challenges.

One must first and foremost be an astute historian initially listening very carefully to the patient. Most often the intricacies, as well as the subtleties, of the neurologic history provide the essential foundation leading to a rational and structured neurologic examination as well as the appropriate diagnostic testing. Although it is easy to define the requisite methodology to examine the neurologic patient, it is much more challenging to similarly address the history acquisition other than making a few generalities. One of the most important elements of neurologic training is the opportunity for the student and the resident to observe senior neurologists evaluate a patient. As a resident, this was absolutely one of our most important learning experiences. Too often the student does not appreciate the elegance illustrated by a carefully derived neurologic clinical history. A major attribute of a skillful and successful neurologist is being an astute listener. This requires the neurologist to bring together various seemingly disparate and subtle data from the patient's various concerns and then focus on this information with specific questions to decide on its relevance to the issues at hand. Understanding the temporal profile of the patient's symptoms is crucial; were the symptoms' onset acute and stable or have they followed an ingravescent course? Very often, this information provides a most important perspective that is one of the very important keys to diagnosis.

Clinical Vignette

A 42-year-old woman with juvenile autoimmune diabetes mellitus came for further investigation of her extremely painful neuropathy initially presumed secondary to diabetes, or possibly to recent chemotherapy for breast cancer. However, her temporal profile was the final clue to her diagnosis. On careful review of the onset of her symptoms, it was found that she had never had the slightest hint of intolerable paresthesiae until awakening from her mastectomy. Her pain had begun precipitously in the recovery room. It was steady from its inception and totally incapacitating in this previously vigorous woman whose favorite pastime was backpacking in mountainous national forests. This temporal profile was in total contradistinction to any

symmetric diabetic or antineoplastic chemotherapy-related polyneuropathy. These disorders always have a clinical course of a subtle onset and very gradual evolution.

With this information, we investigated what transpired at the time of her breast surgery when she awakened with this extremely limiting painful neuropathy. In fact, she had had a general anesthetic with nitrous oxide (N_2O) induction. This N_2O uncovered a second autoimmune disorder, namely vitamin B_{12} deficiency. The anesthetic had precipitously led to symptoms in this previously clinically silent process. Fortunately, vitamin B_{12} replacement led to total resolution of her symptoms.

Comment: In this instance, her initial physicians had let themselves be trapped by what was familiar to them because diabetes is the most common cause for a painful neuropathy. However, only rarely does it lead to a precipitous onset of symptoms. The fine-tuning of this patient's temporal profile, especially the abrupt onset of symptoms, led us to seek a more detailed history as to whether some toxic process was operative. Review of the operative records per se led to the diagnosis when the suspicion of nitrous oxide intoxication was confirmed.

Most neurologic disorders follow a well-defined clinical paradigm. However, it is their very broad clinical perspective that continually challenges the astute neurologic clinician to maintain a vigilant intellectual posture. When these specific clinical subtleties are appreciated, the clinician is rewarded with the knowledge of having done the very best for his or her patient as well as having the intellectual rewards for being on the cutting edge of the clinical neurosciences. The skillful clinician, taking a very careful history, is the one most able to recognize the attributes of something quite uncommon presenting in a fashion more easily confused with more mundane afflictions.

For example, numbness or tingling in a patient's hand most commonly represents entrapment of the median nerve at the wrist, reflecting the presence of a very common disorder known as the *carpal tunnel syndrome*. However symptoms of this type may occasionally represent early signs of a pathologic lesion at the level of the brachial plexus, nerve root, spinal cord, or brain per se. It is imperative for the clinician to always consider a broad anatomic perspective in each patient evaluation. When this approach is not carefully followed, less common, and potentially treatable disorders may not be diagnosed in a timely fashion. It is absolutely imperative that no compromise be made in obtaining a thorough and accurate history when first meeting the patient. This is the most important interchange the physician will have. It needs to be taken in a relaxed, hopefully noninterrupted setting allowing for privacy. Additionally, it is very important to invite the spouse, parent, or significant other into the room. Rarely will a patient object to same; having another close observer of a patient's difficulties available can provide insight that may be essential to diagnosis. A thorough initial evaluation engenders a patient-family sense of trust in the physician as a detailed history, with a careful examination demonstrates a major commitment. Once developed, this clinical setting encourages the patient to communicate openly with their physician as they outline their diagnostic plans and eventually a treatment formulation. This chapter provides a foundation that will serve as an anchor for both the student and resident as they learn the art and science of the performance of detailed neurologic evaluations.

NEUROLOGIC HISTORY AND EXAMINATION

An accurate history requires paying attention to detail, often observing the patient's demeanor while reading the patient's body language, having the opportunity to witness the patient's difficulties, and interviewing family members. History taking is a special art and science in its own right. It is a skill that requires ongoing additions to one's own interviewing techniques. Listening to the patient is a most important part of this exercise; it is something that can be more time consuming than current clinical practice "time allowed guidelines" provide for within various patient settings. This approach provides the diagnostic keystone that often distinguishes an astute clinician's ability to find a diagnosis where others have failed.

A complete neurologic examination also requires carefully honed acquired skills. For example, the ability to decide whether the patient is truly weak and not giving way, or similarly does or does not have a Babinski sign present, often makes the difference between arriving at a correct diagnosis. The ability to define a sensory loss at a spinal cord level is another very crucial exercise.

One of the most challenging clinical scenarios occurs with the patient who has already seen another clinical neurologist and no diagnosis has been made. The patient is frustrated, as often was his or her prior neurologist. To be fair to the patient, as well as oneself, when evaluating such an individual seeking another neurologic opinion it is important to gain one's own initial and totally unbiased history and examination. Furthermore, in order to prevent unwelcome bias, the new neurologist should avoid reading other colleagues' notes or looking at previous neurologic images prior to gaining his or her own history and performing the examinations.

Although time-consuming, the history is the most important factor leading to accurate diagnoses. One of the essential attributes of a skillful neurologist is the ability to be a good listener so as not to miss crucial historic points. It is important to begin the initial meeting by asking patients why they have come; this offers them the opportunity to express concerns in their own words. If at all possible, the neurologist should not interrupt, thus providing the patient the opportunity to provide their primary concerns to the neurologist, emphasizing the symptoms of greatest importance. Rarely, anxious or compulsive patients may speak of their concerns at great length; with experience, physicians learn to make discreet interjections to maintain control of the evaluation and draw the patient back from extraneous tangents.

When the patient's primary concerns are established, specific issues can be explored. Additionally, making careful observations during the review of history allows better focus for subsequent questions. An accurate baseline assessment of mental status and language can be obtained from listening to the patient and observing responses to questions. It is through listening that the clinician gains insight into the patient's real concerns. For example, it is not unusual to see a patient referred to a neurologist for evaluation of headaches, which only became exacerbated with the recent discovery of a brain tumor in someone known to the patient.

Unfortunately, the economics of modern health care has forced primary care physicians and specialists to shorten visit times with patients and their families. One must be fastidious not to use diagnostic tools, such as magnetic resonance imaging (MRI), as substitutes for careful clinical history and examination. The current detailed medical information available on the Internet, in conjunction with a more sophisticated basic health education environment, has indeed enhanced patients' knowledge bases, although not always in a balanced format. Patient expectations sometimes affect the diagnostic approach of physicians. In this environment, it is not surprising that imaging techniques such as MRI and computed tomography (CT) have replaced or supplemented a significant portion of clinical judgment. However, even the most dramatic test findings may prove irrelevant without appropriate clinical correlation. To have patients unnecessarily undergo surgery because of MRI findings that have no relation to their complaints may lead to a tragic outcome. Therein lies the importance of gaining a complete understanding of the clinical issues.

Although neurology may seem in danger of being subsumed by overreliance on highly sophisticated diagnostic studies, this needs to be kept in perspective as many of these innovations have greatly improved our diagnostic skills and therapeutic capacities. For example, much knowledge regarding the early recognition, progression, and response to treatment of multiple sclerosis (MS) depends on careful MRI imaging.

It is essential to make patients feel comfortable in the office, particularly by fostering a positive interpersonal relationship. Taking time to ask about patients' lives, education, and social habits often provides useful clues. A careful set of questions providing a general review of systems may lead to the key diagnostic clue that focuses the evaluation. When the patient develops a sense of confidence and rapport with an empathetic physician, he or she is more willing to return for follow-up, even if a diagnosis is not made at the initial evaluation. Sometimes a careful second or third examination reveals a crucial historic or examination difference that leads to a specific diagnosis. Follow-up visits also allow the patient and physician to have another conversation regarding the symptoms and concerns. Some patients may come to their first office visit with an exhaustive list of concerns and symptoms, whereas others provide minimal information. Subsequent visits are therefore intended not only to discuss the results of tests but also to clarify the symptoms and or response to treatment. If patients feel rushed on their first visit, they may not return for follow-up, thus denying the neurologist a chance at crucial diagnostic observations. The physician–patient relationship must always be carefully nurtured and highly respected.

APPROACH TO THE NEUROLOGIC EVALUATION

Throughout training, examination skills are continually being amplified as the resident is exposed to an ever-evolving clinical experience. One of the most important is the opportunity to observe the varied skill sets demonstrated by academic neurologists as they approach different types of patients. One of the essentials for appropriate interpretation of the neurologic patient evaluation is learning how to elicit important, sometimes subtle, clues to diagnosis; an appreciation of what is "normal" at different ages is also important. A hasty history and examination can be misleading. For example, briskly preserved ankle reflexes in an elderly patient is not normal, whereas moderately diminished vibration sense is normal at the ankles. For example, a diagnosis of early MS may be missed by not asking about such things as previous problems with visual function, shooting electric paresthesiae when bending the neck (Lhermitte sign), or sphincter problems manifested by increasing urgency to urinate.

Even though carpal tunnel syndrome is the most common cause for a patient to experience a numb hand, one must always be fastidious not to overlook other potential pathoanatomic sites, such as within the peripheral nervous system at the level of the more proximal median nerve, the brachial plexus, or the cervical nerve root. In another instance, the failure to undress a patient whom one suspects to have a presumably benign cause for a numb hand, that is, carpal tunnel syndrome, may preclude the examining physician from recognizing the presence of an unexpected positive Babinski response indicative of a central nervous system (CNS) lesion. Similarly, identifying a sensory level is indicative of a myelopathy as the pathophysiologic explanation for the patient's numb hand. Lastly the finding that the sensory loss in the fingers primarily involves position sense and stereognosis becomes the entre to examine the cerebral cortex as the site for these complaints.

Another important outcome from performing a complete neurologic examination at the initial evaluation in almost every patient is that this not only establishes the patient's current status but will provide a baseline for future comparison. There are certain "normal" asymmetries in many individuals, often not previously appreciated by the patient per se or his or her relatives. These may include a patient's slightly asymmetric smile, somewhat irregular pupils, or hint of ptosis. However, at times such findings do take on significant meaning. As an example, a middle-aged woman was thought to have benign tension headaches. This was based on a "normal" neurologic exam elsewhere. However she had an asymmetric smile that previously had not been appreciated. Imaging studies identified a frontal lobe tumor contralateral to her weakness. Thus, the careful observation of seemingly subtle clinical findings may prove to have significant bearing on the issue at hand. Even when these findings are proven to be "normal variants," clear documentation may often be very helpful during the course of the patient's illness or later on when new concerns occur. In that setting, the prior definition of what proves to be a normal asymmetry will prevent erroneous conclusions from being developed.

Formulation

One of the most intellectually challenging aspects of neurology relates to the neurologist's ability to amalgamate the historical and physical findings into a unitary hypothesis. One needs to first consider the multiple neuroanatomic sites that can potentially explain the patient's clinical presentation. Subsequently, this is placed in the perspective of the clinical temporal profile of symptom occurrence. Did all of the patient's symptoms begin abruptly, as usually seen with a stroke but sometimes with a tumor or demyelinating process? Or was there an evolution of degree of clinical loss or did new features gradually get added to the patient's findings as is characteristic of certain neoplastic lesions and sometimes more diffuse vasculitides. Formulation can be hindered by the patient's inability to provide an accurate history or participate in the neurologic examination. One of the more subtle and difficult conditions to recognize is anosognosia to one's illness, as may occur in patients with right parietal brain injury. Under these circumstances, the patient may not have sensory, visual, or motor neglect, but unawareness of cognitive, emotional, and other functional limitations. Family interview is most important in this setting.

Overview and Basic Tenets

The neurologic examination begins the moment the patients get out of their seat to be greeted, the character of their smile or lack thereof, and subsequently as they walk to enter the neurologist's office. An excellent opportunity to judge the patient's language function and cognitive abilities occurs during the acquisition of the patient's history. Concurrently, the neurologist is always attuned to carefully making observations in order to identify various clinical signs. Some are overt movements (tremors, restlessness, dystonia or dyskinesia); others are subtler, e.g., vitiligo, implying a potential for a neurologic autoimmune disorder. Equally important may be the lack of normal movements, as seen in patients with Parkinson disease. By the time the neurologist completes the examination, she or he must be able to categorize and organize these historical and examination findings into a carefully structured diagnostic formulation.

The subsequent definition of the formal examination may be subdivided into a few major sections. Speech and language are assessed during the history taking. The cognitive part of the examination is often clearly defined with the initial history and often does not require formal mental status testing. However there are a number of clinical neurologic settings where this evaluation is very time consuming and complicated; Chapter 2 is dedicated to this aspect of the patient evaluation. However, when there is no clinical suspicion of either a cognitive or language dysfunction, these more formal testing modalities are not specifically required.

Here the multisystem neurologic examination provides a careful basis for most essential clinical evaluations. Neurologists in training and their colleagues in practice cannot expect to test all possible cognitive elements in each patient that they evaluate. Certain basic elements are required; most of these are readily observable or elicited during initial clinical evaluation. These include documentation of language function, affect,

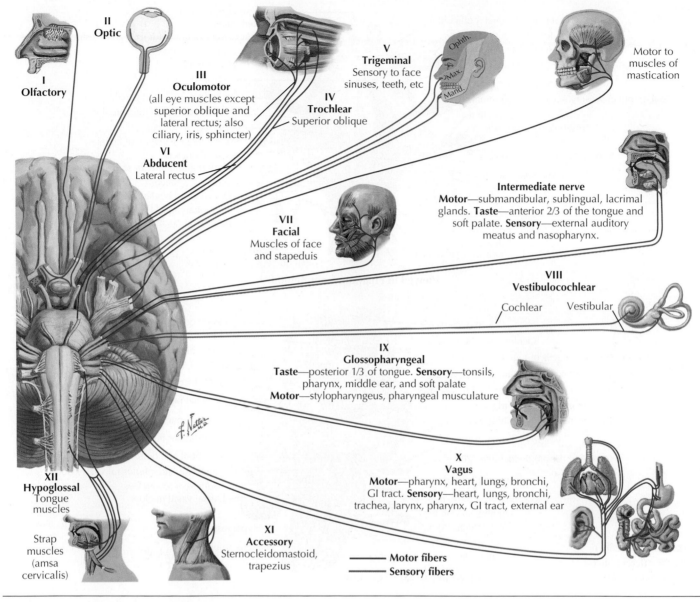

I
Olfactory

II
Optic

III
Oculomotor
(all eye muscles except
superior oblique and
lateral rectus; also
ciliary, iris, sphincter)

IV
Trochlear
Superior oblique

VI
Abducent
Lateral rectus

V
Trigeminal
Sensory to face
sinuses, teeth, etc

Ophth.
Max.
Mand.

Motor to
muscles of
mastication

VII
Facial
Muscles of face
and stapeduis

Intermediate nerve
Motor—submandibular, sublingual, lacrimal
glands. **Taste**—anterior 2/3 of the tongue and
soft palate. **Sensory**—external auditory
meatus and nasopharynx.

VIII
Vestibulocochlear
Cochlear   Vestibular

IX
Glossopharyngeal
Taste—posterior 1/3 of tongue. **Sensory**—tonsils,
pharynx, middle ear, and soft palate
Motor—stylopharyngeus, pharyngeal musculature

X
Vagus
Motor—pharynx, heart, lungs, bronchi,
GI tract. **Sensory**—heart, lungs, bronchi,
trachea, larynx, pharynx, GI tract, external ear

XII
Hypoglossal
Tongue
muscles

Strap
muscles
(amsa
cervicalis)

XI
Accessory
Sternocleidomastoid,
trapezius

—— **Motor fibers**
—— **Sensory fibers**

F. Netter M.D.

Figure 1-1 Cranial Nerves: Distribution of Motor and Sensory Fibers.

concentration, orientation, and memory. When concerned about the patient's cognitive abilities, the neurologist must elicit evidence of an apraxia or agnosia and test organizational skills. Once language and cognitive functions are assessed, the neurologist dedicates the remaining portion of the exam to the examination of many functions. These include visual fields, cranial nerves (CNs) (Fig. 1-1), muscle strength, muscle stretch reflexes (MSRs), plantar stimulation, coordination, gait and equilibrium, as well as sensory modalities. These should routinely be examined in an organized rote fashion in order not to overlook an important part of the examination. The patient's general health, nutritional status, and cardiac function, including the presence or absence of significant arrhythmia, heart murmur, hypertension, or signs of congestive failure, should be noted. If the patient is encephalopathic, it is important to search for subtle signs of infectious, hepatic, renal, or pulmonary disease.

CRANIAL NERVES: AN INTRODUCTION

The 12 CNs subserve multiple types of neurologic function (see Fig. 1-1). The cranial nerves are formed by afferent sensory fibers, motor efferent fibers, or mixed fibers traveling to and from brainstem nuclei (Fig. 1-2A and B).

The special senses are represented by all or part of the function of five different CNs, namely, olfaction, the olfactory (I); vision, the optic (II); taste, the facial (VII) as well as the glossopharyngeal (IX); hearing as well as vestibular function, the cochlear and vestibular (VIII) nerves. Another three CNs are directly responsible for the coordinated, synchronous, and complex movements of both eyes; these include CNs III (oculomotor), IV (trochlear), and VI (abducens). Cranial nerve VII is the primary CN responsible for facial expression, which is important for setting the outward signs of the patient's psyche's representation to his family and close associates, or signs of

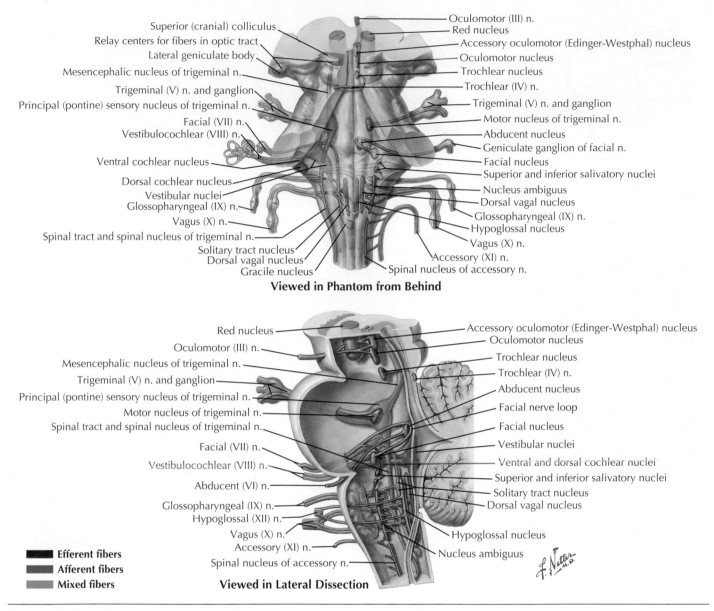

Efferent fibers
Afferent fibers
Mixed fibers

Viewed in Phantom from Behind

Viewed in Lateral Dissection

Figure 1-2 Cranial Nerves: Nerves and Nuclei.

paralysis from a brain or cranial nerve lesion. Facial sensation is subserved primarily by the trigeminal nerve (V); however, it is a mixed nerve also providing primary motor contributions to mastication. The ability to eat and drink depends on CNs IX (glossopharyngeal), X (vagus), and XII (hypoglossal). The hypoglossal and recurrent laryngeal nerves are also important to the mechanical function of speech. Last, CN-XI, the accessory, contains both cranial and spinal nerve roots that provide motor innervation to the large muscles of the neck and shoulder.

Disorders of the CNs can be confined to a single nerve such as the olfactory (from a closed-head injury, early Parkinson disease, or meningioma), trigeminal (tic douloureux), facial (Bell palsy), acoustic (schwannoma), and hypoglossal (carotid dissection). There is a subset of systemic disorders with the potential to infiltrate or seed the base of the brain and the brainstem at the points of exit of the various CNs from their intraaxial origins. These processes include leptomeningeal seeding of

metastatic malignancies originating in the lung, breast, and stomach, as well as various lymphomas, or granulomatous processes such as sarcoidosis or tuberculosis, each leading to a clinical picture of multiple, sometimes disparate cranial neuropathies. Many times, a stuttering onset occurs. The various symptoms are related to individual CNs. These typically develop within just weeks or no more than a few months.

Cranial nerve dysfunctions will commonly bring patients to medical attention for a number of clinical limitations. These include ophthalmic difficulties, such as diminished visual acuity or visual field deficits (optic nerve and peri-cavernous chiasm) and double vision, either horizontal, vertical, or skewed (oculomotor, trochlear, and abducens nerves). Other cranial nerve presentations include facial pain (trigeminal nerve), evolving facial weakness (facial nerve), difficulty swallowing (glossopharyngeal and vagus nerves), and slurred speech (hypoglossal nerves).

CRANIAL NERVE TESTING

I: Olfactory Nerve

The sense of smell is a very important primordial function that is much more finely tuned in other animal species. Here other mammals are able to seek out food, find their mates, and identify friend and foe alike because of their finely tuned olfactory brain. In the human, the loss of this function can still occasionally have very significant consequences primarily bearing on personal safety. If the human being cannot smell fires or burning food, their survival can be put at serious risk. The loss of smell also affects the pleasure of being able to taste, even though, as later noted, taste per se is primarily a function of cranial nerves VII and IX.

Olfactory nerve function testing is relevant despite its only occasional clinical involvement. This may be impaired after relatively uncomplicated head trauma and in individuals with various causes of frontal lobe dysfunction, especially an olfactory groove meningioma. Loss of olfaction is sometimes an early sign of Parkinson disease. Clinical evaluation of olfactory functions is straightforward. The examiner has the patient sniff and attempt to identify familiar substances having specific odors (coffee beans, leaves of peppermint, lemon). Inability or reduced capacity to detect an odor is known as anosmia or hyposmia, respectively; inability to identify an odor correctly or smell distortion is described as parosmia or dysosmia. Bilateral olfactory nerve disturbance with total loss of smell, typically from head trauma, chronic upper airway infections, or medication, is usually a less ominous sign than unilateral loss, which raises the concern for a focal infiltrative or compressive lesion such as a frontal grove meningioma.

II: Optic Nerve

Of all the human sensations, the ability to see one's family and friends, to read, and appreciate the beauties of nature, it is difficult to imagine life without vision, something that is totally dependent on the second cranial nerve. Obviously many individuals, such as Helen Keller, have vigorously and successfully conquered the challenge of being blind; however, given the choice, vision is one of the most precious of all animal sensations. "Blurred" vision is a common but relatively nonspecific symptom that may relate to dysfunction anywhere along the visual pathway (Fig. 1-3). When examining optic nerve function, it is important to identify any concomitant ocular abnormalities such as proptosis, ptosis, scleral injection (congestion), tenderness, bruits, and pupillary changes.

Visual acuity is screened using a standard Snellen vision chart that is held 14 inches from the eye. Screening must be performed in proper light as well as to the patient's refractive advantage using corrective lenses or a pinhole when indicated.

A careful visual field evaluation is the other important means to assess visual function. These tests are complementary, one testing central resolution at the retinal level and the other to

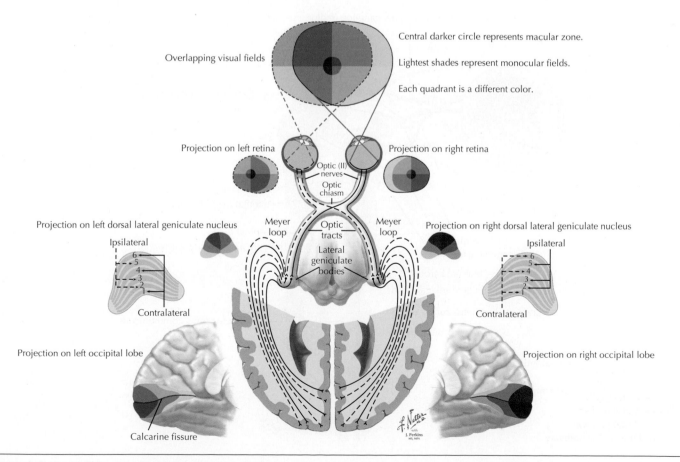

Figure 1-3 Visual Pathways: Retina to Occipital Cortex.

evaluate peripheral visual field defects secondary to lesions at the levels of the optic chiasm, optic tracts, and occipital cortex. Visual fields are evaluated by having the patient sit comfortably facing the examiner at a similar eye level. First, each eye is tested independently. The patient is asked to look straight at the examiner's nose. The examiner extends an arm laterally, equidistant from himself and the patient, and asks the patient to differentiate between one and two fingers. The patient's attention must always be directed back to the examiner as most patients will reflexively look laterally at the fingers. This will require repeated testing. Each quadrant of vision is evaluated separately. After individual testing, both eyes are tested simultaneously for visual neglect, as may occur with right hemispheric lesions. Progressively complex perimetric devices have the advantage of providing valuable data on the health of the visual system.

In *kinetic perimetry*, a stimulus is moved from a non-seeing area (far periphery or physiologic blind spot) to a seeing area, with patients indicating at what point the stimulus is first noticed. Testing is repeated from different directions until a curve can be drawn connecting the points at which a given stimulus is seen from all directions. This curve is the isopter for that stimulus for that eye. The isopter plot has been likened to a contour map, showing "the island of vision in a sea of darkness." The Goldmann perimeter, a half-sphere onto which spot stimuli are projected, is the premiere device for this mapping. The normal visual field extends approximately 90° temporally, 45° superiorly, 55° nasally, and 65° inferiorly. Practically, this

geographic shape mimics the oblique teardrop shape of aviator-style sunglass lenses.

In *static perimetry*, the test point is not moved, but turned on in a specific location. Typically automated, computer testing preselects locations within the central 30° of field. Stimuli are dimmed until they are detected only intermittently on repetitive presentation—this intensity level is called the threshold. The computer then generates a map of numeric values of the illumination level required at every test spot, or the inverse of this level, often called a sensitivity value. Values may also be displayed as a grayscale map, and statistical calculations can be performed—by comparing to adjacent spots or precalculated normal values or noting sudden changes in sensitivity—to detect abnormal areas.

Most visual field changes have localizing value: specific location of the loss, its shape, border sharpness (i.e., how quickly across the field the values change from abnormal to normal). Its concordance with the visual field of the other eye tends to implicate specific areas of the visual system. Localization is possible because details of anatomic organization at different levels predispose to particular types of loss (see Chapter 4).

When one examines the pupils, their shape and size need to be recorded. A side-to-side difference of no more than 1 mm in otherwise round pupils is acceptable as a normal variant. Pupillary responses are tested with a bright flashlight and are primarily mediated by the autonomic innervation of the eye (Fig. 1-4). A normal pupil reacts to light stimulus by constricting with the

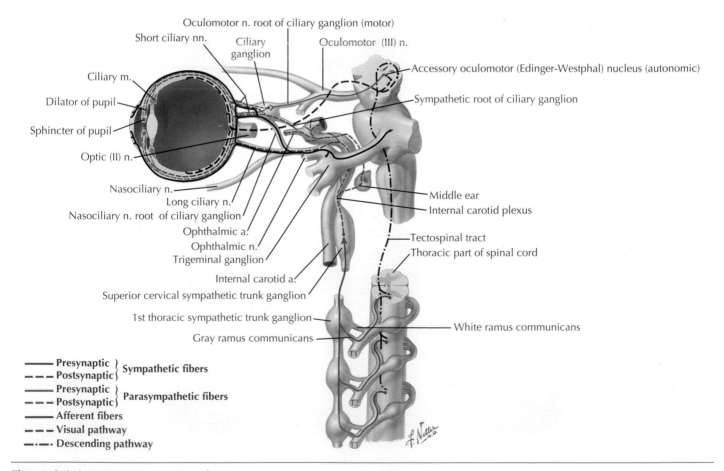

Figure 1-4 Autonomic Innervation of Eye.

Table 1-1 Pupillary Abnormalities

	Argyll Robertson	Horner	Holmes Adie
Response to light	None	Yes	None
Other responses	Brisk reaction to near stimulus	Normal	Tonic reaction to near stimulus
	Converge		Accommodation
Margins	Irregular	Regular	Regular
Associated changes	Iris depigmentation	Ptosis	Loss of MSR
Causes	Tabes dorsalis	Carotid dissection	Ciliary ganglion
		Carotid aneurysm	
		Pancoast tumor	
		Syringomyelia	
Anatomy	Unknown (tectum of midbrain likely)	Loss of sympathetic	Loss of parasympathetic

MSR, Muscle stretch reflex.

contralateral constriction of the unstimulated pupil as well. These responses are called the *direct and consensual reactions*, respectively, and are mediated through parasympathetic innervation to the pupillary sphincter from the Edinger-Westphal nucleus along the oculomotor nerve. The pupils also constrict when shifting focus from a far to a near object (*accommodation*) and during convergence of the eyes, as when patients are asked to look at their nose.

The sympathetic innervation of the pupillary dilator muscle involves a multisynaptic pathway with fibers ultimately reaching intracranially along the course of the internal carotid artery. Branches innervate the eye after traveling through the long and short ciliary nerves. The *ciliospinal reflex* is potentially useful when evaluating comatose patients. In this setting, if the examiner pinches the patient's neck, the ipsilateral pupil should transiently dilate. This provides a means to test the integrity of ipsilateral neuropathways to midbrain structures.

The short ciliary nerve, supplying parasympathetic inputs to the pupil, may be damaged by various forms of trauma. This results in a unilateral dilated pupil with preservation of other third nerve function. Significant unilateral pupillary abnormalities are usually related to innervation changes in pupillary muscles.

A number of pathophysiologic mechanisms lead to mydriasis (pupillary dilatation) (Table 1-1). Atropine-like eye drops, often used for their ability to produce pupillary dilation, inadvertent ocular application of certain nebulized bronchodilators, and placement of a scopolamine anti-motion patch with inadvertent leak into the conjunctiva are occasionally overlooked as potential causes for an otherwise asymptomatic, dilated, poorly reactive pupil. Other medications may also lead to certain atypical light reactions. The presence of bilateral dilated pupils, in an otherwise neurologically intact patient, is unlikely to reflect significant neuropathology. In contrast, the presence of prominent pupillary constriction most likely reflects the use of narcotic analogs or parasympathomimetic drugs, such as those typically used to treat glaucoma.

HORNER SYNDROME

The classic findings include miosis (pupillary constriction), subtle ptosis, and an ipsilateral loss of facial sweating. Here the constricted pupil develops secondary to interference with the

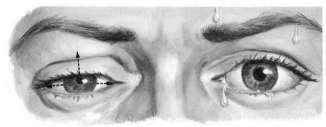

Interruption of the sympathetic fibers outside the brain causes ipsilateral ptosis, anhidrosis, and miosis without abnormal ocular mobility.

Figure 1-5 Right Horner Syndrome.

sympathetic nerves at one of many different levels along its long intramedullary (brain and spinal cord) and complicated extracranial course.

Sympathetic efferent fibers originate within the hypothalamus and traverse the brainstem and cervical spinal cord, then exit the upper thoracic levels and course rostrally to reach the superior cervical ganglia (see Fig. 1-4). Subsequently, these sympathetic fibers track with the carotid artery within the neck to reenter the cranium and subsequently reach their destination innervating the eye's pupillodilator musculature. Typically, patients with Horner syndrome have an ipsilateral loss of sweating in the face (anhidrosis), a constricted pupil (miosis), and an upper lid droop from loss of innervation to Muller's muscle, a small smooth muscle lid elevator (ptosis). The levator palpebra superioris, a striated muscle innervated by the oculomotor nerve CN-III, is not affected (Fig. 1-5).

OPTIC FUNDUS

The ability to peer into the patient's eye is a very unique and fascinating experience as it provides an opportunity to directly examine not only the initial portion of the optic nerve but also tiny arterioles and veins. This is the only portion of human anatomy that provides the physician with such an option. Here one may find signs of increased intracranial pressure or evidences of the effects of poorly controlled hypertension or diabetes mellitus. Today all of these various lesions are much less commonly observed because of much better treatment of systemic illnesses that affect the smaller blood vessels. Similarly the

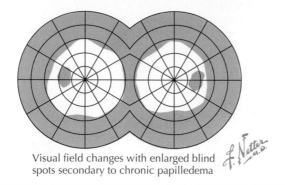

Optic fundus with papilledema

Visual field changes with enlarged blind spots secondary to chronic papilledema

Figure 1-6 Effects of Increased Intracranial Pressure on Optic Disk and Visual Fields.

development of MRI and CT scanning makes it easier to identify intracerebral mass lesions at a much earlier stage of illness. Today as brain tumors no longer reach a critical size, obstructing cerebrospinal fluid flow, creating the increased intracranial pressure that leads to papilledema, this is now a relatively rare finding but one that still demands recognition.

A careful optic funduscopic examination is essential in the evaluation of very many neurologic disorders. This evaluation is best performed in a relatively dark environment that leads to both a reflex increase in pupillary size and improvement in contrast of the posterior chamber structures. Findings that should be documented include optic nerve margins, venous pulsations, and the presence of hemorrhages, exudates, or any obvious obstruction to flow by embolic material (such as cholesterol plaque in patients complaining of transient visual obscuration), and pallor of retinal fields that may reflect ischemia.

Papilledema is characterized by elevation and blurring of the optic disk, absence of venous pulsations, and hemorrhages adjacent to and on the disk (Fig. 1-6). The finding of papilledema indicates increased intracranial pressure of any cause, including brain tumors, subarachnoid hemorrhage, metabolic processes, pseudotumor cerebri, and venous sinus thrombosis.

III, IV, VI: Oculomotor, Trochlear, and Abducens Nerves

Our ability to acutely focus our eyes on an object of interest depends on being able to move the eyes together in a conjugate fashion; this requires three related cranial nerves that take their origin from various juxta midline midbrain and pontine nuclei. These provide us with the ability to astutely focus on an object of interest without concomitantly moving our head. Whether it

is a detective watching a suspect or a teenager taking a furtive glance at a new classmate, these cranial nerves provide us with a broad sweep of very finely tuned motor function. There is no other group of muscles that are so finely innervated as these. Their innervation ratio is approximately 20:1 in contrast to those of large muscles of the extremities with ratios between 400 and 2000 to 1. Certainly, this accounts for the fact that one of the earliest clinical manifestations of myasthenia gravis relates to the extraocular muscles (EOMs), where the interruption of just a few neuromuscular junctions affects the finely harmonized EOM function, leading to a skewed operation and thus double vision.

In order to identify isolated EOM dysfunction, it is most accurate to test each eye individually describing the observed specific loss of EOM function. For example, when the eye cannot be turned laterally, the condition is labeled as an *abduction paresis*, as opposed to CN-VI palsy. This is because the responsible lesion can be at any one of three sites, namely, cranial nerve, neuromuscular junction, or muscle per se. A more detailed assessment of these cranial nerves is available in Section II, Chapter 5.

The medial longitudinal fasciculus (MLF) is responsible for controlling EOM function because it provides a means to modify central horizontal conjugate gaze circuits. The medial longitudinal fasciculus connects CN-III on one side and CN-VI on the opposite side. Understanding the circuit of horizontal conjugate gaze helps clinicians appreciate the relation between the frontal eye fields and the influence it exerts on horizontal conjugate gaze (see Fig. 1-6) as well the reflex relation between the ocular and vestibular systems (Fig. 1-7).

The connection of the vestibular system to the medial longitudinal fasciculus can be tested by two different means. One is the doll's-eye maneuver. Here the patient's head is rotated side to side while the examiner watches for rotation of the eyes. Passive movement of the head to the left normally moves the eyes in the opposite direction, with the left eye adducting and the right eye abducting. The opposite occurs when the head is rotated to the right.

Ice-water caloric stimulation provides another option to study vestibular ocular MLF pathways. This is primarily used for the examination of comatose patients; on very rare occasions, it is extremely helpful for rousing a patient presenting with a suspected nonorganic, that is, feigned coma. Patients are placed at an elevation of approximately 45°. Next, the tympanic membranes are checked for intactness, and then 25–50 mL of ice water is gradually infused into each ear. A normal response in the awake patient, after left ear stimulation, is to observe slow deviation of the eyes to the left followed by rapid movement (nystagmus) to the right (see Fig. 1-10). In contrast, the comatose patient with an intact brainstem has a persistent ipsilateral deviation of the eyes to the site of stimulation with loss of the rapid eye movement component to the opposite side.

The center for vertical conjugate gaze and convergence is also located within the midbrain, although the underlying circuit is not well delineated. The vertical conjugate gaze centers can be tested by flexion of the neck while holding the eyelids open and watching the eye movements. When CNS processes affect conjugate gaze, such as with MS, a prominent nystagmus is often defined. The nystagmus is thought to result from an

Excitatory endings → → → → → →
Inhibitory endings →
Indeterminate endings →

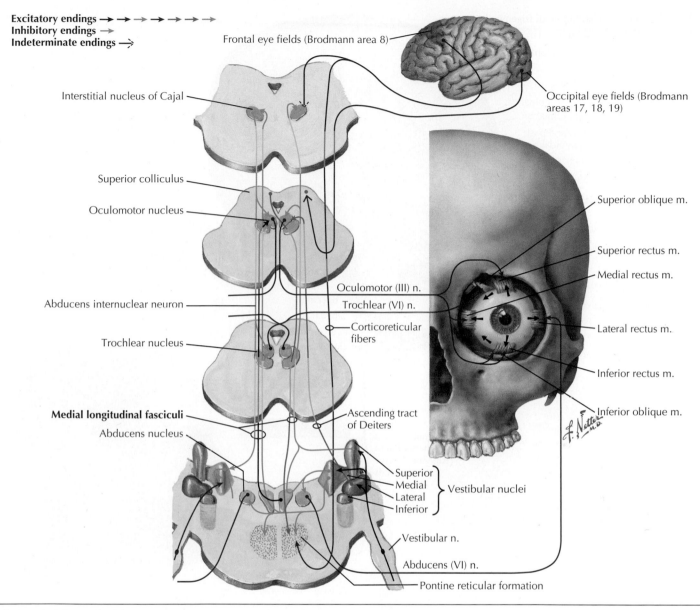

Figure 1-7 Control of Eye Movements.

attempt to maintain conjugate function of the eyes and minimize double images.

V: Trigeminal Nerve

Our ability to perceive various stimuli applied to the face depends almost entirely on this nerve; whether as a warning to protect oneself from subzero cold, something potentially threatening to our eyesight, or the pleasurable sensation from the kiss of a beloved one, all forms of sensations applied to the face are tracked to our brain through the trigeminal nerve (Fig. 1-8). The primary sensory portion of this nerve has three divisions, ophthalmic, maxillary, and mandibular; they respectively supply approximately one third of the face from top to bottom, as well as the anterior aspects of the scalp. The angle of the jaw is spared within the trigeminal mandibular division territory. This provides an important landmark to differentiate patients with conversion disorders or obvious secondary gain as they are not

anatomically sophisticated and will report they have lost sensation in this.

The clinical testing of trigeminal nerve function includes both appreciation of a wisp of cotton and a sharp object on the facial skin per se as well as the corneal reflex. To evaluate the broad spectrum of facial sensation, that is, touch, pain, and temperature, the examiner uses a cotton wisp; the tip of a new, previously unused safety pin; and the cold handle of a tuning fork. In a symmetric fashion, the physician asks whether the patient can perceive each stimulus in the three major divisions of the trigeminal nerve supplying the face.

The *corneal reflex* depends on afferents from the first division of the trigeminal nerve combined with facial nerve efferents. This is also best tested using a wisp of cotton approaching the patient from the side while she or he looks away. Normally, both eyelids close when the cornea on one side is stimulated; this is because this reflex involves multisynaptic brainstem pathways.

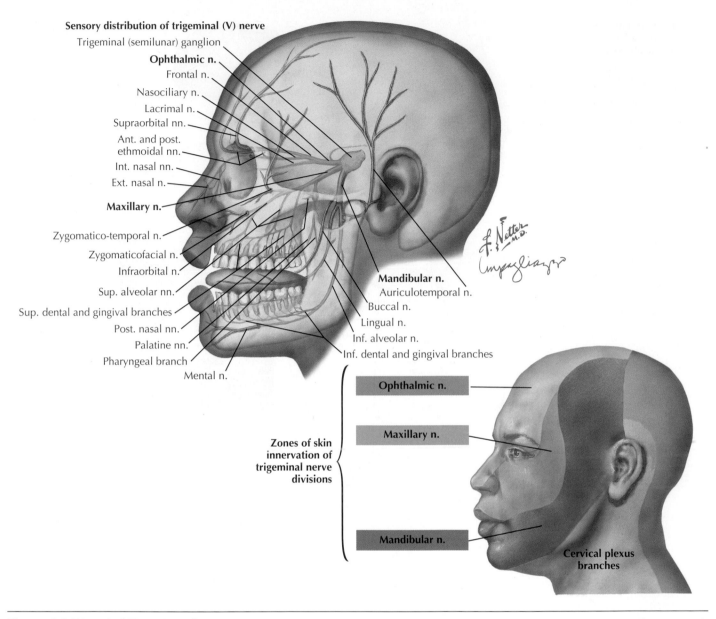

Figure 1-8 Trigeminal Nerve Neuralgia.

Lastly, there is a primary motor portion that is part of the trigeminal nerve. It primarily supplies the muscles of mastication. It is best assessed by having the patient bite down and try to open the mouth against resistance.

VII: Facial Nerve

Facial expression is one of our very important innate human attributes allowing one to demonstrate a very broad spectrum of human emotions, especially happiness and sorrow; these are primarily dependent on the facial nerve (Fig. 1-9). The motor functions of CN-VII are tested by asking patients to wrinkle their forehead, close their eyes, and smile. Whistling and puffing up the cheeks are other techniques to test for subtle weakness. When unilateral peripheral weakness affects the facial nerve after it leaves the brainstem, the face may look "ironed out," and when the patient smiles, the contralateral healthy facial muscle pulls up the opposite half of the mouth while the affected side remains motionless. Patients often cannot keep water in their mouths, and saliva may constantly drip from the paralyzed side. With peripheral CN-VII palsies, patients are also unable to close their ipsilateral eye or wrinkle their foreheads on the affected side. However, although the lid cannot close, the eyeball rolls up into the head, removing the pupil from observation. This is known as the Bell phenomena.

In addition, there is another motor branch of the facial nerve; this innervates the stapedius muscle. It helps to modulate the vibration of the tympanic membrane and dampens sounds. When this part of the facial nerve is affected, the patient notes hyperacusis. This is an increased, often unpleasant perception of sound when listening to a phone with the ipsilateral ear.

Lastly, the facial nerve has a few other functions. These include prominent autonomic function, sending parasympathetic fibers to both the lacrimal and the salivary glands. It also

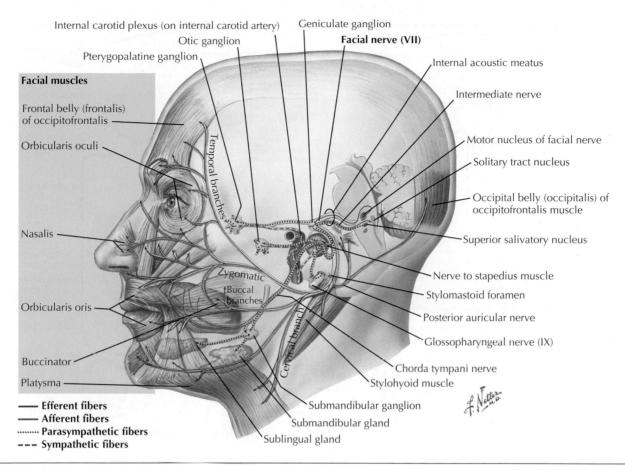

Figure 1-9 Facial Nerve With Its Muscle Innervation.

subserves the important function of taste, another function providing both safety from rancid food and pleasure from a delightful wine. There is also a tiny degree of routine skin sensation represented for portions of the ear.

VIII: Cochlear and Vestibular Nerves (Auditory [Cochlear] Nerve)

Many mornings some of us are blessed by a virtual ornithological symphony in our backyards. This always makes one pause and give thanks once again for this marvelous primary sensation. Here yet another cranial nerve, the cochlear, provides for the emotional highs that auditory sensations bring to the human brain. Whether it is the first cry of a newborn, the reassuring words of a loved one, or Beethoven's seventh symphony, this unique sensation of higher animal life is tracked through this one cranial nerve.

Beyond the simple test of being able to hear at all, more sophisticated clinical evaluation of CN-VIII is often challenging for the neurologist. Fortunately our otolaryngologic colleagues are able to precisely measure the appreciation of specific auditory frequencies in a very sophisticated manner. Barring the availability of these formal audiometric evaluations, simple office-based hearing tests sometimes help us demonstrate diagnostically useful asymmetries. Using a standard tuning fork, it is possible to differentiate between *nerve (perceptive) deafness* caused by cochlear nerve damage and that caused by *middle*

ear (conduction) deafness with two different applications of the standard tuning fork. We are able to test both air and bone conduction.

Initially a vibrating tuning fork is placed on the vertex of the skull, *Weber test*, allowing bone conduction to be assessed. Here the patient is asked to decide whether one ear perceives the sound created by the vibration better than the other (Fig. 1-11). If the patient has nerve deafness, the vibrations are still appreciated more in the normal ear. In contrast, with conduction deafness, the vibrations are better appreciated in the abnormal ear.

The *Rinne test* is carried out by placing this vibrating instrument on the mastoid process of the skull. Here the patient is asked to identify the presence of sound. As the vibrations of the tuning fork diminish, eventually the patient is unable to appreciate the sound. At that instant, the instrument is moved close to the external ear canal to evaluate air conduction. If the individual has normal hearing, air conduction is longer than bone conduction. When a patient has nerve (perceptive) deafness, both bone and air conductions are diminished, but air conduction is still better than bone conduction. In contrast with *conduction deafness*, secondary to middle ear pathology, these findings are reversed. Here, when the patient's bony conduction has ceased, air conduction is limited by the intrinsic disorder within the middle ear. Therefore, the sound can no longer be heard; that is, it cannot pass through the mechanoreceptors that amplify the sound and thus cannot reach the auditory nerve per se.

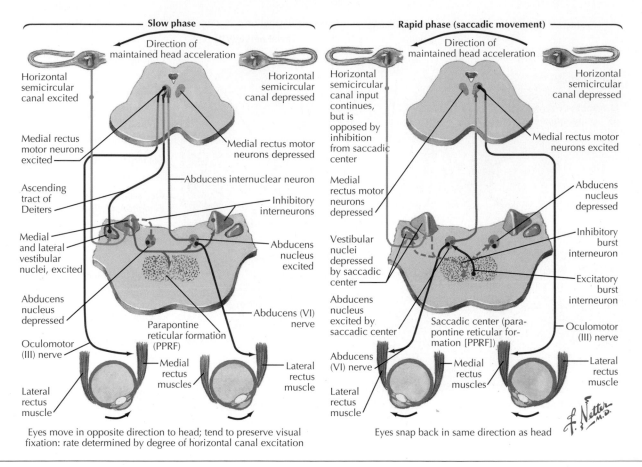

Figure 1-10 Vestibular Eighth Nerve Input to Horizontal Eye Movements and Nystagmus.

VESTIBULAR NERVE

The vestibular system can be tested indirectly by evaluating for nystagmus during testing of ocular movements or by positional techniques, such as the Barany maneuver, that induce nystagmus in cases of benign positional vertigo (BPV) where inner ear dysfunction is caused by otolith displacement into the semicircular canals (Fig. 1-12). Here the patient is seated on an examining table and the eyes are observed for the presence of spontaneous nystagmus. If none is present, the examiner rapidly lays the patient back down, with the head slightly extended and concomitantly turning the head laterally. If after a few seconds' delay, the patient develops the typical symptoms of vertigo with a characteristic delayed rotary, eventually fatiguing nystagmus, the study is positive.

Eye movements depend on two primary components, the induced voluntary frontal eye fields and the primary reflex-driven vestibular–ocular movement controlled by multiple connections (Fig. 1-10; see also Fig. 1-7). The ability to maintain conjugate eye movements and a visual perspective on the surrounding world is an important brainstem function. It requires inputs from receptors in muscles, joints, and the cupulae of the inner ear. Therefore, when the patient has dysfunction involving any portion of the vestibular-ocular or cerebellar axis, the maintenance of basic visual orientation is challenged. Nystagmus is a compensatory process that attempts to help maintain visual fixation.

Traditionally, when one describes nystagmus, the fast phase direction becomes the designated title (see Fig. 1-10). For example, left semicircular canal stimulation produces a slow nystagmus to the left, with a fast component to the right. As a result, the nystagmus is referred to as right beating nystagmus. Direct stimulation of the semicircular canals or its direct connections, that is, the vestibular nuclei, often induces a torsional nystagmus. This is described as clockwise or counterclockwise, according to the fast phase.

A few beats of horizontal nystagmus occurring with extreme horizontal gaze is normal in most individuals. The most common cause of bilateral horizontal nystagmus occurs secondary to toxic levels of alcohol ingestion or some medications, that is, phenytoin and barbiturates.

IX, X, XI: Glossopharyngeal, Vagus, and Accessory Nerves

The most common complaints related to glossopharyngeal-vagal system dysfunction include swallowing difficulties (dysphagia) and changes in voice (dysphonia). A patient with a glossopharyngeal nerve paresis presents with flattening of the palate on the affected side. When the patient is asked to produce a sound, the uvula is drawn to the unaffected side (Fig. 1-13). Indirect mirror examination of the vocal cords may demonstrate paralysis of the ipsilateral cord. The traditional test for gag

Weber Test

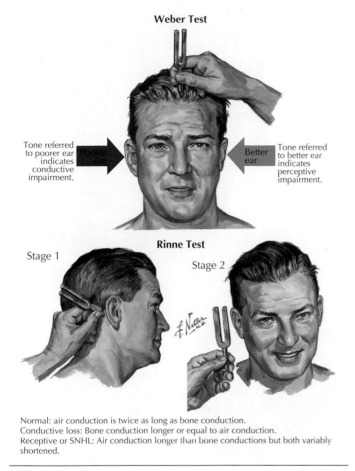

Tone referred to poorer ear indicates conductive impairment.

Poorer ear

Better ear

Tone referred to better ear indicates perceptive impairment.

Rinne Test

Stage 1

Stage 2

Normal: air conduction is twice as long as bone conduction.
Conductive loss: Bone conduction longer or equal to air conduction.
Receptive or SNHL: Air conduction longer than bone conductions but both variably shortened.

Figure 1-11 Auditory Nerve Testing: Weber and Rinne Testing.

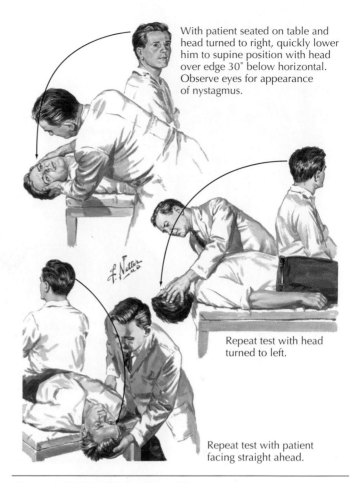

With patient seated on table and head turned to right, quickly lower him to supine position with head over edge 30° below horizontal. Observe eyes for appearance of nystagmus.

Repeat test with head turned to left.

Repeat test with patient facing straight ahead.

Figure 1-12 Test for Positional Vertigo.

reflex, placing a tongue depressor on the posterior pharynx, is of equivocal significance at best, because the gag response varies significantly and patients evidence wide varieties of tolerance to this stimulus. Preservation of swallowing reflexes is best tested by giving the patient 30 mL of fluid to drink through a straw while seated at 90°. Patients with compromised swallowing reflexes develop a "wet cough" and regurgitate fluids through their nose. Intracranial or proximal spinal accessory nerve damage limits the ability to turn the head to the opposite side (weakness of the ipsilateral sternocleidomastoid muscles and trapezius muscle). More distal accessory nerve damage is most commonly seen following surgical misadventures during biopsying a lymph node from the posterior triangle of the neck, sparing the sternocleidomastoid but affecting the trapezius, causing dysfunction and winging of the scapula.

XII: Hypoglossal Nerve

Damage to the hypoglossal nucleus or its nerve produces tongue atrophy and fasciculations The fasciculations usually are seen best on the lateral aspects of the tongue. If the nerve damage is unilateral, the tongue often deviates to that side (see Fig. 1-13). Two means to test for subtle weakness include asking the patient to push against a tongue depressor held by the examiner and having the patient push the tongue into the cheek.

CRANIAL NEUROPATHIES AND SYSTEMIC DISEASE

When one evaluates a patient presenting with any cranial neuropathy, it is important to search for signs of other neurologic and systemic disorders. The patient with recently discovered anosmia may have early Parkinson disease. An acute painful, but pupil sparing, third nerve palsy may be a tip-off to the diagnosis of diabetes mellitus. When one meets an individual with unilateral or bilateral Bell palsies, Lyme disease, as well as sarcoidosis, always requires consideration in the differential diagnosis. When one evaluates patients having multiple cranial neuropathies, leptomeningeal infiltration from metastatic carcinoma or lymphoma, sarcoidosis or chronic infectious processes, such as tuberculosis, always require diagnostic consideration.

CEREBELLAR DYSFUNCTION

Evaluation of posture and gait provides the opportunity to observe the most dramatic clinical manifestations of cerebellar dysfunction. The patient presenting with *midline cerebellar lesions* affecting the vermis characteristically assumes a broad-based stance when walking that typically mimics an inebriated individual. At the extreme, these individuals are unable to maintain a stance. In contrast, when there is a *cerebellar hemisphere problem*, the patient has a tendency to veer to the affected side. With

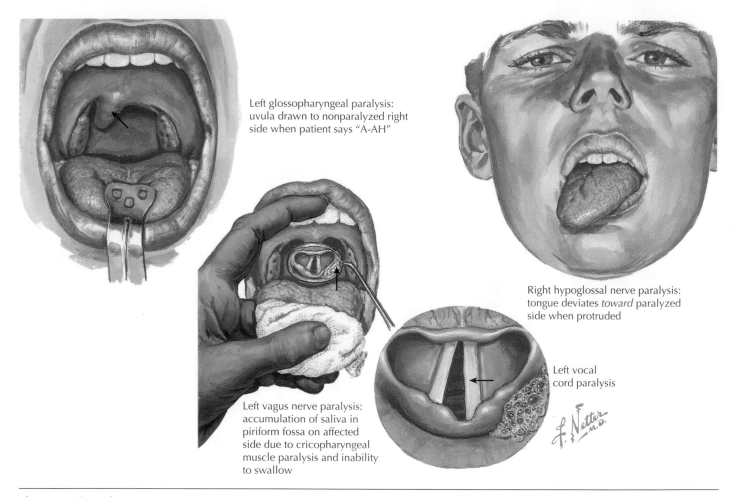

Left glossopharyngeal paralysis: uvula drawn to nonparalyzed right side when patient says "A-AH"

Left vagus nerve paralysis: accumulation of saliva in piriform fossa on affected side due to cricopharyngeal muscle paralysis and inability to swallow

Right hypoglossal nerve paralysis: tongue deviates *toward* paralyzed side when protruded

Left vocal cord paralysis

Figure 1-13 Uvula, Tongue, and Vocal Cord Weakness.

midline lesions, gait is usually unchanged whether the eyes are open or closed, suggesting that this is not the result of disruption of proprioceptive inputs. Patients with unilateral lesions are often able to compensate with their eyes open but deteriorate when they lose visual inputs.

Loss of limb coordination is the result of cerebellar inability to calculate inputs from different joints and muscles and coordinate them into smooth movements. This abnormality is best observed by testing *finger-to-nose* and *heel-to-shin* movements and making bilateral comparisons. When performing the finger-to-nose test, the examiner provides his or her finger as the target; it is sequentially moved to different locations. The patient in turn keeps the arm extended and tries to touch the examiner's finger at each location. When unilateral cerebellar dysfunction is present, the patient *overshoots* the target, so-called *past pointing*. It is important not to misinterpret such findings as always of cerebellar origin, as patients with focal motor or sensory cerebral cortex lesions may present with mild arm weakness and proprioceptive sensory loss affecting that limb. In this setting, a degree of focal limb dysmetria may develop; this is sometimes difficult to distinguish from primary cerebellar dysfunction. One clinical means to distinguish cerebellar from cerebral cortical dysfunction is that the patient with cerebellar hemisphere lesions will have these movements improve after a few trials. In contrast, with cerebral cortical

dysmetria, repeated trials only lead to further deterioration in the attempted action.

Dysdiadochokinesia is a sign of cerebellar dysfunction that occurs when the patient is asked to rapidly change hand or finger movements, that is, alternating between palms up and palm down. Patients with cerebellar dysfunction typically have difficulties switching and maintaining smooth, rapid, alternating movements.

Tremor, *nystagmus*, and *hypotonia* are other important indications of potential cerebellar dysfunction. *Tremors* may develop from any lesion that affects the cerebellar efferent fibers via the superior cerebellar peduncle. This is characterized by coarse, irregular movement. *Nystagmus* may occur with unilateral cerebellar disease; the nystagmus is most prominent on looking to the affected side. *Hypotonia* may be present but is often difficult to document. This is best observed when testing a patient's muscle stretch reflexes at the quadriceps tendon knee jerk. Here, the normal "check" does not occur after the initial movement, so the leg on the affected side swings back and forth a few times after the initial patellar tendon percussion.

GAIT EVALUATION

Whenever possible, the neurologic clinician is encouraged to personally greet the patient, watching them arise from their

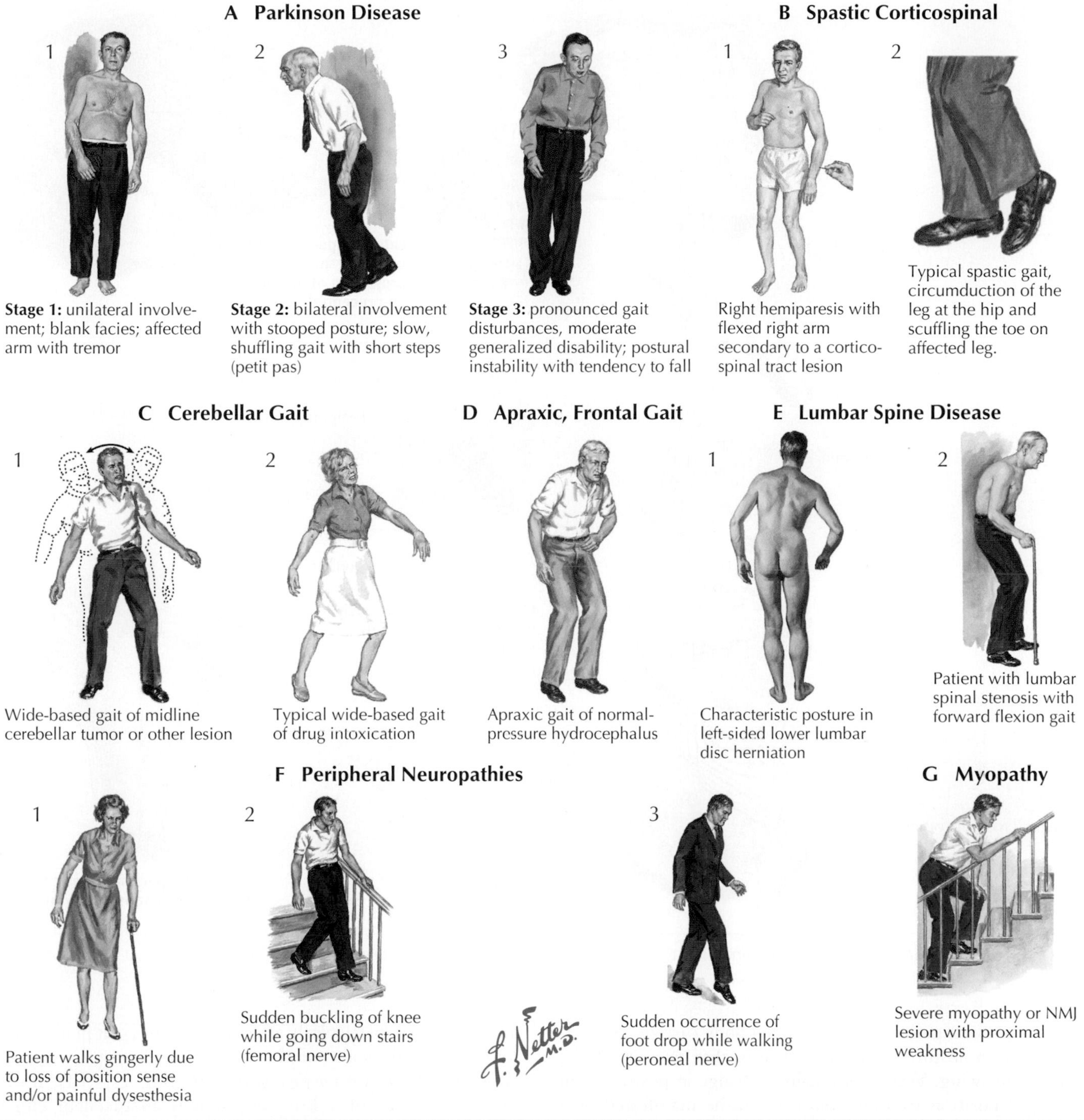

A Parkinson Disease

1

2

3

Stage 1: unilateral involvement; blank facies; affected arm with tremor

Stage 2: bilateral involvement with stooped posture; slow, shuffling gait with short steps (petit pas)

Stage 3: pronounced gait disturbances, moderate generalized disability; postural instability with tendency to fall

B Spastic Corticospinal

1

2

Right hemiparesis with flexed right arm secondary to a corticospinal tract lesion

Typical spastic gait, circumduction of the leg at the hip and scuffling the toe on affected leg.

C Cerebellar Gait

1

2

Wide-based gait of midline cerebellar tumor or other lesion

Typical wide-based gait of drug intoxication

D Apraxic, Frontal Gait

Apraxic gait of normal-pressure hydrocephalus

E Lumbar Spine Disease

1

2

Characteristic posture in left-sided lower lumbar disc herniation

Patient with lumbar spinal stenosis with forward flexion gait

F Peripheral Neuropathies

1

2

3

Patient walks gingerly due to loss of position sense and/or painful dysesthesia

Sudden buckling of knee while going down stairs (femoral nerve)

Sudden occurrence of foot drop while walking (peroneal nerve)

F. Netter M.D.

G Myopathy

Severe myopathy or NMJ lesion with proximal weakness

Figure 1-14 Gait Disorder Characteristics and Etiology.

chair and initiate their gate. Next, before moving to the examination room the patient needs to be observed walking in the hallway. On occasion it is important to observe the patient on stairs particularly if there is a query about proximal weakness. A smooth gait requires multiple inputs from the cerebellum and primary motor and sensory systems. Gait disorders provide a very broad differential diagnostic challenge that results from lesions in any part of the neuraxis (Fig. 1-14).

Frontal lobe (Fig. 1-14,D) processes including tumors and normal-pressure hydrocephalus lead to apraxia, spasticity, and

leg weakness. *Spasticity* per se is a nonspecific marker of corticospinal tract disorders that may arise with various neurologic lesions between the frontal lobe and the distal spinal cord (Fig. 1-15). Various *neurodegenerative* conditions, particularly those affecting the basal ganglia, such as *Parkinson disease* (Fig. 1-15,A1–3), are some of the most common causes of gait difficulties. These are typically manifested by slowness initiating gait, small steps, and eventually gait festination, wherein once patients begin to accelerate their walking, they take increasingly more rapid but paradoxically smaller steps. There is an innate,

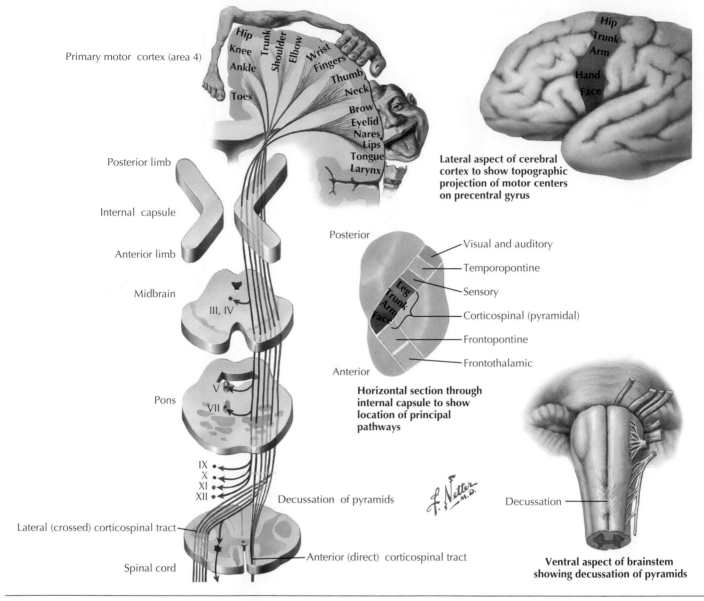

Figure 1-15 Pyramidal System, Corticospinal Tract. Gait Disorders Can Arise From Interruption of These Pathways at Any Level.

almost wax-like rigidity to their stooped body carriage, including the frozen posture of one or both arms that usually lack the normal arm swing. Very occasionally, a change in posture from the seated position to attempted gait will be manifested by a dystonic posturing, which may be indicative of another genetic disorder, dystonia musculorum deformans or paroxysmal choreoathetosis.

Cerebellar disorders related to midline anterior cerebellar *vermis* lesions or various *heredofamilial spinocerebellar* entities lead to a broad-base gait ataxia (Fig. 1-14,C1–2). The patient is asked to walk in tandem, with one foot in front of the other. It is an effective means to elicit a subtle disequilibrium often related to midline cerebellar dysfunction such as with simple entities, including alcohol intoxication.

Myelopathies with posterior column dysfunction, such as vitamin B_{12} deficiency, present with loss of proprioception

function. These particularly affect the patient's gait in dark environments, as do some of the *peripheral neuropathies, especially those with a primary sensory ganglionopathy* (Fig. 1-14,F1). Testing for the presence of a Romberg sign is an excellent clinical marker for these disorders. Here patients are asked to stand in place with their eyes open, gain their equilibrium, and then close their eyes. Individuals with various proprioceptive disorders are unable to maintain their balance when visual clues are withdrawn; such a condition is referred to as a positive Romberg sign. One of the earliest signs, and at times a prominent sign of a myopathy, is needing to push off the arms of a chair when arising to walk. When these individuals do walk their gait may be a broad-based gait mimicking an anterior cerebellar lesion. When viewed from the side the curve of their low back is accentuated, i.e. hyperlordotic. Both the wide base and the hyperlordosis are representative of weakness of the most proximal muscle groups—the iliopsoas, quadriceps, and glutei—as well as the paraspinal axial musculature.

An often overlooked cause of gait difficulties is orthopedic and musculoskeletal problems. A perhaps simplistic perspective on the contribution of this system to gait is the analogy that the musculoskeletal system functions similar to an axle on a car, maintaining alignment and proper, symmetric rotation of the wheels. Our vertebral column is a sophisticated axle that with time loses some of its alignment. The attached muscles, to a misaligned chain of vertebrae, ultimately generates aberrant feedback loops to the spinal cord and the brain.

Many of our *senior citizens* gradually lose precise control of their gait, initially manifested by subtle changes on neurologic exam. Healthy older individuals often have limited ability to perform tandem gait. The very important message here is that this finding in isolation should not be considered abnormal per se among patients living into their eighth decade. Nevertheless, older patients become increasingly limited by a dwindling ability to walk independently.

Very often, in this setting there is not one specific mechanism either operative or identifiable. A number of patients have a multifaceted source related to the gradual *aging* (graying) of multiple neurologic systems. One source that always requires consideration is the possibility of *orthostatic hypotension*. Most commonly, this relates to medications; however, one of the neurodegenerative disorders, multiple system atrophy (see Chapter 34), may present in this fashion. Thus, it is important to carefully check blood pressures in the supine posture, when seated, then immediately on standing, and then every 30 seconds thereafter until the pressure is stabilized. A persistent drop in blood pressure of 20–30/15 mm Hg is usually regarded as significant in this setting.

It is important to ask about the circumstances accompanying the gait decline. Does the individual scuff a foot because of a spastic leg that interferes with a smooth alteration of individual legs? What settings lead to a fall? Does one catch one's toe on a rug as with subtle spasticity (Fig. 1-14,B1–2) or feel a leg give out going downstairs secondary to weakness of the quadriceps femoris muscle (Fig. 1-14,F2)? Having such information, the examiner can then easily try to reproduce the circumstances that lead to the falls.

Typically, gait function is tested under several conditions, including walking straight, walking at least 10 yards in open space, making turns, maneuvering through a tight corridor, attempting tandem gait, or in low light settings as well as on the stairs. The normal degree of foot separation (the base) is widened when proprioception or midline cerebellar vermis function is compromised. Occasionally, having the patient climb stairs reveals a subtle degree of iliopsoas weakness as found in various peripheral motor unit disorders (particularly myopathies) and, less commonly, neuromuscular junction or proximal peripheral neuropathies (Fig. 1-14,G). Finally, the appearance of spasticity may be enhanced by having the patient walk longer distances and even asking him or her to walk several blocks and return to the clinic. Rarely, this uncovers an unsuspected corticospinal tract lesion. Chapter 32 expands on the clinical evaluation of gait disorders.

ABNORMAL ADVENTITIOUS MOVEMENTS

Neurologists are frequently consulted to evaluate various adventitious movements, including tremors, chorea, dyskinesias, and ballismus. The most common movement disorder encountered in the office is "essential tremor," usually a "benign" hereditary condition that generally does not herald a progressive neurodegenerative process. These patients often seek medical attention because they are concerned that their tremors are a sign of Parkinson disease. Therefore, differentiating between different types of tremors is a common and important concern. An essential tremor characteristically occurs during certain voluntary actions, such as when bringing a cup of coffee to the mouth. In contrast, with classic Parkinson disease, the pill-rolling tremor is primarily evident at rest and when the patient is seated or walking and disappears with the spontaneous use of the extremity. A subtle fidgeting may represent the earliest sign of Huntington or Sydenham chorea. Very rarely a patient will present with a more energetic, purposeless, wing beating movement of an extremity referred to as hemiballismus. A full discussion of movement disorders and their presentation is found in Section VII.

MUSCLE STRENGTH EVALUATION

Weakness is one of the most common complaints of patients seeking neurologic care. The motor pathways encompass multiple anatomic areas within the CNS, including the cerebral cortex and important subcortical structures such as the basal ganglia, the brainstem, the cerebellum, the spinal cord, and the peripheral motor unit (Fig. 1-16). Although complaints of generalized weakness, fatigue, or both often are not caused by a specific neurologic condition, the possibility of multiple sclerosis in younger individuals and Parkinson disease in older patients always needs to be considered. When the patient is significantly overweight or has a neuromuscular disorder, sleep apnea needs consideration as a cause of fatigue or a feeling of "weakness." Peripheral motor unit disorders are important considerations for the differential diagnosis of a patient with generalized weakness. These include processes affecting the anterior horn cell (i.e., amyotrophic lateral sclerosis), peripheral nerve (i.e., Guillain–Barré syndrome or chronic inflammatory demyelinating disorders), neuromuscular junction (including Lambert–Eaton myasthenic syndrome [LEMS]), or muscle cells (various myopathies).

Partial limb weakness is referred to as *monoparesis*. Total limb paralysis is referred to as *monoplegia*. Unilateral weakness of the limbs is referred to as hemiparesis or *hemiplegia*. Paraparesis refers to involvement of both legs; if no motor function remains, this is considered *paraplegia*. Similarly, *quadriplegia* relates to total paralysis of all 4 extremities.

Focal weakness often has a subtle character that frequently is not recognized by the patient as loss of motor strength. Dropping objects or clumsy handwriting may represent a single peripheral nerve lesion such as a radial neuropathy leading to a wrist drop. Tripping on rugs or steps may be the expression of a peroneal nerve lesion causing a foot drop (Fig. 1-14,F3). In

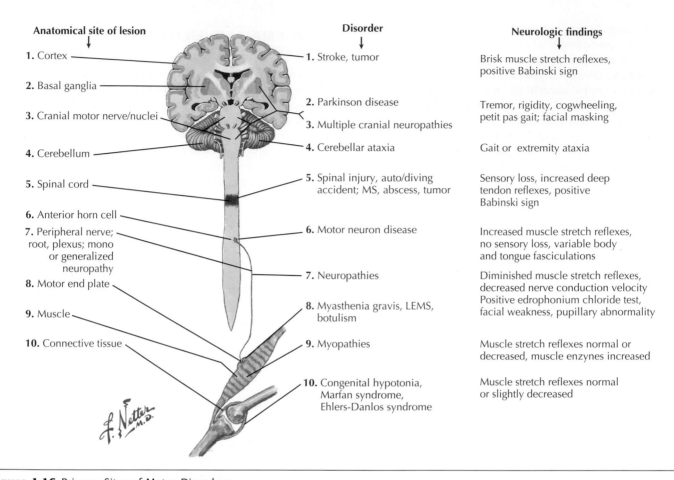

Anatomical site of lesion	Disorder	Neurologic findings
1. Cortex	1. Stroke, tumor	Brisk muscle stretch reflexes, positive Babinski sign
2. Basal ganglia	2. Parkinson disease	Tremor, rigidity, cogwheeling, petit pas gait; facial masking
3. Cranial motor nerve/nuclei	3. Multiple cranial neuropathies	
4. Cerebellum	4. Cerebellar ataxia	Gait or extremity ataxia
5. Spinal cord	5. Spinal injury, auto/diving accident; MS, abscess, tumor	Sensory loss, increased deep tendon reflexes, positive Babinski sign
6. Anterior horn cell	6. Motor neuron disease	Increased muscle stretch reflexes, no sensory loss, variable body and tongue fasciculations
7. Peripheral nerve; root, plexus; mono or generalized neuropathy	7. Neuropathies	Diminished muscle stretch reflexes, decreased nerve conduction velocity Positive edrophonium chloride test, facial weakness, pupillary abnormality
8. Motor end plate	8. Myasthenia gravis, LEMS, botulism	
9. Muscle	9. Myopathies	Muscle stretch reflexes normal or decreased, muscle enzymes increased
10. Connective tissue	10. Congenital hypotonia, Marfan syndrome, Ehlers-Danlos syndrome	Muscle stretch reflexes normal or slightly decreased

Figure 1-16 Primary Sites of Motor Disorders.

contrast, dramatic whole limb weakness is obvious and of greater patient concern, often leading to immediate medical attention as occurs with a stroke. Bilateral motor loss without cognitive or visual difficulties is most commonly due to lesions affecting the spinal cord or the peripheral nervous system and muscle.

When analyzing the complaint of weakness, the physician must consider the presence or absence of associated neurologic complaints or difficulties, such as language, speech, and visual changes; gait dysfunction; difficulty with rising from chairs and associated movements; and alteration in sensation. The neurologist testing for strength must search for evidence of atrophy and fasciculations, or spasticity. Equally important is the need to note the degree of patient effort and cooperation, as well as to consider associated problems that may compromise the testing, such as pain and skin or orthopedic lesions. Formal strength testing must be conducted in a systematic manner evaluating successive areas of the motor unit beginning at the brain and proceeding distally to the individual muscles per se (see Fig. 1-16). Here one places an initial focus on the major muscle groups, such as the flexors and extensors, to seek out any areas of weakness. More specific muscle testing is particularly useful when distinguishing between lesions of the nerve root, plexus, or mononeuropathies (Table 1-2).

When individual muscle testing does not demonstrate specific weakness, other techniques sometimes uncover more less-obvious functional loss. If the patient is instructed to extend the arms with the palms up and the eyes closed, subtle arm weakness may manifest as a pronating downward or lateral drift of the affected extremity. Similarly, moving the fingers as if playing piano or rapidly tapping may demonstrate a subtle in-coordination. Subtle proximal lower extremity weakness may not be appreciated with individual muscle testing. Watching the patient rise from a chair may demonstrate use of furniture arms to "push off" and is a good means to identify early proximal leg weakness. One particularly effective means to uncover proximal leg weakness is to observe the patient climb stairs or squat and attempt to rise without using their arms. Also asking the patient to walk on the heels or the tips of the toes is helpful in uncovering distal leg weakness.

Grading Weakness

The traditional, most widely used British system for quantifying degrees of weakness is based on a scoring range of 0 to 5, with 5 being normal. The extremes of grading are easy to understand, although the subtle grading between 4 and 5 (i.e., >4, 4, >4, or <5) may be slightly different depending on the examiner's own strength (Table 1-3). Other systems judges the patient to have mild (<1), moderate (<2), severe (<3), or total paralysis (<4) strength, and this grading is viewed by some of us to be a simpler and more reproducible methodology. When testing individual muscles of the patient, the examiner must recognize that this is

Table 1-2 Muscle Testing in a Routine Neurologic Examination

Muscle	Action	Nerve	Root
Infraspinatus	External rotation of arm	Suprascapular	C5
Biceps	Flexion of forearm	Musculocutaneous	C5-6
Deltoid	Abduction of arm	Axillary	C5
Triceps	Extension of forearm	Radial	C7
Extensor digitorum	Extension of fingers	Posterior interosseous of radial	C7
Flexor digitorum	Grip	Median	C7-8
APB* and opponens pollicis	Abducting thumb	Median	T1
Dorsal interossei	Spread fingers apart	Ulnar	C8
Iliopsoas	Flexion of thigh	Femoral	L2-3
Quadriceps	Extension of leg	Femoral	L3-4
Hamstring	Flexion of knee	Sciatic	S1
Gluteus medius	Abduction of thigh	Superior gluteal	L5
Gluteus maximus	Extension of thigh	Inferior gluteal	S1
Tibialis anterior	Dorsiflexion of foot	Deep peroneal	L5
Tibialis posterior	Inversion of foot	Tibial	L5
Peroneus longus	Eversion of foot	Superficial peroneal	L5, S1
Gastrocnemius	Plantar foot flexion	Tibial	S1-2

APB, Abductor pollicis brevis.

Table 1-3 Grading System for Clinical Documentation of Degree of Weakness

Grade	Clinical Findings
0	No movement (complete paralysis)
1	Able to move a muscle but no movement of limb
2	Minor movement of limb but inability to overcome gravity
3	Moderate weakness; movement of limb against gravity
4	Mild weakness; some resistance against mild pressure
5	Normal; resistance against moderate pressure

Adapted from Brain. Aids to the Examination of the Peripheral Nervous System. *4th ed. Philadelphia: WB Saunders; 2000.*

not an athletic match but rather a determination of whether the patient has normal strength. There is a significant range of normal, and a sense of that latitude can be gained only by examining multiple individuals.

The examiner assesses the symmetry of function and coexisting changes in tone to formulate appropriate conclusions regarding the significance of subtle changes. The patient's degree of effort also needs to be assessed to distinguish organic disorders from feigned weakness in those with somatoform disorders or individuals with potential for secondary gain, as may occur with workers' compensation or other litigation. One of the most useful methods here is to ask the patient to very briefly put all of his or her effort into just one muscle. Most patients with various emotional nonorganic causes for "weakness" will not move the limb at all or produce very inconsistent (consistently inconsistent) efforts in contrast to a normal person's very firm, persistent motor output. The individual with nonorganic weakness classically *"gives way,"* after just a very brief effort.

In the setting of possible "give way" weakness, one also needs to consider whether there is evidence of posttetanic facilitation, where the patient's initial effort suggests weakness but on a few more tries seemingly normal motor strength is achieved. This is the classic feature of a presynaptic defect in neuromuscular transmission as seen in Lambert-Eaton myasthenic syndrome (LEMS). Occasionally, one sees something like this with early Guillain–Barré syndrome or multiple sclerosis. This is an important and occasionally difficult differentiation. One must always listen carefully to the patient; when one is uncertain, the best study is sometime a careful reexamination of the patient. Today the findings of normal neuroimaging and neurophysiologic modalities are reassuring when considering diagnosis of a functional nonorganic disorder. It is very important to recognize that this is a diagnosis of exclusion. Furthermore, there is no urgency to make such a psychological-based diagnosis. Repeated, careful evaluations may uncover definitive findings leading to an organic diagnosis, or when normal, reassure both physician and patient alike that there is less concern about a serious illness.

Motor Lesions

CEREBRAL CORTEX

When evaluating patients with *focal weakness due to brain lesions*, one should document the evolution of symptoms and any associated changes in sensation or pain. Sudden onset of localized weakness, without preceding trauma or associated pain, suggests ischemic or hemorrhagic cerebral damage. CNS processes cause preferential weakness of the arm extensors and leg flexors. Pure motor weakness of the arm and leg, with slurring of speech, is the hallmark of a stroke in the posterior limb of the internal capsule. Strokes involving the brainstem typically have corticospinal weakness associated with cranial nerve findings. Language deficits usually point to a left hemispheric processes. Neglect of the affected arm or hand, in association with variable degrees of left-sided weakness, often occurs with pathologic processes in the right hemisphere. Visual field deficits may also develop, depending on whether there is concomitant involvement of the optic nerve, chiasm, tract, radiation, or optic cortex.

BRAINSTEM BULBAR WEAKNESS

Rarely, the weakness may be confined to the *brainstem bulbar musculature*, leading to difficulty speaking, chewing, swallowing, or even breathing. Posterior inferior cerebellar artery (PICA) *infarcts* often present with these symptoms accompanied by vertigo, and crossed body sensory loss. Lesions at the *motor neuron* levels such as bulbar amyotrophic lateral sclerosis (ALS), or hypoglossal nerve injury from carotid artery dissection, also require consideration in this setting. Similar symptoms are rarely presenting signs of peripheral *nerve* lesions, including Guillain–Barré and tick paralysis, the *neuromuscular junction*, such as myasthenia gravis and botulism, and rarely *inflammatory myopathies*. Poliomyelitis and diphtheria are always suspected in the rare geographic areas these disorders are still endemic. Fortunately, these are now more of historical interest where modern immunization programs are successful.

MYELOPATHIES

It is necessary to differentiate weakness caused by *spinal cord* lesions from brain disorders. Primary lesions affecting the spinal cord include compressive lesions from progressive spondylosis (thickening of the bony spinal canal), metastases, trauma, demyelinating processes, particularly MS or transverse myelitis, and spinal epidural abscess. Depending on the location and temporal profile, spinal cord lesions often begin with subtle symptoms of gait disturbance, weakness, or both. Concomitantly, spinal cord lesions are usually associated with sensory findings and urinary bladder difficulties. Pain frequently accompanies acute spinal cord lesions; localized spine and or radicular pain from concomitant nerve root involvement is typical of metastatic cancer, epidural abscess, or transverse myelitis. These disorders can rapidly lead to paraplegia.

A very careful examination is crucial in order to define the presence of a sensory level; this is often best documented by using pin and temperature modalities. One must either sit the patient up or turn them on their side, carefully moving the sensory stimulus from the buttocks to the neck to see if there is a sudden change in degree of perception characteristic of a "sensory level." Failure to perform this evaluation may lead to missing a treatable spinal cord lesion. Detailed knowledge of the specific sensory territories of the nerve root dermatomes (Fig. 1-17) is very helpful when assessing potential spinal cord lesions. Looking for a sweat level is also sometimes helpful because the skin below the level of a significant spinal cord lesion will be noticeably drier from loss of autonomic sympathetic innervation. Acute lower extremity weakness is also seen with the Guillain–Barré syndrome or other acute generalized

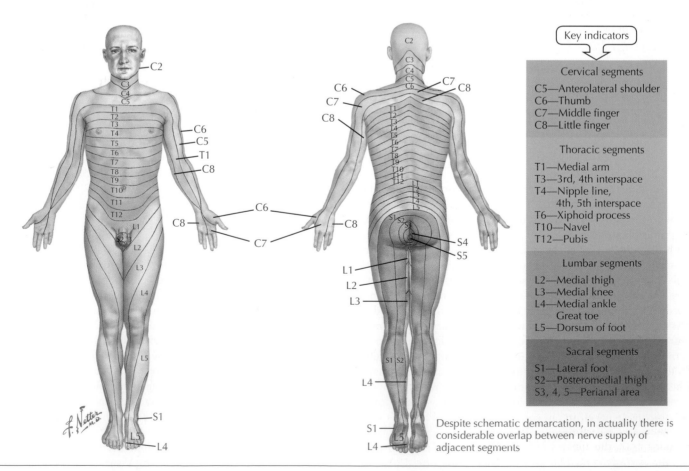

Key indicators

Cervical segments

C5—Anterolateral shoulder
C6—Thumb
C7—Middle finger
C8—Little finger

Thoracic segments

T1—Medial arm
T3—3rd, 4th interspace
T4—Nipple line,
    4th, 5th interspace
T6—Xiphoid process
T10—Navel
T12—Pubis

Lumbar segments

L2—Medial thigh
L3—Medial knee
L4—Medial ankle
    Great toe
L5—Dorsum of foot

Sacral segments

S1—Lateral foot
S2—Posteromedial thigh
S3, 4, 5—Perianal area

Despite schematic demarcation, in actuality there is considerable overlap between nerve supply of adjacent segments

Figure 1-17 Dermatomal Levels.

polyneuropathies. These disorders may mimic a primary spinal cord lesion.

Patients with *painless asymmetric weakness* typically have primary motor neuron or very occasionally motor nerve root, motor nerve level demyelinating lesions. Fasciculations, spontaneous firing of small groups of muscle fibers innervated by a single motor axon (a motor unit), commonly accompany lower motor neuron weakness. Although often perceived by the patient as twitching or jumping, fasciculations may not be easily seen with the naked eye. Sometimes it may be necessary to observe a specific muscle for several minutes to see these signs. Fasciculations are quite common and often benign; when present in isolation with no motor weakness or muscle atrophy, and the patient has a normal EMG, there is little chance that the individual has primary motor neuron disease. Typically lower motor nerve lesions have a concomitant diminution of specific MSRs; however, with ALS the MSRs are exaggerated and often accompanied by Babinski signs.

NERVE ROOT, PLEXUS, OR PERIPHERAL NERVE

The presence of cervical or lumbosacral pain with concomitant focal extremity numbness or weakness is characteristic of a radiculopathy. Interspinal disc herniation and spinal stenosis are the most common processes affecting individual nerve roots. Because sensory examination is the most subjective part of the neurologic examination, occasionally it is difficult to clearly define. Sometimes the patient, per se, can provide the most accurate assessment by using his or her finger to outline the area of diminished sensation. It often then becomes clear that the pattern of sensory loss specifically fits the distribution of a particular peripheral nerve or nerve root dermatome. Knowledge of the cutaneous sensory supply of peripheral nerves is essential to perform an accurate and useful clinical sensory examination (Fig. 1-18).

Some peripheral mononeuropathies, or rarely multifocal motor neuropathies, present with unilateral peripheral weakness; in particular, the wrist drop of radial nerve lesions and foot drop of peroneal nerve lesions are mistaken for processes above the foramen magnum, often mimicking a stroke. Understanding the motor distribution of the major peripheral nerves ultimately aids in the correct diagnosis. Although a peroneal nerve lesion causes a foot drop, similarly an L5 nerve root lesion also presents with a foot drop but usually with associated low back pain. Additionally, the L5 lesion also produces weakness of the posterior tibial muscle innervated by the tibial nerve; this provides the means to make a clinical distinction from a common peroneal nerve lesion. Rarely, lesions as high as the parasagittal frontal lobe within the brain may also present with foot weakness.

Atrophy of muscles innervated by the involved nerve occurs when there is significant denervation. Measuring extremity circumference may document significant side-to-side asymmetries and, by inference, muscle atrophy secondary to anterior horn cell, nerve root, or peripheral nerve damage. It is most important also to carefully search for sensory loss, such as one finds with the ulnar nerve lesion often presenting with painless intrinsic hand muscle atrophy mimicking ALS or syringomyelia.

MUSCLE DISORDERS

Most *myopathic* processes lead to *symmetric proximal weakness*, although such can occur with other disorders, particularly chronic inflammatory demyelinating polyneuropathy or rare neuromuscular transmission defects, such as LEMS. Neck flexor and arm extensor weakness may provide early signs of a myopathic process, especially with myasthenia gravis and the inflammatory myopathies. At its most extreme, these patients may present with a floppy head. On rare occasions, primary myopathies have an asymmetric distribution, particularly inclusion body myositis, that mimics ALS or fascioscapulohumeral muscular dystrophy.

MOTOR TONE

The motor system depends on multiple inputs in order to provide precise, well-synchronized, and smooth muscle function. These include positive inputs from the cerebrum, basal ganglia, cerebellum, brainstem, and spinal cord through the corticospinal tracts. Projections from the pontine reticular formation and reticulospinal tract also have direct connections with motor neurons innervating the proximal and axial body musculature. These fibers also originate from the cerebrum and cerebellum and have a primary inhibitory function that serves to decrease motor tone. Subsequent to damage of structures above the pontine reticular formation, this circuit loses its inhibitory input from the cerebrum and cerebellum, leading to excessive stimulation of motor neurons, especially with antigravity muscles, including arm flexors and leg extensors leading to a flexed and pronated arm posture and an extended and adducted leg position. This increase in tone is referred to as spasticity. This has an interesting paradox in that at rest the spastic muscle has limited tone, but if there is a sudden attempt by the examiner to change the posture the limb is easily moved for a very short distance and then the degree of resistance immediately and rapidly increases up to a maximum and then dissipates. This resembles a "clasp knife," i.e., pocket knife, resistance/relaxation.

Four primary types of changes in tone are found in patients with primary CNS disease: hypotonia, spasticity, flaccidity, and rigidity. It is important to place these observed changes in motor tone within the context of the complete neurologic examination rather than in isolation. The patient's *body tone* is best evaluated when the individual is fully relaxed. Sometimes, it is useful to check tone more than once during the examination. *Tone* is described as the patient's primary level of muscular tension. To become comfortable with this part of the examination, it is important, as with other portions of the neurologic evaluation, to routinely check these parameters in healthy individuals to establish one's normal base of observations.

Hypotonia

This is occasionally demonstrable in patients with cerebellar hemispheric lesions. For example, the distal part of the ipsilateral extremity may not be able to perform rapid alternate

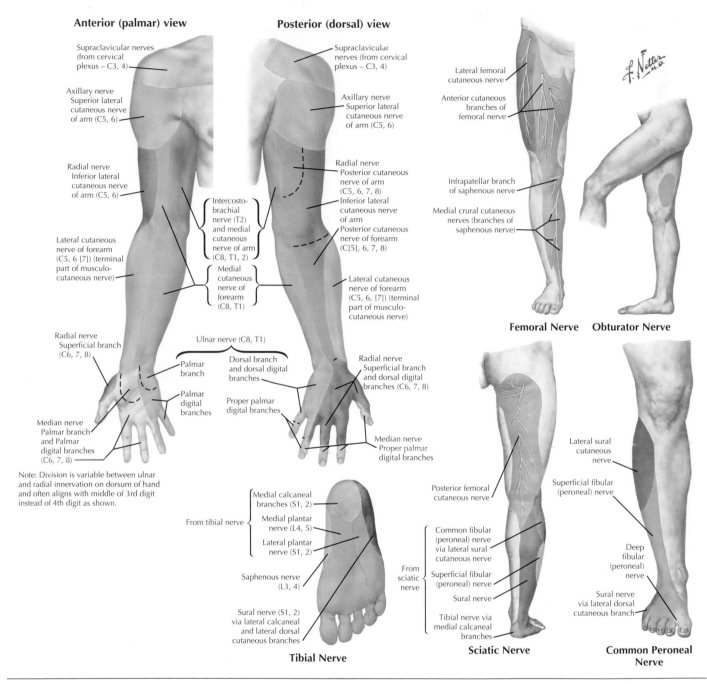

Figure 1-18 Cutaneous Innervations.

movements (called dysdiadochokinesia) because of the inability to maintain a stable posture. Similarly, the smooth, straight pursuit seen when one elicits the knee MSR loses the out-and-back motion that typically has an inhibitory cerebellar check. Instead, on return, there is overshoot with no check, leading to a repetitive pendular response. This classic hypotonic cerebellar tone is a relatively uncommon finding.

A more generalized loss of normal tone is most commonly seen among infants with either central or peripheral motor unit disorders, classically spinal muscular atrophy (Werdnig–Hoffmann disease) or the various congenital myopathies. Although a similar example is seen in adults, rarely, a floppy head syndrome develops in an older patient.

Flaccidity

This is the term for a total loss of tone and is seen in various disease processes affecting the upper motor neurons. Most commonly, this occurs in acute settings such as with a recent stroke or a sudden spinal cord injury, that is, spinal shock. However, with both of these, the flaccidity is temporary and tone increases later to present in the form of varying degrees of spasticity.

Spasticity

Extremes of muscle tone that are maximal at the initiation of the physician's attempt to move the limb and then suddenly release partway through the movement (a clasp-knife, spastic

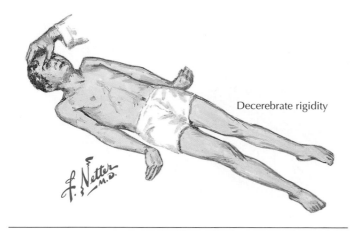

Figure 1-19 Motor Tone Abnormality.

release) are the typical findings seen with a spastic limb. Significant degrees of spasticity are easily elicited with any reasonable stimulation of muscles that induces the stretch reflex. More subtle spasticity may be obvious only with stretching the muscle in a specific direction and at a specific rate. Increased tone, such as may occur with stroke or spinal cord injury, evolves from a flaccid state to spasticity over a matter of days to weeks subsequent to the initial neurologic injury.

Decerebrate Rigidity

When there is total loss of a motor neuron inhibition, as may occur with an upper brainstem injury, the syndrome of decerebrate rigidity develops. Here, a simple noxious stimulus leads to bilateral extension in unison of all four extremities, with the arms pronated and the legs adducted (Fig. 1-19) rotated inward. Most commonly, one sees this in the setting of cardiac arrest or from shear injuries to the brainstem resulting from severe head injuries, most typically from automobile accidents or battlefield injuries. When these patients survive 1 to 3 months, and are otherwise totally unresponsive, they are said to be in a *persistent vegetative state*.

Rigidity

Increasing tone from basal ganglia disorders, as may occur with Parkinson disease, is known as rigidity. Rigidity creates a continuous sense of tightness in the attempt to move the joint through a full excursion from extension to flexion.

MUSCLE STRETCH REFLEXES, CLONUS, AND THE BABINSKI SIGN

Both Ia and Ib peripheral sensory nerve afferents join the posterior columns of the spinal cord, entering through the dorsal root ganglia. Their primary function is to convey information from touch and pressure receptors. Therefore, although the muscle spindles and Golgi tendon organs cannot be specifically tested, some of their spinal cord connections can be clinically evaluated by testing position and vibration sensory modalities. Additionally, the Ia and Ib afferents convey similar information

to the cerebellum via the posterior spinocerebellar tract that travels into the cerebellum through the inferior cerebellar peduncle (Fig. 1-20). In isolation, it is difficult to assess the contribution of each tract specifically to motor control.

With simple passive stretching, such as occurs with tapping the patellar tendon at the knee, the intrafusal muscle spindle is activated, leading to a direct stimulus to the large alpha motor neurons. These in turn stimulate the extrafusal skeletal muscle fibers, leading to the clinically observed muscle contraction (Fig. 1-21). If the afferent sensory or efferent motor limb of this nerve supply is damaged, the muscle stretch reflex (MSR) is affected and may be diminished or lost, as occurs with many peripheral neuropathies. These reflexes are sometimes inappropriately referred to as deep tendon reflexes (DTRs) when in fact their physiologic basis primarily depends on the intrafusal muscle spindle fibers, not the Golgi tendon organs. MSR is a more accurate term.

During the neurologic examination, MSRs (named for the specific muscle stretched) are usually readily elicited by tapping lightly over the muscle insertion tendon or while palpating the tendon and then percussing the palpating digit. Occasionally, it is difficult to obtain MSRs in healthy individuals. In this setting, it is sometimes useful to distract the patient or apply techniques that reinforce the reflex to potentiate the appearance of the MSRs. The most common method is the Jendrassik maneuver, wherein patients flex their fingers, interlocking one hand with the other and pulling on the count of 3 while the clinician percusses the appropriate tendon at the knee or ankle. For the upper extremities, the patient may be asked to clench the contralateral fist as the neurologist percusses over the arm tendons, activating the intrafusal muscle spindle.

When grading MSRs, the extremes are easy to appreciate and range from 0 to 4. A reflex grading of 0 is indicative of complete lack of MSR. A generalized loss of reflexes is pathologic and is known as areflexia; this typically occurs in Guillain–Barré syndrome. Briskly responding MSRs are graded as 4 and are typical of a prior stroke or spinal cord lesion. When the patient has brisk MSRs, a single Achilles tendon percussion sometimes elicits a repetitive series of dorsi and plantar movements in the foot. This is known as *clonus*. This does not commonly occur spontaneously, but clonus may be elicited by giving a quick snap to the dorsiflexed foot as it is held in the palm of the hand. This also occurs, rarely, at the quadriceps tendon. Here the reflex is graded as 4+. The remainder of the grading is very logical. A reflex of 1 is a mere contraction of the muscle; a 2 is a contraction.

The *Babinski sign* is an important pathologic reflex that is elicited at the lateral, plantar surface of the foot using subtle, very careful stroking with a tongue depressor or the base of a key. The great toe extends, and the remaining toes fan out (Fig. 1-22). A more exaggerated response, known as *triple flexion*, includes flexion of the hip, knee, and foot, often with a Babinski response. Because this reflex primarily depends on sensory stimulation of the foot, a kind, gentle, nonirritating stimulus is best to obtain an accurate response. It absolutely does not require excessive or painful pressure. With sensitive or ticklish patients, appropriate responses can usually be obtained from a careful stimulation of the lateral outside, not plantar, surface of the foot. However, some patients have a withdrawal response wherein the

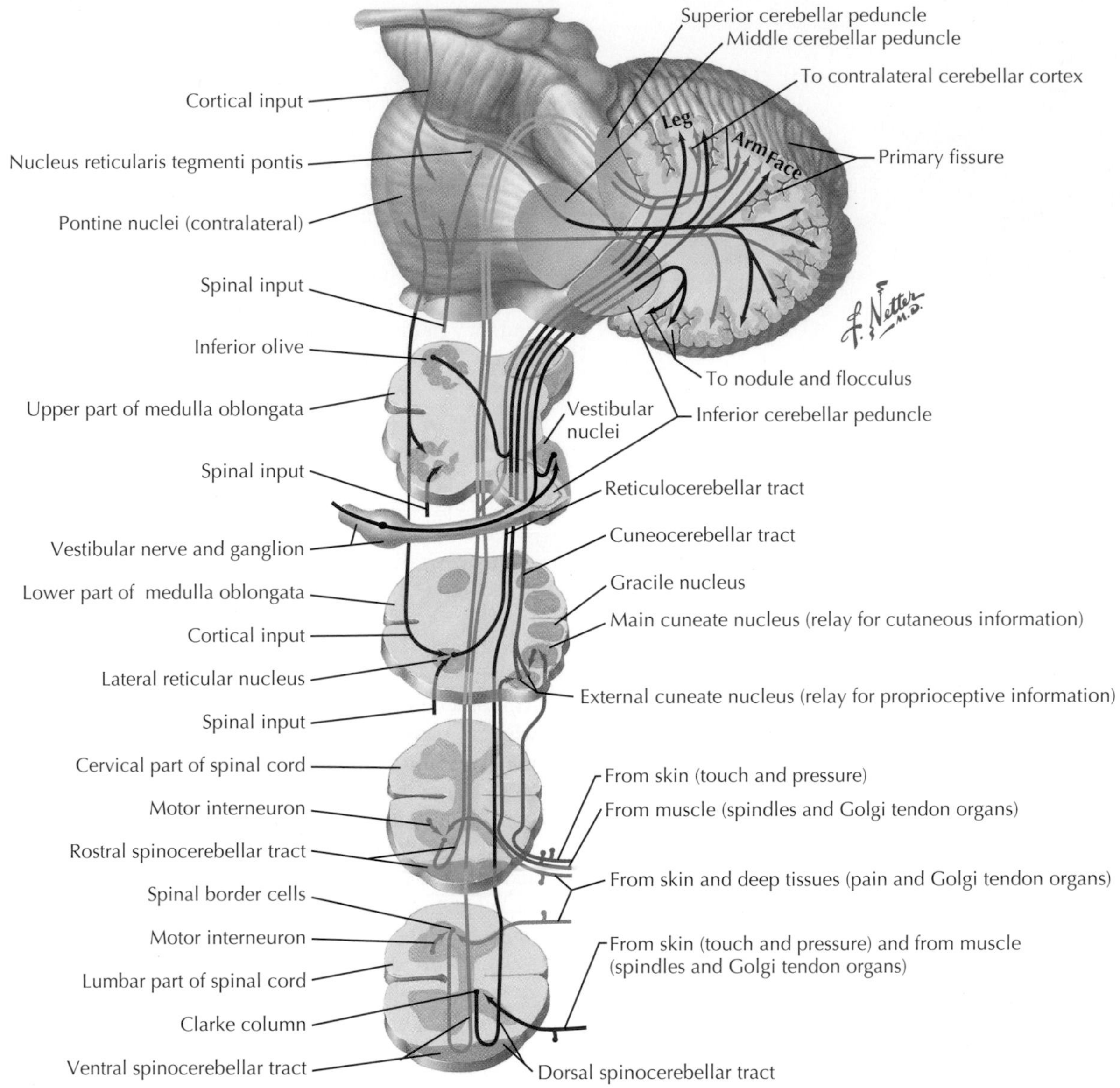

Figure 1-20 Cerebellar Afferent Pathways.

foot and entire set of toes dorsiflex. This is often overcome by separately pulling down on the middle toe while carefully stimulating the sole in traditional fashion.

The clinical circumstance where there is a combination of brisk MSRs, clonus, and a Babinski sign indicates an *upper motor neuron lesion*. These abnormalities result from various pathophysiologic mechanisms originating in the brain or spinal cord. The many possibilities include destructive cerebral lesions, such as stroke, tumor, encephalitis, and spinal cord trauma, or demyelinating disorders such as MS affecting the spinal cord, the brain, or both. Additionally, signs of upper motor neuron lesions are sometimes observed in patients during the postictal period after a seizure or in patients who have toxic or metabolic encephalopathies. Therefore, although brisk MSRs and a Babinski sign are nonspecific regarding the anatomic setting of the CNS abnormality, their presence provides unequivocal evidence of anatomic persistent upper motor neuron pathology, with the exception of the postictal or encephalopathic setting.

SENSORY EXAMINATION

A carefully designed sensory system evaluation is essential to define the presence or absence of normal sensation and, if abnormal, to define the specific anatomic patterns of loss for the affected modalities. Because part of the sensory examination is fairly subjective, the examiner should analyze the consistency of responses. Additionally, the relevance of sensory changes to the patient's complaints and other findings needs to be carefully evaluated. Initially, the examination needs to focus on defining the presence or loss of sensation. One must avoid having the patient be overly zealous trying to define the most subtle differences in sensory appreciation. This often leads to an exhausted patient and a frustrated clinician.

In most clinical settings, it is best to separate the sensory examination into two major categories, that is, those derived from superficial skin receptors or deeper mechanoreceptors. The former are small, unmyelinated, slowly conducting type C

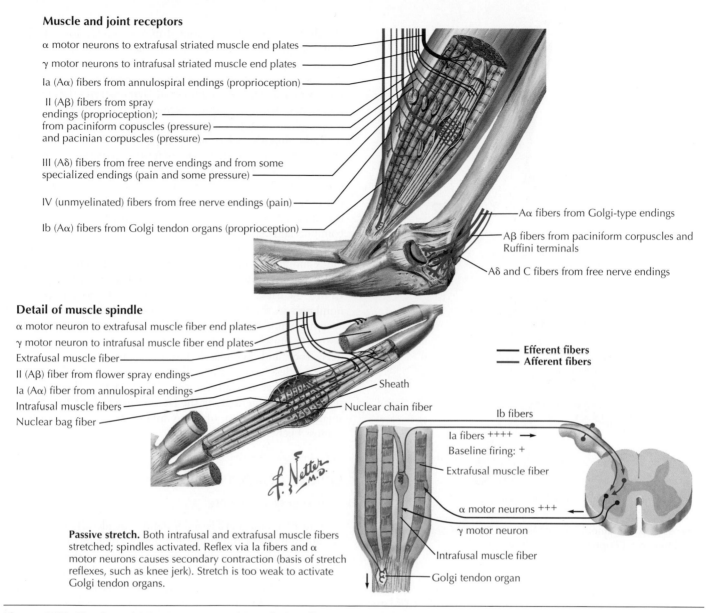

Muscle and joint receptors

α motor neurons to extrafusal striated muscle end plates

γ motor neurons to intrafusal striated muscle end plates

Ia (Aα) fibers from annulospiral endings (proprioception)

II (Aβ) fibers from spray
endings (proprioception);
from paciniform copuscles (pressure)
and pacinian corpuscles (pressure)

III (Aδ) fibers from free nerve endings and from some
specialized endings (pain and some pressure)

IV (unmyelinated) fibers from free nerve endings (pain)

Ib (Aα) fibers from Golgi tendon organs (proprioception)

Aα fibers from Golgi-type endings

Aβ fibers from paciniform corpuscles and
Ruffini terminals

Aδ and C fibers from free nerve endings

Detail of muscle spindle

α motor neuron to extrafusal muscle fiber end plates

γ motor neuron to intrafusal muscle fiber end plates

Extrafusal muscle fiber

II (Aβ) fiber from flower spray endings

Ia (Aα) fiber from annulospiral endings

Intrafusal muscle fibers

Nuclear bag fiber

Sheath

Nuclear chain fiber

—— **Efferent fibers**
—— **Afferent fibers**

Ib fibers

Ia fibers ++++ →

Baseline firing: +

Extrafusal muscle fiber

α motor neurons +++

γ motor neuron

Intrafusal muscle fiber

Golgi tendon organ

Passive stretch. Both intrafusal and extrafusal muscle fibers stretched; spindles activated. Reflex via Ia fibers and α motor neurons causes secondary contraction (basis of stretch reflexes, such as knee jerk). Stretch is too weak to activate Golgi tendon organs.

Figure 1-21 Muscle and Joint Receptors and Muscle Spindles.

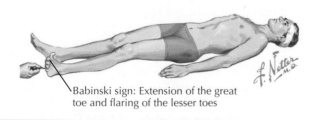

Babinski sign: Extension of the great
toe and flaring of the lesser toes

Figure 1-22 Elicitation of the Babinski Sign.

fibers or larger, slightly myelinated, somewhat more rapidly conducting type A-delta fibers. These small fibers primarily subserve *pain and temperature* (respectively tested using a pin point or a cold object such as the handle of a tuning fork) and gross touch modalities. The large, well-myelinated type A-alpha and A-beta fibers carry the kinesthetic modalities of *position sense* studied by the examiner's passively moving the finger or toe in

the vertical plane and asking the patient which direction the digit was moved, either up or down.

Fine tactile discrimination is evaluated by using a pair of calipers to check their ability to recognize whether one or two points are applied to the digit. *Vibratory sensation* depends on both deep afferent and cutaneous sensory modalities subserved by type A-alpha fibers. It is best tested by a 128-Hz tuning fork that typically has a low frequency rate and longer duration of action. This modality is the one that most commonly diminishes in sensitivity with aging.

Classic Syndromes of Peripheral Sensory Dysfunction

Generalized polyneuropathies typically present with symptoms of numbness and tingling at the tips of the toes and, later, fingers, that is, a stocking-glove distribution (Fig. 1-23). Eventually, this loss will gradually spread proximally past the ankles and wrists into the legs and forearms but usually not above the

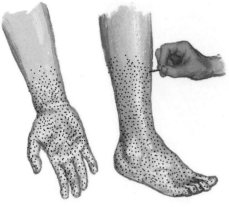

Graduated glove-and-stocking hypesthesia to pain and/or temperature

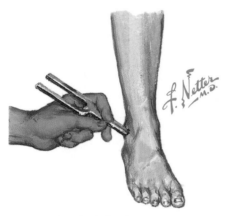

Impaired vibration sense

Figure 1-23 Documentation of Various Types of Sensory Modalities in a Peripheral Neuropathy.

knees and elbows. On examination with a cold object, a pin (for small fiber function), a tuning fork, and position sense (if large fibers are also involved), the examiner notes a distal loss that is maximum in the periphery and gradually reaches normal at a more proximal site.

Individual mononeuropathies are typified by symptoms and findings specific to a single peripheral nerve (see Fig. 1-18). For example, the patient notes numbness in the thumb, index, middle fingers, and adjacent lateral aspect of the fourth finger if the median nerve is involved. In carpal tunnel syndrome with entrapment of the median nerve at the wrist, the examination results are often subtly abnormal, only with loss of fine discriminatory function with subtle diminution of two-point discrimination. Sometimes, one can employ a reflex hammer to percuss directly over the entrapment site. If there is a focal area of peripheral nerve injury, this action commonly elicits brief paresthesiae distal to the percussion site and within the specific distribution of the sensory fibers of that nerve, in this case the median. This maneuver is known as the Tinel sign; the name applies to instances wherein this simple provocative test defines the lesion site for any mononeuropathy.

Plexopathies are usually unilateral in distribution, affecting the brachial or lumbosacral groups of nerves. Typically, these are characterized by a combined motor sensory loss involving multiple peripheral nerves within the affected limbs. These lesions have a broader distribution of motor and sensory loss than do single nerve root or mononeuropathy lesions. Therefore, when a clinical examination demonstrates findings not exclusively defined by one specific peripheral nerve or nerve root, a plexus lesion is likely to be present.

Radiculopathies frequently are characterized by more subjective, often intermittent but sometimes persistent, symptoms confined to the dermatomal patterns of one specific nerve root (see Fig. 1-17). Pain is the most common symptom, starting in the neck, shoulder, and low back, often radiating down along the limb in a specific dermatomal distribution. The most common and classic example in the cervical region is at the C7 nerve root where there are paresthesiae primarily involving the index and middle fingers. Often there is a concomitant diminution in triceps muscle strength as well as loss of the triceps reflex. In the low back, the L5 nerve root is the classic example, with numbness in the first and second toes and the lateral calf and accompanying weakness of both the tibialis anterior and tibialis posterior muscles. However as the knee jerk relates to the L4 nerve root, and the ankle jerk to the S1 root, the examiner has to test a less commonly utilized reflex, namely the internal hamstring that has an L5 root innervation. When there is sensory involvement along the lateral aspect of the foot and the small toe with absence of the Achilles reflex, an S1 root lesion is most likely.

SPINAL CORD SYNDROMES

Transverse Complete

The site of a spinal cord lesion is defined by identifying the exact distribution of specific motor and sensory deficits of the various sensory modalities (Fig. 1-24). A *complete lesion* of the spinal cord leads to total loss of function distal to the site of the abnormality. A distinct level of sensory loss can be discerned with tests for loss of pain and/or temperature sensations, associated with loss of sweating below the lesion level. Concomitantly, all muscles subserved by anterior horn cells distal to the site of the lesion experience paralysis. Distinct partial cord syndromes are briefly described below and discussed further in Section VII (see also Fig. 44-13).

Brown–Séquard

A lesion in the anterior lateral aspect of the spinal cord causes contralateral loss of pain and temperature sensation. If the lesion is more extensive, leading to damage of the anterior and posterior aspects of the cord on one side, the *Brown–Séquard syndrome* occurs; it is characterized by contralateral loss of pain and temperature sensation, ipsilateral loss of position and vibration sensation, and ipsilateral upper motor neuron weakness.

Central Cord

Syringomyelia or a central hemorrhage leads to another anatomically specific lesion referred to as the *central cord syndrome*. The pathology occurs at the center of the cord, destroying fibers

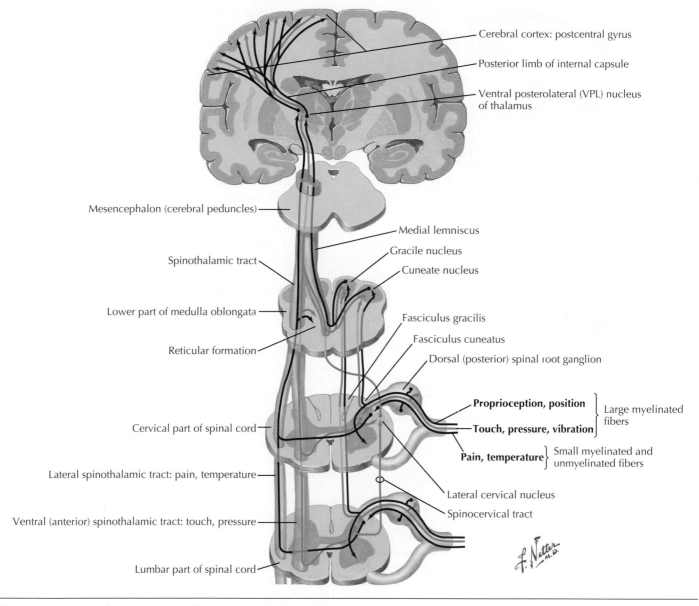

Figure 1-24 Somesthetic System: Body.

carrying pain and temperature sensation from both sides as they cross in the anterior commissure. Because the fibers carrying vibration and position sense do not initially cross at their entry level into the spinal cord, as do the spinothalamic tracts, these ascend within the posterior columns. Therefore a small centrally placed lesion within the cord spares those pathways. This leads to a dissociated sensory loss with isolated loss of pain and temperature sensation, usually in a "cape" distribution, while concomitantly, position sense is preserved.

Anterior Spinal Artery

A patient with an infarction within the territory of this essential artery presents another classic sensory picture. This is related to the inherent territory of supply of the anterior spinal artery; namely, it supplies the anterior two thirds of the cord. Here, there is bilateral damage to the spinothalamic and corticospinal

tracts while the posterior columns are spared because of their dependence on the posterior spinal artery system. Although the patient is paralyzed and has total loss of pain and temperature sensation, position and often vibratory sensory modalities are preserved.

THALAMIC INVOLVEMENT

The ventral posterior lateral and ventral posterior medial thalamic nuclei are the two major sensory relay nuclei (Fig. 1-25). Lesions in these areas can cause loss of sensation to all modalities involving the entire contralateral half of the body. This most commonly occurs in patients with lacunar or hemorrhagic infarcts. Initially presenting with a relatively tolerable numbness, eventually the damage incurred from the stroke may produce an unpleasant, sometimes disabling, hyperpathic sensory alteration known as the thalamic pain syndrome. Rarely, the parietal lobe is the integration of this information with other sensory and motor information to formulate body awareness. In the purest form of cortical sensory dysfunctions, patients are unable to differentiate the location of their toes or fingers in space, make a distinction between one and two points, or employ stereognostic discrimination to allow differentiation of various objects placed in their hands, such as differing coin sizes. In addition, these individuals are unable to recognize numbers traced on the palm (graphesthesia).

Many other sensory abnormalities occur, including "neglect," wherein the patient with a right, nondominant, parietal lesion is unaware of paralysis or sensory loss of the contralateral limbs. These are especially obvious with double simultaneous stimulation (extinction). Here one or two sides of the body are variably stimulated, and the patient is asked to identify the stimulus location. Individuals with a more subtle parietal sensory loss cannot identify the contralateral stimulus when bilateral stimuli are applied. At the extreme a patient sustaining very large hemisphere and subcortical stroke presents with a complete loss of sensation of the contralateral body.

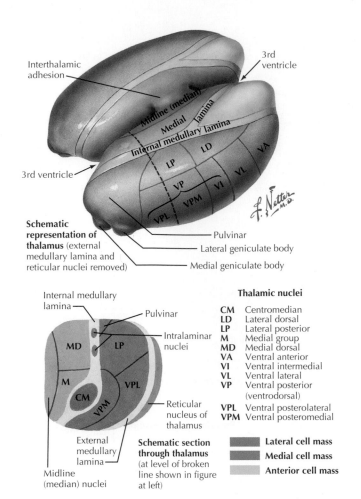

Figure 1-25 Thalamus and Its Multiple Nuclei.

this loss of sensation can lead to a limb deafferentiation sensory choreoathetosis. Lesions within the corona radiata, undercutting the parietal cortex, can cause similar, although often less extensive, findings.

CORTICAL SENSORY INVOLVEMENT

The parietal lobe receives topographically organized sensory inputs from the thalamic nuclei, brainstem, spinal cord, and peripheral nerves (see Fig. 1-24). An important function of

ADDITIONAL RESOURCES

Bates B. A Guide to Physical Examination and History Taking. 4th ed. Baltimore, MD: JB Lippincott Co; 1987.

Bear MF, Connors BW, Paradiso MA. Neuroscience, Exploring the Brain. Baltimore, MD: Lippincott Williams & Wilkins; 2007

Brain. Aids to the Examination of the Peripheral Nervous System. 4th ed. Philadelphia, PA: WB Saunders; 2000.

Brazis P, Masdeau J, Biller J. Localization in Clinical Neurology. 5th ed. Baltimore, MD: Lippincott Williams & Wilkins; 2006.

Kandel, ER, Schwartz JH, Jessell TM. Principles of Neural Science. 4th ed. New York, NY: McGraw-Hill, Health Professions Division; 2000.

Luria AR. Higher Cortical Functions in Man. 2nd ed. New York, NY: Basic Books, Inc; 1980.

Mayo Clinic Department of Neurology. Mayo Clinic Examinations in Neurology. 7th ed. St. Louis, MO: Mosby; 1998.

Benarroch EE, Daube JR, Flemming KD, Westmoreland BF. Mayo Clinic Medical Neurosciences: Organized by Neurologic Systems and Levels. 5th ed. St. Helier, NJ: Informa; 2008.

Miller NR, Newman NJ, Biousse V, Kerrison JB. Walsh & Hoyt's Clinical Neuro-Ophthalmology: The Essentials. Baltimore, MD: Lippincott Williams & Wilkins; 2007.

Parent A. Carpenter's Human Neuroanatomy. 9th ed. Baltimore, MD: Williams & Wilkins; 1996.

Peters A, Jones EG, editors. Cerebral Cortex: Vol 4. Association and Auditory Cortices. New York, NY: Plenum Press; 1985.

Cognitive and Language Evaluation

Yuval Zabar, Dana Penney, and Caitlin Macaulay

2

*T*his chapter provides an overview of the very important neurologic evaluation of higher cortical cognitive and language function. This is predicated on an understanding of frontal, temporal, parietal, occipital lobe and cerebellar function. Detailed anatomic drawings of the cerebral cortex are available for one's review while reading this chapter. It will provide the basics for an introductory mental status examination. In conclusion, the complicated and detailed evaluation of the patient with aphasia is discussed.

Clinical Vignette

A 65-year-old, right-handed, elementary school principal was referred by her primary care physician for evaluation of progressive speech difficulties. The patient reported a 2-year history of insidiously progressive language problems that began with "yes/no unreliability" to the point where she would indicate yes when she meant no, or vice versa. During the next year, she also developed trouble explaining her thoughts. Her speech became variably slurred and "garbled" with mispronounced words, making it increasingly difficult for friends to comprehend. At times she began saying "unexpected" things such as answering the phone stating "yes" versus "hello." Nevertheless, despite using unusual words for certain given situations, in general her speech "made sense." Her voice became gravely as her speech changed in melodic contour, becoming poorly modulated, and more monotone.

Her facial responsiveness became diminished; she frequently appeared angry despite feeling otherwise and her expression seemed "scary" to students. She "lost" her ability to smile and spit while brushing her teeth, developed facial apraxia, and could no longer initiate a smile or eye-blink, although she could spontaneously blink. Mild agraphia developed; in striking contradistinction, she could use the computer and keyboard without difficulty. Her speech and reading comprehension, as well as calculation were normal. She described her mood as "happy"; she denied being depressed. There was no personality change or memory problems. This lady was still independent in her basic activities of daily living (ADLs), being able to live alone, read voraciously easily recalling what she read, hosted dinner parties, pursued her photography hobby, played bridge, and drove her automobile without difficulty.

However, during the next year, she became increasingly apraxic, losing the ability to perform a number of ADLs, including many skilled motor tasks such as removing jar caps and knitting. Her language function further deteriorated and was characterized by an expressive aphasia with markedly dysfluent speech. Concomitantly, she also evidenced increasing verbal and phonemic paraphasic errors, and a stutter with oral lingual dyskinesias that compromised her intelligibility. Interestingly, she relied on texting

(e-mails) for verbal communication, despite the frustration that her typing was becoming increasingly laborious as well. Memory and photography skills remained intact. Personality and mood remained unchanged.

On initial examination, she had only minimal facial animation, characterized by diminished eye-blink frequency. Oral lingual dyskinesia with tongue thrusting and grimacing occurred when she attempted to speak. Speech articulation was effortful, monotonic, and dysarthric. She displayed fine-dexterity problems, such as requiring to pick up her purse using a closed hand with a scooping motion rather than normally grasping her pocketbook with her fingers. Typewritten text was grammatically and semantically normal, yet she had trouble writing. She was able to print her name to command, but was unable to write in cursive. When asked to draw a clock to command, she could not form a reliable circle, drawing an ellipse instead, or could not make an appropriate circle face with correct numbers. Here she demonstrated evidence of mis-sequencing, perseveration, and misplacement of numbers and hands. In contrast, she could copy a clock better than draw one. This suggested impaired organization, planning, and sequencing rather than visuospatial construction impairment. Although she demonstrated inconsistencies in reasoning, she appeared highly intelligent, with intact ability to learn new information.

Comment: This case demonstrates a progressive apraxia of speech. The patient is unable to produce speech but she has relatively normal written language. Comprehension is normal. Other cognitive domains are intact although assessment is limited by the patient's sparse speech production. This is an example of primary progressive aphasia, one of the clinical variants of frontotemporal lobar degeneration.

INTRODUCTION

The initial clinical evaluation of a patient such as this affords the opportunity to assess whether a neurologic patient has overt cognitive or language difficulties. The ability to give a well-organized history provides the experienced neurologist with insight into the patient's general language and cognitive function. In most patient encounters, it is usually clear that intellect and speech are appropriate to the setting, and thus a more formal set of mental status testing is unnecessary. However, in instances of overt intellectual dysfunction, especially when the patient's demeanor suggests such a possibility, or the family expresses concern about an additional problem beyond that of the primary patient complaint, a more detailed cognitive examination is necessary to complement the standard neurologic examination.

One's direct interaction with the patient helps define the behavioral aspects of neurologic function; it is their mood, affect, level of cooperation, and distractibility that are noteworthy. The cognitive part of the neurologic evaluation strives to

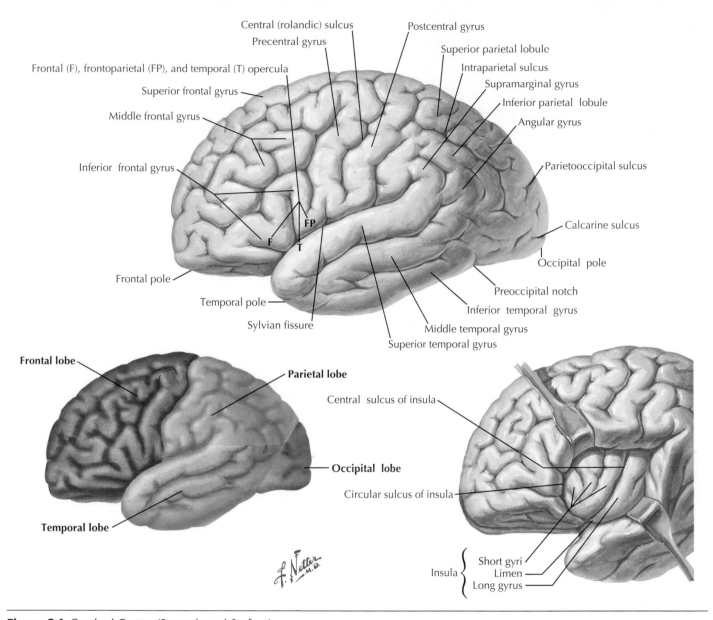

Figure 2-1 Cerebral Cortex (Superolateral Surface).

determine the precise level of various higher cortical functions. The human cerebral cortex, with its multiple gyri and network of many million interconnections, is the most complex part of the brain. Anatomically, the cortex is classified into four major functional areas: frontal, temporal, parietal, and occipital lobes (Fig. 2-1; Table 2-1 and Table 2-2). These anatomic substrates are carefully interconnected in a complex network. Although for the sake of discussion, these cortical areas are typically described in isolation, in reality these interconnections with other cortical and subcortical areas are critical for brain function (Fig. 2-2).

Because some patients are not able to give a history or cooperate with the examiner, the history from reliable family and friends is an essential part of the evaluation. Direct interaction with the patient helps define the behavioral aspects of neurologic function. The patient's mood, affect, level of cooperation, and distractibility are noteworthy. Many individuals with dementia may seem pleasant and jovial, often finding excuses

Table 2-1	Lateral Surface of the Brain: Notable Lateral Sulci	
Structure	**Anatomic Significance**
Lateral (Sylvian) fissure	Separates temporal lobe from frontal and parietal lobes
Central (Rolandic) sulcus	Separates frontal lobe from parietal lobe

From Rubin M, Safdieh J. Netter's Concise Neuroanatomy, Philadelphia, Saunders, 2007, p. 32.

for their inability to answer questions, rarely with any insight into their deficit. In contrast, patients with severe posterior aphasia may seem agitated and uncooperative, and often respond inconsistently to certain commands but not to others. Assessment of cognitive function requires direct testing of various cognitive domains and a structured, hierarchical approach.

Table 2-2 Lateral Surface of the Brain: Cortical Lobes, Lateral View

Lobe	Notable Gyri	Notable Sulci	Notable Functions
Frontal	Superior frontal gyrus Middle frontal gyrus Inferior frontal gyrus Precentral gyrus	Superior frontal sulcus Inferior frontal sulcus Precentral sulcus	Motor control, expressive speech, personality, drive
Parietal	Postcentral gyrus Superior parietal lobule Inferior parietal lobule Supramarginal gyrus Angular gyrus	Postcentral sulcus Intraparietal sulcus	Sensory input and integration, receptive speech
Temporal	Superior temporal gyrus Middle temporal gyrus Inferior temporal gyrus	Superior temporal sulcus Inferior temporal sulcus	Auditory input and memory integration
Occipital		Transverse occipital sulcus Lunate sulcus	Visual input and processing

From Rubin M, Safdieh J. Netter's Concise Neuroanatomy, Philadelphia, Saunders, 2007, p. 32.

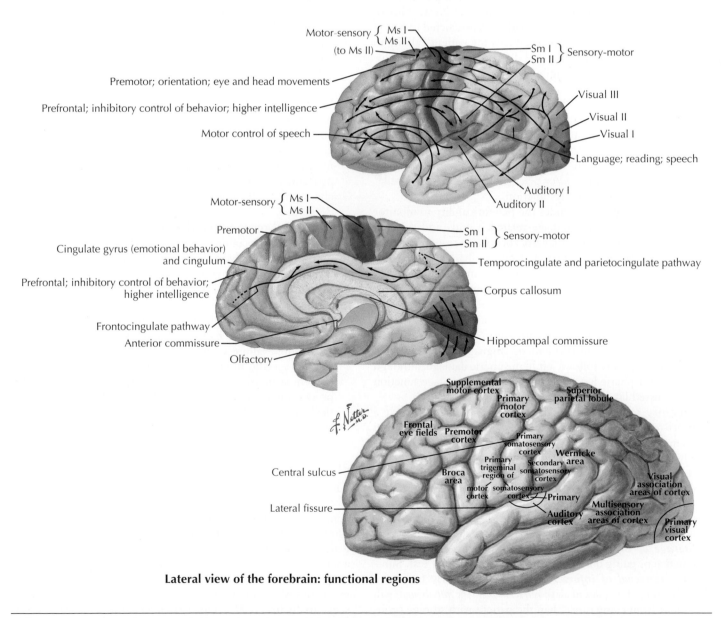

Lateral view of the forebrain: functional regions

Figure 2-2 Cerebral Cortex: Localization of Function and Association Pathways.

COGNITIVE TESTING

The major cognitive domains included in a routine mental status examination include level of consciousness, orientation, attention, language, memory, visuospatial processing, and executive function. These are best defined as follows:

1. **Level of consciousness** underlies all aspects of mental status and must be considered immediately. A stuporous patient often displays attention or language impairment; obviously it is not possible to make a cognitive assessment in a comatose patient.

2. **Attention** allows the individual to focus and register specific information from external and internal environments. Impaired attention may affect the patient's performance in other cognitive tasks, such as reading, writing, or memorizing lists. Digit span testing is a good means to test attention. The examiner gives the patient a list of five digits and asks them to repeat these in the same sequence. Next, a list of three digits is provided and the patient is instructed to repeat these in reverse order. This test elicits the patient's ability to give immediate focus and avoid distraction. Fewer than five digits forward or three digits backward may indicate attention problems.

3. **Orientation** allows an individual to identify when, where, and who they are at any given moment. This requires intact function within widespread cortical regions as well as high-order cognitive processing. Testing this simple modality provides an efficient means to survey general cognitive function. *Disorientation* to time and/or place may occur in either widespread or focal cortical dysfunction.

4. **Language function** includes the patient's ability to monitor and to comprehend language-related sounds and symbols and to generate meaningful verbal or written responses. Most interaction with the patient is language-based, and, therefore, it is crucial to ascertain whether language function is impaired early in the course of the examination. A patient with a nonfluent aphasia may not be able to express three words during memory testing, for example. Such a deficit would not indicate impaired short-term memory or inattention, but primary impairment of language. Impairment of language typically follows left hemispheric damage, although right hemispheric lesions may also impair language function as discussed later in this chapter.

5. **Memory testing** often focuses on the ability to retrieve a short-term recollection of word lists or stories. Short-term memory, of course, involves far more than the ability to recall a list of words. The brain's capacity for memory is enormous. It keeps track of what we hear and see, feel and think, from the moment we awaken to the moment we fall asleep. The use of word lists to test the brain's ability to do this is a very useful bedside tool. The patient must be able to *register* the words, *store* them, and then *retrieve* them from storage. *Storage of information* can be facilitated with repetition/practice or cuing during the learning phase of the test. Similarly, *retrieval of information* may be similarly facilitated with cuing. The patient with *retrieval memory impairment* will benefit from cuing more than the patient with storage problems. The latter patient will not benefit from cuing or practice. *Storage memory deficits* are typical of *medial temporal/hippocampal dysfunction*, such as in early Alzheimer's disease. Whenever a patient has impaired storage function, this must be considered abnormal regardless of age. *Retrieval memory deficits* are more typical of *frontal and subcortical dysfunction*; these limitations are characterized by increasing inefficiency and delay in retrieving information, and occur more frequently with advancing age. The precess of short-term memory is analogous to recording video tapes of various events. The person with impaired retrieval has trouble finding the recordings they made, while the person with impaired storage has trouble recording the tapes in the first place.

6. **Executive function** refers to the brain's ability to coordinate multimodal cortical processes for the purpose of solving problems, planning and executing tasks, and keeping track of multiple tasks at once. This cognitive ability can be likened to that of a conductor of an orchestra where one efficiently plans and coordinates several sections of the orchestra to achieve a cohesive and meaningful whole.

7. **Procedural memory, that is, praxis,** is another important cognitive process that refers to the brain's memory for skilled motor function. This encompasses a host of previously learned motor programs ranging from simple tasks, such as brushing one's teeth or using a spoon, to far more complex motor activities such as playing the piano. When an individual performs these tasks, he or she does not have to precisely recall what to do; rather, once the person initiates the motor program, the task proceeds implicitly. Praxis per se probably involves several cerebral cortical regions, but when abnormal it is most often associated with *dominant frontal lobe dysfunction*.

8. **Nonverbal recognition, that is, gnosis,** refers to the identification and recognition of all aspects of the world around us as well as ourselves. We recognize objects, people, sounds, etc. arranged in very complex sensory environments without needing verbal definition of those items. We can navigate through our world safely and effectively without using language, much like we do while driving home from work, or moving through the hallways of one's workplace. **Agnosia** is an acquired failure to recognize things normally. This may involve specific modalities as in visual agnosia or specific content as in prosopagnosia (loss of facial recognition). This processing likely involves bilateral temporal and parietal cortical regions, although *right hemisphere temporal parietal pathology* predominates.

AN INTRODUCTORY MENTAL STATUS EXAMINATION

This section provides a brief overview for the initial approach to evaluating mental function. Much of this discussion is further amplified in subsequent sections. A brief mental status exam should first include noting the patient's level of consciousness, general appearance, behavior, and affect. In addition, there are a series of brief introductory screening tests that are very useful.

Attention testing: Digit span forwards and backwards is an excellent test for attention problems. Serial 7 subtractions taken sequentially from 100 is often examined at the bedside; however, it is not strictly a test of attention. This modality requires calculation and sustained attention or working memory to reliably keep track of the task and work in progress.

Language testing: There are a few basic and efficient means available to initially screen for such impairments. These include (1) a careful **conversational speech** analysis looking for *paraphasic substitutions* as well as *grammatical errors*, (2) noting the **ability to follow commands**, and (3) **naming**. Other very useful bedside testing modalities include analyzing the patient's ability to **read, write, and repeat sentences**.

Memory is often tested by asking the patient to repeat a list of words immediately after the examiner and then to recall the words after some time delay. Often a 3- or 5-minute delay is employed; however, on occasion subtle problems with storage may require longer delays before recall. **Executive function** may be assessed by asking the patient to draw a clock with all the numbers and to indicate a specific time. The patient's approach to drawing the clock given those instructions may provide hints regarding impairment in **planning and organizing** the task. For example, the circle may be too small, the number placement may be haphazard or incomplete, or the hands may indicate concrete processing, such as pointing to the 10 and the 11 to indicate the time at 11:10. Clock drawing may also demonstrate impairment of spatial processing.

There are several standardized brief assessments of cognition, including the Mini Mental State Exam and the Montreal Cognitive Assessment (MOCA). These studies are particularly useful for assessing memory problems in the elderly. The MOCA is available online at www.mocatest.org along with normative data and translation into multiple languages. It is very useful when screening for very subtle cognitive impairment as seen in Mild Cognitive Impairment or the very earliest stages of dementia. The MMSE may provide a useful tool for staging dementia severity in patients with Alzheimer disease. Additional discussion of such tests is presented in the subsequent dementia chapter (Chapter 18).

FRONTAL LOBE DYSFUNCTION

The frontal lobe comprises the major portion of the adult brain occupying approximately 30% of brain mass. This includes the *motor area* (Brodmann area 4), the *premotor cortex* (Brodmann areas 6 and 8), and *significant prefrontal* areas (Fig. 2-3). A **Brodmann area** is a region of the cortex that is defined by the organization of its cells, or cytoarchitecture, as opposed to gross anatomic landmarks such as sulci or gyri. Reference to Brodmann's areas may provide more precise clinicoanatomic correlation and localization (see Fig. 2-3).

The *significant* **prefrontal** areas are distinct from the adjacent motor and premotor areas, particularly in their connections with other cortical areas and the thalamus (see Fig. 2-2). Most of the prefrontal–thalamic connections are made with the *dorsal medial nucleus*, a prime relay center for limbic projections originating from the amygdala and the basal forebrain. The reciprocal inputs are the most prominent cortical connections, originating from second-order sensory association and paralimbic association areas, including the cingulate cortex, temporal pole, and parahippocampal area. The frontal lobe is an integrator and analyzer of highly complex multimodal cortical areas, including limbically processed information.

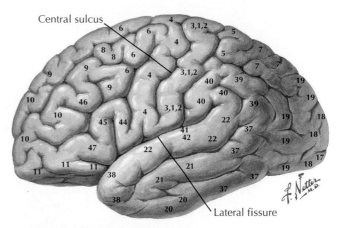

The numbers superimposed on the above brain images are what constitute the Brodmann map of cytoarchitectonics. Brodmann assigned numbers to various brain regions by analyzing each area's cellular structure starting from the central sulcus (the boundary between the frontal and parietal lobes).

Brodmann Functional Brain Cytoarchitecture Areas			
Function	**Primary**	**Secondary**	**Tertiary**
Motor	4	6	9, 10, 11, 45, 46, 47
Speech	44		
Eye Movement	8		
Sensory; Body	1, 2, 3	5, 7	7, 22, 37, 39, 40
Auditory	41	22, 42	
Vision	17	18, 19, 20	21, 37

Table provides a general view of brain function that refers to the Brodmann map shown above.

Figure 2-3 Brodmann Areas: Lateral View of the Forebrain: Cytoarchitecture of the Brain Based on Neuronal Organization.

The ablation of both frontal lobes in experimental animals leads to very unusual observations. Some of the most dramatic symptoms, including automatic nonpurposeful behaviors with a tendency to chew randomly on objects, led to the conclusion that the frontal lobe was important for the integration of goal-directed movement. Investigations in the 1950s began to define the importance of the frontal lobe for analyzing various stimuli. Frontal lobe lesions led to loss of normal social interchange, personal internal reinforcement, and judgment. Therefore, patients sustaining frontal lobe lesions are unable to modify behavior despite the potentially harming or embarrassing effects of their actions. Additionally, these individuals tend to perseverate by repeating automatic behaviors that do not result in conclusive actions; these are identified with perseveration testing.

Humans sustaining frontal lobe disorders develop significant personality changes and "release of animal instincts." One of the earliest descriptions of frontal lobe damage described patients with apathy and disturbed emotions. Elucidation of the frontal lobe connections, particularly the medial-basal portion, demonstrates that the limbic system provides significant input to that area (Fig. 2-4). Autonomic centers originating in the brainstem and hypothalamus also have significant connections with the basal frontal lobe. When these connections are disrupted,

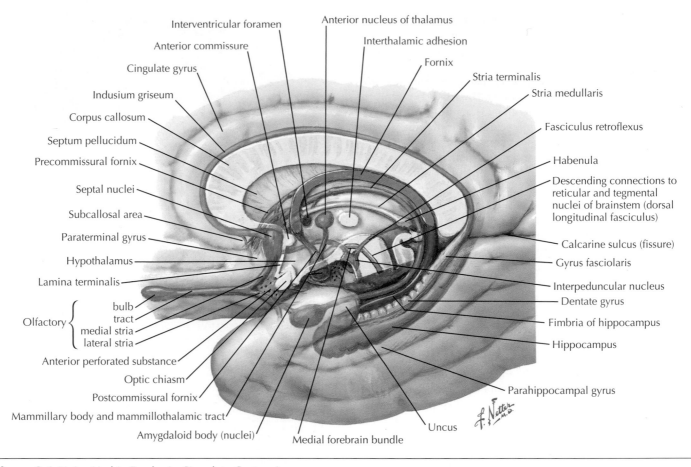

Figure 2-4 Major Limbic Forebrain Cingulate Cortex Areas.

aggressive, impulsive, and uncontrolled behavior results. Subsequent study has revealed an even greater depth and breadth of frontal lobe function.

From a neuropsychological perspective, the frontal lobes are responsible for executive functions. Frontal lobe syndromes typically are classified clinically, anatomically, and neuropsychologically into lateral, medial, and mesial groups. Prefrontal syndromes that affect these anterior areas have been described as dysexecutive, disinhibited, and apathetic-akinetic. From an anatomic perspective, the *dysexecutive syndrome* is due to damage of the dorsolateral prefrontal area. The *disinhibited syndrome* is due to disorders affecting the orbital brain while the *apathetic–akinetic* syndrome is due to medial area dysfunction.

Patients with damage to the *dorsolateral prefrontal* cortex typically exhibit *stereotyped* and *perseverative behaviors* with mental inflexibility (i.e., stuck in set). Additionally, one will note that these patients demonstrate poor self-monitoring, deficient working memory, difficulty generating hypotheses, and reduced fluency. These patients often demonstrate an associated inefficient/unorganized learning strategy, with impaired retrieval for learned information as well as a loss of set. Such individuals are typically apathetic, exhibiting reduced drive, depressed mentation, and motor programming deficits.

Damage to the *orbital–frontal* area is characterized by patients presenting with prominent *personality changes*. They are often disinhibited, impulsive, perseverative, and have potential to be socially inappropriate with poor self-monitoring. Inappropriate

euphoria, affective lability with quick onset, poor judgment, and tendency to confabulate are other characteristic personality changes. Typically, these patients exhibit impaired sustained and divided attention, increased distractibility, and anosmia.

Patients with damage to the *anterior cingulate gyrus* typically experience difficulty reacting to stimuli. They have an impaired initiation of action as well as impaired persistence, reduced arousal, and akinesia/bradykinesia, with loss of spontaneous speech and behavior. Such individuals may present with monosyllabic speech, appear apathetic, have a flat or diminished affect, and may be docile.

Although these various prefrontal lobe syndromes pertain to localized lesions, it is not uncommon for patients to display overlapping behaviors as it is relatively uncommon to have isolated areas of precise frontal lobe pathology. Also, certain behaviors are witnessed that are not due to specific localized deficits. There are some nonspecific frontal signs that sometimes can be elucidated during neurologic examination of the patient with disorders of this nature. These include various frontal release signs, particularly involuntary grasping, and suck reflexes. However, one must take care with interpretation of these findings, especially with elderly individuals, many of whom will have an increased incidence of such findings with normal aging or in the presence of generalized neurologic illness such as with various encephalopathies.

Language dysfunction is a common finding of some frontal lobe lesions. *Broca aphasia* is the classic form of frontal lobe language dysfunction with dominant hemisphere lesions. It is characterized by a nonfluent, effortful, slow, and halting speech. This language dysfunction is typically of reduced length, that is, few words with reduced phrase length, simplified grammar, and impaired naming. Repetition is characteristically intact. These individuals often have associated apraxia (buccofacial, speech, and of the nonparalyzed limb) and right-sided weakness of the face and hand. *Transcortical motor aphasia* is another characteristic of frontal lobe language dysfunction. These patients often have very limited spontaneous speech as well as delayed responsiveness. They also tend to be perseverative, akinetic, and may also have contralateral leg weakness and urinary incontinence because of a mesial lesion. This may result from a lesion either in the distribution of the anterior cerebral artery or in the watershed area between the middle and anterior cerebral artery territories. Proximal extremity weakness very rarely, if ever, occurs with a vascular watershed lesion. Auditory comprehension (barring complex syntax), repetition, and naming are intact in transcortical motor aphasia.

Various diseases or injuries that result in executive dysfunction do not necessarily have to directly affect the frontal lobes per se. This is due to the presence of widespread subcortical–frontal cortical as well as other cortical–frontal cortical connections wherein a distant nonfrontal lesion can impact on primary frontal lobe function. When someone sustains an acceleration/deceleration brain injury wherein the brain strikes the bony prominences of the skull, there is an increased incidence of frontal lobe injury. This is particularly the situation with injuries either at the basal orbital frontal regions lying directly adjacent to the skull's cribriform plate or at the frontal poles adjacent to the frontal bone. Frontal lobe injury may also result indirectly because of shearing of white matter tracts.

Dementing illness, particularly those referred to as frontal-temporal lobar dementias and Lewy Body disease, present with executive dysfunction. This similarly occurs with various subcortical dementias. These occur with Parkinson disease, Huntington disease, AIDS-related dementia, and demyelinating disorders that lead to involvement of subcortical white matter connections. Additionally, there is a high incidence of executive dysfunction with vascular disease, whether due to large vessel stroke, small vessel ischemic disease, or ruptured aneurysm (typically of the anterior communicating artery). The anterior cerebral artery and middle cerebral arteries supply the anterior and medial portions and the lateral dorsal frontal cortex, respectively. Primary brain tumors, for example, gliomas, oligodendrogliomas, meningiomas, and pituitary adenomas, may typically affect executive functioning. Various causes of hydrocephalus, particularly normal-pressure hydrocephalus, may present in a similar fashion although a gait disorder may often presage the dementia-associated normal-pressure hydrocephalus.

TEMPORAL LOBE DYSFUNCTION

Because of the complexity of the temporal lobe regions and the high interconnectivity with other brain regions, damage or injury can result in a wide variety of deficits involving many cognitive functions. It is impossible to assess all of them during an office visit or bedside consult. However, it is important to recognize some of the major symptom complexes that may

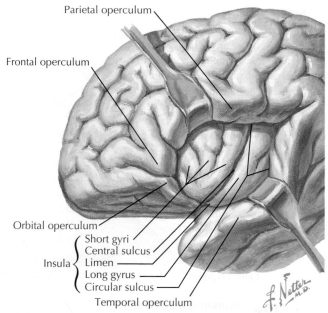

INSULA (INSULAR CORTEX)	
Structure	**Anatomic Notes**
Circular sulcus of the insula	Surrounds and demarcates the insula
Central sulcus of the insula	Divides the insula into anterior and posterior parts
Limen	The apex of the insula at its inferior margin
Short gyri and long gyrus	Gyri of the insula

From Rubin M, Safdieh J. Netter's Concise Neuroanatomy, Philadelphia Saunders, 2007, p. 34.

Figure 2-5 Cerebral Insular Cortex.

occur with lesions in this elegant portion of our brains. One needs to be able to quickly evaluate the patient for lesions at this critical level through specific interview questions with the patient and family or in either the office or bedside setting. The primary manifestations that are addressed here are personality and affect alterations; language and naming deficits; visuoperceptual difficulties; and lastly memory learning problems.

An understanding of temporal lobe anatomy helps one appreciate the various clinical deficits that can arise from lesions at this level. The temporal lobe is defined as encompassing all brain regions below the Sylvian fissure and anterior to the occipital cortex (Figs. 2-1, 2-5, 2-6). These also include subcortical structures such as the hippocampal formation, the amygdala, and limbic cortex. The temporal lobe is divided into three distinct regions: the *lateral area* consisting of the superior, middle, and inferior temporal gyri; the *inferior temporal cortex* containing the auditory and visual areas; and the *medial area* including the fusiform gyrus and parahippocampal gyrus.

The temporal lobe is characterized by a high prevalence of multisite brain connections through efferent projections extending to the limbic system, basal ganglia, frontal and parietal association regions, as well as afferent projections from the sensory areas. The right and left temporal lobes are connected by the corpus callosum and anterior commissure. This

acquired alexia are sometimes taught to use visuospatial techniques to help them relearn to read. The nonlanguage hemisphere role in reading is demonstrated below. One of the groups of lines below represents the word "horses" and the other represents the word "elephant." Can you determine which grouping represents the word "elephant"?

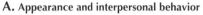

Notice that there are no letters, but because of the right hemisphere contribution you can still identify the word on the left as "elephant" from the contour created by the lines. Similarly, the nonlanguage temporal lobe can also help decode words that are seemingly nonsense if you attend strictly to the letters and rules of phonics. In fact, it deosn't mttaer in waht oredr the ltteers in a wrod are, the olny iprmoetnt tihng is taht the frist and lsat ltteer be at the rghit pclae.

Asking the patient to provide a handwriting sample is very important in order to assess these various problems (Fig. 2-7). Damage to the left temporal region may result in wider right-side margins, spaces, or wide separations between letters or syllables and disrupt the continuity of the writing line. Patients with damage to the left temporal region may also be noted to have a decline in ability to write in script, as opposed to a better-preserved ability to print.

The clock-drawing test that was used to identify frontal lobe deficits is also useful in identifying temporal lobe deficits (see Fig. 2-7). In order to draw a clock, there must be a mental visual representation of what features are essential. Visuospatial abilities are essential to determining the layout and proportions, and for making sure that features are accurate on both sides of space. Visuospatial perception is also a component of evaluating the output and making corrections.

A. Appearance and interpersonal behavior

Pleasant, neatly dressed, good spirits

Depressed, sloppily dressed, careless

Belligerent

B. Language

Good

Defective

Doctor: "Write me a brief paragraph about your work."

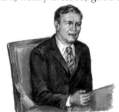
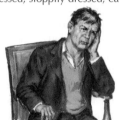

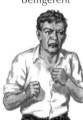

C. Memory

Doctor: "Here are 3 objects: a pipe, a pen, and a picture of Abraham Lincoln. I want you to remember them and in 5 minutes, I will ask you what they were."

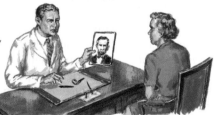
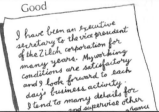
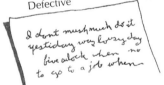

5 minutes later: Patient: "I'm sorry, I can't remember. Did you show me something?"

D. Constructional praxis and visual-spatial function

Doctor: "Draw me a simple picture of a house."

"Draw a clock face for me."

Good   Abnormal   Good   Abnormal

E. Reverse counting

Doctor: "Count backward from 5 to 1 for me." Patient: "5...3...4..., sorry, I can't do it."

Doctor: "Spell the word *worlds* backward for me." Patient: "W..L..R..D..S."

Figure 2-7 Testing for Defects of Higher Cortical Function.

In the clock drawing below, the entire left side is neglected, and the right side is drawn twice because the patient did not attend to his first attempt. This patient had a right temporal lesion causing perceptual problems on the left side of space within the context of intact visual fields.

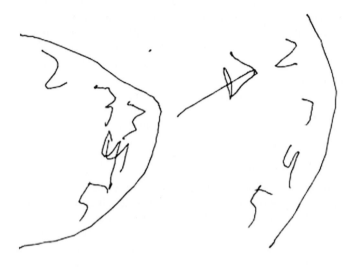

The clock drawing below demonstrates several types of errors associated with the temporal lobes. The patient has added additional structure (lines that look like spokes in a wheel), in an attempt to compensate for perceptual problems in spacing the numbers. There is a numbering error in the upper left quadrant and the hands are missing. These errors are suggestive of right temporal involvement. In addition, the patient wrote a cue to help remember the time, suggesting compensation for a memory problem. Note, too, that the time cue is incorrect: Rather than 10 past 11, the patient wrote 10 to 11, suggesting a language-processing problem. Memory loss, language problem, and time concept error are all suggestive of temporal lobe deficit.

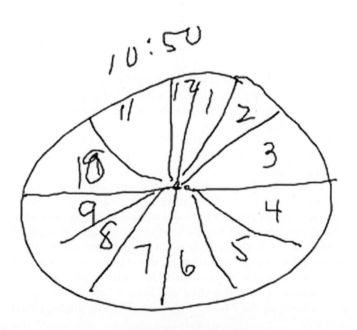

The temporal lobes are essential in the learning of new information. Damage here will affect memory. The ability to retain information starts with *acquisition* (attention, sustaining focus, organization), *encoding* (information processing), *storage* (retention of information through consolidation), and *retrieval* (accessing the information that is in storage) of the information that is stored. *Explicit or episodic memory* is information that can be specifically stated (contextual knowledge, autobiographical information, events, the knowledge in this book). Information that is recalled or influences behavior per se, without conscious intention, that is, procedures such as how to drive a car or ride a bicycle, is called *implicit memory*. Memory deficits may result if any of these complex stages fail. Damage to different regions of the temporal lobe can result in various breakdowns in the memory encoding and storage process. Damage to the mesial temporal regions, the hippocampal complex, can result in profound memory deficits as is well demonstrated by the famous case of HM.

On December 2, 2008, Henry Gustav Molaison, age 82, died of respiratory failure. If the name is unfamiliar, that's because for the last 55 years, he was known to the world only as HM. In 1953 Mr. Molaison underwent temporal lobe surgery for severe epilepsy with uncontrolled seizures. Although the surgery was largely successful in reducing seizure frequency, it left him with a profound memory loss and essentially no ability to learn new things. For fifty five years after the surgery, he could recall almost nothing that happened subsequently: births and deaths of family members, the events of 9-11, or what he did that morning. Each time he met a friend, each time he ate at a restaurant, each time he walked into his own home, it was for him, the first time.

Damage to the *inferior temporal regions* interferes with the intentional retrieval of information. Lesions of the *left hemisphere* tend to preferentially compromise retrieval of *verbal* information (e.g., conversations, word lists), whereas *right hemisphere* damage tends to impair the retrieval of *visual information* (e.g., misplacing items). Assessment of memory is an important aspect of the mental status exam. Patients with memory deficits frequently have difficulty accurately reporting the type and extent of their memory problems. Interviews with the family are the best way to quickly determine the type of memory impairment and the implication of the memory deficit for that patient. The terminology for memory functions may be confusing and may be used differently by different physicians. Effective communication of results and accurate retesting at a later date require both the use of descriptive terms for documenting memory complaints stated by the family, including examples, and a detailed description of the procedures amount and type of information presented, interval delay, and instructions that you use to test memory. One must specify the number of learning trials or types of problems observed during the learning trials, that is, acquisition. It is important to attend to any strategies, for example, rehearsal, that a patient may use to learn the information, that is, encoding. Note how much information is freely recalled after at least a 10- to 15-minute delay retention, and the improvement in the amount of information recalled with cues when compared to the amount freely recalled, that is, retrieval.

Information and orientation questions are useful in assessing episodic memory. Knowing where you are, the date and the time of day, without looking at a clock, have clinical utility. If the patient is not oriented to time, within 30 minutes, then there are likely to be medication compliance problems. The key to assessing information storage is to ensure that registration and encoding have taken place and to allow for sufficient time for memory to decay, that is, forgetting, prior to testing retention. The memory problems in disorders like early Alzheimer disease may not be apparent when tested following a few minutes' delay, but they may be evident when tested 15 minutes later. The MMSE registration and recall of three objects is often used to assess memory function. Although a reasonable brief bedside task for the very impaired patient, it is insensitive to impairment in the young or mildly impaired and can result in the underestimation of memory deficits because of the abbreviated list to be learned and short interval delay between registration and recall. The addition of a second recall condition, 10–15 minutes later, at the completion of your examination affords additional time for storage as well as memory decay. This may be very important for detecting modest memory impairment.

PARIETAL LOBE DYSFUNCTION

The parietal lobe is situated between the frontal and occipital lobes. The central sulcus separates frontal from parietal cortex, while the parietooccipital sulcus separates parietal from occipital cortex (see Fig. 2-1). The Sylvian fissure forms the lateral boundary separating parietal from temporal cortex. The most anterior portion of the parietal lobe, sitting immediately behind the central sulcus, is the primary somatosensory cortex (Brodmann area 3; see Fig. 2-3). More posteriorly, the parietal lobe may be divided into the superior parietal lobule (Brodmann areas 5 and 7) and the inferior parietal lobule (Brodmann areas 39 and 40) (see Fig. 2-3). These areas are separated by the intraparietal sulcus.

The primary role of the parietal lobe is to integrate multimodal sensory information, creating a sensory map of one's self, the perceived world around you, and the relationship of the self within the world. Recent research in primates elucidated the functional anatomy of the parietal lobe. The *posterior parietal lobe* is thought to primarily integrate visual and somatosensory data allowing proper hand–eye coordination, spatial localization of objects, proper targeting of eye movements, and accurate gauging of the shape, size, and orientation of objects. Further functional subdivision identifies that the *posterior (dorsal)* portion provides integration of spatial vision via occipital-parietal connections, the *"where" stream*, whereas the *inferior (ventral)* regions involve *visual recognition* of objects and actions via occipital and temporal connections, the *"what" stream*. There is a further specialization of function within the parietal lobes determined by lateralization. *Number processing and calculation* are primarily represented within the *left* hemisphere whereas *sensory integration* is predominately defined within the *right* hemisphere.

Somatosensory integration begins in the primary somatosensory cortex, where basic tactile localization is appreciated. This is evaluated by testing both joint position and two-point discrimination sensory modalities. Once sensory information is received in the primary somatosensory cortex, this then streams posteriorly toward the somatosensory association cortex (see Fig. 2-2). Here, tactile information is integrated to provide discriminatory sensation over larger areas of the body surface for sensory definition of object weight, size and shape, texture, etc. This allows for specialized tactile sensation, such as graphesthesia and stereognosis. Most importantly, this allows the integrative *mapping* of the spatial, tactile, and visual aspects of one's body. The sensory *mapping* of the external world takes place posteriorly in the parietal lobe. There are two "functional maps," one of the self and the other of the world. These are also integrated, presumably in the heteromodal association area in the right parietotemporal–occipital junction.

Right Parietal Lobe

Patients with lesions at this level develop unilateral neglect of sensory events occurring on their left side when sensory input from those areas seemingly appears to vanish. The patient is unaware of those events, as though they were not happening at all. The patient may be completely unaware of the examiner standing on his left side. Sometimes, this occurs in a milder form, whereby events on the left side of the patient extinguish when competing with sensory events on the right side. Double simultaneous stimulation provides a way to test this at the bedside. When the examiner touches the patient on either side individually, the patient detects each stimulus correctly. However, when the stimuli are presented simultaneously, the patient with neglect will not detect the stimulus on the left side. This may also occur with simultaneous visual stimuli in both visual fields.

A related condition, called *asomatognosia*, involves the patient's inability to recognize his own body part. When viewing his own hand, the patient does not recognize it as his own. Moreover, he may misidentify it as someone else's limb. *Anosognosia* refers to the patient's absent recognition of illness or disability, which is not mediated by psychological denial and is not associated with a disturbance of mood (Fig. 2-8). A milder version of neglect may occur while writing or drawing. The patient may draw a clock and place all the numbers and even the hands within the right hemispace of the clock face. *Visuospatial impairment* is relatively common following right parietal lesions. This may be seen on construction tests, where the patient is asked to copy shapes, such as a clock, a cube, or overlapping geometric figures (see Fig. 2-7).

Dressing apraxia is a fascinating condition though likely a misnomer. This condition involves loss of ability to dress in the absence of weakness or primary sensory loss. This is related to the patient having impaired spatial processing and body mapping and thus losing their ability to dress appropriately. Typically these individuals are unable to distinguish where to place their arm and/or leg within an article of clothing. This is amplified in the office or at the bedside when the examiner takes a shirt, for example, rolling it up, turning a sleeve inside out, and asking the patient to put it on appropriately. Such patients are classically befuddled by this setting and cannot appropriately place the garment on their body; they have difficulty aligning their

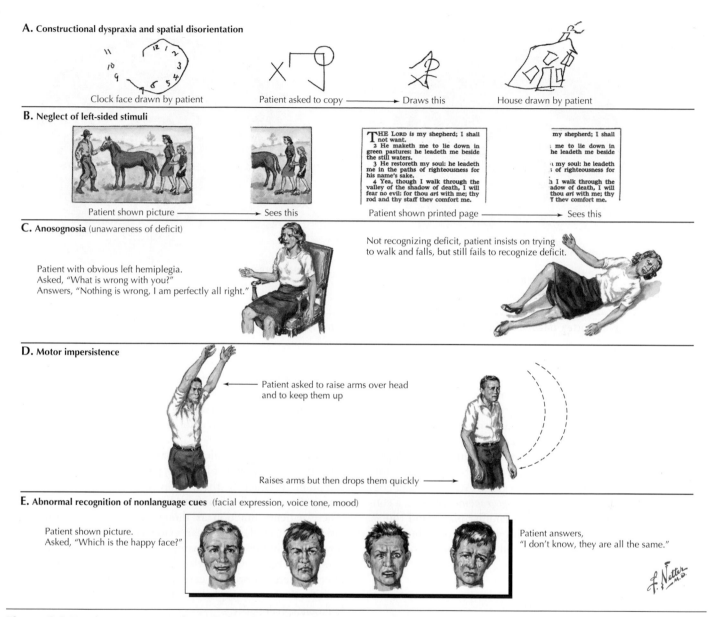

A. Constructional dyspraxia and spatial disorientation

Clock face drawn by patient

Patient asked to copy ⟶ Draws this

House drawn by patient

B. Neglect of left-sided stimuli

Patient shown picture ⟶ Sees this

Patient shown printed page ⟶ Sees this

C. Anosognosia (unawareness of deficit)

Patient with obvious left hemiplegia.
Asked, "What is wrong with you?"
Answers, "Nothing is wrong, I am perfectly all right."

Not recognizing deficit, patient insists on trying to walk and falls, but still fails to recognize deficit.

D. Motor impersistence

Patient asked to raise arms over head and to keep them up

Raises arms but then drops them quickly ⟶

E. Abnormal recognition of nonlanguage cues (facial expression, voice tone, mood)

Patient shown picture.
Asked, "Which is the happy face?"

Patient answers, "I don't know, they are all the same."

Figure 2-8 Nondominant Hemisphere Higher Cortical Function.

clothes properly, rather than forgetting the proper motor sequence for dressing. They cannot rearrange the shirt appropriately to insert their arms correctly into the sleeves. It is not a true apraxia because the motor program for dressing is presumably intact. Sometimes, the dressing difficulty occurs only on the left side with a right parietal lesion. In this circumstance, this finding is considered a part of the neglect syndrome.

Left Parietal Lobe

Gerstmann syndrome is the classic representation of left parietal cerebral dysfunction. This includes four different sets of symptoms that emerge in comparison to those occurring with right-sided parietal lesions. These patients may exhibit an (1) inability to perform arithmetic, *acalculia*; (2) *left–right confusion*, an inability to distinguish left from right side; (3) inability to identify specific fingers such as index, middle, or ring, that is, *finger agnosia*; and (4) inability to write, *agraphia*. When all four of

these symptoms occur together, the condition is known as Gerstmann syndrome. It is debatable whether it ever presents in a pure form given the high proportion of patients with left parietal dysfunction who also have some degree of aphasia. It is intriguing whether the agraphia related to left parietal dysfunction is qualitatively different from agraphia with more anterior lesions, although very difficult to determine in aphasic patients.

Balint syndrome is representative of disorders related to posterior parietal dysfunction and includes three specific forms of visual disorientation. (1) *Simultanagnosia* is evident when the patients are unable to perceive their surroundings as a whole. They literally perceive their environment just one object at a time. Often they have trouble detecting movement. (2) *Optic ataxia* occurs when the patient is unable to shift gaze toward a target accurately. There is a tendency to overshoot or undershoot the target. (3) *Ocular apraxia* is the inability to shift gaze at will toward a new target; this is commonly seen together with simultanagnosia. Cases of Balint syndrome typically follow

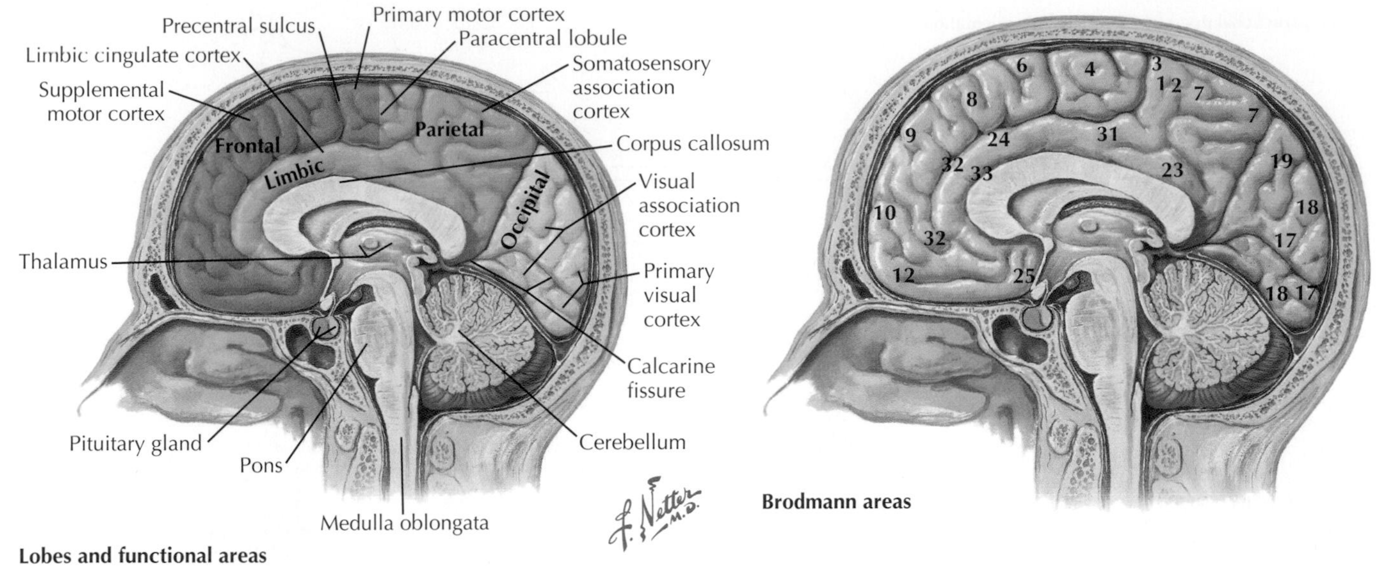

Figure 2-9 Cerebral Cortex (Medial Surface of Brain Lobes and Functional Areas).

bilateral posterior parietal lesions, but there are case reports of unilateral right posterior parietal lesions with Balint syndrome as well.

Classically, these syndromes were described in cases of stroke or tumor. However, a gradual presentation of such symptoms also occurs in cases of *posterior dementia*, a primary neurodegenerative disease affecting posterior parietal lobes initially before spreading to involve other cortical regions. An interesting cognitive syndrome in these patients is *topographical amnesia*, a condition defined by loss of memory of familiar places and routes. In such cases, patients may get lost in their own home but memory for stories, conversations, and lists of things to do may be normal.

OCCIPITAL LOBE DYSFUNCTION

The primary function of the occipital cortex is to process and organize visual information. The *calcarine area*, Brodmann area 17 (Figs. 2-9 to 2-11; Table 2-3), represents the primary visual cortex. It is located within the medial side of the occipital cortex along the calcarine sulcus. This region is also called the *striate cortex* because of prominent myelin striation, called the *Stria of Gennari*. The portion of the occipital cortex that lies beyond the primary visual area is termed *extra-striate* cortex; it subserves higher order visual processing, including color discrimination, motion perception, shape detection, etc. Each visual area contains a full map of the mentally perceived visual world.

The primary visual cortex provides a low-level description of visual object shape, spatial distribution, and color properties. Projections from the extra-striate cortex branch ventrally toward temporal lobes and dorsally toward parietal lobes. The visual information from the ventral stream integrates with temporal lobe association areas to allow recognition of objects, people, and places. Visual information travelling through the dorsal stream merges with parietal association areas to allow proper visual orientation of objects in the environment and of the self within the environment (see Fig. 2-2). There are few cognitive syndromes attributable to disorders placing the occipital lobe in isolation.

Cortical blindness follows bilateral occipital lobe injury. Patients are completely blind but, paradoxically, may deny their symptom. Frequently these individuals describe scenes with extraordinary detail, often with bizarre contextual information. These patients function as though delusional, insisting their vision is intact despite clear evidence to the contrary, lying down, or being unable to manipulate any object they see. This condition, also known as *Anton syndrome*, most commonly occurs after bilateral posterior cerebral artery strokes, progressive multifocal leukoencephalopathy, and posterior reversible leukoencephalopathy.

Pure alexia without agraphia is a *disconnection syndrome* that occurs when a lesion within the left occipital lobe extends to involve fibers traversing across the splenium of the corpus callosum from the right occipital lobe (see Fig. 2-10). This process causes loss of the ability to read while sparing all other language function. All cases include a right homonymous hemianopsia (hemifield cut). Visual information recorded by either or both occipital lobes must be directed to the posterior left temporal lobe per se in order for the individual to detect and process the visual symbols of language. Therefore, the combined left occipital lobe and splenium lesion effectively blocks data—perceived in the left visual field and recorded in the right occipital lobe—from being sent to the contralateral dominant temporal lobe. Thus, even though such individuals can see objects in their left hemifield, utilizing their still intact right occipital lobe, all vision from this cortex effectively has a conduction block vis-à-vis the precise act of reading. This is because any visual symbols of language are no longer being transmitted through the splenium and thus do not reach the dominant language areas. In essence,

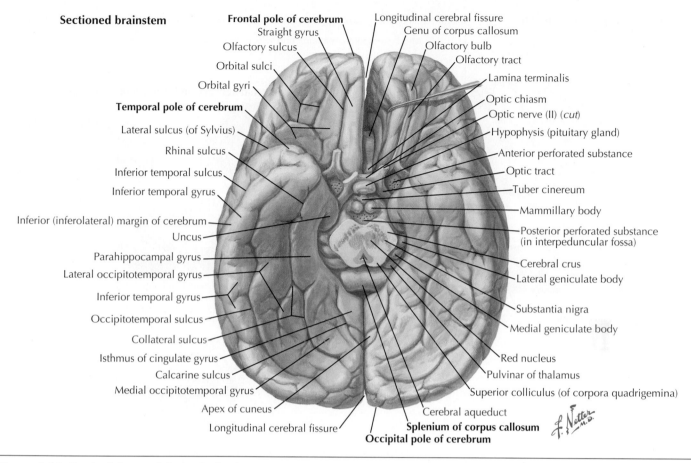

Figure 2-10 Cerebral Cortex (Inferior Surface).

Table 2-3 Inferior Surface of the Brain

	Cortical Structures	
Structure	**Anatomic Notes**	**Functional Significance**
Frontal pole	Anterior-most portion of frontal lobe	Vulnerable to injury during head trauma
Straight gyrus (gyrus rectus)	Most medial and inferior gyrus of frontal lobe	
Olfactory sulcus	Separates straight gyrus from more lateral orbital gyri	Olfactory tract travels with this sulcus
Orbital gyri and sulci	Form the floor of frontal lobes; rest on the roof of orbits	
Temporal pole	Anterior-most portion of temporal lobe	Vulnerable to injury during head trauma
Uncus	Medial-most bulb-shaped projection of temporal lobe	If swollen may compress the ipsilateral midbrain, causing contralateral hemiparesis
Parahippocampal gyrus	Large inferomedial temporal lobe gyrus	Involved in emotion as part of the limbic system
Collateral sulcus	Separates parahippocampal gyrus from medial occipitotemporal gyrus	
Medial occipitotemporal gyrus	Lies lateral to parahippocampal gyrus	
Occipitotemporal sulcus	Separates medial and lateral occipitotemporal gyri	
Lateral occipitotemporal gyrus	Forms inferolateral border of temporal lobe; contiguous with inferior temporal gyrus	
Occipital pole	Posterior-most portion of the occipital lobe	Vulnerable to injury during head trauma

From Rubin M, Safdieh J. Netter's Concise Neuroanatomy, Philadelphia, Saunders, 2007, p. 37.

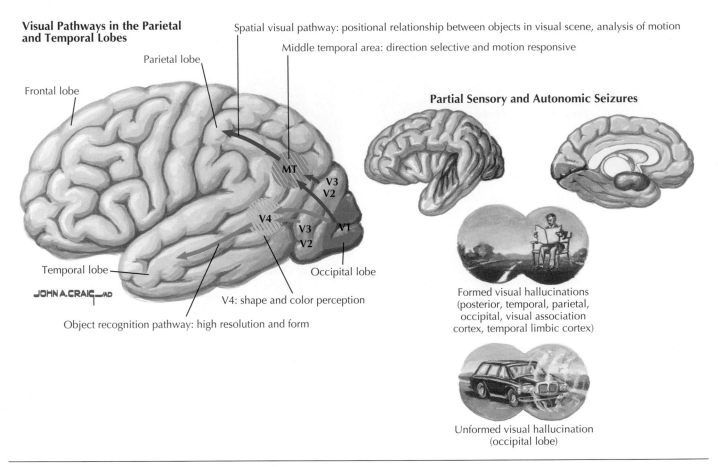

Figure 2-11 Occipital Lobe Functional Anatomy.

this lesion disconnects the right visual cortex visual information from reaching the contralateral language, and writing centers. Although the left hemifield remains intact, its potential language information cannot be "seen" by the dominant left temporal lobe. In effect, this condition could also be called pure word blindness.

In summary, the clinician may use a variety of higher cortical function assessment modalities to evaluate patients with primary cerebral cortex disorders. Some common examples of these methods are outlined in Figure 2-7.

CEREBELLUM

There has been longstanding debate regarding the cerebellum and the role it plays in cognition and behavior. During the 17th century, debates occurred as to whether the cerebellum was critical for vegetative functions and survival. During the 18th century, some considered whether the cerebellum was the center for sexual function or pure motor functioning, a more limited approach. In the 19th century, the sole proposed focus was directed at its role in coordinated movement. More recently, in the latter half of the 20th century, neuroscientists have come to recognize that the cerebellum may be responsible for more than just a balance and coordination function; however, for some this is still a debatable topic. Most think of motor symptoms when considering cerebellar disorders, and these would consist of

ataxia, dysmetria, disordered eye movement, scanning dysarthria, dysphagia, and tremor.

However, the cerebellum is connected to the contralateral cerebral hemispheres, the dorsolateral prefrontal cortex, posterior parietal and superior temporal areas, and occipital lobes, as well as limbic structures. Thus, it is not surprising that there is an increased focus on the cerebellum having an important role in cognitive functioning. Kalashnikova et al. studied 25 patients with isolated cerebellar infarcts and found that 88% exhibited cognitive impairment. Based on the pattern of deficits, they divided them into two groups: dysfunction of the prefrontal and premotor areas and dysfunction of the posterior parietal/temporal/occipital area.

Schmahmann and Sherman have postulated that there is a *cerebellar cognitive affective syndrome*. They attribute this to cerebellar lesions that are connected with the associative zones. *Cognitive affective syndrome* (CAS) is associated with executive dysfunction (e.g., planning, set-shifting, abstract reasoning, divided attention, working memory, perseveration, verbal fluency, and memory deficits due to executive dysfunction), speech disorder (agrammatism, dysprosody, mild anomia), visual spatial dysfunction (difficulty copying and conceptualizing drawings), and personality changes (flat affect, disinhibition, impulsivity, pathologic laughing/crying). However, the degree of impairment tends to depend on the location of cerebellar damage.

Specifically, those with acute cerebellar stroke, slowly progressive cerebellar degenerations, or small strokes within the cerebellum, primarily supplied by the superior cerebellar artery, tended to exhibit very subtle deficits. In contrast, those with bilateral or large unilateral strokes in the territory of the posterior inferior cerebellar arteries, or those with subacute onset of pancerebellar disorders, exhibited more striking deficits. There is a wide range of possible etiologies of cerebellar disorders, including developmental, genetic, toxic, vascular, metabolic, infectious, tumor, trauma, degenerative, and autoimmune. Thus, these patients not only have cerebellar involvement but frequently also have involvement of other areas of the cerebrum.

However, the neurophysiologic role of the cerebellum in cognition is still in relative infancy. It is likely that some study findings will be replicated and it will become more widely accepted that the cerebellum does have a significant role in cognitive functioning. Bedside testing of cerebellar motor dysfunction requires observation of gait and balance, the presence of dysmetria with use of the extremities, tendency to overshoot or overcorrect, and eye movement abnormalities.

Aphasia

Language encompasses multiple cortical regions and is not classifiable within strict cortical anatomic borders. Impairment of language function is a common neurologic symptom presenting acutely, as in stroke, or more insidiously, as in primary progressive aphasia. The classic nomenclature of the aphasia syndromes is largely based on lesion analysis in cases of stroke or tumor. These syndromes postulate distinct cortical regions responsible for the various phases of language processing from comprehension to expression. *Broca syndrome* is characterized by stuttering, agrammatical, effortful, and telegraphic language. This was thought to be an expressive language disorder typical of anterior frontal lesions (so-called motor aphasia). *Wernicke aphasia*, typified as a *receptive comprehension language disorder*, is characterized by the fluent expression of wrong or nonexistent words and syllables that is sometimes referred to as a word salad. Receptive language disorders were thought to be related to lesions of the more posterior temporal parietal cortex (Fig. 2-12).

Other aphasia syndromes, such as conduction aphasia, anomic aphasia, and the transcortical aphasias emerged to describe aphasic syndromes that did not fit neatly into the broader forms of expressive and receptive aphasias. These syndromes were traditionally associated with strokes in various left MCA strokes or tumors and thought to have some localizing value. However, exceptions to the traditional classification of aphasia occur commonly. For example, it is not unusual for a posterior MCA division stroke to produce a nonfluent aphasia. Moreover, the progressive aphasia syndromes often produce

Clinical syndromes related to site of region

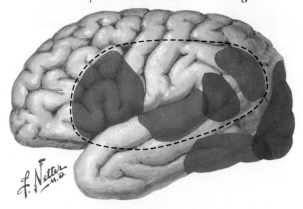

	Broca aphasia	Wernicke aphasia	Angular gyrus	Global aphasia
Pronunciation, speech rhythm	Dysarthria, stuttering, effortful	Normal, fluent, loquacious	Normal	Very abnormal
Speech content	Missed syllables, agrammatical, telegraphic	Use of wrong or nonexistent words	Often normal	Very abnormal
Repetition of speech	Abnormal but better than spontaneous	Abnormal	Normal	Very abnormal
Comprehension of spoken language	Normal	Very abnormal	Normal	Very abnormal
Comprehension of written language	Not as good as for spoken language	Abnormal but better than for spoken	Very abnormal	Very abnormal
Writing	Clumsy, agrammatical, misspelling	Penmanship OK but misspelling and inaccuracies	Very abnormal, spelling errors	Very abnormal
Naming	Better than spontaneous speech	Wrong names	Often abnormal	Very abnormal
Other	Hemiplegia, apraxia	Sometimes hemianopsia and apraxia	Slight hemiparesis, trouble calculating, finger agnosia, hemianopsia	Hemiplegia

Figure 2-12 Dominant Hemisphere Language Dysfunction.

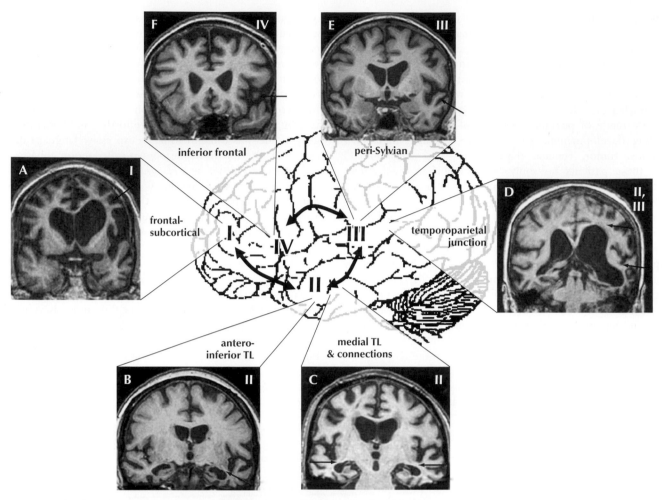

Roman numerals I through IV indicate proposed operational stages in the pathway for language output. Key anatomical areas are indicated along with superimposed MRI images as follows: (A) asymmetric (left greater than right) frontal lobe atrophy, dynamic aphasia; (B) focal left anterior/inferior temporal lobe atrophy, semantic dementia; (C) bilateral mesial temporal atrophy, Alzheimer's disease (anomia); (D) left posterior superior temporal/inferior parietal atrophy, progressive 'mixed', logopenic or jargon aphasia; (E) focal left superior temporal lobe/insular atrophy, progressive nonfluent aphasia; (F) focal left inferior frontal gyrus/frontal opercular atrophy, progressive apraxia of speech. Bidirectional arrows suggest reciprocal communications between key anatomical regions.

From Rohrer JD, Warren JD, Omar R, et al. Brain 2008. January; 131(Pt 1):8-38. By permission of Oxford University Press.

Figure 2-13 Structural Anatomy of Word-Finding Difficulty in Degenerative Disorders.

characteristic language disorders that do not fit any of the traditional aphasia paradigms. Indeed, even in the acute stroke setting, the classification of aphasia as expressive or receptive, motor or sensory, nonfluent or fluent, is too simplistic and often inaccurate. Very few patients present with pure aphasia syndromes.

Often, patients with aphasia present to the neurologist complaining of word-finding difficulty; this is a broad-based symptom that is not always the result of a primary language disorder. Rather, it may be a manifestation of either inattention or a memory impairment. Therefore, the assessment of language must distinguish primary language disorders from other cognitive deficits, that is, *secondary word-finding impairment.* The patient presenting with progressive primary language disturbance often does not fit neatly into the traditional neuroanatomic aphasia classifications (Table 2-4). *Therefore, further discussion of*

language assessment will not focus on the traditional bedside aphasia exam, namely, tests of fluency, comprehension, naming, repetition, writing, and reading. Rather, we will review newer techniques for the examination of language elucidated through study of patients with primary progressive aphasia (Fig. 2-13).

Language may be defined as the attempt to convey a thought in verbal, spoken, or written form. This seems to occur in four stages, including speech initiation, speech content, speech structure, and motor programming of speech.

Stage I: Initiation of speech involves the ability to generate and plan a spoken message. Patients with speech initiation problems are quiet, as though they have nothing to say, so-called *dynamic aphasia.* Responses are terse and elaboration is absent. Patients speak only in response to conversation, not to initiate conversation. Although the amount of speech is reduced, the content and structure of spoken language are normal. This is

Table 2-4 Characteristics of Aphasias

Parameter	Anterior	Posterior	Conduction	Subcortical	Transcortical		
Location	Frontal/ Broca	Temporal/ Wernicke	L. Inferior Parietal	Basal Ganglia/ White Matter	Thalamus/ Anterolateral	Motor	Sensory
Fluency	Poor	Good	Good	Variable	Poor	Poor	Good
Naming	Poor	Poor	Poor-fair	Variable	Poor	Poor	Good
Repetition	Poor	Poor	Poor	Good	Good	Good	Good
Paraphasia	Common	Common	Common	Variable	Variable	Common	Common
Comprehension	Good	Poor	Good	Good	Poor	Good	Poor

often seen in patients with anterior frontal and subcortical abnormalities. These individuals often appear inert and slow to respond in general, sometimes referred to as appearing as a "bump on a log."

Stage II: The content of the message comes next once the mental plan for speech is set. This includes vocabulary and concepts. Content is assessed at the level of single words or in the way words are combined. *Loss of vocabulary* is the major abnormality encountered in this setting. The patient substitutes approximate words or imprecise expressions for words they cannot conjure. *Speech seems vague and deficient of meaning* in more severe cases. Errors of meaning (*semantic paraphasias*) may occur. Stereotyped expressions, such as clichés, are overutilized. This is characteristic of *semantic dementia*, a variant of *fronto-temporal lobar degeneration*.

A variation of this occurs in *Alzheimer disease*, where the patient cannot retrieve words from storage, gradually and progressively developing *logopenic aphasia*. Here the content of the message is impaired because of a loss for words, rather than a loss of the meaning of words. At the level of word combinations, there is a lack of coherence due to incomplete sentences, tangentiality, fragmented phrases, etc. It is hard to follow the patient's train of thought in these cases. This also occurs acutely, most commonly in states of delirium such as alcohol withdrawal.

Stage III: Grammar and phonology is the *basis for the structure* of spoken language. *Grammar* is the ordering of words into normal sentence structure, that is, subject and predicate. It also includes the use of function words such as prepositions and conjunctions. *Phonology* refers to the selection of individual sounds and syllables to form spoken words. Agrammatism leads to telegraphic speech, composed of single words or phrases, often omitting connector words. Phonologic errors lead to errors in particular sounds within words, also known as phonemic paraphasic errors. For example, saying "aminal" for "animal," or "nucular" for "nuclear." These types of errors are *common in progressive nonfluent aphasia*.

Stage IV: Once the structure of the message is defined, *the message is conveyed* to the motor areas for speech where phonetics, articulation, and prosody are applied and the message is spoken. Impairment at this phase is often characterized by *apraxia of speech*, or the loss of learned motor programming for speech production. This often produces great frustration and effortful speech, with severe loss of fluency, phonetic errors, and impaired speech timing and rhythm, as seen in the case vignette at the beginning of this chapter.

The *most important aspect of language assessment* is carefully listening to conversational language during the patient interview. If the patient is not very talkative, the examiner may present him or her with a picture to describe. Further tests of naming, repetition, writing, and reading all provide additional important information. In the case of progressive aphasia, the nature of language disturbance may have significant implication in identifying the underlying neurodegenerative disease. Indeed, assessment of language in this way has proven utility in localizing cortical regions attributed to various primary progressive aphasic syndromes (see Fig. 2-13). This approach elaborates on the classic aphasia exam, providing a better understanding of language processing and improving localization during examination.

ADDITIONAL RESOURCES

Benson DF. Aphasia, Alexia, and Agraphia. New York: Churchill Livingstone Inc.; 1979.

Carey BHM. An Unforgettable Amnesiac, Dies at 82. New York Times Obituaries; December 4, 2008.

Feinberg TE, Farrah MJ. Behavioral Neurology and Neuropsychology. New York, NY: McGraw-Hill; 1997.

Freedman M, Leech L, Kaplan E, et al. Clock Drawing: A Neuropsychological Analysis. New York: Oxford University Press, Inc.; 1994.

Goodglass H, Kaplan E. The Assessment of Aphasia and Related Disorders. 2nd ed. Philadelphia: Lea & Febiger; 1983.

Heilman KM, Valenstein E. Clinical Neuropsychology. 4th ed. New York, NY: Oxford University Press, Inc.; 2003.

Jeffrey P, Nussbaum PD. Clinical Neuropsychology: A pocket handbook for assessment. Washington, DC: American Psychological Association; 1998.

Kalashnikova LA, Zueva YV, Pugacheva OV, et al. Cognitive impairments in cerebellar infarcts. Neuroscience and Behavioral Physiology 2005; 35(8):773-779.

Kaplan E. Right hemisphere contributions to reading: horse and elephant example. Personal communication; 2000.

Kolb B, Whishaw IQ. Fundamentals of Human Neuropsychology. 6th ed. New York, NY: Worth Publishers; 2008.

Kolb B, Whishaw IQ. Fundamentals of Human Neuropsychology. New York, NY: Worth Publishers; 2003.

Lezak MD, Howieson DB, Loring DW. Neuropsychological Assessment Fourth Edition. New York, NY: Oxford University Press, Inc.; 2004.

Mesulam MM. Principles of Behavioral Neurology. Philadelphia: FA Davis; 1985.

Rawlinson G. The Significance of Letter Position in Word Recognition. PhD Thesis, Nottingham University; 1976. http://web.archive.org/web/20080117213646/http://www.mrc-cbu.cam.ac.uk/~mattd/Cmabrigde/rawlinson.html

Rizzo M, Eslinger PE. Principles and Practice of Behavioral Neurology and Neuropsychology. Philadelphia: Saunders; 2004.

Rohrer JD, Knight WD, Warren JE, et al. Word-finding difficulty: a clinical analysis of the progressive aphasias. Brain 131(pt 1):8-38; 2008.

Schmahmann JD, Sherman JC. The cerebellar cognitive affective syndrome. Brain 1998;121:561-579.

Schmahmann JD. Disorders of the cerebellum: Ataxia, dysmetria of thought, and the cerebellar cognitive affective syndrome. Journal of Neuropsychiatry and Clinical Neuroscience 2004;16(3):367-378.

Schmahmann JD, Weilburg JB, Sherman, JC. The neuropsychiatry of the cerebellum—insights from the clinic. The Cerebellum 2007;6: 254-267.

Strauss E, Sherman EMS, Spreen O. A Compendium of Neuropsychological Tests Third Edition. New York: Oxford University Press, Inc.; 2006.

Strub RL, Black FW. The Mental Status Examination in Neurology. Philadelphia: FA Davis; 2000.

Cranial Nerves

Cranial Nerve I: Olfactory

Michal Vytopil and H. Royden Jones, Jr.

Clinical Vignette

This 58-year-old lady, a culinary expert, as well as a neurologist, was hiking when she unexpectedly and forcefully struck her forehead on a low-hanging tree limb that she had not seen because of a very low visor on her hat. She immediately fell backwards powerfully striking her occiput, seeing stars but not losing consciousness. She acutely developed terrible vertigo. Profound spontaneous nystagmus was the only abnormality on a neurologic examination shortly after her fall. Within just a few hours, she noted that potato salad had no smell or taste. Her husband, also a neurologic physician, soon tested her olfactory sensation with perfume; he demonstrated that she had total loss of the sense of smell. Brain and skull computed tomographic (CT) scanning failed to demonstrate a skull fracture or hematoma. This lady maintained a total loss of smell for a few years. Gradually, fleeting inappropriate dysosmias occurred, along with some functional return. Eventually, some appropriate olfactory sense returned, particularly for smells of citrus and cucumber. The normally pleasant smell of raspberries is negatively altered. In contrast, car exhaust now has a paradoxically pleasant perfume-like smell. Currently, she notes that the best thing is a return of her smell and taste for garlic. Despite such effects, this epicurean still has significant difficulties cooking. Most interestingly, she perceives "smells" in her dreams and she still misses her spouse's aroma whenever they are physically close. As a physician, she can no longer appreciate patient odors, such as too much ethanol.

Comment: The olfactory nerves are particularly liable to shearing trauma such as occurs with a closed head injury. Their very thin axons are relatively easily severed. In this instance, the patient experienced two rapidly sequential severe head injuries, first frontal and than occipital. This trauma presumably led to a shearing force totally interrupting the tiny olfactory nerves as they crossed the cribriform plate at the base of the skull prior to entering the olfactory bulb at the base of the frontal lobe. Although there were no overt fractures demonstrated with CT scanning, one can easily suggest that the olfactory nerves were severed at their intracranial point of entry.

The olfactory nerve (CN-I) provides for the sense of smell. This sensory modality provides an important warning system by enabling the identification of spoiled and potentially toxic foods or noxious chemicals. Smell function also contributes to various life qualities as this sensory modality provides awareness of many pleasurable sensations, including appreciation of certain foods and beverages as well as subtle attractions eventually leading to sexual desire and reproduction.

Dysfunction of the olfactory nerve is quite rare, occurring in certain very select circumstances. Examination of olfactory function is not routinely pursued during the average neurologic evaluation (Chapter 1). However, in clinical settings such as in the above vignette, it is essential to routinely evaluate olfactory function by asking the patient to identify a few familiar odors such as coffee, perfumes, tobacco, etc. On occasion, the patient may not be aware of or assign much importance to the loss of his or her smell sensation. This may be particularly true when there is a concomitant neurologic deficit as seen in occasional patients with potentially treatable olfactory groove meningiomas that also compromise frontal lobe function.

ANATOMY

When identifying odors, humans rely on volatile substances entering their nasal cavity to excite receptors. *Olfactory receptor cells* are bipolar sensory neurons whose dendrites form a delicate sensory carpet on the superior aspect of the nasal cavity (Fig. 3-1). The thin, unmyelinated axons of the bipolar sensory cells collectively form the olfactory nerve. These travel through the cribriform plate into the olfactory bulb at the base of the frontoorbital lobe. Within the bulb, CN-I fibers synapse with the dendrites of the large mitral cells, whose axons constitute the olfactory tract passing along the base of the frontal lobe and projecting directly into the primary olfactory cortex within the temporal lobe. In contrast to all other sensory modalities, olfactory sensation does not have a central processing site such as within the thalamic nuclei (Fig. 3-2). This direct pathway to the cerebral limbic structures may have had an important evolutionary function in lower animals and, later, primates.

The human primary olfactory cortex includes the uncus, hippocampal gyrus, amygdaloid complex, and entorhinal cortex (Fig. 3-2). Cortical representation of smell is bilateral. Although most of the olfactory tract fibers supply the ipsilateral olfactory cortex, some fibers decussate in the anterior commissure and terminate in the opposite hemisphere. Consequently, a unilateral lesion distal to the decussation rarely produces any olfactory dysfunction.

CLINICAL EVALUATION AND DIAGNOSTIC APPROACH

Traditionally, olfactory function is tested by relatively crude methods asking a patient to sniff and identify a series of nonirritating odorants (coffee, cinnamon, etc.). A commercially available, standardized, and reliable methodology is available for more precise olfactory definition; however, its practical clinical utility has not been defined. The most widely used of these tests is the University of Pennsylvania Smell Identification Test consisting of 40 microencapsulated odorants embedded in "scratch and sniff" strips. It can be self-administered and takes only several minutes.

Gadolinium-enhanced brain magnetic resonance imaging (MRI) is the modality of choice for the evaluation of intracranial

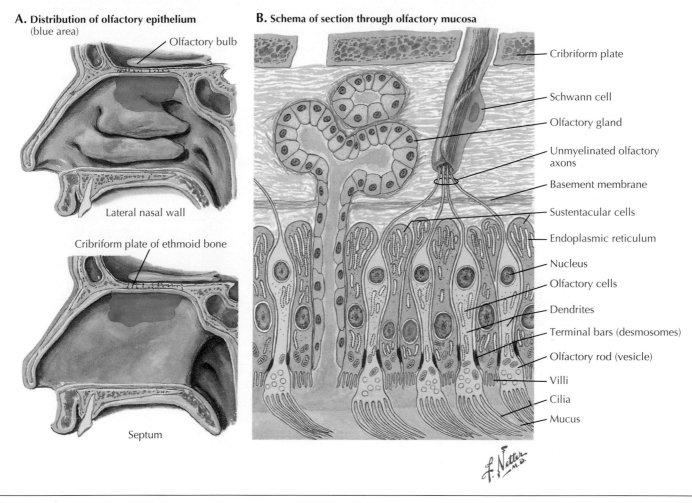

A. Distribution of olfactory epithelium
(blue area)

Olfactory bulb

Lateral nasal wall

Cribriform plate of ethmoid bone

Septum

B. Schema of section through olfactory mucosa

Cribriform plate

Schwann cell

Olfactory gland

Unmyelinated olfactory axons

Basement membrane

Sustentacular cells

Endoplasmic reticulum

Nucleus

Olfactory cells

Dendrites

Terminal bars (desmosomes)

Olfactory rod (vesicle)

Villi

Cilia

Mucus

Figure 3-1 Olfactory Receptors.

causes of olfactory dysfunction. Head CT with contrast is reliable when MRI cannot be performed, or if a bony lesion of anterior fossa is suspected. It is not uncommon with moderately severe head trauma to be unable to define a fracture per se even with detailed CT.

DIFFERENTIAL DIAGNOSIS

Smell dysfunction can be disrupted at any site along the olfactory pathway. Therefore impaired olfaction is not necessarily indicative of first-cranial nerve dysfunction per se. There are some common conditions that interfere with olfactory function without having specific olfactory nerve damage. These particularly include upper respiratory tract infection, especially nasal sinus disease. Primary olfactory bulb, tract, or entorhinal cortex lesions per se are relatively very uncommon. Olfactory impairment is not always apparent to the patient. Instead, he or she may initially complain of a loss of taste because the identification of tasted flavors depends partly on the olfactory system. Disturbances of smell are generally acquired, although there may be a rare patient with a congenital disorder. In general, most patients experiencing olfactory dysfunctions have bilateral loss of function. The rare presence of a unilateral anosmia is an important sign that signals a need for an MRI to exclude an olfactory groove tumor.

Congenital Disorder
KALLMANN SYNDROME

In this condition, anosmia results from a congenital hypoplasia or even absence of the olfactory bulbs. This occurs in conjunction with hypogonadotropic hypogonadism. Although most instances are sporadic, familial cases are reported having variable inheritance patterns: X linked, autosomal dominant, or autosomal recessive. Some of the responsible genes are identified. There is a strong male predilection even with sporadic as well as autosomal forms. It is often first diagnosed at the time of an evaluation for delayed puberty; boys may have a micropenis and girls lack normal breast development. Occasionally, the Kallmann syndrome is associated with other congenital deficits, including cleft palate, lip/dental agenesis, and neural hearing loss.

Acquired Disorders

Upper respiratory infections are the most frequent causes of olfactory dysfunction. Nasal and paranasal sinus disease account for more than 40% of olfactory disturbances. These intranasal processes mechanically prevent volatile chemical stimuli from reaching the olfactory sensory epithelium and activating the receptors. These are defined as *transport* or *conductive olfactory*

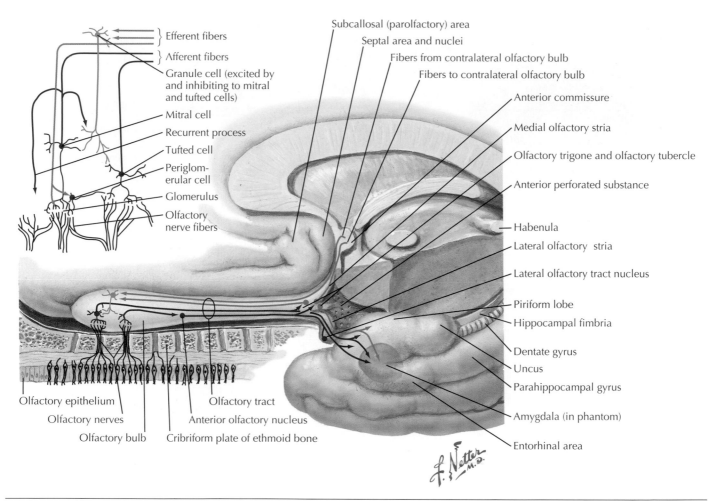

Efferent fibers
Afferent fibers
Granule cell (excited by and inhibiting to mitral and tufted cells)
Mitral cell
Recurrent process
Tufted cell
Periglom-erular cell
Glomerulus
Olfactory nerve fibers

Subcallosal (parolfactory) area
Septal area and nuclei
Fibers from contralateral olfactory bulb
Fibers to contralateral olfactory bulb
Anterior commissure
Medial olfactory stria
Olfactory trigone and olfactory tubercle
Anterior perforated substance
Habenula
Lateral olfactory stria
Lateral olfactory tract nucleus
Piriform lobe
Hippocampal fimbria
Dentate gyrus
Uncus
Parahippocampal gyrus
Amygdala (in phantom)
Entorhinal area

Olfactory epithelium
Olfactory nerves
Olfactory bulb
Olfactory tract
Anterior olfactory nucleus
Cribriform plate of ethmoid bone

Figure 3-2 Olfactory Pathways.

disorders that are not associated with direct damage to the olfactory nerve pathways. The classic temporal profile, characterized by the intermittent occurrence of conductive olfactory dysfunction, provides the most important clinical clue for the diagnosis of a primary nasal source for these common disorders. A thorough otorhinolaryngologic evaluation is indicated for these patients. Conversely, the presence of persistent smell disturbance is the primary characteristic of direct damage to the olfactory nerve pathways.

Head trauma, as noted in the vignette, is responsible for approximately 20% of all cases of smell dysfunction. This is secondary either to direct damage to primary axons of the first cranial nerve or lesions of the associated frontobasal cerebral cortex responsible for olfactory perception. Depending on the severity of the blunt head injury, the incidence of posttraumatic anosmia varies between 7% and 30%. Direct occipital and side injuries to the head are more dangerous to olfaction than are frontally directed injuries. Posttraumatic olfactory dysfunction typically results from shearing of the olfactory nerve as it passes through the cribriform plate. More substantial damage, such as occurs in severe head trauma with anterior fossa fracture, may lead to a contusion of the olfactory bulb or the cortical–subcortical olfactory brain. Posttraumatic anosmia or hyposmia can be either unilateral or bilateral.

Olfactory groove meningiomas are quite infrequent; however, if these remain undiagnosed, these histologically benign tumors may still lead to significant morbidity unless treated early on. Usually meningiomas are slow growing; olfactory groove lesions comprise 8–18% of all intracranial meningiomas (Fig. 3-3). Although unilateral or bilateral olfactory dysfunction is thought to be their first symptom, very few patients present with just a disturbance in their sense of smell. This is probably because their slow and orderly growth leads to a very gradual decline in olfactory function. Furthermore, as most meningiomas are unilateral, they lead to unilateral anosmia and thus patients still retain olfactory function on the contralateral side. Thus, they are usually unaware of any focal loss. Consequently, most orbital meningiomas are not diagnosed until the tumor is large enough (e.g., >4 cm in diameter) to cause other symptoms resulting from pressure on the frontal lobes and optic tracts. These include headache, visual disturbances, personality changes, and memory impairment. Early diagnosis of olfactory groove meningiomas remains challenging. At times, the behavioral changes can be profound and may create a sense the patient is demented or mentally unbalanced.

Very large olfactory groove tumors, typically meningiomas, rarely lead to the development of Foster–Kennedy syndrome. This is characterized by unilateral optic atrophy and

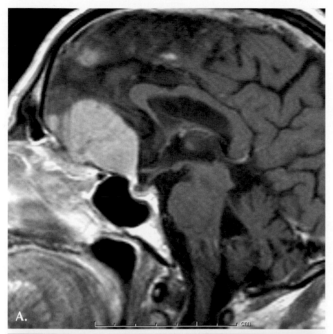

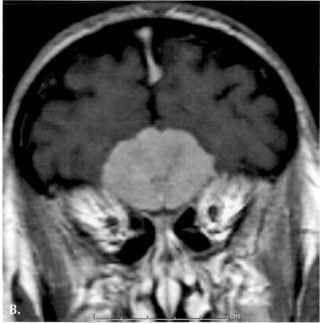

T1-weighted, gadolinium-enhanced sagittal and coronal MR images show a large enhancing mass on the skull base displacing and compressing the olfactory apparatus.

Figure 3-3 Subfrontal Meningioma.

contralateral papilledema. Optic atrophy results from direct pressure of the neoplasm on the optic nerve, whereas increased intracranial pressure produces contralateral papilledema.

Parkinson disease patients often develop olfactory dysfunction as an early clinical feature. In fact, the difficulty with sense of smell may precede the onset of classic striatal motor manifestations by several years. A normal sense of smell in Parkinson disease is such a rare occurrence that its continued normal

function should prompt review of this diagnosis. Alzheimer disease and Lewy body disease are other neurodegenerative disorders commonly associated with olfactory dysfunction.

Other Entities

Normal aging is associated with a progressive decline in the ability to appreciate and discriminate odors.

Olfactory hallucinations are important considerations in the differential diagnosis of any symptomatic positive olfactory dysfunction. Although these events do not occur with primary olfactory nerve disorders per se, most often such symptoms provide the aura for a focal seizure disorder, that is, *uncinate fits*. The typical patient initially experiences a very unpleasant smell of very foul character such as burning garbage. This classically precedes a temporal or frontal orbital lobe focal seizure wherein the patient briefly loses contact with the environment as characterized by staring and various automatisms. Certain patients with psychiatric conditions (depression, psychosis), or alcohol withdrawal syndromes may also experience unusual olfactory symptoms.

Olfactory discrimination is also adversely affected by many medications and drugs, including opiates (codeine, morphine), antiepileptic drugs (carbamazepine, phenytoin), and immuno-suppressive agents, that, similar to radiation, disrupt the physiologic turnover of receptor cells. Cocaine abuse, via intranasal snorting, is particularly prone to cause septal perforation that eventually leads to direct trauma to the olfactory nerve.

PROGNOSIS

Modest recovery is expected in one-third to one-half of patients who experience anosmia. This may be explained by the unique ability of the olfactory neuroepithelium and olfactory bulb to regenerate. Olfactory receptor cells and neurons within the bulb are normally constantly replaced by fresh cells. The olfactory bulb is one of the few brain structures capable of such regeneration.

EVIDENCE

London B, Nabet B, Fisher AR, et al. Predictors of prognosis in patients with olfactory disturbance. Ann Neurol 2008;63:159-166. *In this prospective study, the authors found that many patients experienced improvement of their smell function and that etiology was not the main prognostic determinant.*

Ross Webster G, Petrovitch H, Abbott RD, et al. Association of olfactory dysfunction with risk for future Parkinson's disease. Ann Neurol 2007;63:167-173. *This prospective study suggests that olfactory disturbance can precede the classic features of Parkinson disease by years.*

ADDITIONAL RESOURCES

The Smell and Taste Center at The University of Pennsylvania. Available at: http://www.med.upenn.edu/stc. Accessed in June 2008.
De Kruijk JR, Leffers P, Menheere PP, et al. Olfactory function after mild traumatic brain injury. Brain Inj 2003;17:73-78. *In this study, high prevalence of olfactory dysfunction was found in patients with mild traumatic injury.*
Dode C, Levilliers J, Dupont JM, et al. Loss-of-function mutations in FGFR1 cause autosomal dominant Kallmann syndrome. Nat Genet

2003;33:463-465. *The authors expand our insight into molecular genetics of autosomal dominant Kallmann syndrome.*

Doty RL, Shaman P, Dann M. Development of University of Pennsylvania Smell Identification Test. Physiol Behav 1984;32:489-502. *Authors describe development of the first standardized olfactory test battery (UPSIT). The UPSIT provided the needed scientific basis for many subsequent studies.*

Hawkes Ch. Olfaction in neurodegenerative disorder. Mov Disord 2003;18:364-372. *This excellent review summarizes our knowledge about olfaction in various neurodegenerative conditions, and focuses on the intriguing role of smell disturbance in Parkinson disease and Alzheimer dementia.*

Rubin G, Ben David U, Gornish M, et al. Meningiomas of the anterior cranial fossa floor: review of 67 cases. Acta Neurochir (Wien) 1994;129:26-30. *In this retrospective review, the authors describe the clinical characteristic and prognosis of their large cohort of patients with anterior fossa meningiomas.*

Cranial Nerve II: Optic Nerve and Visual System

Ippolit C. A. Matjucha

INTRAOCULAR OPTIC NERVE

Clinical Vignette

A 48-year-old man was referred for sudden loss of vision in the left eye. He had noted this the morning before while shaving when he could not see the lower half of his chin with the left eye only. He had no pain, and had no preceding systemic symptoms. His past medical history was noteworthy for mild diet-controlled hypercholesterolemia and untreated labile hypertension. The affected eye had 20/40 central acuity, and an inferior central field loss that extended nasally but did not cross into the superior field. The left optic nerve showed acquired elevation and swelling, with mild peripapillary hemorrhages. The fellow nerve was small in diameter, had no physiologic cup, and had mild congenital elevation. The diagnosis of idiopathic (nonarteritic) anterior ischemic optic neuropathy (AION) was made. Over the next 6 weeks, the left optic nerve swelling abated and was replaced by mild pallor noted superiorly. The vision did not recover.

The optic nerve is not a peripheral nerve but rather a central nervous system (CNS) tract containing central myelin formed by oligodendrocytes. It is composed of long axons, whose cell bodies comprise the ganglion cell layer of the inner retina (Figs. 4-1 and 4-2). The axons run in the retina's nerve fiber layer to gather at the optic disk.

The optic nerve nominally begins when the axons of the ganglion cells (the nerve fiber layer of the retina) turn 90°, changing orientation from horizontal along the inner retinal surface to vertical, passing through the outer retina via the scleral canal (Fig. 4-3). The gathering of axons at the canal forms the optic disk (also, *optic nerve head*) of the fundus. Myelin is usually absent from the nerve fiber layer where the nerve exits the globe.

Vascular supply of the retina comes from the ophthalmic artery off the internal carotid artery. Proximal branches from this artery and branches off the muscular arteries constitute the posterior ciliary arteries that form a plexus of vessels around the lamina cribrosa and supply the optic disc, the adjacent optic nerve, and the outer layers of the retina. Cilioretinal branches from this plexus often supply the macula as well. Another branch of the ophthalmic, the central retinal artery, enters the distal optic nerve and emerges out the disc dividing into four arteriolar branches to supply each quadrant of retina. The proximal part of the optic nerve is supplied by a series of small vessels of the ophthalmic while the posterior optic nerve and the chiasm have additional supply from the anterior cerebral and the anterior communicating arteries.

The shape of visual field deficits due to vascular compromise of the inner retina is predictable, being consistent with the specific location of the arterial occlusion. Visual field defects are inverted in relation to the pathologic location: for example, a superior branch occlusion of the retinal artery will cause an inferior field defect. When retinal arteriolar occlusions affect the nerve fiber layer, field defects typically extend beyond the local occlusion in an arcuate or sectoral pattern, following the arc of the nerve fiber layer. Disease of the anterior optic nerve is an important health care problem. Glaucoma alone is suspected to affect 3 million patients, accounting for 120,000 cases of blindness in the United States, with an annual governmental cost of $1.5 billion in expenditures and lost revenue.

Clinical Presentations

Primary open-angle glaucoma (POAG) is a chronic, progressive, degenerative disease of the optic nerve. Its usual hallmark is high intraocular pressure (IOP; above 21 mm Hg), but glaucoma without high IOP (*normal pressure* or *low-tension* glaucoma) is occasionally seen, especially in the elderly. The typical optic nerve finding is cupping atrophy (i.e., enlargement of the disk's central cup as nerve fibers are lost), coupled by progressive visual field loss that often starts nasally, progresses superiorly and inferiorly, and finally extinguishes the central and temporal fields (Fig. 4-4). POAG is usually bilateral and asymmetric and the visual loss is permanent. The time course is measured in years, and because of the slow pace and the late involvement of the central field, patients may remain asymptomatic until the disease is quite advanced. It is essential that all standard eye examinations include screening IOP measurements and optic disk inspection.

Glaucoma has other forms besides POAG, which may be congenital, secondary to systemic disease (e.g., diabetes), or other acquired eye conditions (e.g., trauma). Among these, **acute narrow-angle glaucoma** (also, *acute angle closure glaucoma*) may present dramatically with nausea, unilateral headache, and ipsilateral monocular visual loss. The diagnosis and treatment of glaucoma forms a significant subspecialty within ophthalmology, but treatment efforts revolve around lowering of IOP, whether by medical or surgical means. There are no restorative or neuroprotective treatments.

Central retinal artery occlusion (CRAO) results from interruption of the central retinal artery circulation with ischemia to the entire retina. If only a portion of the inner retinal circulation is affected, a more limited version, **branch retinal artery occlusion (BRAO)**, is present. BRAO and CRAO are in effect retinal strokes, affecting the nerve fiber and ganglion cell layers. The presentation is one of sudden, painless, complete or partial monocular visual loss often described as a "curtain" obscuring the involved area. Retinal infarcts are commonly caused by emboli, and in BRAO the embolus is typically visible in the affected retinal vessel. Episodes of temporary monocular visual loss (TMVL; transient monocular blindness or TMB and also, *amaurosis fugax*) often herald retinal infarcts and represent temporarily compromised flow of the inner retinal arteries usually by passing clot.

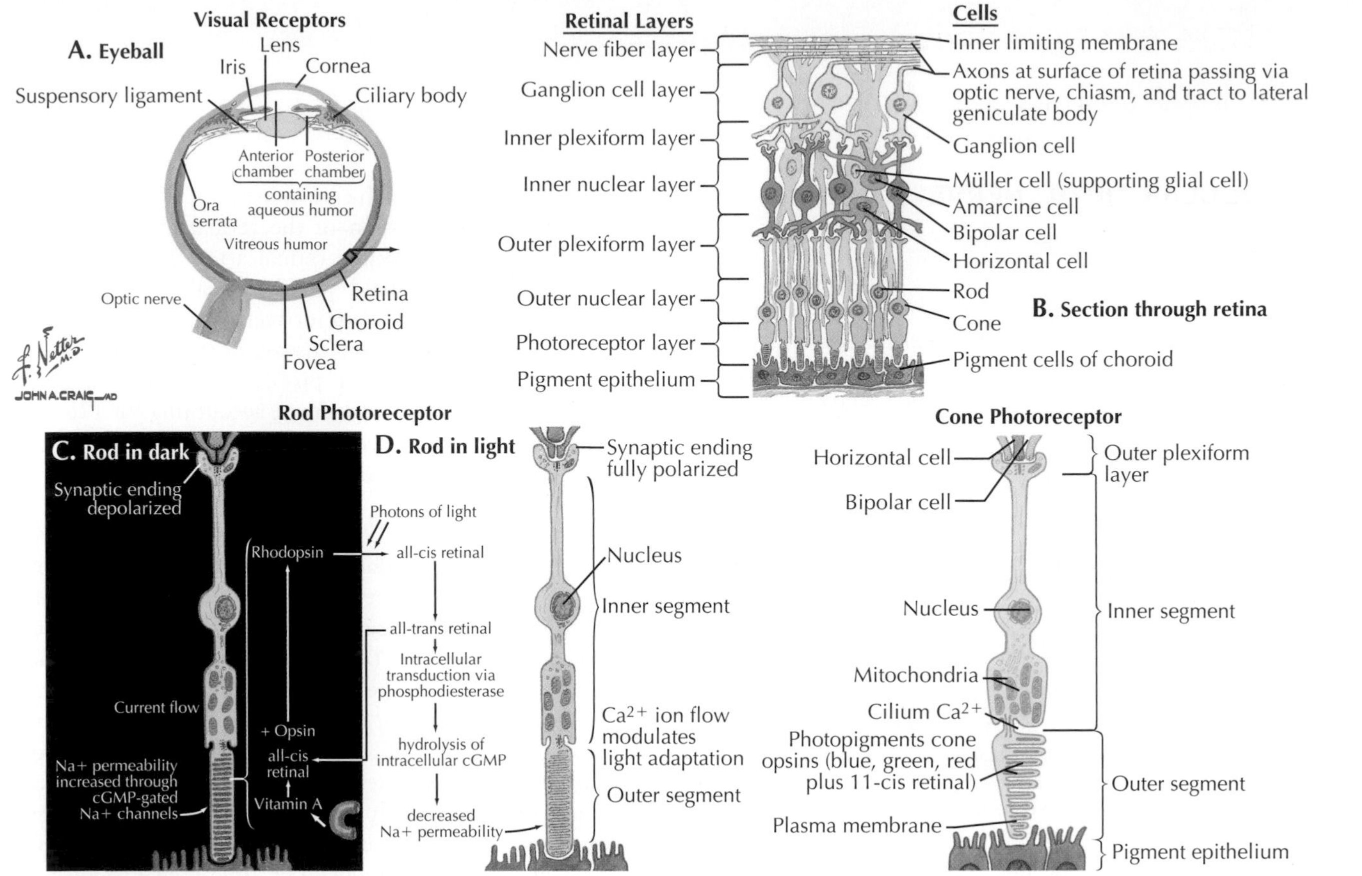

Visual Receptors

A. Eyeball

Lens
Iris
Cornea
Suspensory ligament
Ciliary body
Anterior chamber
Posterior chamber
containing aqueous humor
Ora serrata
Vitreous humor
Optic nerve
Retina
Choroid
Sclera
Fovea

F. Netter M.D.
JOHN A.CRAIG_MD

Retinal Layers

Nerve fiber layer
Ganglion cell layer
Inner plexiform layer
Inner nuclear layer
Outer plexiform layer
Outer nuclear layer
Photoreceptor layer
Pigment epithelium

Cells

Inner limiting membrane
Axons at surface of retina passing via optic nerve, chiasm, and tract to lateral geniculate body
Ganglion cell
Müller cell (supporting glial cell)
Amarcine cell
Bipolar cell
Horizontal cell
Rod
Cone
Pigment cells of choroid

B. Section through retina

Rod Photoreceptor

C. Rod in dark

Synaptic ending depolarized

Current flow

Na+ permeability increased through cGMP-gated Na+ channels

D. Rod in light

Photons of light

Rhodopsin → all-cis retinal

all-trans retinal
Intracellular transduction via phosphodiesterase

hydrolysis of intracellular cGMP

+ Opsin
all-cis retinal
Vitamin A

decreased Na+ permeability

Synaptic ending fully polarized
Nucleus
Inner segment
Ca^{2+} ion flow modulates light adaptation
Outer segment

Cone Photoreceptor

Horizontal cell
Bipolar cell
Outer plexiform layer

Nucleus
Inner segment

Mitochondria
Cilium Ca^{2+}
Photopigments cone opsins (blue, green, red plus 11-cis retinal)
Plasma membrane
Outer segment
Pigment epithelium

Figure 4-1 The Retina and the Photoreceptors.

Patients who present for care within the first hours after the onset of CRAO or large BRAO are usually treated with intermittent ocular massage and lowering of IOP (either by topical agents or by paracentesis of the anterior chamber) to promote movement of the embolus to a more distal arteriolar branch. Oxygen, alone or in combination with 5% CO_2 to promote arteriodilation, can also be used. Based on animal studies, it is felt that such interventions are unlikely to be helpful after 100 minutes of retinal ischemia, and in general the outlook for recovery is bleak; nevertheless, significant recovery of vision, even beyond the 100-minute window, is occasionally seen.

CRAO, BRAO, and TMVL may also serve as a warning sign of impending hemispheric stroke. Identification and treatment of the embolic source, if one can be identified, becomes the main focus of therapy after the window for acute treatment of the involved eye has passed. CRAO is often a sign of carotid stenosis, the appropriate management of which will significantly reduce long-term stroke risk (see Chapter 55, "Ischemic Stroke"). Heart embolism is another cause and a full stroke investigation is usually required. Nevertheless, up to 40% of cases remain without a definite identifiable cause with the presumed mechanism relating to intrinsic narrowing of the retinal artery due to atherosclerosis or, less commonly, other arteritides or compression.

Anterior ischemic optic neuropathy can be divided into nonarteritic and arteritic (associated with temporal arteritis [TA]) and is caused by loss of blood flow in the short posterior ciliary arteries. Patients usually experience sudden and severe painless monocular visual loss, often on awakening. Examination classically reveals an altitudinal (superior or inferior) visual field loss, with a unilaterally swollen, hemorrhagic disk (Fig. 4-5). The disk loses its swelling and becomes pale within weeks. The visual loss in most cases does not change following the event but 20% may show measurable change for better or worse over days. In contrast to retinal artery occlusions, embolic AION is extremely rare. In most cases, AION occurs in middle-aged individuals who have a congenitally small, elevated ("crowded") optic disk, or in those with one or more vascular disease risk factors, such as diabetes, hypertension, or sleep apnea. In these cases, a transient fall in blood pressure causes hypoperfusion of the posterior ciliary circulation and subsequent ischemic damage to the optic nerve head.

There is no proven treatment for AION, although a recent retrospective study suggests that acute treatment with oral steroids may improve outcome. There is a 50% risk of eventual involvement of the fellow eye. Strategies to reduce this risk have focused on identifying and treating cerebrovascular risk factors, daily aspirin, preventing systemic hypotension, and avoiding certain drugs, such as sildenafil, which may be associated with higher risk.

In older patients, AION can be a complication, and sometimes the presenting sign, of TA (also, *giant cell arteritis*), a systemic inflammatory process of the medium-sized arteries. TA can also produce TMVL and CRAO. Funduscopic appearance

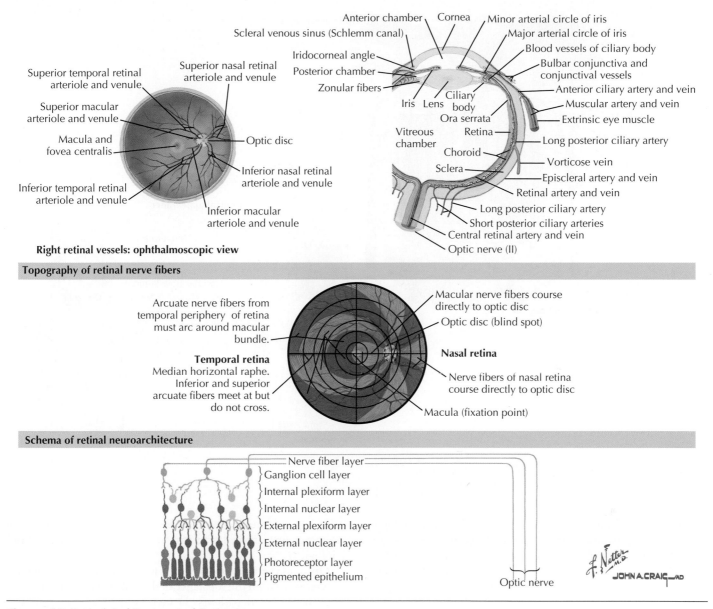

Right retinal vessels: ophthalmoscopic view

Topography of retinal nerve fibers

Arcuate nerve fibers from temporal periphery of retina must arc around macular bundle.

Macular nerve fibers course directly to optic disc

Optic disc (blind spot)

Temporal retina
Median horizontal raphe. Inferior and superior arcuate fibers meet at but do not cross.

Nasal retina

Nerve fibers of nasal retina course directly to optic disc

Macula (fixation point)

Schema of retinal neuroarchitecture

Nerve fiber layer
Ganglion cell layer
Internal plexiform layer
Internal nuclear layer
External plexiform layer
External nuclear layer
Photoreceptor layer
Pigmented epithelium

Optic nerve

Figure 4-2 Retinal Architecture and Perimetry.

in arteritic AION often consists of pallid swelling of the disk, in contrast to the hyperemic swelling seen in idiopathic AION. In addition to an altitudinal visual loss, patients will have arteritic symptoms, including headache, scalp tenderness, jaw claudication, neck pain, malaise, loss of appetite, fevers, and morning stiffness of proximal muscles (i.e., polymyalgia rheumatica). Only rarely will a patient with arteritic AION have little or no systemic symptoms.

Untreated, TA may lead rapidly to blindness from bilateral AION, or to other serious complications including aortic dissection, myocardial infarction, renal disease, and stroke. Therefore, in any patient older than age 50 years with AION, clinical suspicion for TA is raised especially in the presence of systemic symptoms, or physical exam findings (pallid disk swelling or abnormal greater superficial temporal arteries). A high erythrocyte sedimentation rate (ESR, >45 mm/hour), high C-reactive protein (CRP, >2.45 mg/L), normocytic anemia, and thrombocytosis are supportive, but the diagnosis is established by

temporal artery biopsy that reveals inflammation in the media of the arteries with disruption of the internal elastic membrane. The presence of characteristic multinucleated giant cells within the affected areas is diagnostic.

TA is treated with high-dose corticosteroids, started urgently and usually tapered over many months. Other anti-inflammatory medications, especially methotrexate, have been used in those at high risk for corticosteroid complications, but the efficacy of nonsteroidal agents has been questioned. Steroid dosage is gradually reduced over time, with the patient monitored for disease recrudescence by following symptoms and the ESR or CRP.

Papilledema (see Fig. 1-6) is bilateral optic nerve elevation and expansion due to high intracranial pressure (ICP). In mild cases, patients may have no visual symptoms. Moderate papilledema is typically accompanied by transient binocular visual obscurations, either spontaneously or during coughing, straining, or abrupt postural change. Other symptoms of high ICP may be present and include headaches (worse with

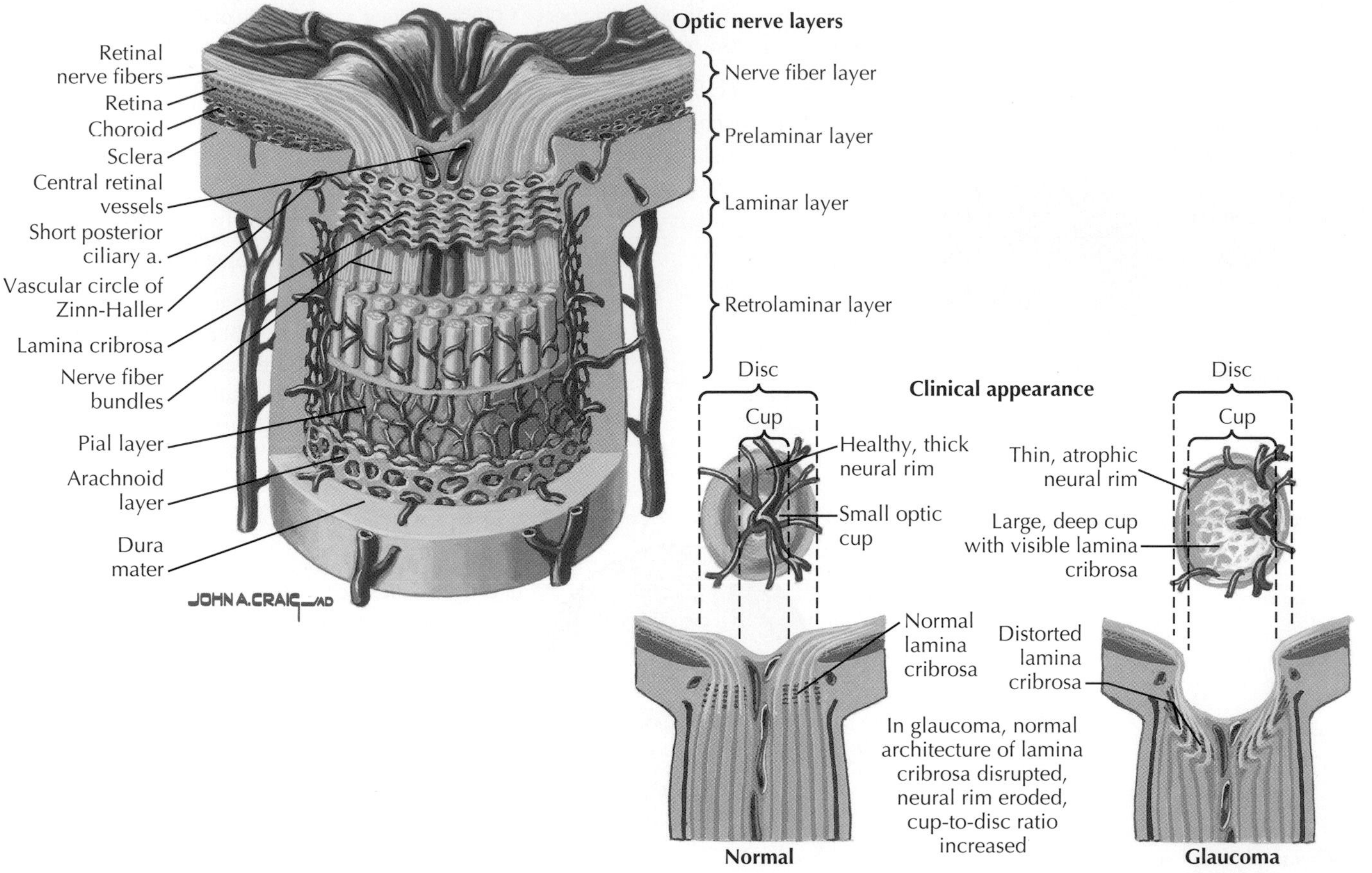

Figure 4-3 Anatomy of Optic Nerve (Clinical Appearance).

recumbency) and diplopia (resulting from nonlocalizing abducens palsy; see Chapter 5). When visual loss occurs, it starts with blind spot enlargement (see Fig. 1-6), a nonspecific and often reversible change. Visual field loss resembling that of glaucoma can ensue, often over a period of many weeks. However, papilledema due to very high ICP can progress rapidly, with severe permanent visual loss within days.

Many pathophysiological mechanisms are associated with papilledema, including CNS tumor with mass effect or edema, obstructive hydrocephalus, meningitis, certain medications (e.g., tetracycline or vitamin A), and intracranial venous thrombosis or obstruction. Papilledema is occasionally seen without explanation in obese women of childbearing age and is then termed **idiopathic intracranial hypertension** (IIH; also, *pseudotumor cerebri*; see Chapter 11). Treatment involves only weight loss if the condition is mild and there is no evidence of progressive visual loss or debilitating headache. In progressive IIH, in addition to weight loss, carbonic anhydrase inhibitors such as acetazolamide (typically 1–2 g/day in divided doses) are used to reduce cerebrospinal fluid (CSF) production and optic nerve edema. When medical treatment fails, two surgical options exist: optic nerve sheath fenestration or CSF shunting either with lumboperitoneal or ventriculoperitoneal shunts.

Papilledema can be mimicked by the rare entity of **optic perineuritis**, which consists of monocular or bilateral optic disk swelling without central visual loss or raised ICP. Its usual cause is idiopathic optic nerve sheath swelling or inflammatory orbital pseudotumor but may be due to a systemic arteritis (Wegener or giant cell arteritis) or of an infectious (syphilitic) etiology.

Optic nerve drusen are small, translucent, usually bilateral concretions within the substance of the disk that may be observed in perhaps 1% of patients. Drusen contain calcium and can therefore be demonstrated on ultrasound and computed tomographic (CT) examinations. It is speculated that a very small scleral canal may inhibit proper axonal metabolism, causing extracellular debris to be deposited as drusen over time. Drusen of the optic nerve is often associated with visual field loss, and treatment to retard such loss is uncertain. Drusen of the nerve head are occasionally seen in patients with certain retinal disorders, such as retinitis pigmentosa.

Congenital dysplasia of the optic nerve can be seen as an isolated monocular or binocular finding, or as part of a larger disorder. The mildest form of dysplasia is "tilted" optic disks: nerve heads that are overall small with the nasal portions appearing elevated; superior temporal visual field loss (sometimes mimicking *bitemporal hemianopia*) is often encountered. Septo-optic dysplasia combines optic nerve hypoplasia with dysgenesis of midline brain structures, often with pituitary dysfunction. Up to a quarter of patients with fetal alcohol syndrome will have disk hypoplasia with associated inferior visual field loss, among other ocular manifestations. Optic nerve coloboma (congenital incomplete or malfusion of the globe structures including the retina and optic nerve) can be part of Aicardi

Early

Right eye
nasal side

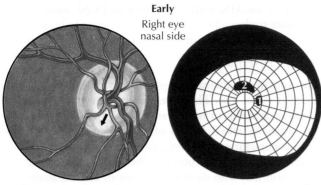

Funduscopy: notching of contour of physiologic cup in optic disc with slight focal pallor in area of notching; occurs almost invariably in superotemporal or inferotemporal (as shown) quadrants

Perimetry: slight enlargment of physiologic blind spot (1); development of a secondary, superonasal field defect (2) which corresponds to nerve fiber damage in area of inferotemporal notching

Minimally advanced

Right eye
nasal side

JOHN A.CRAIG—MD

Funduscopy: increased notching of rim of cup; thinning of rim of cup (enlargement of cup); deepening of cup; lamina cribrosa visible in deepest areas

Perimetry: localized constriction of superonasal visual field (3) because of progressive damage to inferotemporal fibers; superior arc-shaped scotoma (Bjerrum scotoma) develops (4)

Figure 4-4 Optic Disc and Visual Field Changes in Glaucoma.

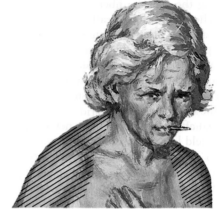

Senior citizen with sudden monocular visual blurring or blindness, associated with malaise, scalp tenderness, and myalgia. The erythrocyte sedimentation rate is very elevated, usually 60 to 120 mm/hr.

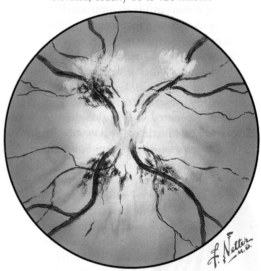

Anterior ischemic optic neuropathy

Figure 4-5 Giant Cell Arteritis: Ocular Manifestations.

syndrome, and the "morning glory" disk anomaly has been associated with several developmental syndromes.

Diagnostic Approach

As all pathologic entities in this group display abnormalities of the disc and/or retinal vessels, careful fundus examination is the essential step in diagnosis. Visual field testing typically reveals patterns of visual loss (arcuate, altitudinal, and nasal losses with a "step" at the horizontal meridian) that localize the lesion to the anterior optic nerve, does not often guide the diagnosis. Sector losses can suggest branch arterial occlusion (any location), optic nerve hypoplasia (typically inferior), optic disk tilt, or coloboma (these last two often producing superior losses).

Additional information can be obtained by special imaging of the ocular fundus. Fluorescein angiography of the fundus reveals vascular occlusions and areas of edema caused by incompetent blood vessels. Optical coherence tomography, scanning laser ophthalmoscopy, and scanning laser polarimetry provide precise measurement of the nerve fiber layer in the peripapillary retina and can help define subtle cases of disk edema or atrophy and changes in disk appearance over time.

ORBITAL AND INTRACANALICULAR OPTIC NERVE

Clinical Vignette

A 26-year-old woman presented with right monocular visual loss and headache after a car accident. She said she had suffered "whip-lash," without bruising impact to the head. The visual loss had started 2 days after the accident. The headache was centered at the right orbit, with eye movement among its aggravating factors. Subjective visual acuity was 20/80 right eye, and visual field testing revealed nonphysiologic responses, indicating the patient was inattentive to the test, in both eyes. Fundus examination of both eyes was entirely normal; however, pupillary examination suggested a mild relative afferent papillary defect on the right. A magnetic resonance imaging (MRI) examination was obtained revealing multiple white-matter lesions. A diagnosis of multiple sclerosis (MS) presenting as optic neuritis was eventually confirmed based on spinal fluid assays and subsequent clinical course.

indentation with posterior chorioretinal folds, or signs of chronic central retinal vein compression and optociliary venous shunting. MRI with gadolinium is generally preferred for imaging of orbital masses, although bone structure and abnormalities (hypertrophy with meningioma, destruction with cancers, and remodeling with large benign tumors) are better seen on CT scanning.

Typical orbital tumors compressing the optic nerve are cavernous hemangioma (the most common benign orbital tumor), optic nerve sheath meningioma, and optic nerve glioma. Cavernous hemangiomas are relatively easy to address surgically, except when at the orbital apex. Optic nerve meningioma generally cannot be removed surgically without severe loss of vision, and the preferred treatment, once optic nerve compression begins, is fractionated stereotactic external beam radiation to limit tumor growth. Glioma of the optic nerve cannot be resected short of excising the nerve, causing immediate blindness in the affected eye. Therefore, the gliomas are generally left in place, with excision indicated only if severe proptosis with eye exposure or extension of the glioma toward the chiasm, threatening vision in the other eye, occurs. Stereotactic radiation can be used. Attention to the possibility of rare, aggressive gliomas requiring early excision is a cause for frequent reimaging initially when following these tumors. Multiple gliomas, typically slow-growing, are a common feature of von Recklinghausen neurofibromatosis (NF-1).

The enlarged extraocular muscles of *thyroid-related orbitopathy* are a common cause of proptosis, but in rare instances may also cause optic nerve compression. Patients with thyroid-related orbitopathy are monitored by serial central vision and visual field testing. Thyroid-related optic nerve compression is often treated initially with systemic corticosteroids, with definitive treatment of orbital decompression to quickly follow.

Orbital cellulitis produces an obvious clinical picture with acute pain, proptosis and periorbital edema. Because of the risk to vision posed by this acute disease, patients are often hospitalized for close monitoring and intravenous antibiotic therapy. Etiology of orbital cellulitis in adults is typically from recent penetrating periorbital trauma, from contiguous spread of facial sinusitis or from hematogenous seeding from facial soft tissue infections. *Idiopathic orbital inflammation* (also, *orbital pseudotumor*) resembles orbital cellulitis, but does not respond to antibiotic therapy, and lacks clear traumatic or infectious prodrome. A dramatic response to systemic corticosteroids is a key diagnostic feature. Orbital cellulitis can also be mimicked by Wegener granulomatosis or invasive fungal sinusitis.

Diagnostic Approach

The orbit represents the most anterior location where examination of the eye itself may not provide clues to the etiology of visual loss. Nevertheless, complete eye examination, with attention to central acuity, visual fields, pupil, and optic disk, remain central to diagnosis. External examination of the orbit, looking for proptosis, resistance to retropulsion of the globe, and limitation of ocular movement, may suggest an orbital tumor or mass. Details in the history of present illness (abruptness of onset, accompanying pain, etc.) will suggest the most likely etiologies.

In some diseases of the orbital optic nerve, optic disk changes may be present, as in the disk hyperemia of LHON. Additional fundus imaging may then be appropriate to better define the abnormalities

However, for the orbit—and for all more posterior etiologies of visual loss—eye examination must be coupled with appropriate imaging. MRI of the orbits is usually recommended, and is done with fat-suppression and gadolinium paramagnetic contrast to enhance tumors such as hemangiomas and meningiomas. Inclusion of the brain, especially fluid-attenuated inversion recovery (FLAIR) sequences, in cases of optic neuritis, helps to assess for additional white-matter lesions, suggestive of MS. However, as mentioned above, CT scanning can reveal diagnostic orbital bone changes missed by MRI. Timing of imaging is usually predicated on the acuteness of the visual loss.

When a specific diagnosis is suggested, additional studies may be indicated, as spinal fluid analysis for optic neuritis or mitochondrial genetic testing in LHON. In cases where examination and imaging do not suggest specific etiology, screening for systemic disease may be needed.

OPTIC CHIASM

Clinical Vignette

A 51-year-old woman presented with worsening vision over many months. She reported no other significant medical history. While confirming normal central acuity, the examiner discovered that the patient could see only the left half of the eye chart with her right eye and only the right half with her left eye. A gross confrontation visual field check confirmed a dense bitemporal hemianopia. The examiner also noted that the woman had facial hypertrichosis and enlargement of her brow, nose, lips, and jaw and that the patient's rings and shoes no longer fit properly. Acromegaly, from abnormally high circulating levels of human growth hormone produced by a pituitary tumor, was diagnosed. MRI confirmed the lesion compressing the optic chiasm.

Bitemporal hemianopia is the characteristic field abnormality of optic chiasm disease. The chiasm (from the Greek letter x) represents the "Great Divide" of the afferent visual system, separating clinical field defects into three anatomic areas. **Prechiasmatic** defects affect the visual field of the ipsilateral eye only and typically result from retinal or optic nerve pathology. **Chiasmatic** disorders classically lead to bitemporal hemianopia (also, *hemianopsia*), with loss of the right lateral field in the right eye and left lateral field in the left eye. **Postchiasmatic** defects produce homonymous hemianopias, with defects appearing more congruous (equal for both eyes) the farther posteriorly the lesion is located.

The optic chiasm is the intersection of the optic nerves from each eye and is located above the pituitary body that lies within the sella turcica of the sphenoid bone, and covered by the diaphragm sellae (Fig. 4-7). The chiasmatic cistern is located between the chiasm and the diaphragm sella. Superior to the chiasm is the third ventricle. The internal carotid arteries flank

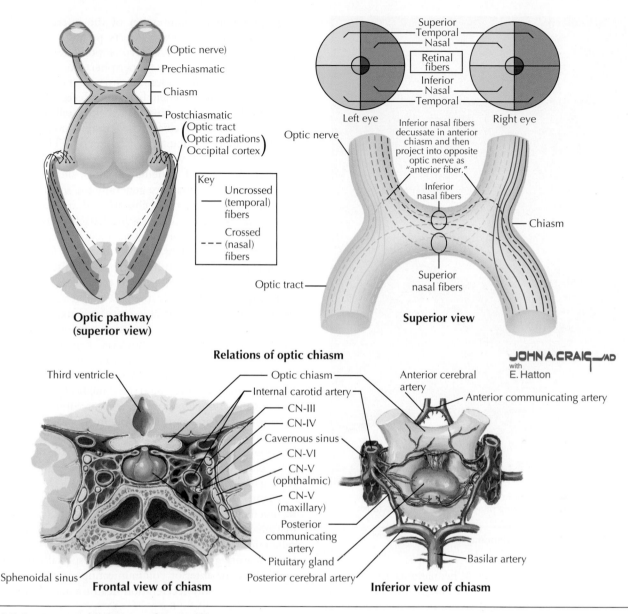

Optic pathway (superior view)

Key
Uncrossed (temporal) fibers
Crossed (nasal) fibers

(Optic nerve)
Prechiasmatic
Chiasm
Postchiasmatic
(Optic tract
Optic radiations
Occipital cortex)

Superior
Temporal
Nasal
Retinal fibers
Inferior
Nasal
Temporal
Left eye   Right eye

Optic nerve
Inferior nasal fibers decussate in anterior chiasm and then project into opposite optic nerve as "anterior fiber."
Inferior nasal fibers
Chiasm
Optic tract
Superior nasal fibers

Superior view

Relations of optic chiasm

JOHN A. CRAIG_AD with E. Hatton

Third ventricle
Optic chiasm
Internal carotid artery
CN-III
CN-IV
Cavernous sinus
CN-VI
CN-V (ophthalmic)
CN-V (maxillary)
Posterior communicating artery
Pituitary gland
Posterior cerebral artery
Sphenoidal sinus
Frontal view of chiasm

Anterior cerebral artery
Anterior communicating artery
Basilar artery
Inferior view of chiasm

Figure 4-7 Anatomy and Relations of Optic Chiasm.

the optic chiasm laterally and then bifurcate into the anterior and middle cerebral arteries. The anterior cerebral arteries and the anterior communicating artery are anterior to the optic chiasm.

Within the chiasm, axons from the temporal retina (nasal field) comprise its lateral aspect and remain ipsilateral as they pass through the chiasm to the optic tract. In contrast, the nasal retinal fibers decussate, carrying temporal visual field information to the contralateral side. Inferior nasal fibers decussate within the chiasm more anteriorly than superior ones. As the inferior nasal retinal fibers approach the posterior aspect of the chiasm, the fibers shift to occupy the lateral aspect of the contralateral optic tract (see Fig. 4-7).

The arterial blood supply of the optic chiasm is derived from the circle of Willis, particularly, the superior hypophyseal arteries, derived from the supraclinoid segment of the carotid arteries. A "prechiasmatic plexus," the hypophyseal portal system, and branches of the anterior cerebral arteries also contribute to

the chiasmatic blood supply. Venous drainage goes to two primary areas: blood from the superior chiasm flows into the anterior cerebral veins, whereas the inferior aspect drains into the infundibular plexus and thus to the paired basal veins of Rosenthal.

The location of the chiasm renders it vulnerable to compression from vascular structures (e.g., aneurysm near the origin of the anterior communicating artery or the ophthalmic artery), from tumors of the meninges, from sphenoid sinus masses, and most important from the pituitary (Fig. 4-8).

Clinical Presentations

Central chiasmatic lesions most commonly produce a bitemporal hemianopia (Fig. 4-9A) that ensues when the optic chiasm is compressed or damaged midsagittally at its decussation. Such lesions preferentially affect the crossing nasal retinal fibers responsible for temporal vision, as in the vignette in this chapter.

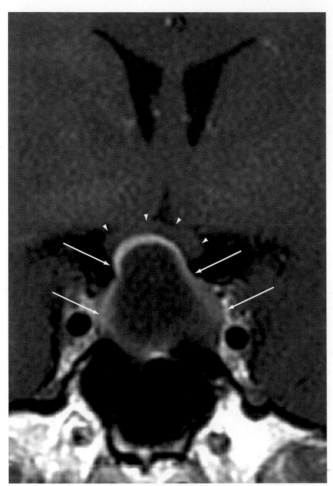

Coronal postcontrast pituitary MR: Optic chiasm (arrowheads) compressed by rim enhancing pituitary macroadenoma (arrows).

Figure 4-8 Pituitary Macroadenoma.

Variants on the classic bitemporal hemianopia are seen with compression of the optic nerve at its entrance to the anterior chiasm, resulting in a **junctional scotoma**, with central visual loss in the ipsilateral eye and a superotemporal defect in the other. The field loss in the contralateral eye reflects involvement of the opposite inferior nasal optic nerve fibers that swing forward into the ipsilateral anterior chiasm (Willebrand knee) before decussating to the optic tract (Fig. 4-9B).

Posterior optic chiasm lesions lead to a **posterior junctional scotoma**, which displays the features of chiasmatic and optic tract lesions. The classic finding is **incongruous** (less dense in the ipsilateral eye) **hemianopic visual field loss** contralateral to the lesion from involvement of the anterior optic tract and an inferotemporal visual field loss in the ipsilateral eye—from pressure on the posterior chiasm affecting the late-crossing superotemporal retinal fibers (Fig. 4-9C). Such defects occur in lesions located near the anterior aspect of the third ventricle that approach the chiasm posteromedially. The incongruous nature of the hemianopsia is caused by the incomplete intermixing of the decussating fibers entering the optic tract with their corresponding uncrossed fibers from the contralateral eye.

Progressive visual field loss from an expanding sellar tumor characteristically begins in the upper temporal fields, likely

from preferential compression of the inferior chiasm as the underlying pituitary tumor exerts pressure through the diaphragm sellae. Early, the superotemporal defects may be paracentral with sparing of the far periphery. As the tumor enlarges, the superotemporal quadrantanopsia extends to the periphery, and the inferotemporal field becomes affected. Later, the inferonasal quadrant, and eventually all vision, will be lost.

Most commonly, chiasmatic compression results from a benign pituitary adenoma (see Chapter 52). These are common brain tumors, and with high-resolution MRI imaging are detected in 10% of patients. Tumors smaller than 10 mm, termed microadenomas, are generally too small to place significant pressure on the optic chiasm. and are usually discovered because of the effects of excess pituitary hormone (e.g., prolactin) secretion. Small nonsecreting adenomas can be found as an incidental finding on brain MRI obtained for other reasons. Once a tumor grows sufficiently and obliterates the 10 mm distance from diaphragm sella to the chiasm, the potential for visual loss exists. Typically, the chiasm can accommodate slowly growing tumors, so that chiasmatic impingement or displacement by such tumors may be seen without any field defect. When the macroadenoma, however, reaches 20–25 mm, field defects are likely. The usual indications for surgical excision are continued tumor growth or the presence of visual compromise. Prolactinomas can often be treated medically using bromocriptine or cabergoline to shrink the tumor. Similarly, mitotane has been used for adrenocorticotropic hormone–secreting tumors, and somatostatin analogues for tumors secreting human growth hormone. Failure of medical therapy leaves the options of transsphenoidal surgical excision, or perhaps precision radiotherapy (e.g., gamma-knife).

Many other sellar masses cause bitemporal hemianopia and include benign or malignant intrinsic tumors (glioma and glioblastoma), extrinsic tumors (benign meningioma and craniopharyngioma or malignant chordoma and lymphoma), and inflammatory granulomas. Aneurysm (especially of the carotid, ophthalmic, or anterior communicating artery), demyelinating disease or MS, and deceleration head trauma are other important etiologies.

Pituitary apoplexy is defined as sudden expansion of a pituitary tumor from infarction or hemorrhage, with subsequent edema and necrosis. Patients typically present with rapid and painful visual loss, often accompanied by alteration of consciousness and ocular motor palsy. Death from pituitary insufficiency can supervene if replacement corticosteroids are not instituted. Prompt surgical decompression of the chiasm is recommended, although improved visual outcomes has not been rigorously proven.

MRI scanning with attention to the sella is recommended in any patient presenting with bitemporal hemianopia. Patient presenting with acute bilateral visual loss should receive urgent MRI or CT scanning to look for pituitary apoplexy or aneurysm.

POSTERIOR VISUAL AFFERENT SYSTEM: OPTIC TRACTS, LATERAL GENICULATE NUCLEUS, OPTIC RADIATIONS

The axons comprising the optic tract are still those emanating from the retinal ganglion cells, which have yet to synapse.

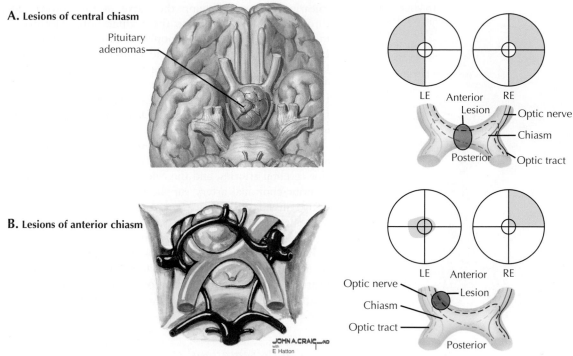

A. Lesions of central chiasm

Pituitary adenomas

LE Anterior RE
Lesion
Optic nerve
Chiasm
Posterior Optic tract

B. Lesions of anterior chiasm

JOHN A. CRAIG—AD
with
E Hatton

LE Anterior RE
Optic nerve
Lesion
Chiasm
Optic tract
Posterior

Anterior chiasm tumor compressing optic nerve at its entrance to chiasm results in junctional scotoma consisting of a central visual field loss in eye ipsilateral to lesion and a superior temporal defect in the opposite eye.

C. Lesions of posterior chiasm

Aneurysm

LE RE
Optic nerve
Anterior
Chiasm
Lesion
Optic tract
Posterior

Posterior communicating artery aneurysm affecting posterior chiasm combines features of both a chiasmatic and an optic tract lesion, resulting in a posterior junctional scotoma—an incongruous (less dense in ipislateral eye) hemianopic field loss contralateral to lesion.

Figure 4-9 Disorders Affecting Optic Chiasm.

Nevertheless, after they leave the chiasm for the optic tract, they nominally become part of the "posterior visual pathway" (Fig. 4-10). Axons of the optic tract course via the anterior limb of the internal capsule, between the tuber cinereum and the anterior perforated substance, then continue posteriorly as a band of flattened fibers around the cerebral peduncles to synapse in the lateral geniculate nucleus (LGN) within the thalamus. The LGN is a thalamic relay nucleus that serves as the synapse point of the retinal ganglion cells. It comprises six gray matter layers separated by five white matter layers. The layers are folded over, forming a bend or small knee. Each layer has a retinotopic organization, creating a map of the contralateral hemifield (Fig. 4-11). The ratio of geniculate cells to retinal axons is approximately 1:1. Retinal input to the LGN comprises only one fifth of its afferent fibers. The remainder comes from the mesencephalic reticular formation, posterior parietal cortex, occipital cortex, and other thalamic nuclei. The LGN may use these nonretinal elements to "screen" the visual input, gating certain inputs to the visual cortex while blocking other signals, depending on the relevance of the inputs.

A relatively small number of nonvisual retinal fibers within the optic tract accompany the optic nerve and chiasm, but remain extrageniculate to supply the afferent stimulus to the pupillomotor center within the pretectal nucleus.

The same vessels that supply the posterior chiasm nourish the anterior one third of the optic tract: the internal carotid, middle cerebral, and posterior communicating arteries. The blood supply of the posterior two thirds of the optic tract is derived from the anterior choroidal artery, a branch of the internal carotid that runs posteriorly near the optic tract. The lateral geniculate body receives blood from the posterior cerebral artery and the posterior communicating arteries.

The optic radiations are myelinated axons emanating from LGN and course to the primary visual cortex. After they leave the LGN, they continue through the posterior limb of the internal capsule. Most fibers take a fairly direct path to the

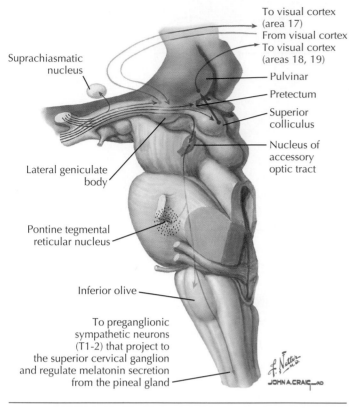

Suprachiasmatic nucleus

To visual cortex (area 17)

From visual cortex

To visual cortex (areas 18, 19)

Pulvinar

Pretectum

Superior colliculus

Nucleus of accessory optic tract

Lateral geniculate body

Pontine tegmental reticular nucleus

Inferior olive

To preganglionic sympathetic neurons (T1-2) that project to the superior cervical ganglion and regulate melatonin secretion from the pineal gland

Figure 4-10 Posterior Visual Pathway and Connections.

calcarine cortex, following the curve of the corona radiata through the parietal lobe to the occipital lobe. However, the most inferior axons (Meyer loop) that carry visual information from the opposite superior field detour laterally around the lateral ventricles and through the posterior temporal lobe (Fig. 4-11). Therefore, stroke or injury confined to this portion of the temporal lobe affects only this portion of the optic radiations. Meyer loop fibers rejoin the rest of the optic radiations after their detour.

Five primary arteries supply blood to the optic radiation: the anterior and posterior choroidal arteries, the middle and posterior cerebral arteries, and the calcarine artery (Fig. 4-12). The anterior choroidal artery supplies the anterior portion of the optic radiations, the optic tract, and the lateral geniculate body. The anterior optic radiations are also fed by a meshwork of branches from the posterior choroidal arteries. The middle portion of the optic radiations, however, is fed via the deep optic branch of the middle cerebral artery, which lies lateral to the ventricle. The posterior portion of the optic radiation is fed by the posterior cerebral artery and one of its branches, the calcarine artery.

Clinical Presentations

Posterior to the chiasm, any insult to the afferent visual system is immediately recognizable by the resulting contralateral homonymous (same laterality and region in each eye) visual loss. It

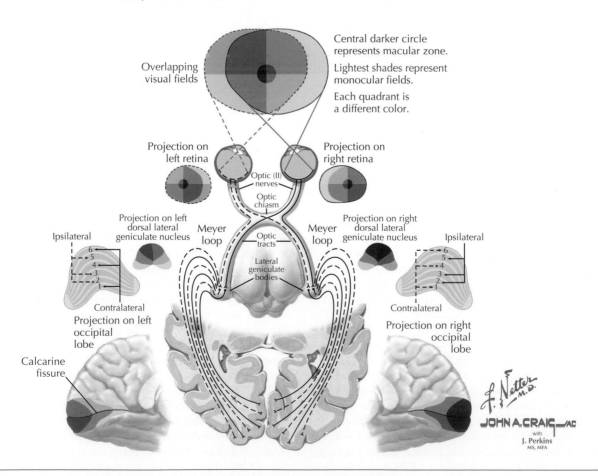

Overlapping visual fields

Central darker circle represents macular zone.

Lightest shades represent monocular fields.

Each quadrant is a different color.

Projection on left retina

Projection on right retina

Optic (II) nerves

Optic chiasm

Projection on left dorsal lateral geniculate nucleus

Meyer loop

Optic tracts

Meyer loop

Projection on right dorsal lateral geniculate nucleus

Ipsilateral

6
5
4
3
2
1

Lateral geniculate bodies

Ipsilateral

6
5
4
3
2
1

Contralateral

Projection on left occipital lobe

Contralateral

Projection on right occipital lobe

Calcarine fissure

Figure 4-11 Topographic Representation of the Visual Fields Across the Optic Pathway.

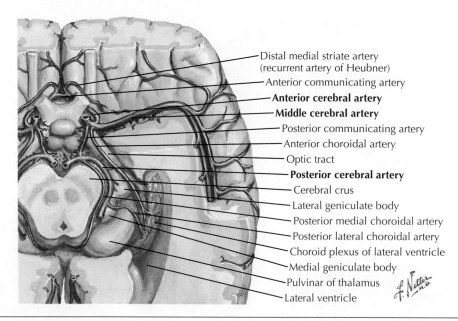

Distal medial striate artery
(recurrent artery of Heubner)
Anterior communicating artery
Anterior cerebral artery
Middle cerebral artery
Posterior communicating artery
Anterior choroidal artery
Optic tract
Posterior cerebral artery
Cerebral crus
Lateral geniculate body
Posterior medial choroidal artery
Posterior lateral choroidal artery
Choroid plexus of lateral ventricle
Medial geniculate body
Pulvinar of thalamus
Lateral ventricle

Figure 4-12 Arteries of Brain: Inferior Views.

is commonly found that in pure hemianopias without optic nerve or chiasm contribution, central visual acuity for individual letters is unaffected; however, the "macular splitting" that results from total hemianopia can cause difficulty with reading text.

Optic tract lesions are unique in that they cause homonymous hemianopias combined with pupillary abnormalities and optic disk pallor. Total lesions of the optic tract affect the pupillary afferents within the tract and produce a mild relative afferent pupillary defect in the contralateral eye because more crossed fibers exist within the tract from the contralateral eye than uncrossed fibers from the ipsilateral eye. When wallerian degeneration ensues, pallor characteristic of optic tract lesions develops in the optic disks. The ipsilateral eye, losing axons from the retina temporal to the fovea, has chiefly superior and inferior polar atrophy, whereas the contralateral eye, losing the interior of the papillomacular bundle and the axons from the retina nasal to the optic nerve, has pallor in the temporal and nasal poles (**"bow-tie" atrophy**).

For the optic tract, the field loss affects both eyes and is contralateral to the affected tract. The loss depends on the extent of the tract lesion and is either a complete or incomplete homonymous hemianopia. Incomplete tract hemianopias are often incongruous (i.e., the defects in each eye do not match exactly) wedge-shaped defects, with the point of the wedge encroaching on the center, a "dagger into fixation" or "sectoranopia." As with the chiasm, neoplasms, aneurysms, and trauma are the typical lesion in this region; strokes are relatively uncommon.

Posterior to the optic tract, visual field loss is not accompanied by pupillary change or optic atrophy. However, specifics of the hemianopia can assist in localizing the lesion. LGN lesions produce field defects similar to those of the optic tract. Lesions confined to the temporal lobe can reach only the Meyer loop portion of the optic radiations, with the resulting visual field defect typically as a homonymous, incongruous superior wedge—one side located at the vertical meridian and the second edge being less sharp. This defect, resembling a "slice" removed

from the superior visual field, has been termed the *pie-in-the-sky defect*. When encountered, it provides strong evidence of a temporal lobe pathogenesis. Often, other findings of temporal lobe dysfunction confirm the localization.

Conversely, if a parietal lesion affects the optic radiations anteriorly, an inverse lesion sparing the temporal lobe "wedge" occurs; however, such lesions are rarely encountered. Occasionally, larger or far posterior parietal lesions can affect all of the optic radiations after the Meyer loop has rejoined the other fibers, producing a complete homonymous hemianopia. Pathologic entities affecting the posterior visual afferents are most commonly stroke, tumor, demyelination, and trauma.

Differential and Diagnostic Approach

Complete homonymous hemianopias cannot be reliably localized as to the level of the optic tract, lateral geniculate body, parietal lobe, or occipital lobe. Other than the visual fields, a broader ophthalmologic examination may provide hints to the site of the lesions. For example, optic tract lesions produce a mild contralateral relative afferent pupil defect and bow-tie atrophy of the optic disks. The parietal lobe contributes to pursuit eye movements, and patients with a complete homonymous hemianopia from a parietal lesion may show altered or absent optokinetic nystagmus in the direction of the lesion.

As with any visual loss, the diagnostic course for hemianopic visual loss includes complete eye examination, visual fields with attention to assessment of central acuity, pupillary reactions, pursuit movements, and funduscopy. The presence of additional neurologic or systemic symptoms and the speed of onset may help both localize the lesion and suggest an etiology. Review of past medical history may reveal if the patient has known risks for some etiologies, such as stroke, demyelination, or metastasis. The most important ancillary test is diagnostic imaging. Typically, MRI examination is recommended as best able to detect, and distinguish among, the potential pathologies. Diffusion-weighted images can be particularly useful in defining recent

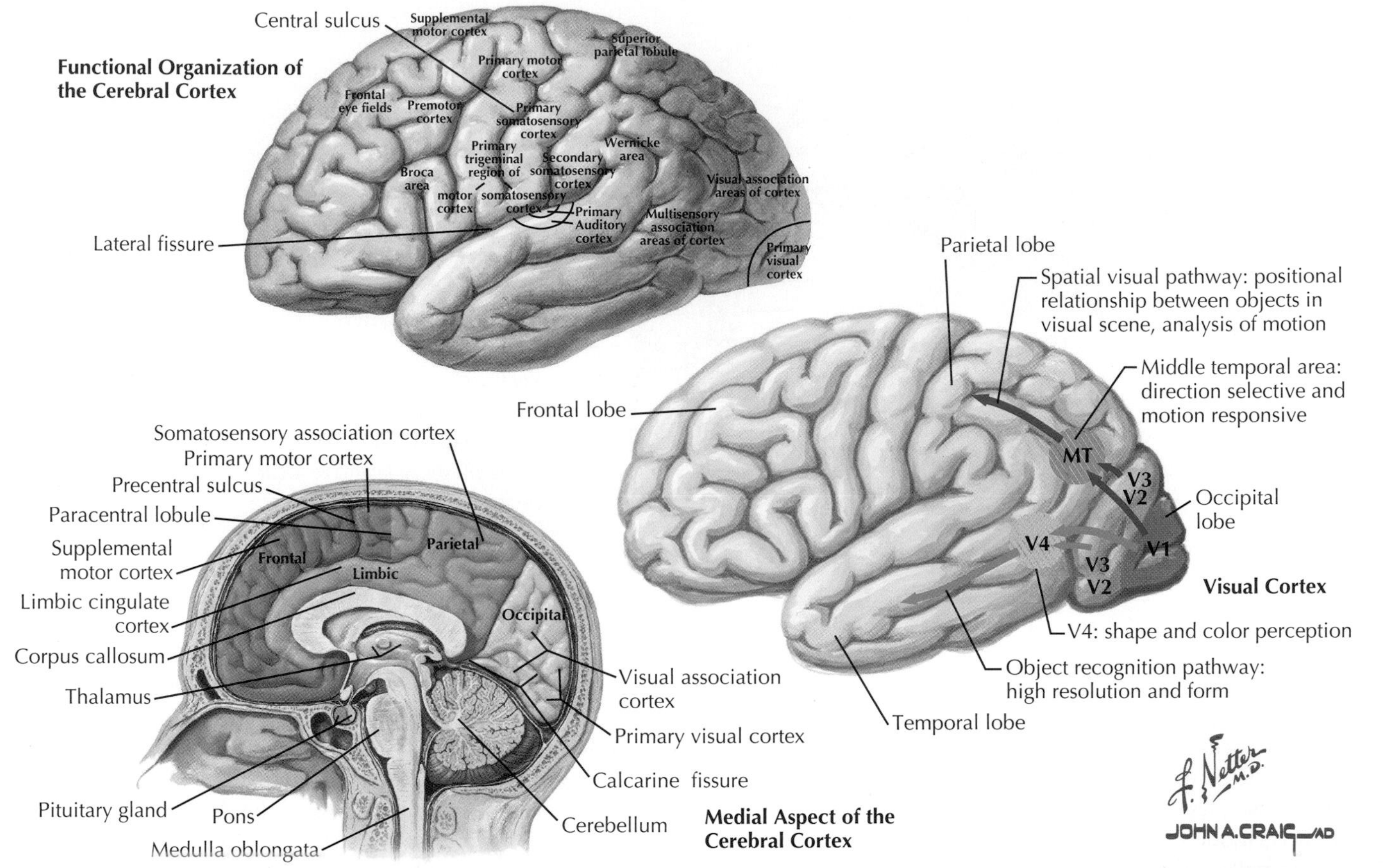

Figure 4-13 Occipital Cortex and Projections.

stroke (see Chapter 55). Management and therapy are dictated by the etiology.

PRIMARY VISUAL CORTEX AND VISUAL ASSOCIATION CORTICES

Clinical Vignette

A 64-year-old gynecologist, while operating, suddenly had difficulty seeing to the right. He had to turn his head to see the full operative field. The next day, he saw his ophthalmologist, who found evidence of a dense right homonymous hemianopia.

A subsequent neurologic consultation was otherwise unremarkable. MRI demonstrated a positive diffusion-weighted lesion in the left occipital lobe. ECG and transesophageal echocardiography results were normal. A 48-hour Holter monitor documented seven periods of intermittent atrial fibrillation. Anticoagulation was initiated. The patient was advised to stop driving.

Axons of the optic radiations synapse with the primary visual cortex. A unique white stripe or stria (*stripe* or *line of Gennari* for the discovering anatomist) represents a myelin-rich cortical layer; it is easily seen in gross sections through the cortex and bespeaks the layered, highly structured organization of **V1** (also known as the *primary visual cortex*, the *striate cortex*, or *Brodmann area 17*). Primarily located on the mesial surface of the occipital lobe within and surrounding the calcarine fissure, the most posterior aspect of V1 typically wraps around the posterior (occipital) pole for a short distance (Fig. 4-13).

Microscopically, the visual cortex is arranged in six laminae, running from the surface to a depth of slightly greater than 2 mm. The most superficial, layer I, primarily contains glial cells. Layers II and III contain pyramidal cells and small interneurons. The thickest stria is layer IV, comprising almost half the depth of the visual cortex. Highly branched stellate cells exist superficially within layer IVa. The Gennari stripe comprises layer IVb, containing myelinated axons from afferent visual (geniculate) cells and cortical association fibers. Pyramidal and granule cells and giant pyramidal (Meynert) cells occur more deeply at IVc. Layer V is a densely cellular region with variously sized pyramidal cells. Layer VIa is a less cellular superficial portion, and layer VIb contains a varied neuronal population.

The blood supply of the striate cortex primarily derives from the **calcarine artery**, a branch of the **posterior cerebral artery**, and sometimes the **middle cerebral artery**, or anastomoses from it (Fig. 4-14). The calcarine artery is a major supply to the visual area; however, in 75% of cases, other arteries contribute as well: the posterior temporal or parietooccipital arteries, and, occasionally, anastomotic connections from the middle cerebral artery.

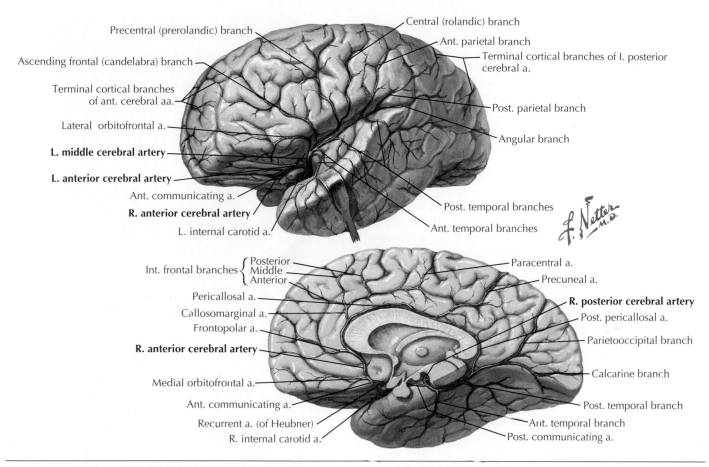

Figure 4-14 Arteries of Brain (Lateral and Medial Views).

Specific anatomic correlations are the primary clinical features pertinent to the striate cortex: visual information from the left visual field in each eye is projected to the right visual cortex (and conversely); the superior visual field is projected into the inferior half of V1 (and conversely); and the most central visual field is projected most posteriorly, whereas the peripheral field is located anteriorly within V1.

"Cortical magnification" in V1 results in much more cortex dedicated to the central area than to the periphery. Up to 50% of the cortex may correspond to the central 10° of vision; in fact, the most central 1° of vision uses as much cortex posteriorly as the most peripheral 50°. Cortical magnification is considered a reflection of the evolutionary importance of precise central vision to human survival.

Ocular dominance columns run at right angles to the cortical surface. Within a column, visual input is derived from one eye only; in the immediate neighboring cortical surface, perhaps 0.5 mm away, another column deriving input from the other eye is encountered.

Monocular occlusion in animal experiments during the early postnatal period demonstrates that the columns of the occluded eye grow smaller, whereas the columns of the open eye enlarge. Subsequent uncovering of the occluded eye does not restore the equality of the columns, which is considered central to understanding critical periods in visual development. The failure of that development is designated *amblyopia*.

A hierarchy exists to the processing of visual information at a cellular level. The striate cortex has different cell types that respond to increasingly specific stimuli. **Simple cells** have the same light–dark, center–surround response profile as retina and LGN cells. **Complex and hypercomplex cells** respond best to a light stimulus that is not a spot but a line at a particular angle or a specific length to achieve an optimal cell response.

This hierarchical structure suggests that additional cell types, probably located in extrastriate association cortices, respond to more specific and complex stimuli until, eventually, there may be "higher" association cortices, with groups of cells producing specific **patterns of neuronal activation** that represent the anatomic correlate for a specific perceptual recognition.

Brodmann areas 18 and 19, immediately adjacent to area 17, in the area surrounding the calcarine fissure, were termed the *parastriate* or *association visual cortex* on the assumption that they function to "associate" the visual data from V1 with brain areas regarding spatial orientation, recognition, and language.

The economic implications of hemianopic visual loss can be estimated by looking at its primary etiology, stroke. It has been estimated that 15% of stroke patients suffer homonymous visual loss. Overall, stroke costs in the United States will reach $2.2 trillion in the next 45 years, with hemianopia representing perhaps $300 billion.

Clinical Presentations

The vignette at the beginning of this section typifies an embolus to the left posterior cerebral artery causing a left occipital lobe infarct. Although occasionally such patients improve, often individuals have no substantial resolution of function. Driving restriction is essential in this case because of the total inability to perceive objects in the densely lost field.

Striate cortex lesions, like other neurologic lesions, can be classified into ischemic, neoplastic, demyelinating disease, and rare infections. Clinical characteristics of V1 visual field defects provide diagnostic anatomic localization even before imaging procedures are done. Incomplete hemianopias from V1 lesions show congruent deficits in each eye's visual field. The small size and close proximity of the left and right ocular dominance columns make it impossible to selectively damage the visual field of only one eye.

Features of homonymous hemianopias that suggest occipital lobe origin include extremely congruous partial defects between eyes, macular sparing, central homonymous defects, keyhole defects, as well as temporal crescent defects. Because of the specialized nature of V1, lesions in it affect only the vision, without other neurologic dysfunction (except, occasionally, headache). In addition to the above, striate cortex lesions produce no signs of anterior visual pathway involvement such as optic pallor or relative afferent papillary defect. Typically, central acuity in the preserve field is normal (Fig. 4-15).

The extreme temporal visual field of each eye represents an exception to the above principle of symmetric homonymous defects. Because the nasal visual field extends only approximately 65°, the remaining 25% of the lateral field on each side is supplied solely by the ipsilateral eye. This "temporal crescent" of the visual field corresponds to the most anterior aspect of V1, abutting the occipitoparietal fissure, where ocular dominance columns are absent, because all input comes solely from the contralateral nasal retina. Therefore, lesions of the anterior striate cortex may result in a "monocular temporal defect."

Rarely, bilateral occipital cortical lesions occur simultaneously or in quick succession. Generalized systemic hypotension, such as from a cardiac arrest or basilar or bilateral posterior cerebral artery occlusion, can cause bilateral ischemic damage. Similarly, both occipital poles can be injured by direct trauma or contrecoup mechanisms during skull injury. Initially, bilateral occipital pole lesions may be confused with bilateral optic nerve lesions because an apparent "central scotoma" is found in each eye. However, careful visual field mapping along the vertical axis demonstrates a discontinuity, or a vertical step. The vertical step is expected because cortical injuries should not be absolutely symmetric and the extent of clinical visual field loss should vary in size between the left and right hemifields. The size difference is easily recognized at the vertical meridian, resulting in a "keyhole defect." Like temporal crescent defects, keyhole defects are characteristic of occipital lobe lesions.

The most central visual field is represented widely on the posterior pole rather than only in the mesial occipital surface of V1 and is often supplied by the middle rather than the posterior cerebral artery. This means that even lesions affecting most of V1 may miss the most anterior, central vision area and produce a pattern of *macular sparing* in homonymous hemianopia with

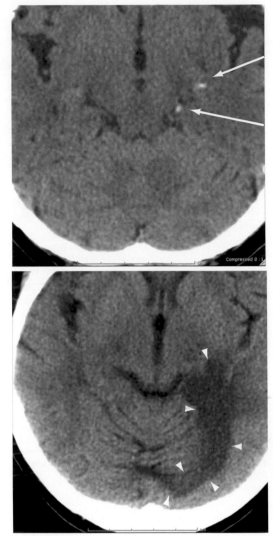

Axial noncontrast brain CT: Left posterior cerebral intraluminal thrombus (arrows) with subsequent evolution of left posterior cerebral cortically based infarct (arrowheads).

Figure 4-15 Left Posterior Cerebral Infarction.

incomplete striate cortex lesions. However, when there is total loss of the cortex (e.g., surgical removal), macular sparing is not expected.

Parietal lesions differ from the isolated loss of visual field seen in V1 occipital disease in that both homonymous contralateral field loss and abnormal eye movements are usually detected. The loss of visually guided horizontal saccades to the side away from the lesion is best seen as an abnormal opticokinetic nystagmus response: when the drum is rotated toward the side of the lesion, the eyes, unable to saccade and pick up the next stripe on the drum, drift toward the affected side.

The clinical presentations of extrastriatal cortical lesions continue to be defined. Cerebral achromatopsia (impaired color perception due to occipital insult) has been described. The pathologies producing more complex visual deficits, typically termed visual agnosias, reach beyond the parastriate cortices. Prosopagnosia, for example, is typically caused by lesions encompassing the occipital and temporal lobes.

Diagnostic Approach

Visual fields, ocular, and neurologic examinations will often serve to localize the visual problem to the occipital cortex. The etiology is suggested by the tempo of onset, accompanying symptoms, and presence of risk factors for a specific disease entity. MR imaging however remains standard for better specifying the pathologic process.

Cases of diffuse cerebral dysfunction may occasionally present with poor vision as the chief complaint. Electroencephalography and positron emission tomographic (PET) scanning may help in diagnosing patients with the Heidenhain variant of Creutzfeldt–Jakob disease, where visual symptoms predominate and MRI is normal in the early course. In the visual variant of Alzheimer disease, however, neuropsychological testing and PET scanning with hypometabolism of the bilateral parieto-occipital cortices and the frontal eye fields probably provide the best diagnostic strategy.

Treatment

Treatment for most types of homonymous hemianopia is unavailing. If there is no improvement in visual deficits after the first 2 weeks, visual loss due to stroke is generally permanent. Surgical removal of an arteriovenous malformation or tumor is usually expected to leave significant residual visual loss.

Therefore, mainstays of treatment are stabilization of vision (e.g., stroke prevention if stroke was the etiology) and visual rehabilitation. Rehabilitation efforts resemble those in other areas of post-stroke rehabilitation, with focus on developing strategies to return to activities of daily living (e.g., reading and avoiding obstacles while ambulating) in spite of the hemianopic visual loss. Much of the improvement generally seen over time is usually attributed to increased visual scanning on the side of the blind hemifield, utilizing saccades and head turns to that side. Protection of the patient who is unable to see obstacles in one hemifield may be improved by use of a cane on the hemianopic side and a brimmed or billed hat to detect obstacles before collision.

The possibility of "visual restoration" after stroke or traumatic brain injury using a computer-based, stimulus-detection paradigm is being explored. Data suggesting an average of 12% increase in "stimulus detection" after 6 months of therapy have been reported, but how and whether such testing improvement translates into practical functional improvement or reorganization on a neuronal basis remains unclear.

The use of a split prismatic spectacle correction, which presents part of the "blind" hemifield to the patient's remaining vision with less head turning, may aid selected patients by providing a way to monitor the area of visual loss more easily. Except in cases of quite minor loss, returning to driving after hemianopic visual loss is generally impossible, even if prismatic spectacles or visual restoration attempts are employed.

FUTURE DIRECTIONS

The preceding chapter covers a wide range of diseases that have an impact on vision. Research on improved diagnosis, prevention, treatment, genetics, and risk factors is active on all fronts.

As seen, current controversy attends the possibility of therapy for homonymous hemianopia. With the large number of patients affected by hemianopia, establishing the presence and significance of any improvement becomes an important economic, as well as medical, issue.

ADDITIONAL RESOURCES

INTRAOCULAR OPTIC NERVE

Beck RW, Servais GE, Hayreh SS. Anterior ischemic optic neuropathy. IX. Cup-to-disc ratio and its role in pathogenesis. Ophthalmology 1987 Nov;94(11):1503-1508. *Cites disk morphology as risk factor in AION.*

Douglas DJ, Schuler JJ, Buchbinder D, et al. The association of central retinal artery occlusion and extracranial carotid artery disease. Ann Surg 1988 Jul;208(1):85-90. *Shows risk of ipsilateral stoke after CRAO.*

Hayreh SS, Kolder HE, Weingeist TA. Central retinal artery occlusion and retinal tolerance time. Ophthalmology 1980 Jan;87(1):75-78. *Establishes retinal viability at 100 minutes after retinal artery occlusion.*

Hayreh SS, Podhajsky PA, Raman R, et al. Giant cell arteritis: validity and reliability of various diagnostic criteria. Am J Ophthalmol 1997 Mar;123(3):285-296. *Offers guidance regarding confirmatory testing in TA.*

Hayreh SS, Zimmerman MB. Non-arteritic anterior ischemic optic neuropathy: role of systemic corticosteroid therapy. Graefes Arch Clin Exp Ophthalmol 2008 Jul;246(7):1029-1046. *Suggests benefit to 65-day oral steroid course in vision recovery after AION.*

Salomon O, Huna-Baron R, Steinberg DM, et al. Role of aspirin in reducing the frequency of second eye involvement in patients with non-arteritic anterior ischaemic optic neuropathy. Eye 1999 Jun;13 (Pt 3a):357-359. *Suggests benefit of aspirin in this context.*

ORBITAL AND INTRACANALICULAR OPTIC NERVE

Alabduljalil T, Behbehani R. Paraneoplastic syndromes in neuro-ophthalmology. Curr Opin Ophthalmol 2007 Nov;18(6):463-469. *Review of available data for paraneoplastic optic neuropathy.*

Beck RW, Cleary PA, Anderson MM Jr, et al. A randomized, controlled trial of corticosteroids in the treatment of acute optic neuritis. The Optic Neuritis Study Group. N Engl J Med 1992 Feb 27;326(9):581-588. *Established benefits of early intravenous methylprednisolone on recovery time and interval to next MS episode.*

Hayreh SS. Posterior ischaemic optic neuropathy: clinical features, pathogenesis, and management. Eye 2004 Nov;18(11):1188-1206. *Characteristics of 42 cases of PION.*

Sadda SR, Nee M, Miller NR, et al. Clinical spectrum of posterior ischemic optic neuropathy. Am J Ophthalmol 2001 Nov;132(5):743-750. *Divides 72 cases into three etiological categories.*

Wallace DC, Singh G, Lott MT, et al. Mitochondrial DNA mutation associated with Leber's hereditary optic neuropathy. Science 1988;242:1427–1430. *First description of mitochondrial DNA mutation in an LHON pedigree.*

Wingerchuk DM, Weinshenker BG. Neuromyelitis optica. Curr Treat Options Neurol 2008 Jan;10(1):55-66. *Review of current diagnosis and treatment.*

OPTIC CHIASM

Thomas R, Shenoy K, Seshadri MS, et al. Visual field defects in non-functioning pituitary adenomas. Indian J Ophthalmol 2002 Jun;50(2):127-130. *Relates visual field defects to tumor size.*

POSTERIOR VISUAL AFFERENT SYSTEM: OPTIC TRACTS, LATERAL GENICULATE NUCLEUS, OPTIC RADIATIONS

Bowers AR, Keeney K, Peli E. Community-based trial of a peripheral prism visual field expansion device for hemianopia. Arch Ophthalmol 2008 May;126(5):657-664. *Showed long-term tolerance and functional improvement in 47% of patients using prismatic spectacles for hemianopic loss.*

Brazis PW, Lee AG, Graff-Radford N, et al. Homonymous visual field defects in patients without corresponding structural lesions on neuroimaging. J Neuroophthalmol 2000 Jun;20(2):92-96.

Horton JC, Hoyt WF. The representation of the visual field in human striate cortex: a revision of the classic Holmes map. Arch Ophthalmol 1991;109:816-824. *Discusses anatomic basis of cortical magnification, temporal crescent, etc.*

Lee AG, Martin CO. Ophthalmology. Neuro-ophthalmic findings in the visual variant of Alzheimer's disease. Ophthalmology 2004 Feb;111(2):376-380; discussion 380-381. *These two articles propose diagnostic strategies for patients with visual loss and underlying progressive dementia.*

Pambakian AL, Mannan SK, Hodgson TL, et al. Saccadic visual search training: a treatment for patients with homonymous hemianopia. J Neurol Neurosurg Psychiatry 2004 Oct;75(10):1443-1448. *Results of 29 patients.*

Pelak VS, Dubin M, Whitney E. Homonymous hemianopia: A critical analysis of optical devices, compensatory training, and NovaVision. Curr Treat Options Neurol 2007 Jan;9(1):41-47. *This reference discusses issues in the NovaVision data, tempering claims of visual improvement.*

Rathore SS, Hinn AR, Cooper LS, et al. Characterization of incident stroke signs and symptoms: findings from the atherosclerosis risk in communities study. Stroke 2002 Nov;33(11):2718-2721. *Showed 15% prevalence of homonymous hemianopia among 474 stroke patients.*

ACKNOWLEDGMENT

The author thanks Professor Thomas R. Hedges III, MD, for his help in organizing and clarifying this chapter.

Cranial Nerves III, IV, and VI: Oculomotor, Trochlear, and Abducens Nerves: Ocular Mobility and Pupils

Ippolit C. A. Matjucha

CRANIAL NERVE III: OCULOMOTOR

Clinical Vignette

A 37-year-old woman presented with a 2-day history of "blurry" vision on upward gaze, and headache. One month previously, when she had experienced the same symptoms, sinusitis was diagnosed, and an antibiotic was prescribed; symptoms had resolved in 5 days.

Examination demonstrated impaired upward, downward, and medial movement in the right. There was mild right-sided ptosis, and the pupil was slightly larger and reacted poorly compared with the left.

Magnetic resonance imaging (MRI) yielded normal results, but catheter angiography demonstrated a posterior communicating artery (p-com) aneurysm. At craniotomy the same night, the neurosurgeon reported fresh and old clot around a 10-mm aneurysm compressing the right oculomotor nerve. The aneurysm was clipped, and patient had an uneventful recovery with gradual resolution of the neuro-ophthalmologic findings.

*O*culomotor palsy is most often associated with microvasculopathy due to diabetes mellitus, hypertension, or advanced age, so that its pool of potential victims is large. It is sometimes the harbinger of urgent, dangerous disease such as expanding berry aneurysm. Even in idiopathic cases, the diplopia it typically produces is not only distressing for the patient but also disrupts daily activities. Even in cases where ptosis is severe enough to eliminate diplopia by blocking the vision of the affected eye, the impact on patients, both on an emotional and practical level, is severe.

The oculomotor nerves course from the ventral midbrain to the orbits. CN-III provides the general somatic motor efferent innervation controlling upper lid elevation and most of the extraocular movements upward, medially, and downward. In addition, CN-III carries the general visceral motor (parasympathetic) efferent innervation responsible for pupillary constriction and accommodation (near focus) of the crystalline lens.

CN-III begins at its nucleus in the midline upper midbrain. The nucleus is a lepidopteroid collection of nine subnuclei located in the center of the rostral midbrain at the level of the superior colliculi (Fig. 5-1). The most ventral of these subnuclei is the central caudate nucleus, a midline structure that innervates both levator palpebrae muscles. Uniquely, axons from the medial subnuclei or columns decussate completely to innervate the contralateral superior rectus muscles. The other six subnuclei, three left-and-right pairs, innervate ipsilateral extraocular

muscles. The ventral subnucleus, intermediate column, and dorsal subnucleus, respectively, control the medial rectus (eye adduction), inferior oblique (intorsion and some elevation), and inferior rectus (depression).

Sometimes considered a subnucleus of CN-III, the Edinger–Westphal nucleus abuts the others rostrodorsally, residing at the ventral edge of periaqueductal gray matter. The Edinger–Westphal nucleus supplies the cholinergic efferents producing pupillary constriction and ciliary muscle contraction (lens accommodation). Afferents from the pretectal nuclei mediate the pupillary light reflex, whereas inputs influencing pupil constriction and lens accommodation in response to near visual stimulus originate from striate and prestriate cortex and the superior colliculus. When the pupillary fibers join the oculomotor nerve, they move exteriorly and dorsally within the nerve, a clinical continuation of the spatial relation of the Edinger–Westphal nucleus to CN-III.

The CN-III nucleus receives numerous afferents, including inputs from the paramedian pontine reticular formation for horizontal eye movement, the rostral interstitial nucleus of the medial longitudinal fasciculus for vertical and torsional movements, and the vestibular nuclei. Other afferents come from the superior colliculi, the occipital cortex, and the cerebellum.

Axons from the CN-III nucleus gather into a fascicle that sweeps ventrally in an arc curving toward the medial surface of the cerebral peduncle, then passes through the red nucleus.

The nascent oculomotor nerve emerges from the medial surface of the cerebral peduncle to enter the interpeduncular cistern. It crosses the cistern for approximately 5 mm, passing under the posterior cerebral artery. The fibers subserving pupillary constriction are located externally at the caudal aspect of the nerve and are less prone to microvascular changes as deeper fibers are. This arrangement is thought to explain the pupil's resilience to ischemia affecting CN-III and to its susceptibility in compression. The nerve follows beneath the posterior communicating artery (p-com) for 10 mm and then pierces the dura underneath the p-com before it passes the internal carotid artery (ICA) en route to the cavernous sinus.

The cavernous sinus is part of the intracranial venous system. It receives blood from the ophthalmic vein and sphenoparietal sinus, transmitting this flow to the superior and inferior petrosal sinuses. The left and right cavernous sinuses are connected via the intracavernous plexus; they also communicate with the basilar sinus and the pterygoid and foramen ovale plexuses. The cavernous sinus resides lateral to the pituitary gland, resting atop the roof and lateral wall of the sphenoid sinus. Besides venous blood, the space contains the intracavernous portions of CN-III, -IV, and -VI; the ophthalmic branch of CN-V and its

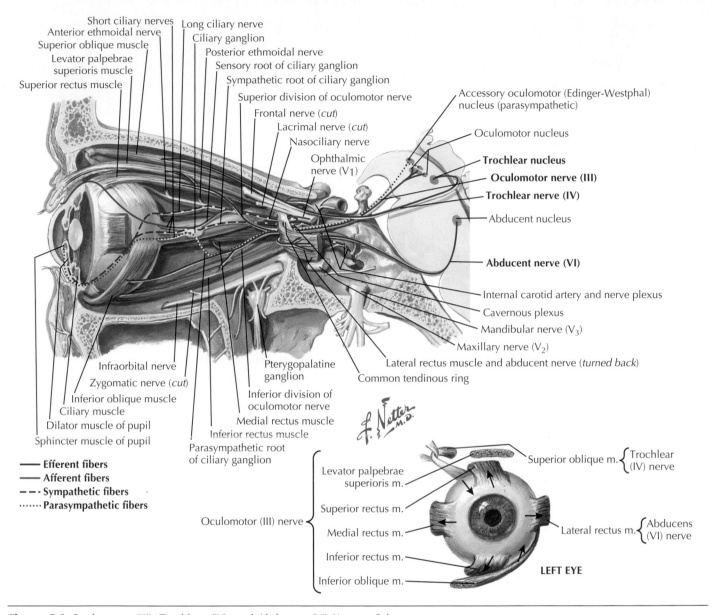

Figure 5-1 Oculomotor (III), Trochlear (IV), and Abducent (VI) Nerves: Schema.

maxillary nerve posteriorly; the ICA; and the sympathetic nerve fibers investing the adventitia of the ICA. CN-III, -IV, and -VI and the ophthalmic nerve all leave the cavernous sinus to enter the orbit via the superior orbital fissure.

Given the confluence of multiple structures into this relatively small sinus, cavernous lesions are prone to produce multiple cranial nerve palsies often with pain or numbness in the ophthalmic distribution of CN-V. If the pathologic process is extensive, signs of venous obstruction in the orbit also develop (proptosis and chemosis).

CN-III typically divides into superior and inferior branches within the anterior cavernous sinus, thus entering the orbit as two distinct structures. The superior branch supplies the superior rectus and levator palpebrae muscles. The inferior branch provides somatic innervation to the medial and inferior recti and the inferior oblique, and it supplies the parasympathetic pupillary input to the ciliary ganglion, located superolaterally to the optic nerve. The parasympathetic axons from the

Edinger–Westphal nucleus synapse here, with the postsynaptic neurons providing visceral motor control to the iris sphincter and the ciliary muscles via the short ciliary nerves.

Etiology and Pathogenesis

Etiologies for CN-III are broadly divided into two groups: those due to microvascular nerve infarction (e.g., diabetes mellitus) and those due to compression. There are also other, less frequent etiologies.

In the patient presenting with acute, severe headache and pupil-involved CN-III palsy, an expanding *aneurysm*, usually of the posterior communicating artery (p-com), is the most important cause (Fig. 5-2). The location of these aneurysms is the origin of p-com at the ICA (Fig. 5-3) and 90% of these aneurysms present with CN-III palsy. Aneurysm in other nearby arteries can likewise present as CN-III palsy, with up to 30% of acquired CN-III palsies being caused by aneurysms.

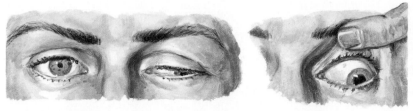 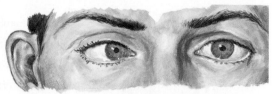

Oculomotor palsy: Ptosis, eye turns laterally and inferiorly, pupil dilated; common finding with cerebral aneurysms, especially carotid-posterior communicating aneurysms

Abducens palsy: Affected eye turns medially. May be first manifestation of intracavernous carotid aneurysm. Pain above eye or on side of face may be secondary to trigeminal (V) nerve involvement.

Superior cerebellar artery aneurysm with CN III and IV compression

Basilar a.
R. trochlear (IV) n.
R. oculomotor (III) n.
Posterior clinoid process
Middle fossa
R. internal carotid a.
R. ophthalmic a.
R. optic (II) n.
R. anterior cerebral a.
R. middle cerebral a.
R. posterior communicating a.
Temporal lobe (elevated)
Tentorium (divided)
R. trigeminal (V) n.
Pons
Cerebellum
R. superior cerebellar a.
Aneurysm
R. posterior cerebral a.

Retinal changes

Optic atrophy may develop as a result of pressure on the optic (II) nerve from a supraclinoid carotid, ophthalmic, or anterior cerebral aneurysm.

Papilledema may be caused by increased intracranial pressure secondary to rupture of a cerebral aneurysm.

Hemorrhage into optic (II) nerve sheath after rupture of aneurysm may result in subhyaloid hemorrhage with blood around disc.

Figure 5-2 Ophthalmologic Manifestations of Cerebral Aneurysms.

However, the majority of acquired CN-III palsies will be due to vascular compromise of some portion of CN-III, commonly affecting patients with known risk factors for vasculopathy or microvascular disease. In 60–80% of microvascular CN-III palsy cases the pupil is spared. Typically, these palsies have a favorable prognosis and uncomplicated recovery within 2–4 months. Although common vasculopathies secondary to diabetes and hypertension are seen most frequently, attention should be paid to the possibilities of other systemic vasculitides, temporal arteritis, clotting disorder, and infiltrative processes.

Third-nerve palsies due to lesions of the nucleus or fascicle within the midbrain are usually part of a larger midbrain syndrome (see below). The usual etiologies of such palsies are stroke for older patients and inflammatory or demyelinating disease (i.e., multiple sclerosis) in the young.

Open or closed head injuries may lead to *traumatic oculomotor nerve palsy*. The suspected mechanism is traction or shearing where the third-nerve root is relatively fixed at its origin and at its entrance into the dura.

Typically, traumatic CN-III palsy is associated with severe frontal deceleration impact with loss of consciousness and, usually, skull fracture (e.g., unrestrained occupant in a motor vehicle accident). In cases where pupil-involving CN-III palsy is discovered after seemingly trivial injury, neurovascular imaging to detect a possible underlying skull base tumor, often meningioma, or aneurysms should be performed.

Cavernous sinus thrombosis may produce a cranial polyneuropathy that features CN-III palsy. Often it is a septic complication of central facial cellulitis and a dreaded clinical entity typically producing proptosis, ophthalmoplegia, and optic neuropathy. Septic phlebitis of the facial vein or pterygoid plexus is the usual intermediary between cellulitis and infectious thrombosis.

Tolosa–Hunt syndrome is a painful ophthalmoplegia caused by idiopathic cavernous sinus inflammation, with most instances

Internal carotid a.

Cavernous sinus

Oculomotor (III) n. (divided)

Trochlear (IV) n.

Trigeminal (V) n.

Abducens (VI) n.

Oculomotor (III) n. (divided)

Posterior communicating a.

Posterior cerebral a.

Basilar a.

**Posterior Communicating Artery Aneurysm
Compressing Cranial Nerve III**

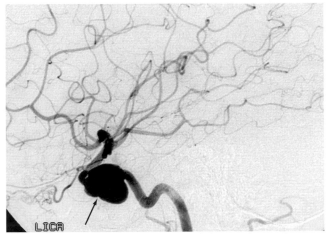

Intracranial Aneurysm: Lateral projection left internal carotid arteriogram: Large fusiform cavernous internal carotid aneurysm (arrow).

Figure 5-3 Aneurysms Causing Oculomotor Nerve Palsy.

considered within the spectrum of inflammatory pseudotumor. It typically involves multiple cranial nerves and varies in degree over days. MRI of the cavernous sinus is needed to confirm the diagnosis, and treatment with high-dose corticosteroids is indicated once tumor and infection have been excluded.

Intrinsic, extrinsic, and metastatic tumors can cause third-nerve palsy. Carcinomatous or granulomatous meningitis can affect multiple cranial nerves in succession, often simulating Tolosa–Hunt syndrome.

Clinical Presentations

The classic presentation of a complete CN-III palsy is unmistakable: because of the unopposed actions of the superior oblique and lateral rectus muscles, the eye is turned outward and usually down. Upper-lid ptosis often requires that the lid be held up by the examiner to assess ocular motility.

The presence or absence of ipsilateral mydriasis ("pupil-involvement" or "pupil-sparing," respectively) has traditionally been considered a major diagnostic consideration. CN-III palsies of compressive origin have pupillary involvement in the vast majority of cases and, if acute with severe headache, strongly suggest aneurysm as the etiology. Pupil-sparing usually implies temporary CN-III palsy due to microvascular ischemia. Patients with microvascular oculomotor palsy may report a mild ache in the ipsilateral brow, but occasionally the pain can be severe.

Motor involvement of CN-III palsies are generally characterized as complete, incomplete (where the innervated muscles show subtotal palsy), and, since the CN-III divides into superior and inferior rami just before its entrance into the orbit, divisional. "Superior division" CN-III palsy involves ipsilateral dysfunction of the superior rectus and levator palpebrae muscles, whereas an "inferior division" palsy has impaired downgaze, medial gaze, and on occasion, loss of pupillary constriction. Divisional palsies would seem to imply an orbital or anterior cavernous sinus pathologic site; however, more proximal

intracranial disease is often responsible. Many cases will have negative imaging and recover well, and are then assumed microvascular in etiology.

Incomplete CN-III palsies show partial losses of up-, down-, and medial-gaze, along with partial ptosis with some CN-III-innervate muscles more affected than others. In such cases—as the clinical vignette illustrates—recognition that the patient's ocular misalignment is a form of third-nerve palsy can be challenging. It is generally agreed that the presence of the pupil-sparing in such cases does not rule out compressive etiology.

A patient with an *isolated medial rectus dysfunction* (inability to adduct the eye) should not be considered to have an incomplete CN-III palsy. Most often, this condition is caused by *internuclear ophthalmoplegia* (see below). It may also be seen in cases of myasthenia gravis or from orbital disease involving the horizontal rectus muscles.

When the origin of third nerve palsy is at the nucleus, the presentation is one of ipsilateral medial rectus, inferior rectus, and inferior oblique dysfunction, with contralateral superior rectus weakness because of the decussation of axons from the medial column subnucleus. Because of bilateral lid innervation by the central caudate subnucleus, the eyelids exhibit either bilateral blepharoptosis or are normal, depending on the extent of the insult. In clinical practice, such cases are exceedingly rare.

With insult to the third-nerve fasciculus, clinical localization is often aided by the presence of other signs of midbrain dysfunction. CN-III fasciculus lesions at the red nucleus present as oculomotor palsy with crossed hemitremor, *Benedikt syndrome*. If the lesion extends to the medial lemniscus, there is also contralateral hypesthesia. Similar lesions with caudal extension into the brachium conjunctivum produce ipsilateral cerebellar ataxia or *Claude syndrome*. When damage extends ventrally into the basis pedunculi and the corticospinal tract, hemiplegia contralateral to the CN-III palsy occurs (*Weber syndrome*).

In comatose patients, unilateral mydriasis ("*blown*" or Hutchinson pupil) is indicative of supratentorial increased intracranial pressure (ICP), sufficient to force the uncus of the temporal lobe laterally and caudally to compress the third nerve against the anterior edge of the tentorial foramen (*uncal herniation*). In fact, using oculocephalic maneuvers, additional evidence of compressive CN-III palsy can be uncovered. Pupil checks and oculocephalic maneuvers need to be monitored frequently in any unresponsive patient, since uncal herniation can be rapidly fatal if not detected and addressed at its earliest sign. The laterality of the blown pupil does not always correlate with the side of the lesion.

Although a few cases exist of mydriasis as a possible sign of compressive third-nerve palsy in patients who are awake and alert, this remains exceedingly unlikely without evolving signs of altered consciousness and usually indicates another etiology, such as pharmacologic pupillary mydriasis or *Adie tonic pupil* (below).

Whereas microvascular CN-III palsy is generally followed by full recovery, the prognosis for traumatic or postoperative compressive CN-III palsy is guarded. If recovery occurs, it is usually marked by aberrant regeneration and *synkinesis*. The best-known example is the pseudo–von Graefe sign: the branch of CN-III that normally innervates the inferior rectus now synkinetically innervates the levator palpebrae, causing the upper lid to lift on downward gaze (clinically simulating the lid lag, or von Graefe sign, of Graves orbitopathy). Internal motor efferents can likewise be involved, resulting in a change of pupil size as gaze is shifted.

Occasionally, *primary aberrant regeneration* (aberrant regeneration without history of prior palsy) will be encountered. This finding is due to chronic compression of the third nerve, typically within or near the cavernous sinus usually due to meningioma and occasionally from an aneurysm of the intracavernous ICA. Adie tonic pupil is another example of aberrant regeneration affecting a facet of CN-III function with a probable intraorbital location within the ciliary ganglion and is discussed further in the section pertaining to pupils.

As opposed to the preceding discussion of isolated CN-III disease, the oculomotor nerve can be involved in cranial polyneuropathies, in which case the accompanying deficits typically help localize the etiology. *Cavernous sinus syndrome* typically affects CN-III, -IV, and -VI and the ophthalmic branch of CN-V. When the intracavernous carotid artery wall is also involved, sympathetic pupil dysfunction (Horner pupil) will result, producing miosis; the Horner pupil will be unnoticeable if CN-III-related mydriasis obscures it. The clinical history in the case of slowly expanding tumor in the cavernous sinus often includes chronically increasing diplopia, sometimes with pain or numbness in the CN-V ophthalmic distribution; in cases of inflammation or infection, the onset is usually dramatic and painful. *Superior orbital fissure syndrome* is often indistinguishable from cavernous sinus syndrome.

Lesions producing diminished vision, internal (i.e., pupillary involvement) or external ophthalmoplegia, orbital pain, and corneal hypesthesia characterize *orbital apex syndrome*. In simplified terms, this syndrome is clinically characterized by findings of superior orbital fissure syndrome with a concomitant compressive optic neuropathy. It must be distinguished from *pituitary apoplexy* where sudden, painful visual loss due to chiasmal compression by pituitary hemorrhage is often accompanied by

unilateral or bilateral CN-III palsy as impingement upon the adjacent cavernous sinuses evolves.

Differential Diagnosis

Myasthenia gravis, a disorder of somatic neuromuscular junction failure that does not affect the pupil, will occasionally simulate pupil-sparing third-nerve palsy. A history of diurnal variability, findings of inducible fatigability, and resolution of the "palsy" during intravenous administration of edrophonium chloride is often sufficient to expose the diagnosis, which can then be confirmed by serum antibody testing and electromyography.

Chronic, progressive external ophthalmoplegia (CPEO) presents as slowly progressive bilateral ptosis and loss of extraocular movements, usually without diplopia. CPEO has been associated with specific mutations of mitochondrial and nuclear DNA and can be part of a larger syndrome, oculopharyngeal dystrophy. The Kearns–Sayre variant of CPEO includes pigmentary retinopathy with nyctalopia, and hormonal dysfunction.

The Miller Fisher variant of Guillain–Barré syndrome produces an external ophthalmoplegia that may be initially confused with CN-III palsy; the presence of viral prodrome, ataxia, areflexia, cerebrospinal fluid albuminocytologic dissociation, and positive serum anti-GQ1b IgM and IgG antibodies will confirm the diagnosis.

Patients with *internuclear ophthalmoplegia* have inability to move the ipsilateral eye into adduction when attempting horizontal gaze to the contralateral side. The responsible lesion is in the medial longitudinal fasciculus, interrupting the interneurons traveling from the CN-VI nucleus to the CN-III ventral subnucleus that innervates the medial rectus (see discussion of CN-VI anatomy, below). Such patients are often assumed to have a "medial rectus palsy"; however, such a variant of CN-III palsy is rarely if ever seen clinically, and the preservation of adduction during convergence to near stimulus (mediated by the mesencephalon) in internuclear ophthalmoplegia serves to confirm its central nervous system supranuclear origin.

Duane syndrome is an example of a congenital aberrant innervation. In affected individuals, prenatal abducens nerve dysgenesis or injury causes subsequent misdirected CN-III innervation of the lateral rectus. Therefore, attempted lateral eye movement results in simultaneous stimulation of the medial and lateral recti, causing variable eye movement, measurable globe retraction into the orbit, and consequent pseudoptosis. In type II Duane syndrome, the combination of poor adduction and pseudoptosis during globe retraction may simulate CN-III palsy. The congenital nature of this condition is most easily deduced by the absence of symptomatic diplopia in lateral gaze despite the presence of incomitant strabismus.

Patients with isolated ptosis are often screened for the presence of CN-III palsy. The most common cause of ptosis, typically encountered in patients older than age 50 years—but occasionally seen in younger patients with a history of frequent eye rubbing—is *aponeurotic ptosis*, a lengthening of the tendon (aponeurosis) connecting the levator palpebrae muscle to the upper lid. Aponeurotic ptosis is particularly common in patients who have undergone cataract surgery. In those patients who, in addition, experienced intraoperative iris injury with postoperative mydriasis, erroneous suspicion of a partial compressive CN-III palsy can be easily prompted.

Marcus Gunn jaw-winking is a syndrome of congenital aberrant innervation of the levator palpebrae muscle by the motor neurons of CN-V that innervate the pterygoid muscles of the mandible. The typical patient will have ptosis that partially resolves with lateral and forward jaw movements with costimulation of the levator.

In the traumatic setting, ophthalmoplegia due to CN-III palsy must be distinguished from that due to orbital disease (e.g., orbital floor fracture with entrapment of the inferior rectus muscle).

Diagnostic Approach

Whether a spared pupil in otherwise complete CN-III palsy reliably excludes an aneurysm deserves discussion. Certainly, with instances of an incomplete extraocular CN-III palsy, the absence of pupil involvement must not be considered evidence of a benign etiology; however, total pupil-sparing in otherwise complete CN-III palsy due to acute compression seems exceedingly rare.

In 1985, neurovascular imaging of patients with isolated, complete, pupil-sparing CN-III palsy was not recommended for patients older than age 50 years. This recommendation was based in part on the frequency of microvascular palsies in this age group, the relative danger of intracranial catheter angiography, and the lack of noninvasive neurovascular imaging modalities. With the emergence of detailed CTA and gadolinium-enhanced magnetic resonance angiography, the number of patients with acute CN-III palsy who should be excluded from imaging is vanishingly small.

Once aneurysm has been excluded in those patients without clear precipitants, testing for diabetes mellitus, hypertension, vasculitis and other inflammatory disease, clotting disorders, spirochetal disease (syphilis and Lyme disease) and myasthenia gravis is recommended. Even in patients with microvascular CN-III palsy without evidence of causative disease, consideration may be given to reevaluate already defined cerebrovascular risk factors.

Any patient presenting with diplopia, initially thought to be related to a cranial mononeuropathy, must have careful examination of the adjacent cranial nerve to exclude their involvement. Also, patients with apparently isolated CN-III palsy should be checked for signs of ataxia, areflexia, or contralateral rubral tremor, hemiparesis, or hypesthesia. Similarly, patients presenting with new upper facial pain or numbness must always be checked for impaired eye movements and corneal hypesthesia to exclude early cavernous sinus syndrome.

Management and Therapy

The management of symptomatic intracranial aneurysm is usually urgent, via endovascular or surgical intervention if the general state of the patient permits (see Chapter 57). Management of microvascular palsy usually centers on prevention of recurrent events via reduction of risk factors. Optimization of any causative disease, such as diabetes, is crucial, and daily aspirin is often recommended. Therapy for other underlying causes of CN-III palsy will vary, appropriate to etiology.

Visual management of nonhealing CN-III palsies is complicated by the number of paretic extraocular muscles involved, as ocular misalignment changes significantly depending on the direction of gaze. Prismatic spectacles are often unavailing, except in cases of minimal residual misalignment. Strabismus surgery, often involving two or three staged procedures, has the limited goal of stable relief of diplopia in primary gaze only. Often the simplest management tool, if acceptable to the patient, is a patch on the affected eye to eliminate diplopia, if the ptosis does not already accomplish that.

CRANIAL NERVE IV: TROCHLEAR

Clinical Vignette

A workman, bent over his work, sustained left occiput blunt head trauma and scalp laceration when a coworker dropped a tool from above. Diplopia and headache subsequently developed.

Examination revealed poor depression of the right eye in leftward gaze. Prismatic spectacle lenses were prescribed to alleviate the diplopia. After a few months, the patient reported that his vision had returned to normal.

This vignette describes isolated trochlear nerve (CN-IV) injury with relatively mild closed head trauma. Often the most benign of the cranial neuropathies, particularly those related to extraocular muscle function, it tends to recover fully over a period of weeks or months.

The CN-IV nuclei are located at the level of the inferior colliculi in the lower midbrain off midline at the ventral edge of the periaqueductal gray. The nuclei are crossed; the left trochlear nucleus innervates the right superior oblique and vice versa.

Axons emanating from the trochlear nucleus arc dorsally around the periaqueductal gray into the tectum of the midbrain, where they cross the midline and then emerge laterally beneath the inferior colliculus at the medial border of the brachium conjunctivum as CN-IV. It then completely decussates and exits the brainstem from its dorsal aspect, a unique feature among the cranial nerves. It passes through the quadrigeminal and ambient cisterns and then runs along the free edge of the tentorium. It enters the orbit via the superior orbital fissure and innervates a singe extraocular muscle, the superior oblique.

The superior oblique is chiefly a depressor of the globe and is most active when the eye is adducted and depressed. It has a secondary function of intorting the eye during ipsilateral head tilt and is a weak abductor of the eye in downgaze (Fig. 5-4). Therefore, CN-IV palsy will produce ipsilateral loss of depression (hyperopia) and excyclotorsion of the globe.

Etiology and Pathogenesis

Trauma is the most frequent cause of CN-IV palsies. Traumatic palsies may be bilateral, but most often one side is spared or

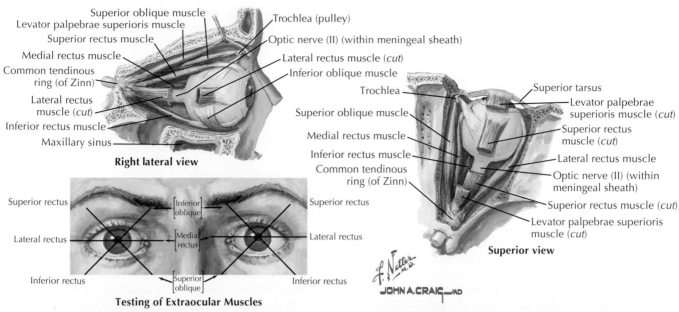

Testing of Extraocular Muscles

Superior view

Muscle	Origin	Insertion	Innervation	Main Actions
Levator palpebrae superioris	Sphenoid bone, anterosuperior optic canal	Tarsal plate and skin of upper eyelid	Oculomotor nerve (superior tarsal muscle supplied by sympathetic fibers)	Elevates upper eyelid
Superior rectus (SR)	Common tendinous ring (annulus of Zinn)	Sclera just posterior to cornea	Oculomotor nerve	Elevates, adducts, and rotates eyeball medially
Inferior rectus (IR)	Common tendinous ring (annulus of Zinn)	Sclera just posterior to cornea	Oculomotor nerve	Depresses, adducts, and rotates eyeball medially
Medial rectus	Common tendinous ring (annulus of Zinn)	Sclera just posterior to cornea	Oculomotor nerve	Adducts eyeball
Lateral rectus	Common tendinous ring (annulus of Zinn)	Sclera just posterior to cornea	Abducent nerve	Abducts eyeball
Superior oblique (SO)	Body of sphenoid bone	Passes through a trochlea and inserts into sclera	Trochlear nerve	Medially rotates, depresses, and abducts eyeball
Inferior oblique (IO)	Floor of orbit	Sclera deep to lateral rectus muscle	Oculomotor nerve	Laterally rotates, elevates and abducts eyeball

From Hansen JH. Netter's Clincial Anatomy, 2e. Saunders, Philadelphia, 2010, p. 380.

Figure 5-4 Extraocular Muscles and General Function.

recovers so that patients are left with unilateral dysfunction. The frequent association of trauma with CN-IV palsy may imply that the thin dorsal tectum is vulnerable to traumatic forces causing shear between the emerging nerves and the colliculi or the cerebellar tentorium or direct injury from a hydraulic pressure wave transmitted through the aqueduct. MRI demonstration of tectal subarachnoid hematoma in traumatic trochlear palsy supports this theory. In addition, a pathologic study has shown that, with sufficient force, avulsion of the CN-IV root from the pons can occur.

The nucleus and fasciculus of the trochlear nerve lie within the pons; in this location, CN-IV palsies may result from stroke, demyelination, and tumor. Lesions of the fascicle, rarely seen clinically, produce a contralateral CN-IV palsy and an ipsilateral Horner syndrome due to coinvolvement of the descending first-order pupillary sympathetic axons passing through the pontine tegmentum. The trochlear nerve fasciculi decussate just dorsal to the sylvian aqueduct, and

tumors or stroke in this area will produce bilateral trochlear palsies.

In the subarachnoid space, CN-IV can be affected by carcinomatous meningitis, by aneurysm (especially of the superior cerebellar artery; Fig. 5-2), or by dolichoectasia of the basilar artery. The nerve itself may be the site of schwannomas. Once within the dural canal leading to the cavernous sinus, the nerve may be affected by tumor, especially meningioma. Compression of CN-IV can occur at the cavernous sinus itself, by dissections or aneurysm of the carotid artery, by extension of sellar and orbital tumors, and by metastases. Typically CN-IV, -III, -VI, and the ophthalmic branch of CN-V are involved in cavernous sinus lesions.

In cases where imaging reveals no structural cause of CN-IV palsy and where there is no history of trauma, microvascular ischemia is the usual assumed etiology. Patients with diabetes, hypertension, vasculitis, sarcoidosis, or treponemal infection may present with seemingly "idiopathic" palsies.

Clinical Presentations

Patients with trochlear palsy have hypertropia or impaired ability to depress the eye on the involved side. Weakness of depressor function of the superior oblique is exaggerated with medial downward gaze or when the head is tilted toward the side of palsy

Normally during head tilt to one side, the ipsilateral superior oblique is activated to accomplish incyclotorsion of the eye, keeping the retina relatively level despite the head shift. The medial rectus is activated simultaneously, so that the incyclotorsion of the superior oblique is not accompanied by usual depressing of the globe. In trochlear palsy, then, when the head is tilted toward the palsied side, abnormal excyclotorsion is emphasized, magnifying both the hypertropia and diplopia. This pattern of incomitant strabismus is summarized as "hypertropia worse with gaze away and with tilt toward the affected side."

Patients with CN-IV palsy often adopt a secondary torticollis, offering a diagnostic clue. Patients prefer a chin-down posture with the head tilted away from the palsy, so that the affected eye is in up and out, where the superior oblique normally has the least action, and its palsy matters the least. Because this posture minimizes the visual consequences of a CN-IV palsy, congenital CN-IV palsies are often undiagnosed for decades. A diagnosis in adulthood may be made after intermittent diplopia develops from progressive asthenopia or when treatment for torticollis is sought. The presence of the characteristic head tilt in childhood photographs often confirms the congenital nature of the palsy.

In most cases of CN-IV palsy, there is a history of trauma. A high frontal head impact with contrecoup forces at the dorsal tectum, occipital impact producing more direct injury, or coccygeal impact transmitted up a straight spinal column are all encountered. Occasionally, the appearance of vertical diplopia after frontal head trauma will prompt suspicion of *orbital floor "blow-out" fracture* before CN-IV palsy is uncovered.

The amount of force needed to produce traumatic CN-IV palsy seems variable, and, in contradistinction to traumatic CN-III palsy, impact sufficient to produce alteration in consciousness is not required. An acquired trochlear palsy after minor head trauma should still, however, prompt suspicion of an undiagnosed mass lesion, producing a "pathologic" palsy in an already damaged nerve.

Patients with bilateral CN-IV palsy complain of rotational instead of vertical diplopia. Loss of incyclotorsion for both eyes causes images seen by the left eye to rotate clockwise compared with those seen by the right eye. Most patients with bilateral involvement will note occasional vertical diplopia: right eye image above left eye image with left head tilt or rightward gaze, and vice versa. Often, esotropia is seen in downgaze as well, because of loss of the abducting action of the superior obliques. They may adopt a chin-down head position without horizontal tilt.

A lesion interrupting both the predecussation trochlear fasciculus and the ipsilateral central tegmental (pupillary sympathetic) tract within the tectum produces an ipsilateral Horner syndrome with crossed CN-IV palsy. CN-IV palsy has occurred in the setting of idiopathic intracranial hypertension and after lumbar puncture—presumably because of tractional mechanisms—both with CN-VI coinvolvement. It can also occur in conjunction with CN-III involvement in spontaneous intracranial hypotension.

Perhaps because of their relatively fixed location within the lateral wall of the cavernous sinus, the trochlear and trigeminal nerves can be injured concomitantly. Patients with a posteriorly draining carotid–cavernous fistula may present with painful superior oblique dysfunction along with an oculomotor nerve palsy, presumably due to local cavernous distention.

Differential Diagnosis

Other entities that produce vertical binocular diplopia with hypertropia may be initially confused with CN-IV palsy; myasthenia gravis is one such mimic. However, the pattern of changing misalignment in different directions of gaze will usually serve to distinguish true trochlear palsies from its simulators.

Restrictive diseases affecting the inferior rectus muscle (such as thyroid-related orbitopathy, orbital floor fracture with entrapment of the muscle, or injury from local anesthetic for cataract surgery) produce vertical diplopia; such diplopia, however, worsens in upgaze. Restrictive disease of the inferior oblique is a far better mimic, as patients would have ipsilateral hyperopia with excyclotorsion and worsening on attempted downgaze.

Injury to the orbital trochlea (through which the superior oblique tendon passes) typically produces *Brown tendon sheath syndrome*, with the eye shooting into downgaze on adduction because the tendon remains tight even when the muscle relaxes; however, on occasion, the injured trochlea will not allow the tendon to retract in response to superior oblique retraction, perfectly simulating CN-IV palsy. History of orbital trauma and trochlear abnormality on orbital imaging will serve to clarify the diagnosis.

Skew deviation due to imbalance of the otolithic inputs to the vestibulo-ocular system can also produce vertical misalignment. In such cases, reclining the patient to a supine position may eliminate the hypertropia.

Diagnostic Approach

Diagnosis of unilateral CN-IV palsy is made when ipsilateral hypertropia is demonstrated to worsen in downward gaze, contralateral gaze, and ipsilateral head tilt. Cases of bilateral trochlear palsies may present the seeming paradox of no hypertropia in primary gaze when the head is straight. However, these patients demonstrate a left hypertropia on right gaze and left head tilt, and right hypertropia on left gaze with a right head tilt.

Blood testing for infection, abnormal clotting, and systemic inflammation is usually done in nontraumatic cases. Patients with isolated CN-IV palsies may be observed for spontaneous improvement over 3 to 4 months if the history indicates a likely etiology (e.g., trauma or known diabetes); otherwise, neuroimaging is done upon diagnosis. Even in cases with a presumed etiology, nonresolution over time usually prompts imaging unless congenital CN-IV palsy is strongly suggested by history and examination findings (e.g., vertical fusional amplitude greater than 4 diopters and photographic evidence of life-long compensating head tilt).

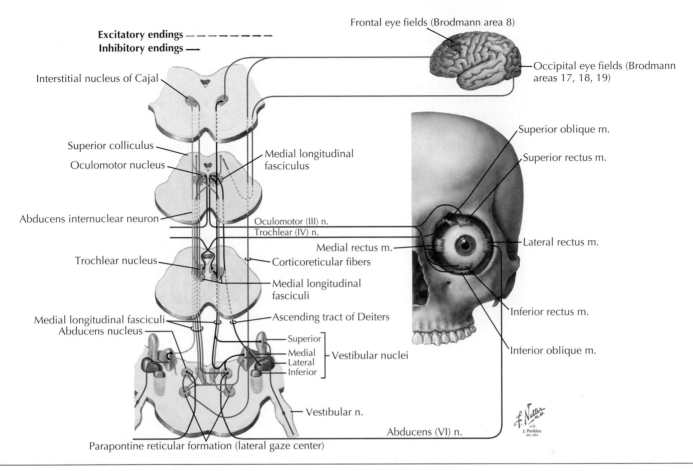

Figure 5-5 Central Control of Eye Movements.

Management and Therapy

Therapy directed at the cause of CN-IV palsy (when a cause other than trauma can be identified) will be dependent on the pathologic entity encountered. Symptomatic diplopia in non-healing trochlear palsies may be reduced by the use of prismatic glasses to shift "second images" to line up with primary images. However, the utility of prismatic glasses in CN-IV palsy may be limited because such spectacles do not correct image tilt and because only one prismatic strength can be ground into the spectacles, but different strengths are needed for different gaze directions. Many patients prefer strabismic surgical treatment of nonresolving palsies; it offers correction of excyclotorsion and greater range of gaze without diplopia.

CRANIAL NERVE VI: ABDUCENS

Clinical Vignette

A 68-year-old hypertensive, diabetic patient presented with isolated sixth cranial nerve (CN-VI) palsy, manifesting as inability to abduct the involved eye. No imaging was initially requested, given the presumed microvascular etiology. Four days later, the patient developed severe headache, and 2 days after that presented to the emergency room where computed tomographic scan revealed a hemorrhagic pituitary fossa mass.

Two days later the patient expired due to hyperthermia from hypothalamic compression. It is argued that the sellar hemorrhage was in fact present at the time of the patient's initial symptoms and that this patient represents a case of pituitary apoplexy presenting with painless, isolated CN-VI palsy.

The sixth cranial nerve (CN-VI) innervates a single extraocular muscle, the lateral rectus, which is the primary abductor for the eyes.

The CN-VI nucleus, located just beneath the facial colliculi in the inferior pons is enveloped by the turning CN-VII fascicular fibers of the facial genu and contains two physiologically—but not topographically—distinct groups of neurons (Fig. 5-5). One group innervates the ipsilateral lateral rectus; the other sends axons across the midline to the contralateral medial longitudinal fasciculus (MLF). These latter axons ascend in the MLF to the ventral nucleus of the contralateral CN-III nuclear complex. These internuclear neurons connect the nuclei of CN-VI and -III, producing the almost simultaneous stimulation of the contralateral medial rectus during ipsilateral abducens nerve stimulation to produce lateral horizontal gaze.

From its position laterally abutting the paramedian pontine reticular formation, the CN-VI fasciculus first travels medially (toward the MLF, temporarily with the interneuron axons) and then turns ventrally, passing through the paramedian pontine reticular formation and the undecussated corticospinal tract to reach the ventral surface of the brainstem at the inferior lip of the pons.

On exiting the ventral pons, the abducens nerve ascends between the pons and the clivus within the subarachnoid pontine cistern. After it enters the dura, CN-VI continues up the clivus to the posterior clinoid. It travels over the petrous ridge to lie beneath the inferior petrosal sinus and then enters the cavernous sinus via the Dorello canal just medial to the Meckel cave, which houses the gasserian ganglion.

After CN-VI is within the cavernous sinus, it passes forward, adjacent to the internal lateral aspect of the carotid artery. Here, it likely carries the majority of the tertiary sympathetic pupillary axons the short distance from the carotid artery to the ophthalmic branch of the trigeminal nerve. The sympathetics then follow the ophthalmic nerve via its nasociliary branch to the ciliary ganglion; the sympathetic fibers pass through the ganglion without synapsing, entering the eye via the short ciliary nerves. Additional sympathetic fibers bypass the ciliary ganglion, entering the eye as the long ciliary nerves.

Etiology and Pathogenesis

Microvascular palsy, associated with risk factors such as hypertension or diabetes, is the most common cause of acquired, isolated CN-VI palsy. In some cases, advanced age is the only identifiable risk factor and the palsy is considered idiopathic. However, occasionally sixth-nerve palsy will be the presenting sign of other vasculitides such as *temporal arteritis* or treponematosis.

Within the brainstem, cranial nerve palsies can be caused by tumor, stroke, and demyelination. Often, other neurologic signs localizing to the pons will be present, but isolated abducens palsies can be seen.

The sixth nerve has the longest intracranial course of all the cranial nerves. It may suffer compression along this path from tumors at a number of locations, including at the cerebello-pontine angle, the clivus, the petrous bone, and the cavernous sinus. Tumors include acoustic neuroma, meningioma, hemangioma, lymphoma, chondrosarcoma, eosinophilic granuloma, and nasopharyngeal carcinoma, as well as various other carcinomas, both local and metastatic. Midline tumors of the skull base, such as chordoma, can cause bilateral CN-VI palsies by compressing both nerves as they ascend the clivus. Isolated unilateral palsy is, in rare cases, due to abducens schwannoma.

Within the cavernous sinus, the sixth nerve is often involved by disease of the carotid artery, including aneurysm, dissection, dolichoectasia, and carotid–cavernous fistula. The cavernous sinus is also a frequent location of hemangiomas, septic thrombosis, idiopathic inflammation (*Tolosa–Hunt syndrome*), and metastatic carcinoma that can affect the sixth nerve. Pituitary apoplexy can cause CN-VI palsy by compressing against the cavernous sinus. Often, the other cranial nerves of the cavernous sinus will also be involved, along with the tertiary pupillary sympathetic neurons.

Traumatic CN-VI palsy is seen in the setting of a significant impact, severe enough to cause change of consciousness or bone fracture. CN-VI can also be injured during skull-based neurosurgery and can be seen after percutaneous radiofrequency ablation of CN-V for trigeminal neuralgia.

Vincristine produces CN-VI palsies, presumably from direct neuropathic action on the nerve. Reports of CN-VI in patients using vitamin A and its analogs must probably relate to increased ICP secondary to retinoid-induced pseudotumor cerebri.

Raised ICP alone, whether due to medication, tumor, obstructive hydrocephalus, meningitis, or idiopathic intracranial hypertension, can produce unilateral or bilateral CN-VI palsy. Such abducens palsy is a *falsely localizing sign*, suggesting impinging upon the sixth nerve, when in fact the causative tumor may be remote from the CN-VI territory, or there may be no tumor at all. The course of CN-VI between the internal auditory artery and the anterior inferior cerebellar artery makes it vulnerable to such palsy. As ICP begins to rise, downward brainstem herniation causes stretching of CN-VI, and perhaps compression against either artery. Similarly, downward shift of the pons in relation to the petrous ridge is thought to account for CN-VI palsies sometimes seen in spontaneous or post–lumbar puncture intracranial hypotension.

Clinical Presentations

Patients with CN-VI paresis have an inward deviation of the affected eye and a noncomitant esotropia. Temporal eye movement beyond midline is lost or reduced. Patients with partial or mild abducens palsies adopt a posture with the head turn toward the affected side to minimize diplopia by keeping the eye adducted. In more severe palsies, this strategy often fails or is uncomfortable, so patients present with one eye shut, or covered.

The typical patient with microvascular CN-VI palsy will report painless, sudden-onset, horizontal binocular diplopia. Such patients typically show complete, spontaneous resolution within 2–4 months of onset.

Patients with unilateral or bilateral CN-VI palsy from high ICP will present with the symptoms of headache, worsening with recumbency, and visual symptoms ranging from mild dimming to 1–2 seconds of bilateral visual obscurations to profound visual field loss. In cases of *obstructive hydrocephalus*, gait instability, urinary incontinence, and change in mental status are present. Primary nuclear CN-VI lesions typically have concomitant ipsilateral facial nerve involvement, because of the contact between the abducens nucleus and the genu of the facial fasciculus. For example, stroke of the inferior medial pons produces both ipsilateral gaze palsy and CN-VII as part of *Foville syndrome*. These deficits are accompanied by contralateral hemiplegia from more extensive involvement of the corticospinal tract prior to its decussation.

As Foville syndrome demonstrates, lesions of the CN-VI nucleus do not, in fact, result in clinical CN-VI palsy but rather an ipsilateral *gaze palsy* with inability to move both eyes to the affected side. This gaze palsy occurs because the CN-VI nucleus contains both the motor neurons headed for the lateral rectus muscle and the interneurons going to the contralateral third-nerve nucleus via the MLF. The pontine localization of the gaze palsy can be inferred from the finding that such "lower" gaze palsies, in contradistinction to "higher" gaze palsies from frontal lobe disease, cannot be overcome with vestibulo-ocular reflex (e.g., doll's-eyes maneuver), caloric labyrinthine stimulation, or optokinetic stimulation.

Larger lesions affecting the CN-VI nucleus and extending rostrally into the ipsilateral MLF interrupt the crossed internuclear neurons from the opposite CN-VI nucleus coursing up toward the CN-III nucleus, with consequent inability to adduct the ipsilateral eye in horizontal gaze. This combined lesion of ipsilateral gaze palsy and internuclear ophthalmoplegia is known as the *Fisher "one-and-a-half" syndrome*: As with other internuclear ophthalmoplegia variants, convergence (the ability to adduct both eyes simultaneously for near vision) is spared as neither the upper midbrain pathways producing convergence nor the CN-III nuclei are affected.

Paramedian basilar artery branch occlusion causes infarction of the medial and ventral structures of the inferior pons, producing ipsilateral gaze palsy (paramedian pontine reticular formation involvement), hemifacial paralysis (CN-VII), limb ataxia and nystagmus (involvement of middle cerebellar peduncle and possibly vestibular nuclei efferents), crossed paralysis (corticospinal tract), and crossed tactile hypesthesia (medial lemniscus). More focal lesions may produce *Raymond syndrome* (abduction palsy and crossed hemiplegia) from abducens fascicular injury at the corticospinal tract in the basis pontis, whereas similar lesions with some lateral extension also involve the facial fasciculus, adding ipsilateral facial palsy to the presentation (*Millard–Gubler syndrome*).

Anterior inferior cerebellar artery occlusion typically produces more lateral damage characteristically to the vestibular nuclei, the auditory nerve, CN-VII, the paramedian pontine reticular formation, the spinothalamic tract, and the middle cerebellar peduncle and possibly extending dorsally to the cerebellar hemisphere and rostrally to the CN-V nucleus. The combined deficits produce a lateral inferior pontine syndrome of nystagmus (with beats or fast phase directed ipsilaterally), vertigo, gaze palsy, facial paralysis and hypesthesia, deafness, and ataxia, all with crossed body analgesia.

CN-VI, the carotid artery, and sympathetic pupil fibers are situated closely within the cavernous sinus, and an expanding *intracavernous carotid dissection or aneurysm* can compress these structures, producing painful abducens palsy with an ipsilateral Horner syndrome. Other pathologic processes, such as carotid cavernous fistula (CCF) and granulomas within this region sometimes produce a similar clinical picture. Patients with CCF may have additional feature of headache, enlarged conjunctival vessels, proptosis, and an audible bruit over the orbit.

Processes that affect the anterior midline brainstem also deserve consideration in the differential diagnosis, including various posterior fossa tumors or inflammatory processes that affect the abducens nerve during its ascent of the clivus. Chordomas, slowly growing tumors that favor the midline skull base, occasionally present as isolated or bilateral CN-VI palsy as do durally based meningiomas.

Gradenigo syndrome is characterized by a painful abducens palsy resulting from mastoiditis and petrositis complicating chronic otitis media. The infectious process erodes the bone, affecting the abducens nerve and the gasserian ganglion and, at times, the CN-VII as it passes through the mastoid bone en route to the stylomastoid foramen. A combined trigeminal-abducens-facial nerve syndrome can be produced by other entities, particularly tumors, that affect this region.

Differential Diagnosis

Möbius syndrome is a congenital, bilateral CN-VI and CN-VII palsy. MRI typically shows pontine hypoplasia in the region of the affected CN nuclei. The characteristic elongated, expressionless lower facies of these patients is usually sufficient to suggest the diagnosis, and such patients usually do not have symptomatic diplopia. However, Chiari malformation with syringomyelia can produce a similar, acquired picture.

Duane syndrome, a congenital condition of misdirected CN-III innervation of the lateral rectus, can also simulate abducens palsy. In patients with type I Duane syndrome, attempted lateral gaze reveals lack of abduction. Again, the chief clues to this diagnosis are life-long history and absence of symptomatic diplopia in lateral gaze despite the presence of noncomitant strabismus.

Inability to abduct the eyes, a seeming bilateral CN-VI palsy, can be seen in Wernicke encephalopathy resulting from thiamine depletion. Confusion, confabulation, ataxia, and history of alcoholism suggest the diagnosis, which is confirmed by low serum thiamine levels. Occasionally, sudden onset of esotropia simulating bilateral CN-VI palsy occurs because of divergence palsy, probably due to microvascular ischemia at the putative mesencephalic "divergence center." Spontaneous improvement in 2–3 months is expected. Divergence palsy can be differentiated from the more common, frequently psychogenic, convergence spasm by the miosis that accompanies convergence spasm as in normal close vision.

Myasthenia gravis may simulate CN-VI palsy but can be diagnosed by history of diurnal variation, variable ocular misalignment, presence of serum antibodies to acetylcholine receptors or striated muscle, and positive response to intravenous edrophonium chloride.

Traumatic fracture of the medial orbital wall (the lamina papyracea of the ethmoid sinus) with entrapment of the medial rectus muscle produces a restrictive esotropia that may at first suggest traumatic CN-VI palsy. Similarly, thyroid-related ophthalmopathy, which often preferentially restricts the medial rectus muscle, or orbital tumor may lead to restrictive esotropia and consideration of abducens palsy. *Force duction testing* (see below) will be normal in myasthenia, but positive—the eye resists the attempted movement—in cases of restrictive strabismus. Orbital imaging will confirm restrictive esotropia.

Diagnostic Approach

Complete palsies if CN-VI are usually evident, with cursory examination revealing esotropia that lessens with gaze away from the affected side (direction in which the lateral rectus is usually least active). Abduction of the affected eye past midline is not possible, and the movement from adducted to midline position is slow.

Partial abducens palsies can be subtler, especially as only one muscle, and one plane of eye movement, is affected. Having the patient describe the diplopia will usually clarify that it is the

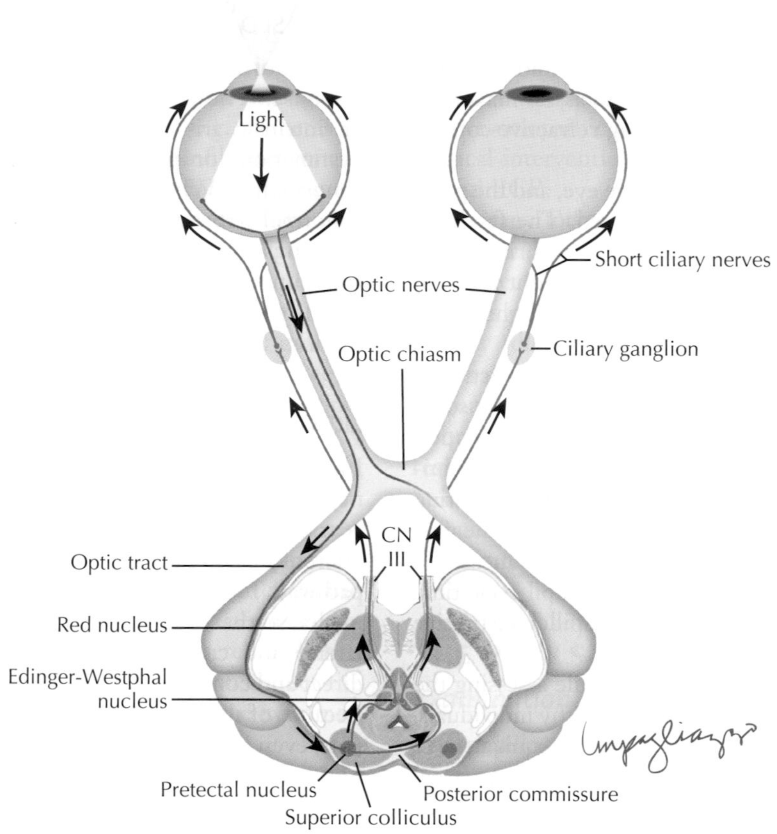

Figure 5-6 Parasympathetic Pupillary Innervation and the Light Reflex Pathway.

Rarely, one encounters disease that has affected the extrageniculate pupillary afferent fibers only, after they separate from the geniculate-bound vision fibers. In those cases, the patient will show a clear afferent pupillary defect without any visual defect. A reverse case, with unilateral visual loss, optic atrophy, and no RAPD, has not yet been reported.

EFFERENT LIMB ABNORMALITIES: PARASYMPATHETIC

The pretectal nuclei receive input from both optic nerves, and in turn send efferents to both Edinger–Westphal nuclei. These nuclei send efferent pupilloconstrictive fibers via the oculomotor nerve (CN-III) to the ciliary ganglion, where they synapse with the short ciliary nerves carrying motor efferents to the pupillary sphincter (see Fig. 5-6).

Typically located on the exterior of the nerve, the pupilloconstrictive fibers of CN-III are particularly vulnerable to compression, but relatively resistant to microvascular ischemia (e.g., from diabetes mellitus). Hence, this leads to the classic (but occasionally inaccurate) clinical observation that ischemic CN-III palsies spare the pupil, whereas those due to compression palsies add pupillary dilation to the external oculomotor abnormalities.

Idiopathic, painless loss of pupillary constriction (and lens accommodation) is occasionally seen as an "acute *Adie pupil*." Over weeks, such patients experience partial recovery of pupillary constriction, but with persistent abnormalities due to

incomplete healing and aberrant regeneration. A typical (chronic) *Adie tonic pupil* will be mid-dilated, irregular with areas of atonic iris sphincter, and showing asynchronous, segmental sphincter contraction (vermiform movement). The pupil shows *light-near dissociation*, with absent light reflex, and slow, strong constriction to near stimulus that persists for many seconds after gaze is redirected to distance (tonic constriction). Similar aberrant regeneration features can also be seen when a compressive, pupil-involving CN-III palsy recovers but absent in the few rare cases of ischemic CN-III palsy with pupillary involvement.

EFFERENT LIMB ABNORMALITIES: SYMPATHETIC

The sympathetic innervation of the pupillary dilator muscle involves a three-chain pathway. The primary neuron runs from the hypothalamus to the ciliospinal center of Budge and Waller at the junction of the thoracic and cervical spinal cord; the secondary neuron starts there, crosses over the lung apex and synapses in the superior cervical ganglion; and the tertiary neuron follows the ICA to the cavernous sinus, eventually reaching the eye after passing through the ciliary ganglion without synapsing (Fig. 5-7).

A pupil that has lost its sympathetic innervation will sluggishly redilate when light stimulus is removed (redilation lag), and will not open past mid-dilation even in darkness; in mesopic lighting, it is miotic compared to a normal pupil. The sympathetics innervating the facial arteries, sweat glands, and the

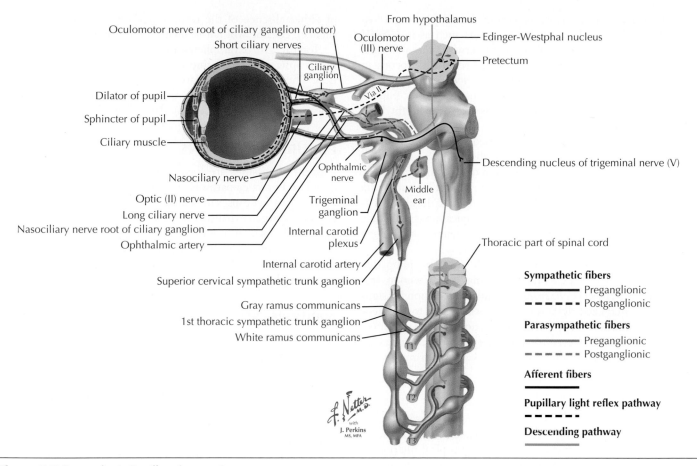

Figure 5-7 Sympathetic Pupillary Innervation.

Mueller muscle of the lid travel with the pupillary sympathetic; therefore, sympathetic-denervation leads to miosis often accompanied by ipsilateral ptosis and hemifacial anhydrosis (Horner syndrome). Hemifacial flushing can also be present (harlequin syndrome).

LIGHT-NEAR DISSOCIATION

As has already been mentioned, light-near dissociation is the blunting or absence of the pupils' light response while the near response is preserved. Afferent pupil defect and the aberrant regeneration of Adie tonic pupil have already been given as two examples.

Two additional well-known examples will be discussed. The *Argyll Robertson pupil* was at one time a renowned feature of tertiary syphilis. In this condition, the pupils are miotic, irregular, and show absent or minimal reaction to light, but a brisk reaction to near-stimulus, however without the tonicity seen in Adie pupil. It has been proposed that Argyll Robertson pupil is due to a specific lesion of the pathway between the pretectal nucleus and the Edinger–Westphal nucleus, but the exact mechanism remains unknown.

Finally, in *Parinaud dorsal midbrain syndrome*, there is loss of pupillary light reflex, likely due to direct injury to the pretectal nuclei but with sparing of the presumably more ventral structures producing the near-response.

PUPIL ABNORMALITIES IN COMA

Patients who have suffered intracranial catastrophe can also display characteristic pupillary syndromes. In patients with severe supratentorial edema or hemorrhage, the uncus is forced down upon the tentorial edge, compressing CN-III and producing mydriasis. It is often referred to as a "blown pupil," or *Hutchinson pupil*. The laterality of the mydriasis usually, but not invariably, indicates an ipsilateral location of the responsible mass.

In patients with pontine hemorrhagic stroke, "pontine pinpoint pupils" are encountered. Although very small, close examination, sometimes with a magnifying glass, shows that they do react to light stimulus. However, it should be kept in mind that the findings of miosis with stupor or coma may also suggest opiate poisoning.

LATERALITY

Systemic disease, toxic exposure, and bilateral ocular or neuropathic conditions will cause bilateral pupillary dysfunction, but the pupils remain equal, or show only minimal *anisocoria*. By contrast, obvious anisocoria suggests focal trauma, inflammation, ischemia, or compression (or perhaps topical pharmacologic exposure) as the likely etiology.

When anisocoria is present, the question arises: is the smaller or the larger pupil abnormal? When accompanying external signs are present (i.e., mydriasis with ipsilateral ptosis and loss of medial and vertical external movements such as in CN-III palsy), the answer may be obvious. Otherwise, the abnormal pupil can be determined by comparing the relative anisocoria in dark and light conditions. Anisocoria that is worse in dark conditions suggests a defect of dilation, and that the miotic pupil is abnormal; conversely, anisocoria that is worse in bright light suggests the larger pupil is abnormal.

Physiological anisocoria is the term used to describe neurally based anisocoria which is not due to disease. The difference between the pupils is most often 0.5 mm or less, and very rarely exceeds 1 mm. It may vary from day to day. The anisocoria remains fairly constant in differing illumination levels, and is eliminated by bilateral administration of topical pharmacologic miotic or mydriatic agents (confirming neural origin—see below).

Unilateral Adie tonic pupil is a fairly common idiopathic cause of anisocoria. When bilateral, it may (with tendon areflexia) form the *Holmes-Adie syndrome*, and investigation for signs of a more generalized dysautonomia, perhaps due to paraneoplastic autoantibodies or spirochetal infection, may be indicated. Bilateral tonic pupil, or even total pupillary areflexia, can be seen in the Miller Fisher variant of Guillain–Barré syndrome.

Pharmacologic Diagnosis of Pupillary Dysfunction

The diagnosis of anisocoria or of bilateral pupillomotor abnormality can be sharpened by the use of topical pharmacologic agents. Strong mydriatics or miotics override neural influences, so that any remaining anisocoria (or subnormal response) indicates iris disease, whereas elimination of anisocoria (or normal response) indicates a neural cause of the pupillary dysfunction.

For example, incomplete (or asymmetric) response to standard pharmacologic dilation (phenylephrine 2.5–10% with tropicamide 1%) suggests an iris structural abnormality, which may be more easily detected at slit-lamp after attempted dilation. Conversely, incomplete miotic response to pilocarpine 1–2% may suggest previous pupillary sphincter trauma, or recent exposure to an anticholinergic agent (topically to the eye if unilateral, and perhaps systemically if bilateral).

In contrast, weak mydriatic or miotic agents can be used to highlight denervation supersensitivity when it exists. Within days of sympathetic denervation of the iris, the dilator muscle will exhibit supersensitivity to weak alpha-1 adrenergic agonists (epinephrine 0.1%, phenylephrine 1%, or most recently apraclonidine 0.5–1%); such agents (or cocaine, below) are often used to distinguish Horner pupil from physiological anisocoria. Similarly, a weak cholinergic agonist (pilocarpine 0.06–0.12%) can demonstrate the cholinergic supersensitivity found in Adie tonic pupil.

Two additional agents are classically employed in the diagnosis of Horner pupil. Cocaine 10% solution has the unique property of preventing presynaptic norepinephrine reuptake; because of the steady baseline release of small amounts of norepinephrine into the neuromuscular cleft of the pupillary dilator muscle, the normal response to topical cocaine is pupillary dilatation. When baseline norepinephrine release is absent (because of either absence of the tertiary neuron or its neurochemical silence), cocaine will fail to dilate the Horner pupil.

Topical hydroxyamphetamine 1% causes release of stored presynaptic norepinephrine at the dilator's neuromuscular junction. Therefore, lack of dilation in response to hydroxyamphetamine suggests absence of the tertiary neuron, helping to "localize" the lesion in the pupillary sympathetic chain.

FUTURE DIRECTIONS

Current discussions are focused upon developing better paradigms and practice pathways for proper and timely diagnosis of the many varied causes of ocular motor palsies and their mimics. Balance between exhaustiveness on one hand and cost-efficiency on the other seems at all times problematic. As the availability of good noninvasive neuroimaging increases, best-practice patterns may be trending away from diagnostic decision making and toward universal imaging.

ADDITIONAL RESOURCES

OCULOMOTOR

Arle JE, Abrahams JM, Zager EL, et al. Pupil-sparing third nerve palsy with preoperative improvement from a posterior communicating artery aneurysm. Surg Neurol 2002;57:423-426. *Reports pupil-sparing in aneurysmal incomplete CN-III palsy.*

Eyster EF, Hoyt WF, Wilson CB. Oculomotor palsy from minor head trauma. An initial sign of basal intracranial tumor. JAMA 1972 May 22;220(8):1083-1086. *Notes frequent association of CN-III palsy after low-force head trauma with skull-base meningiomas.*

Hamilton SR. Neuro-ophthalmology of eye-movement disorders. Curr Opin Ophthalmol 1999 Dec;10(6):405-410. *Discusses attempts to reach a best-practices approach to diagnosis of CN-III palsy.*

Heinze J. Cranial nerve avulsion and other neural injuries in road accidents. Med J Aust 1969 Dec 20;2(25):1246-1249. *Describes avulsion of CN-III and CN-IV nerve roots in trauma.*

Lustbader JM, Miller NR. Painless, pupil-sparing but otherwise complete oculomotor nerve paresis caused by basilar artery aneurysm. Case report. Arch Ophthalmol 1988 May;106(5):583-584. *Presents the only clear case of pupil-sparing in aneurysmal complete CN-III palsy.*

Trobe JD. Isolated pupil-sparing third nerve palsy. Ophthalmology 1985 Jan;92(1):58-61. *Articulates standard at that time regarding which third-nerve palsies need imaging.*

TROCHLEAR

Hara N, Kan S, Simizu K. Localization of post-traumatic trochlear nerve palsy associated with hemorrhage at the subarachnoid space by magnetic resonance imaging. Am J Ophthalmol 2001 Sep;132(3):443-445. *Offers MRI evidence regarding the probable locus minoris resistentiae in traumatic CN-IV palsy.*

Moster ML, Bosley TM, Slavin ML, et al. Thyroid ophthalmopathy presenting as superior oblique paresis. J Clin Neuroophthalmol 1992 Jun;12(2):94-97. *Presents worsening in upgaze as the distinguishing feature of this diagnosis.*

Parulekar MV, Dai S, Buncic JR, et al. Head position-dependent changes in ocular torsion and vertical misalignment in skew deviation. Arch Ophthalmol 2008 Jul;126(7):899-905. *Suggests that a decreased vertical misalignment with face-up head position in skew deviation can distinguish it from CN-IV palsy.*

ABDUCENS

Cushing H. Strangulation of the nervi abducentes by lateral branches of the basilar artery in cases of brain tumour. Brain 1910;33:204-235. *Classic reference regarding the possible mechanism of non-localizing CN-VI palsy.*

Flanders M, Qahtani F, Gans M, et al. Vertical rectus muscle transposition and botulinum toxin for complete sixth nerve palsy. Can J Ophthalmol 2001 Feb;36(1):18-25. *Presents a treatment option for non-healing CN-VI palsies.*

Miller RW, Lee AG, Schiffman JS, et al. A practice pathway for the initial diagnostic evaluation of isolated sixth cranial nerve palsies. Med Decis Making 1999 Jan-Mar;19(1):42-48. *Articulation of the traditional standard of not initially imaging patients with presumptive vasculopathic CN-VI palsy, based on review of 407 cases.*

Ouanounou S, Saigal G, Birchansky S. Möbius syndrome. AJNR Am J Neuroradiol 2005 Feb;26(2):430-432. *MRI finding of pontine hypoplasia in Möbius syndrome.*

Pilon A, Rhee P, Newman T, et al. Bilateral abducens palsies and facial weakness as initial manifestations of a Chiari 1 malformation. Optom Vis Sci 2007 Oct;84(10):936-940. *Syringomyelia producing "acquired" Möbius syndrome.*

Warwar RE, Bhullar SS, Pelstring RJ, et al. Sudden death from pituitary apoplexy in a patient presenting with an isolated sixth cranial nerve palsy.

J Neuroophthalmol 2006 Jun;26(2):95-97 . *Report of the case used in this section's clinical vignette.*

PUPILS

Girkin CA, Perry JD, Miller NR. A relative afferent pupillary defect without any visual sensory deficit. Arch Ophthalmol 1998 Nov;116(11):1544-1545. *Clinical description of a lesion of the extrageniculate pupillary afferent pathway.*

Miller SD, Thompson HS. Pupil cycle time in optic neuritis. Am J Ophthalmol 1978;85:635–642. *Description of this clinical test.*

Morales J, Brown SM, Abdul-Rahim AS, et al. Ocular effects of apraclonidine in Horner syndrome. Arch Ophthalmol 2000 Jul;118(7):951-954. *First description of the usefulness of this agent in the diagnosis of Horner pupil.*

Thompson HS, Kardon RH. The Argyll Robertson pupil. J Neuroophthalmol 2006 Jun;26(2):134-138. *Modern neuro-anatomic review of a classic pupillary syndrome.*

Thompson S, Pilley SF. Unequal pupils (A flow chart for sorting out the anisocorias). Surv Ophthalmol 1976;21:45-48. *The diagnostic paradigm that has become a classic.*

ACKNOWLEDGMENT

I am grateful and indebted for the suggestions of Professor Thomas R. Hedges III, MD, on modifying the form and content of this chapter.

6

Cranial Nerve V: Trigeminal

H. Royden Jones, Jr., and Michal Vytopil

Clinical Vignette

A 58-year-old car salesman presented to his physician noting recent onset of a subtle numbness on his left cheek first apparent while shaving or washing his face. He pointed to a "dead area about the size of a dime" over his left zygoma. This patient had a minor pea-sized skin lesion removed from that same area of his face 2 years earlier and the wound healed uneventfully. He otherwise enjoyed perfect health. Twenty months later, he first noted the numbness, describing it as a minor sense of something crawling under his skin. He first mentioned this symptom during a routine checkup with his internist, who could not find any abnormalities such as skin induration, tenderness, or lymphadenopathy. A referral to his previous surgeon also failed to demonstrate any abnormalities; his examination was "totally benign." For completeness, the surgeon had the tissue pathology reviewed by a pathologist, who reassured that total removal of the tumor was achieved and tumor margins were "clean."

The area of numbness was described as "dead skin." These symptoms had an insidious onset. When the patient's symptoms persisted and became more well defined, he was referred to a neurologist. A very small area of subjective sensory loss, the size of a dime, was noted; the remainder of his neurologic examination was normal. MRI scan of the face and skull base was normal. The patient was advised to return for follow-up examinations every 6 months. Although the small degree of sensory loss persisted, no new clinical or MRI findings were defined during the next 2.5 years. The patient did not return for his 3-year follow-up despite his neurologist advising him to do so. Almost 3.5 years after the onset of his facial numbness, the area of sensory loss enlarged and the patient's wife felt that his left eye was more prominently seen within the orbit. Repeat neurologic exam confirmed the presence of a larger "quarter-sized" sensory loss. MRI now demonstrated a large infraorbital mass. Biopsy demonstrated metastatic squamous cell skin cancer.

Comment: Invasion of trigeminal nerve perineural spaces is a rare but well appreciated complication of various facial skin malignancies. As this case dramatically illustrates, these can have an insidious onset, with no more than subtle sensory loss at the onset. Excellent but nondiagnostic imaging studies can lead to a false sense of security for the patient and inexperienced clinician alike. Eventually the tumor may metastasize along a peripheral cutaneous nerve per se, in this case the maxillary nerve (second division of the trigeminal), to the base of the brain, where the tumor penetrated the foramen rotundum. This centripetal spread along the trigeminal nerve and its gasserian ganglion is rare. Any epithelial squamous cell carcinoma (SCC) has this discrete potential for a perineural spread with potential central nervous system dissemination. The indolent progression of a cranial nerve palsy in any patient with history of a resected cutaneous SCC of the head and neck must raise clinical suspicion of perineural spread, even in the absence of positive findings on detailed and repeated MRI imaging.

ANATOMY

The trigeminal cranial nerve (CN-V) has three major divisions: ophthalmic, maxillary, and mandibular (Figs. 6-1 and 6-2). CN-V is the major sensory nerve of the face, mouth, and nasal cavity. It also supplies motor and proprioceptive fibers to the muscles of mastication. The trigeminal nerve sensory and motor roots are derived from a large sensory and smaller motor nucleus within the pons. These roots converge to emerge at the midlateral pons, then continue toward the trigeminal (Gasserian) ganglion at the base of the middle cranial fossa. General sensory fibers are derived from their cell bodies of origin within this ganglion. Distal to the trigeminal ganglion, three sensory divisions respectively exit the skull through the superior orbital fissure, foramen rotundum, and foramen ovale. The motor component passes through the trigeminal ganglion into the mandibular division.

CN-V Nuclei

The **sensory nucleus** is the largest of the trigeminal pontine complex. This begins rostrally within the midbrain, and extends caudally through the pons and medulla into the second segment of the cervical spinal cord (Fig. 6-3). It is subdivided into three portions: (1) the *spinal tract nucleus* primarily dedicated to pain and temperature fibers; (2) the *principal sensory nucleus*, the pontine trigeminal portion, which primarily receives tactile stimuli and, therefore, principally subserves light touch; (3) the *mesencephalic sensory nucleus*, which contains cell bodies of sensory fibers carrying proprioceptive information from the masticatory muscles. Lastly, there is a **motor nucleus** located within the pons medial to the large sensory nucleus.

Principal Sensory Component

This component of CN-V conveys general sensation from the facial skin and scalp to the top of the head, tragus of the ear, and anterior wall of the external auditory meatus (Fig. 6-4). Also, it provides general sensation from the mouth, including the tongue and teeth, nasal and paranasal sinuses, and meninges lining the anterior and middle cranial fossae.

Trigeminal (Gasserian, Semilunar) Ganglion

The cell bodies of almost all sensory CN-V fibers are located within the trigeminal ganglion (Fig. 6-5). This is contained within a skull-based depression, the *Meckel cave*, that is located

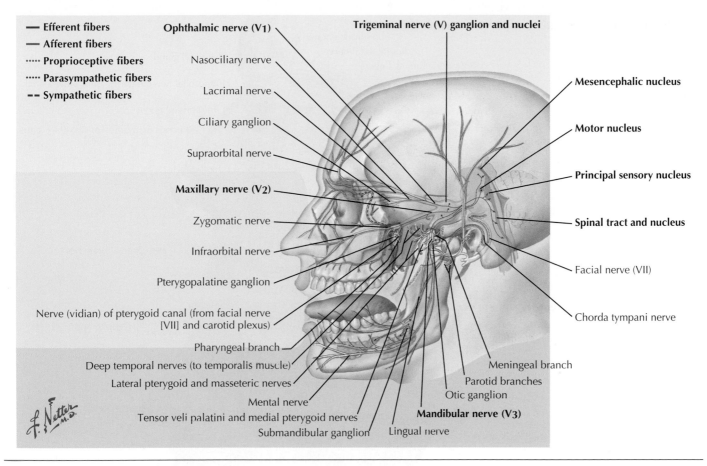

Figure 6-1 Trigeminal Nerve (V): Schema.

in the floor of the middle cranial fossa. Central processes of neuronal cell bodies constitute the large sensory root that enters the pons and projects into the pontine trigeminal main sensory nucleus and spinal tract nucleus. The peripheral processes of this nerve divide into the three sensory divisions that exit the skull through the superior orbital fissure, the foramen rotundum, and the foramen ovale.

Sensory Divisions

The **ophthalmic division** collects touch, pain, temperature, and proprioceptive information from the upper third of the face, including the top of the nose, adjacent sinuses, and scalp regions. These nerve branches course posteriorly in the orbit toward the superior orbital fissure, where they enter the skull.

The **maxillary division** carries sensory information from the skin overlying the maxilla, side of the forehead, medial cheek, and side of the nose, upper lip, palate, upper teeth, nasopharynx, and meninges of the anterior and middle cranial fossae.

The **mandibular division** primarily provides sensory innervation for the skin overlying the lower jaw (with the exception of the angle of the jaw innervated by both the second and third cervical nerves), cheeks, chin and lower lip, mucous membrane of the mouth, gums, inferior teeth, anterior two thirds of the tongue, side of the head, anterior wall of the external auditory meatus, external wall of the tympanic membrane, and temporomandibular joint.

Motor Component

The *motor nucleus*, originating within the mid pons, receives its major input from primary proprioceptive neurons in the mesencephalic subnucleus, creating a monosynaptic reflex arch similar to spinal reflexes, assessable by eliciting the jaw jerk. Motor nucleus axons exit the pons as the motor root medial to the sensory root, passing through the trigeminal ganglion and exiting the skull via the foramen ovale. Extracranially, this root combines with the sensory mandibular division forming the mandibular nerve, which provides branches innervating the muscles of mastication: the masseter, temporalis, medial and lateral pterygoid, mylohyoid, and anterior digastric muscles.

CN-V LESIONS

Clinical Presentation and Diagnostic Approach

Trigeminal neuralgia is the most common fifth cranial nerve disorder as discussed in ***Primary and Secondary Headache,*** **Chapter 11.** In contrast, a primary trigeminal neuropathy, as illustrated in this chapter's vignette, is very uncommon.

Facial numbness is the classic symptom of a primary trigeminal (CN-V) neuropathy. Patients with this complaint may have a lesion at any site along the trigeminal nerve sensory pathway, including the nuclei within the brainstem, sensory root, trigeminal ganglion, or primary divisions of CN-V. To determine

Ophthalmic (V₁) and Maxillary (V₂) Nerves, Sensory

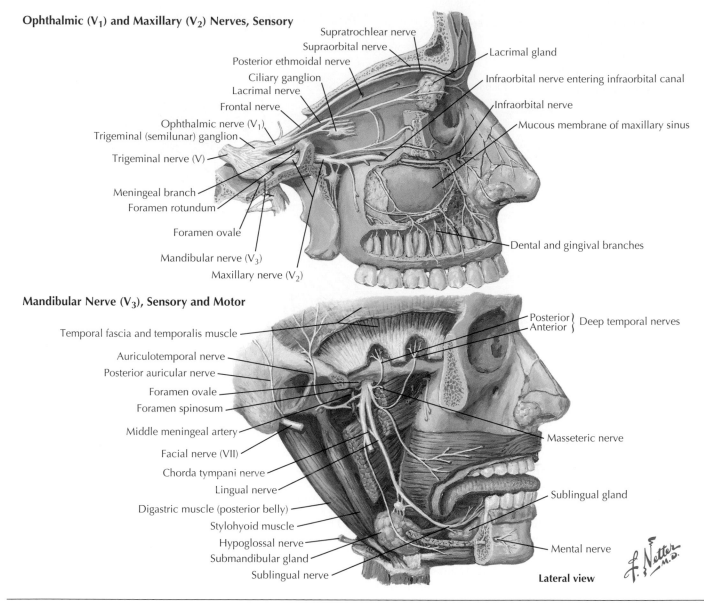

Mandibular Nerve (V₃), Sensory and Motor

Figure 6-2 Ophthalmic (V1), Maxillary (V2), and Mandibular (V3) Nerves.

precisely which portion of the trigeminal nerve complex is affected, the examiner needs to initially test touch, temperature, and pain sensation within the distribution of each of the three major divisions. Examining the corneal reflex provides another useful clinical tool. Application of a wisp of cotton to the cornea normally leads to an eye blink, provided the facial nerve is intact, permitting a blink to occur when the sensory portion of this reflex arc is preserved. When there is a significantly asymmetrical corneal response or actual unilateral loss of this reflex, there is evidence of ophthalmic division CN-V neuropathy.

Both general and special sensation to the tongue and palate are necessary for fully functional taste. Impairment of general sensation from the tongue and palate carried by CN V may also cause taste disturbances, even though the special sensory fibers providing primary taste sensation are supplied by the facial and glossopharyngeal nerves. Masticatory weakness is often very difficult to test when the change is subtle. Normally both lateral

pterygoid muscles pull the jaw anteriorly or forward. When there is a unilateral motor fifth nerve lesion, the healthy unopposed pterygoid pulls the jaw across the midlines, thus leading to a deviation of the jaw to the side of the paretic motor fifth. This occurs when the motor nucleus, root, or mandibular division of the fifth cranial nerve is damaged.

Differential Diagnosis

Facial pain, numbness, or both are the hallmarks of most CN-V lesions. *Facial trauma*, particularly secondary to vehicular accidents or rarely invasive **dental treatments**, accounts for the majority of trigeminal nerve injuries. CN-V divisions and branches are exposed to *trauma* especially from **fractures of facial bones** within the face and neck and other clinically invasive procedures, particularly from dental work. Typically, these injuries lead to anesthesia within the specific distribution of whichever trigeminal branch is compromised.

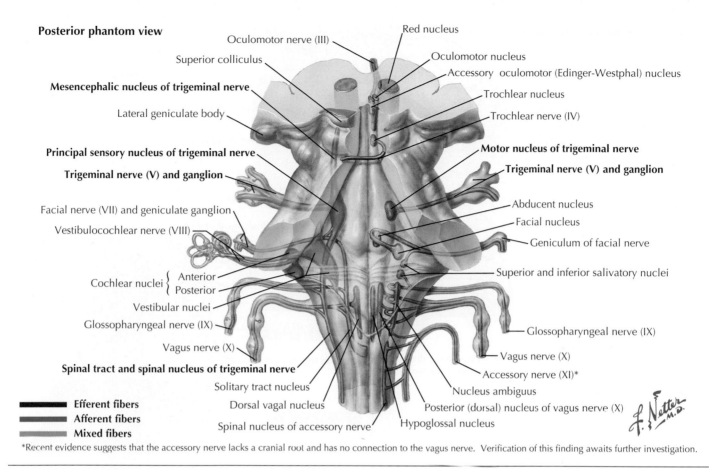

Figure 6-3 Cranial Nerve Nuclei in Brainstem: Schema.

In the Western world, ***Herpes zoster*** is the most common infectious cause of a trigeminal neuropathy (Fig. 6-6). **Herpes zoster ophthalmicus** occurs when latent varicella zoster virus infection within the trigeminal ganglion becomes reactivated, almost always affecting the ophthalmic division. However, very rarely, the maxillary or mandibular divisions may be primarily affected. Most patients present with a characteristic periorbital vesicular rash and severe neuralgic pain within the ophthalmic division (see Fig. 6-6). Similar to other herpes zoster syndromes, the pain may precede the eruption of cutaneous lesions. Permanent visual impairment is the most serious outcome of ophthalmic zoster infection. Antiviral agents such as acyclovir are the main therapy. Corticosteroid eyedrops are shown to decrease pain and hasten corneal healing and are sometimes prescribed by ophthalmologists if there are no other ocular or systemic diseases that might contraindicate their use. Rarely, an ipsilateral middle cerebral artery infarction may subsequently develop in these patients as the virus travels within the trigeminal nucleus and affects the adjacent intracavernous portion of the carotid artery or its branches with a granulomatous angiitis of the brain. CSF varicella zoster virus antibodies are frequently found, and antiviral treatment is felt to be helpful.

Worldwide, leprosy or ***Hansen disease*** is a more common cause of CN-V neuropathy. This primarily occurs in economically depressed countries. It generally affects the coolest areas of the skin. Thus, if sensory loss is confined to the tip of the

---

Box 6-1 Differential Diagnosis of CN-V Lesion Origin

Brainstem: stroke, brainstem gliomas, multiple sclerosis, or syringobulbia
Intracranial: trigeminal neurinoma, acoustic neurinoma, meningioma, granuloma, metastasis, herpes zoster, carotid or basilar aneurysms, trigeminal sensory neuropathy
Skull base lesions: metastasis, nasopharyngeal carcinoma, lymphoma, basilar meningitis
Trigeminal divisions and nerve branches: trauma, metastasis, spreading skin tumor, salivary tumor, vasculitis, leprosy (Hansen disease)
Drug intoxication: trichloroethylene, hydroxystilbamidine

---

nose or the pinna of the ear, Hansen disease is a primary consideration (Box 6-1).

Trigeminal sensory neuropathy occurs when the trigeminal ganglion cell bodies are the primary pathologic target. Although the pathogenesis of this ganglionopathy is frequently enigmatic, an association with connective tissue disorders, particularly ***scleroderma or Sjögren*** syndrome, is recognized. Patients with these disorders typically have numbness that begins around the mouth and spreads slowly over months involving all CN-V divisions, unilaterally or bilaterally, with the ophthalmic division at times spared. In Sjögren syndrome, trigeminal neuropathy is common and is usually representative of a more widespread sensory ganglionopathy. Presumably,

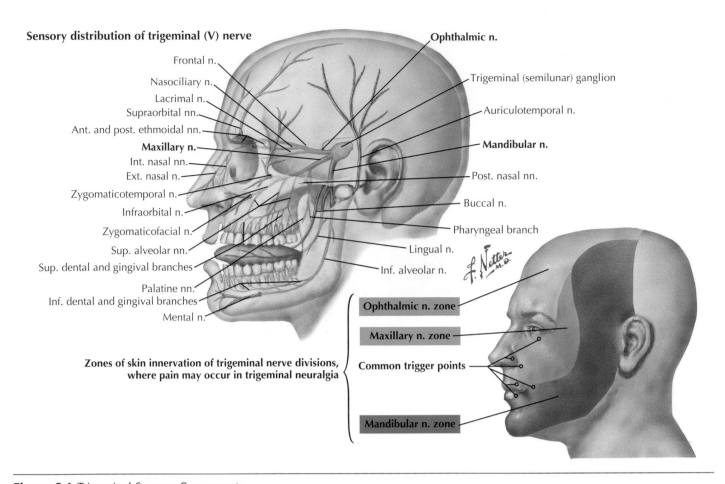

Sensory distribution of trigeminal (V) nerve

Frontal n.
Nasociliary n.
Lacrimal n.
Supraorbital nn.
Ant. and post. ethmoidal nn.
Maxillary n.
Int. nasal nn.
Ext. nasal n.
Zygomaticotemporal n.
Infraorbital n.
Zygomaticofacial n.
Sup. alveolar nn.
Sup. dental and gingival branches
Palatine nn.
Inf. dental and gingival branches
Mental n.

Ophthalmic n.
Trigeminal (semilunar) ganglion
Auriculotemporal n.
Mandibular n.
Post. nasal nn.
Buccal n.
Pharyngeal branch
Lingual n.
Inf. alveolar n.

Zones of skin innervation of trigeminal nerve divisions, where pain may occur in trigeminal neuralgia

Ophthalmic n. zone
Maxillary n. zone
Common trigger points
Mandibular n. zone

Figure 6-4 Trigeminal Sensory Components.

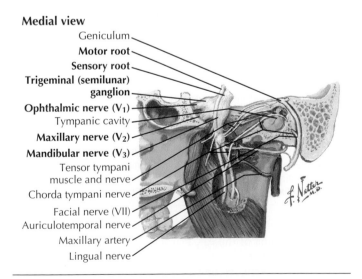

Medial view

Geniculum
Motor root
Sensory root
Trigeminal (semilunar) ganglion
Ophthalmic nerve (V₁)
Tympanic cavity
Maxillary nerve (V₂)
Mandibular nerve (V₃)
Tensor tympani muscle and nerve
Chorda tympani nerve
Facial nerve (VII)
Auriculotemporal nerve
Maxillary artery
Lingual nerve

Figure 6-5 Mandibular Nerve (V3) Sensory and Motor.

circulating autoantibodies attack the ganglion cells, where the blood–brain barrier is more permeable to large molecules than is the blood–brain barrier elsewhere in the peripheral nervous system.

A specific medication reaction is another exceedingly uncommon cause of a trigeminal neuropathy. The two best-recognized offenders are the industrial solvent trichloroethylene and the biological tracer hydroxystilbamidine.

The possibility of a *metastatic neoplasm* infiltrating a fifth nerve branch must always be included in the differential diagnosis of a persistent, but not always severe, facial numbness or pain. This is very well illustrated in this chapter's vignette. Tumors involving the face, such as **squamous cell carcinoma**, microcystic adnexal (sweat gland) carcinoma, and keratoacanthoma, have a proclivity for invading cutaneous nerves because of their innate neurotropism.

Primary trigeminal neurinomas are rare, usually benign, well-demarcated, and slowly growing neoplasms. These comprise 0.2% of intracranial tumors and 2–3% of intracranial neurinomas. Most frequently, these tumors arise near the trigeminal ganglion, usually extending into the middle and posterior cranial fossae. Rarely, they arise exclusively from one of the sensory divisions and spread extracranially. Rare instances of malignant schwannomas originating within the trigeminal ganglion also occur. Most neurinomas have very slow growths, and reach a 2.5 cm diameter before a specific diagnosis is made. Initially, these patients typically report developing numbness and paresthesiae within the CN-V distribution. It is very rare for typical trigeminal neuralgia pain or even intermittent burning pain to be the presenting sign of a primary trigeminal tumor. Rarely, these sensory findings are accompanied by other neurologic symptoms resulting from damage to adjacent structures. For example, tumors growing downward into the posterior fossa may lead to cerebellar ataxia and lesions of CN-VII and CN-VIII, manifesting with facial palsy, tinnitus, or hearing loss.

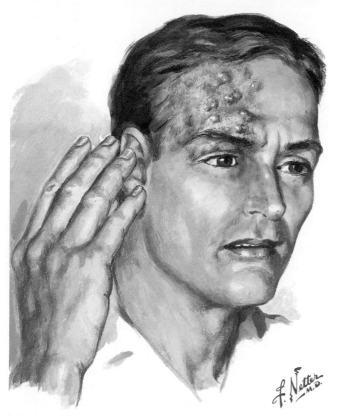

Herpes zoster: Maculopapular erythematous rash with formation of vesicles that rupture, then encrust over days.

Figure 6-6 Varicella Zoster with Probable Keratitis.

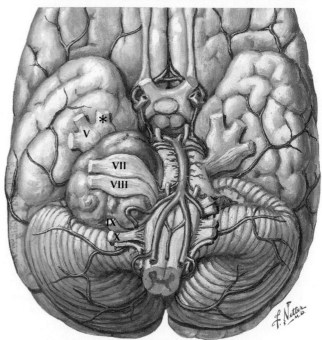

Large acoustic neurinoma filling cerebellopontine angle, distorting brainstem and cranial nerves V, VII, VIII, IX, X

Figure 6-7 Acoustic Neurinoma Compressing Trigeminal Nerve.

In contrast, neurinomas exert pressure upward on the lateral wall of the cavernous sinus, leading to CN-II, -III, -IV, and -VI lesions.

Cerebellopontine angle tumors, typically acoustic neurinomas arising form CN-VIII (Fig. 6-7), may enlarge and compress the trigeminal sensory root and lead to facial numbness or pain with subsequent ipsilateral loss of the corneal reflex. Other neoplasms include meningiomas, epidermoids, lymphomas, hemangioblastomas, gangliocytomas, chondromas, and sarcomas. Similarly, certain skull base tumors, such as **nasopharyngeal carcinoma**, **salivary gland adenocarcinoma**, and **metastatic disease**, may invade various trigeminal divisions. The *numb chin syndrome* consists of unilateral numbness of the chin and adjacent lower lip. Although seemingly harmless, it is usually an ominous sign of primary or metastatic cancer involving the mandible, skull base, or leptomeninges. **Lymphoproliferative malignancies** and **metastatic breast cancer** are the most common etiologies.

Lastly one may find that some primary trigeminal neuropathies defy specific definition and thus are labeled as *idiopathic*. However, one must emphasize the need for a vigilant approach with frequent follow-up as illustrated in the above vignette, especially with patients with prior known facial malignancies such as SCC or other masses.

ADDITIONAL RESOURCES

Chan WO, Madge S, Dodd TJ, et al. Multiple cranial nerve palsies as a result of perineural invasion by squamous cell carcinoma. Br J Hosp Med (Lond) 2008 Aug;69(8):476-477.

Elias WJ, Burchiel KJ. Trigeminal neuralgia and other neuropathic pain syndromes of the head and face. Curr Pain Headache Rep 2002;6:115-124.

Hughes RAC. Diseases of the fifth cranial nerve. In: Dyck PJ, Thomas PK, Griffin JW, et al, editors. Peripheral Neuropathy. 3rd ed. Philadelphia, Pa: WB Saunders Co; 1993. p. 801-817.

Loeser JD. Tic douloureux. Pain Res Manag 2001;6:156-165.

Maillefert JF, Gazet-Maillefert MP, Tavernier C, et al. Numb chin syndrome. Joint Bone Spine 2000;67:86-93.

Nager GT. Neurinomas of the trigeminal nerve. Am J Otolaryngol 1984;5:301-333.

Rosenbaum R. Neuromuscular complications of connective tissue diseases. Muscle Nerve 2001;24:154-169.

Rowe JG, Radatz MW, Walton L, et al. Gamma knife stereotactic radiosurgery for unilateral acoustic neuromas. J Neurol Neurosurg Psychiatry 2003;74:1536-1542.

Severson EA, Baratz KH, Hodge DO, et al. Herpes zoster ophthalmicus in Olmsted County, Minnesota: have systemic antivirals made a difference? Arch Ophthalmol 2003;121:386-390.

Starr CE, Pavan-Langston D. Varicella-zoster virus: mechanisms of pathogenicity and corneal disease. Ophthalmol Clin North Am 2002;15:7-15.

Sweeney PJ, Hanson MR. The cranial neuropathies. In: Bradley WG, Daroff RB, Fenichel GM, et al, editors. Neurology in Clinical Practice: Principles of Diagnosis and Management. 2nd ed. Boston, Mass: Butterworth-Heinemann; 1996. p. 1721-1732.

Zhu JJ, Padillo O, Duff J, et al. Cavernous sinus and leptomeningeal metastases arising from a squamous cell carcinoma of the face: case report. Neurosurgery 2004 Feb;54(2):492-498; discussion 498-499.

Cranial Nerve VII: Facial

Michal Vytopil and H. Royden Jones, Jr.

7

Clinical Vignette

A 62-year-old judge became aware of subtle weakness of his left lower face that he first noted while shaving. Two months later, he noted that he could no longer close his left eye lid fully and he was having increasing weakness of the remainder of his left face. He was referred to a neurologist, who reassured him that he had a "benign" Bell palsy. He sought a second opinion when his facial weakness continued to worsen over another month with an inability to close the eye and to form a symmetrical smile.

Neurologic examination demonstrated weakness in all divisions of the left CN-VII with total inability to close his eye or form a left-sided smile. Palpation of the cheek demonstrated some fullness in the left parotid gland, with the remainder of his head and neck examination being normal. Complete neurologic and otoscopic examinations were unremarkable. Audiologic test results were normal, including the left acoustic/stapedius reflex. A corneal reflex was sluggish on the left but present bilaterally.

A left parotid gland biopsy demonstrated a malignant adenocarcinoma with extension beyond the capsule at surgery. He died of metastatic cancer 20 months later.

Comment: Fortunately, this case represents a relatively rare occurrence. However, it emphasizes that what may initially look routine and benign indeed may have a much more serious pathophysiologic mechanism. The issue in this case is to appreciate the history of a gradual evolution of the neurologic deficits in contrast to the relatively acute onset of idiopathic Bell palsy. Furthermore, Bell palsy is typically preceded by retroauricular pain and often associated with hyperacusis and loss of taste on the anterior two thirds of the tongue. When these symptoms are lacking, as in this instance, the pathoanatomic site is distal to the styloid foramen and potentially within the parotid gland as the facial nerve passes through its body. In addition, the gradual progression of this patient's symptoms provided a strong suspicion of a neoplasm.

*F*acial nerve (CN-VII) lesions are the most common cranial mononeuropathy. This is one of the most complex cranial nerves having multiple functions (Fig. 7-1). It has a long and somewhat circuitous course with four primary components. (1) **Motor fibers**, which constitute the major division and serve the primary function of CN-VII: innervating the muscles of facial expression (unilateral, complete facial weakness is the hallmark of almost all facial neuropathies); (2) **autonomic fibers**, which are responsible for lacrimal, salivary, and mucous secretions; (3) **special sensory fibers**, which provide taste from the anterior two thirds of the tongue; and (4) **general sensory fibers**, which innervate the external auditory canal and a small area behind the ear.

When a patient presents with facial weakness, differentiation should be made between peripheral facial nerve lesions and CNS processes. With the latter, when the patient is relaxed, subtle suggestions of a facial nerve lesion may be appreciated by nasolabial fold flattening on the affected side. Brain lesions such as cerebral infarction, tumor, inflammation, or demyelination are often associated with other findings that can help with localization. For example, a small lesion near the Broca area may result in motor aphasia and facial weakness. Larger lesions affecting a significant portion of a hemisphere, as with large hemispheric strokes, cause a constellation of symptoms, including face, arm, and leg weakness and sensory loss; gaze deviation; and neglect or aphasia. Posterior limb lesions of the internal capsule result in face, arm, and leg weakness without sensory, visual, or cognitive changes. While peripheral facial weakness involves the upper and lower part of the face to the same degree, **upper motor neuron lesions** typically present with a gradient of weakness (Fig. 7-2), with relative preservation of movement in the brow and forehead (orbicularis oculi and frontalis muscles). This is due to presumed dual hemispheric innervation of the forehead muscles. In addition, corticobulbar tract involvement, as in various suprabulbar palsies, leads to absence of *voluntary* facial movement but retained reflexive movements such as in response to emotional stimuli.

ANATOMY

Intrapontine Portion

CN-VII consists of two primary roots (Fig. 7-1). The larger division carries **somatic motor fibers** and has its origin within the facial nucleus in the caudal pons, where it lies adjacent to the spinal tract of the trigeminal nerve (CN-V). It then passes dorsally and rostrally to curve around the abducens nerve (CN-VI) nucleus (internal genu) and exits the brainstem at the bulbopontine angle between CN-VI and CN-VIII. Its smaller component, the **nervus intermedius** (intermediate nerve of Wrisberg), contains a combination of **autonomic**, **special sensory (taste)**, and **general sensory** fibers. Its preganglionic parasympathetic fibers arise from the superior salivatory nucleus, relay through the pterygopalatine and submandibular ganglions, and eventually provide efferent function for lacrimation and salivation. The remaining intermediate nerve fibers carry taste and general somatic sensation and have their primary cell bodies in the geniculate ganglion and ultimately terminate within the nucleus solitarius and the spinal tract of CN-V, respectively.

Peripheral CN-VII

Both roots of CN-VII leave the brainstem to enter the temporal bone via the internal auditory meatus, where they accompany the auditory nerve (CN-VIII) passing through the internal auditory canal (Fig. 7-1, bottom). CN-VII continues to the periphery through the facial canal; this segment has five parts, based on their relation to surrounding anatomic structures. (1) The

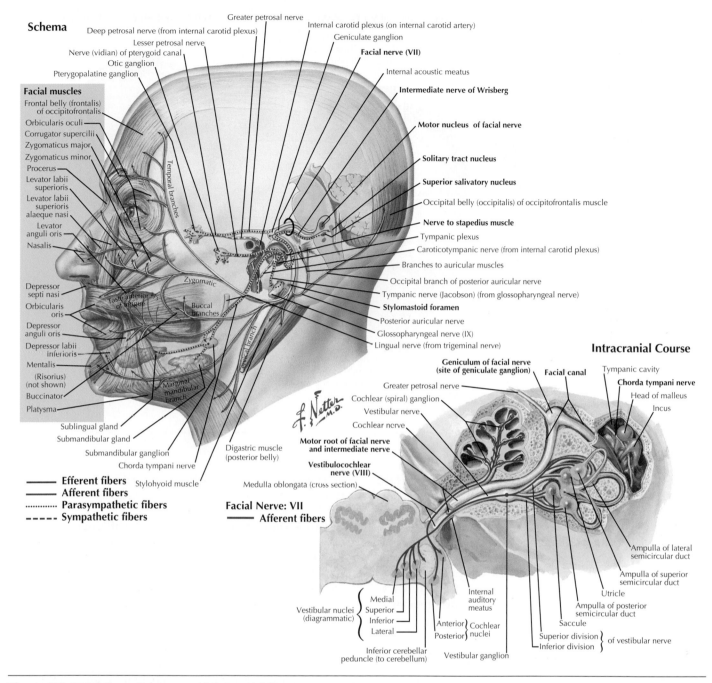

Figure 7-1 Facial Nerve Schema and Intracranial Course.

labyrinthine segment passes above the labyrinth and leads anterolaterally to the *geniculate ganglions* that contain the cell bodies of CN-VII afferents. (2) At this site, the canal abruptly turns posteriorly and forms the *external genu of CN-VII*. (3) The *greater petrosal nerve* originates here; it carries preganglionic parasympathetic fibers to the pterygopalatine ganglion, where they synapse and subsequently direct postganglionic fibers to the lacrimal gland. (4) The *tympanic segment* of CN-VII travels posteriorly and laterally along the medial wall of the middle ear. At the posterior wall of the middle ear, the facial canal changes its course and travels inferiorly toward its exit at the stylomastoid foramen. (5) The vertical portion is named the *mastoid segment* and has two important branches:

proximally, the *stapedius nerve* arises to innervate the stapedius muscle; more distally, the *chorda tympani* branches and exits the facial canal and, after traversing the middle ear, joins the lingual nerve belonging to the third division of CN-V. The chorda tympani contains preganglionic parasympathetic fibers that synapse within the submandibular ganglion to innervate the submandibular and sublingual glands. The chorda tympani also carries taste fibers. Their cell bodies originate within the geniculate ganglion, mediating taste sensation from the anterior two thirds of the tongue.

Soon after leaving the skull at the stylomastoid foramen, the distal CN-VII gives rise to several small motor branches innervating the posterior auricular, occipital, digastric, and stylohyoid

Hyperacusis

Left Peripheral VII Facial Weakness

Left Central VII Facial Weakness

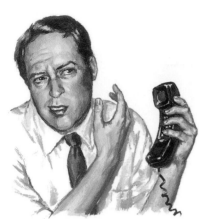

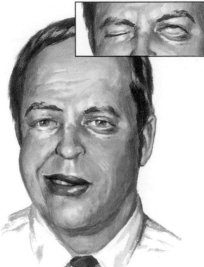

Attempt to close eye results in eyeball rolling superiorly exposing sclera (Bell phenomenon) but no closure of the lid per se.

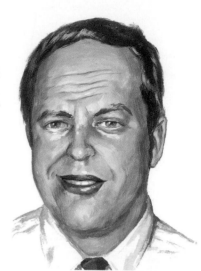

This may be early or initial symptom of a peripheral VII nerve palsy: patient holds phone away from ear because of painful sensitivity to sound. Loss of taste also may occur on affected side.

Patient unable to wrinkle forehead; eyelid droops very slightly; cannot show teeth at all on affected side in attempt to smile; and lower lip droops slightly.

Incomplete smile with very subtle flattening of affected nasolabial fold; relative preservation of brow and forehead movement.

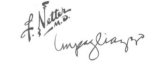

Figure 7-2 Central Versus Peripheral Facial Paralysis.

muscles (Fig. 7-1, top). The ***main motor trunk of CN-VII*** then passes through the parotid gland to terminate as the temporal, zygomatic, buccal, mandibular, and cervical branches. The first two innervate the muscles involved in moving the forehead, closing the eyes, and wrinkling the nose. Muscles of the lower face and neck are primarily innervated by the latter two branches. CN-VII subserves all muscles of facial expression except the levator palpebrae superioris and, therefore, CN-VII impairment, with a resultant asymmetric facies, is a major social and cosmetic impediment.

CLINICAL CORRELATIONS AND ENTITIES

The facial nerve can be damaged at any level along its complex course. Paralysis of the facial musculature is the hallmark of seventh cranial nerve lesions no matter what the lesion's anatomic site. The clinical presence or absence of symptoms related to the various other components of the facial nerve is very important in identifying the lesion site.

The patient with a ***peripheral seventh (facial) nerve*** palsy in most instances, with the exception of an early very distal branch lesion within the parotid gland, loses function of the entire ipsilateral side of their face and cannot smile, close their eyelid (orbicularis oculi), or wrinkle (frontalis) their forehead.

When ***intrapontine*** (Fig. 7-3, #1) lesions affect the facial motor nucleus per se, as well as its exiting fibers, involvement of neighboring brainstem structures is typically seen. The association of peripheral facial paralysis with ipsilateral conjugate gaze palsy (paramedian pontine reticular formation lesion),

ipsilateral lateral rectus palsy (sixth cranial nerve lesion), or paresis of the opposite arm and leg (corticospinal tract lesion) usually indicates a pontine localization.

Extramedullary lesions (Fig. 7-3, #2) affecting the seventh nerve as it enters its intracranial course primarily occur within the cerebellopontine (CP) angle. Most commonly these are benign, relatively large acoustic neuromas that initially involve the eighth nerve and later extend to produce a seventh-nerve lesion. Thus, diminished hearing, sometimes initially presenting with tinnitus, usually precedes the onset of this type of peripheral facial paresis (see Fig. 7-4). Occasionally, with very large CP angle tumors there is concomitant involvement of the ipsilateral fifth cranial nerve (trigeminal nerve V) with unilateral facial numbness or initially only loss of the corneal reflex.

A relatively ***proximal pregeniculate, intracanicular facial nerve*** lesion (Fig. 7-3, #3) characteristically leads to diminished lacrimation from greater petrosal nerve involvement as well as hyperacusis (an increased sensitivity to sound that is particularly noticeable while using a telephone), due to associated stapedius muscle paresis. These lesions also lead to diminished salivation, absent or altered taste sensation for the anterior two thirds of the tongue, and affected somatic sensation for the external auditory canal.

When a facial nerve lesion is more distally situated, ***between the geniculate ganglion and the stapedius nerve*** all of the above findings occur, but lacrimation is spared as the greater petrosal nerve has already exited the geniculate ganglion. If damage occurs in the ***facial canal***, involvement of the ***stapedius nerve and the chorda tympani*** (Fig. 7-3, #4) leads to hyperacusis

Course and distribution of facial (VII) nerve

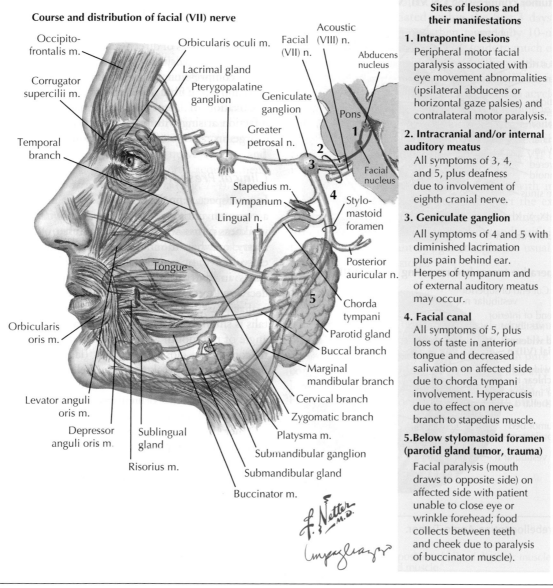

Occipito-frontalis m.

Corrugator supercilii m.

Temporal branch

Orbicularis oris m.

Levator anguli oris m.

Depressor anguli oris m.

Risorius m.

Sublingual gland

Orbicularis oculi m.

Lacrimal gland

Pterygopalatine ganglion

Geniculate ganglion

Greater petrosal n.

Stapedius m.

Tympanum

Lingual n.

Tongue

Facial (VII) n.

Acoustic (VIII) n.

Abducens nucleus

Pons

Facial nucleus

Stylo-mastoid foramen

Posterior auricular n.

Chorda tympani

Parotid gland

Buccal branch

Marginal mandibular branch

Cervical branch

Zygomatic branch

Platysma m.

Submandibular ganglion

Submandibular gland

Buccinator m.

Sites of lesions and their manifestations

1. Intrapontine lesions
Peripheral motor facial paralysis associated with eye movement abnormalities (ipsilateral abducens or horizontal gaze palsies) and contralateral motor paralysis.

2. Intracranial and/or internal auditory meatus
All symptoms of 3, 4, and 5, plus deafness due to involvement of eighth cranial nerve.

3. Geniculate ganglion
All symptoms of 4 and 5 with diminished lacrimation plus pain behind ear. Herpes of tympanum and of external auditory meatus may occur.

4. Facial canal
All symptoms of 5, plus loss of taste in anterior tongue and decreased salivation on affected side due to chorda tympani involvement. Hyperacusis due to effect on nerve branch to stapedius muscle.

5. Below stylomastoid foramen (parotid gland tumor, trauma)
Facial paralysis (mouth draws to opposite side) on affected side with patient unable to close eye or wrinkle forehead; food collects between teeth and cheek due to paralysis of buccinator muscle).

Figure 7-3 Bell Palsy.

and impaired salivation and taste but no change in lacrimation. When the seventh-nerve lesion is *distal to the chorda tympani*, it is characterized by a pure ipsilateral facial weakness (Fig. 7-3, # 5). Very rarely, a lesion of this type occurs after the facial nerve exits the skull through the stylomastoid foramen. On occasion, this can cause diagnostic difficulty early on as it may initially involve just individual motor branches, with limited weakness of individual facial muscles before a complete palsy develops. Facial trauma is the most common cause for acute pure motor CN-VII lesions; however, an insidious progressive course suggests that a parotid adenocarcinoma, as illustrated in the vignette on p. 98, is the most likely cause.

Clinical Vignette

A vigorous 18-year-old woman awakened with a mild dull ache behind her left ear. While washing her face she noted an inability to smile on that side and that her left eye lid could not close. As a grandparent had recently had a stroke presenting with facial weakness, she rushed to the local emergency room for immediate physician evaluation. Her clinical examination demonstrated that she was unable to smile, close her eyelid, or wrinkle the forehead on the left. Her left eye was slightly injected and dry secondary to diminished tearing. She had no taste sensation on the anterior of the left tongue. The remainder of her neurologic examination was normal. No imaging studies were indicated.

A diagnosis of idiopathic Bell palsy was made; this patient was most relieved to have not had a stroke. As she lived in an endemic area for Lyme disease, specific antibodies were obtained before discharge on oral prednisone treatment. Over the next 2 months, she experienced a gradual and total return of her facial muscle function.

axon loss, and therefore, recovery is prompt, complete, and without synkinesis. The remaining patients have axonal damage with wallerian degeneration, and improvement requires regenerating axons to reinnervate paralyzed muscles, resulting in slow and incomplete recovery.

The recovery rate from Bell palsy follows two patterns: most patients begin to regain facial strength within 3 weeks after onset, but in some, the initiation of recovery is delayed for at least 3–6 months. The overall prognosis is good; most patients (80–85%) recover completely, but the rest may have various residual effects. These include synkinesis, residual weakness, tearing, or contracture. Synkinesis, the most frequent permanent sequel, clinically manifests as synchronized movement of different muscles that normally do not contract together. Typically, there is subtle eye closure with smiling, or a lip or chin twitch with blinking. Synkinesis occurs when there is a misdirection of regenerating axons into muscles that they originally did not innervate. This is rarely disabling but can be disfiguring and cause involuntary eye closure at inopportune times. Botulinum toxin injections have emerged as a symptomatic treatment of these abnormal movements. Another rare phenomenon following recovery of facial nerve injury is excessive lacrimation when eating ("crocodile tears") and results from aberrant regeneration of salivatory fibers to the lacrimal glands.

An EMG provides valuable prognostic information, especially in those individuals not beginning to demonstrate improvement within the first few months after onset of Bell palsy. It should never be performed until approximately 3 weeks after onset. By then, it is possible to distinguish between nerve fibers that have undergone wallerian degeneration and those that are only temporarily blocked. A significantly reduced amplitude of the facial nerve compound muscle action potential and abundant fibrillation potentials in facial muscles indicates severe axonal damage, whereas a demyelinating conduction block is typically partially resolved by that time, evidenced by absent or scarce fibrillation potentials.

Infectious Facial Palsies

VARICELLA-ZOSTER VIRUS

The Ramsay–Hunt syndrome, caused by reactivation of the varicella-zoster virus (VZV) within the geniculate ganglion, is the second most common cause of atraumatic facial palsy. Clinically, it is characterized by the triad of acute facial palsy, neuralgic pain, and eruption of herpetic vesicles within the external auditory canal, ipsilateral palate, and anterior two thirds of the tongue. The areas of pain and rash are appropriate to the general sensory innervation of the afferent facial nerve branches. The geniculate ganglion cell bodies host the latent varicella-zoster virus infection. The close proximity of the geniculate ganglion to the vestibulocochlear nerve in the bony facial canal explains the concomitant otologic symptoms such as tinnitus, vertigo, and hearing loss in some patients. The detection of VZV IgM antibody in blood and cerebrospinal fluid (CSF), or VZV DNA in CSF, saliva, or blood is often helpful in assigning a viral etiology.

The prognosis for Ramsay–Hunt syndrome is worse than that of idiopathic Bell palsy, with frequent complete paralysis,

incomplete recovery, and residual synkinesis. Therefore, aggressive treatment with acyclovir (30 mg/kg daily IV or 4000 mg daily oral) is indicated. A course of prednisone similar to the one used for Bell palsy is probably reasonable, although no evidence-based data exist to support this treatment. The best long-term results are obtained when treatment is started within 3 days of onset.

LYME DISEASE

Clinical Vignette

Five weeks after returning from her family's summer home in Old Lyme, Connecticut, this 32-year-old woman presented with left facial drooping and arm pain. Three days prior, she had woken up with severe pain behind the neck shooting down her right arm to the thumb. She noted difficulty holding a coffee mug to her lips.

Her temperature was 38°C (100.6°F). There was a 10-cm circular rash on the medial aspect of her right thigh. Her neck was slightly rigid; no intra-auricular vesicles were noted. Neurologic examination results demonstrated severe left facial weakness associated with loss of taste. On attempted eye closure, her left eyelids remained 6 mm apart. Her right biceps, brachioradialis, and pronator teres were weak. Right brachioradialis reflex was absent.

Brain computed tomography (CT) results were unremarkable. Lumbar puncture revealed a white blood cell count of 23/mm³, primarily lymphocytes, with a normal protein level and a slightly decreased glucose level. CSF and serum Lyme antibody test results were positive.

Comment: This vignette is typical of facial palsy secondary to Lyme disease (neuroborreliosis). At times, as in this case, facial weakness occurs with concomitant, often very painful, nerve root lesions. Although relatively uncommon, this classic syndrome of Lyme meningoradiculitis should always be considered, particularly in endemic areas.

Facial paralysis is the most common focal manifestation of neuroborreliosis; 40% of these patients have cranial neuropathies, and approximately 80% have CN-VII involvement. Multiple cranial nerves are affected in one fifth of those with a cranial neuropathy; two thirds with multiple cranial neuropathies primarily have bilateral facial palsy. Patients with an acute facial palsy in the presence of systemic signs, such as erythema migrans, or a history of possible exposure to disease-transmitting ticks warrant further studies for neuroborreliosis.

Standard CSF analysis usually demonstrates a pleocytosis with lymphocytic predominance. Confirmatory studies include titers of anti-*Borrelia burgdorferi* antibodies, and polymerase chain reaction detection of bacterial DNA in blood and CSF. Western blot improves sensitivity of serologic studies by identifying the specific antigens against which the patient generates antibodies. Facial paralysis may also occur before seroconversion, e.g., early in the disease before antibody testing results become positive. When clinical suspicion of Lyme disease is high, follow-up serologic tests are indicated.

Optimal treatment is still debated; the use of IV antibiotics is probably appropriate in severe cases with other manifestations such as headache or radiculitis, in the presence of CSF pleocytosis, or when parenchymal brain or cord involvement is suspected. Typical regimen consists of ceftriaxone (2 g daily) or cefotaxime (6 g daily) for 2 weeks. In mild cases with an isolated facial neuropathy, oral doxycycline (200 mg daily) for 2 weeks is felt to be an acceptable option. Once treated, the prognosis of facial palsy in Lyme disease is excellent, with most patients recovering completely.

OTHER INFECTIONS

Peripheral facial paralysis may occur with infectious mononucleosis, caused by Epstein–Barr virus, and poliomyelitis, caused by an enterovirus.

Infectious conditions involving the temporal bone can cause peripheral facial paralysis, such as acute and chronic otitis media and osteomyelitis of diverse etiologies, including tuberculosis and syphilis. Acute bacterial and particularly tuberculous meningitis may affect multiple cranial nerves including CN-VII. Leprosy is a common cause of facial palsy in endemic areas.

Granulomatous Disorders

Sarcoidosis is a disease of unknown etiology characterized by histopathologic findings of nonnecrotizing granulomas within multiple organs. Unilateral or bilateral CN-VII palsy with hyperacusis and dysgeusia, thought to result from granulomatous meningitis, is the most frequent neurologic manifestation. The prognosis is favorable, and most patients recover completely after steroid treatment.

Wegener granulomatosis is a systemic disease characterized by necrotizing granulomatous lesions of the upper and lower respiratory tract, glomerulonephritis, and systemic necrotizing vasculitis. Of the primary systemic vasculitides, only Wegener granulomatosis is associated with a significant frequency of cranial neuropathies. CN-VII involvement, usually occurring in conjunction with other cranial neuropathies, may reflect granulomatous invasion of the temporal bone or granulomatous basilar meningitis. The 2-year fatality rate of untreated Wegener granulomatosis is greater than 90%, and aggressive immunotherapy is warranted immediately upon diagnosis.

Traumatic Facial Palsy

Clinical Vignette

A 40-year-old man was brought to emergency room after being hit by a motorcycle while crossing a busy street. He received a blow to the forehead as he fell on the pavement, and was knocked unconscious for 2 minutes. In the emergency room, he complained of headache and decreased hearing on the right side. Urgent ENT evaluation found fresh blood in the right meatus and a ruptured tympanic membrane. Neurologic exam demonstrated incomplete right peripheral facial weakness and loss of taste over the right anterior two thirds of the tongue. A high-resolution CT of the skull base revealed a transversely oriented fracture through the petrous bone, as well as right

hemotympanum, pneumocephalus, and occipital soft tissue swelling. The patient was treated conservatively with complete resolution of the hearing loss and facial weakness within 3 months.

Comment: This is a rather typical case of traumatic incomplete facial paralysis and thus has a good prognosis in contrast to those who present with complete loss of facial nerve function.

Nearly all patients with facial palsy after blunt head trauma have a temporal bone fracture. Concomitant damage to CN-VIII, cochlea, labyrinth, or middle ear structures may produce hearing loss and vestibular dysfunction. Contusion, compression, and edema of the CN-VII have all been proposed as possible mechanisms of traumatic facial paralysis. Some of these processes can evolve gradually and lead to delayed facial palsy after several days. Immediate and complete facial palsy often indicates that the nerve has been transected, and portends a poor prognosis for functional recovery. In such cases, surgical exploration should be considered. Conversely, patients with incomplete weakness and with early signs of improvement, similar to the one in this vignette, usually achieve good recovery within months with conservative management alone.

Neoplasms

Several primary and metastatic malignancies may cause a facial palsy. Carcinomatous meningitis usually affects multiple cranial nerves; the most common sources are the lung, the breast, gastrointestinal cancers, and lymphomas. Typically, these tumors have an aggressive clinical course; those that present with an isolated CN-VII lesion soon demonstrate signs of multiple cranial or spinal nerve root involvement or both.

Certain benign tumors may exert chronic extrinsic pressure on the facial nerve. Schwannomas from the vestibular portion of CN-VIII, typically occurring within the acoustic meatus at the CP angle, or less commonly meningiomas at similar sites, affect CN-VII very gradually over time. When they eventually do so, they tend to predominantly and subtly affect sensory fibers over the motor fibers that are more resilient to chronic deformation. Therefore, the only sign of early CN-VII involvement may be relatively minor numbness behind the ear, on the floor of the ear canal, in the posterior inferior quadrant of the eardrum (Hitzelberger sign), or a combination of these. The change in hearing, however, usually leads to the diagnosis. Signs of a motor CN-VII lesion do not occur until these lesions become large.

Malignant distal infiltration of CN-VII is seen with parotid tumors (see Fig. 7-5).

Uncommon Mass Lesions

Cholesteatomas are rare mass lesions at the CP angle that deserve consideration in patients with slowly evolving facial paralysis. Other uncommon entities include pontine gliomas, arachnoid cysts, lipomas, and hemangiomas (Fig. 7-6).

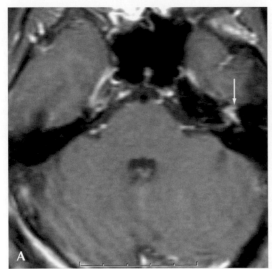

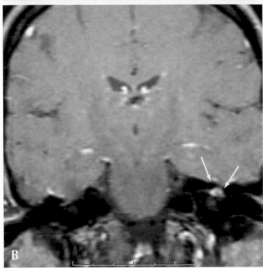

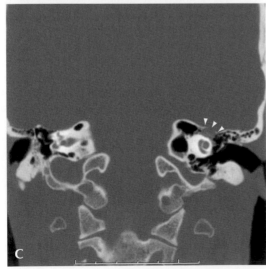

A and B, Axial and coronal post-gadolinium-enhanced, T1-weighted, fat-saturated MR images demonstrate enlargement and enhancement of the geniculate ganglion (thin arrows). C, Coronal thin section CT of petrous bone shows smooth enlargement of the geniculate region (arrowheads).

Figure 7-6 Seventh Nerve Hemangioma.

Neuromuscular Disorders with Facial Weakness

The motor portion of the CN-VII nucleus as well as the respective brainstem nuclei of CN-V, -IX, -X, -XI, and -XII may be involved in various motor neuron diseases, particularly amyotrophic lateral sclerosis and bulbospinal muscular atrophy (Kennedy disease).

CN-VII is affected in 33–50% of Guillain–Barré syndrome cases and often bilaterally. Although usually evident when limb weakness is severe, CN-VII lesions may develop at any stage, including as the presenting sign. The Miller–Fisher syndrome, a variant of Guillain–Barré syndrome, is characterized by ophthalmoplegia, ataxia, and areflexia. However, involvement of cranial nerves other than CN-III, -IV, and -VI occurs in many cases. Facial weakness has been reported in nearly half of the Miller–Fisher syndrome cases, underscoring the important clinical overlap between classic ascending Guillain–Barré syndrome and Miller–Fisher syndrome.

Neuromuscular junction disorders (NMJDs), particularly myasthenia gravis (MG), often lead to bifacial weakness. This is a common finding in the majority of MG patients where there is associated ptosis and extraocular muscle involvement. Interestingly, although some patients with the less common Lambert–Eaton myasthenic syndrome have diplopia, ptosis, dysphagia, and dysarthria, facial nerve weakness is not found in this presynaptic NMJD.

Some primary myopathies may cause bilateral facial weakness, typically accompanied by wasting. In adult-onset myotonic dystrophy, muscles innervated by CN-III and CN-V, such as the levator palpebrae superioris and the temporalis, are also involved. Therefore, ptosis and jaw weakness often also occur. Congenital myotonic dystrophy may present with bilateral facial diplegia and is sometimes associated with severe neonatal hypotonia. Facial weakness occurs in 95% of patients with facioscapulohumeral (FSH) dystrophy who are younger than 30 years. It affects predominantly the orbicularis oris and is often asymmetric. Although facial weakness is rarely the presenting problem, most patients with FSH dystrophy reveal long histories of difficulties whistling or blowing balloons. Therefore, facial involvement is likely to be an early, slowly progressing sign.

Recurrent CN-VII Palsy

Recurrence occurs in approximately 10% of Bell palsy cases, a circumstance necessitating careful diagnostic evaluation to exclude underlying causes, especially neoplasms and basilar meningeal involvement.

Melkersson–Rosenthal syndrome, an autosomal dominant hereditary disorder, is characterized by a triad of facial palsy, facial edema, and a furrowed tongue (lingua plicata). This often exhibits an incomplete penetrance. Each component may occur independently or in combination. Patient history is characterized by recurrent attacks of facial paralysis, often beginning during childhood. Attacks can also include facial swelling, particularly affecting the upper lip. The tendency to recur is the only feature of facial paralysis that distinguishes it from most Bell palsy cases.

Hereditary liability to pressure palsies is an allelic disorder with the Charcot–Marie–Tooth IA neuropathy, caused by deletion of the region containing the peripheral-myelin-protein 22 gene. It manifests with recurrent acute painless palsies from nerve lesions at sites of compression or increased exposure. Although the typical presentation is of peroneal or ulnar neuropathy, recurrent facial paralysis occasionally occurs.

CN-VII Hyperactivity

Several positive symptoms occur from excessive reactivity of CN-VII; synkinesis, facial myokymia, and hemifacial spasm are the most frequent.

Synkinesis is frequently observed subsequent to aberrant reinnervation in patients with antecedent severe Bell palsy; an inappropriate facial movement results, for example, concomitant blinking while smiling. Ephaptic transmission, or "artificial synapse," may arise at a lesion site where depolarization of the injured fibers acts as a stimulus to the intact portion of the nerve.

Facial myokymia is characterized by subtle, continuous, undulating movement of facial muscles. The movements are usually unilateral, subtle, often confined to one to two facial muscles, and sometimes accompanied by facial contracture or weakness. Observed mainly in multiple sclerosis, it much less commonly reflects an intrinsic brainstem tumor, particularly pontine gliomas. In the former, it is usually self-limited and abates after several weeks. Some cases of facial myokymia are thought to be caused by antibody to a specific subtype of voltage-gated potassium channels. The specific antibody identified in some patients with facial myokymia also occurs with Isaac syndrome.

Hemifacial spasm consists of intermittent paroxysms of rapid, irregular, clonic twitching facial movements. The attack typically starts around the eyes and spreads to other ipsilateral facial muscles, especially in the perioral region. It is strictly confined to muscles innervated by CN-VII; preceding CN-VII lesions are rare. Paroxysms are often induced by voluntary or reflex facial movements, stress, and fatigue and may persist during sleep. The most common pathogenic mechanism for hemifacial spasm seems to be vascular compression of CN-VII by an aberrant arterial loop near the brainstem. Therefore, detailed imaging studies including MR angiography are essential for diagnosis of hemifacial spasm. Less frequent pathophysiologic mechanisms include tumors and localized infectious processes. Botox injections are an effective symptomatic treatment. Surgical decompression is an alternative sometimes leading to remission.

DIAGNOSTIC MODALITIES

Diagnostic modalities include imaging studies that may define direct involvement of CN VII or the presence of contiguous lesions. Other specialized testing modalities are used to study the various functions of CN-VII. Cerebrospinal fluid analysis is important in infections, Guillain–Barré syndrome, and if meningeal infiltration (usually cancerous) is suspected. The use of EMG in Bell palsy is discussed earlier in this chapter.

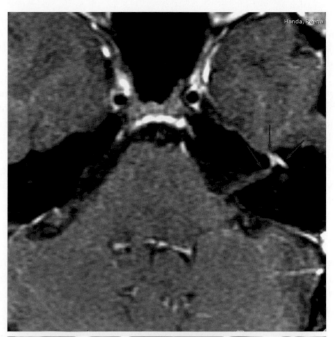
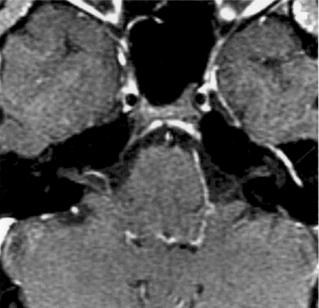

Axial T1-weighted, post-gadolinium MR image showing marked enhancement of fundal, geniculate, and tympanic segments of cranial nerve VII (arrows).

Figure 7-7 Imaging of Bell Palsy.

Imaging Studies

The two primary imaging options are MRI and CT. MRI is best at imaging the intracranial facial nerve, CP angle, and the parotid gland (Fig. 7-7). CT is the choice to image the temporal bone and its facial (fallopian) canal. MRI must include primary and gadolinium enhancement images. There may be unexpected relatively diffuse leptomeningeal enhancement when a facial neuropathy is the inciting lesion leading to a diagnosis of metastatic carcinoma or lymphoma.

The very rare primary facial neuromas also strongly enhance with contrast. It is crucial that the ordering physician indicate a diagnosis of facial palsy, requesting an evaluation of CN-VII along its entire course, not just the intracranial portion.

Extracranial lesions must also be considered in the imaging evaluation of facial weakness/palsy. If the neoplasm appears to be distal to the stylomastoid foramen, as with a highly malignant adenocarcinoma of parotid gland, MRI of the face may identify this tumor. Bone erosion or destruction versus remodeling is another important distinction that can be evaluated only on a bone window CT. Slow-growing benign lesions remodel bone, whereas bone erosion is more indicative of an aggressive or malignant process.

Intrinsic CN-VII Topognostic Testing Studies

Intrinsic CN-VII topognostic testing studies are based on the presence or absence of specific anatomic branch-point functions. With modern imaging studies, these are used less often but are occasionally valuable.

The Schirmer test of lacrimal flow depends on an intact geniculate ganglion, the site of the most proximal anatomic branch point along the course of CN-VII, giving rise to the greater superficial petrosal nerve. The greater superficial petrosal nerve carries autonomic fibers to the lacrimal gland. Decreased lacrimation based on Schirmer testing suggests involvement of the greater superficial petrosal nerve, or CN-VII proximal to the ganglion. An associated facial palsy eliminates the former two possibilities.

EVIDENCE

Allen D, Dunn L. Aciclovir or valacyclovir for Bell's palsy (idiopathic facial paralysis). Cochrane Database Syst Rev 2004;(3):CD001869. *Review of data from three randomized studies including 246 patients found inconclusive evidence in regard to antiviral use in Bell palsy.*

Engström M, Berg T, Stjernquist-Desatnik A, et al. Prednisolone and valacyclovir in Bell's palsy: a randomised, double-blind, placebo-controlled, multicentre trial. Lancet Neurol 2008 Nov; 976-977, 993-1000. *A randomized, double-blind, placebo-controlled, multicenter trial of patients aged 18–75 years* who sought care directly or were referred from emergency departments or general practitioners within 72 hours of onset of acute Bell palsy. Prednisone was effective but acyclovir was of no value.

Grogan PM, Gronseth GS. Practice parameter: steroids, acyclovir, and surgery for Bell's palsy (an evidence-based review): report of the Quality Standards Subcommittee of the American Academy of Neurology. Neurology 2001;56:830-836. *This review summarizes available evidence for the treatment of Bell palsy.*

Halperin JJ, Shapiro ED, Logigian E, et al. Practice Parameter: Treatment of nervous system Lyme disease (Evidence-based review). Report of the Quality Standards Subcommittee of the American Academy of Neurology. Neurology 2007;69:91-102. *This review summarizes available evidence on treatment of neuroborreliosis and issues evidence-based recommendations. Some of the controversies are also discussed.*

Sullivan FM, Swan IRC, Donnan PT, et al. Early treatment with prednisolone or acyclovir in Bell's palsy. N Engl J Med 2007;357:1598-1607. *This well-conducted randomized, multicenter, placebo-controlled trial compares effectiveness of early treatment with corticosteroids, acyclovir, or both, on outcome of patients with Bell palsy.*

ADDITIONAL RESOURCES

Ang KL, Jones NS. Melkersson-Rosenthal syndrome. J Laryngol Otol 2002;116:386-388. *Differential diagnosis of MRS is discussed.*

Finsterer J. Management of peripheral facial palsy. Eur Arch Otorhinolaryngol 2008;265:743-752. *This paper provides an excellent up-to-date review of idiopathic peripheral facial paralysis.*

Grose C, Bonthius D, Afifi AK. Chickenpox and the geniculate ganglion: facial nerve palsy, Ramsay Hunt syndrome and acyclovir treatment. Pediatr Infect Dis J 2002;21:615-617. *This review suggests that facial palsy associated with VZV infection has poorer outcome than Bell palsy, and recommends the use of acyclovir.*

Keane JR. Bilateral seventh nerve palsy: analysis of 43 cases and review of the literature. Neurology 1994;44:1198-1202. *Differential diagnosis of facial diplegia is discussed.*

Yanagihara N, Hato N, Murakami S, et al. Transmastoid decompression as a treatment of Bell's palsy. Otolaryngol Head Neck Surg 2001;124(3):282-286. *In this study, 58 patients with severe palsy underwent transmastoid decompression after steroid treatment and had better outcomes compared to 43 patients treated conservatively.*

8

Cranial Nerve VIII: Auditory and Vestibular

Kinan K. Hreib, Ellen Choi, and Peter J. Catalano

AUDITORY NERVE

Clinical Vignette

A 68-year-old man presented with sudden onset of unilateral right-sided hearing loss. He stated that this was preceded by several months of constant ringing in his right ear. He had a history of hypertension and type 2 diabetes mellitus that was well controlled by oral hypoglycemic agents. He had no recent head trauma or previous surgeries. His only medications included atenolol and glyburide. There was no family history of hearing loss. He did not have a history of excess noise exposure or recent travel. No other otolaryngologic symptoms were reported.

On examination, his tympanic membranes (TMs) were normal. The Weber test lateralized the tuning fork to the side opposite the hearing loss. Rinne's test results were normal. The rest of the head and neck examination was unremarkable.

Complete blood count was normal, and a fluorescent treponemal antibody absorption blood test was negative. The patient received a baseline audiogram demonstrating a right ear sensorineural hearing deficit predominantly in the higher frequencies. Brain MRI failed to demonstrate any mass lesion. A brainstem auditory evoked response (BAER) study was performed and revealed a prolonged interaural wave I–III latency, compatible with a retrocochlear process.

S udden unilateral hearing loss, such as in the above vignette, in the absence of a tumor or lesion involving the vestibular nerve and with a history of diabetes is often attributable to microvascular infarction of the auditory nerve. However, sudden unprovoked hearing loss is not uncommon in patients without microvascular risk factors and the cause, in many cases, remains unknown.

ANATOMY

The eighth cranial nerve (CN-VIII) is actually composed of two separate portions: the vestibular and cochlear nerves (vestibulocochlear nerve). The vestibular nerve is responsible for efferent and afferent fibers that control balance and equilibrium (see next section). The cochlear nerve, also called the auditory nerve, carries efferent and afferent fibers for hearing. To understand dysfunction of the auditory nerve, a brief description of the human hearing mechanism is required.

Sound waves travel through the external auditory canal and vibrate the TM, which in turn produces motion of the middle ear ossicles (incus, malleus, and stapes). The vibrations are transmitted through the oval window at the footplate of the stapes, causing a wave to travel through the endolymphatic fluid of the cochlea of the inner ear. The fluid waves vibrate the organ of Corti's basilar membrane, stimulating inner and outer hair cells (Fig. 8-1). Hair cells, receptors of the sensorineural system, transmit action potentials to bipolar neurons, the bodies of which are in the spiral ganglion.

Afferent fibers projecting toward the CNS comprise the auditory nerve (Fig. 8-2). They travel to the dorsal and ventral cochlear nuclei located in the caudolateral pons. Most of the secondary neurons project contralaterally across the midline to the superior olivary nucleus and then travel up the lateral lemniscus into the inferior colliculus of the midbrain. Decussating fibers from the cochlear nucleus to the superior olivary nucleus are located in the trapezoid bodies and also in the base of the pons. Fibers from the inferior colliculus continue to travel rostrally to the medial geniculate body of the thalamus and then terminate in the auditory cortex located in the transverse temporal gyri of Heschl.

CLINICAL PRESENTATION

History

Hearing loss can result from pathologic conditions anywhere along the anatomic pathway for hearing. It may spare the auditory nerve, such as in middle ear pathology (e.g., serous otitis media) or involve the auditory nerve (e.g., acoustic tumors). Sensorineural hearing loss (SNHL) is a hearing deficit from dysfunction of the cochlea (sensory), the auditory nerve (neural), or any part of the central auditory pathway. Auditory nerve dysfunction usually results in tinnitus, SNHL, or both. A targeted history and physical examination narrow the diagnosis. The temporal profile of symptom onset (i.e., sudden, progressive, fluctuating, or stable) is critical.

Tinnitus presents with or without concomitant SNHL and is classified into two groups. *Subjective tinnitus*, the most common, is heard solely by the patient. It can range from soft fluctuating ringing noise to loud constant debilitating roar. The cause of subjective tinnitus is usually unknown but it can often be associated with exposure to loud noise, ototoxic drugs (such as aspirin, cisplatinum, and aminoglycosides), acoustic tumors, Ménière disease, and cochlear otosclerosis. *Objective tinnitus* is heard by the patient and the examiner and is usually not a sign of auditory nerve dysfunction. Pulsatile tinnitus is usually secondary to vascular causes, such as arteriovenous malformations or glomus tumors. Middle ear effusions, as in serous otitis media, can magnify vascular pulsations from the nearby internal carotid artery and produce vascular tinnitus. Clicking tinnitus is secondary to temporomandibular joint disease, palatal myoclonus, or spontaneous contraction of the middle ear muscles.

Determining the laterality of hearing loss is essential. Bilateral deficits occur in processes such as ototoxicity, noise exposure, and hearing loss related to aging (presbycusis). Unilateral hearing loss raises the concern of neoplastic, vascular, neurologic, or infectious etiologies. Fluctuation of hearing is seen in

Weber Test

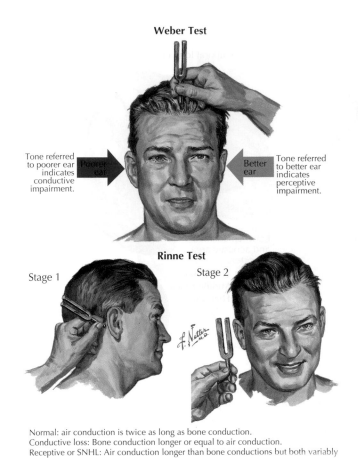

Tone referred to poorer ear indicates conductive impairment.

Poorer ear

Better ear

Tone referred to better ear indicates perceptive impairment.

Rinne Test

Stage 1

Stage 2

Normal: air conduction is twice as long as bone conduction.
Conductive loss: Bone conduction longer or equal to air conduction.
Receptive or SNHL: Air conduction longer than bone conductions but both variably shortened.

Figure 8-3 Hearing Tests: Weber and Rinne.

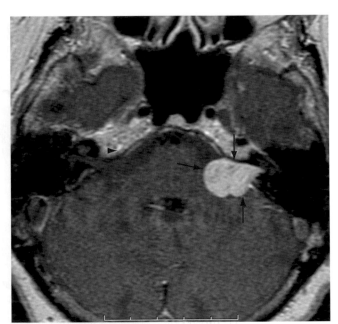

Axial T1-weighted, post-gadolinium-enhanced fat-saturated MR image shows an enhanced mass (arrows) widening the medial left internal auditory canal and extending into the CP angle with distortion of the pons. The right side is normal (arrowhead).

Figure 8-4 Vestibular Schwannoma.

peaks characterize the BAER, corresponding to specific anatomic points within the auditory pathway: I, CN-VIII action potential; II, cochlear nucleus; III, olivary complex; IV, lateral lemniscus; and V, inferior colliculus. A change in peak morphology and latency helps localize the pathologic condition.

DIFFERENTIAL DIAGNOSIS

Idiopathic, sudden SNHL is generally defined as loss that develops over 12 hours or less. However, a broad differential of sudden SNHL includes Ménière disease, neoplasms, vascular disorders, viral infections, MS, and rarely, hematologic disorders.

Ménière Disease

Ménière disease is an idiopathic process characterized by a combination of episodic vertigo, fluctuating SNHL, tinnitus, and aural fullness. Vestibular symptoms are usually the main complaint. Patients with Ménière disease likely constitute less than 5% of all patients with SNHL. However, a condition called cochlear Ménière produces only SNHL and is considered a "diagnosis of exclusion" as there are no specific tests for it.

Neoplasms

In any case of sudden, unilateral hearing loss, neoplastic lesions, although rare, should be considered in the differential until

excluded by diagnostic or radiologic testing. Vestibular schwannomas (also known as acoustic neuromas) are benign tumors arising from the Schwann cells of CN-VIII and account for 6% of all intracranial tumors (Fig. 8-4). These occur on the vestibular portion of CN-VIII and involve the adjacent cochlear division by compression against the bony walls of the internal auditory canal. Less commonly, neuromas can also arise directly from the cochlear nerve.

Hearing loss is the most commonly reported symptom, occurring at some point in approximately 95% of patients with vestibular schwannoma. Progressive hearing loss generally results from stretching or compression of the cochlear nerve as the tumor grows. In contrast, when hearing loss is precipitous, it is thought to be secondary to occlusion of the internal auditory artery supplying the cochlea. Tinnitus with acoustic neuromas is typically high pitched, continuous, and unilateral. Paradoxically, vestibular symptoms are not frequently seen with vestibular nerve schwannomas because as these lesions grow, the contralateral vestibular system gradually adjusts to the imbalance, preventing any significant or longstanding vestibular symptomatology. Larger tumors occasionally lead to facial or trigeminal nerve involvement with symptoms of facial paralysis or paresthesias, respectively.

Before MRI, BAERs were the diagnostic test of choice for acoustic neuromas, with a sensitivity of 93–98%. The sensitivity is significantly lower with tumors less than 1 cm (58%). MRI will detect smaller tumors in patients who have had normal BAERs.

Vascular Etiologies

Vertebrobasilar stroke is another cause of sudden, unilateral SNHL with potentially devastating effects. Distinguishing whether hearing loss results from microvascular disease or a brainstem infarct is vital. The anterior inferior cerebellar artery supplies blood to the inferolateral portion of the pons, CN-VII, the spinal trigeminal tract, and the inferior cerebellum. A stroke from occlusion of this artery causes an infarct of the ipsilateral pons, creating a myriad of symptoms: ipsilateral hearing loss and vestibular symptoms, gait ataxia, conjugate gaze palsy, ipsilateral facial paralysis and often contralateral loss of pain and temperature sensation in the extremities (see Chapter 55).

Computed tomography is usually the initial imaging study and excludes hemorrhagic infarction within the cerebellum and brainstem. MRI and MR angiography, however, provides better definition when available and concomitant imaging of the major vessels of the circle of Willis.

Unilateral hearing loss also occurs secondary to occlusion of the cochlear blood supply from the internal auditory artery, a terminal branch of the anterior inferior cerebellar artery, or the basilar artery. This usually occurs secondary to compression by an acoustic neuroma in the internal auditory canal, but a thrombotic, vasculitis, or rarely embolic event can also be the cause.

Microvascular disease due to diabetes and hypertension is linked to sudden, unilateral hearing loss, and the mechanism is thought to be similar to other diabetic cranial neuropathies with involvement of the vaso nervosum and nerve microinfarction.

Multiple Sclerosis

Sensorineural hearing loss appears as a retrocochlear manifestation in approximately 4–10% of patients with MS. However, it is rare for SNHL to be the initial or sole presentation. Usually, hearing loss is sudden but resolves within weeks of treatment. If MS is suspected, CSF evaluation may be helpful; increased IgG index and oligoclonal bands in gel electrophoresis suggest MS. Audiometric testing can show normal or decreased speech discrimination in proportion with pure-tone threshold. MRI is the radiologic study of choice and can show periventricular white matter lesions on T2-weighted images within the inferior colliculus or cochlear nucleus.

Infections

Various viral and bacterial infections can cause sudden hearing loss. Herpes zoster oticus usually affects the sensory portion of the facial nerve, creating herpetic skin eruption around the auricle and in the external auditory canal with secondary inflammation and edema. Measles and mumps, previously a relatively common cause of hearing loss in children, have now been largely eliminated as a result of widespread vaccination in economically privileged countries.

Sudden deafness following a flu-like illness or nonspecific viral processes are considered a common cause of sudden hearing loss, especially when no vestibular symptoms coexist. The mechanism of action is unknown and it, therefore, should be considered a "diagnosis of exclusion."

Otosyphilis is defined as a positive syphilis serologic result in the setting of unexplained SNHL. The hearing loss, usually a late manifestation of the disease, begins at higher frequencies and can progress to bilateral cochlear and vestibular dysfunction. The exact causal mechanism is unknown; however,

proposed theories include microvascular disease, direct spirochetal infiltration of the perilymph, and temporal bone osteitis. Diagnostic tests for syphilis, a treatable cause of SNHL, include the fluorescent treponemal antibody absorption blood test.

Hematologic Disorders

Leukemia, sickle cell anemia, polycythemia, and macroglobulinemia can cause sudden SNHL, usually from sludging, hemorrhage into the inner ear, or microthrombi. A careful history, a complete blood count and coagulation studies can exclude hematologic causes.

Presbycusis

The most common cause of slowly progressive, bilateral, symmetric, high-frequency hearing loss that develops with increasing age, presbycusis originates from a pathologic condition that decreases the number of hair cells within the organ of Corti. It has an almost universal incidence in the elderly. Multiple factors determine its progression rate. Three of the most common are genetic predisposition, nerve toxins, particularly medications, and history of long exposure to loud noises.

Otosclerosis

Otosclerosis is the most common cause of conductive hearing loss in young adults and often affects both ears. It occurs as a result of abnormal ossicle growth followed by sclerosis of bone in the middle ear and often affects the stapedial connection to the oval window, thus hindering transmission of sound waves to the inner ear. Rare cases of associated cochlear sclerosis and SNHL have been described. Hearing loss is gradual, and individuals report hearing better in noisy environments. Some patients may have tinnitus and dizziness. There are familial tendencies but with variable expression, and middle-aged women are most at risk. An audiogram and tympanogram help in making a diagnosis, and stapedectomy usually improves hearing.

TREATMENT

When the primary cause of hearing loss is identified, such as an acoustic neuroma or syphilis, therapy is straightforward and potentially remediable depending on when the lesion is diagnosed in the illness course. There is no treatment of vascular lesions with infarction of the auditory nerve. However, for common disorders such as presbycusis, a variety of high-technology hearing-enhancing modalities can be designed, with the aid of an otologist, to meet the patient's needs.

VESTIBULAR NERVE

Clinical Vignette

A 65-year-old woman came to the emergency department with a chief complaint of "dizziness." At 3:00 AM, she had awoken to an odd feeling in her head, which was

ETIOLOGIC CLASSIFICATION OF PERIPHERAL VESTIBULOPATHIES

Etiologic classification of peripheral vestibulopathies is initially based on symptoms and the presence of hearing loss. When symptoms persist for days to weeks with concomitant cochlear symptoms, such as hearing loss and tinnitus, a diagnosis of **labyrinthitis** is made once other causes are excluded. Although labyrinthitis is presumably of viral origin, certain structural pathologic conditions, including erosive cholesteatoma, temporal bone trauma or fistula, and central pathophysiologic mechanisms, need to be excluded.

Ménière disease is characterized by recurrent vertigo, fluctuating sensory neural hearing loss, tinnitus, and aural fullness. The prevalence of the disease ranges from 500 to 1000 per million, with no difference in regard to gender. Patients often present in their fourth decade, usually with unilateral symptoms, although many will develop bilateral symptoms within a few years. Initial presentation can simply be aural fullness or short bouts of vertigo that resolve spontaneously. Vertigo, even in advanced stages, rarely lasts more than 2 hours and is nonpositional. Patients can have multiple attacks per month or only one every few years. In the early stages of the disease, symptoms often appear in isolation, and the hearing deficit is not initially noticeable, rendering diagnosis difficult. As the disease progresses, prominent low-frequency hearing loss appears, and the symptoms are more prolonged and recur more frequently. Some patients are left with a chronic sense of imbalance.

The underlying pathophysiology of Ménière disease is presumably related to either excessive production or decreased absorption of endolymph. An autoimmune etiology has been proposed, but the exact mechanism remains unclear. Diagnostic tests such as glycerol dehydration test and audiometry have high sensitivity for Ménière disease, especially if performed during an attack. Other tests such as electrocochleography and vestibular evoked myogenic potentials can be helpful for diagnosis or staging the disease. Serologic tests to exclude co-morbid conditions include thyroid function test, antinuclear antibody, rheumatoid factor, complement antibodies, serum immunoglobulin levels, anticardiolipin antibodies, C-reactive protein, syphilis, and Lyme treponemal titer. Symptomatic treatment includes antiemetics, benzodiazepines, diuretics, and a low salt diet. Avoidance of alcohol, caffeine, nicotine, and stress may help. Reports have suggested a role for antiviral medications and immunosuppressant drugs, at least for short-term control of symptoms. Intratympanic instillation of drugs such as dexamethasone may be helpful to control vertigo for months but has less effect on hearing loss. Intratympanic gentamicin and streptomycin, strong vestibular toxins, are used as a last resort to eliminate residual vestibular function in cases of intractable vertigo. Endolymphatic sac decompression and shunting, as well as surgical labyrinthectomy and vestibular neurectomy, have also been used in refractory cases.

Vestibular neuritis is characterized by prolonged vertigo without hearing loss. This is a cranial mononeuropathy limited to the vestibular division of CN-VIII. Diagnosis is often difficult in patients with recurrent true vertiginous episodes lasting hours, without associated cochlear symptomatology.

Initially, it is important to exclude vertebrobasilar TIAs, particularly in those with vascular risk factors or in young persons with associated recent neck injury and possible vertebral artery dissection. However, it is rare for vertigo to be the sole manifestation of a TIA, emphasizing the importance of a careful history, as patients may overlook seemingly less important symptoms that could lead to a central diagnosis and may focus on the vertigo. Occasionally, early Ménière disease is diagnosed in some patients when hearing loss eventually develops.

TYPES OF VERTIGO AND DISORDERS

Benign paroxysmal positional vertigo (BPPV) is the most common cause of vertigo in the elderly. The typical presentation is that of recurrent bouts of position-dependent vertigo with either a transient spinning sensation or an illusion of side to side movement. Spells are brief, lasting seconds to minutes, and often associated with nausea and sometimes vomiting. Symptoms occur with sudden shift in position, when turning in bed, or with neck extension, as while looking up or while in a dentist or hairdresser chair. Often patients become anxious and guard against fast movements. Episodes become gradually shorter and symptoms improve over 72 hours but can occasionally linger for many days. BPPV results from otolith debris errantly entering the semicircular canals, usually the posterior canal, rendering them gravitationally sensitive with the solid material acting as a plunger or weight within the fluid-filled system. Symptoms become less defined when the horizontal or superior canal is involved or bilateral vestibular disruptions are present. Although many cases can be diagnosed in the emergency department or outpatient clinic, BPPV patients are often referred either to neurology or otolaryngology specialists. When the presentation is not typical, tests such as brain MR and electronystagmograms are done to exclude other pathology. Recurrent symptoms can lead to vascular evaluations to rule out possible vertebral artery compromise. Although unusual, vertigo as the sole manifestation of vertebrobasilar disease has been reported, especially with posterior inferior cerebellar artery ischemia, and caution is advised when vascular risk factors are present in those with atypical presentations. However, distinct positionally inducible isolated vertigo remains more a feature of a peripheral vestibulopathy than of cerebral ischemia.

The diagnosis of BPPV in large part depends on the clinical history and bedside testing. The Dix-Hallpike maneuver, when performed and interpreted properly is diagnostic. Studies suggest that the Dix-Hallpike maneuver has a sensitivity and specificity of approximately 75%. In our experience the ability to perform the maneuver properly in anxious patients fearful of provocative maneuvers is a major limiting factor for accurate evaluation. Risk factors for BPPV include recent head trauma (which can be relatively minor); otologic surgery or disease; habitual unusual positioning such as is a daily occurrence for plumbers, mechanics, and yoga enthusiasts; or advanced age. Particle repositioning maneuvers or canalith repositioning maneuver is the main treatment for benign paroxysmal positional vertigo (Fig. 8-7). Another maneuver known as the liberatory maneuver, developed by Semont et al., relies on rapidly swinging the patient from lying initially on the involved side

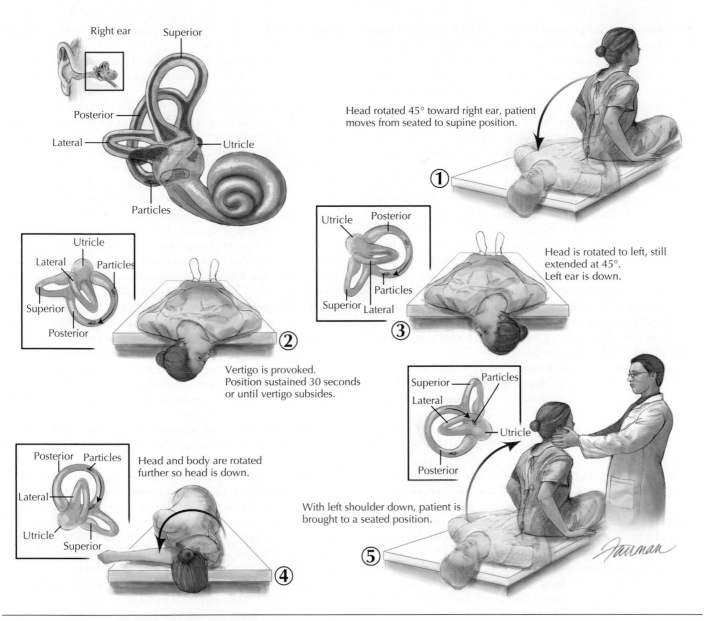

Right ear Superior

Posterior

Lateral

Utricle

Particles

Head rotated 45° toward right ear, patient moves from seated to supine position.

①

Utricle

Lateral Particles

Superior

Posterior

Vertigo is provoked.
Position sustained 30 seconds or until vertigo subsides.

②

Utricle Posterior

Particles

Superior Lateral

Head is rotated to left, still extended at 45°.
Left ear is down.

③

Posterior Particles

Lateral

Utricle

Superior

Head and body are rotated further so head is down.

④

Superior Particles

Lateral

Utricle

Posterior

With left shoulder down, patient is brought to a seated position.

⑤

Figure 8-7 Canalith Repositioning (Epley) Maneuver.

through 180 degrees to the opposite, uninvolved side. Unfortunately any repositioning maneuver can be limited by the inability of the patient to physically participate (musculoskeletal and orthopedic limitations, especially of the head and neck) or when induced symptoms are intolerable. In 5% of patients, symptoms may worsen with repositioning maneuvers in part due to conversion from posterior to horizontal canal involvement. Outcome studies regarding the effectiveness of the canalith repositioning maneuver provide a range of reported success, as most studies rely on subjective reporting, which is inherently unreliable because patients quickly develop adaptive behavior spontaneously. Overall, however, there is evidence to favor repositioning maneuvers, with some studies demonstrating resolution of symptoms in 90% of patients after only one treatment. Self-administered maneuvers in combination with guided treatments can often help expedite improvement in the remaining patients. Successful treatment with the repositioning

maneuvers does not influence recurrence rate, which averages around 20% over a 20-month period. Persistent vertigo or frequent recurrences of BPPV is uncommon, but under such circumstances surgical occlusion of the posterior semicircular canal with bone grafts and fibrin glue is an effective treatment. Medications can provide temporary relief by controlling nausea and suppressing the vestibular responses. Meclizine and benzodiazepines are the most frequently prescribed medications but can be sedating and should be used only for a few days.

Chronic vestibulopathies are less likely to cause vertigo, because their duration allows for CNS compensation. Acoustic neuromas and other slow-growing neoplasms affecting CN-VIII may cause unilateral tinnitus, hearing loss, and abnormal hypoactive caloric responses on electronystagmogram. However, these tumors rarely present with vertigo.

Bilateral vestibulopathy typically do not cause vertigo or a sensation of turning. However, bilateral vestibular disruption does affect the vestibular–ocular reflex, which stabilizes visual perception during head motion. The main symptoms in these cases are a sense of imbalance, especially when visual cues are altered (unequal surface, dim illumination, and quick head movements), and oscillopsia (see below). Vestibulotoxic agents, such as aminoglycosides, alcohol, and heavy metals, can lead to transient or permanent vestibular damage, but bilateral vestibular hypo-function can also occur in otherwise healthy adults (idiopathic) or can result from a genetic predisposition.

Oscillopsia, or failure to stabilize vision during head movement, can cause bobbing visual perception and loss of dynamic visual acuity while walking. Because some patients call this "dizziness," a close history is needed to help differentiate it from true vertigo. In addition to bilateral peripheral vestibulopathies, oscillopsia can be seen with central lesions involving the brainstem and cerebellar, particularly mass lesion around the foramen magnum. It is typically seen in patients with the Arnold–Chiari syndrome, a developmental condition often associated with syringomyelia and syringobulbia, and is rarely observed in patients with multiple sclerosis. This phenomenon is usually binocular, and monocular symptoms raise the possibility of ocular muscle myokymia instead.

Canal dehiscence syndrome, first described in 1998 by Lloyd B. Minor, is caused by thinning or developmental absence of part of the temporal bone overlying the superior semicircular canal leading to an extra direct conduit for impulses into the inner ear in addition to normal conduction through the oval window. Canal dehiscence presents with a variety of symptoms including a sensation of ear blockage that is relieved with Valsalva maneuver, hyperacusis, sound distortion, conductive hearing loss, and chronic imbalance. Abrupt vertigo, disequilibrium, nystagmus, oscillopsia, and nausea induced by external sounds and even one's own voice or pulsations occur in some cases and is known as the Tullio phenomenon. Clinical diagnosis, however, can be difficult, as symptoms may often be nonspecific or occur in isolation. Some seemingly bizarre complaints, such as hearing louder than usual gastric noises and being aware of the eyeballs moving in the socket, are reported. Pulsatile tinnitus is also common and often leads to a suspicion of vascular causes.

A combination of tests helps establish the diagnosis of canal dehiscence and differentiates it from conditions such as Ménière disease or perilymphatic fistulas. A normal vestibular-evoked myogenic response in the presence of temporal bone abnormalities seen on high-resolution CT scan has more than 90% sensitivity and specificity. Low frequency conductive hearing with normal tympanometry and an intact acoustic reflex provides further support. A variety of surgical techniques to repair or plug the bone around the superior semicircular have been developed.

DIAGNOSTIC APPROACH

A **complete neurologic examination** is of the utmost importance in the evaluation of dizziness or vertigo. When one sensory vestibular mechanism is absent, the remaining sensory inputs are used to elicit corrective postural reactions. Superimposed neurologic disorders, including stroke, Parkinson disease, cerebellar pathology, or peripheral neuropathy, may affect the potential of the nervous system to compensate, and symptoms are amplified significantly.

Electronystagmogram (ENG): This test is intended to evaluate the effects of vestibular input on the ocular system. Disorders of both the otoliths and the vestibular nerve can cause abnormalities on the ENG. The two basic elements of the ENG include the equivalent of cold calorics and the second is rotatory chair testing. Vestibular nerve abnormalities can manifest as a delay in conduction of the vestibular–ocular reflex via the medial longitudinal fasciculus. Otolith dysfunction is not easily detected by this test, however, and false-negative results are common. Rotatory chair testing, on the other hand, may elicit abnormal responses in patients with otolith dysfunction as well as in those with vestibular nerve dysfunction. The tests are affected by medications and patient cooperation and depend on comparison to standard tables or to the normal side. The results should be interpreted with the clinical presentation and potential confounding variables taken into account.

Dynamic posturography is a complex testing modality that defines the extent to which a patient is able to use visual, somatosensory, and vestibular input for postural control. The patient stands on a shifting platform in front of a simulated visual field presented at different angles. The postural response to various shifts can be assessed and quantitated. To date, however, the value of this test is still questionable, although it is sometimes used for designing rehabilitation strategies.

The clinical test of sensory interaction and balance uses a combination of two visual (eyes open or closed) and two support surface (soft unstable, firm stable) conditions to clinically measure a patient's sensory interaction for postural stability. The **Romberg (stationary) and sharpened Romberg (tandem stance) test** with eyes open and eyes closed, and unilateral standing with eyes open and eyes closed are not specific for postural deficits secondary to vestibular pathologic conditions. However, patients with vestibular damage may demonstrate increased sway or falling during these tests.

Dynamic tests, such as floor walking with the eyes closed, measure tandem walking for up to 10 steps. Persons with acute or chronic vestibular disorders may fail this test based on established age-related norms.

Several performance tests are used to establish a baseline function analysis and measure outcome in individuals with impairments of static and dynamic postural control. These include the Timed Up and Go Test, the Dynamic Gait Index, and the Berg Balance Scale.

The **Timed Up and Go** test measures the time required to rise from a standard chair, walk 10 feet, return to that chair, and sit. The norm for neurologically intact older adults is 10–12 seconds. The results may be a predictor for falls in community-dwelling elders. There is a maximum of 14 seconds for elders at minimal risk for falls and less than 30 seconds for elders who are dependent on assistance for ambulation in the community. There is no threshold established for patients with vestibular disorders.

The Dynamic Gait Index measures the ability to modify gait in response to eight different tasks during ambulation. Each task is given a score of 0 to –3. A score of 11 ± 4 is found in older adults with a history of falls but no neurologic disorders.

The Berg Balance Scale uses 14 test-specific items rated 0–4 that measure postural control during functionally related tasks. These require anticipatory abilities and are performed only while sitting and standing. Test scores are a good predictor of elderly fall risk. Scores less than 45 were associated with an increased risk for falls; scores less than 36 were associated with a 100% risk of falls.

GENERAL TREATMENT CONSIDERATIONS

Rehabilitation

Many vestibular rehabilitation programs provide a range of treatment modalities aimed to facilitate acute recovery and ongoing compensation programs for patients with varying degrees of residual vestibular deficit. Some are useful for acute or chronic vestibular lesions and are equally applicable to vertigo, dizziness, and dysequilibrium in general.

Pharmacologic Therapy

Recent studies suggest that methylprednisolone significantly improves the recovery of peripheral vestibular neuritis, whereas valacyclovir does not. Treatment is begun with 100 mg daily with reduction by 20 mg every third day, eventually down to 10 mg daily. Vestibular suppressant medications such as meclizine, scopolamine, and benzodiazepines are useful for relief of acute symptoms of vertigo, dizziness, and dysequilibrium from any vestibular process. However, long-term use interferes with central vestibular compensation mechanisms and should preferably be avoided.

Nonpharmacologic Therapy

Vestibular compensation results from active neuronal changes in the cerebellum and the brainstem in response to sensory conflicts created by vestibular pathology. Despite spontaneous "recovery," patients still experience disequilibrium, motion-provoked vertigo, or both because the vestibular system, inhibited to a certain degree by the cerebellum, is unable to respond appropriately to labyrinthine input produced by normal head movement.

Because movement provokes a sense of dysequilibrium and vertigo, patients with vestibular disorders may restrict their activity level and trunk and head movements to avoid these symptoms. This provides for greater short-term compensatory stability but interferes with long-term recovery if patients are not challenged to increase movement to facilitate vestibular compensation. Educating patients about vestibular function encourages and reassures them to safely increase their activity level even though early recovery movement provokes symptoms.

Initially, an assistive device such as a cane or walker may be recommended. Sensory input through the upper extremity from a cane or light touch through fingertips can reduce postural sway in patients without proper vestibular function.

Motor organization exercises help to improve standing, ambulation, and functional activities such as moving at various speeds, changing directions, and maneuvering around obstacles.

Weekly therapy visits for 4–12 weeks help to monitor the effectiveness of assigned home exercise programs. Treatment success depends on the nature of the primary underlying neurologic dysfunction. Peripheral vestibular disorders such as BPPV and stable vestibular hypofunction are most amenable to treatment. In contrast, individuals with primary CNS disorders have poorer outcomes but still demonstrate reduced symptomatology with treatment.

Other factors influencing treatment effectiveness include the degree of initial disability and a more recent time of onset. Comorbidities, such as underlying musculoskeletal dysfunction and other neurologic impairments, and patient compliance also affect outcomes. Elderly patients often require longer treatment times to reach maximum benefit.

ADDITIONAL RESOURCES

AUDITORY

Duck SW, Prazma J, Bennett PS, et al. Interaction between hypertension and diabetes mellitus in the pathogenesis of sensorineural hearing loss. Laryngoscope 1997;107:1596-1605.

Ho SY, Kveton JF. Acoustic neuroma: assessment and management. Otolaryngol Clin N Am 2002;35:393-404.

Rudick RA. Multiple sclerosis and demyelinating conditions of the central nervous system. In: Goldman L, Ausiello D, editors. Cecil Textbook of Medicine. 22nd ed. Philadelphia, Pa: WB Saunders Co; 2004. p. 2320-2327.

Schmidt RJ, Sataloff RT, Newman J, et al. The sensitivity of auditory brainstem response testing for the diagnosis of acoustic neuromas. Arch Otolaryngol Head Neck Surg 2001;127:19-22.

Sismanis A. Pulsatile tinnitus. Otolaryngol Clin N Am 2003;36:389-402.

VESTIBULAR

Furman J, Cass S. Benign paroxysmal positional vertigo. N Engl J Med 1999;341:1590-1596.

Furman J, Whitney S. Central causes of dizziness. Phys Ther 2000;80:179-187.

Helminski JO, Zee DS, Janssen I, Hain TC. Effectiveness of particle repositioning maneuvers in the treatment of benign paroxysmal positional vertigo: a systematic review. Phys Ther 2010;90:663-678.

Herdman S. Advances in the treatment of vestibular disorders. Phys Ther 1997;77:602-618.

Horak FB, Jones-Rycewiccz C, Black FO, et al. Effects of vestibular rehabilitation on dizziness and imbalance. Otolaryngol Head Neck Surg 1992;106:175-180.

Hotson J, Baloh R. Acute vestibular syndrome. N Engl J Med 1998;339:680-685.

Norrving B, Magnusson M, Holtas S. Isolated acute vertigo in the elderly: vestibular or vascular disease? Acta Neurol Scand 1995;91:43-48.

Podsialdo D, Richardson S. The timed "Up & Go": a test of basic functional mobility for frail elderly persons. J Am Geriatr Soc 1991;39:142-148.

Shumway-Cook A, Brauer S, Woollacott M. Predicting the probability for falls in community-dwelling older adults using the timed up and go test. Phys Ther 2000;80:896-903.

Strupp M, Zingler VC, Arbusow V, et al. Methylprednisolone, valacyclovir, or the combination for vestibular neuritis. N Engl J Med 2004;351:354-361.

Vassiliou A, Vlastarakos PV, Maragoudakis P, et al. Meniere's disease: still a mystery disease with difficult differential diagnosis. Ann Indian Acad Neurol 2011;14:12-18.

Zhou G, Gopen Q, Poe DS. Clinical and diagnostic characterization of canal dehiscence syndrome: a great otologic mimicker. Otol Neurotol 2007;28:920-926.

Cranial Nerves IX and X: Glossopharyngeal and Vagus

9

Eva M. Michalakis, Allison Gudis Jackson, Peter J. Catalano, and Timothy D. Anderson

CRANIAL NERVE IX: GLOSSOPHARYNGEAL NERVE AND SWALLOWING

Clinical Vignette

A 70-year-old man with a history of hypertension and paroxysmal atrial fibrillation presented to the emergency department with acute onset of slurred speech, left-sided paresis, left neglect, and a left inferior quadrantanopsia. MRI revealed a right middle cerebral artery stroke. An initial oral peripheral and cranial nerve examination revealed bilateral depressed gag reflex and diminished soft palate elevation, left central facial weakness, reduced labial retraction, and mild tongue deviation to the right side with protrusion. The patient was to receive nothing per mouth (NPO) and was referred to a speech pathologist.

Clinical swallowing evaluation demonstrated hoarse and moderately dysarthric speech that retained fair intelligibility. Graduated sized boluses of thin liquids, nectar thick liquids, and purees were administered. The patient had significant difficulty with oral containment, bolus formation, and posterior transport through the oral cavity, on the left more than on the right. Posterior placement on the right side facilitated oral swallowing. Reduced orolabial seal benefited from the use of a straw. Attempts to administer a soft solid bolus were unsuccessful because of delayed triggering of oropharyngeal swallow. Mild voice changes after liquids, characterized by a wet vocal quality, indicated laryngeal penetration and possible silent aspiration. The patient was able to clear with cues and to use a throat clear/reswallow strategy. Use of a chin tuck swallowing posture with nectar thick liquids eliminated clinical signs of aspiration.

He was placed on a modified pureed diet with nectar thick liquids, and medications were crushed in applesauce. Aspiration precautions included remaining upright 90° during and 45 minutes after oral intake and single, small boluses. Swallowing strategies included a chin tuck posture and right posterior placement of food in the oral cavity to decrease anterior leakage and to assist in oral transport. A flexible endoscopic evaluation demonstrated bilateral vocal cord movement, but sensory testing revealed severe left laryngopharyngeal sensory deficit and silent aspiration.

Swallowing malfunctioning, or dysphagia, prevents adequate nutrition intake and may predispose to significant aspiration with a risk for potentially fatal pneumonia. Dysphagia occurs in a variety of central and peripheral neurologic disorders and can rarely be the presenting sign of neurologic disease. It is seen with central disorders including acute cerebral infarction, brainstem stroke, Parkinson disease, and demyelinating disease such as multiple sclerosis. Dysphagia may be a prominent and progressive problem in motor neuron disease, syringobulbia, or primary pontomedullary meningeal-based tumors. Peripheral disorders of the nerve (e.g., Guillain-Barré syndrome), neuromuscular junction (e.g., myasthenia gravis), and hereditary or acquired muscle disease (e.g., oculopharyngeal dystrophy, myotonic dystrophy and dermatomyositis) can also compromise swallowing function.

PHYSIOLOGY

Swallowing is a complex process involving motor control with sensory feedback from many anatomic structures within the oral cavity, pharynx, larynx, and esophagus (Fig. 9-1). The trigeminal (CN-V), facial (CN-VII), glossopharyngeal (CN-IX; Fig. 9-2), vagus (CN-X; Fig. 9-3), and hypoglossal (CN-XII) cranial nerves are involved. A "normal swallow" comprises two major components, bolus transport and airway protection. The swallowing process is typically classified into four phases (Fig. 9-4).

1. The **oral preparatory phase** involves voluntary motor function during which food or liquid is taken into the mouth, masticated (CN-V), and mixed with saliva to form a cohesive bolus (Fig. 9-4, nos. *1* and *2*). This phase requires coordination of several cranial nerves and corresponding structures. Tension in the labial and buccal musculature closes the anterior and lateral sulci (CN-VII) while rotary mandible motion produces chewing (CN-V$_3$). Lateral rolling tongue motion (CN-XII) and bulging of the soft palate forward (widening the nasal airway, and sealing the posterior oral cavity) properly positions the bolus for the swallowing (CN-IX). Tongue mobility is the most important neuromuscular function involved in this first phase. The mid and lower divisions of CN-V provide sensory feedback for positioning the bolus. Saliva derived from the parotid, sublingual, and submandibular glands (innervated by secretomotor fibers of CN-IX and -VII) contain digestive enzymes that act as an emollient to soften and shape the bolus.

2. The **oral swallowing phase** is initiated when the tongue (CN-XII) sequentially squeezes the bolus posteriorly against the hard palate and initiates propulsion into the oropharynx (Fig. 9-4, nos. *3* and *4*). Lips and buccal muscles contract (CN-V and CN-VII) with elevation of the velum (CN-V and CN-X) providing the valving process that generates pressure to seal the nasopharynx, preventing reflux and nasal regurgitation. CN-V is responsible for the afferent (sensory) feedback for the entire oral cavity and tongue. The soft palate (CN-IX), critical to containing the bolus within the oral cavity during the oral preparatory phase, now moves posteriorly to allow the bolus to pass through the faucial arches and simultaneously prevent the bolus from entering the nasopharynx. The swallowing reflex is triggered as the bolus passes the anterior tonsillar pillars, which initiates the pharyngeal phase.

Taste for the anterior two thirds of the tongue is carried by CN-VII, whereas the afferent CN-IX controls taste for the posterior one third of the tongue and the posterior pharyngeal wall. CN-X supplies primary innervation to the palatal muscles, pharyngeal constrictors, laryngeal musculature, and cricopharyngeus. Afferent fibers also provide critical sensory feedback from the larynx and esophageal inlet.

3. The **pharyngeal phase** begins with the bolus passing into the throat, triggering the swallowing reflex and causing several pharyngeal physiologic actions to occur simultaneously, allowing food to pass into the esophagus (Fig. 9-4, nos. 5–7). Once pharyngeal swallowing is elicited, essential functions of airway protection occur. Intrinsic laryngeal muscles innervated by CN-X close the larynx at the aryepiglottic, false vocal, and at the true vocal folds, creating a seal that separates the airway from the digestive tract protecting the laryngeal vestibule from foreign material aspiration. The tongue (CN XII) is the major force pushing the bolus through the pharynx. Synergistic actions with CN-X produce pharyngeal peristalsis as it innervates the pharyngeal constrictors and carries afferents from the lower pharynx.

CN-IX mediates the sensory portion of the pharyngeal gag but innervates just 1 muscle, the stylopharyngeus. The absence of the gag reflex is not the sole indicator of a patient's swallowing abilities. A study of the risk of aspiration in patients with dysphagia and absent gag reflexes demonstrated that the majority could tolerate a modified diet. Additionally, the gag reflex was absent in 10–13% of nondysphagic individuals in the control group.

Poor airway protection and delayed triggering of pharyngeal swallow may cause aspiration. When swallowing is inefficient and aspiration occurs, a reflexive cough needs to occur as a respiratory defense against foreign matter. The cough reflex is induced by irritation of afferent CN-IX and CN-X sensory fibers in the larynx, trachea, and larger bronchi (Figs. 9-2 and 9-3). If a reflexive cough is not elicited in response to foreign material within the airway, **silent aspiration** results; it is radiographically documented in 50% of aspiration cases.

CN-IX is the primary afferent of the swallowing response, whereas CN-X is the secondary afferent; both nerves terminate in the **swallowing center** located in the medulla within the nucleus solitarius. Sensory events initiating swallowing occur with stimulation to jaw, posterior tongue, faucial pillars, and upper pharynx and are mediated through CN-V, CN-IX, and CN-X. These afferent fibers converge on the nucleus solitarius in the medulla and communicate with the nucleus ambiguous via interneurons stimulating the motor response.

4. The **esophageal phase** occurs with the passage of the bolus through the cricopharyngeal sphincter, moving over the closed airway and passing the pharyngoesophageal segment into the esophagus via the cricopharyngeal sphincter at the proximal esophagus (Fig. 9-4, nos. 8–10). This area contains the cricopharyngeus muscle that normally keeps the esophagus closed. CN-X mediates the action of the cricopharyngeus, which relaxes to allow food to pass from the hypopharynx into the esophagus.

Elevation and anterior movement of the larynx is the significant mechanical force contributing to the opening of the cricopharyngeal sphincter which, in conjunction with the relaxation of the cricopharyngeus muscle, opens the pharyngoesophageal segment, permitting the passage of food into the esophagus. The sphincter must otherwise remain closed to prevent the entrance of air into the stomach and reflux from the esophagus

into the hypopharynx. CN-X, specifically the efferent fibers from the dorsal nucleus, innervate the involuntary muscles of the esophagus, stomach, small intestine, and portions of the large intestine.

CLINICAL PRESENTATION

Dysphagia, or difficulty swallowing, can result from many causes, including neurologic disorders, both peripheral and central; viral, bacterial, or fungal infections of the upper airway; surgeries or disease processes that directly involve the oral, pharyngeal, or laryngeal structures; and psychogenic mechanisms. Aging and medications may exacerbate dysphagia. A number of antidepressant medications cause xerostomia (reduced salivary flow), affecting bolus formation. Sedative medications may significantly affect swallowing by reducing oropharyngeal coordination for bolus formation and airway protection. Common signs of dysphagia include pocketing of food in the oral cavity, drooling, wet vocal quality during meals, episodes of coughing and throat clearing, and shortness of breath during meals.

Aspiration, the primary concern when dealing with dysphagia, is technically defined as the entry of a foreign substance below the level of the vocal cords into the trachea. Aspiration is a dangerous precursor of aspiration pneumonia. Risk factors include chronic obstructive pulmonary disorders, congestive heart failure, feeding tubes, dependence for oral care and feeding, decreased laryngopharyngeal sensation, medications, and a reduced level of alertness. Any patient with aspiration risk needs to be placed on aspiration precautions and referred for swallowing evaluation before oral intake is initiated.

DIAGNOSTIC APPROACH

Formal assessment of swallowing function through various examinations serves to define the severity of dysphagia and to identify therapeutic strategies to minimize the risk of aspiration. Clinical swallowing evaluation includes the patient history; observations regarding mental awareness and ability to cooperate; oral, peripheral, and cranial nerve examinations; and the overall respiratory status. Various food consistencies are administered with close monitoring of the oral preparatory and pharyngeal phases of swallowing. Based on this initial evaluation, swallowing strategies may be implemented or the need for objective studies may be identified.

Flexible endoscopic evaluation of swallowing with sensory testing (FEES) allows direct evaluation of motor and sensory aspects of the pharyngeal swallow. It requires transnasal passage of a fiberoptic laryngoscope into the hypopharynx to view the larynx and surrounding structures. Laryngeal airway protection and the integrity of the oropharyngeal swallow are assessed by giving various food consistencies tinted with coloring to enhance visualization. Similar to the modified barium swallow (MBS), compensatory strategies and postures are attempted to facilitate improved swallowing function and decrease the risk of aspiration. Velopharyngeal closure, anatomy of the base of the tongue and hypopharynx, abduction and adduction of the vocal folds, pharyngeal musculature, and the patient's ability to manage secretions are assessed. Laryngopharyngeal reflux can also be visualized.

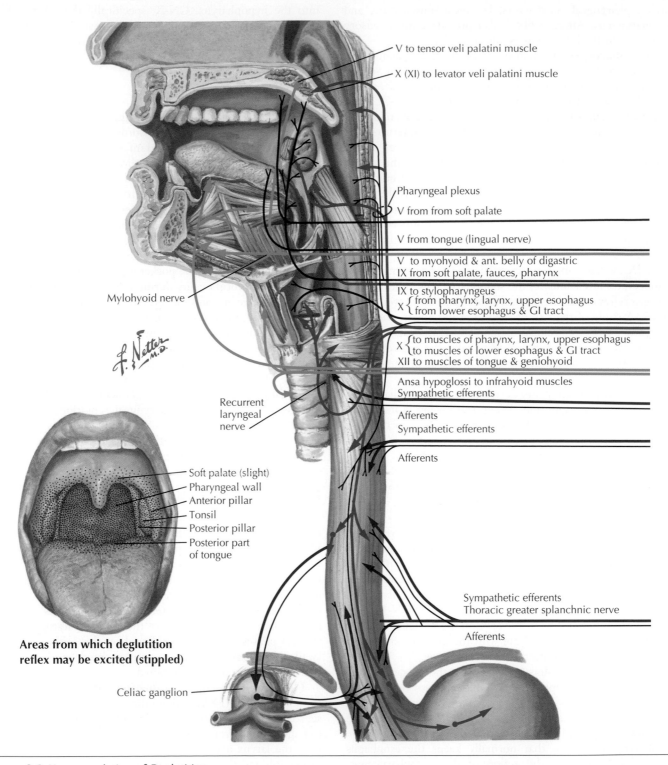

V to tensor veli palatini muscle

X (XI) to levator veli palatini muscle

Pharyngeal plexus

V from from soft palate

V from tongue (lingual nerve)

V to myohyoid & ant. belly of digastric
IX from soft palate, fauces, pharynx

IX to stylopharyngeus
X { from pharynx, larynx, upper esophagus
X { from lower esophagus & GI tract

X { to muscles of pharynx, larynx, upper esophagus
X { to muscles of lower esophagus & GI tract
XII to muscles of tongue & geniohyoid

Ansa hypoglossi to infrahyoid muscles
Sympathetic efferents

Afferents
Sympathetic efferents

Afferents

Sympathetic efferents
Thoracic greater splanchnic nerve

Afferents

Mylohyoid nerve

Recurrent
laryngeal
nerve

Soft palate (slight)
Pharyngeal wall
Anterior pillar
Tonsil
Posterior pillar
Posterior part
of tongue

**Areas from which deglutition
reflex may be excited (stippled)**

Celiac ganglion

Figure 9-1 Neuroregulation of Deglutition.

Modified barium swallow (MBS), also called **videofluoroscopy** or **videopharyngogram**, is a functional evaluation requiring active patient participation. Before scheduling MBS, laryngopharyngeal sensation should be evaluated via FEES to assess the risk of barium aspiration. MBS is performed in conjunction with radiologic examination but differs from the standard barium swallow in that patients ingest graduated sized boluses of various consistencies mixed with barium in the upright position. The primary purpose of MBS is to determine appropriate therapeutic intervention strategies to facilitate safe

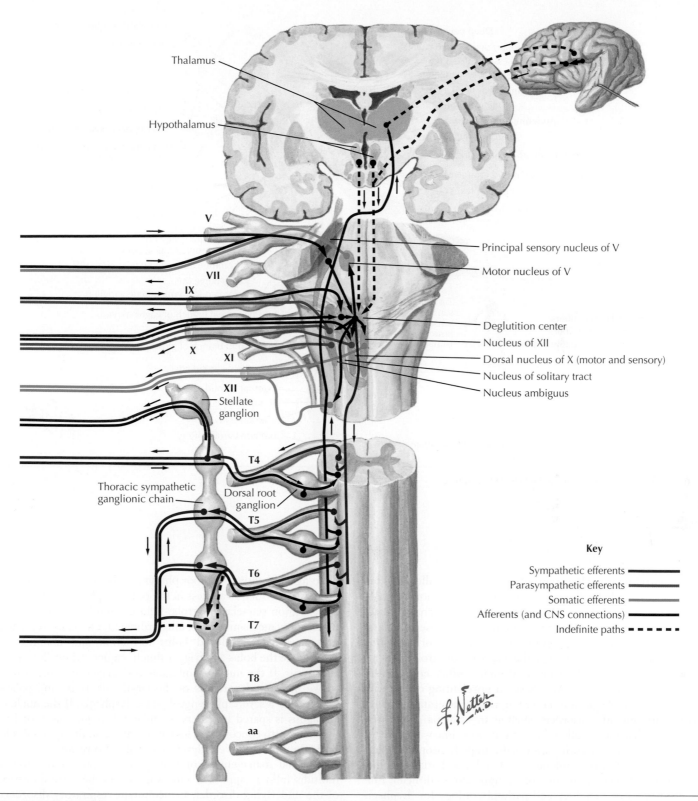

Thalamus

Hypothalamus

V

Principal sensory nucleus of V

Motor nucleus of V

VII

IX

X

XI

Deglutition center

Nucleus of XII

Dorsal nucleus of X (motor and sensory)

Nucleus of solitary tract

Nucleus ambiguus

XII

Stellate
ganglion

Thoracic sympathetic
ganglionic chain

Dorsal root
ganglion

T4

T5

T6

T7

T8

aa

Key

Sympathetic efferents

Parasympathetic efferents

Somatic efferents

Afferents (and CNS connections)

Indefinite paths

Figure 9-1, cont'd

and efficient swallowing function. Aspiration and silent aspiration can also be detected. Images are taken in lateral and anterior–posterior projections to focus on oropharyngeal swallowing anatomy and physiology, and to screen for esophageal motility and pharyngeal reflux. The patient need not be NPO for an MBS.

CLINICAL CONSIDERATIONS AND OUTLOOK

There are three major considerations for resumption of oral intake in dysphagic patients: safety of swallow, ability to maintain oral nutritional support, and quality of life. In patients

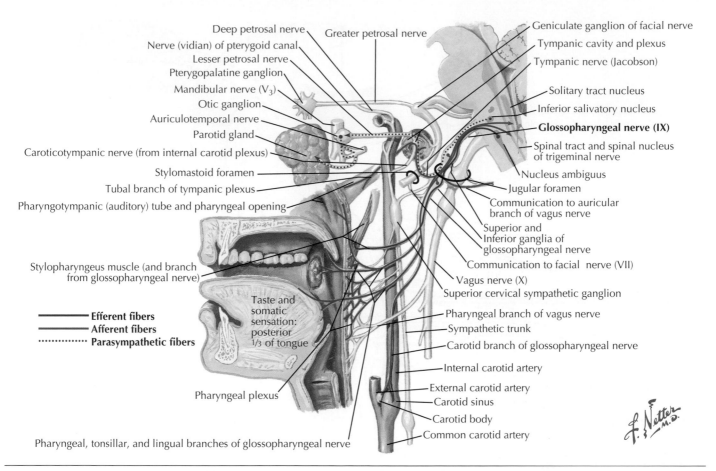

Deep petrosal nerve
Nerve (vidian) of pterygoid canal
Lesser petrosal nerve
Pterygopalatine ganglion
Mandibular nerve (V₃)
Otic ganglion
Auriculotemporal nerve
Parotid gland
Caroticotympanic nerve (from internal carotid plexus)
Stylomastoid foramen
Tubal branch of tympanic plexus
Pharyngotympanic (auditory) tube and pharyngeal opening
Stylopharyngeus muscle (and branch from glossopharyngeal nerve)

Greater petrosal nerve

Geniculate ganglion of facial nerve
Tympanic cavity and plexus
Tympanic nerve (Jacobson)
Solitary tract nucleus
Inferior salivatory nucleus
Glossopharyngeal nerve (IX)
Spinal tract and spinal nucleus of trigeminal nerve
Nucleus ambiguus
Jugular foramen
Communication to auricular branch of vagus nerve
Superior and Inferior ganglia of glossopharyngeal nerve
Communication to facial nerve (VII)
Vagus nerve (X)
Superior cervical sympathetic ganglion

Taste and somatic sensation: posterior ⅓ of tongue

Efferent fibers
Afferent fibers
Parasympathetic fibers

Pharyngeal branch of vagus nerve
Sympathetic trunk
Carotid branch of glossopharyngeal nerve
Internal carotid artery
External carotid artery
Carotid sinus
Carotid body
Common carotid artery

Pharyngeal plexus

Pharyngeal, tonsillar, and lingual branches of glossopharyngeal nerve

Figure 9-2 Glossopharyngeal Nerve (IX): Schema.

with central neurologic compromise, safety of swallow is often grossly impaired and the risk of aspiration pneumonia significantly increased. Additionally, many of these patients are bedridden and have cognitive impairment or decreased levels of alertness. In this setting, even small amounts of aspiration cannot be tolerated. Although the majority of stroke patients improve over time and resume oral intake, other neurodegenerative disorders such as ALS have an unrelenting course with progressive dysphagia and increasing risk of aspiration. Others with neuromuscular disorders, such as myasthenia gravis, may present with a good swallow, but fatigue over time with chewing and consecutive swallowing eventually impede proper deglutition and the potential to tolerate a full oral diet. Eating becomes effortful, making consumption of enough calories difficult. Elucidating the exact etiology and pathophysiology for dysphagia in each case helps direct the treatment approach and predict outcome.

Damage to descending corticobulbar fibers can occur from stroke, head injury, or multiple sclerosis. Stroke can result in mild to severe dysphagia depending on the site and size of the lesion the accompanying deficits. Unilateral hemispheric stroke is a common but usually temporary cause of dysphagia. Delayed oral transit times, delayed or absent triggering of the

pharyngeal swallow, and poor pharyngeal bolus propulsion with decreased sensory awareness in the oral and pharyngeal cavities are common sequelae of stroke-induced dysphagia. Apraxia of the swallow mechanism with uncoordinated muscle movements, characterized by reduced bolus formation and inability to manipulate the bolus and trigger timely sequenced swallow, may also occur. If the nucleus ambiguus is damaged in a brainstem stroke, ipsilateral paralysis of the larynx, pharynx, and palate may lead to a severe pharyngeal phase dysphagia. If the nucleus ambiguus is spared but there is unilateral tongue, face, or jaw weakness with concomitant loss of sensation on the affected side of the oral cavity, severe dysphagia could also result.

Optimal management of neurogenic dysphagia requires a multidisciplinary approach and awareness of the natural history of the underlying disorder. Concomitant respiratory disorders and psychosocial aspects of eating should also be considered.

Placement of a percutaneous esophagogastrostomy can be lifesaving in neurologic disorders associated with severe dysphagia that have significant potential for recovery, such as strokes. Even in terminal illnesses such as amyotrophic lateral sclerosis, a percutaneous esophagogastrostomy can provide sustained comfort and maintain nutrition intake while significantly lessening the risk aspiration pneumonia.

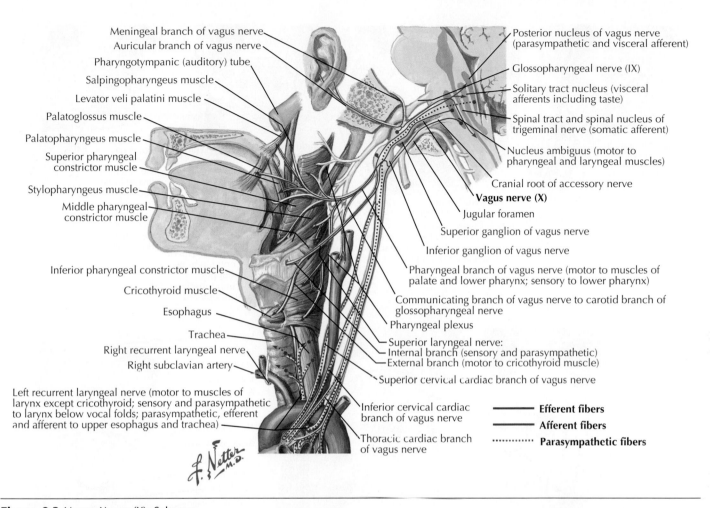

Figure 9-3 Vagus Nerve (X): Schema.

CRANIAL NERVE X, VAGUS: VOICE DISORDERS

Clinical Vignette

A 33-year-old female computer programmer with no prior medical problems presented with abrupt onset of a weak, breathy voice. She woke up without a voice 3 days prior to her visit. In addition to the weak voice, she has noted coughing and choking when drinking thin liquids and frequently feels that small particles of food become stuck in the left side of her throat. Physical examination reveals a healthy female with a very breathy, weak voice and asymmetric elevation of the palate. The otolaryngology consultant finds a complete left vocal fold paralysis, with the vocal fold in the paramedian position. Workup, including a chest x-ray and CT of the neck, reveals no lesions or masses along the course of the left vagus nerve. Idiopathic vocal fold paralysis is diagnosed, and the patient defers temporary injection of the vocal fold to improve voice and swallowing. Over the next 12 weeks, the patient notes a slow but steady return of her voice, and reexamination of the larynx 4 months after symptom onset shows near-normal function of the left vocal fold.

Although the larynx is usually considered the source of speech, speech production requires precise coordination of multiple organ systems. Contraction of the abdominal musculature, diaphragm, and chest wall provides a power source for the voice. The larynx acts as a pressure regulator and vibratory source. The pharynx, tongue, nose, and mouth shape these vibrations into recognizable speech and singing. However, the larynx is the most easily injured of these systems, and most vocal problems originate within it.

ANATOMY OF THE LARYNX

The framework of the larynx consists of thyroid and cricoid cartilages. The arytenoid cartilages articulate with the posterior portion of the cricoid. Vocal ligaments stretch from the arytenoids to the thyroid cartilage. Muscles inserting on the arytenoids move the arytenoids and vocal folds together for speech and swallowing, and apart for respiration. Although the arytenoids' motion is multidimensional, knowledge of the intrinsic laryngeal muscles and their functions is important for diagnosis (Table 9-1; Fig. 9-3). Note that the cricothyroid muscle is the only intrinsic laryngeal muscle innervated by the superior laryngeal nerve (SLN), and the posterior cricoarytenoid is the only vocal fold abductor.

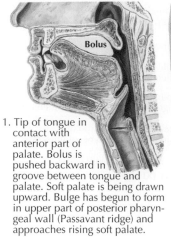

1. Tip of tongue in contact with anterior part of palate. Bolus is pushed backward in groove between tongue and palate. Soft palate is being drawn upward. Bulge has begun to form in upper part of posterior pharyngeal wall (Passavant ridge) and approaches rising soft palate.

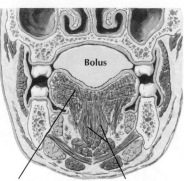

Transverse intrinsic musculature of tongue

Genioglossus muscles

2. Bolus lying in groove on lingual dorsum formed by contraction of genioglossus and transverse intrinsic musculature of tongue.

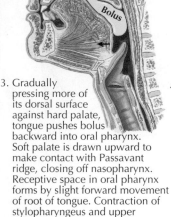

3. Gradually pressing more of its dorsal surface against hard palate, tongue pushes bolus backward into oral pharynx. Soft palate is drawn upward to make contact with Passavant ridge, closing off nasopharynx. Receptive space in oral pharynx forms by slight forward movement of root of tongue. Contraction of stylopharyngeus and upper pharyngeal constriction muscles draws pharyngeal wall upward over bolus.

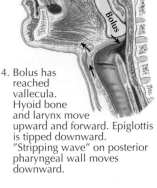

4. Bolus has reached vallecula. Hyoid bone and larynx move upward and forward. Epiglottis is tipped downward. "Stripping wave" on posterior pharyngeal wall moves downward.

Soft palate

Root of tongue

Epiglottis turned down

Laryngeal aditus

Bolus

5. Epiglottis is tipped down over laryngeal aditus but does not completely close it. Bolus flows in two streams around each side of epiglottis to piriform fossae. Streams then unite to enter esophagus. Trickle of food may enter laryngeal aditus (viewed from behind).

F. Netter M.D.

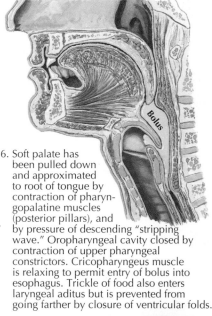

6. Soft palate has been pulled down and approximated to root of tongue by contraction of pharyngopalatine muscles (posterior pillars), and by pressure of descending "stripping wave." Oropharyngeal cavity closed by contraction of upper pharyngeal constrictors. Cricopharyngeus muscle is relaxing to permit entry of bolus into esophagus. Trickle of food also enters laryngeal aditus but is prevented from going farther by closure of ventricular folds.

Soft palate

Root of tongue

Vallecula

Epiglottis turned down (*sectioned*)

Thyroid cartilage

Aryepiglottic fold

Ventricular fold

Ventricle of larynx

Vocal fold

Cricoid cartilage

Residuum of bolus

7. Laryngeal vestibule is closed by approximation of aryepiglottic and ventricular folds, preventing entry of food into larynx (coronal section: AP view).

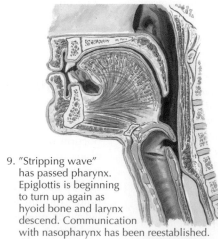

8. "Stripping wave" has reached vallecula and is pressing out last of bolus therefrom. Cricopharyngeus muscle has relaxed and bolus has largely passed into esophagus.

9. "Stripping wave" has passed pharynx. Epiglottis is beginning to turn up again as hyoid bone and larynx descend. Communication with nasopharynx has been reestablished.

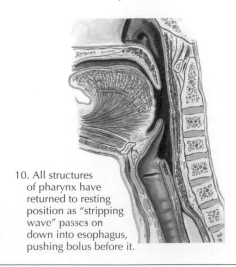

10. All structures of pharynx have returned to resting position as "stripping wave" passes on down into esophagus, pushing bolus before it.

Figure 9-4 Deglutition.

Table 9-1 Laryngeal Muscle Innervation, Action, and Vocal Function*

Muscle	Innervation	Action	Vocal Function
Lateral cricoarytenoid	RLN	Adduction	Speech
Posterior cricoarytenoid	RLN	Abduction	Respiration
Thyroarytenoid	RLN	Adduction and shortening	Fine voice control
Cricothyroid	SLN	Lengthening	Increase pitch

*RLN indicates recurrent laryngeal nerve; SLN, superior laryngeal nerve.

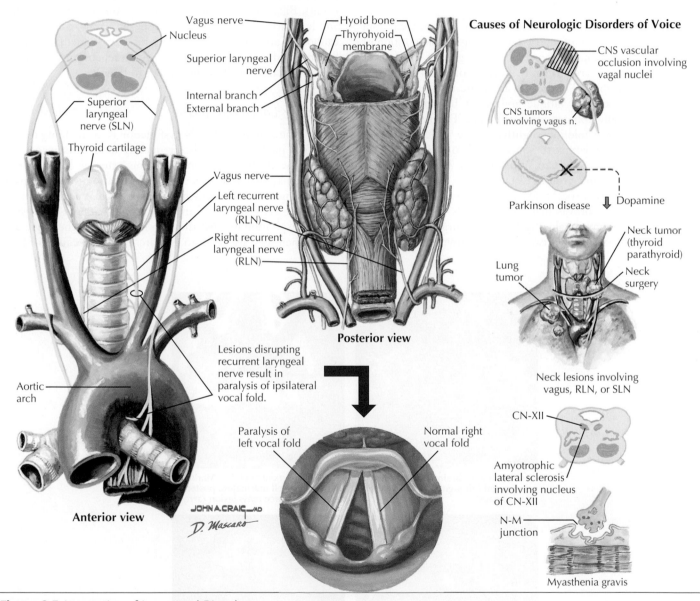

Figure 9-5 Innervation of Larynx and Disorders.

The motor supply of the laryngeal muscles begins in the nucleus ambiguus (see Fig. 9-3). These fibers travel within the vagus nerve (CN-X) as it exits the cranium via the jugular foramen, traveling through the neck within the carotid sheath (Fig. 9-5). High in the neck, the SLN splits from CN-X and travels medially and inferiorly. It splits again into internal and external branches. The internal branch pierces the thyrohyoid membrane and provides sensory innervation to the pharynx and larynx. The external branch travels lower in the neck past the superior pole of the thyroid gland to innervate the cricothyroid muscle.

The recurrent laryngeal nerve (RLN) takes a more tortuous path. It separates from CN-X, loops around the aortic arch on the left and the brachiocephalic artery on the right, and travels back toward the larynx in the tracheoesophageal groove bilaterally. It passes under the thyroid gland and inserts into the larynx under the thyroid cartilage, innervating all other intrinsic laryngeal muscles. Both these nerves are vulnerable to injury and have distinct symptoms when injured.

DISORDERS OF VOICE

Recurrent Laryngeal Nerve

Recurrent laryngeal nerve damage usually causes vocal fold immobility on the side of injury. Depending on the position of the vocal fold, symptom severity varies greatly. The most common symptoms are a breathy, hoarse voice and ineffective cough. If the paralyzed vocal fold is in the midline, the only symptom may be vocal fatigue and slight breathiness. Most patients eventually compensate somewhat. The normal vocal fold may cross the midline slightly, or the patient may use muscles around the larynx to squeeze the vocal folds shut. If accessory muscles are used to speak, muscle fatigue and neck pain may develop after prolonged talking.

Common causes of vocal fold paralysis include thyroid, lung, or neck tumors; cerebrovascular accidents; CN-X tumors (paragangliomas or glomus vagale [Fig. 9-6]); and surgery near CN-X or the RLN. Less common causes include thyroiditis (causing

inflammation of the RLN), infectious diseases, diabetes, or other neuropathies.

Diagnostic evaluation of vocal fold paralysis may include imaging of the brain, neck, and chest, serologic testing, and thyroid function tests; electromyography of the laryngeal muscles may confirm the diagnosis. Even with extensive investigation, the cause of vocal fold paralysis sometimes cannot be determined. Treatment is usually directed at moving the paralyzed vocal fold to the midline. Reinnervation procedures have been described but are not widely used because of inconsistent results. Bilateral vocal fold paralysis is a rare but severe problem and leads to respiratory compromise: the paralyzed vocal folds cannot be abducted and generally move to a medial position. Severe stridor generally results, and tracheostomy is almost always required to allow the patient to breathe.

Superior Laryngeal Nerve

The classic symptom of SLN dysfunction is the inability to raise the vocal pitch. Patients also frequently have weak voices that tire easily. If the injury includes the external SLN branch, patients may also have poor laryngeal sensation leading to aspiration. High CN-X lesions and cerebrovascular accidents cause combined SLN and RLN injuries. These patients are at high risk for aspiration because they can neither close the larynx nor sense when they are about to aspirate. Common causes of SLN

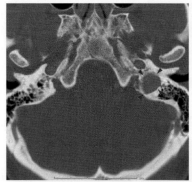

Axial skull base brain CT: Smoothly marginated left jugular fossa expansion (arrowheads).

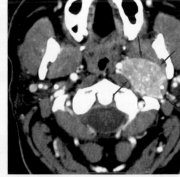

Postcontrast axial neck CT: Markedly enhancing, well marinated, posterior left carotid space mass lesion (arrows).

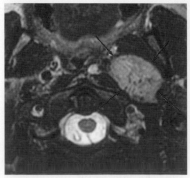

Axial T2 neck MR: Discrete, left posterior carotid space mass with "salt and pepper" signal pattern (arrows).

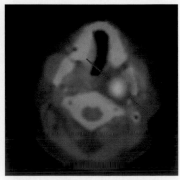

Axial octreotide scan of the neck: Markedly avid uptake left carotid space mass lesion (arrows).

Figure 9-6 Glomus Tumor of Vagal Nerve.

dysfunction include thyroiditis and thyroid surgery. However, most cases of SLN paresis are idiopathic.

Other Neurologic Disorders of the Larynx

Spasmodic dysphonia is a task-specific dystonia affecting the larynx. Patients have irregular voice breaks when trying to speak, but many can sing normally. Its cause is unknown. Treatment involves identifying the involved muscles and paralyzing them with injections of botulinum toxin.

Patients with laryngeal tremor have regular voice breaks and a tremulous voice. Laryngeal examination reveals regular contractions of the laryngeal muscles at rest and during phonation. Singing is not spared. It can be difficult to distinguish spasmodic dysphonia from tremor.

Although most common in Parkinson disease, vocal fold bowing can occur in several other neurologic disorders. The voice is weak and breathy, and accessory muscle compensation is common, causing neck pain and vocal fatigue. Medical treatment of the underlying disease is the first therapy. Speech therapy is also frequently successful. Surgery is sometimes necessary to straighten and bulk the bowed vocal folds.

Neuromuscular disorders, most commonly myasthenia gravis, can affect the laryngeal muscles. A rare form of myasthenia gravis isolated to the laryngeal muscles has been described. The most common symptom is vocal fatigue. Patients generally respond to medical therapy.

Other Neurologic Voice Disorders

Neurologic damage to other portions of the vocal production system can create voice complaints. Tongue dysarthria, from cerebrovascular accident, amyotrophic lateral sclerosis, or hypoglossal nerve damage, is one of the most common. Paralysis of the palatal muscles can give a hypernasal voice. Although tongue and pharyngeal neurologic disorders can cause voice problems, swallowing problems associated with these disorders are often more problematic and require urgent diagnosis and management.

ADDITIONAL RESOURCES

CRANIAL NERVE IX

Hughes TAT, Wiles CM. Clinical measurement of swallowing in health and in neurogenic dysphagia. Q J Med 1996;89:109-116.

Langmore SE, Skarupski KA, Park PS, et al. Predictors of aspiration pneumonia in nursing home residents. Dysphagia 2002;17:298-307.

Larson C. Neurophysiology of speech and swallowing. Semin Speech Lang 1985;6:275-289.

Logemann JA. Evaluation and Treatment of Swallowing Disorders. 2nd ed. Austin, Tex: Pro-Ed; 1998.

McConnell FMS, Cerenko D, Mendelson MS. Manofluorgraphic analysis of swallowing. Otolaryngol Clin N Am 1988;21:625-635.

Zemlin WR. Speech and Hearing Science: Anatomy and Physiology. 4th ed. Boston, Mass: Allyn and Bacon; 1998.

CRANIAL NERVE X

Hill AN, Jankovic J, Vuong KD, et al. Treatment of hypophonia with collagen vocal cord augmentation in patients with parkinsonism. Mov Disord 2003 Oct;18(10):1190-1192.

Lorenz RR, Esclamado RM, Teker AM, et al. Ansa cervicalis-to-recurrent laryngeal nerve anastomosis for unilateral vocal fold paralysis: experience of a single institution. Ann Otol Rhinol Laryngol 2008 Jan;117(1):40-45.

Mao VH, Abaza M, Spiegel JR, et al. Laryngeal myasthenia gravis: report of 40 cases. J Voice 2001;15:122-130. *The largest series of patients with laryngeal manifestations of myasthenia gravis.*

Paniello RC, Barlow J, Serna JS. Longitudinal follow-up of adductor spasmodic dysphonia patients after botulinum toxin injection: quality of life results. Laryngoscope 2008 Mar;118(3):564-568.

Rosen CA, Gartner-Schmidt J, Casiano R, et al. Vocal fold augmentation with calcium hydroxylapatite: twelve-month report. Laryngoscope 2009 May;119(5):1033-1041.

Roy N, Smith ME, Dromey C, et al. Exploring the phonatory effects of external superior laryngeal nerve paralysis: an in vivo model. Laryngoscope 2009 Apr;119(4):816-826.

Rubin AD, Sataloff RT. Vocal fold paresis and paralysis. Otolaryngol Clin North Am 2007 Oct;40(5):1109-1131, viii-ix.

Sulica L. The natural history of idiopathic unilateral vocal fold paralysis: evidence and problems. Laryngoscope 2008 Jul;118(7):1303-1307. *Meta-analysis of 717 cases of idiopathic unilateral vocal fold paralysis regarding duration and outcome of the paralysis.*

Cranial Nerves XI and XII: Accessory and Hypoglossal

Michal Vytopil and H. Royden Jones, Jr.

10

CRANIAL NERVE XI: THE SPINAL ACCESSORY NERVE

Clinical Vignette

A 23-year-old medical student noted swollen lymph nodes in the left posterior triangle of his neck. He was otherwise asymptomatic. The student health service told him that he was overly concerned and there was nothing wrong. Within a period, he became quite fatigued with bouts of fever and sought another opinion from a respected internist. Except for the presence of abnormal left posterior cervical and axillary lymphadenopathy, his clinical examination was normal. Results of a mononucleosis spot test were normal but liver function studies revealed elevated transaminases. Excision of cervical lymph nodes was performed.

During the procedure, the surgeon queried the student about the risks of this minor operation. The student replied that it is important to exercise caution so as not to cut the spinal accessory nerve (CN-XI) because paralysis of the trapezius muscle would result. When he returned to his rotation on the chief of surgery's service, the student was informed by the intern that the chief, on hearing about his missing student, commented that there was a 50% 5-year mortality rate among his patients undergoing this procedure.

The professor of pathology could not arrive at a diagnosis and sent the node to the Armed Forces Institute of Pathology and to the Mayo Clinic for more definitive opinions. They did not believe it represented a lymphoma; 6 weeks later, the test for infectious mononucleosis was positive. The senior editor of this text notes that it is now 49 years since he had this biopsy.

The lymph node revealed cellular hyperplasia and atypia but general preservation of lymph node architecture. It was felt that the pathology likely represented a reactive process without evidence of a definitive malignancy or lymphoma. A repeat monospot now returned positive and he was instructed to convalesce, with little physical activity, over 2 weeks. A similar case was encountered by the author soon after. However, in this case, upon returning to exercise, sagging of the left shoulder, restricted shoulder movements, and pain (especially when elevating the arm) were noted by the patient. An evaluation revealed atrophy and weakness of the trapezius on the left with downward and outward winging of the scapula upon arm extension. An electromyography (EMG) confirmed an accessory nerve lesion with denervation potentials isolated to the upper trapezius.

Comment: This vignette exemplifies that physicians always need to give careful consideration to every patient complaint, especially those in the medical profession. The patient was labeled with "medical studentitis," and a peer created further emotional turmoil for him by suggesting he might die within 5 years. Fortunately, a benign mechanism was established.

Occasionally, patients undergoing similar procedures experience iatrogenic laceration to the spinal accessory nerve. Such leads to significant shoulder pain and atrophy of the unilateral trapezius muscle and residual scapular winging. The more proximally innervated sternocleidomastoid muscle (SCM) is spared. Cervical lymph node biopsies may be the most common cause of CN-XI palsy.

Cranial nerve CN-XI, or the spinal accessory nerve (SAN), serves primarily a motor function for the neck and shoulder. It has an intriguing functional array with one of the two major muscles it innervates, the SCM, inserting on the ipsilateral occiput. When one side contracts, it turns the head in the opposite direction; for example, a right SCM contraction turns the head to the left and vice versa. Both SCM muscles contracting simultaneously results in neck flexion.

The seemingly paradoxical function of the SCM is also of interest and used in rare circumstance of a *hysterical pseudohemiparesis* or *functional somatization* with secondary gain. Patients feigning a right hemiparesis will give way when asked to turn their head against resistance to the right, not realizing that it is the left SCM that turns the head contralaterally. Thus when asked to turn their head to the asymptomatic left, they use the right SCM without difficulty.

ANATOMY

The SAN is primarily a motor nerve innervating the SCM and trapezius muscles in the neck and back (Fig. 10-1). In contrast to the other cranial nerves, its lower motor neuron cell bodies are located primarily within the spinal cord. The accessory nucleus is a cell column within the lateral anterior gray column of the upper five or six cervical spinal cord segments. Proximally it lies nearly in line with the nucleus ambiguus and caudally within the dorsolateral ventral horn. Originating from the accessory nucleus, the rootlets emerge from the cord and unite to form the trunk of CN-XI. This extends rostrally through the foramen magnum into the posterior cranial fossa. Intracranially, it accompanies the caudal fibers of the vagus nerve (CN-X) exiting the skull through the jugular foramen. The SAN then descends in close proximity to the internal carotid artery and internal jugular vein (Fig. 10-2).

Once the spinal accessory nerve is extracranial, it is joined by fibers derived from the third and fourth upper cervical ventral rami. Some of these cervical fibers may innervate the caudal trapezius, whereas the proximal trapezius and the entire SCM muscle are primarily innervated by CN-XI. The spinal accessory nerve then emerges from the midpoint of the posterior border of the SCM, to cross the posterior triangle of the neck superficial to the levator scapulae. It is here that this cranial nerve is in close proximity to the superficial cervical lymph

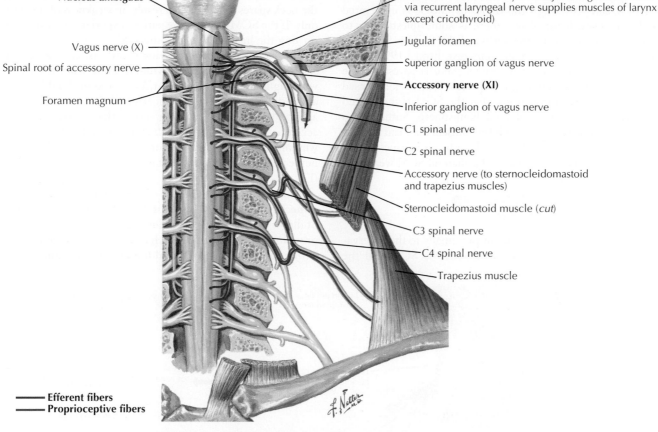

Nucleus ambiguus

Vagus nerve (X)

Spinal root of accessory nerve

Foramen magnum

Cranial root of accessory nerve (joins vagus nerve and via recurrent laryngeal nerve supplies muscles of larynx except cricothyroid)

Jugular foramen

Superior ganglion of vagus nerve

Accessory nerve (XI)

Inferior ganglion of vagus nerve

C1 spinal nerve

C2 spinal nerve

Accessory nerve (to sternocleidomastoid and trapezius muscles)

Sternocleidomastoid muscle (*cut*)

C3 spinal nerve

C4 spinal nerve

Trapezius muscle

——— **Efferent fibers**
——— **Proprioceptive fibers**

Figure 10-1 Accessory Nerve (XI): Schema.

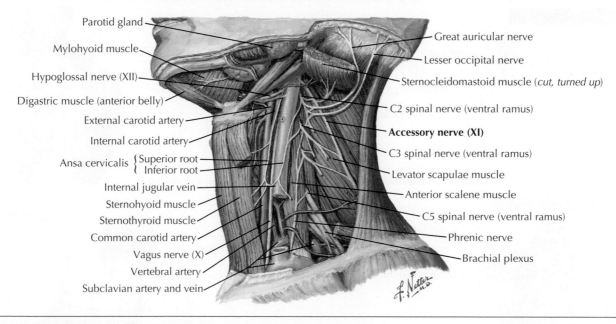

Parotid gland

Mylohyoid muscle

Hypoglossal nerve (XII)

Digastric muscle (anterior belly)

External carotid artery

Internal carotid artery

Ansa cervicalis { Superior root
Inferior root

Internal jugular vein

Sternohyoid muscle

Sternothyroid muscle

Common carotid artery

Vagus nerve (X)

Vertebral artery

Subclavian artery and vein

Great auricular nerve

Lesser occipital nerve

Sternocleidomastoid muscle (*cut, turned up*)

C2 spinal nerve (ventral ramus)

Accessory nerve (XI)

C3 spinal nerve (ventral ramus)

Levator scapulae muscle

Anterior scalene muscle

C5 spinal nerve (ventral ramus)

Phrenic nerve

Brachial plexus

Figure 10-2 Cervical Plexu in Situ.

nodes. Further caudally, approximately 5 cm above the clavicle, it passes into the anterior border of the trapezius muscle, which it also innervates.

There is a minor afferent component to the SAN that carries primary proprioceptive function for the two muscles it

innervates. Also, a minor cranial root contribution to the spinal accessory consists of a few fibers originating in the caudal portion of the nucleus ambiguus. These fibers traverse with the intracranial spinal accessory nerve and exit through the jugular foramen.

The supranuclear innervation of the CN-XI nuclei is still a matter of debate. Although the trapezius muscle is innervated from the opposite hemisphere, there is some question as to whether the supranuclear innervation of the SCM is also contralateral. One standard neuroanatomy text, Brodal 1998, states that with clinical corticobulbar lesions there is paresis of the contralateral SCM as well as the trapezius. Others note, based on intracarotid Amytal injections, that the SCM is innervated predominantly from the ipsilateral hemisphere. Suffice it to say that the most proximal and midline musculature can be activated bilaterally. Therefore, one needs to be circumspect when attempting to lateralize the source of unilateral SCM weakness.

CLINICAL PRESENTATION AND DIAGNOSTIC APPROACH

SAN lesions located intracranially or proximally to the innervation of the SCM cause weakness of both the SCM and the trapezius. Damage to this nerve within the posterior triangle of the neck spares the SCM and results in weakness of the trapezius only. If the SCM is weak, the patient experiences weakness when turning the head to the opposite side.

Involvement of the trapezius manifests as drooping of the shoulder and mild scapular winging away from the chest wall with slight lateral displacement. Weakness in shoulder elevation and arm abduction above horizontal is typical. Winging is apparent with arms hanging along the trunk, and becomes accentuated when patients abduct the arms. In contrast, scapular winging from serratus anterior weakness due to long thoracic nerve palsy is most prominent on forward elevation of the arms (Fig. 10-3).

Most individuals with CN-XI palsies present with shoulder or neck pain or both. The painful paresis can be sudden, because of direct injury during procedures as seen in the above vignette or with trauma or delayed, such as with entrapment of the nerve within scar tissue or structural lesions such as tumors. As in all

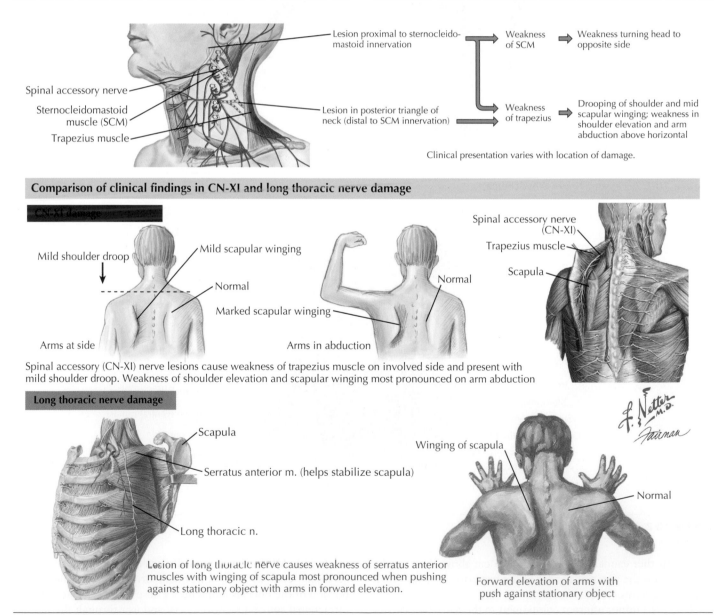

Figure 10-3 Clinical Findings with Cranial Nerve XI Damage.

patients with neck and shoulder pain, careful exam and history are necessary to exclude lesions at the level of the cervical nerve roots or brachial plexus.

Electromyography is important for confirming that the lesion is confined to the distribution of CN-XI. In addition, a gadolinium-enhanced magnetic resonance imaging (MRI) is appropriate if any question exists of a more widespread lesion other than a simple CN-XI neuropathy.

DIFFERENTIAL DIAGNOSIS

The most common site of isolated CN-XI neuropathy is within the neck. The close association of CN-XI with superficial cervical lymph nodes renders it vulnerable to iatrogenic damage during lymph node biopsy or a radical neck surgical dissection. The spinal accessory nerve can also be directly compressed by swollen lymph nodes or other solid tumors. Rarely, CN-XI neuropathy occurs after blunt or penetrating **neck trauma**, or due to **radiation injury** with treatment of adjacent tumors. Although it is not part of the brachial plexus, CN-XI can be involved in patients with **brachial plexitis** (neuralgic amyotrophy). Damage also rarely occurs after carotid endarterectomy or jugular vein cannulation because of the nerve's proximity to large neck vessels.

Intraspinal and intracranial portions of CN-XI may be affected by **intrinsic spinal cord lesions**, posterior fossa **meningiomas**, or **metastases**. Benign tumors such as an en plaque meningioma at the base of the brain or **metastatic tumors** at the jugular foramen or foramen magnum may impinge on the SAN; however, these various lesions usually affect concomitantly the glossopharyngeal, vagal, and sometimes even the hypoglossal nerve exiting through the adjacent hypoglossal foramen. Very rarely, varied pathologic lesions of the SAN occur just after it leaves the skull and courses through the space behind the parotid gland and pharynx. Cranial nerves IX, X, XI, XII, and adjacent sympathetic chain fibers, causing Horner syndrome, are potentially involved in variable combinations with primary or metastatic tumors.

Various disorders at the anatomic level of the anterior horn cell are within the differential of CN-XI neuropathy, including **motor neuron disease**, **syringomyelia**, and **poliomyelitis**. In these cases, one finds prominent atrophy and fasciculations affecting both the SCM and trapezius muscles.

PROGNOSIS

For patients with benign traumatic lesions, the likelihood of reinnervation is good unless the proximal and distal SAN segments are widely separated. Sometimes surgical exploration is helpful. The time frame for reinnervation is similar to that for any peripheral nerve: 1 mm per day or 3 cm per month.

CRANIAL NERVE XII: HYPOGLOSSAL

Despite being the most distal of the 12 paired cranial nerves, the hypoglossal nerve (CN-XII) controls what is teleologically an important human function: the final common pathway for verbal language implementation. Phylogenetically, the hypoglossal nerve has major significance because of its role in food intake. As with any cranial nerve, CN-XII is susceptible to numerous pathologic processes.

ANATOMY

CN-XII carries motor fibers that supply all intrinsic and most extrinsic tongue muscles, that is, the hyoglossus, styloglossus, genioglossus, and geniohyoid (Fig. 10-4). Its fibers originate from the hypoglossal nucleus beneath the floor of the fourth ventricle (Fig. 10-5). In its intramedullary course, CN-XII axons pass ventrally and lateral to the medial lemniscus emerging from the medulla in the ventrolateral sulcus between the olive and the pyramid. The rootlets unite to form CN-XII, which exits the skull through the hypoglossal foramen adjacent to the foramen magnum within the posterior cranial fossa (Fig. 10-6).

After exiting the skull, CN-XII runs medial to CN-IX, -X, and -XI. It continues between the internal carotid artery and internal jugular vein, and deep into the posterior belly of the digastric muscle. It then loops anteriorly, coursing on the lateral surface of the hyoglossus muscle, and later, it divides to supply the intrinsic and extrinsic muscles of the ipsilateral tongue (see Fig. 10-4).

The anterior primary ramus of the spinal nerve C1 sends fibers to accompany CN-XII for a short distance; these fibers later connect with the fibers of C2 and C3 anterior primary rami, forming a loop called the *ansa cervicalis*. This innervates the infrahyoid muscles, that is, sternohyoid, omohyoid, sternothyroid, thyrohyoid, and geniohyoid. These small muscles aid in head flexion.

Clinical Vignette

This 64-year-old lady presented with a 2-month history of unrelenting, increasingly disconcerting left occipital headache. This occasionally radiated with brief jabs toward her left ear. Whenever she bent her head forward the pain became unbearable. Although she was initially diagnosed with occipital neuralgia, two local nerve blocks were ineffective. She admitted that her tongue also felt "leathery" and "numb." One year earlier she was treated for adenocarcinoma of the breast with a partial mastectomy and axillary node dissection. Sampled lymph nodes were negative for cancer.

Neurologic exam demonstrated atrophy and fasciculations of the left half of the tongue. This was best observed with the tongue at rest inside the mouth. Upon protrusion, the tongue deviated to the left. The head pain was aggravated by neck flexion and suboccipital palpation.

Contrast-enhanced computed tomography (CT) of the skull base revealed an infiltrating lesion eroding the left occipital condyle. Further imaging showed multiple metastases in the ribs and thoracic vertebrae, as well as liver and lungs. The lesions were assumed to represent metastatic carcinoma. Radiation therapy led to resolution of her headache; however, her hypoglossal neuropathy persisted. Subsequently, she was placed on systemic chemotherapy for disseminated cancer.

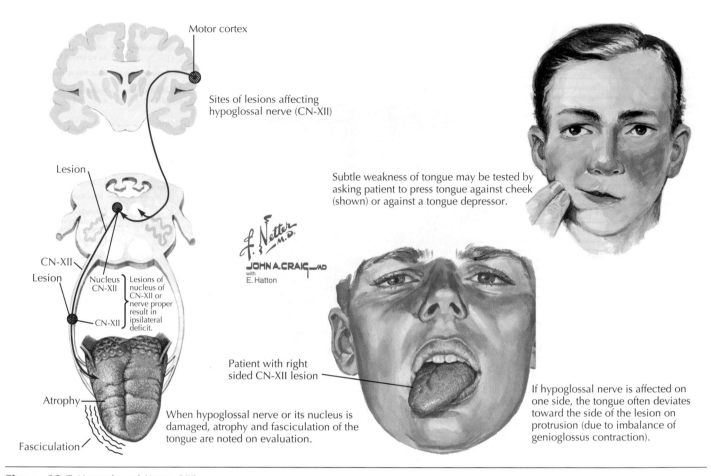

Motor cortex

Sites of lesions affecting hypoglossal nerve (CN-XII)

Lesion

CN-XII

Lesion

Nucleus CN-XII

Lesions of nucleus of CN-XII or nerve proper result in ipsilateral deficit.

CN-XII

Atrophy

Fasciculation

When hypoglossal nerve or its nucleus is damaged, atrophy and fasciculation of the tongue are noted on evaluation.

Subtle weakness of tongue may be tested by asking patient to press tongue against cheek (shown) or against a tongue depressor.

Patient with right sided CN-XII lesion

If hypoglossal nerve is affected on one side, the tongue often deviates toward the side of the lesion on protrusion (due to imbalance of genioglossus contraction).

JOHN A. CRAIG
with
E. Hatton

Figure 10-7 Hypoglossal Nerve (XII).

to evaluate for fasciculations is to keep the tongue at rest on the floor of the mouth. Sometimes, fasciculations may be enhanced by stroking the lateral aspect of the resting tongue with a standard wooden tongue blade. A *unilateral upper motor neuron lesion* may on occasion result in deviation of the tongue; however, this is contralateral to the central lesion, and there is never any accompanying atrophy or fasciculations. In certain disorders, particularly amyotrophic lateral sclerosis, both upper and lower motor neuron components may be present, with the combination leading to some initial diagnostic confusion if this area is the first to become clinically affected.

DIFFERENTIAL DIAGNOSIS

Anterior horn cell disorders frequently affect the hypoglossal nucleus, particularly with **motor neuron disease**, spinal muscular atrophy, or **poliomyelitis**. Other intramedullary processes such as **syringobulbia**, **intramedullary tumors**, **cavernomas**, or **multiple sclerosis** may also lead to tongue paresis. Because of the close midline proximity of the two hypoglossal nuclei, these structural intramedullary lesions often lead to bilateral tongue paralysis.

When there is a precipitous onset of tongue weakness, this is usually caused by rare atherosclerotic occlusion within a midline penetrating branch of the vertebral basilar system and stroke. This leads to damage of the hypoglossal nucleus and its

emerging fibers, the corticospinal tract, and the medial lemniscus. This **medial medullary syndrome** is clinically characterized by an ipsilateral lower motor tongue weakness accompanied by a contralateral hemiparesis and loss of proprioception and vibration. The more proximally innervated face is spared.

The intracranial course of the 12th cranial nerve can also be damaged by lesions, typically neoplasms, at the basal meninges and skull base. **Metastatic** bronchial or breast carcinomas, lymphomas, or benign lesions such as **meningiomas**, **chordomas**, or **cholesteatomas** occasionally affect the hypoglossal nerve. The proximity of hypoglossal and jugular foramina explains frequent concomitant involvement of other lower cranial nerves (CN-IX, -X, and -XI) in these cases. Both neoplastic and infectious–inflammatory lesions may lead to a basal meningitis affecting multiple cranial nerves, including the hypoglossal. Rarely other non-neoplastic, primary bony processes, such as platybasia and Paget disease, may be implicated.

The close spatial relation between the hypoglossal nerve and the carotid artery makes this nerve vulnerable to primary carotid pathology within the neck. Very rarely, *dissection of the internal carotid artery* is accompanied by a CN-XII neuropathy, most likely related to nerve compression by the increased circumference of the dissected vessel. Occasionally, an iatrogenic hypoglossal neuropathy occurs subsequent to a *carotid endarterectomy* or other types of neck surgery. A **nasopharyngeal cancer** may damage CN-XII along its intracranial course or within the neck

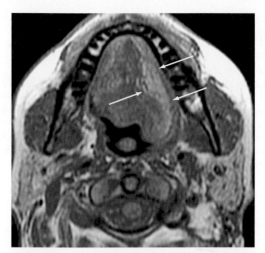

A. Axial neck MR: Denervation atrophy left hemitongue (arrows).

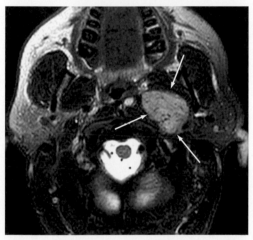

B. Axial T2 neck MR: Discrete, large, left carotid space mass with distinctive "salt and pepper" signal pattern (arrows).

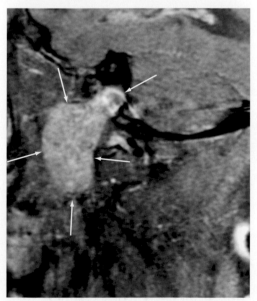

C. Sagittal T2 neck MR: large jugular fossa and carotid space mass with "salt and pepper" signal pattern (arrows).

Figure 10-8 Glomus Jugulare with Hypoglossal Palsy.

per se; this is usually in conjunction with involvement of other cranial nerves. **Glomus jugulare tumor** is a rare hypervascular malignancy that arises from the paraganglionic tissue at the jugular foramen and can compress CN-XII either at the base of the brain or conceivably within the neck (Fig. 10-8A–C). Similar to other cranial nerves, the CN-XII may also be affected by *radiation therapy* and *neck trauma*. Most uncommonly, the hypoglossal nerve is affected as part of two primary demyelinating peripheral nerve syndromes, namely, **hereditary neuropathy with liability to pressure palsies (HNPP)** or a variant of chronic inflammatory demyelinating polyneuropathy (CIDP), the **Lewis–Sumner syndrome**.

Glossodynia is a controversial syndrome with no specific etiology as yet defined. This is characterized by an uncomfortable burning pain within the tongue unassociated with any tongue weakness or atrophy. The condition occurs more frequently in women. Vitamin B_1, or B_{12}, deficiency, as well as Sjögren syndrome, have been suggested as pathophysiologic mechanisms. Unfortunately, many of these patients with idiopathic tongue pain are subsequently suspected of having a psychogenic basis, but this may simply reflect our lack of full understanding of this often distressing complaint.

DIAGNOSTIC APPROACH

Magnetic resonance imaging of the brain, skull base, and neck are the diagnostic tests of choice. If these imaging studies do not define evidence of a specific mass lesion, a careful search for leptomeningeal enhancement is in order. This is typically seen with metastatic tumors, sarcoidosis, or other rare leptomeningeal infiltrating lesions such as tuberculosis. Contrast-enhanced CT with thin slices through the skull base may also be useful to identify very discrete bony lesions.

Cerebrospinal fluid (CSF) analysis is indicated if an infiltrative process is clinically suspected or suggested from MRI. CSF analysis must include routine studies and cytologic analysis for malignant cells.

Electromyography of the genioglossus as well as anatomically adjacent muscles are indicated when the above studies are unremarkable. Unfortunately, an asymmetrically atrophied tongue is commonly the presenting sign of motor neuron disease.

ADDITIONAL RESOURCES

Berger PS, Bataini JP. Radiation-induced cranial nerve palsy. Cancer 1977;40:152-155. *This classic paper describes 25 patients with cranial nerve palsies following radiation therapy for head and neck cancer; the spinal accessory nerve was involved in 5 patients.*

Brodal P. The Central Nervous System, Structure and Function. 2nd edition. Oxford: Oxford University Press; 1998. p. 452-453.

Brown H. Anatomy of the spinal accessory nerve plexus: relevance to head and neck cancer and atherosclerosis. Exp Biol Med (Maywood) 2002;227:570-578. *This article provides a detailed review of surgical anatomy of spinal accessory nerve and its relationship to cervical and brachial plexus as well as other neck structures. Special attention is given to the nerve's vascular supply.*

DeToledo JC, Dow R. Sternomastoid function during hemispheric suppression by Amytal: insights into inputs to the spinal accessory nerve nucleus. Mov Disord 1998;13:809-812. *Weakness of the SCM ipsilateral to the Amytal carotid injection argues that ipsilateral hemisphere is the one more involved in supranuclear innervation of the SCM.*

Friedenberg SM, Zimprich T, Harper CM. The natural history of long thoracic and spinal accessory neuropathies. Muscle Nerve 2002;25:535-539. *This retrospective review of 56 cases seen at Mayo Clinic over 22 years provides insight into the natural history, outcome predictors, and role of electrophysiology in spinal accessory nerve lesions.*

Greenberg HS, Deck MD, Vikram B, et al. Metastasis to the base of the skull: clinical findings in 43 patients. Neurology 1981;31(5):530-537. *In this classic paper, the combination of occipital headache and unilateral hypoglossal palsy due to a skull base metastasis was first described as the occipital condyle syndrome.*

Gutrecht JA, Jones HR. Bilateral hypoglossal nerve injury after bilateral carotid endarterectomy. Stroke 1988;19:261-262. *This instructive case points out the often dramatic difference between the clinical presentation of bilateral versus unilateral hypoglossal neuropathy.*

Keane JR. Twelfth-nerve palsy. Analysis of 100 cases. Arch Neurol 1996;53:561-566. *In this large series, nearly half of the cases of hypoglossal neuropathy were due to a neoplasm.*

Kim DH, Cho YJ, Tiel RL, et al. Surgical outcomes of 111 spinal accessory nerve injuries. Neurosurgery 2003;53:1106-1112. *This is a retrospective review of injury mechanisms, operative techniques and surgical outcomes of 111 cases of spinal accessory neuropathy that underwent surgical repair.*

Wesselmann U, Reich SG. The dynias. Semin Neurol 1996;16:63-74. *In this review of "dynias," authors discuss the controversial syndrome of glossodynia.*

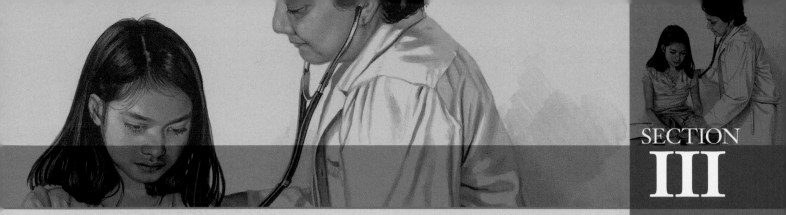

Headache and Pain

Primary and Secondary Headache

11

Carol Moheban, Matthew Tilem, and Jose A. Gutrecht

Clinical Vignette

A 50-year-old woman is referred to a neurologist because of severe headaches. She first developed headaches during adolescence, and they worsened in the setting of menopause. A typical headache is unilateral and localized to the right frontotemporal and periorbital regions. The pain is described as throbbing and pulsating. When severe, her headaches are associated with nausea, vomiting, photophobia, phonophobia, and visual symptoms. Her headaches had increased in frequency and were occurring a few times a month, lasting for at least 12 hours, and causing her to miss work. Her examination was normal. Blood work and a magnetic resonance imaging (MRI) of the brain were normal.

Headache is one of the most common symptoms in medicine and is often the primary complaint presented to the internist, neurologist, or emergency room physician. Despite this, like many pain syndromes, headaches are underdiagnosed and undertreated. Accurate headache diagnosis is important before specific treatment can be initiated. It can be the presenting symptom in many primary neurologic illnesses and in a number of serious systemic disorders. The preceding vignette is typical of migraines, one of the most common headache syndromes. Distinguishing features of more serious causes, such as brain tumors, ruptured aneurysms, low cerebrospinal pressure syndromes, subdural hematoma, meningitis, and temporal arteritis, are often present but should be deliberately inquired of and must not be overlooked. Assessment of a patient presenting with headache starts with a detailed history. Essential characteristics should be defined: any premonitory symptoms, manner of onset (e.g., precipitous or gradual), diurnal variation, provoking and alleviating factors, location, pain characteristics, duration, medical and psychiatric comorbidities, and degree of disability. Family and social history, current medications, drug allergies, and review of systems are also paramount. A detailed neurologic and general medical examination is essential to the evaluation, particularly with individuals having a recent or precipitous onset or experiencing changes in headache characteristics. Ancillary laboratory and neuroradiologic testing are often indicated.

Headache syndromes must first be classified as primary, without significant underlying neurologic pathology, or secondary due to intracranial pathology. The differentiation between primary and secondary headache is critical; it dictates the diagnostic approach and guides treatment and prognosis.

PRIMARY HEADACHE DISORDERS

MIGRAINE

Migraine, often underdiagnosed, is the most common type of headache that leads patients to seek medical care. According to the US Headache Consortium, an estimated 6% of men and 15–17% of women in the United States have migraine, but only 3–5% of them receive preventive therapy. First-degree relatives of patients with migraine are at higher risk. Migraine can occur at any age but frequently begins during puberty. It is most prevalent in individuals aged 25–55 years and is one of the leading causes of chronic suffering and disability in this population. They tend to diminish or totally disappear in the older population but have been known to transiently flare up again in women around the time of menopause.

Migraine pathophysiology includes a combination of cortical hyperexcitability and discharge followed by cation and neurotransmitter release with secondary activation of trigeminal pathways, and subsequent release of vasoactive neuropeptides and proinflammatory substances. These promote meningeal blood vessel dilatation and neurogenic inflammation in the primary pain nerve endings of the head lying in the arteries, leptomeninges, and nasal sinuses (Figs. 11-1 and 11-2). In migraine with aura, the pathophysiology of the aura is thought to be related to slow neuronal discharge of the cortex in a sequential pattern or "spreading depression" followed by a concomitant decrease in cerebral blood flow.

Patients with migraine often have prodromal symptoms that herald the oncoming headache. These include fatigue, thirst, anorexia, fluid retention, food cravings, gastrointestinal symptoms, and emotional or mood disturbances such as irritability, elation or depression. Approximately 15% of migraine patients have an aura preceding the pain phase. This presentation known presently as migraine with aura (formerly classic migraine) comprises focal neurologic symptoms, most commonly visual (>95% of all auras), that typically evolve and then regress over minutes before headache onset. These visual phenomena can occur in a homonymous or hemifield distribution. Typical migraine scotomata include scintillating flashes or stars (phosphenes) and geometric patterns known as fortification spectra (Fig. 11-3). Auras may also involve sensory, motor or rarely higher cortical pathways, including language. Most auras develop slowly over several to 20 minutes, last less than 1 hour, and may spread over different anatomic areas. For example, the patient may initially experience numbness in the fingers that gradually spreads up the arm to the face and sometimes even down the leg. In some individuals, the auras may not be necessarily followed by the headache phase. Less commonly, the aura phase consists of complex symptomatology with a more abrupt onset. For example, in basilar artery migraine, symptoms may include dysarthria,

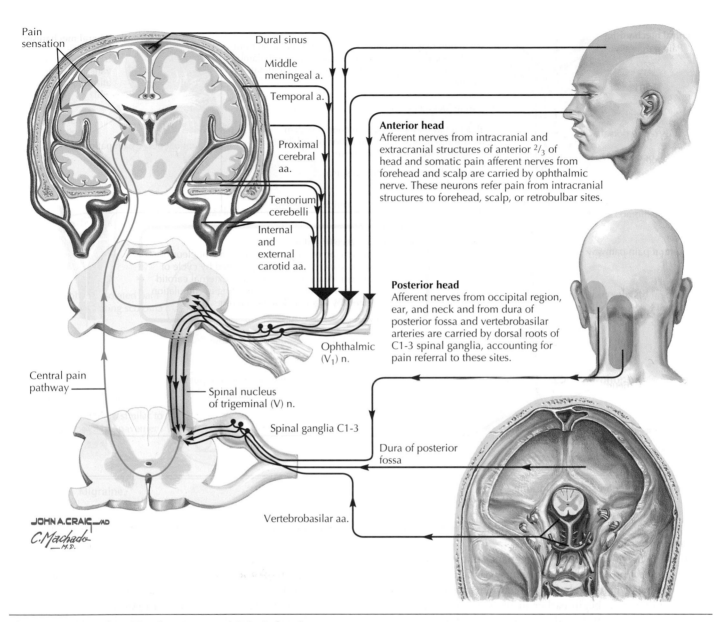

Figure 11-1 Pain-Sensitive Structures and Pain Referral.

vertigo, ataxia, diplopia, hearing deficits, and even altered mentation or loss of consciousness. In confusional migraine, cognitive deficits are more prominent. Ocular nerve palsies are the hallmark of ophthalmoplegic migraine. Hemiplegic migraine is associated with variable but prominent unilateral weakness, and there is often a family history with an inherited voltage-dependent calcium channelopathy.

Careful neurologic evaluation is mandatory before migraine can be safely diagnosed in individuals with a focal aura, and it is usually a diagnosis of exclusion. Although auras are thought to typify migraine and help differentiate it from other headaches, most migraine patients never experience an aura.

The pain phase and its associated symptoms support the clinical classification of headaches as migraine. The most widely used headache classification system was developed in 1988 by the Headache Classification Committee of the International Headache Society, and it was revised in 2004. Recurrent headaches may be classified as migraines, if they last 4–72 hours (either untreated or unsuccessfully treated) and are associated with one of the two features: nausea and/or vomiting, or photophobia and phonophobia. The headaches are characterized by two of the following four symptom characteristics: unilateral location, pulsating quality, moderate to severe intensity, and aggravation by routine physical activity. It remains crucial, however, for the physician to ensure that specific secondary causes are excluded before confirming a diagnosis of migraine. Therefore, careful evaluation of the patient presenting with new-onset headaches is essential. Similarly, any change in the character of previously experienced headaches warrants a fresh investigation of any potential underlying mechanism.

Special Considerations

Two thirds of women with migraine primarily experience them just before or during menses. These headaches are often associated with other premenstrual dysphoric symptoms.

daily activities or responsibilities. Tricyclic antidepressants, β-blockers, calcium channel blockers, sodium valproate, gabapentin, and topiramate are the most frequently used migraine prophylactic medications. Experimentation with different agents may be needed to determine which medication is the most effective for any individual patient. The initial choice may be directed by existing comorbidities or considerations. For instance, difficulty with sleep may prompt prescribing medications that are more sedating and help sleep initiation. Topiramate may be preferable over valproic acid for those in whom weight gain is a concern. A concomitant mood disorder may prompt the use of antidepressants or medications with mood-stabilizing properties. β-Blockers may help in controlling coexisting hypertension in some patients but should be avoided in those with reactive-airway disease or in athletes. Elucidating and avoiding potential dietary and environmental triggers is an important part of non-pharmacological migraine prevention. Sleep deprivation, dehydration, and erratic meals are strong triggers, and proper general health habits should be encouraged.

Future Directions

Half of migraine patients report dissatisfaction with therapy, despite the above options. A comprehensive approach to treatment of migraine headache is important, and must also address contributing factors such as hypertension or other medical problems, mood and sleep disorders, psychosocial stressors, and excessive use of caffeine, alcohol, and nicotine. Avoidance of rebound headache from overuse of analgesics is essential. Adjunct treatment with certain vitamins and supplements (riboflavin or vitamin B_2 and magnesium sulfate), exercise, biofeedback, cognitive–behavioral management training, and acupuncture can also be beneficial. Botulinum toxin type A is showing promise for migraine prevention as are clonazepam and some of the newer antiepileptic medications.

CLUSTER HEADACHE

Clinical Vignette

A 34-year-old man presents to his internist for evaluation of severe pain above and behind his right eye. The pain began a few days ago and is intermittent. It occurs several times a day, usually lasting for 30–60 minutes, and often awakens him at night. The pain is associated with ipsilateral tearing, conjunctival injection, and nasal congestion. Alcohol triggers or exacerbates the pain. His wife reports that he has been irritable and agitated. On exam, he has right-sided periorbital edema and mild ptosis. He reports having similar symptoms 2 years ago and is concerned because that episode lasted for several weeks.

Cluster headaches are much less common than migraines, to which they are unrelated, affecting only 0.1% of adults. However, they are usually more severe and debilitating and have been referred to as the "suicide headache." Although cluster headaches are very distinctive and stereotyped, they tend to be underdiagnosed. Cluster headaches usually respond well to the appropriate therapy and, therefore, a very careful history that aids in making the correct diagnosis is important. They usually first occur in the third decade, affecting men more often than women, although the ratio has decreased over the past several years (male-to-female ratio is 2–4 : 1).

The distinctive clinical features, as summarized in the clinical vignette, assist in diagnosing cluster headaches (Fig. 11-5). The underlying pathophysiology is related to activation of the trigeminal vascular and parasympathetic systems. The first two divisions of the trigeminal pathway are more commonly involved. Recent positron emission tomographic scan studies by Goadsby and colleagues revealed activation of the medial hypothalamic gray matter, an area involved in the control of circadian rhythms. It is felt that dysfunction of neurons in this area leads to activation of a trigeminal-autonomic loop in the brainstem. These pathophysiologic mechanisms would explain the cardinal symptoms of cluster headache that include the episodic/circadian nature of the attacks, the distribution and quality of pain, and associated autonomic symptoms.

According to the International Headache Society's revised classification of cluster headache, there must be recurrent attacks of at least severe unilateral pain lasting 15-180 minutes. The pain must be orbital, supraorbital, and/or temporal. The headaches must be accompanied by at least one of the following: restlessness or agitation, ipsilateral conjunctival injection and/or lacrimation, nasal congestion and/or rhinorrhea, eyelid edema, forehead and facial sweating, ipsilateral miosis and/or ptosis. Attacks have a frequency of one every other day to eight a day. Finally, other causes must be ruled out.

Management and Therapy

Like migraine, the treatment algorithm includes short-term and preventive therapy. The two most effective abortive therapies for cluster headache are sumatriptan 6 mg subcutaneous and high-flow oxygen inhalation at 7–10 L/min for 15–20 minutes. Other triptan preparations, oral indomethacin three times daily, ergotamines (particularly intravenous dihydroergotamine), and intranasal lidocaine are often beneficial. Melatonin and intranasal capsaicin are showing promise for treatment of episodic cluster headache. Preventive therapy must also be used. Verapamil 240 mg daily is the drug of choice for prophylaxis of cluster headaches. Other beneficial drugs include sodium valproate, lithium, topiramate, short-term corticosteroids, and methysergide, although now in short supply. Ten percent of cluster headache patients develop chronic or relentless symptoms, and combined-drug therapy may be needed. Very rarely, and only in well-selected medically refractory patients, is surgical ablation or radiofrequency rhizotomy of the trigeminal nerve necessary.

OTHER TRIGEMINAL AUTONOMIC CEPHALGIAS

Paroxysmal Hemicranias

These are unusual primary headaches—unilateral and short-lived (2–45 minutes), which occur in a chronic or episodic

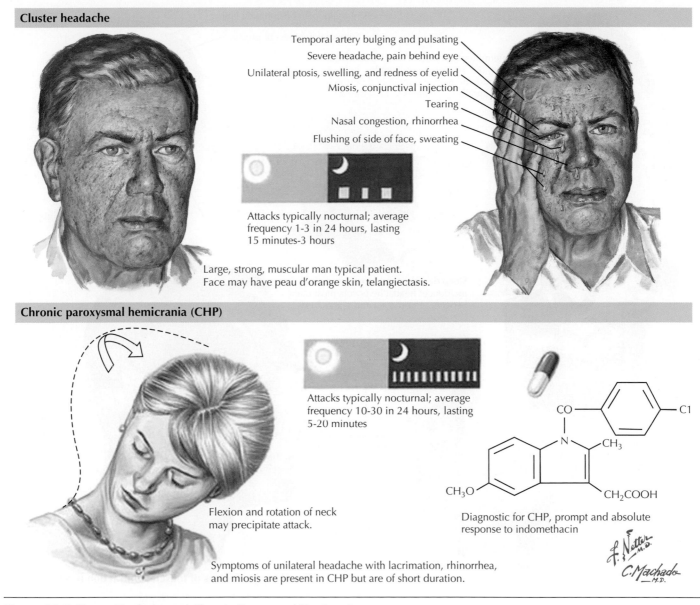

Cluster headache

Temporal artery bulging and pulsating
Severe headache, pain behind eye
Unilateral ptosis, swelling, and redness of eyelid
Miosis, conjunctival injection
Tearing
Nasal congestion, rhinorrhea
Flushing of side of face, sweating

Attacks typically nocturnal; average frequency 1-3 in 24 hours, lasting 15 minutes-3 hours

Large, strong, muscular man typical patient. Face may have peau d'orange skin, telangiectasis.

Chronic paroxysmal hemicrania (CHP)

Attacks typically nocturnal; average frequency 10-30 in 24 hours, lasting 5-20 minutes

Flexion and rotation of neck may precipitate attack.

Diagnostic for CHP, prompt and absolute response to indomethacin

Symptoms of unilateral headache with lacrimation, rhinorrhea, and miosis are present in CHP but are of short duration.

Figure 11-5 Cluster Headache and Chronic Paroxysmal Hemicrania.

manner. Typically, the pain has a severe throbbing or boring quality and often recurs several times during the same day. These headaches are associated with ipsilateral cranial autonomic dysfunction but, unlike cluster headaches, occur more often in women than in men. Furthermore, these headaches have daily recurrences and tend not to conglomerate over a few days such as in cluster headaches. They usually respond well to 25–50 mg indomethacin 2–3 times daily for at least 48 hours. These headaches by definition are "indomethacin responsive," and a trial is always warranted if there are no medical contraindications to its use (Fig. 11-5). There are reports of good response as well to acetazolamide. Calcium channel blockers, such as verapamil, are used for long-term prophylactic treatment.

Short-Lasting Unilateral Neuralgiform Headache Attacks with Conjunctival Injection and Tearing

This is a syndrome of strictly unilateral headache attacks with the pain confined to the ocular/periocular area. Most episodes are moderate to severe in intensity with a burning, stabbing, or electrical quality. The duration of the paroxysms usually ranges from 10 to 120 seconds. Prominent, ipsilateral conjunctival injection and lacrimation are present. Nasal stuffiness or rhinorrhea and ipsilateral forehead perspiration may also be present. In contrast to paroxysmal hemicranias, this headache syndrome predominates in middle-aged men and is not responsive to indomethacin. In fact, treatment efforts with numerous medications have been frustrating, with little or inconsistent responses. Lately, lamotrigine promises to be of some benefit.

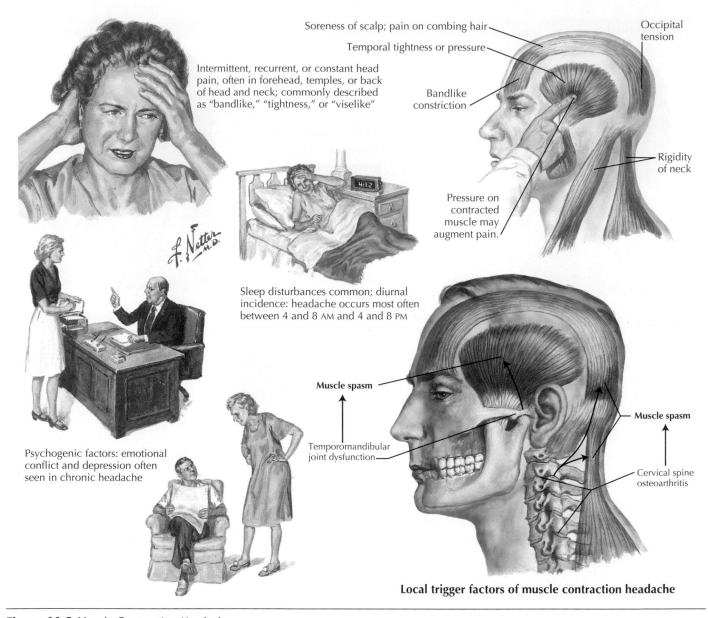

Soreness of scalp; pain on combing hair

Temporal tightness or pressure

Occipital tension

Intermittent, recurrent, or constant head pain, often in forehead, temples, or back of head and neck; commonly described as "bandlike," "tightness," or "viselike"

Bandlike constriction

Rigidity of neck

Pressure on contracted muscle may augment pain.

Sleep disturbances common; diurnal incidence: headache occurs most often between 4 and 8 AM and 4 and 8 PM

Psychogenic factors: emotional conflict and depression often seen in chronic headache

Muscle spasm

Temporomandibular joint dysfunction

Muscle spasm

Cervical spine osteoarthritis

Local trigger factors of muscle contraction headache

Figure 11-6 Muscle Contraction Headache.

TENSION-TYPE HEADACHE

Tension headache is the most common headache type. In 2004, the Headache Classification Committee of the International Headache Society reaffirmed that a diagnosis of tension headache requires the presence of at least two of the following pain characteristics: a nonpulsatile steady pressure-like quality, a nondisabling mild to moderate intensity, bilateral location, and no aggravation with routine physical activity. In addition, these patients do not experience nausea or vomiting and do not have photophobia or phonophobia. Tension-type headaches last less than 7 days. Their frequency varies from occasional to daily. If they occur more than 15 days per month, the diagnosis of chronic tension-type headache applies.

Careful evaluation is indicated in every patient suspected of having tension-type headache. Exclusion of structural, infectious, or metabolic disorders is essential. Although sometimes features of migraine are present, they are a minor part of the clinical picture. Specific triggers are less common than with migraine. The precise pathophysiology is unknown. It is likely a heterogeneous disorder with various etiologic factors that ultimately lead to pericranial and nuchal muscular tension or spasm (Fig. 11-6). Disrupted sleep, psychosocial stress, anxiety, depression, and analgesic drug overuse are contributing factors. The treatment of tension headache usually requires only over-the-counter analgesics and NSAIDs, nonpharmacologic intervention, that include relaxation and biofeedback techniques massage, and heat application. Prophylactic medication is indicated for frequent recurrence or when abortive therapies are ineffective or contraindicated. The best available evidence supports the use of tricyclic antidepressants, specifically amitriptyline. This medication is best tolerated when started at a nightly low dose (10–25 mg) and increased gradually if needed.

CHRONIC DAILY HEADACHES

Clinical Vignette

A 45-year-old man complains of daily headache for 10 years. His headache lasts all day but is worse on awakening. He notes a dull, sometimes pulsatile, moderate, bifrontal head pain with mild nausea that responds to an over-the-counter combination of aspirin, acetaminophen, and caffeine. He currently takes two of these pills every 6 hours around the clock while awake. He has had numerous cranial scans and consultations for this problem. There is a long-standing history of intermittent headaches beginning in childhood. He is placed on a weaning schedule with eventual discontinuation of over-the-counter headache medications over 4 weeks and is advised to avoid all other forms of caffeine. His daily headache initially worsens, but then gradually improves. When seen in follow-up, he is improved and reports only intermittent, thrice-weekly tension-type headache. He is counseled on the hazards of medication and caffeine overuse and started on amitriptyline for prophylaxis.

The heterogeneous nature and numerous comorbidities associated with chronic daily headache represent a diagnostic and therapeutic challenge. The syndrome of chronic daily headache may evolve from a variety of primary and/or secondary headache types, with tension and migraine headaches being the most common. Frequent headaches of any type may lose their clinical distinctiveness and lead to an ill-defined vague head pain whose characteristics defy specific definition. The clinician must then uncover any previous history of intermittent or episodic headaches that may have transformed over time. Anxiety, mood, and sleep disorders are just a few of the common comorbid conditions. Medication overuse frequently contributes to chronic daily headache Almost any short-acting analgesic may lead to "rebound" headaches, but vasoactive medications such as caffeine, triptans, and ergotamines are the most likely to cause this phenomenon. Special care must be taken when patients overuse substances whose abrupt withdrawal may prove dangerous or life threatening, including butalbital, benzodiazepines, and opioids.

The treatment of chronic daily headache first requires that overused substances are weaned or discontinued. Many patients may resist this intervention out of fear that headaches will worsen. Careful education is necessary to explain the association between medication overuse and the chronic headaches. Support mechanisms to control anxiety and a clear management plan for headache recurrence are needed. Comorbid etiologic factors—depression, psychosocial stresses, and poor sleep—require attention. Nonpharmacologic interventions include emotional support, counseling, physical therapy, relaxation techniques, heat, and massage. The choice of prophylactic medication should be based on the underlying headache type and comorbidities. For example, the patient above suffers from transformed tension-type headache, and therefore amitriptyline is recommended. The use of botulinum toxin type A as a prophylactic agent for chronic daily headache has not been supported by randomized control trials. A recent trial has shown significantly decreased frequency of chronic headaches in patients receiving botulinum toxin injections compared to placebo and supports its future use as an adjuvant treatment for chronic headache syndromes in selected patients.

PRIMARY HEADACHE SYNDROMES WITH DEFINED TRIGGERS

Exertional Headache

Physical exercise is always the precipitating factor in primary exertional headaches. They may develop during acute straining, such as weight lifting, or after sustained exercise, such as running. These headaches are characterized by throbbing pain for minutes or hours after discontinuation of activity. They often respond to 25–50 mg of indomethacin three times daily taken either after the exercise or prophylactically once a typical pattern is established. β-Blockers may also be used for prophylaxis. However, the possibility of serious disorders such as arterial dissection, aneurysmal rupture, and even an intracranial mass must be excluded. Computed tomography (CT), MRI, and MR angiography may be appropriate.

Headache Associated with Sexual Activity (Coital Headache)

Typically, these headaches develop as dull, generalized pain during sexual activity or as an acute, sometimes explosive, pain during orgasm. The headache lasts for minutes to hours after the cessation of sexual activity. Patients with coital headache often suffer from exertional headache as well. Clinicians may find patients suffering from this condition to be less than forthcoming about the circumstances surrounding the onset of headache. A careful history including questions about sexual symptoms is needed. Embarrassment and an unwillingness to address sexual concerns with a physician may lead patients with coital headache to go undiagnosed for years. As with other paroxysmal headaches, a search for underlying systemic or intracranial pathology, particularly a ruptured aneurysm, is needed before diagnosing a benign process. NSAIDs, particularly indomethacin (25–50 mg), may be helpful when administered before sexual activity.

Others

Hypnic headaches tend to occur more in women 50 years or older during rapid eye movement sleep and can recur several times at night. The pain is usually unilateral but can be bilateral and lasts 20–120 minutes after awakening. NSAIDs with caffeine or lithium have been used to control them. *Cough headaches* in contrast are sudden acute bilateral headaches occurring in older men and induced by straining or coughing. They last from seconds to 30 minutes and tend to be indomethacin responsive. Cough-induced headache is common in Arnold–Chiari type I malformations and this as well as cerebrovascular dissection or a rupture intracranial aneurysm should be excluded before making a diagnosis of a primary cough-induced headache.

SECONDARY HEADACHE DISORDERS

Although most headaches occur in the absence of underlying intracranial or systemic pathology, some result from more serious illness. The neurologist is often the initial physician contacted, and a careful history is mandatory to achieve an accurate diagnosis and to institute proper management. The headache's temporal profile, pain characteristics, and precipitating factors as well as patient's age, gender, family history, and associated systemic symptoms require analysis. The history is followed by a careful neurologic and general examination. Often, immediate laboratory evaluation and neuroimaging are indicated. With the widespread availability and relatively inexpensive nature of cranial CT, it is judicious to image patients who have experienced recent onset of a significant headache, including those with normal clinical examinations. Significant pathology, such as subarachnoid hemorrhage, subdural hematoma, and neoplasm provide examples wherein cranial CT may diagnose serious neurologic conditions when even the most careful neurologic examination may, at times, be normal.

GIANT CELL (TEMPORAL) ARTERITIS

Clinical Vignette

A 78-year-old man reports a constant, global headache for more than a month. He has felt generally unwell, with poor appetite, fatigue, and a 10-pound weight loss over the same time period. He experiences stiffness and pain in his shoulders and hips on awakening. A week prior to evaluation, he noticed a transient blurring of vision in his left eye for 20 minutes. His neurologic examination is normal, except for questionable temporal artery tenderness on the left. His sedimentation rate is found to be elevated, at 85 mm/hour. He is placed on prednisone 60 mg daily with rapid improvement of his symptoms. A left temporal artery biopsy, performed several days later, demonstrates findings typical for giant cell arteritis (transmural inflammatory response with occasional multinucleated giant cells and areas of internal elastic lamina disruption). Eight months later, he remains on 5 mg of prednisone to control his stiffness and pain.

Headache is the most common and prominent presenting symptom of giant cell or temporal arteritis, a serious disorder of the elderly with potentially devastating complications such as permanent blindness. As in the above vignette, early identification and prompt treatment prevents blindness from developing. The pain of temporal arteritis is usually bilateral and nonspecific, being throbbing or continuous, and with variable intensity, at times so mild that its potential significance is easily overlooked. Systemic complaints including anorexia, general malaise, myalgias, and arthralgias are common, and severe as important diagnostic clues. Polymyalgia rheumatica, a condition characterized by proximal musculoskeletal pain and morning stiffness, frequently accompanies the headache. Jaw or tongue claudication and rarely facial tissue ischemia have been described and

reflect external carotid artery involvement. Patients may have subtle and intermittent visual blurring or frank episodes of monocular visual loss mimicking transient ischemic attacks. Although often present, temporal artery tenderness may be relatively minor (Fig. 11-7). Early diagnosis is paramount as arteritis may precipitously cause unilateral or sequential bilateral anterior ischemic optic neuropathy with permanent visual loss. Although posterior ciliary arteries are most commonly involved, visual loss may less commonly result from ophthalmic artery involvement and rarely retinal artery arteritis. Furthermore, the arteritis may be widespread with involvement beyond the temporal arteries to the aorta and its branches. Infrequently, ischemic stroke may occur as arteritis affects the extracranial carotid or vertebral arteries. The intracranial circulation is generally spared. Erythrocyte sedimentation rate (ESR) and C-reactive protein provide the laboratory means to support the diagnosis. Typically, the ESR is significantly increased to 60–110 mm/hour, although there are exceptions. Biopsy of a long temporal artery segment is indicated in every patient suspected of having temporal arteritis. Because the arteritis is patchy, a unilateral biopsy may fail to show the inflammatory changes of giant cell arteritis and bilateral biopsies may be required to make the diagnosis. A mixed infiltrate of neutrophils and T lymphocytes involves the media with concurrent intimal hyperplasia and gradual luminal narrowing. Granulomatous, inflammatory arteritis with giant cell formation and marked disruption of the internal elastic lamina are classic for temporal arteritis (see Fig. 11-7).

Treatment

Because temporal arteritis is a chronic disorder, it requires relatively long-term oral corticosteroid treatment. Prompt diagnosis and treatment are required to prevent serious complications. Treatment must not be delayed because corticosteroids do not alter the pathologic findings if the biopsy is done within a few days of initiating therapy. Prednisone is begun at 40–60 mg/day, followed by a very gradual taper. When transient visual or neurologic symptoms occur, higher initial dosages of corticosteroid may be indicated. Steroids may be needed for 1–2 years at smaller doses to control associated symptoms. Treatment must be individualized, with frequent monitoring of sedimentation rate and symptoms. Long-term steroid side effects, such as truncal weight gain, glucose intolerance, electrolyte imbalance, hypertension, osteoporosis, potential immunosuppression, and cataract formation, to name just a few, need to be followed closely.

Future Directions

Giant cell arteritis is a chronic disease that requires prolonged immunosuppression. In selected patients with longstanding disease, the use of corticosteroid-sparing drugs like methotrexate, azathioprine, and tumor necrosis factor-α inhibitors have been explored.

BRAIN HEMORRHAGE, INFECTIONS, AND TUMORS

Subdural hematoma, intracerebral hemorrhage, subarachnoid hemorrhage, meningitis, and brain tumors are causes of secondary headaches. Each of these entities needs consideration in

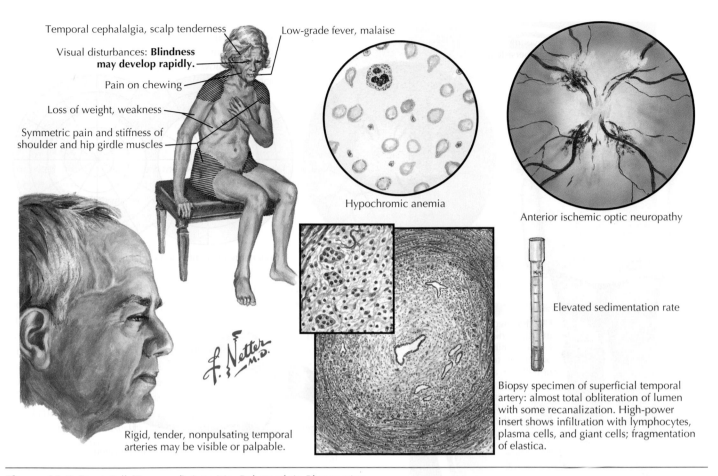

Temporal cephalalgia, scalp tenderness

Visual disturbances: **Blindness may develop rapidly.**

Pain on chewing

Loss of weight, weakness

Symmetric pain and stiffness of shoulder and hip girdle muscles

Low-grade fever, malaise

Hypochromic anemia

Anterior ischemic optic neuropathy

Elevated sedimentation rate

Rigid, tender, nonpulsating temporal arteries may be visible or palpable.

Biopsy specimen of superficial temporal artery: almost total obliteration of lumen with some recanalization. High-power insert shows infiltration with lymphocytes, plasma cells, and giant cells; fragmentation of elastica.

Figure 11-7 Giant-Cell (Temporal) Arteritis, Polymyalgia Rheumatica.

patients who experience the recent onset of headache without prior history or of a changing pattern of headache. Each of these important disorders is discussed elsewhere in this text; however, a few comments are warranted.

Every individual with a precipitous onset of "the worst headache of my life" warrants immediate careful medical and neurologic evaluation by their physician or in the emergency room. Funduscopic examination should evaluate for papilledema or subhyaloid hemorrhages. Regardless of the findings, emergency imaging is indicated. Cranial CT offers a rapid and readily available means to evaluate for hemorrhage and mass lesions. MRI and MR angiography may be indicated but are generally not required for the urgent evaluation of thunderclap headache. If no mass lesion is found on imaging, CSF analysis is indicated to evaluate for subarachnoid hemorrhage and infection (Chapters 48, 49, and 57).

IDIOPATHIC INTRACRANIAL HYPERTENSION

Clinical Vignette

A 38-year-old overweight woman presented with a recent onset of headaches and blurred vision. The headaches were increasingly severe and more bothersome to her when she bent forward. She noted intermittent double vision on lateral gaze.

Neurologic examination demonstrated limitation of lateral eye movements compatible with CN-VI paresis and modest papilledema. Brain imaging demonstrated diminished size of the lateral ventricles. Spinal fluid pressure was 350 mm CSF; its hematologic, cytologic, and chemical components were normal.

Idiopathic intracranial hypertension, also called pseudotumor cerebri, is a unique syndrome of relatively severe poorly defined and often progressive headaches with associated horizontal diplopia. In addition, transient visual obscurations and pulsatile tinnitus may be part of the clinical picture. It primarily presents in healthy, usually overweight, young women. Pseudotumor cerebri is associated with increased intracranial CSF pressure about 250 mm H_2O (Fig. 11-8).

Clinical Presentation and Diagnostic Studies

Neurologic examination demonstrates papilledema, with eventual optic nerve atrophy and visual field loss. Because of increased ICP, lateral rectus muscle weakness (pseudo–sixth nerve palsy) may be seen but patients are otherwise awake, alert, and have no focal neurologic deficits.

autologous blood patch injected at the lumbar puncture site, theoretically sealing the leak, almost universally improves post–lumbar puncture headaches, providing credence to the theory that they are secondary to a CSF leak. Other options for treatment include prolonged bed rest and continuous intrathecal or epidural saline infusions. Surgical intervention is rarely necessary. In spontaneous cases, a blood patch in the lumbar region often provides relief despite no identifiable tear in that region. Occasionally, such headaches are resistant to therapy and become disabling.

In the above vignette, a diagnosis of traumatic leptomeningeal tear with CSF leak and subsequent low-pressure syndrome was made. A therapeutic trial of an autologous blood dural patch was successful, with relief of the headaches and associated symptoms within a week.

CRANIAL NEURALGIAS

This group of patients experiences brief but severe paroxysms of head pain in the distribution of a specific cranial nerve, particularly the trigeminal nerve.

Trigeminal Neuralgia

Clinical Vignette

A 50-year-old woman develops pain in her left cheek. The pain begins as a dull ache, similar to a toothache. Soon she develops recurrent attacks of sudden sharp pain in the same distribution. The attacks are brief, lasting only a few seconds, but she describes them as the worst pain of her life. Brushing the teeth, a cold breeze, or any physical contact to the left side of her face frequently triggers the pain. She visits her dentist on several occasions, and eventually has two teeth extracted but without significant relief of symptoms. An MRI demonstrates tortuosity of the vertebrobasilar circulation with left trigeminal nerve neurovascular impingement. She is treated with varying dosages of carbamazepine and gabapentin, with only partial relief and side effects of lethargy and drowsiness. After 5 years, she undergoes microvascular decompression surgery and feels immediate relief. A year later the pain recurs, and she meets with her surgeon to discuss percutaneous radiofrequency ablation.

A careful history is the key to the diagnosis of this uncommon but eminently treatable facial neuralgia. Trigeminal neuralgia, also called tic douloureux, is a disabling, lancinating, or electrical facial pain that occurs in the trigeminal nerve distribution (see also Chapter 6). It is one of the worst pains humans experience. This condition is not defined by any test but requires the clinician to recognize it by its primary historical attributes. There are no associated neurologic deficits.

The patient, almost always an adult and usually a woman, experiences paroxysmal and frequently provocable intermittent unilateral pain that rarely occurs during sleep. The stereotyped attacks are very brief, lasting anywhere from an indefinable instant to several minutes. In between sudden attacks, the patient may experience a more constant dull or aching pain, which may lead them to believe the problem is dental in origin. The frequency of attacks may fluctuate markedly, disabling a patient for weeks or months at a time before going into a remission.

It primarily involves the second or third divisions of the trigeminal nerve and occasionally the first division. Triggers include talking, chewing, shaving, drinking hot or cold liquids, or any form of sensory facial stimulation. The pain is usually unilateral; when it affects both sides of the face, it does not do so concomitantly.

In perhaps the majority of individuals, an idiopathic loss of myelin insulation within the posterior root of the trigeminal nerve causes the pain. When it occurs in a young adult, the demyelination from multiple sclerosis is often the mechanism. Another cause is a tortuous or ectatic artery, often a branch of the superior cerebellar artery, compressing or pulsating against the trigeminal posterior rootlets. Trigeminal neuralgia results from other conditions compressing the trigeminal nerve, such as acoustic neuroma (vestibular schwannoma), meningioma, arteriovenous malformation, and rarely a carotid-posterior communicating or distal anterior inferior cerebellar artery aneurysm. Cranial scanning with MRI is indicated for all patients with trigeminal neuralgia. Bilateral symptoms, trigeminal sensory finding, and loss of corneal reflexes are a strong indicator of secondary trigeminal neuralgia and should raise concern.

Anticonvulsants are the mainstay of medical therapy for trigeminal neuralgia. Most patients respond to the use of carbamazepine, which stabilizes cell membranes and raises the threshold of neural stimulation. Carbamazepine and oxcarbazepine carry the best scientific evidence for efficacy. Phenytoin, gabapentin, lamotrigine, topiramate, and pregabalin may be useful but these agents are not studied as well. Baclofen, an antispasmodic, may provide some relief as may certain antidepressants, including amitriptyline. Baclofen is advocated by some as an adjuvant treatment to carbamazepine if higher doses alone are inadequate or cause side effects. The effectiveness of any agent may diminish over time.

Several surgical approaches are available for patients who cannot tolerate medical therapy. Percutaneous approaches include trigeminal radiofrequency lesioning, glycerol injection, and balloon compression. Available open procedures such as posterior cranial fossa microvascular decompression open trigeminal rhizotomy are much more invasive and may be less appropriate for elderly patients or those in poor health. Focused-beam radiosurgery by gamma knife or linear particle accelerator (Linac) is also available for this condition. Microvascular decompression often relieves the tick pain and causes less sensory loss than other procedures.

Trigeminal neuralgia can recur after any procedure at a lifetime rate of 15–20%. Recurrences can be treated with subsequent radiofrequency ablation. Ipsilateral hearing loss is occasionally a complication of decompressive surgery, relating to the delicate anatomic relationship between the auditory and trigeminal nerves. The operation carries a 1% risk of death or stroke.

Accurate diagnosis is essential to successful surgical relief. Steady nonparoxysmal pain, posttraumatic pain, pain after dental procedures, and pain that is not in the trigeminal zone will not be effectively treated by radiofrequency ablation or other procedures mentioned above. Knowledge of trigeminal nerve anatomy, its facial distribution, and an appreciation of the paroxysmal, provocable, and unilateral character of trigeminal neuralgia is essential for accurate diagnosis and management.

Glossopharyngeal Neuralgia

Glossopharyngeal neuralgia is less common than trigeminal neuralgia and generally located in the ear, tonsillar area, or deep within the throat in the CN-IX sensory distribution. The pain is paroxysmal, recurrent, and severe, usually with swallowing as the primary triggering mechanism. Occasionally, patients experience bradycardia during the pain paroxysms and, sometimes, loss of consciousness. Medical treatment is similar to that of trigeminal neuralgia. Rhizotomy or decompression of CN-IX may be necessary in severe, medically intractable cases.

Occipital Neuralgia

Although similar in pain characteristics to trigeminal neuralgia, occipital neuralgia is differentiated by location to the posterior scalp innervated by the greater and lesser occipital nerves from the C2 dermatome (Fig. 11-10). Occipital neuralgia is probably underdiagnosed. Pain is generally localized to the base of the skull but may extend to the vertex, behind the ear or into the neck and upper back. Pain may be initially incited by hyperextension of the neck or whiplash injury. Patients are commonly seen after motor vehicle accident, sports trauma, or work-related injury. The neuralgia is usually unilateral, at times bilateral, and occurs in brief paroxysms of jabbing pain superimposed on a more chronic dull occipital ache.

Diagnosis is assisted by the identification of an occipital trigger point at the base of the skull between the mastoid process and the occipital protuberance. Although the pain and disability may be similar to trigeminal neuralgia, occipital neuralgia is more easily treated. Infiltration of the greater and lesser occipital nerves with a local anesthetic and steroid compounds may prove both diagnostic and therapeutic. When ineffective, carbamazepine and other drugs commonly used in the treatment of neuropathic pain are often employed.

OBSTRUCTIVE SLEEP APNEA

Headache may be the presenting symptom in sleep apnea. Patients frequently complain of daily headaches that are worse upon awakening. Invariably, these patients are fatigued and experience excessive daytime sleepiness. A careful history, including discussion of snoring, may prove vital in making this diagnosis. The neurologic examination is generally normal, although certain clues on physical exam may include obesity and

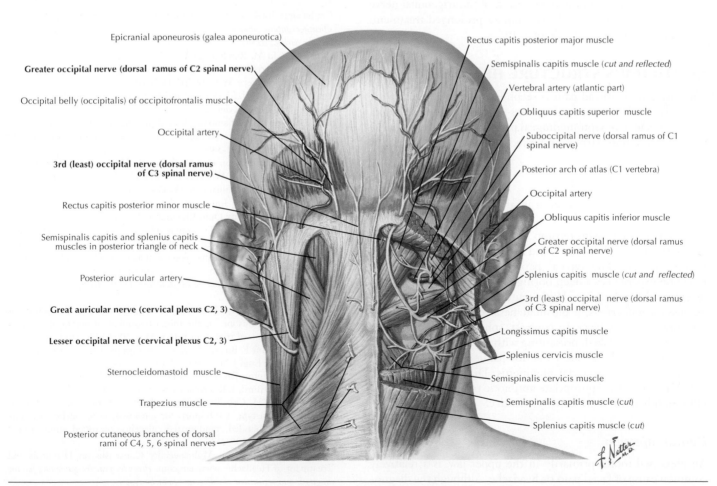

Figure 11-10 Suboccipital Triangle.

abnormalities or tissue redundancy of the palate, uvula, or tongue. When correctly identified, this headache syndrome may improve dramatically with nocturnal continuous positive airway pressure treatment. Sleep apnea is discussed in more detail in Chapter 15.

INFECTIOUS MECHANISMS

Meningitis must be considered in anyone experiencing an acute-onset headache. Typically, these individuals have a concomitant fever and stiff neck (meningismus) as detailed in Chapter 48.

Cranial herpes zoster (shingles) is a "reactivation" of the varicella-zoster virus within the gasserian ganglion or upper cervical dorsal root ganglion. Typically, these patients report severe, sometimes excruciating, boring head pain or neuralgia. The rash usually precedes the onset of the headache, but, in some instances, intense head pain can antedate skin lesions by a few days. The classic vesicles can vary from a few easily overlooked lesions to an extensive vesicular rash. After the dermatologic changes appear, treatment with antiviral medications, such as acyclovir, valacyclovir, and Famvir, is indicated. When herpes zoster ophthalmicus occurs, an ophthalmology consultation should be obtained and along with antivirals, coadministration of corticosteroids may be considered, when no contraindication exists. There is an increased incidence of shingles in the elderly and the immunosuppressed. Postherpetic neuralgia may occur in the distribution of the trigeminal nerve or upper cervical roots and may require prolonged treatment. Treatment is discussed in Chapter 49.

CONTIGUOUS STRUCTURE HEADACHES

The last group of head pain is secondary contiguous anatomic structures such as the nasal sinuses or teeth. Inherent brain, cerebrovascular, or leptomeningeal pathology is discussed in the sections on tumors, stroke, and infectious diseases, respectively.

Nasal Sinus Infection

This entity must be considered in all patients presenting with headache.

Often, a patient with tension headache presents with a self-diagnosis of "sinus headache" and a careful history and examination is needed. The typical patient with active nasal sinus infection experiences a deep boring discomfort in the maxillary or ethmoid facial region. With acute infections, there is often percussion tenderness, a purulent nasal discharge, and, if the infection is severe, fever. In contrast, sphenoid sinus infections are more easily masked, presenting with only deep-seated headaches, and pose the greatest risk for parameningeal seeding of the meninges and bacterial meningitis. Diagnosis depends on CT, MRI, or both. Appropriate antibiotic treatment, decongestants, and hydration are usually effective.

Dental Infection

An abscessed tooth, primarily in the upper jaw, is a relatively common cause of facial pain or headache. Although the diagnosis is usually obvious to patients, on occasion they may present

to a physician first. The neurologist must consider a primary dental source as an unusual cause for some instances of head and facial pain. A careful dental evaluation may be diagnostic when no other mechanism is identified. Temporomandibular joint dysfunction causes referred periorbital, temporal, zygomatic, and mandibular pain and is often mistaken for a primary or secondary headache syndrome. Joint clicking or crepitance, focal tenderness, limited jaw movement, and an altered bite are hints to its diagnosis.

ADDITIONAL RESOURCES

Attal N, Cruccu G, Haanpaa M, et al. EFNS guidelines on pharmacological treatment of neuropathic pain. Eur J Neurol 2006;13:1153-1169.

Bennetto L, Patel N, Fuller G. Trigeminal neuralgia and its management. Br Med J 2007;334:201-205.

Bigal ME, Lipton RB, Tepper SJ, et al. Primary chronic daily headache and its subtypes in adolescents and adults. Neurology 2004;63:843-847.

Cady R, Dodick DW. Diagnosis and treatment of migraine. Mayo Clin Proc 2002;77:266-261.

Chole R, Patil R, Degwekar S, et al. Drug treatment of trigeminal neuralgia: a systemic review of the literature. J Oral Maxillofac Surg 2007;65:40-45.

Dodick D. Chronic daily headache. N Engl J Med 2006;354:158-165.

Headache Classification Committee of the International Headache Society. Classification and diagnostic criteria for headache disorders, cranial neuralgia, and facial pain. Cephalalgia 1988;8(Suppl. 7):1-96. *Classic reference providing a framework from which to approach headache and treatment.*

Headache Classification Subcommittee of the International Headache Society. The International Classification of Headache Disorders. 2nd ed. Cephalalgia 2004;24(Suppl. 1):9-160. *This second edition of headache classification contains some minor changes reflecting recent advances in understanding the pathophysiology and therapeutics of headaches.*

Hoffman G, Cid M, Rendt-Zagar K, et al. Infliximab for maintenance of glucocorticosteroid-induced remission of giant cell arteritis: a randomized trial. Ann Intern Med 2007;146:621-630.

Lance JW, Goadsby PJ. Mechanism and Management of Headache. 7th ed. Philadelphia, PA: Elsevier; 2005.

Lipton RB, Bigel ME, Diamond M, et al, for the AMPP Advisory Group. Migraine prevalence, disease burden, and the need for preventive therapy. Neurology 2007;68:343-349.

Loder E, Rizzoli P. Tension-type headache. Br Med J 2008;336:88-92.

Olesen J, Tfelt-Hansen P, Welch KMA. The Headaches. 2nd ed. Philadelphia, Pa: Lippincott Williams & Wilkins; 2000.

Pipitone N, Salvarani C, Improving therapeutic options for patients with giant cell arteritis. Curr Opin Rheumatol 2008;20(1):17-22.

Ramadan NM, Silberstein SD, Freitag FG, et al. for the US Headache Consortium. Evidence-based guidelines for migraine headache in the primary care setting: pharmacological management for prevention of migraine. Available from: www.aan.com/professionals/practice/pdfs/gl0090.pdf. *Provides evidence-based guidelines for the treatment of migraine headache.*

Salcarani C, Macchioni P, Manzini C, et al. Infliximab plus Prednisone or Placebo plus prednisone for the initial treatment of polymyalgia rheumatica: a randomized trial. Ann Intern Med 2007;146(9):631-639.

Salvarani C, Cantini F, Boiardi L, et al. Polymyalgia rheumatica and giant cell arteritis. N Engl J Med 2002;347(4):261-271.

Silberstein SD, Lipton RB, Dalessio DJ. Wolff's headache and other head pain. 7th ed. Oxford, UK: Oxford University Press; 2001.

Straube A, Empl M, Ceballos-Baumann A, et al. Pericranial injection of botulinum toxin type A (Dysport) for tension-type headache—a multicentre, double-blinded, placebo-controlled study. Eur J Neurol 2008;15(3):205-213.

US Headache Consortium. Multispecialty Consensus on Diagnosis and Treatment of Headache. www.aan.com. *Provides practice guidelines for the diagnosis and treatment of different headache types.*

Wareham D, Breuer J. Herpes zoster. Br Med J 2007;334:1211-1215.

Pain Pathophysiology and Management

John Markman

12

Clinical Vignette

A 53-year-old woman with type 2 diabetes mellitus presented with burning pain in both feet. This was persistent throughout the day, and began to make it rather uncomfortable to stand or walk for any prolonged period of time. This was particularly worse at night, often preventing her from getting to sleep. Eventually this pain became so intense that this middle-aged lady had to stop working as a hair stylist, despite being the sole wage earner for her family. She had been noncompliant with her diabetic monitoring and her various medications as evidenced by wide fluctuations in her serum glucose. Her neurologic examination demonstrated a stocking hypoesthesia in both feet with loss of her Achilles muscle stretch reflexes. She also has an asymptomatic plantar ulcer under her right great toe.

Comment: This very common clinical scenario illustrates the toll that chronic pain can have on an otherwise healthy individual, as well as the potential social and economic repercussions of untreated chronic pain.

NEUROPATHIC PAIN SYNDROMES

Neuropathic pain encompasses an array of chronic debilitating nerve injury syndromes that specifically have an adverse impact on the quality of life. To capture the diversity of etiologies, the International Association for the Study of Pain has defined neuropathic pain rather broadly as a "pain initiated or caused by a primary lesion or dysfunction in the nervous system." These syndromes originate at every level of the neuraxis and include diabetic polyneuropathy, HIV neuropathy, postsurgical pain, postherpetic neuralgia (PHN), trigeminal neuralgia, complex regional pain syndrome (CRPS), spinal cord injury pain, poststroke pain, multiple sclerosis, and phantom limb pain.

Neuropathic pain may be subdivided into two broad neuroanatomic subgroups based on the localization of nerve injury. *Central nervous system syndromes* result from pathology of the brain and spinal cord such as that associated with a demyelinating plaque in multiple sclerosis or stroke. *Peripheral neuropathic pain* syndromes are the far more common group and include processes such as reactivation of the varicella-zoster virus giving rise to PHN and painful diabetic polyneuropathy.

Pathophysiology

The understanding of the relationship between the clinical features of neuropathic pain and underlying molecular mechanisms in humans remains in its infancy. Following nerve injury, neuronal remodeling occurs, with microscopic structural changes in the neuronal membrane and individual membrane bound ion channels. Animal models suggest that neuronal remodeling alters the membrane electrical properties, resulting in a state of hyperexcitability wherein thresholds are lowered, action potentials are propagated more easily, and the duration of nerve impulses is prolonged. These aberrant action potentials are reproduced at multiple anatomic levels: from the primary sensory neuron, to the sensory ganglia, and neurons within the dorsal horn of the spinal cord (Fig. 12-1). Such a pattern of aberrant nerve discharges may account for the positive symptoms of neuropathic pain. The cognizant perception of painful symptoms is based on the neural pathways commencing in the periphery at the primary sensory nerve ending, transmitted through the dorsal root ganglia, the spinal cord, up to the thalamus and finally the somatosensory parietal cerebral cortex (Fig. 12-2). During the passage of nerve potentials along this pathway, a number of opportunities are available at the various synapses for modulation of the impulses per se and thus the eventual perception of the original stimulus.

When chronic pain syndromes develop, there is evidence to support the conjecture that different ion channels are involved in both remodeling and ectopic neuronal signaling. The variability in symptomatology as well as the response to pharmacologic treatment may depend on the specific type of channel involved. An example of this correlation is the expression of the acid- and heat-sensitive capsaicin/vanilloid receptor (TRPV1) in nociceptive C-fibers. Inflammation and focal tissue acidity following nerve injury may activate this receptor, enhancing exaggerated pain responses. On the other hand, continuous activation of this receptor may desensitize these fibers and account for the analgesic efficacy of capsaicin.

In addition, an alteration of central nervous system signal transduction also occurs in some patients suffering from neuropathic pain. Following nerve injury, retrograde transport of growth factors from the distal neuron to the cell body is impaired or lost. Disruption of intercellular signaling cascades causes structural changes in second- and third-order neurons, altering the expression of neuromodulators such as brain-derived natriuretic factor and substance P in nociceptive A-fibers. Simultaneously, ectopic activity and injury discharge may cause preferential death of inhibitory interneurons located in the superficial laminae of the dorsal horn. These changes ultimately lead to decreased inhibition of pain signaling within the spinal cord. In addition to changes in inhibitory pathway signaling, the preferential loss of C-fiber neurons as observed in animal models may lead to remodeling of synaptic architecture. Following denervation, A-fiber neurons from deep laminar loci sprout new afferents to form functional synapses in portions of the spinal column formerly occupied by C-fiber termini. This expansion of neuronal receptive fields may play a key role in the zones of hyperalgesia adjacent to the territory of primary nerve injury.

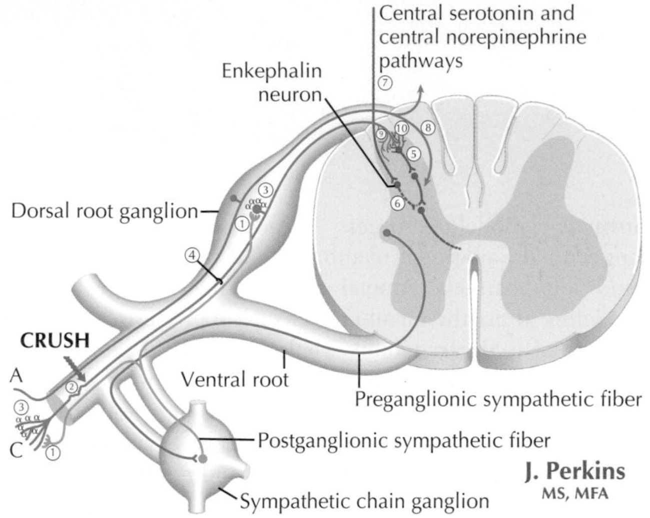

Mechanisms of Neuropathic Pain

1. Sprouting of sympathetic postganglionic nerve fibers on 1° afferent endings and 1° sensory cell bodies
2. Lowered threshold for firing of C fibers (hyperesthesia) and A delta fibers (allodynia)
3. Proliferation of alpha (α)-adrenergic receptors on 1° sensory afferent endings and 1° sensory cell bodies
4. Possible ephaptic afferent activation
5. Permanent hyperactivation of wide dynamic range neurons
6. Glutamate excitotoxic cell death of inhibitory neurons (glutamate storms)
7. Inadequacy of central descending serotonin, norepinephrine, opioid peptide pathways to control nociception
8. Immobilization by pain decreases gating of nociceptive input, limiting physical therapy to initiate gating
9. Sprouting of C fibers in spinal cord
10. Extension of interneuron dendrites into additional spinal cord laminae

Figure 12-1 Mechanisms of Neuropathic Pain.

Diagnosis and Clinical Manifestations

The diagnosis of neuropathic pain syndromes requires a thorough exam and careful consideration of a patient's medical history. *Neuropathic pain* symptoms are distinct from nonneuropathic (nociceptive) pain. The following criteria have been proposed to define and differentiate neuropathic pain from nociceptive pain:

1. Pain and sensory symptoms that persist beyond the healing period.
2. Presence of neurologic sensory signs manifesting as negative and positive sensory phenomena.
3. Presence of other neurologic signs, including motor, manifesting as negative and positive motor phenomena, or autonomic signs.

Using this schema, there are four forms of pain that are characterized by positive sensory phenomena:

dysesthesia (unpleasant abnormal sensation),
paresthesia (abnormal sensation),
hyperalgesia (exaggerated response to painful stimulus), and
allodynia (pain caused by nonnoxious stimulus).

In contrast, negative phenomena refer to loss of sensation. Differences in quality and spatial characteristics of pain symptoms may also be used to distinguish *neuropathic pain* from nonneuropathic pain, with symptoms of stimulus-evoked pain, shooting pain, electric shock, burning, and cold significantly more common in patients with neuropathic pain. *Neuropathic pain* also tends to be perceived as a superficial sensation, whereas other forms of pain are felt in deeper tissues, muscles, and joints. Motor as well as other nonsensory neurologic symptoms may also occur in neuropathic pain syndromes. These include weakness, spasticity, tremor, ataxia, apraxia, spasticity, hypotonia, muscle spasms, and muscle tenderness. The concordance of these nonsensory symptoms with positive and negative phenomena is strongly suggestive of the presence of a neuropathic pain syndrome.

The quality, intensity, and duration of symptoms should always be carefully assessed in any chronic pain patient, and the characteristics and distribution of aberrant sensory phenomena can be used to guide the focused neurologic examination. Standard neurologic physical exam tools such as cotton wisps, tuning forks, and warm and cold objects may be used to evaluate evoked pain and, when coupled with a thorough neurologic examination, may help to localize the lesion. In the presence of confirmatory history and laboratory data, positive and negative phenomena (evoked or spontaneous) occurring in the territory of a localized lesion confirms the clinical diagnosis.

In addition to the history and physical examination, ancillary studies may aid in diagnosis. These are very important for confirming or excluding the presence of underlying etiologies for neuropathic pain. Magnetic resonance imaging is used to assess the integrity of central neuroanatomic structures involved in pain signaling pathways. These include the spinal cord, brainstem, thalamus, and cortices (see Fig. 12-1). Peripheral sources for the pain can sometimes be defined by electromyography and nerve conduction studies. The latter particularly assess the function of large myelinated nerve fibers. Nonneurologic tests such as oral glucose tolerance, Tzanck prep (a rapid test previously performed to diagnose infections caused by herpes viruses) and enzyme-linked immunosorbent assay. This can be used to confirm or exclude the presence of a number of underlying diseases that may lead to sequelae of neuropathic pain. Psychiatric evaluation is also useful in evaluating possible somatization disorders in patients with multisystem complaints that may date back into early developmental stages.

Treatment

Gauging the efficacy of treatment protocols represents a significant challenge in the treatment of neuropathic pain. Severity of pain is typically assessed at the time of exam, as well as over short time intervals, and subjectively graded by the patient on the 0–10 numeric rating scale, with a score of 0 representing "no pain" and a score of 10 representing "worst possible pain." Research suggests that clinically important pain relief is achieved with a 30% reduction in score on this scale, corresponding to a categoric rating of "moderate relief" or "much improved." In addition, counseling patients and families about reasonable expectations for symptom improvement is crucial. Patients

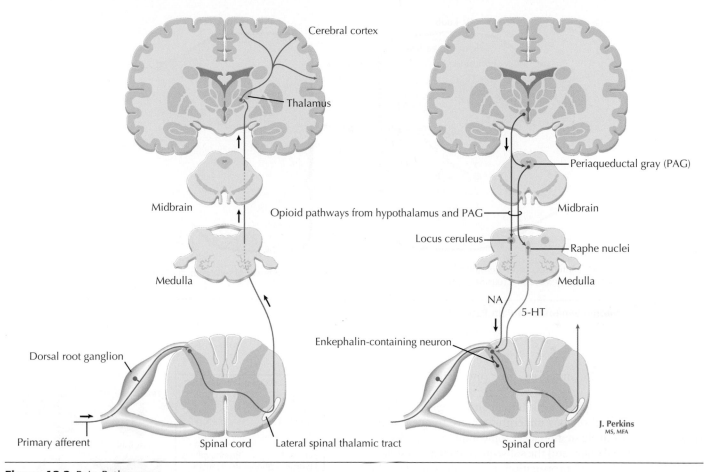

Figure 12-2 Pain Pathway.

must understand that *partial reduction* in pain intensity *is the norm* with pharmacotherapy. Furthermore, successful treatment will require a program of *adaptive coping* by the patient per se. A comprehensive approach that calls on close monitoring of side effects of medications used to treat neuropathic pain is essential, as many of these drugs have significant adverse events, especially when used in older patients.

MULTITIERED APPROACH TO PAIN MANAGEMENT

The International Association for the Study of Pain has developed a multitier approach to managing neuropathic pain. This is centered around patient communication and a number of available pharmacotherapeutic agents. The first step in this system involves a thorough clinical evaluation and discussion of a patient's underlying disease state as outlined above. The second step in the multitiered approach to managing NP is the prescription of a "first-line" pharmaceutical agent. Following prescription, the third step in treatment is reevaluation of the patient's pain intensity and its response to therapy. Therapy is continued if the patient's response has been complete. In contrast, if the patient has not responded to this medication, or the side effect profile is unacceptable, another first-line therapy needs to be initiated. Finally, if the patient reports a partial response, the initial therapy is continued and another first- or second-line medication is combined with this. If acceptable

symptom resolution does not occur with this approach, then the physician needs to consider introducing a third-line pharmaceutical agent.

FIRST-LINE PRESCRIPTION AGENTS

These include topical lidocaine, calcium channel α2-δ ligands (gabapentin, pregabalin), tricyclic antidepressants (TCAs) and serotonin norepinephrine reuptake inhibitors.

Putative calcium channel ligands such as gabapentin inhibit presynaptic calcium channel α2-δ subunits activity in the superficial laminae of the dorsal horn of the spinal cord. Their exact site of action within the central nervous system as antiepileptic agents and for their other benefits remains unclear.

Tricyclic antidepressants historically are thought to modulate pain signaling by affecting both serotonergic and noradrenergic reuptake in descending inhibitory supraspinal pathways (Fig. 12-3). Desipramine and nortriptyline are preferred for neuropathic pain because of their favorable side-effect profiles relative to amitriptyline. Although their anticholinergic side effects demand careful consideration when these are used in patients with comorbidities, TCAs will relieve pain in PHN, postmastectomy pain syndrome, and painful diabetic neuropathy (PDN) and nondiabetic peripheral neuropathy. These agents should be tried alone initially, and then may be used in combination to pursue symptomatic improvement if necessary, provided that

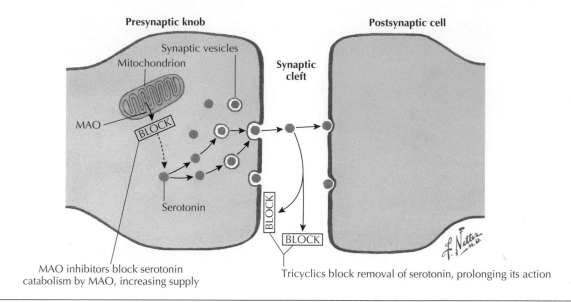

Presynaptic knob

Postsynaptic cell

Synaptic vesicles

Mitochondrion

Synaptic cleft

MAO

BLOCK

Serotonin

BLOCK

BLOCK

MAO inhibitors block serotonin catabolism by MAO, increasing supply

Tricyclics block removal of serotonin, prolonging its action

Figure 12-3 Serotonin Synapses of Pain Pathways.

the clinician carefully monitors their interactions and side effects.

Lidocaine preferentially inhibits voltage gated sodium channels in neuronal regions undergoing more frequent depolarization. It effectively suppresses ectopic impulses that develop following neuronal injury and the subsequent increase in sodium channel production and propagation at the affected site. This selectivity allows lidocaine to be safely used at low enough doses that avoid disrupting normal impulse conduction while still suppressing hyperexcitability. Infusion has proven an efficacious route for delivery in the treatment of both PHN and DPN (diabetic polyneuropathy), but its use is limited because of dosing and delivery issues arising with intravenous administration. Lidocaine is mainly used in the 5% patch form for the treatment of PHN and, in contrast, has a low probability for drug interactions and systemic side effects.

Opioid analgesia (Fig. 12-4) is considered by many experts to be a first-line agent as well, although considerable debate surrounds its role in management of neuropathic pain because of issues of tolerability, long-term efficacy, and the risks of misuse and abuse. Multiple trials support the use of these various pharmacologic modalities in chronic conditions such as PDN and PHN with evidence of superior efficacy and reduced side-effect burden when prescribed in combination with a calcium channel modulator. In clinical trials, opioid side effects, including nausea, sedation, and constipation, contributed to significant patient dropout, despite reported reductions in pain. *Tramadol* exerts its analgesic effects through both opioid and descending inhibitory pathways; it has been shown to be effective in reducing pain associated with nerve injury and improving quality of life.

A **Ten-Step Process** for **opioid therapy** utilized over the long term has been suggested by the International Society of Interventional Pain Physicians (Box 12-1). This provides the clinician with responsible guidelines for maintaining careful control of a potentially very useful therapeutic modality.

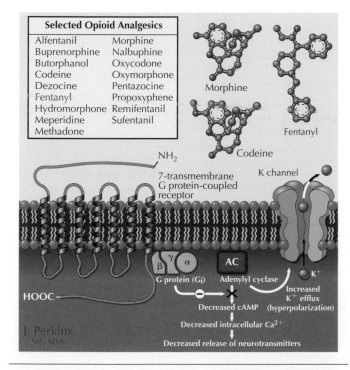

Selected Opioid Analgesics	
Alfentanil	Morphine
Buprenorphine	Nalbuphine
Butorphanol	Oxycodone
Codeine	Oxymorphone
Dezocine	Pentazocine
Fentanyl	Propoxyphene
Hydromorphone	Remifentanil
Meperidine	Sufentanil
Methadone	

Morphine

Fentanyl

Codeine

NH_2

7-transmembrane G protein-coupled receptor

K channel

HOOC

β γ α

G protein (G_i)

AC

Adenylyl cyclase

K^+

Increased K^+ efflux (hyperpolarization)

Decreased cAMP

Decreased intracellular Ca^{2+}

Decreased release of neurotransmitters

J. Perkins
MS, MFA

Figure 12-4 Opioid Receptor-Transduction Mechanism. Inhibits adenylyl cyclase by decreasing nociceptive neurotransmitter release from presynaptic terminals. Inhibits postsynaptic hyperpolarization by increasing K+ channel conductance.

SECOND-LINE PHARMACOTHERAPY

When an acceptable response to treatment is not achieved with the use of first-line agents, a number of less well substantiated second-line agents may be used. These include the anticonvulsant *lamotrigine* that blocks voltage-gated sodium channels implicated in hyperexcitability states, resulting in decreased net

Box 12-1 Ten-Step Process for Long-Term Opioid Therapy in Chronic Pain

Step I: Perform comprehensive initial evaluation
Step II: Establish diagnosis
   X-rays, MRI, CT scan
Step III: Establish medical necessity
   Physical diagnosis
   Therapeutic interventional pain management
   Physical modalities
   Behavior therapy
Step IV: Assess risk-to-benefit ratio
   Treatment is beneficial
Step V: Establish treatment goals
Step VI: Obtain informed medical consent and agreement
Step VII: Institute initial dose adjustment (up to 8–12 weeks)
   Start low dose
   Utilize opioids, nonsteroidal anti-inflammatory drugs, and adjuvants
   Discontinue because of side effects
      Lack of analgesia
      Side effects
      Lack of functional improvement
Step VIII: Assess stable phase
   Assess for the four A's
      Analgesia
      Activity
      Aberrant behavior
      Adverse effect
Step IX: Monitor adherence
   Prescription monitoring program
   Random drug screen
   Pill counts
Step X: Assess outcomes
   Successful: continue
      Stable doses
      Analgesia, activity
      No abuse, side effects
   Failed: discontinue if
      No analgesia
      Noncompliance
      Abuse
      Side effects
      Complications

Adapted from Trescot AM, Boswell MV, Atluri SL, et al: Opioid guidelines in the management of chronic non-cancer pain. Pain Physician 9:1-39, 2006.

Ca$^+$ influx. Lamotrigine is clinically effective in managing pain from PDN, HIV neuropathy, trigeminal neuralgia, some spinal cord injuries, and central poststroke pain, although its use is limited by the risk of severe rash and Stevens–Johnson syndrome.

Carbamazepine is the first anticonvulsant that the FDA approved for the treatment of trigeminal neuralgia. The research that supports its use for the treatment of PHN and PDN predated the era of large, multicenter clinical trials. Unfortunately, side effects and strength of evidence has relegated it to a second-line therapy. Initial trials of oxcarbazepine and other second-generation anticonvulsants for the treatment of trigeminal neuralgia and other neuropathic pain syndrome have demonstrated some favorable results, but further studies are required to establish their role, if any, in managing neuropathic pain.

THIRD-LINE PRESCRIPTION AGENTS

A large number of other pharmacologic agents have been or are currently under investigation for the treatment of neuropathic pain, including *N*-methyl-D-aspartate (NMDA) receptor blockers, selective serotonin reuptake inhibitors, bupropion, clonidine, dextromethorphan, mexiletine, capsaicin, and cannabinoids. Although clinical research has not demonstrated widespread efficacy of these agents, many have proven effective in individual cases of NP syndromes, and further research is warranted. As with any pharmacologic agent, special attention should be paid to patient education and adverse effect profile before initiating therapy with any of the third-line agents.

PAINFUL DIABETIC NEUROPATHY

Clinical Vignette

Julia, a 53-year-old woman, presents complaining of burning pain in her lower extremities. The pain started 18 months earlier beginning in her toes and has progressively ascended to involve her feet to the ankles bilaterally. She describes the pain as a persistent burning and tingling throughout the day, stating that her feet feel like "they're asleep all the time," and says the pain is worse at night. Her past medical history is significant for type 2 diabetes mellitus diagnosed 5 years prior for which she takes oral medications, including metformin and a glitazone. When questioned, she describes a pattern of poor medication compliance, erratic home blood glucose values, and denies performing regular foot inspections.

On exam, her muscle strength, patellar muscle stretch reflexes, and proprioceptive sensation as well as pedal pulses are normal, but she demonstrates diminished light tough, pinprick, and vibratory sensation below the mid-calf bilaterally and absent ankle muscle stretch reflexes. She had an antalgic (painful gait) and had recently been fitted with a prosthetic boot. She also has an asymptomatic plantar ulcer surrounded by callus on the first metatarsal head of the right foot, of which she denies knowledge.

Laboratory values are significant for an HbA$_1$C of 8.7% and creatinine of 1.1, but are otherwise normal. Nerve conduction studies (NCS) demonstrate no abnormalities, including detailed sensory nerve testing. However, these studies did not exclude a small-fiber sensory neuropathy as these unmyelinated type C fibers cannot be separately distinguished from the large-fiber responses with standard NCS.

Overview

This is an increasingly common complication of diabetes mellitus, developing in up to 66% of insulin-dependent (type 1) and 59% of non–insulin-dependent (type 2) diabetics. Of these patients, studies suggest that up to 20% will experience symptoms of pain, loss of sensation, numbness, and tingling of at least 3 months' duration, meeting the criteria for symptomatic peripheral neuropathy. Diabetic polyneuropathies also occur in other divisions of the nervous system and may present as

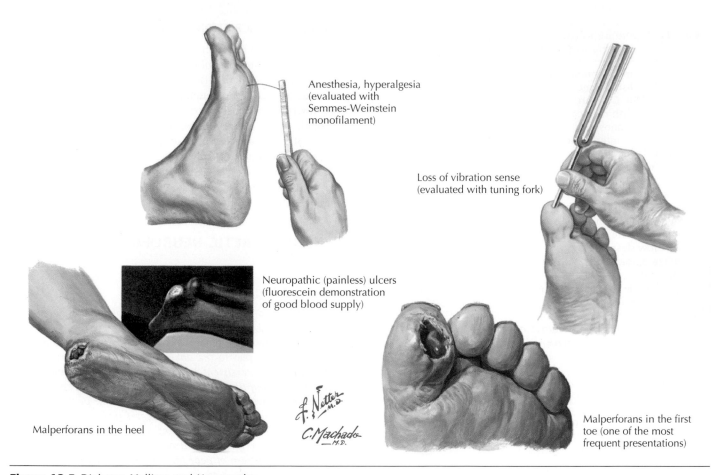

Anesthesia, hyperalgesia
(evaluated with
Semmes-Weinstein
monofilament)

Loss of vibration sense
(evaluated with tuning fork)

Neuropathic (painless) ulcers
(fluorescein demonstration
of good blood supply)

Malperforans in the heel

Malperforans in the first
toe (one of the most
frequent presentations)

Figure 12-5 Diabetes Mellitus and Neuropathy.

autonomic neuropathies involving the gastrointestinal, cardio-vascular, or genitourinary system, or as amyotrophic neuropa-thies with focal motor involvement especially in the thigh. Long-term complications of diabetic neuropathy include foot ulcers, which occur in 15% of diabetic patients and account for 85% of amputations in the same group (Fig. 12-5). PDN is a serious condition responsible for debilitating pain as well as serious long-term sequelae (Fig. 12-6), with early diagnosis and management crucial in preventing long-term complications and reductions in quality of life.

Pathophysiology

The pathophysiology of PDN is complex, involving an imper-fectly understood interaction of metabolic and vascular factors present in diabetes mellitus. Hyperglycemia and increased flux through the polyol pathway leads to intracellular accumulation of sorbitol and fructose, with reduction in Na^+/K^+-ATPase activ-ity, as well as the accumulation of nonenzymatic advanced glyca-tion end products on neural and vascular proteins. These metabolic derangements, coupled with protein kinase C activa-tion, derangements in fatty acid metabolism, and oxidative stress driven by hyperlipidemia and hyperglycemia are responsible for gradual damage and impairment of microvascular endothelial function. Hypoperfusion follows, with hyalinization and mal-adaptive hyperplasia of microvascular vasa nervorum accounting

for progressive dysfunction of both small and large nerve fibers. This hypoxia also damages small unmyelinated fibers innervat-ing arterioles responsible for arteriovenous shunting in endo-neurium and perineurium, further exacerbating ischemic nerve injury. Patients experiencing painful symptoms also demon-strate neovascularization on the surface of nerves in affected regions, mirroring hypoxia-induced neovascularization seen in diabetic retinopathy. This expansion of vascular territories may lead to a hyperperfusion state, with paradoxically less hypoxia in painful neuropathy and, although poorly understood, sug-gests a hemodynamic etiology to the development of painful symptoms in diabetic polyneuropathy.

Clinical Features and Diagnosis

Painful diabetic polyneuropathy generally occurs as a symmetri-cal sensory neuropathy, initially involving the distal lower extremities and spreading proximally. At the time of midcalf involvement, patients typically begin to experience symptoms in their hands as well, developing into the typical "stocking glove" sensory distribution of the disease. Although a number of systems have been proposed to screen for and diagnose diabetic neuropathy, most have proven to be poorly reproducible, and the diagnosis remains dependent on interpreting a constellation of clinical symptoms and signs. As discussed above, a thorough history and physical examination with assessment of pain

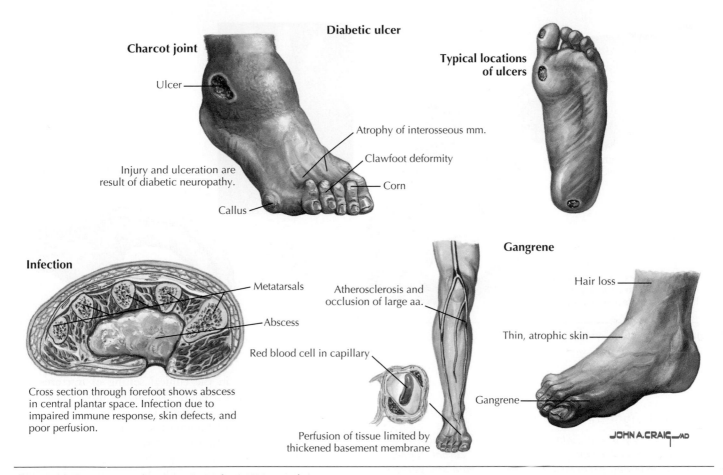

Figure 12-6 Foot Complications in Diabetic Neuropathy.

characteristics as well as neurosensory testing is necessary to make the diagnosis. In the context of diabetes, the occurrence of positive symptoms overlapping regions of sensory deficit is strongly suggestive of PDN.

Nerve conduction velocity very gradually diminishes in PDN and can be used to track disease progression to some extent; however, it does not correlate with the degree of symptoms as it only evaluates large myelinated fibers. NCS are frequently normal during the early phases of the disease, owing to initial involvement of predominantly small, unmyelinated fibers. Poor glycemic control is a risk factor for developing PDN and may be reflected by high hemoglobin A_1C levels, an indication of average glucose levels over a period of 2 to 3 months.

Treatment

The mainstay of treatment in painful diabetic polyneuropathy is proper glycemic control targeting an HbA_1C at or below 6.5%. Although intense diabetes management cannot completely arrest the development of neuropathy, it has been shown to significantly delay the onset of symptoms in type 1 diabetes and may have some benefit in type 2 diabetes.

Symptomatic treatment of pain is a mainstay of diabetic neuropathy management, as it has significant impact on quality-of-life issues such as sleep and daily comfort. The assessment of symptoms per se and communication regarding treatment

outcome expectations is the first step in managing any chronic neuropathic pain syndrome, followed by prescription of a first-line pharmaceutical agent. Among the first-line agents previously reviewed, the **serotonin–norepinephrine reuptake inhibitor** duloxetine has shown particular promise in PDN, demonstrating superior efficacy compared to placebo (number needed to treat [NNT] = 4.9–5.3) and comparable safety compared to standard care (gabapentin, amitriptyline, and venlafaxine) in a number of double-blind clinical trials. Duloxetine's frequent side effects included nausea, somnolence, dizziness, reduced appetite, and dry mouth. This is started at 30 mg/day and titrated to 60–120 mg/day after 4–5 days to minimize side effects. TCAs may also be used to treat painful diabetic polyneuropathy, with relatively lower NNTs compared to other agents (amitriptyline, 2.1; desipramine, 2.2; imipramine, 1.3; clomipramine, 2.1; and nortriptyline with fluphenazine, 1.2.)

Dosage of these agents begins at 10 mg/day and can be titrated upward to 150 mg/day as needed. Gabapentin and pregabalin may also be used at dosage ranges of 900–3600 mg/day and 300–600 mg/day, respectively, with NNTs of 3.8 and 5.9 and maximum dose. Oxycodone may also be used adjunctively in pain-resistant standard pharmacotherapy, but careful consideration of the risks and benefits should be undertaken prior to initiation because of the potential for dependence and abuse.

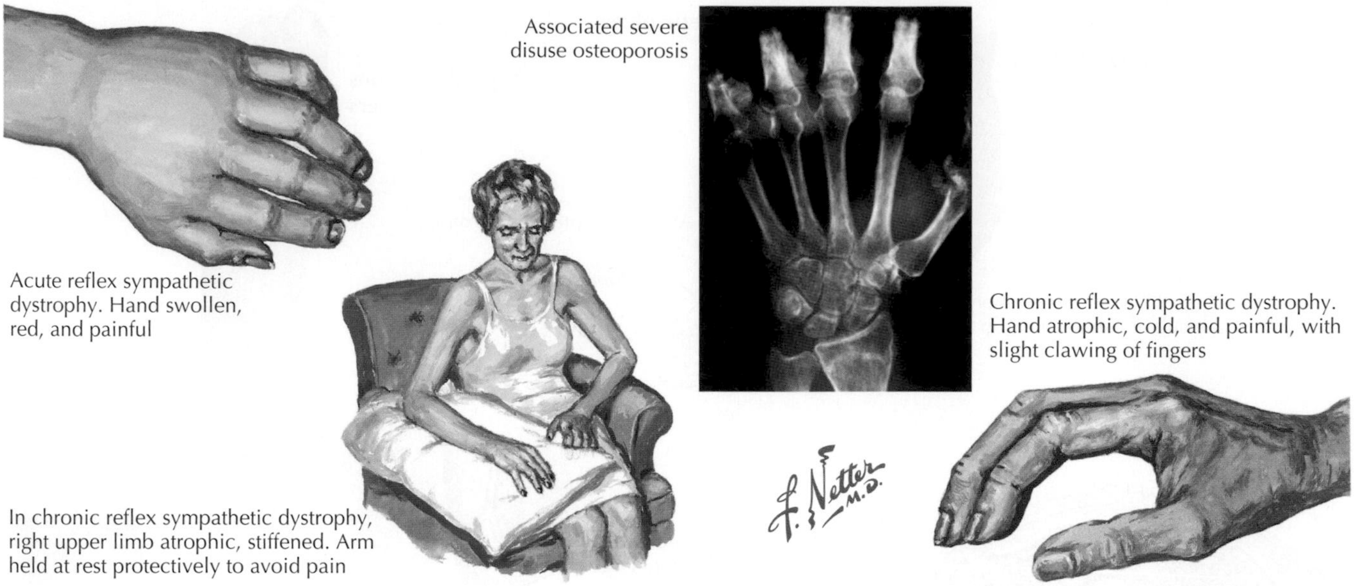

Acute reflex sympathetic dystrophy. Hand swollen, red, and painful

Associated severe disuse osteoporosis

Chronic reflex sympathetic dystrophy. Hand atrophic, cold, and painful, with slight clawing of fingers

In chronic reflex sympathetic dystrophy, right upper limb atrophic, stiffened. Arm held at rest protectively to avoid pain

Figure 12-7 Reflex Sympathetic Dystrophy.

COMPLEX REGIONAL PAIN

Clinical Vignette

Tracy, a 65-year-old right-hand-dominant receptionist is referred to orthopedic surgery for right carpal tunnel release following progressively worsening pain and paresthesia in her right hand. Surgery is performed under conscious sedation without complications, and the patient is discharged home that afternoon to follow up with physical therapy for rehabilitation. However, the patient fails to keep her physical therapy appointment and returns to work 4 weeks later.

Seven weeks postoperatively, the patient presents back to the orthopedic surgeon complaining of swelling, redness, and stiffness of her right hand. She also notes that her hand has become more sensitive to painful stimuli and that she experiences significant discomfort when her hand contacts virtually anything. On exam, the hand is warm, red, and swollen, with hyperhydrosis noted on the palmar surface (Fig. 12-7).

Despite admission to the hospital for empiric treatment of postoperative infection, the patient fails to improve and develops exquisite pain even to light touch.

Overview

Previously known as reflex sympathetic dystrophy, causalgia, and several other names, complex regional pain syndrome (CRPS) is an increasingly recognized chronic and often debilitating neuropathic pain condition characterized by autonomic and somatic neurologic dysfunction following various injuries. This often leads to chronic pain, trophic tissue changes, and motor impairment. Frequently, the clinical dysfunction often expands beyond the distribution of one peripheral nerve, and may be grossly disproportionate to the inciting event. CRPS occurs predominantly in the clinical setting of fractures and surgical trauma to the extremities, including distal radial fractures, carpal tunnel release, tibial fractures, total knee replacement, hip arthroplasty, and numerous arthroscopic procedures. It has been reported in mild trauma such as joint sprains, and nontraumatic conditions, including stroke, pregnancy, and neoplastic disease. This is occasionally documented with visceral trauma, but is much less common in this setting.

Although the epidemiology of CRPS is poorly characterized, studies closely evaluating pain symptoms suggest incidence rates of 20–25% in fractures, predominantly affecting the extremities. This occurs more frequently in females at a 2–3 : 1 ratio to males, tending to more frequently affect the upper extremities in adults and the lower extremities in children.

Pathophysiology

Although the precise pathophysiology of CRPS remains imperfectly understood, a number of studies have advanced promising and increasingly well-developed theories. Some evidence indicates that diminished sensory input, reduction of central modulation, or end organ hypersensitivity results in increased sympathetic nervous system activity following injurious stimuli. These changes may be caused by impaired transport of nerve growth factors by damaged axons or by alterations in the membrane channel populations following nerve injury. A number of studies support the assertion that catecholamine sensitivity develops in peripheral cutaneous and deep tissue nociceptors following nerve injury.

Expansion of neuronal fields may also occur after peripheral nerve injury, with formation of artificial synapses between somatic and sympathetic fibers, dorsal root ganglia resulting in autonomic dysfunction, and aberrant sources of pain signaling. Supporting this theory is the fact that sympathetic blockade may sometimes alleviate pain symptoms, although there is tremendous variability in clinical response to these treatments.

Loss of nociceptive small-fiber axons following nerve injury may also contribute to CRPS. Limited studies have demonstrated a 30% reduction in neurite density of skin biopsies compared to ipsilateral control sites in patients experiencing allodynia and hyperalgesia at CRPS-affected sites, strongly supporting this theory. Disproportionate inflammatory reaction following injury may occur, with free radical damage to tissues, anoxia, and subsequent dysregulation of vascular function and blood flow. Langerhans cell proliferation following denervation has also been documented, suggesting a significant inflammatory component in CRPS. Proinflammatory and chemotactic cytokines TNF-α, IL-1, and IL-6 released from these cells may play a role in the exaggerated local inflammatory response as well as the trophic changes in nails, hair, and bony tissues.

Although psychological influences in the development of CRPS have been postulated, current evidence increasingly suggests that psychological symptoms are more likely secondary to the syndrome rather than the primary cause. Overall, characterization of pathophysiological factors contributing to the development of CRPS is in its infancy, and further research is an area of high priority.

Clinical Features and Diagnosis

The major clinical features of CRPS are spontaneous pain, allodynia, hyperalgesia, edema, vasomotor instability, autonomic dysfunction, and progressive trophic changes. CRPS occurs as two subtypes, with the presence of an identifiable noxious stimulating event delineating between the two. *Type I CRPS* develops in the absence of an identifiable focal nerve lesion, whereas *type II CRPS* occurs in the presence of identifiable nerve damage. CRPS has historically been considered a multiphasic disorder, with an early "acute" phase characterized by vasomotor instability and edema, a late "atrophic" phase defined by atrophy and contracture, with an intermediate phase between the two. More recent research, however, suggests that the different symptoms of CRPS are more likely variant subtypes as opposed to stages of the disease. The vast majority of CRPS patients experience only the "acute" phase symptoms, typically with spontaneous resolution over time, and only 2% go on to develop the atrophic symptoms associated with chronic CRPS.

The predominant features of CRPS are pain symptoms such as allodynia, hyperalgesia, and spontaneous sensations of burning, shooting, aching, or other discomfort. The pain is typically experienced in a distribution beyond the initially affected nerve(s) and may spread to involve the entire affected limb and, rarely, the contralateral limb as well. These symptoms are generally constant in nature and frequently worsen over time, leading to significant impairment of quality of life and psychological distress.

Additionally, sympathetic dysfunction is present, mediating pain symptoms as well as autonomic instability (see Fig. 12-7). Patients may initially experience a warm, anhydrotic, edematous extremity with progression to a cold, hyperhidrotic limb and resolving edema. Trophic changes in the affected limb also occur, with hypertrophic or atrophic hair and nail growth and degeneration of the skin and subcutaneous fat. Connective tissues may become adherent to each other, leading to contractures and loss of function in the affected extremity. Rapid

bone loss also develops, resulting in demineralization and osteoporosis. Finally, weakness, tremor, and other motor anomalies may occur in the affected extremity, with profound loss of function.

Diagnosis of CRPS is a clinical one; there are no specific diagnostic tests for CRPS. When the typical symptoms of CRPS occur in the context of surgery, fracture, or other noxious stimulus, these are very suggestive of the diagnosis. Initially one must exclude various primary neurologic, infectious, and autoimmune etiologies. *Plain bony radiographic* testing may help to demonstrate unilateral demineralization and cortical erosions suggestive of CRPS, and Tc 99m-labeled bisphosphonate *bone scan techniques* demonstrate an 80% sensitivity and specificity in detecting osseous changes typical of CRPS.

Infrared thermography demonstrating greater than 1°C difference in temperature between the affected and contralateral extremity is 93% sensitive and 89% specific in the diagnosis of CRPS, although it is rarely employed because of the specialized equipment required. In patients simultaneously experiencing severe pain and sympathetic dysfunction, stellate ganglion and lumbar paravertebral sympathetic blocks have also been used to diagnose and treat CRPS, with greater than 50% reduction in pain considered significant enough to warrant this diagnosis. However, more recent studies show that sympathetic block is neither sensitive nor specific. Nevertheless, some clinicians still perform this procedure because of the dual prospect of diagnosis and treatment coupled with low morbidity when performed by skilled professionals. Ultimately, the diagnosis of CRPS remains challenging, and further research is warranted because of its marked limitation in the patient's ability to carry on activities of daily living (ADLs).

Treatment

This requires a multidisciplinary approach to managing symptoms and preserving function. Progressive pain and loss of function account for significant morbidity in these patients, and especially in cases of chronic CRPS. Psychological interventions merit consideration for developing adaptive coping modalities for the affected patient. Symptom management is divided into two broad categories, pharmacotherapy and interventional therapy.

Pharmacotherapy includes several classes of agents, including neuropathic drugs, opioids, bisphosphonates, ketamine, and calcitonin. A large range of neuropathic agents are used to treat CRPS, including TCAs, calcium channel α2-δ ligands, tramadol, and local anesthetics. These have had a varying success.

Amitriptyline is perhaps the most frequently prescribed of these agents, with dosage starting at 10 mg and titrating upwards to a target of 75 mg QHS. In part because of the complexity of CRPS classification and symptoms, prospective studies of these agents are lacking or are very limited, and further characterization is needed. The *bisphosphonate* alendronate 40 mg/day has been shown in a small trial to improve joint mobility, pain, and hyperalgesia in patients with CRPS through unclear mechanisms.

Ketamine acts as an NMDA antagonist, and is reported to demonstrate promise in the treatment of CRPS. However, larger studies evaluating optimal dosing and duration are needed. Initial retrospective studies have shown drastic reductions in subjective pain scores following subanesthetic ketamine infusion, with a number of patients remaining pain free beyond 3 years after multiple infusions. A further open-labeled study at anesthetic doses of ketamine over 5 days demonstrated complete symptom relief in 79% of patients at 6 months and significant pain relief in all patients who did experience relapse.

A number of *interventional therapeutic approaches* to CRPS have been studied. Local anesthetic sympathetic blockade is accomplished by infiltrating an agent such as lidocaine in the vicinity of the stellate ganglion for upper-extremity CRPS or the lumbar sympathetic chain for lower-extremity CRPS. This technique aims to address both autonomic and somatic symptoms by disrupting the sympathetic-afferent coupling postulated to account for CRPS symptoms. Although previously considered the gold standard in the treatment of CRPS, clinical study of these techniques has been complicated by difficulty with blinding, variations in technique, and small numbers of patients. The benefit of these techniques is often of limited duration. These may be optimized when used in conjunction with physiotherapy to improve functional status and strength. With a similar therapeutic rationale, sympathetic denervation has also been used in the treatment of CRPS. Only one third of patients undergoing surgical sympathectomy report persistent symptom relief at 5 years. These procedures are associated with major side effects, including increased neuropathic symptoms, spinal cord injury, and Horner's syndrome.

Spinal cord stimulation has also shown promise for treatment of CRPS. However, further study of its long-term benefit and improved methods of identifying the subpopulation of patients most likely to benefit are needed. Recent studies demonstrate that the initial high cost of these systems may be offset over the long term if medication and other utilizations are reduced. Spinal cord stimulation may improve ADL not only by reducing pain, but improving other domains of function impaired by CRPS.

Physiotherapy is also considered a first-line therapy in the treatment of CRPS, with aggressive range-of-motion and strengthening exercises shown to improve pain symptoms and reduce overall disability. Careful attention to initial pain management before beginning physiotherapy is very important to make it possible for the patient to physically participate. This underscores the importance of a multimodal approach to CRPS management.

ADDITIONAL RESOURCES

Eisenberg E, McNicol ED, Carr DB. Efficacy and safety of opioid agonists in the treatment of neuropathic pain of nonmalignant origin: systematic review and meta-analysis of randomized controlled trials. JAMA 2005 Jun 22;293(24):3043-3052.

Miller A. Neuropathic Pain. In: American Academy of Neurology. Continuum. Philadelphia, PA: Lippincott Williams & Wilkins; 2009. p. 15:No 5.

O'Connor AB, Dworkin RH. Treatment of neuropathic pain: an overview of recent guidelines. Am J Med 2009 Oct;122(Suppl. 10):S22-S32.

Treede RD, Jensen TS, Campbell JN, et al. Neuropathic pain: redefinition and a grading system for clinical and research purposes. Neurology 2008 Apr 29;70(18):1630-1635.

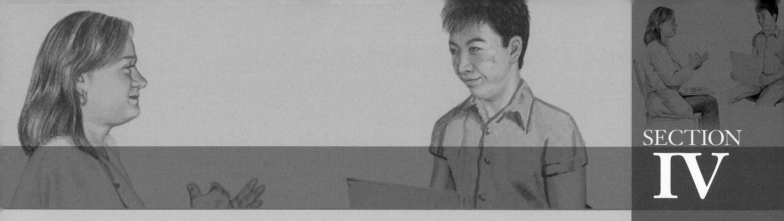

Attention and Consciousness

Autonomic Disorders and Syncope

13

Jose A. Gutrecht and Jayashri Srinivasan

Clinical Vignette

A 65-year-old man presented with subacute onset of severe unexplained orthostatic dizziness and light-headedness. Over the next 2 months, he developed dry mouth, dry eyes, urinary hesitancy, erectile dysfunction, and severe constipation. His previous medical history was unremarkable. His only medication was aspirin. He smoked one pack per day and drank sparingly. His family history was noncontributory. The patient's blood pressure was 124/76 mm Hg supine and 66/40 mm Hg standing at 2 minutes, with normal heart rates of 72 and 76 beats per minute while supine and standing. His remaining general examination was normal. There were impaired pupillary responses to light and accommodation and dry mucous membranes. Sensory examination revealed distal sensory loss to proprioception in both hands and feet.

Tilt-table testing revealed orthostatic hypotension. Sweat testing demonstrated profound anhidrosis. Paraneoplastic autoantibody studies revealed positive anti-HU (antineuronal) antibodies. Chest computed tomography demonstrated left hilar mass. Small-cell lung carcinoma was diagnosed after bronchoscopic biopsy. The patient's orthostatic intolerance improved after the third course of chemotherapy. Remission has persisted.

Comment: Development of signs and symptoms related to parasympathetic and sympathetic dysfunction in the absence of central nervous system abnormalities was compatible with an autonomic neuropathy.

ANATOMY OF THE AUTONOMIC SYSTEM

The primary role of the autonomic system is the maintenance of homeostasis and this is done by two separate but complementary systems: the sympathetic and the parasympathetic systems. The central regulation of the autonomic system is mediated by neurons in the frontal lobe, limbic system and the hypothalamus. The preganglionic neurons of the sympathetic nervous system arise from the intermediolateral column of the thoracic spinal cord. These axons form the white communicating rami that synapse with the neurons of the sympathetic ganglia in the paravertebral chain; postganglionic fibers form the gray communicating rami that travel along with the spinal nerves to blood vessels and sweat glands (Fig. 13-1). Sympathetic innervation of the adrenal medulla is the exception as it receives preganglionic sympathetic fibers; the adrenal medulla is considered the equivalent of a sympathetic ganglion, and it secretes epinephrine and norepinephrine directly into the blood stream (Fig. 13-1).

The parasympathetic system consists of the cranial and sacral output; the cranial output arises in the visceral nuclei of the cranial nerves III, VII, IX, and X, and the axons travel along with the respective cranial nerves to innervate target organs. The preganglionic fibers from the Edinger–Westphal nucleus travel in the oculomotor nerve (III) and synapse in the ciliary ganglion innervating the ciliary and pupillary muscles (Fig. 13-2). The preganglionic fibers from the superior salivatory nuclei travel along with the facial nerve (VII) as greater petrosal nerve and the chorda tympani, synapse in the sphenopalatine and submandibular ganglion, and innervate the lacrimal, submandibular, and sublingual glands (Fig. 13-3). The preganglionic fibers from the inferior salivatory nuclei travel along with the glossopharyngeal nerve (IX) and synapse in the otic ganglion and innervate the parotid gland (Fig. 13-4). The preganglionic fibers from the dorsal motor nucleus of the vagus travel along with the vagal nerve (X) and synapse in the ganglia in the walls of the viscera and innervate the visceral organs of the gastrointestinal, cardiac, and renal systems (Fig. 13-5). The sacral part of the parasympathetic system arises from the sacral spinal cord, synapses in the ganglia in the walls of the organs, and innervates the colon, bladder, and pelvic organs (Fig. 13-6).

Autonomic functions are mediated through neurotransmitters released by the sympathetic and parasympathetic neurons. *Acetylcholine* is the most important neurotransmitter. This is released by preganglionic sympathetic and parasympathetic neurons as well as all postganglionic parasympathetic neurons and some postganglionic sympathetic neurons (e.g., sweat glands). *Norepinephrine* is the other important autonomic neurotransmitter. It is secreted by the remaining postganglionic sympathetic neurons directing its action on both α- and β-adrenergic receptors.

DIAGNOSTIC APPROACH

Patients with dysautonomic symptoms require careful, and complete, neurologic examinations to find concomitant features of central and peripheral nervous system involvement. Electromyography is often valuable in patients who have concomitant sensorimotor neuropathy findings. Heart rate responses to Valsalva maneuvers and deep breathing are used to assess cardiovagal parasympathetic function.

Commonly used parameters to assess sympathetic competency include blood pressure responses to standing and to Valsalva maneuvers and quantitative measurements of sweat production in response to cholinergic stimuli. The latter is typically done at four standardized locations to detect the abnormality pattern. Quantitative sensory testing, comparing thresholds for vibration to cold- and heat-pain thresholds, is helpful for detecting small myelinated and unmyelinated somatic peripheral nerve dysfunction. Quantitation of intraepidermal nerve fiber density by skin punch biopsy and subsequent immunostaining directed at axons is performed at some centers to assess the severity of small-fiber loss. Comprehensive screening for all recognized paraneoplastic antibodies is recommended in acute

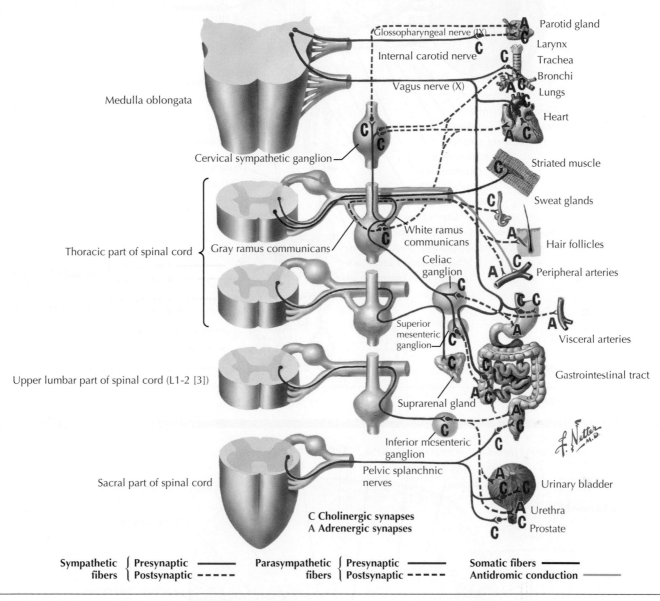

Medulla oblongata

Parotid gland

Glossopharyngeal nerve (IX)

Internal carotid nerve

Larynx

Trachea

Bronchi

Lungs

Vagus nerve (X)

Heart

Cervical sympathetic ganglion

Striated muscle

Thoracic part of spinal cord

Gray ramus communicans

White ramus communicans

Sweat glands

Hair follicles

Celiac ganglion

Peripheral arteries

Superior mesenteric ganglion

Visceral arteries

Upper lumbar part of spinal cord (L1-2 [3])

Gastrointestinal tract

Suprarenal gland

Inferior mesenteric ganglion

Sacral part of spinal cord

Pelvic splanchnic nerves

Urinary bladder

Urethra

Prostate

C Cholinergic synapses
A Adrenergic synapses

| Sympathetic fibers | Presynaptic ——— Postsynaptic - - - - - | Parasympathetic fibers | Presynaptic ——— Postsynaptic - - - - - | Somatic fibers ——— Antidromic conduction ——— |

Figure 13-1 Cholinergic *(C)* and Adrenergic *(A)* Synapses: Schema.

to subacute cases where paraneoplastic autonomic neuropathy is possible.

CLINICAL PRESENTATIONS

Typically, patients have combinations of both parasympathetic and sympathetic dysfunction (Fig. 13-7). The former is characterized by dry mucous membranes, particularly noticeable in the eyes and mouth, with varying gastrointestinal involvement manifested as early satiety, nausea, vomiting, constipation, diarrhea, urinary bladder dysmotility, and erectile dysfunction.

Disorders of sweating and sudden feelings of severe lightheadedness or syncope when assuming an upright posture are usual symptoms of impaired sympathetic function. Combinations of parasympathetic (erection) and sympathetic (ejaculation) disorders affect sexual function. Signs of autonomic

dysfunction include fixed heart rates, tonic pupils, and orthostatic hypotension, with normal strength and sensory examination (i.e., sparing the somatic nerves). Autonomic disorders may be classified as peripheral or central autonomic disorders and may present acutely or in a chronic fashion.

Acute Peripheral Autonomic Disorders

Acute or subacute autonomic neuropathies are usually related to toxic, metabolic, or autoimmune disorders. In the absence of toxic or metabolic influences, autoimmune and paraneoplastic disorders should be considered the primary mechanism. Primary autonomic polyneuropathies represent an uncommon subgroup of disorders. However, many length-dependent polyneuropathies have various degrees of autonomic fiber involvement, occasionally with important implications. Impotence is a prime example in young patients with diabetic polyneuropathies.

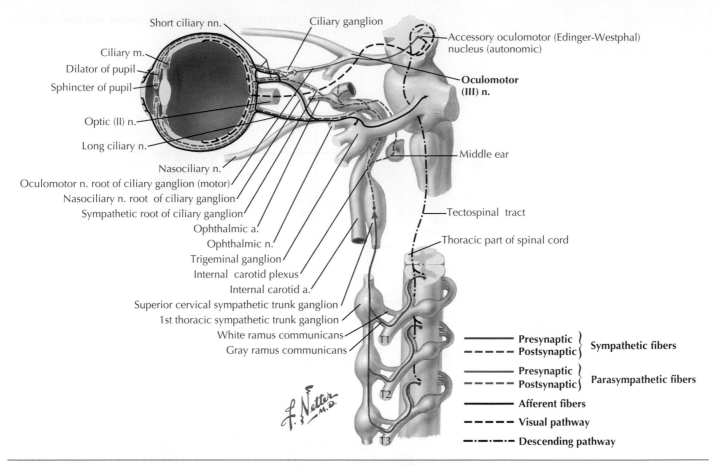

Figure 13-2 Eye: Autonomic Innervation.

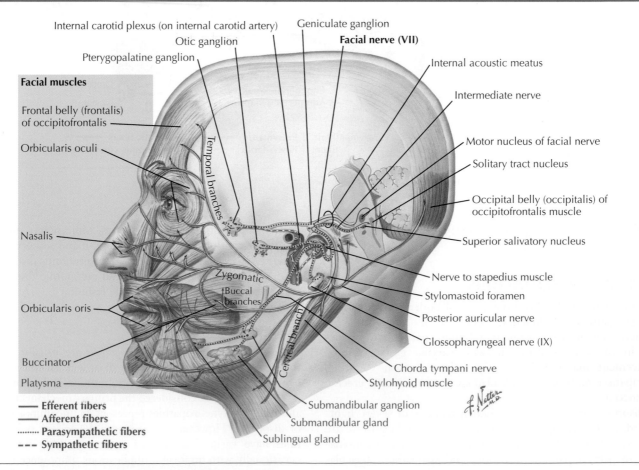

Figure 13-3 Facial Nerve: Autonomic Innervation.

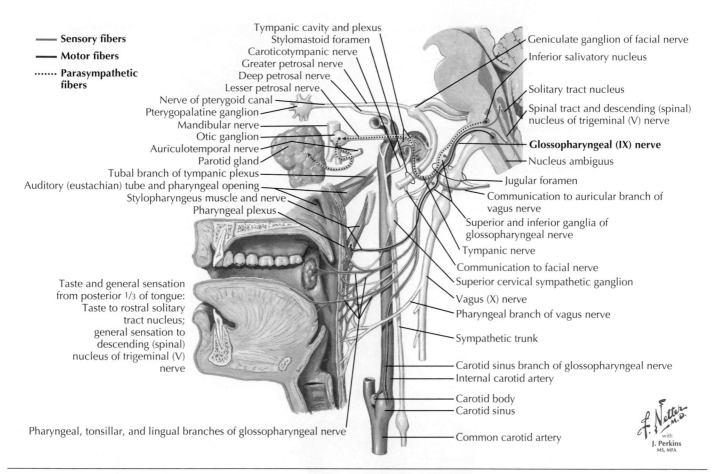

Figure 13-4 Glossopharyngeal Nerve: Autonomic Innervation.

Antecedent viral infections occur in more than half of patients with *autoimmune autonomic neuropathy*, suggesting that it may be a Guillain–Barré syndrome variant. The very rare patient with acute pandysautonomic neuropathy often presents with rapid onset of sympathetic and parasympathetic dysfunction. They most often have severe generalized disorders, but restricted milder forms also occur. Orthostatic intolerance and gastrointestinal dysmotility are common presentations. Autonomic tests are almost always abnormal. Nerve biopsies demonstrate inflammatory infiltrates supporting an immune-mediated hypothesis. Recovery is slow and often incomplete. High titers of ganglionic nicotinic acetylcholine receptor antibodies are reported in approximately half of these patients, supporting the presumed autoimmune basis.

Guillain–Barré syndrome preferentially involves somatic motor fibers but also causes dysautonomia in two thirds of cases, especially affecting the cardiovascular and gastrointestinal systems. Bladder dysfunction is less common. Autonomic complications may be life threatening; patients often must be monitored in the ICU.

Paraneoplastic autonomic neuropathy is often indistinguishable from primary autoimmune autonomic neuropathy. Gastrointestinal dysmotility is a common presenting manifestation. Antineuronal nuclear antibody type 1 is associated with small cell lung cancer. It is the most frequently demonstrated abnormal paraneoplastic neurologic antibody.

Hereditary porphyria presents with acute attacks of dysautonomic symptoms (abdominal pain, vomiting, constipation, hypertension, and tachycardia) in addition to predominantly motor polyneuropathies. Diagnosis requires demonstration of increased urinary excretion of porphobilinogen.

Toxins: Chemicals, including various medications, particularly cisplatinum and vinca alkaloids cause peripheral neuropathies with autonomic features. Other specific nerve toxins such as organophosphates, heavy metals (e.g., thallium and arsenic), hexacarbons, and acrylamide may produce acute autonomic peripheral neuropathies.

Chronic Peripheral Autonomic Disorders

Diabetic autonomic neuropathies are common accompaniments of diabetic peripheral neuropathies and often correlate with the duration and control of diabetes. Early clinical autonomic testing often reveals evidence of cardiovagal dysfunction manifested by impairment of heart rate response to Valsalva maneuver or to deep breathing. Autonomic dysfunction due to uncontrolled diabetes can cause considerable morbidity.

Postural orthostatic tachycardia syndrome (POTS) is seen predominantly in young women. It is characterized by orthostatic symptoms associated with significant rise in heart rate on standing without orthostatic hypotension or other clinical or

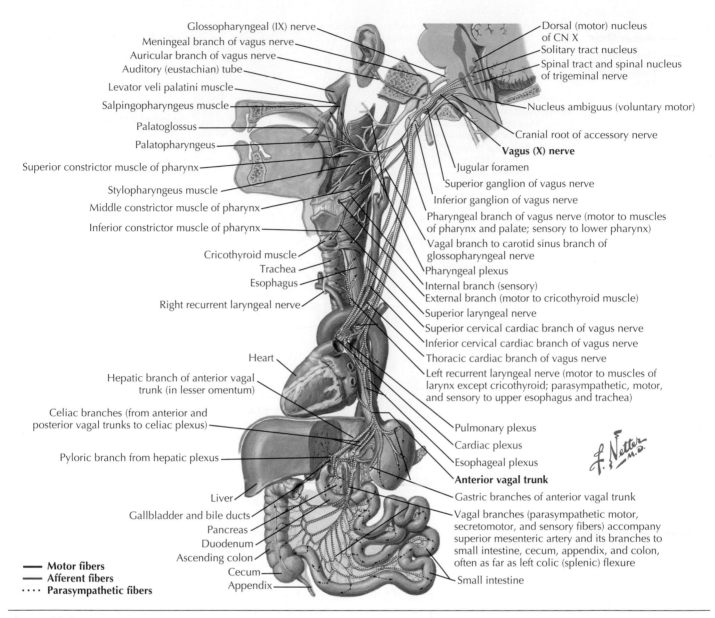

Glossopharyngeal (IX) nerve
Meningeal branch of vagus nerve
Auricular branch of vagus nerve
Auditory (eustachian) tube
Levator veli palatini muscle
Salpingopharyngeus muscle
Palatoglossus
Palatopharyngeus
Superior constrictor muscle of pharynx
Stylopharyngeus muscle
Middle constrictor muscle of pharynx
Inferior constrictor muscle of pharynx
Cricothyroid muscle
Trachea
Esophagus
Right recurrent laryngeal nerve
Heart
Hepatic branch of anterior vagal trunk (in lesser omentum)
Celiac branches (from anterior and posterior vagal trunks to celiac plexus)
Pyloric branch from hepatic plexus
Liver
Gallbladder and bile ducts
Pancreas
Duodenum
Ascending colon
Cecum
Appendix

Dorsal (motor) nucleus of CN X
Solitary tract nucleus
Spinal tract and spinal nucleus of trigeminal nerve
Nucleus ambiguus (voluntary motor)
Cranial root of accessory nerve
Vagus (X) nerve
Jugular foramen
Superior ganglion of vagus nerve
Inferior ganglion of vagus nerve
Pharyngeal branch of vagus nerve (motor to muscles of pharynx and palate; sensory to lower pharynx)
Vagal branch to carotid sinus branch of glossopharyngeal nerve
Pharyngeal plexus
Internal branch (sensory)
External branch (motor to cricothyroid muscle)
Superior laryngeal nerve
Superior cervical cardiac branch of vagus nerve
Inferior cervical cardiac branch of vagus nerve
Thoracic cardiac branch of vagus nerve
Left recurrent laryngeal nerve (motor to muscles of larynx except cricothyroid; parasympathetic, motor, and sensory to upper esophagus and trachea)
Pulmonary plexus
Cardiac plexus
Esophageal plexus
Anterior vagal trunk
Gastric branches of anterior vagal trunk
Vagal branches (parasympathetic motor, secretomotor, and sensory fibers) accompany superior mesenteric artery and its branches to small intestine, cecum, appendix, and colon, often as far as left colic (splenic) flexure
Small intestine

— Motor fibers
— Afferent fibers
···· Parasympathetic fibers

Figure 13-5 Vagus nerve: Autonomic Innervation.

laboratory evidence of autonomic neuropathy, except for distal sweat loss. The pathophysiology of POTS is heterogeneous. It may include limited autonomic neuropathies, hypovolemia, and deconditioning and often there may be an associated anxiety or depressive disorder.

Amyloidosis is a multisystem disorder that may be sporadic or familial. Autonomic neuropathy often occurs presenting with symptoms of somatic small fiber dysfunction, orthostatic intolerance, and constipation alternating with diarrhea.

Pure autonomic failure is also known as idiopathic autonomic hypotension. It is an insidious process with typical signs of disordered autonomic function. The absence of parkinsonian features helps differentiate this disorder from multiple systems atrophy. It results from postganglionic sympathetic neuron degeneration.

Hereditary autonomic neuropathies are rare disorders. Hereditary sensory and autonomic neuropathy type III, also known as

Riley Day syndrome, is an autosomal recessive disorder, presenting with defective control of blood pressure, sweating, temperature, and lacrimation in children. Dysautonomic manifestations are less pronounced in the other hereditary sensory and autonomic neuropathies.

Central Disorders

Parkinson disease is associated with significant autonomic dysfunction, particularly in long-standing disease. There is a loss of pigmented substantia nigra dopaminergic cells and other pigmented nuclei, including the locus ceruleus and the dorsal vagal nucleus, and this may partially explain the autonomic symptoms. Peripheral sympathetic heart denervation is common, resulting in orthostatic hypotension in severe cases.

Multiple systems atrophy is a degenerative disorder characterized by parkinsonian features with autonomic, cerebellar, and

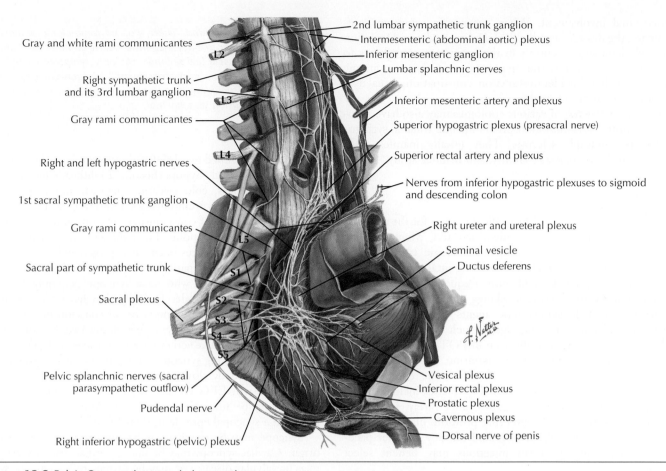

Figure 13-6 Pelvic Organs: Autonomic Innervation.

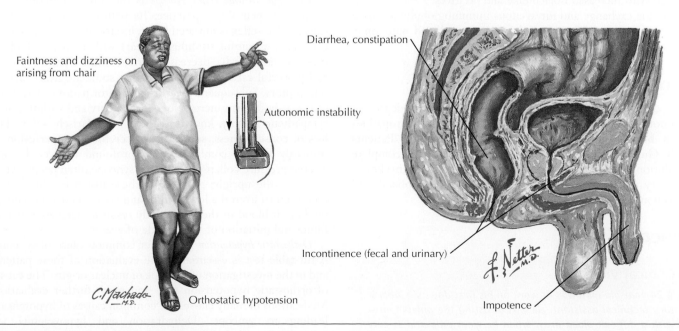

Figure 13-7 Symptoms of Dysautonomia.

corticospinal involvement. When autonomic symptoms predominate, the disorder is called *Shy–Drager syndrome*. Depletion of catecholaminergic neurons in the brainstem contributes to development of orthostatic hypotension. Other autonomic symptoms include bladder dysfunction, constipation, sexual dysfunction, and laryngeal stridor.

Spinal cord disorders of various etiologies may also have autonomic symptoms. Common disorders include trauma, syringomyelia, and multiple sclerosis. They usually manifest with arrhythmias, blood pressure lability, and bladder atony.

THERAPY

Primary treatment consists of specific therapies for the underlying disorders, when these are identified and, when possible, symptomatic relief per se. Nonpharmacologic treatments of orthostatic hypotension include increasing intake of dietary salt and water, eating smaller and more frequent meals, avoiding alcohol, and wearing elastic stockings or abdominal binders. Medications include sympathetic agents such as midodrine and fluid- and salt-conserving agents such as fludrocortisone. Orthostatic symptoms typically seen in POTS may respond to low-dose β-blockers or low-dose midodrine.

Bladder dysfunction in most dysautonomic conditions is characterized by failure to empty. Treatments include timed voiding, intermittent catheterizations, and, rarely, indwelling catheters. Pharmacologic agents that promote bladder emptying, such as bethanechol, have limited efficacy. Bladder pacemakers and botulinum toxin injections may benefit select patients.

Treatment of erectile dysfunction includes agents such as sildenafil, yohimbine, topical nitroglycerin or minoxidil, injections of prostaglandins, or penile implants.

Gastrointestinal dysfunction is best aided by strategies to maintain hydration and nutrition. Gastroparesis is treated with prokinetic agents such as metoclopramide; constipation is treated with increased fiber intake and laxatives.

Plasma exchange and intravenous immunoglobulin are used for the treatment of suspected immune-mediated autonomic neuropathy with variable success.

PROGNOSIS

This depends on the etiology, severity, and overall degree of autonomic dysfunction. Autoimmune autonomic neuropathies often have a limited, unsatisfactory improvement. Patients with Guillain–Barré syndrome usually experience complete resolution of autonomic dysfunction in parallel with clinical recovery of strength. Prognosis for chronic peripheral and central autonomic disorders is less favorable.

SYNCOPE

Clinical Vignette

A 24-year-old man was at work on his first day as a laboratory technical assistant. He was assisting the phlebotomist with a difficult blood draw when he went pale and sweaty and fell to the ground. There was no tonic–clonic activity, tongue biting, or urinary incontinence. He came around and was alert in just a few seconds. His only symptom when he came around was "embarrassment." His general physical examination including blood pressure and pulse and neurologic examination was normal.

Syncope is defined as a brief and transient loss of consciousness from cerebral hypoperfusion. Lightheadedness, visual dimming, paleness, cold sweating, nausea, and a feeling of warmth are common premonitory symptoms (Fig. 13-8). These are followed by loss of consciousness and postural muscle tone, and, if the patient is standing, he or she will usually fall. Significant trauma and fractures occur in approximately 5% of these patients. In contrast to patients who lose consciousness from a convulsion, individuals who have syncope generally have no confusion after the episode. Typically, they have good recollection of premonitory symptoms. Loss of consciousness lasts just a few seconds. Occasionally, a few clonic twitches or a brief generalized seizure-like activity occurs at the end of the episode. EEG recorded during syncope demonstrates early depression of activity followed by slow wave activity in the theta and delta range. Transient EEG voltage depression may follow. Elderly patients may be amnestic for the event. Almost 20% of people have had a syncopal episode in their lifetime.

Syncope may be classified as having cardiac or noncardiac origin. Cardiac syncope may be due to cardiac disease (arrhythmias or valvular disease) or may be cardiac reflex syncope from orthostatic hypotension. Noncardiac syncope is subclassified as neurologic, metabolic, or idiopathic.

The most common type, cardiac reflex syncope, has three subtypes: vasovagal (called neurocardiogenic or vasodepressor), situational (e.g., micturition, Valsalva, ocular compression, venipuncture, fear, exertion), and carotid hypersensitivity.

Vasovagal cardiac reflex syncope is the most commonly seen syncope in neurologic practice. Its pathophysiology is unresolved. The reflex is initiated by an intense sympathetic activation (e.g., a painful stimulus or fear) with increase of blood pressure, tachycardia, decreased cardiac filling ("empty heart"), and powerful cardiac contractions that stimulate heart mechanoreceptors. Subsequently, cardiac inhibitor pathway activation causes a short-term increase of vagal activity and withdrawal of sympathetic activity, known as the Bezold–Jarisch reflex. The loss of consciousness, secondary to cerebral hypoperfusion, is primarily from a combination of profound bradycardia and arterial pressure collapse. Vasovagal syncope often occurs while assuming the upright posture. In these instances, diminished blood return from the lower limbs and viscera and a subsequent pooling of blood in the lower body result in decreased cardiac filling and initiation of the cascade of events.

Orthostatic hypotension is another common cause of syncope. A tilt-table test is essential to the evaluation of these patients and in the investigation of syncope of unclear origin. The causes of orthostatic hypotension vary and merit further evaluation. Medications of many classes are common causes of hypotension leading to syncope. Dehydration and hypovolemia are other, easily excluded, common pathophysiologic mechanisms.

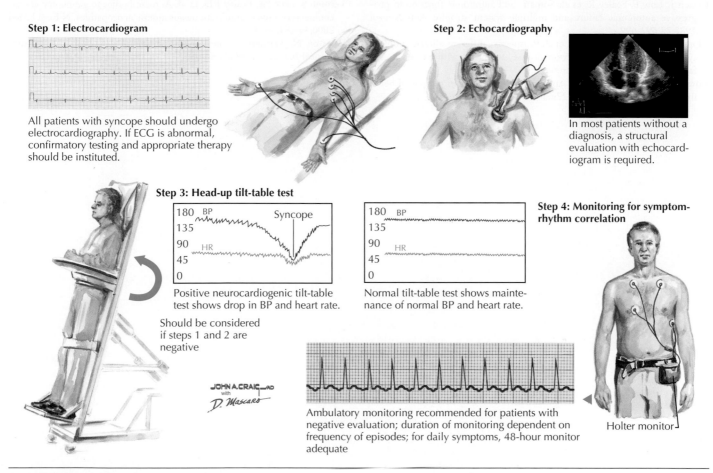

Step 1: Electrocardiogram

All patients with syncope should undergo electrocardiography. If ECG is abnormal, confirmatory testing and appropriate therapy should be instituted.

Step 2: Echocardiography

In most patients without a diagnosis, a structural evaluation with echocardiogram is required.

Step 3: Head-up tilt-table test

Positive neurocardiogenic tilt-table test shows drop in BP and heart rate.

Should be considered if steps 1 and 2 are negative

Normal tilt-table test shows maintenance of normal BP and heart rate.

Step 4: Monitoring for symptom-rhythm correlation

Ambulatory monitoring recommended for patients with negative evaluation; duration of monitoring dependent on frequency of episodes; for daily symptoms, 48-hour monitor adequate

Holter monitor

Figure 13-8 Syncope: Four-Step Management Approach.

Hyperventilation with associated hypocapnia is a rare cause of syncope. Metabolic causes of syncope include hypoglycemia and hypoxia. *Psychogenic syncope* sometimes can be difficult to document. It is best excluded by a careful history, witnessing the event, or both.

Primary neurologic causes of syncope are uncommon and usually have other associated symptoms. *Peripheral neuropathies* are the most common neurologic causes of syncope associated with orthostatic hypotension, particularly in patients with neuropathies secondary to diabetes and rarely primary amyloidosis. *Central nervous system disorders* such as multiple system atrophy with parkinsonian, cerebellar, or mixed features, previously called Shy–Drager disease, and pure autonomic failure must be considered despite their rare occurrence. Transient ischemic attacks in the vertebrobasilar system or basilar migraine are conditions that rarely produce syncopal episodes. There is no evidence that unilateral or bilateral critical carotid stenosis can cause syncope. The drop attacks of epileptic seizures are infrequently confused with syncope; although these patients lose postural tone and "drop," they do not lose consciousness.

The clinical examination of a patient with presumed syncope aims first to exclude serious illnesses, including structural heart disease, such as valvular aortic stenosis, cardiac rhythm disturbances, such as brady arrhythmias, coronary artery disease, and cardiomyopathies with compromised cardiac output. Patients with syncope from heart disease have a higher mortality rate than individuals with other causes of syncope. Evaluation must include a detailed history and physical examination with particular attention to the heart, an ECG, Holter monitor, other forms of cardiac event monitoring, echocardiography, stress test, and occasionally invasive electrophysiologic testing. Autonomic testing including quantitative sweat testing, heart rate responses to deep breathing and Valsalva maneuver and tilt-table tests are indicated in patients where autonomic dysfunction is suspected.

The management of syncope focuses on the underlying disease process, often requiring specialized medical or surgical treatments. Cardiac, neurologic, and situational mechanisms must be addressed. The therapy of reflex vasovagal syncope is problematic. Analysis of whether syncope is primarily from cardiac inhibition or hypotension is sometimes difficult because these often occur together. Education, increased salt and fluid intake, β-blockers, blood volume expanders such as mineralocorticoids (fludrocortisone), α-adrenergic agonists such as midodrine, and serotonin reuptake inhibitors are recommended. Antiarrhythmic agents and pacemakers are also sometimes indicated.

ADDITIONAL RESOURCES

Benarroch EE, Smithson IL, Low PA, et al. Depletion of catecholaminergic neurons in the rostral ventrolateral medulla in multiple system atrophy with autonomic failure. Ann Neurol 1998;43:56-163.

Cohen J, Low P, Fealey R, et al. Somatic and autonomic function in progressive autonomic failure and multiple system atrophy. Ann Neurol 1987;22:692-699.

Lipp A, Sandroni P, Ahlskog JE, et al. Prospective differentiation of multiple system atrophy from Parkinson disease, with and without autonomic failure. Arch Neurol 2009 Jun;66(6):742-750.

Low PA, Vernino S, Suarez G. Autonomic dysfunction in peripheral nerve disease. Muscle Nerve 2003;27:646-661.

Vernino S, Low PA, Fealey RD, et al. Autoantibodies to ganglionic acetylcholine receptors in autoimmune autonomic neuropathies. N Engl J Med 2000;343:847-855.

Winston N, Vernino S. Autoimmune autonomic ganglionopathy. Front Neurol Neurosci 2009;26:85-93.

Epilepsy

14

Joel M. Oster, Jose A. Gutrecht, Ritu Bagla, Jeffrey E. Arle, and G. Rees Cosgrove

*E*pilepsy is generally defined as an illness of recurrent seizures. The prevalence of epilepsy is estimated at 1 in 200 persons. It affects all ages and is generally a chronic problem with significant personal, social, and economic impact, often affecting the ability to hold jobs and drive. Poor epilepsy control and the seizures themselves can lead to significant cognitive and personality changes as well as chronic depression. The incidence is about 200,000 new cases yearly in the United States. The clinical manifestations are initiated by abnormal electrical discharges within the brain. The underlying pathophysiology is complex and not completely defined, but ultimately involves repetitive cortical potentials leading to altered modulation of excitatory inputs and suppression of inhibitory feedback circuits (Fig. 14-1). The diagnosis of epilepsy is primarily clinical, based on patient and witness history of the events and on the neurologic examination. An abnormal electroencephalograph (EEG) may substantiate a suspected diagnosis with specific EEG patterns, particularly focal or generalized spikes or spike-and-wave discharges, being highly associated with seizures. Many other EEG changes are not specific for seizures and are of little help in differentiating epileptic from nonepileptic events. Epilepsy is a treatable disease, often with a specific correctable medical or surgical pathology. Accurate diagnosis must be the predominant goal in approaching a patient with seizures of recent onset. Magnetic resonance imaging (MRI) and neuroimaging studies are critical to define any potentially treatable structural brain disease (Fig. 14-2). Laboratory testing may assist in the evaluation and treatment. Patients with chronic forms of epilepsy require long-term medical treatment. Failure of medical therapy or quality-of-life issues may necessitate intensive patient evaluation for potential seizure surgery. Surgical removal of carefully selected areas of diseased brain may provide improvement and often a cure.

DIFFERENTIAL DIAGNOSIS

All paroxysmal disorders of consciousness or perception may be included in the differential of seizures. Migraine with aura (classic migraine) is differentiated by generally distinct and recurrent positive visual or sensory phenomenon evolving gradually, then resolving over minutes and followed by a throbbing often unilateral headache. Transient ischemic attacks are characterized by negative (loss of function) neurologic symptoms often consistent with a single vascular territory that start maximally, then resolve gradually over seconds to minutes. Syncope is usually preceded by prodromal symptoms of lightheadedness, limpness, pale complexion, and diaphoresis. Once the patient falls or lies down and cerebral circulation is restored, full consciousness is regained with little or no persistent confusion or

disorientation, unlike the postictal period following seizures. Parasomnias with stereotyped nocturnal movements and psychiatric disorders can also be confused with seizures. One disorder that continues to be difficult to classify is transient global amnesia (TGA). It is considered by most to be a distinct benign entity that does not warrant any specific long-term treatment. A brief discussion follows.

TRANSIENT GLOBAL AMNESIA

Transient Global Amnesia is a term that was first used by Fisher and Adams in the 1960s to denote a syndrome of abrupt onset of severe anterograde amnesia with other elements of neurologic function remaining intact or unchanged from baseline. Retrograde amnesia may be present to a variable degree. Patients appear anxious or even agitated but are able to communicate and often ask the same exact questions repeatedly even when answered promptly. Patients recover fully without residual memory problems but have no recollection of the spell and do not normally evoke any precipitating event. Associated altered level of consciousness, ataxia, dysarthria, visual changes, headache, abnormal movements, and vomiting strongly suggest a basilar ischemic etiology or seizure and should be absent. Several etiologies have been proposed including seizure, migraine, ischemia, venous congestion, and psychogenic disturbances.

In 1985 Caplan proposed to reserve the term TGA for patients who do not have epilepsy. Case reports of documented seizures causing memory dysfunction mimicking TGA have been described. However, attacks in these cases tend to recur more frequently and are generally briefer, lasting minutes as opposed to hours with classic TGA. Unlike TGA, these attacks may be associated with EEG abnormalities and respond to antiepileptic medications. TGA cases rarely recur and there have been no consistently associated EEG epileptiform abnormalities. A theoretical concern however is that surface EEG may not detect deep mesial temporal seizures. To date, there have not been any reports of invasive or implanted electrodes monitoring during a typical spell of TGA.

A review of the TGA literature suggests associated subtle neuroimaging changes with transient intense diffusion-weighted imaging (DWI) signal seen within the hippocampus. This has led to the speculation of a vascular cause of the syndrome. However, similar DWI changes and transient hippocampal dysfunction have been seen in the perictal period and is due to excitotoxicity rather than ischemia.

Therefore, for now, the exact etiology of TGA remains unknown and without an identifiable purely vascular or an ictal mechanism; more research will be needed to settle the issue.

Normal firing pattern of cortical neurons

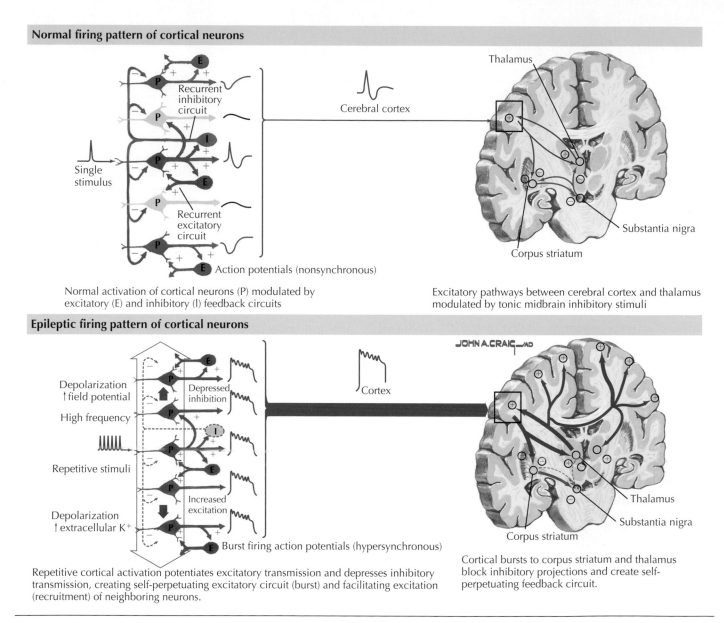

Normal activation of cortical neurons (P) modulated by excitatory (E) and inhibitory (I) feedback circuits

Excitatory pathways between cerebral cortex and thalamus modulated by tonic midbrain inhibitory stimuli

Epileptic firing pattern of cortical neurons

JOHN A.CRAIG—AD

Repetitive cortical activation potentiates excitatory transmission and depresses inhibitory transmission, creating self-perpetuating excitatory circuit (burst) and facilitating excitation (recruitment) of neighboring neurons.

Cortical bursts to corpus striatum and thalamus block inhibitory projections and create self-perpetuating feedback circuit.

Figure 14-1 Origin and Spread of Seizures.

PARTIAL SEIZURES

Simple Partial Seizures

Clinical Vignette

A 40-year-old woman experiences episodic numbness that spreads from the left thumb to the hand, arm, and then to the face over a period of about 30 seconds. These occur sporadically and are stereotypical in nature. She maintains alertness throughout the events. Since starting antiepileptic medications, these events have abated.

This history represents typical simple partial seizure (SPS). During the episodes, patients are conscious, aware of their surroundings, and able to respond appropriately. Partial seizures originate and develop within a discrete area of the cerebral cortex (Fig. 14-3). They may have a "Jacksonian march" wherein the cortical epileptic discharges spread along contiguous cortical regions. The brain area involved determines the clinical signature of the event. Symptoms may be somatosensory, as in the above vignette, when the origin is in the parietal lobe, motor when discharges arise from the frontal or motor cortex, and visual when they begin in the occipital lobe. However, the relation of focal cortical location to clinical expression is not absolute. Seizures may start in a "silent" cerebral cortical area with the manifest ictal symptoms representing the result of the discharge spreading to neighboring cortical areas. SPSs may occasionally have autonomic, psychic, or cognitive manifestations. Other seizure types may start off as SPS and then evolve into broader disruptions. By definition, these simple ictal events do not include any change in level of consciousness and it is this preserved responsiveness to the external environment that characterizes SPSs. Auras, a warning that a patient experiences prior to altered or loss of consciousness, are, in effect, SPS.

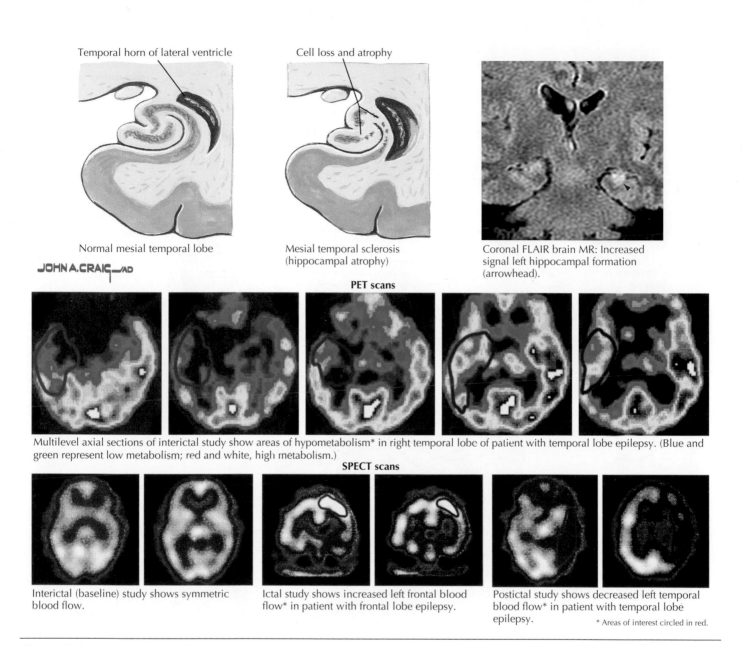

Temporal horn of lateral ventricle

Cell loss and atrophy

Normal mesial temporal lobe

Mesial temporal sclerosis
(hippocampal atrophy)

Coronal FLAIR brain MR: Increased
signal left hippocampal formation
(arrowhead).

JOHN A. CRAIG—AD

PET scans

Multilevel axial sections of interictal study show areas of hypometabolism* in right temporal lobe of patient with temporal lobe epilepsy. (Blue and green represent low metabolism; red and white, high metabolism.)

SPECT scans

Interictal (baseline) study shows symmetric blood flow.

Ictal study shows increased left frontal blood flow* in patient with frontal lobe epilepsy.

Postictal study shows decreased left temporal blood flow* in patient with temporal lobe epilepsy.   * Areas of interest circled in red.

Figure 14-2 Neuroimaging Studies.

Clonic phases of partial motor seizures that continue uninterrupted for prolonged periods, with no progression into other body segments, are known as epilepsia partialis continua, or Kojevnikov syndrome, and are discussed below.

The clinical evaluation of patients with partial epilepsy must include an EEG, a neuroimaging test, and laboratory testing. Although routine EEG recordings may often be normal in patients with unequivocal seizure disorders, it remains of paramount importance for the correct diagnosis and classification of the ictal events. Even when the neurologist suspects a seizure disorder from the clinical description, the EEG, if positive, may serve as an important confirmatory test when the episode is not well described. It should be remembered, however, that a routine EEG represents only a limited time sample and that sporadically firing interictal discharges can, therefore, be easily missed in patients with unequivocal seizure disorders. Long-term seizure telemetry units and ambulatory EEG monitoring are now

available to increase recording time and enhance detection rates. The EEG hallmark of partial epilepsy is focal spikes or spike-and-wave discharges. Because delta-wave non-REM sleep activates or disinhibits epileptiform discharges, the EEG is preferably recorded during both wakefulness and sleep to increase the probability of making the correct diagnosis and defining the focal origin (Fig. 14-4). A definitive result is often obtained only during sleep recordings. Repeated recordings may be necessary if the nature of the episode is unclear or if psychogenic nonepileptic seizures are suspected. In contrast, the EEG in patients with epilepsia partialis continua contains spike-wave discharges in a variably continuous manner, often in the contralateral frontal lobe. A small number of individuals in the healthy population have abnormal EEG containing focal spikes but do not go on to have seizures later in life. This emphasizes that an abnormal EEG can only be interpreted in light of the presenting clinical symptoms and that it does not, on its own, define a

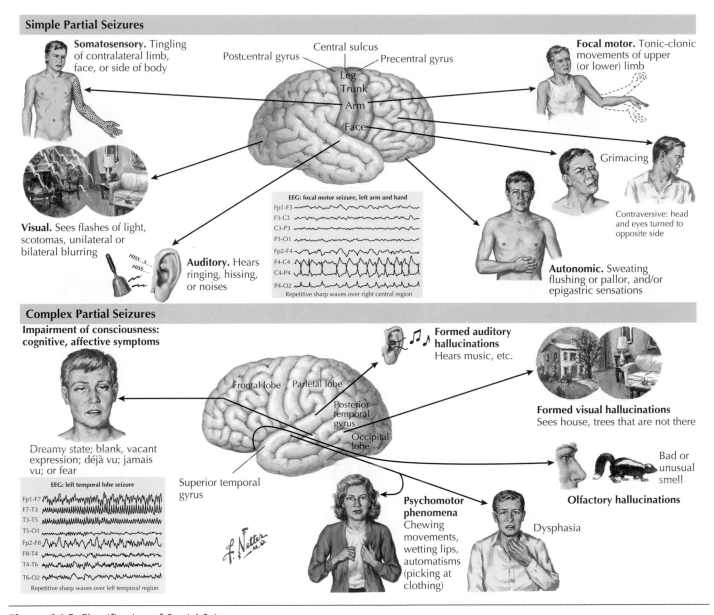

Simple Partial Seizures

Somatosensory. Tingling of contralateral limb, face, or side of body

Visual. Sees flashes of light, scotomas, unilateral or bilateral blurring

Auditory. Hears ringing, hissing, or noises

HISS...S...
HISS...

Postcentral gyrus
Central sulcus
Precentral gyrus
Leg
Trunk
Arm
Face

EEG: focal motor seizure, left arm and hand
Fp1-F3
F3-C3
C3-P3
P3-O1
Fp2-F4
F4-C4
C4-P4
P4-O2
Repetitive sharp waves over right central region

Focal motor. Tonic-clonic movements of upper (or lower) limb

Grimacing

Contraversive: head and eyes turned to opposite side

Autonomic. Sweating flushing or pallor, and/or epigastric sensations

Complex Partial Seizures

Impairment of consciousness: cognitive, affective symptoms

Dreamy state; blank, vacant expression; déjà vu; jamais vu; or fear

EEG: left temporal lobe seizure
Fp1-F7
F7-T3
T3-T5
T5-O1
Fp2-F8
F8-T4
T4-T6
T6-O2
Repetitive sharp waves over left temporal region

Frontal lobe
Parietal lobe
Posterior temporal gyrus
Occipital lobe
Superior temporal gyrus

Formed auditory hallucinations
Hears music, etc.

Formed visual hallucinations
Sees house, trees that are not there

Bad or unusual smell

Olfactory hallucinations

Psychomotor phenomena
Chewing movements, wetting lips, automatisms (picking at clothing)

Dysphasia

F. Netter M.D.

Figure 14-3 Classification of Partial Seizures.

seizure syndrome or dictate treatment. At best, the EEG may capture an ongoing seizure and greatly clarify its origin. It may also help to localize the epileptogenic pathology, guiding surgery if medical treatment fails.

Neuroimaging studies, especially MRI, are vital to the evaluation of new-onset or changing-pattern seizures. Brain computed tomography is a useful screening technique when MRI is not available. The onset of new partial seizures strongly suggests the development of a new pathologic process, including tumors (primary or metastatic) or abscess in the adult population, stroke from emboli or rarely vasculitis in older age groups, and focal encephalitis such as Rasmussen encephalitis in children, herpes simplex encephalitis in children or adults, or head trauma (Fig. 14-5). However, sometimes a patient with a lesion, for example, mesial temporal sclerosis or an AVM, does not present with partial seizures until adulthood. Rarely, acute-onset partial seizures may be caused by metabolic abnormalities, such as non-ketotic hyperglycemia or hypoglycemia.

Complex Partial Seizures

Clinical Vignette

A 37-year-old patient experiences episodic events that start with a rising feeling in the stomach followed by a blank stare with loss of awareness. Subsequently, he has nonpurposeful movements of the hands lasting several minutes followed by somnolence.

This patient's history represents a typical example of complex partial seizures (CPSs). The clinical manifestations of this seizure type include changes in alertness or level of consciousness, partial amnesia, and automatisms (Fig. 14-3). Patients often perform simple motor tasks and even may walk during the seizure. CPSs usually arise from mesial temporal structures but

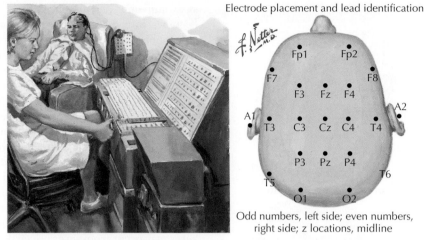

Electrode placement and lead identification

Odd numbers, left side; even numbers, right side; z locations, midline

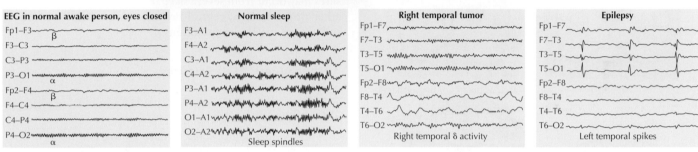

Figure 14-4 Electroencephalography.

can also originate in other extralimbic temporal structures or the inferior frontal lobe and spread via the uncinate fasciculus and other pathways to the mesial temporal area.

Partial seizures of frontal lobe origin are frequently confused with a CPS of temporal origin but are distinguished by brief auras with rapid generalization or versive head and eye movements with tonic posturing of the arms. Rarely, a fall is the only clinical feature. Nocturnal frontal lobe seizures often produce odd complex behaviors suggestive of psychogenic nonepileptic seizures but should be kept in mind in those with fairly consistent patterns and no obvious secondary gain.

Because complex seizures are of focal origin, patient evaluation is similar to that undertaken for SPS. Typically, the interictal EEG (i.e., obtained between seizures) reveals spike discharges in one or both anterior temporal lobes. The ictal EEG is usually abnormal, with recurrent focal spikes or rhythmic activity. Brain MRI with special attention given to the temporal lobes shows that these patients often have mesial temporal lobe sclerosis with cell loss and atrophy (see Fig. 14-5).

Partial Seizures with Secondary Generalization

At times, an SCS or a CPS develops into a generalized tonic–clonic convulsion. Careful attention to the history is necessary to distinguish this secondarily generalized seizure from a primary generalized convulsion, especially when the event goes unwitnessed or the initial partial symptom may be brief or not recalled. Capturing a seizure with continuous EEG recordings may be the only way to differentiate them.

GENERALIZED SEIZURES

Tonic–Clonic (Grand Mal) Seizures

Clinical Vignette

A 40-year-old patient experiences events in which he suddenly stiffens, cries out, loses consciousness, and progresses to have rhythmic tonic–clonic movements of all four extremities lasting several minutes. The events are associated with incontinence, tongue bites, muscle soreness, and ultimately a state of somnolence. Several hours later, the patient was awake and back to normal but had no recollection of the event.

This type of seizure represents the classic picture that the public and medical community generically perceives as epilepsy. Generalized seizure begin with simultaneous and almost equal involvement of both hemispheres from the onset and, unlike partial seizures with focal cortical abnormalities, involve the deeper thalamic, subcortical, and brainstem structures in a feedback loop to the cortices. Tonic–clonic (grand mal) seizures are often preceded by nonspecific, vaguely defined prodromes lasting at times up to hours or have no promontory symptoms at all. Seizures with specific auras, on the other hand, usually are of a focal origin with secondary generalization.

Grand mal seizures start with loss of consciousness, a cry, generalized tonic muscle contraction, and a fall (Fig. 14-6). Autonomic signs are often present during the tonic phase, including tachycardia, hypertension, cyanosis, salivation,

Primary

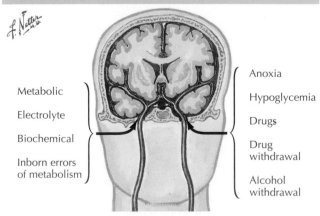

Unknown (genetic or biochemical predisposition)

Intracranial

Focal onset seizures with or without secondary generalization

Tumor

Vascular (infarct or hemorrhage)

Arteriovenous malformation

Trauma (depressed fracture, penetrating wound)

Infection (abscess, encephalitis)

Congenital and hereditary diseases (tuberous sclerosis)

Extracranial

Metabolic

Electrolyte

Biochemical

Inborn errors of metabolism

Anoxia

Hypoglycemia

Drugs

Drug withdrawal

Alcohol withdrawal

Figure 14-5 Causes of Seizures.

sweating, and incontinence. The tonic muscle contraction becomes interrupted relatively soon and is followed by the clonic phase of the seizure with brief relaxation periods progressively lengthening until the seizure eventually abates. Patients may remain stuporous for a moment and eventually awaken confused with postictal headaches, lethargy, disorientation, and myalgia that may persist for up to a few days.

A single generalized grand mal seizure does not warrant the diagnosis of epilepsy. In the vignette above, the patient later admitted that during the previous year, he was worried about his business and had been abusing alcohol and sedatives. He had recently discontinued these and had not had alcohol or sedatives for 48 hours. EEG and neuroimaging studies were normal. The seizure described above represents a reactive type of generalized grand mal seizure secondary to drug withdrawal. Similar seizures may occur from severe sleep deprivation, withdrawal from other drugs, trauma, central nervous system (CNS) infection, and various metabolic conditions.

Absence (Petit Mal) Seizures

Clinical Vignette

A 10-year-old boy is noted to have abrupt and brief (~10-second) episodes of impaired alertness. These can be brought out particularly when he hyperventilates. Eye fluttering is often noted during the episodes and occasional lip movements. The child returns to normal right after the episodes and the neurologic examination is normal.

This is the typical history of a child with generalized absence (petit mal) seizures. Petit mal epilepsy is the classic example of benign primary generalized epilepsy, which tends to remit in adulthood. Brief lapses in consciousness without an aura or any postictal symptoms are the main features (Fig. 14-7). Automatic movements may be observed but are generally simple and brief. The neurologic examination is usually normal.

EEG provides the best diagnostic confirmation and typically demonstrates brief generalized bilaterally synchronous 3-Hz spike-and-wave discharges. Hyperventilation may precipitate petit mal seizures and the classic EEG changes describe above. There is neither focal interictal EEG epileptic activity nor focal initiation of the spike-and-wave pattern.

ATYPICAL ABSENCE SEIZURES

Atypical absence seizures differ from typical absence seizures because motor symptoms are more prominent and sometimes have a focal preponderance. Additionally, some patients have postictal confusion. Usually beginning during childhood, atypical absence seizures tend to occur over a longer lifetime period than classic petit mal seizures. Children with atypical absence seizures tend to have multifocal or generalized cerebral pathology, clinically associated with a lag in attaining normal developmental milestones

The EEG demonstrates a slow (1.5- to 2.5-Hz) spike-and-wave pattern. This clinical constellation with its associated

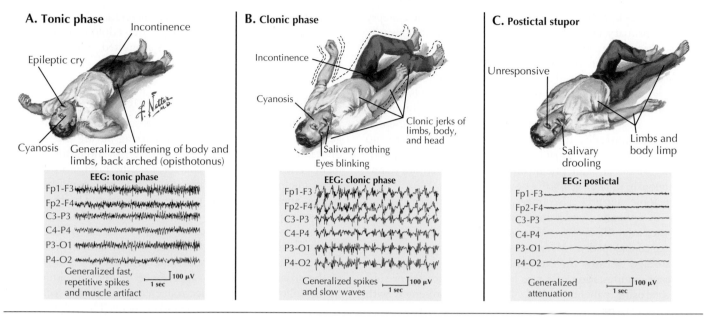

A. Tonic phase

Incontinence

Epileptic cry

Cyanosis   Generalized stiffening of body and limbs, back arched (opisthotonus)

EEG: tonic phase

Fp1-F3
Fp2-F4
C3-P3
C4-P4
P3-O1
P4-O2

Generalized fast, repetitive spikes and muscle artifact   100 μV / 1 sec

B. Clonic phase

Incontinence

Cyanosis

Clonic jerks of limbs, body, and head

Salivary frothing
Eyes blinking

EEG: clonic phase

Fp1-F3
Fp2-F4
C3-P3
C4-P4
P3-O1
P4-O2

Generalized spikes and slow waves   100 μV / 1 sec

C. Postictal stupor

Unresponsive

Limbs and body limp

Salivary drooling

EEG: postictal

Fp1-F3
Fp2-F4
C3-P3
C4-P4
P3-O1
P4-O2

Generalized attenuation   100 μV / 1 sec

Figure 14-6 Generalized Tonic–Clonic Seizures.

seizures and EEG pattern are characteristic of the Lennox–Gastaut syndrome. Generally, these patients also have other seizure types, and treatment of the seizures is difficult, usually requiring multiple anticonvulsants.

Myoclonic Seizures

Clinical Vignette

A 20-year-old college student reports a history of muscle jerks involving either arm for the past several years, which tended to occur in the morning. She also had two recent unexplained falls, without lapse of consciousness during the falls. Her neurologic examination results were normal. On two occasions, once after staying up late studying for exams, and another after drinking alcohol to excess and missing her medications, she had a generalized tonic–clonic seizure.

One of the most frequently observed settings for myoclonus is the postanoxic syndrome (Lance–Adams syndrome) following prolonged cardiac arrest and resuscitation. Prognosis for full recovery in those who display myoclonus is generally poor. In the adult population, myoclonus is one of the classic findings in the prion-induced dementing illness or transmissible spongiform encephalopathy (Creutzfeldt–Jakob disease). This disease usually occurs in middle to late life. The EEG in Creutzfeldt–Jakob disease has a classic appearance with periodic sharp and slow wave complexes recurring usually at 1–2 Hz. The background EEG is abnormal. Myoclonus is also a nonspecific term that describes brief nonepileptic muscle jerks. They may involve a body segment or be generalized, may be single or repetitive, and may be spontaneous or provoked by sensory stimulation (reflex) or limb action. Myoclonus may be mediated by cortical, subcortical, brainstem, or spinal cord mechanisms.

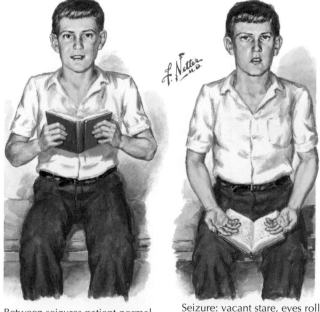

Between seizures patient normal

Seizure: vacant stare, eyes roll upward, eyelids flutter (3/sec), cessation of activity, lack of response

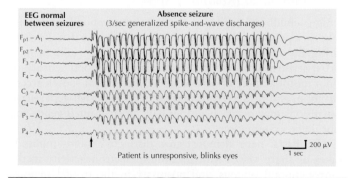

EEG normal between seizures   Absence seizure (3/sec generalized spike-and-wave discharges)

Fp1 – A1
Fp2 – A2
F3 – A1
F4 – A2
C3 – A1
C4 – A2
P3 – A1
P4 – A2

Patient is unresponsive, blinks eyes   200 μV / 1 sec

Figure 14-7 Absence (Petit Mal) Seizures.

The above-described patient has juvenile myoclonic epilepsy (JME), a primary generalized epilepsy syndrome that usually begins during the teenage years and is associated with morning myoclonic jerks soon after awakening. Many of these patients have occasional generalized seizures, especially under period of physiologic stress. The EEG typically demonstrates bilaterally synchronous, irregular spike-wave or polyspike discharges at variable 4- to 6-Hz repetition rates but no focal epileptic discharges. Paradoxically, the EEG discharges usually have no clinical myoclonic accompaniment. This condition responds generally well to antiepileptic medication and sometimes remits spontaneously in later years.

Myoclonic seizures also may occur in children with a variety of epileptic syndromes such as the Lennox–Gastaut syndrome, infantile spasms (West syndrome), and early myoclonic encephalopathy. Myoclonus also may be a part of CNS storage diseases. In the past, myoclonus occurred as a significant manifestation of a rare late form of measles or subacute sclerosing panencephalitis. This illness presented with poor school performance, mental changes, and myoclonus in teenagers, with periodic EEG complexes occurring regularly every several seconds.

EPILEPTIC SYNDROMES

Stereotypic seizures at a particular age and associated with fairly distinct EEG abnormalities or a symptom complex constitute the epileptic syndromes. The seizures in these syndromes may be classified into reactive, the best known being benign febrile convulsions; primary or idiopathic, exemplified by childhood absence (petit mal) epilepsy; and secondary or symptomatic, for example, infantile spasms or West syndrome.

Benign Febrile Convulsions

Benign febrile convulsions occur in otherwise healthy children at the age of 6 months to 5 years. Up to 5% of healthy children in the United States experience at least one febrile convulsion, usually early during a benign febrile illness. The seizures are brief, simple, and without localizing or lateralizing preponderance. Interictal EEGs are always normal. If not, other seizure mechanisms should be considered. The long-term prognosis is usually excellent if no seizures occur in nonfebrile settings.

Benign Childhood Epilepsy With Centrotemporal (Rolandic) Spikes

Benign childhood epilepsy with centrotemporal (rolandic) spikes is a primary (idiopathic) epileptic syndrome that develops during the first decade of life. Typically, these children have partial seizures characterized by unilateral perioral sensory or minor motor activity associated with dysarthria or speech arrest, salivation, and preserved consciousness. Nocturnal generalized convulsions may occur. Children have normal intelligence and neurologic examination.

The EEG here demonstrates distinctive high-amplitude spikes or sharp waves with maximum electronegativity in the centrotemporal regions, and positivity in the frontal regions. These epileptiform discharges, which increase during sleep, are commonly bilateral, shifting in preponderance from side to side or occur independently. Although the etiology is unknown, autosomal dominant inheritance is suggested. The prognosis is excellent for this benign type of epilepsy.

Infantile Spasms (West Syndrome)

West syndrome is an example of a secondary (symptomatic) generalized epileptic syndrome occurring during the first year of life. There is a concomitant arrest of psychomotor development. These seizures are characterized by brief jerks followed by a tonic phase and a subsequent period of generalized atonia lasting approximately 1 minute or associated with flexion–extension spasms.

The chaotic appearance of a typical EEG, called hypsarrhythmia, shows high-amplitude slow-wave activity with mixed high-amplitude sharp or spike discharges. The EEG correlate of the spasm is a sudden appearance of high-amplitude slow waves followed by an electrodecremental period with low-voltage fast activity. The prognosis is poor. The primary treatment is corticotropin administration.

STATUS EPILEPTICUS

Clinical Vignette

A 60-year-old patient has a witnessed tonic–clonic seizure. 911 is called, and en-route to the local hospital, he has repeated tonic–clonic seizures, without regaining consciousness between episodes. He becomes cyanotic with labored breathing and requires emergent intubation.

Generalized convulsive status epilepticus (GCSE) is defined as recurrent seizures without recovery of consciousness lasting more than 30 minutes or when seizure activity becomes unremitting (Fig. 14-8). One of the most common and life-threatening neurologic emergencies, GCSE mandates immediate treatment because of the potential for irreversible CNS damage, that is, neuronal loss secondary to anoxia and systemic metabolic and autonomic dysfunction. Medical complications such as cardiac arrhythmias, pulmonary edema, and renal failure sometimes occur in association with GCSE. The GCSE mortality rate approaches 30%. Unfortunately, the history in the above vignette in this chapter is common in patients with partial seizures with secondary generalization who do not comply with antiepileptic therapy and progress to status epilepticus.

Treatment of GCSE treatment requires the maintenance of an adequate airway, ventilation, and circulatory support and the termination of seizures. Etiologic mechanisms include anticonvulsant or other medication withdrawal, illicit toxic drugs, hypoglycemia, hyponatremia, and hypocalcemia. GCSE may be the first manifestation of acute cerebral pathology.

The initial therapy, a benzodiazepine or phenytoin, often depends on whether the patient is actively seizing. Both first-line medications are frequently utilized within a short time. Intravenous lorazepam at 1–2 mg every 1–2 minutes up to 8 mg or diazepam 5 mg up to 20 mg is most often the initial therapy. An infusion of phenytoin (at 50 mg/minute) or fosphenytoin (at

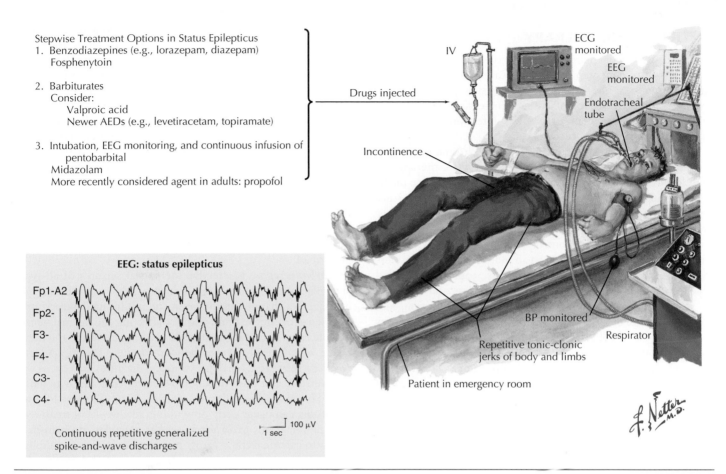

Stepwise Treatment Options in Status Epilepticus
1. Benzodiazepines (e.g., lorazepam, diazepam)
   Fosphenytoin

2. Barbiturates
   Consider:
      Valproic acid
      Newer AEDs (e.g., levetiracetam, topiramate)

3. Intubation, EEG monitoring, and continuous infusion of
      pentobarbital
   Midazolam
   More recently considered agent in adults: propofol

Drugs injected

ECG monitored
EEG monitored
Endotracheal tube
IV
Incontinence
BP monitored
Respirator
Repetitive tonic-clonic jerks of body and limbs
Patient in emergency room

EEG: status epilepticus

Fp1-A2
Fp2-
F3-
F4-
C3-
C4-

100 μV
1 sec

Continuous repetitive generalized
spike-and-wave discharges

Figure 14-8 Status Epilepticus.

150 mg /minute) up to 20 mg/kg must also be started promptly because of the short-term effect of benzodiazepines. Phenytoin is given with normal saline and not with glucose as it precipitates out of solution in this vehicle. ECG monitoring is required to monitor the effects of phenytoin on cardiac conduction, especially if infused too rapidly. Hypotension is also a serious side effect, especially in patients showing evidence of hemodynamic instability. The propylene glycol and alcohol content of the intravenous preparation is thought to be partially responsible for these effects and is dependent on the infusion rate. Fosphenytoin, a water-soluble phosphate ester rapidly converted to phenytoin, can be administered at a more rapid rate (150 mg/minute of phenytoin equivalent) while minimizing the risk of cardiovascular instability in unstable patients. Fosphenytoin also has a lower incidence of pain and burning at the infusion site but its routine use remains restricted because of its high cost. If seizures persist and serum phenytoin levels drawn 20 minutes after the initial infusion are less than 20 mg/dL then additional phenytoin or fosphenytoin (5–10 mg/kg) to control seizure and maintain the level around 20–30 mg/dL may be given. Sodium valproate IV, at a loading dose of 10–15 mg/kg, has also been used successfully to control status epilepticus, especially in patients on regular regimens of oral valproic acid.

Barbiturates have been traditionally used as second-line agents in status epilepticus. Long-acting phenobarbital

(at 50–100 mg/minute, up to 20 mg/kg) or short-acting pentobarbital (3–5 mg/kg loading dose, followed by an infusion of 3–5 mg/kg/hour) may be added. Intubation for airway protection and continuous EEG monitoring are usually required at this stage. Over the years, however, many centers have shifted to using continuous infusions of other agents, such as the short-acting benzodiazepine midazolam or the hypnotic propofol (decreases excitatory effect of glutamate) for control of recurrent seizures. Many centers now use continuous infusion of benzodiazepines such as midazolam or propofol before barbiturate anesthesia is initiated.

Nonconvulsive status epilepticus or absence status epilepticus is another form of continued seizures without motor accompaniments. Typically, patients are poorly responsive with decreased alertness or obtundation. EEG reveals mostly continuous generalized spike-and-wave activity, the so-called spike–wave stupor. Intravenous benzodiazepine administration, the treatment of choice, is generally effective.

Complex partial seizures may occasionally evolve into complex partial status epilepticus, in which patients do not regain full consciousness between seizures. Prompt treatment as prescribed for GCSE is necessary. An SPS may evolve into epilepsia partialis continua, as described above. Long-term anticonvulsant therapy is usually needed in patients who have experienced status epilepticus.

ANTIEPILEPTIC THERAPY

The goal of antiepileptic treatment is the control of seizures. The most important step in seizure treatment is identification and treatment of the primary pathophysiologic mechanism. Examples include resection of a tumor, correction of a metabolic imbalance, and treatment of a CNS infection. Appropriate therapy may stop seizure recurrence.

Unfortunately, most seizures occur with chronic neurologic processes and are not amenable to specific curative therapy and therefore require long-term treatment. The ideal seizure medication would have high efficacy across a broad range of seizure types, with no adverse effects and little interaction with other drugs. Unfortunately, no such anticonvulsant exists, and treatment must balance seizure control with quality of life. Choosing an anticonvulsant must be done on an individual basis, considering seizure or epilepsy type, side effects, comorbidities, and psychosocial factors such as age, sex, ease of use, and cost.

There is no single approach to medication selection, and good knowledge of the available drugs and their basic properties is essential. As of 2005, phenytoin and carbamazepine are still the most commonly prescribed medications; however, seizure-free rates have recently been shown to be similar between the older and newer antiseizure medications. Newer agents are well tolerated, require less monitoring, and may be safer in the long term. With time and increasing regulatory approval, these anticonvulsants, initially approved for use as adjunctive agents, may soon replace the older ones as first-line agents in seizure management. Still, the newer medications are often more costly and may present various drug-specific side effects or issues. In addition, the therapeutic ranges are not as well established as compared to the older agents. With the exception of levetiracetam and lacosamide, the newer agents are not available in parenteral form. The variety of mechanisms of action of the newer medications has allowed these preparations to be possibly useful in other neurologic conditions such as for bipolar disease, headache, and neuropathic pain.

Phenobarbital and primidone are among the oldest antiseizure medication and are effective in all types of partial seizures and generalized tonic–clonic seizures. It binds to the beta-2 subunit of the γ-aminobutyric acid (GABAa) receptor, allowing GABA to bind to the beta-1 subunit and increase chloride conductance. It is metabolized by the hepatic cytochrome p-450 system. The half-life is about 72 hours; doses of 90–180 mg/day can be given once a day. The therapeutic blood level is between 20 and 40 µg/mL. Adverse effects are sedation and rash. Sedation is the prevalent adverse effect and has contributed to their decreased use.

Phenytoin is another long-established anticonvulsant used for more than 50 years initially as a superior less-sedating alternative to barbiturates. It is effective for partial onset seizures of all types and generalized tonic–clonic seizures. Phenytoin's presumed mechanism of action is through the blockade of membrane voltage-dependent sodium channels to increase transmembrane potential recovery time and limit high-frequency firing. At higher concentrations, phenytoin delays efflux of potassium and prolongs neuronal refractory periods. It is metabolized by the hepatic cytochrome p-450 system and its half-life is 12–36 hours, thus allowing twice-a-day dosing (5–7 mg/kg or about 300–500 mg a day). Optimum seizure control occurs with blood levels of 10–20 mg/mL. When plasma levels are higher there is a shift from first-order to zero-order kinetics with a longer half life and with rapid increases in concentration levels and subsequent toxicity caused by small increases in the dose. Acute side effects mimic alcohol intoxication with dizziness, nystagmus, ataxia, slurred speech, and confusion. Prolonged use may produce coarsening facial features, gingival hyperplasia, acne, hirsutism, cerebellar impairment, megaloblastic anemia, and, at times, polyneuropathy. Acute idiosyncratic reactions occur in approximately 10% of patients, and vary from a mild morbilliform rash to a rare severe exfoliative dermatitis. As with other anticonvulsants, teratogenic effects may occur. Phenytoin interacts with numerous drugs of many classes and close monitoring of the levels is advised whenever such medications are prescribed.

Carbamazepine is effective for partial seizures of all types and generalized tonic–clonic seizures. It acts presumably by blocking Na channels in the brain and inhibiting depolarization of seizure foci in the brain without affecting the normal neuronal function. The usual dose is 600–1000 mg/day and the therapeutic blood serum level is between 4 and 12 mg/L. Adverse reactions relate to CNS depression and dizziness, nausea, as well as reversible and dose-dependent neutropenia and hyponatremia. Hypersensitive allergic reactions and Stevens–Johnson Syndrome can occur early on within a few weeks of treatment.

A newer agent, *oxcarbazepine*, has a similar mechanism of action to carbamazepine via its rapid and complete metabolism to an active 10-monohydroxy derivative. Oxcarbazepine has linear pharmacokinetics, no autoinduction, minimal interaction with other seizure medications, and does not cause neutropenia. Hyponatremia sometimes occurs. Adverse reactions include psychomotor slowing and sedation but, on the whole, it may be better tolerated than carbamazepine. The typical starting dosage is 300 mg twice daily, increased gradually to 600 mg twice daily. Occasionally, higher dosages are used but should not exceed 2400 mg daily.

Divalproex sodium is an extremely effective drug for absence, myoclonic, and generalized tonic–clonic seizures. It inhibits calcium ion influx through T-type calcium channels and inhibits sodium ion influx through voltage-gated sodium channels. The therapeutic blood level ranges from 50 to 150 µg/mL, and it is given in doses of 1000–3000 mg/day. Divalproex sodium inhibits the hepatic cytochrome p-450 system and will therefore diminish the metabolism of other drugs. Adverse effects are gastrointestinal upset, somnolence, dizziness, tremor, weight gain, and hair loss. More serious effects include hepatotoxicity, pancreatitis, thrombocytopenia, polycystic ovarian disease, and teratogenic effects (neural tube defects and lowered IQ). *Ethosuximide* is the first antiseizure drug used to treat absence (petit mal) seizures. It is thought to inhibit calcium ion influx through T-type calcium channels. Adverse effects are gastrointestinal and CNS related, but this drug is generally well tolerated. A common dose is 250–2000 mg/day according to age and response. The therapeutic blood level is 40–100 µg/mL.

Felbamate blocks voltage-dependent sodium channels and N-methyl-D-aspartate (NMDA) receptors and was found to be more effective than divalproex sodium in partial seizures and had a significant benefit for Lennox–Gastaut syndrome. It is better tolerated than other drugs, with relatively minor gastrointestinal and cognitive adverse effects. Unfortunately, its relatively high rates of (at times fatal) hepatoxicity and aplastic anemia have severely restricted its use to those with severe epilepsy, such as Lennox–Gastaut syndrome.

Several other newer agents such as lamotrigine, gabapentin, topiramate, levetiracetam, tiagabine, and zonisamide are recommended as adjunctive to the first-line medications of carbamazepine, phenytoin, phenobarbital, primidone, or valproate. Because they have different mechanisms of action, they may complement the traditional first-line drugs.

Lamotrigine is a newer antiepileptic drug recommended as an adjunct medication for partial seizures, primary generalized tonic–clonic seizures patients of all ages and Lennox–Gastaut syndrome. It is indicated for conversion to monotherapy in adults with partial seizures treated with the older anticonvulsants, carbamazepine, phenytoin, phenobarbital, primidone, or valproate. Lamotrigine blocks voltage-gated sodium and calcium channels and inhibits the presynaptic release of glutamate and aspartate. Metabolized by glucuronidation, it is not an enzyme inducer or inhibitor. When prescribed with an enzyme-inducing antiseizure medication, lamotrigine serum concentration may decrease by up to 40%. Frequent monitoring is therefore needed when switching to lamotrigine monotherapy. It has a half-life of about 12–60 hours, and typical adult doses are 300–500 mg/day divided twice a day. It must be introduced at low doses with slow titration to the desired maintenance level over months to reduce the risk of Stevens–Johnson syndrome. Adverse effects are gastrointestinal and CNS related. There is a 10% risk of an idiosyncratic rash and a 3 in 1000 risk of Stevens–Johnson syndrome in adults, especially in those taking valproic acid. There are no known long-term effects.

Levetiracetam is another newer antiepileptic medication whose mechanism of action is not completely understood but may involve modulating neurotransmitter release at the SV2A binding receptor complex. It is indicated for partial seizures and generalized seizures. The usual adult maintenance dose is between 1000 and 2000 mg/day in divided doses. An intravenous formulation is also available. It is not an enzyme inducer or inhibitor and has few drug interactions with other medications. Levetiracetam is eliminated renally with a half-life of 6–8 hours. Adverse effects include sedation, lethargy, or ataxia. Not to be overlooked are behavioral changes seen at higher doses around 3000 mg/day with aggression, depression, suicidal ideation, and, in extreme cases, frank psychosis.

Gabapentin is usually used as adjunctive therapy for partial seizures with or without secondary generalization. There is concern that it may worsen absence and myoclonic seizure and should generally be avoided in primary generalized epilepsy syndromes. It is an analogue of GABA; however, its exact mechanism of action is unknown. It is not an enzyme inducer or inhibitor and is eliminated through the renal system with a half-life of about 5–6 hours. It is given in doses of 900–3600 mg/day in divided doses. Adverse effects are somnolence, dizziness, ataxia, fatigue, weight gain, and behavioral changes, especially in children.

Topiramate blocks voltage-gated sodium channels, enhances GABA-mediated synaptic inhibition, and antagonizes the excitatory effect of glutamate on NMDA receptors. It has limited hepatic metabolism with a half-life of about 20 hours, and typical doses are 100–400 mg/day divided twice a day. Topiramate can increase phenytoin levels. It is indicated as an adjuvant treatment or monotherapy of partial and primary generalized tonic–clonic seizures and in Lennox-Gastaut syndrome. Adverse effects are CNS related, including cognitive impairment or word-finding difficulty, weight loss, decreased sweating, glaucoma, and a 1–1.5% risk of kidney stones.

Zonisamide blocks voltage-gated sodium channels and inhibits calcium ion influx through T-type calcium channels. It is not an enzyme inducer or inhibitor, has hepatic metabolism followed by glucuronidation, and has a half-life of about 63 hours. It is given in doses of 300–400 mg once a day, or higher doses divided twice a day. Adverse effects are CNS related, rash, decreased sweating, weight loss, and a 0.6% risk of kidney stones. *Tiagabine* is indicated for use as adjunctive therapy for refractory partial seizures. It is a GABA uptake inhibitor, is not an enzyme inducer or inhibitor, has hepatic metabolism, and a half-life of about 7–9 hours. Adverse effects are CNS related, rash, and nonconvulsive status. *Pregabalin* is usually used as adjunctive therapy for partial seizures. Its exact mechanism of action is not known, is not an enzyme inducer or inhibitor, has renal metabolism, and has a half-life of about 6 hours. Adverse effects are CNS related, weight gain, and peripheral edema. Lacosamide is the newest antiseizure medication approved as adjuvant therapy for partial-onset seizures. It is available in oral and IV formulation and is thought to work by the unique mechanism of selectively modulating the slow inactivation of voltage-gate sodium channels. It is renally excreted, has few drug interactions, and is dosed at 100–400 mg/day. CNS and behavioral adverse effects have been described but are thought to be less frequent than with levetiracetam.

Ideally, a single antiepileptic drug is used. If adequate control of seizures is not achieved with one drug, another drug is substituted. Discontinuing antiseizure medications should be done gradually over 2–3 months to avoid withdrawal seizures from rebound.

Anticonvulsant Treatment Considerations

The decision to treat with antiepileptic drugs a first-time unprovoked seizure remains an individualized process that takes into account the structural integrity of the brain, the EEG findings, the circumstances surrounding the seizure, past history of provoked or unprovoked seizures, as well as the potential side effects of medications prescribed.

The incidence of recurrence after a single unprovoked seizure varies widely from 10% to 70%. Predictors of recurrent seizures are an abnormal EEG demonstrating epileptiform discharges (especially generalized patterns), focal spikes or sharp waves, abnormal MRI scans, and an abnormal neurologic examination. Although only about 30% or fewer of EEGs done in adults will yield significant abnormalities, these have a strong predictive power of recurrent seizures in up to 50–60% of patients within 2–3 years. Any patient presenting with a first-time seizure will require, in addition to a detailed neurologic history and examination, imaging of the brain (preferably an MRI) and an EEG in the awake and sleep state (preferably within the first 24–48 hours). Other studies such as a toxic screen and lumbar puncture have a low general yield but may be helpful in specific clinical situations.

Immediate short-term anticonvulsant treatment reduces the likelihood of recurrent seizures by half to two thirds but does not affect the long-term recurrence rate over 1–2 years. Patients who are younger than 16, and those with partial onset seizures, either witnessed or inferred from a postictal Todd paralysis, have a significantly higher risk of recurrence. Other factors that may increase the likelihood of developing recurrent seizure or epilepsy after a first-time unprovoked seizure included a history of perinatal or congenital neurologic difficulties, a family history of epilepsy, and previous unprovoked seizures.

It is recommended that patients remain seizure free for about 2–5 years before considering discontinuation of antiepileptic drugs (AEDs). The recurrence rate and the predictive factors are similar to those mentioned above for first-time seizures. However, strong consideration should be given to the impact that a recurrent seizure, no matter how unlikely, may have on the life of active and productive patients under good seizure control and the impact on those who rely on them.

WOMEN WITH EPILEPSY

There are special considerations regarding management of women with epilepsy. Seizures and AEDs may impact menstruation, contraception, bone health, menopause, pregnancy, and breast feeding. The majority of women with epilepsy have routine pregnancies and deliver healthy babies. However, detailed discussions with patients about the potential teratogenic effects and the risks of seizures must begin prior to conception. About 25% of women experience an increase in seizures during pregnancy because of poor compliance, lowered anticonvulsant levels and protein binding, hormonal changes, or sleep deprivation. The incidence of preeclampsia (pregnancy-induced hypertension), preterm delivery, intrauterine bleeding, hyperemesis gravidarum, and abruptio placenta is increased twofold in women with epilepsy.

Generalized tonic–clonic seizures are harmful to a developing fetus and can cause seizure-related trauma, intrauterine death, and miscarriage. The risk of major fetal malformations for women with epilepsy is 4–6% compared to 2–3% in the healthy population. The major congenital anomalies include cleft lip or palate and urogenital, cardiac, and neural tube defects. Most antiseizure medications have potential teratogenic effects caused by varying degrees of folate deficiency. The risk is highest with valproic acid and increases with polypharmacy as well as higher concentration levels of antiseizure medication. The risk of major malformations, particularly neural tube defects, with valproic acid is 10.7%; phenobarbital, 6.5%; and with lamotrigine monotherapy, 2.6%. The newer antiseizure medications have pharmacokinetic advantages over the older agents and may be safer, but data are limited.

Some women with medically refractory epilepsy consider epilepsy surgery in order to attain seizure freedom before planning pregnancy. In many circumstances, seizure-free women may be tapered off their antiseizure medication before conception. Women may choose not to take antiepileptic medications in the first trimester during organogenesis, especially if the seizure type is minor and infrequent. Not all patients can do this safely and there is evidence to suggest adverse effects of recurrent complex partial seizures on fetal growth and development. The goal throughout pregnancy is to remain seizure free while exposing the fetus to the least number of drugs and the lowest possible levels of antiseizure medication.

The neural tube closes between the 24th and the 27th day after conception. Folate reduces the risk of neural tube defects in the general population. Because neural tube closure defects occur early, before many women may realize they are pregnant, prophylaxis with folic acid is recommended in all epileptic women of childbearing age. The optimal dose of folic acid is not known but ranges from 0.4 to 5 mg/day. Tests to assess for neural tube and other anticonvulsant-induced congenital defects should be considered routine prenatal care.

Antiepileptic medications during pregnancy require close monitoring and often frequent adjustments to maintain the desired therapeutic levels. Serum levels decrease during pregnancy because of accelerated hepatic metabolism, changes in plasma volume, absorption, and protein binding. With the exception of lamotrigine, the newer antiseizure medications are less prone to fluctuating levels during pregnancy. Pregnant women with epilepsy should be under the care of a high-risk obstetrician. Maternal serum alpha fetoprotein and a high-level ultrasound is recommended at 14–18 weeks and may be repeated at 22–24 weeks to screen for anomalies. About 3–4% of epileptic women experience a seizure around delivery. The risk is highest in women with subtherapeutic drug levels, idiopathic generalized epilepsy, or a history of seizures during pregnancy.

Mothers taking enzyme-inducing antiseizure medications are prescribed vitamin K 10 mg/day orally in the last month of pregnancy, and their infants should be given 1 mg of vitamin K intramuscularly at birth to prevent maternal and fetal hemorrhage. Antiseizure levels need to be monitored postpartum because levels will gradually return to baseline 8–10 weeks after delivery. Lamotrigine levels decrease markedly during pregnancy because of increased clearance and need to be monitored closely after delivery to avoid postpartum toxicity. The concern of exposing nursing infants to antiseizure medication should be discussed with the mother. Most antiseizure medications have a milk-to-plasma ratio of less than one, but the serum level below which there are no clinical effects on the neonate is unknown. Other than congenital malformations, children exposed in utero to phenobarbital and valproic acid may be at increased risk of cognitive deficits with lower verbal IQ and greater need for special education. The Neurodevelopmental Effects of Antiepileptic Drugs study is currently underway to assess children's neurobehavioral outcomes in mothers with epilepsy and those exposed to antiseizure medications.

Estrogen may have proconvulsant effects by reducing GABAa inhibition, whereas progesterone may have anticonvulsant effects by increasing GABAa inhibition. Women are prone to seizures during ovulation because of the rapid decline of progesterone that triggers menstruation. Seizures may increase a few days before or occur during the first days of menses. Seizures can also increase in midcycle as a result of increased estrogen midcycle. Women with anovulatory cycles fail to form a progesterone-secreting corpus luteum and can experience an increase in seizures during the second half of their cycle because of low progesterone levels. If a pattern can be documented, an increase in the daily dose of medication at the expected time of seizures may help control seizures. Use of acetazolamide, around the time of expected increase in seizures, has had some limited success.

Contraceptive pills are less effective in women taking hepatic enzyme–inducing antiseizure medications (carbamazepine, oxcarbazepine, phenobarbital, phenytoin, primidone) with a 6% failure rate. Topiramate in doses of >200 mg/day increases the clearance of estradiol and thus reduces its effectiveness. The American Academy of Neurology suggests that women on the above-mentioned antiseizure medication take higher doses of estradiol, but the lower progesterone dose may still lead to hormonal failure. Depo-Provera may be an alternative if given every 10 weeks instead of 12 weeks. Patients should be referred to their gynecologist to discuss and manage these issues long term. On the other hand, oral contraceptives in their turn may reduce lamotrigine and valproic acid levels. Levels should be monitored when oral contraceptives are initiated or discontinued. Intrauterine devices are effective in patients taking enzyme-inducing drugs and may be a safer alternative to oral contraceptives in preventing pregnancy.

Women with epilepsy may experience early menopause. There is some concern that estrogen replacement therapy might be associated with increased seizures. Although estrogen is not strictly contraindicated in women with epilepsy, selective estrogen receptor modulators may be a better alternative.

Patients with epilepsy are at increased risk for osteoporosis and fractures. Bone loss is caused by virtually all the anticonvulsants and is not restricted to the hepatic enzyme–inducing drugs. The mechanism remains obscure and no clear data exists as to which agent may be preferable. A dual-energy x-ray absorptiometry (DEXA) scan is generally recommended after 2 years of treatment with an anticonvulsant. Patients with osteopenia are advised calcium 1200 mg/day and vitamin D 800 IU/day, and lifestyle changes that include weight-bearing exercise, decreased alcohol consumption, and smoking cessation. Patients with osteoporosis should be referred to a specialist and followed closely.

All pregnant women with epilepsy, whether or not taking any antiseizure medication, should be encouraged to enroll in the North American Pregnancy Registry (www.aedpregnancyregistry.org), a prospective study to assess the risk of major fetal malformations. These data may provide the comparative teratogenic risk for individual antiseizure drugs and will help make more rational treatment decisions for pregnant women with epilepsy.

SURGICAL TREATMENTS FOR EPILEPSY

Surgical treatment may be an option for individuals whose seizures are unresponsive to medical therapy or those who cannot take medications because of significant adverse effects or quality-of-life issues. Some of the first craniotomies on record were performed to treat refractory seizure disorders. Cerebral localization was grossly defined by the specific characteristics of a seizure, and cerebral tumors were localized and removed based on these techniques. Many aspects of cortical mapping and function were derived from work related to surgery for epileptic activity.

Surgical Candidates

Clinical Vignette

A 36-year-old woman had febrile seizures as an infant followed by a latent period of about 12 years. Complex partial seizures characterized by a rising epigastric sensation and staring with oral automatisms and unresponsiveness returned at menarche, and continued 2–4 times monthly despite several medication trials. The patient could not drive, experienced medication side effects, and worsening short-term memory. MRI identified right mesial temporal sclerosis without any other overt structural abnormality.

Inpatient video EEG monitoring revealed interictal right temporal spikes and concordant complex partial seizures. Positron emission tomographic imaging revealed right temporal lobe hypometabolism.

The above vignette identifies the typical clinical scenario of a patient with medically refractory mesial temporal lobe epilepsy with hippocampal sclerosis. Seizures are not fully controlled by medical therapy in about 30–40% of patients with epilepsy. Once a patient fails to respond to two antiseizure drugs, the chance of achieving control on a third drug is small. The initial response to medication seen in the above vignette does not mean permanent seizure control. In a randomized controlled study of patients with refractory temporal lobe epilepsy, patients that underwent temporal lobectomy were more likely to be seizure free than the patients randomized to AED therapy (58% vs 8%). Patients who underwent surgery had a significant improvement in their quality of life. Successful surgery not only can provide seizure control in patients, but also can arrest or reverse cognitive decline, lower the mortality, and relieve psychiatric disorders. Any patient in whom seizures persist after trials of two appropriate AEDs should be referred to a tertiary epilepsy center for surgical evaluation. Surgical evaluation consists of confirming a diagnosis of epilepsy and defining the location and extent of the epileptogenic zone. The above vignette represents a patient who is likely a candidate for an anterior temporal lobectomy that can often stop or completely cure the epilepsy.

Preoperative Assessments

Video EEG analysis is one of the mainstays of preoperative evaluations and is used to localize the ictal onset zone. The video is used to determine if the ictal semiology represents seizure origin or propagation. Often, seizures cannot be localized to one region of the brain but can be lateralized to one hemisphere, requiring invasive monitoring prior to surgical resection (Fig. 14-9). Invasive monitoring can also be utilized for functional mapping to define the boundaries of the epileptogenic zone in relation to eloquent cortex or key somatomotor regions that may be close to the potential resective zone. MRI is one of the most important structural neuroimaging tool in the presurgical evaluation of patients with medically refractory epilepsy. The presence of a structural abnormality may suggest site of seizure origin and surgical pathology. It can suggest a more favorable surgical outcome and help tailor the resection. The most

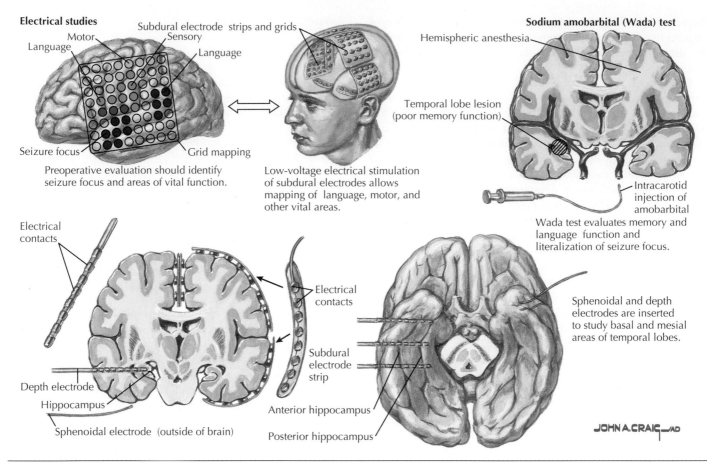

Figure 14-9 Preoperative Evaluation.

common imaging finding in patients undergoing surgical evaluations is hippocampal atrophy best seen using T1-weighted coronal images and an increased mesial temporal signal intensity on T2-weighted or FLAIR coronal images. Magnetic resonance spectroscopy, positron emission tomography, single photon emission computed tomography, functional MRI, and magnetoencephalography are functional imaging tests that could better define the epileptogenic zone. In select cases, a Wada test can be performed for language and memory lateralization. Neuropsychological testing is performed to determine a patient's risk for postoperative memory decline. Ultimately, a decision regarding surgical treatment is based on a convergence of all these neurodiagnostic tests.

Types of Surgery

TEMPORAL LOBECTOMY

Temporal lobectomy is the most common operation for epilepsy. When coupled with anatomic evidence of mesial temporal sclerosis, it has the best chance (approximately 85%) for eliminating seizures. Typically, the resection includes a 3- to 6-cm section of neocortex from the superior, middle, inferior, and basal temporal gyri and the amygdalohippocampal complex (Fig. 14-10). Smaller-sized resections, usually less than 5 cm, should be considered on the dominant side, whereas a larger

6- or 7-cm segment may be removed from the nondominant temporal lobe. Larger resections risk damage to the optic radiation fibers (Meyer loop) and can result in contralateral superior quadrantanopsia.

The precise location of the resected edge in the temporal cortex is often determined visually by appreciating the venous anatomy of the cortical surface, cortical arteries, and the sulcal pattern. A hippocampal resection, often performed separately, typically removes 3–4 cm of the hippocampus.

FOCAL RESECTION

If a relatively small area of the nontemporal cortex can be defined as a specific seizure focus (typically with subdural grid electrodes, intraoperative cortical recordings of interictal spikes, or both), its removal can successfully eliminate focal seizures. Functionally relevant brain tissue, such as the visual or language cortex, known as the "eloquent" *cortex*, must be distinguished from less functional or "noneloquent" areas. It is important that the focus to be resected is in a relatively "noneloquent" region of cortex, such as part of the anterior frontal lobe, and intraoperative mapping of motor or language areas may help avoid undue significant neurologic postoperative morbidity. Epileptogenic lesions such as cavernous malformations, or small tumors, may be removed using similar techniques.

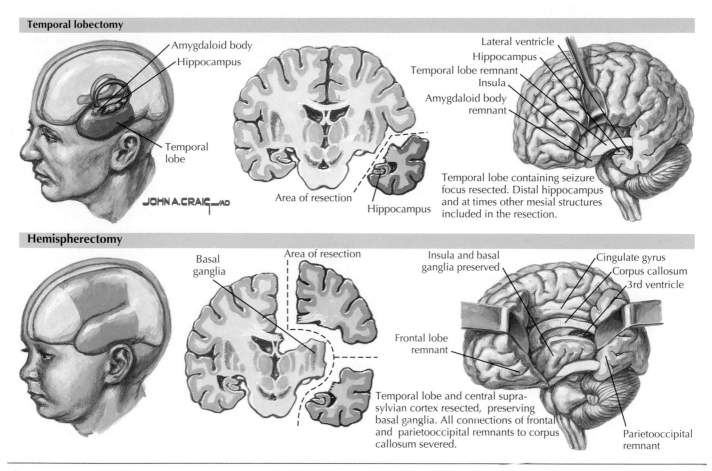

Temporal lobectomy

Amygdaloid body
Hippocampus
Temporal lobe

Area of resection
Hippocampus

Lateral ventricle
Hippocampus
Temporal lobe remnant
Insula
Amygdaloid body remnant

Temporal lobe containing seizure focus resected. Distal hippocampus and at times other mesial structures included in the resection.

JOHN A.CRAIG—AD

Hemispherectomy

Basal ganglia
Area of resection

Insula and basal ganglia preserved
Cingulate gyrus
Corpus callosum
3rd ventricle

Frontal lobe remnant

Temporal lobe and central suprasylvian cortex resected, preserving basal ganglia. All connections of frontal and parietooccipital remnants to corpus callosum severed.

Parietooccipital remnant

Figure 14-10 Resective Surgery.

Clinical Vignette

A 40-year-old patient with mental retardation has tonic and generalized tonic–clonic seizures, many of which result in falls with serious injuries. Video EEG reveals interictal slow generalized spike and wave and paroxysmal fast activity, and nonlocalized seizure onset. The seizures and falls continue despite medication trials.

CORPUS CALLOSOTOMY

Occasionally, surgical division of this important interhemispheric connector is helpful for controlling seizures that spread quickly from one side to the other. Drop attack seizures are good examples. The extent of surgery is debatable; generally an approximate 60–80% resection is appropriate for the best outcome and the lowest degree of deficit. Left-handed patients with potential crossed dominance should undergo Wada's test before surgery because significant behavioral or language deficits may occur if language and handedness are entirely in opposite hemispheres.

FUNCTIONAL HEMISPHERECTOMY

Functional isolation of specific cerebral regions within each hemisphere is possible by dividing the fiber connections between frontal, temporal, and parietal lobes while avoiding

large resection of cortex and sparing the deeper nuclei and structures such as the basal ganglia (see Fig. 14-10). Typically, these patients already have widespread contralateral neurologic deficits. Although this procedure is primarily used only in extremely severe generalized seizure disorders, such as Lennox–Gastaut syndrome, some children often regain significant neurologic function as new pathways develop in the years after surgery.

MULTIPLE SUBPIAL TRANSECTIONS

The multiple subpial transection procedure was developed to treat seizure foci localized to eloquent cortex. Surgical incisions with specially angled blades are made parallel to each other, 5 mm apart, across the cortex of interest, to section horizontally connected u-fibers while preserving many of the vertically oriented output fibers. Theoretically, it prevents spread of seizures through the cortex from this area. Although clinical outcomes vary, it may provide significant seizure control in settings where resection would be neurologically devastating. Often in the immediate postoperative period, a profound focal deficit occurs that resolves during a period of hours to weeks.

VAGUS NERVE STIMULATOR

Stimulation of afferent fibers within the left vagus nerve can modify seizure activity. (The left contains approximately 80%

afferent fibers, whereas stimulation of the right interferes with the cardiac cycle and may provoke asystole.) A set of three electrodes are coiled around the nerve after it has been dissected free within the carotid sheath in the neck. The electrodes are connected to a battery/pulse generator placed under the skin just below the clavicle. This appealing methodology does not require an intracranial procedure, although it is still prone to complications such as infection, bleeding, occasional hoarseness or coughing, and breathing dysregulation such as dyspnea and sleep apnea. Results vary, but some patients have excellent seizure control or are seizure free. Cure rates of VNS are approximately 5–15% but may offer many patients the opportunity to reduce medications and enhance seizure control. This procedure warrants consideration in poorly controlled patients without a well-defined or accessible focus for resection.

DEEP BRAIN STIMULATOR

Other procedures being evaluated require placing electrodes in deep brain structures such as the anterior nucleus of the thalamus or hippocampus to control seizures. The requisite electrodes have been successfully used for treating tremors and Parkinson disease. For patients with uncontrolled epilepsy, the electrodes may be programmed or activated automatically when seizure activity is recorded. Less invasive procedures such as this may become more effective than focal resective procedures, with fewer risks of postoperative deficits in the future.

Common Pathologies Found in Surgical Resections

Mesial temporal sclerosis, appreciated histologically as a gliosis and cell loss within the mesial temporal structures, indicates previous long-term damage. There is usually no inciting event predisposing to this pathologic finding. However, it is often seen in patients who have had temporal lobe seizures for years, birth trauma, evidence of anoxic damage, or previous head injuries. Hippocampal atrophy is often seen with mesial sclerosis.

Cortical dysplasia is a general term covering many cortical developmental architectural variants. Classified by the etiology of the dysplasia (proliferation, migration, or reorganization), up to 20–30% of the normal population have such changes. Dysplastic abnormalities are often found microscopically in idiopathic cases in which no overt lesion is identified by MRI. Such alterations may comprise up to 40% of extramesial seizure foci.

Dysembryoplastic neuroectodermal tumor and low-grade glioma are two tumor types often associated with seizure generation. Typically slow growing, they can be barely perceptible on MRI or other imaging modalities. With complete resection, patients often become seizure free.

FUTURE DIRECTIONS

Future directions in the treatment of epilepsy include the development of more-sensitive MRI techniques and multimodal imaging that will combine anatomic detail with functional and metabolic mapping delineating dysfunctional regions of the brain likely responsible for the pathogenesis of seizures and

potential surgical targets. Many genetic components are being investigated that could have potential for therapies. Clinical trials are currently underway with implantable stimulators and sensing devices that may detect, modulate, and prevent seizure discharges.

ADDITIONAL RESOURCES

Akanuma N, Koutroumanidis M, Adachi N, et al. Presurgical assessment of memory-related brain structures: the Wada test and functional neuroimaging. Seizure 2003;12:346-358.

American Academy of Neurology; American Epilepsy Society. Practice Parameter: evaluating an apparent unprovoked first seizure in adults (an evidence-based review): report of the Quality Standards Subcommittee of the American Academy of Neurology and the American Epilepsy Society. Neurology 2007 Nov 20;69(21):1996-2007. *An evidence-based guide to the workup of a first-time unprovoked seizure and analysis of the predictive value of each finding.*

Asadi-Pooya AA, Sperling M. Antiepileptic Drugs: A Clinician's Manual. Oxford University Press; 2009. *This handbook provides practical, up-to-date information on how to select, prescribe, and monitor AEDs.*

Engel J Jr, Wiebe S, French J, et al. Practice parameter: temporal lobe and localized neocortical resections for epilepsy: report of the Quality Standards Subcommittee of the American Academy of Neurology, in association with the American Epilepsy Society and the American Association of Neurological Surgeons. Neurology 2003;60:538-547.

Engel J Jr, Pedley TA, editors. Epilepsy: A Comprehensive Textbook. Philadelphia, Pa: Lippincott–Raven; 1998.

Engel J Jr. Seizures and Epilepsy. Philadelphia, Pa: FA Davis Co; 1989.

Harden CL. The adolescent female with epilepsy: mood, menstruation, and birth control. Neurology 2006;66(S3). *An excellent supplement that addresses the challenges in treating women with epilepsy including the link between epilepsy and depression, risk of reproductive disorders, efficacy of hormonal contraceptives, and interactions between oral contraceptives and AEDs.*

Kwan P, Brodie MJ. Early identification of refractory epilepsy. N Engl J Med 2000;342(5):314-319.

Meador KJ, Baker GA, Finnell RH, et al. In utero antiepileptic drug exposure: fetal death and malformations. Neurology 2006;67(3):407-412. *More adverse outcomes were observed with in utero exposure to valproate compared to other AEDs suggesting that valproate poses the greatest risk to the fetus.*

Morrell MJ. In: Levy RH, et al, editors. Antiepileptic Drugs. 5th ed. Lippincott Wilkins & Williams; 2002. p. 132-148. *An excellent reference of the mechanisms of action, chemistry, biotransformation, pharmacokinetics, interactions, use and adverse effects of AEDs.*

Motamedi GK, Meador KJ. Antiepileptic drugs and neurodevelopment. Cur Neurol Neurosci Rep 2006;6(4):341-346. *Children with in utero exposure to valproate had a higher incidence of additional educational needs, showed a significantly lower verbal IQ, developmental delays, memory impairment, and dysmorphic features compared to other AEDs.*

Porter RJ, Meldrum BS. Antiseizure Drugs. In: Katzung BG, editor. Basic & Clinical Pharmacology, Lange Medical Book, McGraw-Hill. 10th ed. Chapter 24. 2006. p. 374-394. *An up-to-date and complete pharmacology textbook.*

Rosenow F, Luders H. Presurgical evaluation of epilepsy. Brain 2001;124:1683-1700.

Siegel AM. Presurgical evaluation and surgical treatment of medically refractory epilepsy. Neurosurg Rev 2004;27:1-18.

Sperling MR, Feldman H, Kinman J, et al. Seizure control and mortality in epilepsy. Ann Neurol 1999;46(1):45-50.

Wiebe S, Blume WT, Girvin JP, et al. A randomized controlled trial of surgery for temporal lobe epilepsy. N Engl J Med 2001;345(5):311-318.

Working Group on Status Epilepticus. Treatment of convulsive status epilepticus. JAMA 1993;270:854-859.

Zahn CA, Morrell MJ, Collins SD, et al. Management issues for women with epilepsy. A review of the literature. Neurology 1998;51:949-956. *A review of the recommendations concerning contraception, folate supplementation, vitamin K use in pregnancy, breast feeding, bone loss, catamenial epilepsy, and reproductive endocrine disorders.*

Sleep Disorders

Paul T. Gross and Joel M. Oster

15

Primary sleep disorders, such as sleep apnea syndrome, narcolepsy, periodic limb movements, and rapid eye movement (REM) behavior disorder are common and underdiagnosed. They are important because of the sleep-related symptoms they produce (excessive sleepiness and/or disrupted sleep) and because they may have a profound effect on quality of life, and on other illnesses, particularly cardiovascular disease. Many people living in Western societies are sleep deprived. Excessive daytime sleepiness plays a significant role in automobile accidents and lost work productivity.

NEUROTRANSMITTERS AND SLEEP

The primary neurochemical/physiology of the sleep-wake cycle is well defined (Fig. 15-1). Sleep onset depends on GABAergic circuitry within the anterior hypothalamus. In contrast, the posterior hypothalamus contains histamine and orexin or hypocretin pathways that promote wakefulness. Wakefulness and consciousness are mainly acetylcholine dependent; however, contributions are also made by norepinephrine, glutamate, and serotonergic pathways. REM sleep is modulated by the serotonergic, noradrenergic system and promoted by acetylcholine and glutamate. Additionally, specific cell populations either activate or inhibit REM.

Within the brainstem several nuclei make up the REM sleep center. These normally provide inhibition of spinal motor neurons through the neurotransmitter glycine. Concomitantly these nuclei alter the electroencephalogram with rostral projections that impact thalamocortical systems.

The pineal gland releases melatonin when light-detecting cells within the retina identify the onset of darkness and transmit data to the hypothalamic suprachiasmatic nucleus (SCN). Melatonin has direct effects on the transcription of genes in the SCN that are involved in modulating the biologic clock and the circadian system. Prostaglandins and other neuropeptides may also be important in the modulation of the sleep-wake cycle. Progressive sleep deprivation leads to accumulation of adenosine within the basal forebrain and preoptic hypothalamus; going to sleep reverses this. Caffeine blocks the effects of adenosine. This provides a neurologic basis for why humans have cultivated coffee and our use of caffeine socially to promote wakefulness.

Numerous cholinergic pathways originate from the basal forebrain that project throughout the cortex along with widespread connections from the reticular activating system of the brainstem via thalamocortical projections that promote consciousness and wakefulness as witnessed by an activated EEG. In contrast, cellular networks at the thalamic level inhibit sensory stimuli from causing arousal during sleep. Generally sedatives enhance the activity of GABA, which promotes sleep by inhibiting pathways that promote wakefulness and activates pathways enhancing slow-wave sleep.

INSOMNIA

Insomnia, the most common sleep disorder, is defined as the inability to initiate or maintain sleep. Typically, adults require 7–9 hours of sleep daily. Disorders such as depression, musculoskeletal pain, and heart failure may significantly interfere with sleep and produce secondary insomnia. This section focuses on insomnia as a primary illness.

A small percentage of people with a complaint of insomnia have a **sleep state misperception** disorder. These individuals believe that they do not have an adequate amount of sleep but, when tested, they do not lack appropriate sleep. Another small subset of individuals sleeps reasonably well at night, but for a more limited period of time, perhaps 5–7 hours. Although they may feel restored and function reasonably well during the day, they are unlikely to be functioning at their best.

Among true sleep disorders, the most common insomnias are **primary insomnia** and **psychophysiologic insomnia**. Patients with **primary insomnia** have a history of sleeping poorly since early childhood. They are unable to sleep enough to meet their needs, and this is not secondary to depression, anxiety, or an underlying illness. Good sleep hygiene, such as avoidance of stimulants and daytime naps, with adequate daily exercise and mental stimulation may help some of these individuals to sleep longer. However, medication may also be needed to achieve adequate sleep.

Psychophysiologic insomnia is the most common cause of the inability to initiate or maintain sleep. It is defined as the inability to relax sufficiently to fall asleep, which, through repetition, then becomes reinforced as a behavior. Multiple factors contribute to this condition, including anxiety, stress, and inability to relax, resulting in a learned behavior of poor sleep. Relaxation and good sleep hygiene are important treatment modalities. Some patients sleep well when given a prescription for a hypnotic that, even if never filled or taken, removes the anxiety about sleep. For others, a program of taking a hypnotic on three predetermined nights each week, such as every Sunday, Tuesday, and Thursday, allows for sleep on some nights. This may eventually lead to reasonably good sleep without any need for medication.

SLEEP APNEA SYNDROME

Clinical Vignette

A 37-year-old man was seen at the request of his wife, for loud snoring. She noticed occasional snoring when they were first married 10 years earlier. Since then, however, he gained 15 pounds, and his shirt collar size had increased from 16 to 17. If he has two or more alcoholic beverages and sleeps on his back, the snoring can be heard in a room down the hall. The patient's wife was not certain whether he stops breathing in his sleep. He initially denied daytime sleepiness, but his wife reminded him that he tended to

Numerous neurotransmitters, nuclei, and fiber projections mediate arousal and cortical activation, as well as the sleep-wake cycle.

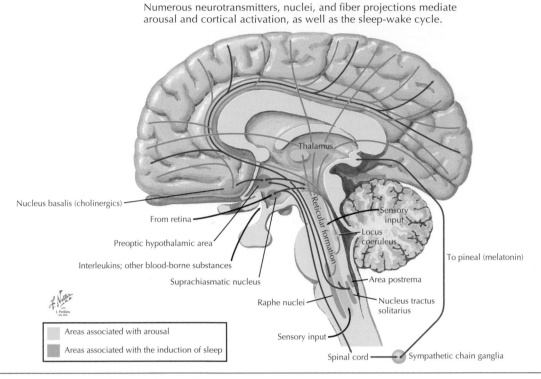

Figure 15-1 Primary Networks Involved in Sleep-Wake Cycle.

fall asleep with visitors present, and he confessed that he was having trouble staying awake during his 30-minute drive to work. He had hypertension and a family history of stroke in both parents.

On examination, he appeared fatigued and modestly overweight. He was 5 feet 11 inches tall, and weighed 220 pounds (body mass index of 30.7). His blood pressure was 154/95.

An all-night sleep test demonstrated 245 apneas, with an apnea index (number of apneas/hour) of 33. His oxygen saturation during the apneas decreased to 88 from a baseline of 92, although occasionally it was as low as 81. Subsequently, he had a second night in the sleep laboratory for continuous positive airway pressure (CPAP) titration. A repeat all-night sleep test demonstrated that a CPAP of 9 cm H_2O eliminated.

After using CPAP, he and his wife noted a distinct change in his alertness. He commented that he had not realized how sleepy he was until he saw how well he could feel under treatment.

Disorders causing excessive daytime sleepiness are a result of either sleep disruption at night, such as sleep apnea syndrome or periodic limb movements in sleep, or a disorder of the brain's sleep–wake system, such as narcolepsy or idiopathic hypersomnolence. The patient in the preceding vignette had severe obstructive sleep apnea. Many similar patients deny or minimize their symptoms. Often they come at the bed partner's insistence, or the patient may present with nonspecific fatigue and weakness.

During an episode of obstructive sleep apnea, the soft palate and tongue relax excessively, producing upper airway obstruction, which results in snoring, apneas, and hypopneas (partial apneas). Predisposing factors include male gender; excessive weight; abnormal structure of the palate, uvula, tongue, and jaw; increasing age; use of alcohol; use of testosterone or reduction in female hormones; and positive family history.

Clinical Presentation

Loud snoring, caused by upper airway tissue vibration, is a warning sign of sleep apnea syndrome. When the obstruction becomes complete, an apneic event occurs. Concomitantly, blood oxygen saturation decreases and carbon dioxide increases. When this develops, a sleep arousal occurs. Although the patient is usually unaware of the event, often the partner is aroused and frightened by the individual's having ceased to breathe. Loud snoring, in combination with daytime sleepiness, raises the suspicion of clinically significant obstructive sleep apnea (Fig. 15-2A). Paradoxically, the majority of patients with obstructive sleep apnea do not report choking or gasping for breath, are unaware of their apneas, and often believe that they have had an adequate night's sleep.

The cumulative effect of hundreds of such nighttime arousals is excessive daytime sleepiness. Patients with severe (≥30 episodes per hour), and possibly, those with moderate (15–29 episodes per hour) sleep apnea are at increased risk for cardiovascular complications of hypertension, myocardial infarction, arrhythmias, and stroke.

Sleep fragmentation may lead to arousal in which there are higher levels of catecholamines present on average through the night; in turn this may lead to hypertension. The amount of respiratory effort is increased in compensation as oxygen desaturation is detected. Increase in central negative intrathoracic pressure may lead to increased secretion of aldosterone or catecholamines. Ultimately this promotes increased intravascular fluid volume and central venous pressure.

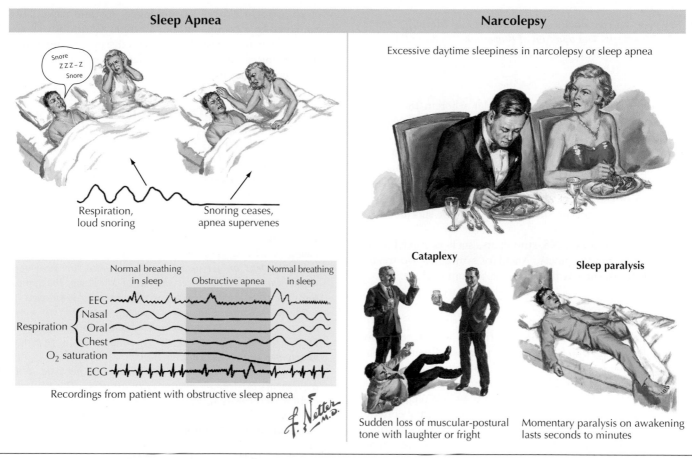

| Sleep Apnea | Narcolepsy |

Figure 15-2 Sleep Disorders with Hypersomnia.

The associated elevated mean intrathoracic negative pressure may also lead to abnormal transmural forces affecting the heart, leading to remodeling of central cardiovascular structures and in turn leading to release of additional humoral factors contributing to various cardiac arrhythmias. A metabolic syndrome develops with resultant insulin resistance and further weight gain; its pathogenesis has yet to be defined. In turn this leads to progressive worsening of hypertension. Fortunately, many patients treated with continuous positive airway pressure (CPAP) subsequently are now able to control both their hypertension and its associated cardiovascular risks. CPAP allows the airway to be maintained by pneumatic pressure, eliminating airway collapse; oxygen desaturation no longer occurs, and the above-defined pathophysiologic cascade is aborted and treated.

Diagnosis and Treatment

An **all-night sleep study** is the best means to detect and quantitate apneic events. Treatment with CPAP is used to reduce daytime sleepiness and reduce cardiovascular risk. Healthy people may experience up to 4 apneas per hour of sleep at night. Patients with severe and even moderate sleep apnea will significantly benefit from CPAP use by improving daytime alertness and reducing cardiovascular risk. Reduction of risk factors, such as obesity and use of alcohol in the evening, may help.

Although surgical efforts to restructure the oropharynx are often helpful for relieving snoring, they are not as useful for obstructive sleep apnea and, therefore, are considered secondary treatment measures for the patient with sleep apnea. Respiratory stimulant medications but generally have minimal clinical usefulness.

NARCOLEPSY

Clinical Vignette

A 22-year-old man began having difficulty staying awake during college. Even with 8–9 hours of sleep at night, he fell asleep during class or when he was trying to study at home. Sometimes, he had a "second wind" and would be alert later in the evening. He found that a 5–10-minute nap was moderately refreshing, at least for an hour or two.

The patient had noticed that he would lean against a wall or sit when he was laughing, as he otherwise might precipitously drop to the floor as his legs unexpectedly collapsed. On another occasion, he had a very frightening episode, when he woke from a nap but was unable to move. At that time, he had the sense of an evil stranger peering over him and tried to scream, but could not. After 45 seconds, he was able to move and talk.

*Results of an all-night sleep test were normal, aside from a borderline early REM latency of 51 minutes. A **multiple sleep latency test** (MSLT), containing five daytime naps, showed an average latency to sleep onset of 3.2 minutes, and three of the naps contained REM sleep. He was treated with modafinil, with some improvement in his sleepiness.*

> *However, he continued to have episodes of cataplexy and sleep paralysis. The addition of fluoxetine, 10–20 mg daily, helped to ameliorate those symptoms.*

Narcolepsy is a primary sleep disorder wherein the central nervous system regulation of sleep, and particularly REM sleep, is impaired. Patients with narcolepsy tend to be much sleepier than the average person, although even in narcolepsy it is unusual to fall asleep under extreme circumstances, such as when crossing a street or answering a question. Depending on the severity of the illness, the external circumstances, and the patient's willpower, he or she may or may not succumb to a severe urge to sleep.

Treatment includes CNS stimulants, such as modafinil or amphetamines, for sleepiness. Ancillary symptoms are treated with SSRI drugs, such as fluoxetine or sodium oxybate.

Clinical Presentation

The symptoms of the **narcolepsy tetrad** include excessive daytime sleepiness, which is present in almost all patients, and the ancillary symptoms of cataplexy, sleep paralysis, and hypnagogic hallucinations (Fig. 15-2B). One or more of these ancillary symptoms are present in about 50–60% of narcoleptics, and they are due to the inappropriate occurrence of partial episodes of REM sleep. During REM sleep, healthy individuals are often dreaming, and except for the extraocular and respiratory musculature, most muscles are paralyzed. This paralysis is subclinical in healthy individuals because it occurs while they are asleep.

In contrast, patients with narcolepsy may enter partial REM sleep at inappropriate times. Typically these events occur in two specific settings: *cataplexy*, which is sudden paralysis occurring in response to strong emotions including laughter or anger, and *sleep paralysis*, which includes waking with paralysis and often hallucinations. *Hypnagogic hallucinations* are realistic—often frightening—dreams that occur at sleep onset while the patient retains some degree of consciousness. The etiology of narcolepsy is multifactorial. There is an association with reduced hypocretin levels in the hypothalamus, and genetic and environmental factors may also play a role.

Diagnosis

Narcolepsy is diagnosed clinically by the combination of a classic history of excessive daytime sleepiness relieved by brief naps, associated in about half of cases with other portions of the narcolepsy tetrad: cataplexy, sleep paralysis, and hypnagogic hallucinations. By measuring the average latency to sleep onset and the appearance of REM sleep on MSLT during the naps in a sleep lab, a diagnosis of narcolepsy can be supported. An all-night sleep test needs to be done on the night preceding a MSLT, because the MSLT cannot be properly interpreted unless the quality and quantity of the preceding night's sleep is assessed.

Idiopathic hypersomnolence is a disorder seen in a small percentage of patients who have excessive daytime sleepiness but do not have narcolepsy or a nocturnal sleep disturbance. In contrast to narcolepsy, these individuals have prolonged periods of sleep at night as well as prolonged daytime naps. This is documented by a combination of all-night sleep study showing adequate sleep and no significant sleep disruption and a MSLT demonstrating excessive daytime sleepiness but no daytime REM sleep. Similar to narcolepsy, it is treated with stimulants.

PERIODIC LIMB MOVEMENTS

Clinical Vignette

A 45-year-old woman saw her physician for excessive daytime sleepiness. She was tired much of the day but, if necessary, could stay awake. Soft snoring was noted if she slept on her back. Her husband noted that she had trouble sitting still in the evening. She remarked that if she was trying to sit and read or watch television, she needed to move her legs or get up and walk around. This provided momentary relief, but after she sat or lay down, the symptoms recurred. Her sister has similar evening symptoms.

Physical examination and neurologic examination were unremarkable. Blood tests demonstrated a low ferritin level, but no anemia. Depression or hypothyroidism were ruled out by her primary care physician.

An all-night sleep test showed frequent periodic limb movements of sleep associated with arousals. The Periodic Limb Movement (PLM) index was 59 episodes per hour, 46/hour of which were associated with arousals. A diagnosis of restless leg syndrome (RLS) and periodic limb movement syndrome (PLMS) was made. Treatment with iron resulted in 50% symptomatic improvement. Treatment with 0.25 mg pramipexole at 6:00 PM and again at 9:00 PM led to additional significant improvement.

Periodic limb movements are another important consideration in the differential diagnosis of excessive daytime sleepiness. They consist of repeated brief episodes of movements of the lower extremities. These movements range from simple dorsiflexion of the great toe to violent movements of the whole lower extremity. Many patients and their bed partners are unaware that they have PLMs during sleep. Individuals with PLMS present with excessive daytime sleepiness because each episode disrupts their sleep.

Many of these patients also have RLS (an irresistible urge to move the legs while sitting or lying down), especially those with iron deficiency, and treatment with iron may help. Symptoms are also treated with dopamine agonists, benzodiazepines, or narcotics. Antidepressants and stimulants may exacerbate RLS and PLMS.

PARASOMNIAS

Clinical Vignette

An 82-year-old man was brought to the neurologist by his wife for violent activity in his sleep that concerned her for both of their safety. She recently noted him waving his fists, kicking, and occasionally banging his head against the headboard, all in his sleep. On one occasion, he fell out of bed, but, fortunately, did not hurt himself. Once, she had to wake him because he was punching her, completely contrary to his character and past behavior. When she woke him after this episode, he told her that he had dreamt that someone was trying to attack him. During the day, he was becoming more clumsy, took a long time to dress, and occasionally had a tremor of his right hand at rest.

On exam, he had findings of subtle right hemiparkinsonism. An all-night sleep test demonstrated abundant tonic muscle activity during REM sleep. The diagnosis of REM behavior disorder was made on the basis of the wife's history and the abnormal all-night sleep study. He was treated with clonazepam 0.5 mg nightly, and the spells resolved by approximately 90%. A diagnosis of possible Parkinson disease was also entertained, with a plan to follow him for any additional Parkinson symptoms.

Parasomnias, characterized by certain unusual or unwanted symptoms occurring during nighttime sleep, are another major category of sleep disorders.

REM Behavior Disorder

The vignette above has a typical history for REM sleep behavior disorder (RBD). The patient is unaware of the episodes during sleep. Treatment with clonazepam is usually successful. Some of these patients have RBD as a first manifestation of degenerative neurologic disease, and in this case, the patient may have early Parkinson's disease.

Most healthy individuals are paralyzed and dreaming during REM sleep. The characteristic paralysis, sparing both eye movements and respiratory muscles, is from activation of inhibitory reticulospinal pathways, which results in an inhibition of anterior horn cells within the spinal cord, preventing patients from acting out dreams. In sleep paralysis, this otherwise normal phenomenon occurs while the patient is awake. In RBD, this activation fails to occur, resulting in the patient acting out a dream (Fig. 15-3).

After age 70 years, some people lose this ability to be paralyzed during REM sleep. Subsequently, they begin to act out their dreams by talking, yelling, kicking, or in extreme cases, attacking their bed partner. If awakened, they relate that they are in the middle of a violent dream. A third or more of patients with RBD have, or will develop, a neurodegenerative disease, such as Parkinson disease or Lewy body disease. Most of the patients are male and respond positively to treatment with 0.5 mg clonazepam at bedtime.

Night Terrors

Night terrors are common in children and occasionally persist into adult life. The patient suddenly sits up in bed, has dilated pupils, a frightened expression, and a rapid pulse. Occasionally affected individuals dash from the bed, sustaining injury. Children often return to sleep without memory of the event. If awakened, they describe a frightened feeling or image but not a complex dream, because these episodes arise during stage 3 or

Patients with REM sleep behavior disorder lack reticulospinal inhibition that normally induces paralysis during REM sleep. Patients act out their dreams without any recollection in the morning. The episodes are usually witnessed by the spouse.

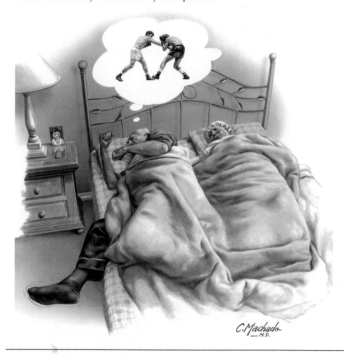

Figure 15-3 REM Sleep Behavior Disorder.

4 sleep, in which dreams do not usually occur. Somnambulism tends to occur in the same patients, also during stage 3 or 4 sleep. Often an explanation of the problem is sufficient, but tricyclic antidepressants or benzodiazepines may be helpful.

Delayed Sleep Phase Syndrome

Delayed sleep phase syndrome is a **circadian rhythm disorder.** Individuals are not able to adjust their circadian clock to the time used by the rest of the world.

Most people can delay their sleep–wake cycle 1 hour or more daily and can advance it to an earlier time by approximately a half-hour daily. Therefore, it is commonly easier to sleep and awaken later, than to sleep and awaken earlier.

Some people have particular difficulty advancing to an earlier time. For example, a student with delayed sleep phase syndrome who spends 2 weeks staying up late may find it impossible to learn to go to bed early and wake up early for a summer job. She will report insomnia because she cannot fall asleep at night, or daytime sleepiness because she cannot awaken before 11:00 AM. Treatments include medication, light therapy, or a program to delay sleep by 3 hours every day until sleep time returns to the new desired bedtime.

ADDITIONAL RESOURCES

Barion A, Zee PC. A clinical approach to circadian rhythm sleep disorders. [Review] [120 refs] Sleep Medicine 2007 Sep;8(6):566-577.

Monti JM, Pandi-Perumal SR, Sinton CM, eds. Neurochemistry of Sleep and Wakefulness. Cambridge: Cambridge University Press; 2008.

Wise MS, Arand DL, Auger RR, et al. American Academy of Sleep Medicine. Treatment of narcolepsy and other hypersomnias of central origin. [Review] [91 refs] Sleep 2007 Dec 1;30(12):1712-1727.

Coma, Vegetative State, Brain Death, and Increased Intracranial Pressure

Gregory J. Allam

16

COMA

Clinical Vignette

A 57-year-old man with coronary artery disease develops severe chest pain and heaviness on exertion and then loses consciousness while working in the garden with his wife. Emergency Medical Service is called immediately and arrives at the scene within minutes. The man is found pale, unresponsive, and flaccid. The systolic blood pressure is low, about 70–85 mm Hg, and he is found to be in ventricular tachycardia, but he promptly reverts to sinus rhythm with electroconversion. In the hospital, he is found to have roving eyes, grimaces and withdraws his limbs to painful stimuli, but has no directed responses to verbal commands. Over a 3-day period, he is awake and conversant but has poor short-term memory and ataxia. These symptoms gradually resolve over a 3-week period.

Clinical Vignette

A 76-year-old man was found unconscious in bed at home. His wife informed the emergency physician that he had a history of prostate cancer but no risk factors for vascular disease. She denied knowledge of any recent head injury. He was totally unresponsive to verbal and painful stimuli. Neurologic examination showed he was comatose with pinpoint pupils. Eye movements to doll's-eyes maneuvers were full and conjugate, and cold caloric stimulation of the ear canals produced ipsilateral tonic deviation of the eyes without nystagmus. There were bilateral withdrawal responses of his extremities to noxious stimuli, and bilateral Babinski signs.

Intravenous administration of 0.4 mg naloxone produced dramatic change, with full awakening within a few minutes. Results of a subsequent brain computed tomography (CT) were normal, confirming that there was no evidence of intracerebral, subarachnoid, or subdural hemorrhage, cerebral infarction, or mass lesions. When asked about narcotic use, the patient stated that he was no longer able to tolerate the pain of metastatic prostate cancer; he had taken an overdose of an opioid analgesic.

The first vignette reflects a common scenario for anoxic–ischemic brain injury secondary to cardiac arrest. The degree of recovery usually depends on a number of factors that include age, extent, or duration of the ischemic insult and the initial presenting neurologic examination. A detailed history, review of in-field records, and serial examinations is an essential first step in guiding prognostic predications and determining the need for further workup. The second vignette illustrates the classic case of "toxic-metabolic" induced coma. Despite profound unresponsiveness and very miotic pupils, neurologic examination demonstrated retained brainstem reflexes and CT results were normal. Although pontine hemorrhage is often suspected in a comatose septuagenarian with pinpoint pupils, intact reflexive eye movement strongly indicated a metabolic cause. The prognosis in such cases, in the absence of secondary hypoperfusion or anoxia, is overwhelmingly favorable.

Consciousness is the state of awareness of internal and external stimuli and is manifested by the ability to react to these stimuli through thought or by directed physical movement. Coma is the loss of awareness of stimuli and the ability to react voluntarily to them. Full consciousness of one's self and the surroundings can be disrupted partially without total loss of arousal or wakefulness and is sometimes referred to as a state of stupor. Varying degrees of consciousness can therefore be roughly delineated by the specificity or accuracy of the response to a particular stimulus, and terms such as *confusion*, *obtundation*, or *stuporous* are used to reflect this. However, the most useful tool in following patients with altered mentation remains the exact description of patient behavior and reactions to specific stimuli. For example, it is preferable to indicate that a patient stays alert without stimulation but is unable to give the exact date and location or follow two sequential commands than to only say that the patient is *confused* or *clouded*. Nevertheless, defining terms may provide uniformity in meaning when encountered in patient records. *Obtundation* describes a condition in which repeated stimuli are needed to draw the patients' attention back to a task. *Stupor* is a state of extreme inattention in which wakefulness and minimal interaction with the examiner can be achieved only by repeated or constant stimulation. *Delirium* is an acute confusional state often involving sympathetic nervous system overactivity with attention marred by hyperexcitability. Tachycardia, perspiration, hypertension, and hallucinations may all be features of delirium.

Because the examining physician can only infer thought from patients' actions (e.g., speech or movement), a reliable and reproducible physical examination is essential in evaluating the comatose or stuporous patient. The neurologist must make every effort to establish the presence or absence of a directed nonreflexive response and judge its quality. For example, in basilar occlusion when the lesion is restricted to the basis pontis a "locked-in" syndrome occurs with the patient seemingly having no directed response to stimuli, yet on close examination may blink in an exact fashion to instructions and indirectly answer questions appropriately. Partially preserved voluntary vertical eye movements may also be present. Similarly, in patients with severe acute polyneuropathies such as Guillain–Barré syndrome, consciousness is preserved but difficult to assess and quantify secondary to profound peripheral weakness.

The Glasgow Coma Scale assesses and quantifies the degree of consciousness across three measures: response to verbal commands, response of eye opening, and the nature of motor movements in response to verbal or physical stimuli. Those not responding to verbal commands or opening their eyes with a Glasgow Coma Scale score of 8 or less are defined as being in a coma (Fig. 16-1). The Glasgow Coma Scale is one of the primary predictors of long-term outcomes, especially in cases of head trauma.

Prevalence of the different etiologies of coma varies depending on the population surveyed. For example, head trauma and intoxicants are the major causes in registries based on densely populated high-crime areas. Stroke and cardiac events are the leading etiologies in suburban areas with retirement communities. Overall, trauma, stroke, diffuse anoxic–ischemic brain insult (secondary to cardiorespiratory arrest), and intoxicants are the leading mechanisms for coma. Infections, seizures, and metabolic–endocrine disorders account for the remaining cases (Fig. 16-2).

States that affect cognition and attention without affecting wakefulness such as the various degenerative dementias (characterized by progressive cognitive deterioration) and focal brain lesions (which cause restricted cortical dysfunction) do not fit the definition of coma. Sleep is a normal patterned physiologic disconnection of the cortex from external stimuli and is discussed elsewhere (Chapter 15).

EVALUATION AND TREATMENT OF THE COMATOSE PATIENT

The initial evaluation of a patient in coma must occur simultaneously with its management. Any delay in treatment while waiting to determine the exact cause is not acceptable. Clearing the airway and ensuring adequate ventilation and oxygenation with a bag mask or intubation, if needed, must be addressed immediately. Management of hypotension must be prompt, especially in suspected cases of increased intracranial pressure (ICP). Hemodynamic collapse should never be attributed to an intracranial process, and cardiac or circulatory causes need to be sought. These form the "ABCs of coma management": airway, breathing, and circulation (Fig. 16-3). Immobilizing the neck until a cervical spine injury is excluded is also important in cases of suspected trauma.

Emergent evaluation of comatose patients requires the following blood studies: a full blood count, glucose level, serum chemistry, toxicology screen, liver profile, thyroid function tests, arterial blood gases, and cultures. Creatine kinase and troponin measurements, in conjunction with electrocardiography, are important for excluding myocardial infarction and transient

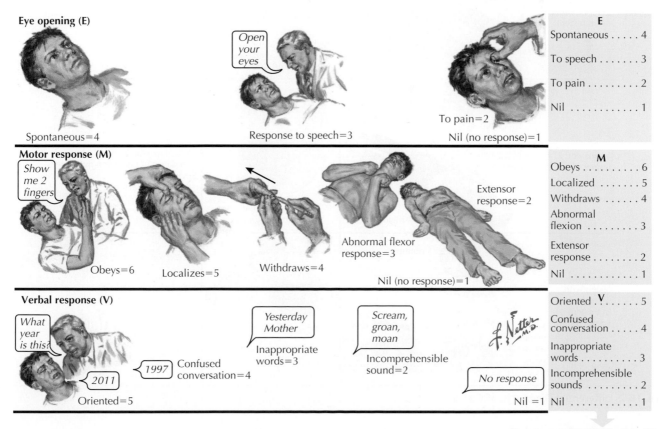

Figure 16-1 Glasgow Coma Scale.

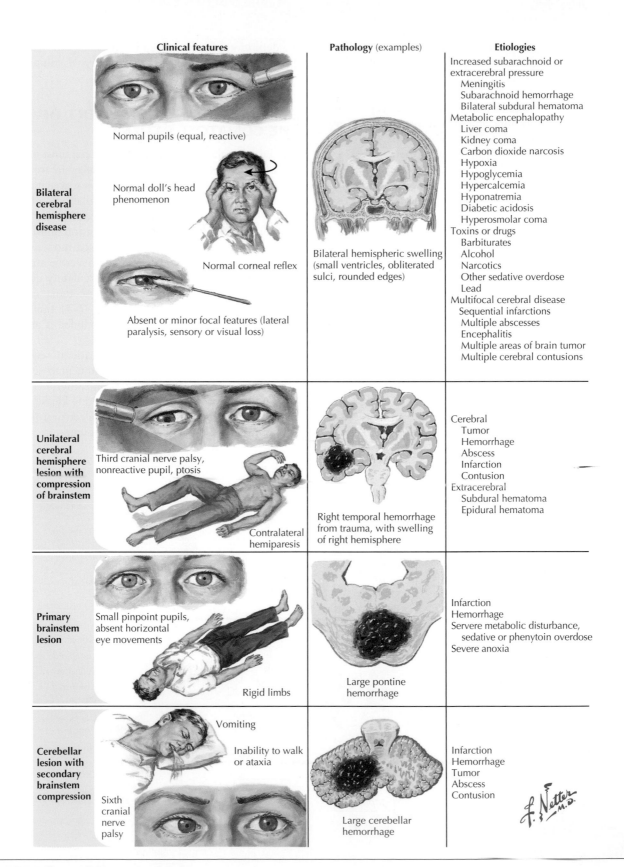

	Clinical features	Pathology (examples)	Etiologies
Bilateral cerebral hemisphere disease	Normal pupils (equal, reactive) — Normal doll's head phenomenon — Normal corneal reflex — Absent or minor focal features (lateral paralysis, sensory or visual loss)	Bilateral hemispheric swelling (small ventricles, obliterated sulci, rounded edges)	Increased subarachnoid or extracerebral pressure Meningitis Subarachnoid hemorrhage Bilateral subdural hematoma Metabolic encephalopathy Liver coma Kidney coma Carbon dioxide narcosis Hypoxia Hypoglycemia Hypercalcemia Hyponatremia Diabetic acidosis Hyperosmolar coma Toxins or drugs Barbiturates Alcohol Narcotics Other sedative overdose Lead Multifocal cerebral disease Sequential infarctions Multiple abscesses Encephalitis Multiple areas of brain tumor Multiple cerebral contusions
Unilateral cerebral hemisphere lesion with compression of brainstem	Third cranial nerve palsy, nonreactive pupil, ptosis — Contralateral hemiparesis	Right temporal hemorrhage from trauma, with swelling of right hemisphere	Cerebral Tumor Hemorrhage Abscess Infarction Contusion Extracerebral Subdural hematoma Epidural hematoma
Primary brainstem lesion	Small pinpoint pupils, absent horizontal eye movements — Rigid limbs	Large pontine hemorrhage	Infarction Hemorrhage Severe metabolic disturbance, sedative or phenytoin overdose Severe anoxia
Cerebellar lesion with secondary brainstem compression	Vomiting — Inability to walk or ataxia — Sixth cranial nerve palsy	Large cerebellar hemorrhage	Infarction Hemorrhage Tumor Abscess Contusion

Figure 16-2 Differential Diagnosis of Coma.

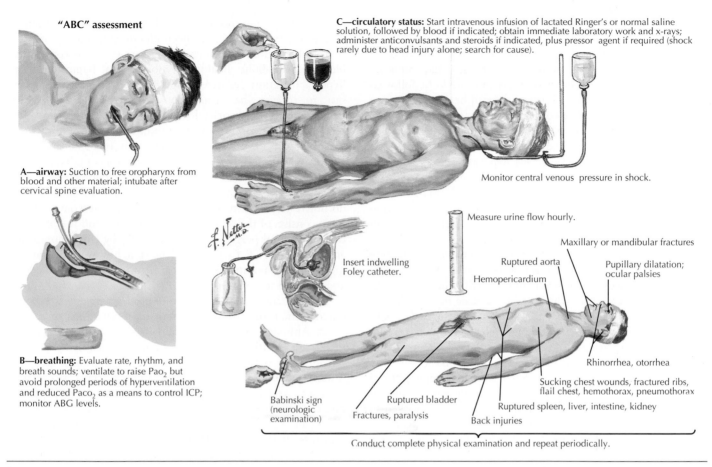

"ABC" assessment

C—circulatory status: Start intravenous infusion of lactated Ringer's or normal saline solution, followed by blood if indicated; obtain immediate laboratory work and x-rays; administer anticonvulsants and steroids if indicated, plus pressor agent if required (shock rarely due to head injury alone; search for cause).

A—airway: Suction to free oropharynx from blood and other material; intubate after cervical spine evaluation.

Monitor central venous pressure in shock.

Measure urine flow hourly.

Insert indwelling Foley catheter.

Maxillary or mandibular fractures

Ruptured aorta

Hemopericardium

Pupillary dilatation; ocular palsies

B—breathing: Evaluate rate, rhythm, and breath sounds; ventilate to raise Pao₂ but avoid prolonged periods of hyperventilation and reduced Paco₂ as a means to control ICP; monitor ABG levels.

Babinski sign (neurologic examination)

Fractures, paralysis

Ruptured bladder

Back injuries

Ruptured spleen, liver, intestine, kidney

Rhinorrhea, otorrhea

Sucking chest wounds, fractured ribs, flail chest, hemothorax, pneumothorax

Conduct complete physical examination and repeat periodically.

Figure 16-3 Initial Management of Coma and Severe Head Injuries.

cardiac arrest. Anticonvulsant drug levels and an electroencephalograph (EEG) can help identify patients with nonconvulsive status epilepticus.

The immediately treatable causes of coma are hypoglycemia and narcotic intoxication. These can be managed promptly, once oxygenation and hemodynamic status are stable. Infusion of 100 mg thiamine must precede the infusion of 50 mL of 50% dextrose in water as a precaution against Wernicke encephalopathy. This is postulated to be due to osmotic or metabolic damage to the mammillary bodies and the medial thalamus exerted by glucose, which, in the absence of thiamine, cannot be transported and metabolized in the tissue. When narcotics overdose is suspected, such as in comatose patients with miotic pupils, 0.4 mg intravenous (IV) naloxone, a central opioid antagonist, improves the level of consciousness within minutes. Repeated doses may be needed to maintain wakefulness and reverse respiratory depression. Caution should be exercised for known or suspected opioid dependency as abrupt or complete reversal of opioid effects by repeated doses may precipitate an acute withdrawal state. In such instances, only supportive care should be provided once the diagnosis is made. Administration of flumazenil, a pure benzodiazepine antagonist (0.2 mg IV), given three to four times, can improve the mental state and reverse respiratory depression in benzodiazepine overdose. As with naloxone, it should be used cautiously in those with a history of long-term benzodiazepine use or dependency as it can

precipitate seizures. It should generally be avoided in patients with epilepsy and those at risk of seizures.

Urgent intravenous antibiotic coverage is indicated for febrile patients because time is crucial in treating meningitis and septicemia (Chapter 48). Lumbar puncture should be performed only after brain imaging has excluded mass lesions that could lead to herniation.

Assessment of the comatose patient should include examination of the skin. Rashes may indicate streptococcal or staphylococcal meningitis, bacterial endocarditis, or systemic lupus erythematosus. Purpura may indicate meningococcal meningitis, a bleeding diathesis, or aspirin intoxication. Skin dryness suggests anticholinergic or barbiturate overdose, whereas excessive perspiration indicates cholinergic poisoning, hypoglycemia, and other causes of sympathetic overactivity. Dark pigmentary changes in the axillary and genital areas suggest adrenal insufficiency, whereas doughy pale skin is typical of myxedema. Renal failure may present with urea salt crystal skin condensations or "urea frost." Facial or basal skull fractures often cause ecchymosis around the eyes (raccoon eyes or panda bear sign) or in the mastoid area (Battle sign). Extremities must be examined for needle and track marks that indicate intravenous drug abuse.

The patient's breath may be uremic, fruity as in ketoacidosis, or have the musty fishy odor of hepatic failure. Fever may indicate meningitis or encephalitis but also occurs with sympathomimetic or tricyclic (anticholinergic) overdose and drug or alcohol withdrawal. Occasionally a low-grade fever occurs with subarachnoid hemorrhage or brainstem lesions.

Focal neurologic signs on initial examination may implicate a structural lesion as the cause of coma and should be followed closely for signs of evolving herniation until brain imaging can be performed. Other causes of focal presentation are compensated old brain injuries clinically reemerging as a result of seizures, toxins, or metabolic derangements. However, metabolic disorders including nonketotic hyperosmolar hyperglycemia, hypoglycemia, and hepatic coma may cause focal seizures or lateralizing neurologic signs without focal brain lesions. Evolving signs of increased intracranial pressure or herniation must be treated promptly regardless of cause; there is no use in waiting for brain CT results or other tests.

Electroencephalography is often helpful in evaluating patients with altered consciousness or coma. An abnormal tracing makes psychogenic coma unlikely. EEG detects nonconvulsive or absence status, which can present de novo without a history of epilepsy. Although nonspecific, diffuse EEG background slowing correlates with metabolic derangements and focal slowing with localized structural brain disease. Hepatic and other metabolic encephalopathies may show triphasic waves. In herpes simplex encephalitis, periodic lateralized epileptiform temporal lobe discharges are often seen and support the clinical diagnosis. Finally, when a basis pontis lesion with the "locked-in syndrome" is suspected, a normal EEG shows that the patient is alert despite limited or no obvious response to stimuli.

PROGNOSIS

Determining the prognosis of an individual comatose patient is a difficult task. Statistical numbers given to patients' families as measures of outcome probabilities often are difficult to apply in relation to their loved one. The focus usually shifts to the chances of recovery, no matter how limited, rather than the likelihood of severe disability. A statistical grid or flow chart cannot be relied on to decide each individual case, and numerous factors, including cause of the coma, the evolution of the neurologic examination, age, comorbidities, and the religious or philosophical beliefs of the patient and the family must be considered.

Recovery from drug intoxication, barring ischemic brain injury from secondary hypoxemia or circulatory collapse, is usually good, with rare mortality or instances of severe disability. In hepatic and likely other metabolic comas, only brainstem dysfunction, with disruption of oculocephalic reflexes and loss of pupillary reactivity, increases the likelihood of poor prognosis or death. The duration of the coma and absent localizing motor responses do not exclude a good recovery and probably only reflect persistent metabolic derangement. Hepatic encephalopathy, to a large extent, is caused by the accumulation in the portal system of ammonia derived primarily from enzymatic activity of intestinal bacteria upon nitrogenous material and amino acids. Liver failure leads to shunting of portal vein ammonia into the systemic circulation and the brain not having proper detoxification. The effects of ammonia and other toxic elements on the brain include astrocyte swelling with cytotoxic brain edema, altered cerebral blood flow (CBF), and the accumulation

of inhibitory neurosteroids and inflammatory cytokines. Numerous precipitants have been identified (anemia, constipation, dehydration, excessive dietary protein, gastrointestinal bleeding, metabolic alkalosis, hypoglycemia, hypothyroidism, hypoxia, infection, sedatives) and aggressive treatment is necessary to reverse the encephalopathy. Removal of intestinal ammonia with nonabsorbable disaccharides (lactulose) and antibiotics such as neomycin or metronidazole are commonly used and relatively effective. The mechanism of coma and brain edema in acute fulminate hepatic failure is less understood but likely involves some of the same pathophysiologic mechanism already described. However, a large proportion of these patients do not respond to treatment and have poor outcomes. Treatment consists of the above outlined measures and the preservation of cerebral perfusion pressure (CPP) by close monitoring and control of ICP. Liver transplantation, however, remains the most effective and immediate treatment to control brain edema and ICP and to reverse coma.

In most instances, coma from head trauma has a better outcome than that from nontraumatic mechanisms or cardiac arrest. Although severe head trauma has a mortality of approximately 50% within the first 48 hours, few surviving patients remain in a permanent vegetative state and most progress toward some degree of functional improvement. Those who remain vegetative usually succumb within 3–5 years. There are rare reports of patients who awaken after a prolonged vegetative period and show some return of functionality. None, however, return to their premorbid status or even an independent state. Signs that correlate with a poor prognosis after head trauma are age older than 60, bilateral pupillary abnormalities or absent oculocephalic reflexes at initial examination in a relatively stable patient. Large volumes of contused brain, large intra- or extraaxial hematomas, and lack of intracranial pressure response to conventional medical treatment (usually associated with compression of basal cisterns on CT) also betoken a poorer prognosis (Fig. 16-4).

Anoxic–ischemic causes of coma have a mortality rate of up to 60–70%, with generally only 10–15% of patients returning to a good functional status. The lack of bilateral pupillary responses for more than 6–12 hours correlates highly with poor functional outcome and death. Absent oculocephalic (vestibule–ocular or caloric) responses after 24 hours likely have the same prognostic value. In patients who do retain or regain pupillary reactivity, the absence of at least reflexive flexor motor movements on day 1, or some withdrawal movement on day 3, also holds a poor prognosis, with less than 10% chance of recovery to a state of even moderate disability. Lack of spontaneous eye opening or of localizing motor movements on day 7 holds the same grim prognostic significance. Myoclonus status epilepticus (generalized multifocal unrelenting myoclonus) correlates with severe ischemic damage to the cortex, brainstem, and spinal cord and is strongly associated with in-hospital mortality or a vegetative state.

Other laboratory findings have been shown to reliably predict a poor prognosis and can be used to assist in the evaluation. These include EEG tracings (without sedatives or metabolic abnormalities) showing patterns of complete suppression, burst suppression or periodic discharges upon a generalized flat background, absent N20 somatosensory evoked responses after 24

	Poorer	**Better**
Glasgow Coma Scale	3–8	9–15

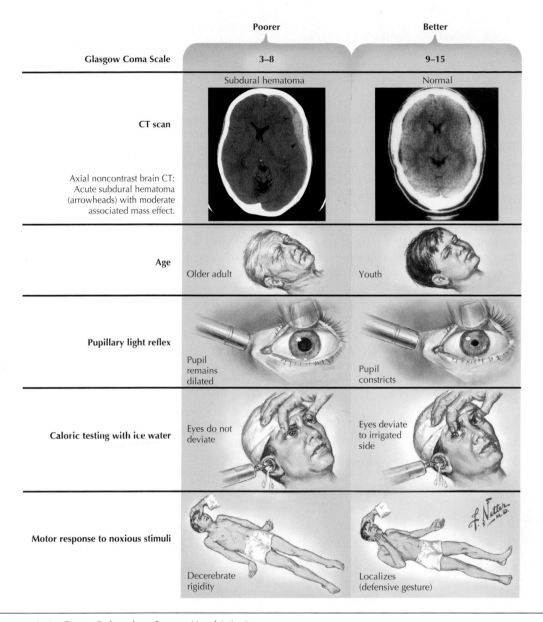

CT scan Axial noncontrast brain CT: Acute subdural hematoma (arrowheads) with moderate associated mass effect.	Subdural hematoma	Normal
Age	Older adult	Youth
Pupillary light reflex	Pupil remains dilated	Pupil constricts
Caloric testing with ice water	Eyes do not deviate	Eyes deviate to irrigated side
Motor response to noxious stimuli	Decerebrate rigidity	Localizes (defensive gesture)

Figure 16-4 Prognosis in Coma Related to Severe Head Injuries.

hours, and neuron-specific enolase >33 μg/L beyond the first day.

Vocalizations or any verbal response early within the first day of the causative event indicates a relatively good chance of functional improvement within a year.

These observations can guide families and staff toward the best course of action for each patient. Often the examination is changing or unclear. Consequently, further waiting and repeated evaluations, although stressful for the family, result in more certainty in the appropriateness of the eventual decisions taken. Those showing unfavorable prognostic signs on day 1 and who show no improvement or evolution in their neurologic examination are not likely to do well. However, for individuals who exhibit evolving neurologic function, the duration of observation needs to be extended and the final determination of outcome delayed, even if the initial examination shows no major interactive or directed function.

PERSISTENT VEGETATIVE STATE

Clinical Vignette

A 23-year-old woman was an unrestrained driver in a "head-on" automobile accident. She was ejected 30 feet through the windshield and sustained major head trauma. On arrival in the emergency department, she was totally unresponsive, hypotensive, and tachycardic. Brain CT demonstrated generalized cerebral edema and diffuse subarachnoid hemorrhage. Neurologic examination showed her to be unresponsive even to painful stimuli, other than some rare nonpurposeful right leg movements. Pupils were minimally and inconsistently reactive, and she had a dense left hemiplegia. Subsequent magnetic resonance imaging (MRI) demonstrated bilateral focal contusions of the cerebral hemispheres, shear injury of the splenium of the corpus callosum and brainstem edema. Four months later, after no improvement in her clinical state, she was diagnosed with persistent vegetative state (PVS).

Cases of PVS frequently involve young individuals with healthy cardiovascular and pulmonary systems. Before the recognition of these patients' hopeless outcomes after a few months of no improvement, some were maintained in chronic care facilities or their parents' homes for years, with the unrealistic hope that they might someday regain the ability to meaningfully interact.

The vegetative state, minimally conscious states, or post-coma unawareness are terms that describe a state of preserved brainstem and hypothalamic functions with absent or insufficient cortical function to sustain awareness of environment and self. Wakefulness is by definition preserved, and patients may cycle through sleep stages. There is no behavioral evidence of even the simplest reproducible response. Patients may startle, look about, occasionally move a limb, shift position, or yawn, but none of these actions are consistently in response to a specific stimulus (Fig. 16-5). Even the most basic voluntary actions, such as chewing and swallowing, are lost. Once reversible metabolic or exogenous causes have been eliminated, the condition

Condition is called *persistent* when it lasts without change for more than 1 month.

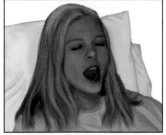

Patients may startle, look about, or yawn, but none of these actions are in conscious response to a specific stimulus.

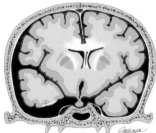

Subarachnoid hemorrhage

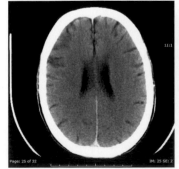

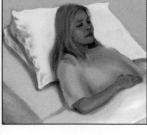

Non-contrast brain CT demonstrating ominous sign of diffuse brain injury and possible prelude to a persistent vegetative state: sulcal effacement (diffuse edema) and subtle disappearance of normal differentiation between gray and white matter.

Figure 16-5 Persistent Vegetative State.

is called persistent when it lasts without change for more than 1 month. It is considered permanent when lasting more than 12 months for traumatic brain injury and more than 3 months for nontraumatic causes. After these time limits, the chance of recovery is exceedingly low and at best progresses to severe disability.

As with coma, individuals in a posttraumatic PVS have better chances of recovery than cases due to medical causes. Nevertheless, one third of all these patients die within the first year. Of patients with head trauma, one third regains consciousness after 3 months and approximately one half in a year. Overall, one fourth of all patients with traumatic PVS recover to a level of moderate disability, mostly those who regain awareness within 3 months.

Of patients with nontraumatic PVS, more than 50% die within a year and only approximately 10–15% regain consciousness by the third month. Most remain severely disabled, with rare improvement in functional status. If the condition persists longer, there is minimal chance of any significant functional recovery. Neither age nor cause seems to correlate with eventual recovery, but of those recovering, the younger patients show somewhat better outcomes than older patients, at least in locomotion and self-care. After 3 months, once PVS is considered permanent, withdrawal of nutritional support and hydration can be discussed with the family. Many physicians consider such withdrawal acceptable, based on the contention that nutritional support in such cases constitutes medical treatment that is neither alleviating suffering nor improving the overall condition. When viewed as a human or legal rights issue, such reasoning becomes more complex and less applicable as a general principle.

INCREASED INTRACRANIAL PRESSURE AND CEREBRAL HERNIATION

Clinical Vignette

A 46-year-old man was found lying on the floor at home. Examination in the emergency department (ED) demonstrated a left hemiplegia, with conjugate eye deviation to the right. He was awake but had profound neglect for his left arm and denied any difficulties with his limbs. Brain CT demonstrated a large right middle cerebral artery and anterior cerebral artery territory stroke, with incipient potential for significant brain edema and increased ICP ("malignant brain swelling"). During the next 2 days, the patient became obtunded and progressively less responsive to external stimulation. Repeat brain CT scan showed loss of sulcal markings and a right cerebral shift across the midline falx and downward through the cerebellar tentorium, with distortion of the midbrain.

The patient underwent intubation for airway protection and, soon afterward, could not be aroused. He had right-sided flexed arm posturing and left-sided extension, with tonic leg extension and plantar flexion. His pupils were irregular and sluggishly reactive to light. Conjugate eye movements to the doll's-eyes maneuver were lost. He did not respond to osmotic agents or hyperventilation. A

Anatomic Considerations

The skull is a rigid closed cavity that serves as a basin in which the brain is suspended and protected from traumatic injury. The brain comprises approximately 90% of intracranial volume, with the remaining 10% blood and CSF. The ability to compensate for increased intracranial volume is therefore limited, and when maximum accommodation occurs, any further volume increase causes an exponential increase in ICP. Eventually, arterial and arteriolar perfusion is compromised, and ischemic tissue damage with swelling ensues, causing an even greater increase in ICP. If the exerted force on the brain is asymmetric (e.g., focal brain tumor, lobar bleed, or a unilateral stroke), then shifts in brain tissue against or across fixed structures may occur. Extrusion of shifted brain across fixed intracranial structures (falx cerebri, cerebellar tentorium, and the skull) is called herniation. Whether brain dysfunction occurs as a result of shift without actual herniation is unclear. Shift and herniation likely represent progressive stages in an evolving continuum, starting with reversible tissue dysfunction and ending with eventual cell ischemia and death.

Rostrocaudal Signs of Brain Compromise

As pressure from a hemispheric lesion increases, patients gradually move from being easily roused, but inattentive, to sleepy and unable to maintain wakefulness, then to coma—a state of absent voluntary or directed response to external or internal stimuli.

The ascending reticular formation, excited by sensory input, mediates arousal and consciousness to the cortex via the thalamic nuclei. Lesions that cause coma are at one of three levels along the neuraxis: bilateral cerebral cortex, the thalami, or the upper brainstem. The classic concept of herniation and coma produced by brain mass lesions pertains to a hemispheric process that ultimately causes "rostrocaudal" deterioration of function, gradually coursing down the hemispheres into the medulla. Although these "stages" rarely manifest symmetrically in a strict and clearly delineated sequential pattern, this paradigm remains useful for evaluating deteriorating patients with evolving neurologic signs. In addition to the level of consciousness, important physical examination elements include pupillary size and reactivity, reflexive eye movements, limb posturing, and breathing pattern (Fig. 16-4, Table 16-1).

PUPILLARY REACTIVITY AND EYE MOVEMENTS

When pressure onto or across the diencephalon exists, loss of wakefulness results, but patients may transiently continue to withdraw appropriately from uncomfortable stimuli and to resist

Table 16-1 Stages of Coma

	Hemispheric/Diencephalon	Mesencephalon	Pontine	Medullary
Respiratory pattern	Cheyne–Stokes Sighs and yawning	Hyperventilation; Central neurogenic hyperventilation	Rapid and shallow	Irregular and shallow Gasps and apneas
Pupils				
Central	Reactive small	Irregular midposition, poorly or nonreactive	Midposition, nonreactive	Absent response
Uncal	Ipsilateral: irregular and dilated with poor reactivity	Ipsilateral: pupil dilated and nonreactive Contralateral: irregular, dilated, and poorly or nonreactive	Bilateral dilated and nonreactive	Bilateral dilated and nonreactive
Oculocephalogyric				
Central	Preserved; no nystagmus	Impaired/ dysconjugate, internuclear ophthalmoplegia	Absent	Absent
Uncal	Ipsilateral partial or complete CN-III palsy; opposite eye moves fully	Contralateral eye may move laterally only; ipsilateral eye does not move and may be abducted and downwardly deviated	Absent: eyes dysconjugate	Absent: eyes dysconjugate
Motor				
Central	Resistance to movement or paratonia, then decorticate	Decerebrate	No posturing other than Babinski signs and brief flexor knee responses with stimulation	Absent or flexor responses in leg with stimulation
Uncal	Contralateral paratonia and ipsilateral withdrawal; ipsilateral hemiplegia is seen in Kernohan notch phenomena	Decerebrate	As above	As above

passive limb movements. Pupils are small and retain reactivity, although at times blunted and subtle to detect. Although there is no visual fixation, eye movements are conjugate and full. As pressure mounts across the thalami onto the mesencephalon, pupillary and eye movement abnormalities appear. Involvement of CN-III or its nucleus initially causes irregular and poorly reactive pupils (corectopia). Eventually, eye movements are disrupted by CN-III or CN-VI lesions or from involvement of the medial longitudinal fasciculus (MLF). The MLF, a paracentral dorsally located tract coursing up the vestibular nuclei to the CN-III nucleus, maintains conjugate eye movements either initiated voluntarily in the waking state or induced reflexively from cervical or vestibular inputs in comatose patients. This pathway provides the basis of doll's-eyes testing or caloric stimulation testing of the semicircular canals. An intact MLF system keeps the eyes from moving passively when the examiner rolls the head to one side. The eyes remain in their primary position in relation to the examiner or seem to move to the opposite side

in relation to the head rolling. With unilateral caloric stimulation of the ears, the eyes deviate conjugately to one side or another, depending on the water temperature used for irrigation. The direction of the convection current induced in the semicircular canals by different temperatures determines the direction of eye movement. With the head maintained in the neutral position, cold water causes the eye to deviate to the side of the stimulated ear while warm water causes deviation away from the stimulated ear. Disruption of the MLF system causes an abnormal or absent responses of these reflexive eye movements (Fig. 16-6). Therefore oculocephalic testing checks the integrity of a large portion of the brainstem from the vestibular nuclei to the mesencephalic third-nerve nucleus.

MOVEMENT

If the motor pathways of the brainstem are disconnected from corticothalamic input, certain primitive tonic postures appear in

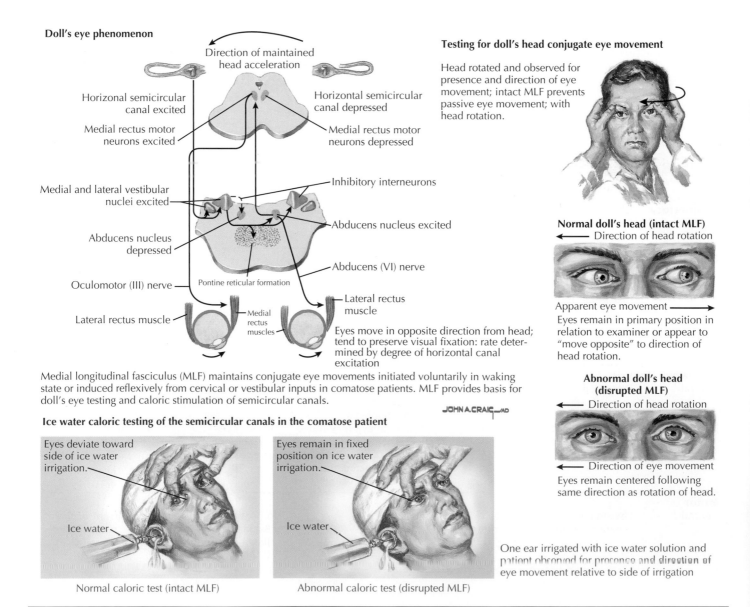

Doll's eye phenomenon

Direction of maintained head acceleration

Horizonal semicircular canal excited

Medial rectus motor neurons excited

Horizontal semicircular canal depressed

Medial rectus motor neurons depressed

Medial and lateral vestibular nuclei excited

Inhibitory interneurons

Abducens nucleus excited

Abducens nucleus depressed

Oculomotor (III) nerve

Pontine reticular formation

Abducens (VI) nerve

Lateral rectus muscle

Medial rectus muscles

Lateral rectus muscle

Eyes move in opposite direction from head; tend to preserve visual fixation; rate determined by degree of horizontal canal excitation

Medial longitudinal fasciculus (MLF) maintains conjugate eye movements initiated voluntarily in waking state or induced reflexively from cervical or vestibular inputs in comatose patients. MLF provides basis for doll's eye testing and caloric stimulation of semicircular canals.

JOHN A. CRAIG—AD

Ice water caloric testing of the semicircular canals in the comatose patient

Eyes deviate toward side of ice water irrigation.

Ice water

Normal caloric test (intact MLF)

Eyes remain in fixed position on ice water irrigation.

Ice water

Abnormal caloric test (disrupted MLF)

Testing for doll's head conjugate eye movement

Head rotated and observed for presence and direction of eye movement; intact MLF prevents passive eye movement; with head rotation.

Normal doll's head (intact MLF)
◄— Direction of head rotation

Apparent eye movement ——►
Eyes remain in primary position in relation to examiner or appear to "move opposite" to direction of head rotation.

Abnormal doll's head (disrupted MLF)
◄— Direction of head rotation

◄— Direction of eye movement
Eyes remain centered following same direction as rotation of head.

One ear irrigated with ice water solution and patient observed for presence and direction of eye movement relative to side of irrigation

Figure 16-6 Eye Movements in Coma.

succession and reflect the level of central nervous system (CNS) damage. Depending on the area of cerebral cortex involved, patients may show unilateral signs of upper motor neuron dysfunction, with the typical triad of increased flexor tone, hyperreflexia, and paralysis. The opposite side may still show semivoluntary or directed movements, such as consistently withdrawing away from noxious stimuli or breaking the fall of a limb held against gravity. When damage progresses below the diencephalon or to the upper reticular activating system, a decorticate posture appears, characterized by rigid arm adduction, forearm pronation with flexion of the elbow and wrist, and leg extension at the hips and knees. With further rostrocaudal deterioration, decerebrate rigidity evolves, with arm extension at the elbows, hyperextension of the trunk and legs, and prominent plantar flexion of the feet. Arm adduction, wrist flexion, and forearm pronation persist. Animal models suggest that decerebrate rigidity corresponds to mesencephalic lesions at the level of the red nucleus. With ischemia to the lower pons and medulla, the body becomes flaccid, with no reactivity except for occasional bilateral toe extensor responses with knee and hip flexion.

BREATHING

Respiratory patterns also change with worsening levels of consciousness in coma (Fig. 16-7). The earliest breathing alterations are Cheyne–Stokes respirations. Hemispheric forebrain structures serve to regulate breathing by mechanisms independent of CO_2 accumulation. With bilateral cerebral cortex damage, this breathing control is lost, and CO_2-driven breathing is accentuated with only modest CO_2 accumulations, thus inducing an increased rate and depth of respiration. This reactive hyperpnea leads to an eventual decrease in arterial CO_2 and, again without forebrain control, loss of respiratory drive. The ensuing apnea then allows CO_2 to reaccumulate and the cycle to repeat itself, resulting in hyperpnea of a crescendo–decrescendo pattern, alternating with intervening episodes of brief apnea.

Midbrain and upper pons lesions cause hyperventilation with a constant rate and amplitude, without periods of apnea. The reasons for the so-called "central neurogenic hyperventilation" are unclear but are unlikely to be of purely neuronal origin. Lung congestion caused by immobility and poor airway protection likely play a major role. Hypothalamic and midbrain lesions engender increased sympathetic activity, which in turn promotes capillary fluid seepage, worsening lung congestion and, in extreme cases, pulmonary edema.

Injury to the lower half of the pons damages the respiratory control system, possibly generating apneustic breathing; a pattern of prolonged end inspiratory pauses alternating with end-expiratory pauses of several seconds, without the crescendo–decrescendo pattern of Cheyne–Stokes breathing. Further damage causes this pattern to fragment into an irregular, unpredictable rhythm of varying amplitude, intermixed with pauses

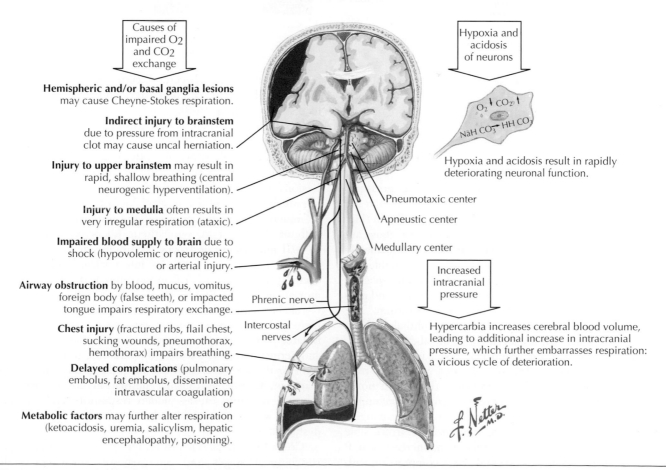

Figure 16-7 Respiratory Exchange in Head Injury.

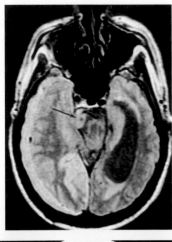

A. Axial FLAIR Brain MR:
Uncal herniation (arrow)
with mesencephalic compression.

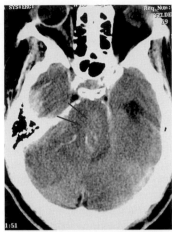

B. Axial Noncontrast Brain CT:
Pontine hemorrhages (arrows).

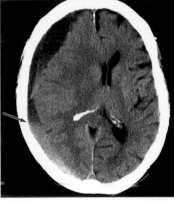

C. Subacute Subdural Hematoma.
Axial noncontrast brain CT: Layering
subdural blood products (arrow) with
frontal and parieto-occipital mass
effect.

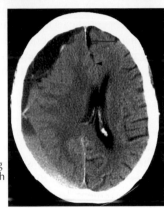

**D. Complications of Increased
Intracranial Pressure:** Cingulate
gyrus (arrowhead) herniation
beneath the falx cerebri (arrow).

Figure 16-8 MR and CT Images Showing Cerebral Herniation Patterns.

of variable length. Ultimately, destruction of the centrally located dorsomedial medullary respiratory center causes total cessation of breathing, even before circulatory collapse occurs.

Variation from the Classic Rostrocaudal Paradigm

Unilateral cerebral lesions can cause asymmetric pressures leading to medial temporal lobe (uncal) herniation through the tentorial incisure, with direct compression of the midbrain (Fig. 16-8). In this case, the diencephalic features described above are not seen; instead, rapid loss of consciousness is immediately followed by a decerebrate posture. This is usually heralded by a compressive palsy of CN-III as it exits the ventral aspect of the midbrain and runs between the superior cerebellar and posterior cerebral arteries across the top of the tentorium. The initial sign is pupillary dilation, followed by ophthalmoplegia and ptosis with downward displacement of the abducted globe. Hemiplegia ipsilateral to the lesion may result from compression of the contralateral anteriorly located pyramidal tract against the anterior edge of the tentorium (Kernohan notch phenomenon). Further increase in pressure causes stretching of the pontine penetrators off the basilar artery or venous congestion with paramedian hemorrhages and usually irreversible worsening (Fig. 16-8). A sudden worsening and increase in ICP may also result from posterior cerebral artery compression with occipital lobe infarction. Finally, the cingulate gyrus may herniate beneath the falx cerebri, compressing the ipsilateral or contralateral anterior cerebral artery and causing infarction in its distribution (Fig. 16-8).

Infratentorial lesions within the brainstem tegmentum or secondary to brainstem compression, such as with cerebellar mass lesions, cause coma abruptly as a result of the almost immediate involvement of the reticular activating system. Lesions involving the midbrain result in oculomotor- or infranuclear-type ophthalmoplegia or both, with fixed irregular or midposition dilated pupils. If the lesion involves the pons without the midbrain, sympathetic fibers running up to the CN-III nucleus are destroyed, and pupils are pinpoint in size but still reactive to light. An internuclear ophthalmoplegia occurs from bilateral MLF lesions, but vertical oculocephalic movements, controlled by the tectal midbrain, are preserved. Cerebellar mass lesions can cause forward brainstem displacement and may produce findings similar to those described for isolated pontine lesions or may cause cerebellar tissue crowding and herniation upward around the midbrain through the tentorium or downward around the medulla through the foramen magnum. Cerebellar tonsillar herniation down through the foramen magnum causes sudden respiratory and circulatory arrest, without gradual signs of evolving brainstem dysfunction.

Coma from metabolic disease rarely conforms to the typical rostrocaudal stages and often shows concurrent findings pertaining to different nervous system levels. For example, hypoglycemia can cause unconsciousness with decerebrate posturing but preserved oculocephalic responses and pupillary reactivity. In metabolic comas from opioid overdose, pupils are tiny but reactive, even though respiratory drive may be obliterated. Also, the oculocephalics are intact, despite drug-induced pinpoint pupillary changes mimicking a pontine hemorrhage, as the vignette at the beginning of this chapter illustrates. Finally, pupillary reactivity remains relatively resistant to metabolic effects; when other brainstem signs are absent, the presence of brisk pupillary reactivity suggests a nonstructural metabolic or toxic cause.

Treatment of Increased Intracranial Pressure

When signs of increased ICP are evident, emergent treatment is needed to halt progressive obtundation or coma and to avoid herniation and irreversible brain injury. Delaying treatment to first determine the underlying pathophysiologic mechanism is of minimal benefit. An invasive, but highly effective, method to decrease ICP is CSF drainage through an external ventricular drain if applicable. Noninvasive therapeutic modalities available to acutely control increasing ICP act mainly by three mechanisms: vascular, osmotic, and metabolic. With induced vasoconstriction, cerebral blood flow (CBF) diminishes, reducing total cerebral blood volume with a subsequent decrease in ICP. Agents that create a hyperosmolar intravascular compartment in relation to brain tissue induce water movement down a gradient from cells and the interstitium into plasma, reducing total brain water content, volume, and pressure. This affects both normal and, likely to a lesser extent, damaged edematous brains. Osmotic agents may have other beneficial actions, such as preserving cerebral perfusion pressure (CPP), decreasing blood viscosity, decreasing CSF production, and the scavenging of free radicals.

Increased metabolic demand from injury or illness may increase blood flow and enhance the delivery of oxygen, which, in turn, may cause increased free radical production and cell injury. Decreasing the metabolic drive helps limit blood flow and decreases the need for tissue oxygen delivery.

HYPERVENTILATION

The least invasive, most effective, and fastest mechanism to decrease ICP is induced hypocapnia produced by active hyperventilation. Intact brain tissue with preserved cerebrovascular autoregulation mediates this effect. Autoregulation is abolished in damaged tissue or ischemic areas, which do not respond to hyperventilation. The goal of intact cerebrovascular autoregulation is to keep CBF stable under conditions of normal slight fluctuations in systemic pressures. Factors such as fever, hypoxemia, and ischemia induce the need for increased CBF and are mediated through the vasodilatory effect of hydrogen ions from lactic and carbonic acid accumulation. The brain is therefore sensitive to CO_2 levels, and increased CO_2 pressure produces an almost linear increase in CBF. Similarly, decreased CO_2 pressure causes vasoconstriction and a decrease in CBF. Correspondingly, intracranial blood volume and ICP decrease, provided that enough intact tissue exists to mediate this response.

The response to hyperventilation is almost immediate, with its peak effect occurring within 30 minutes. Effectiveness diminishes over the course of hours to a day, limiting the utility of hyperventilation as a long-term option to control increased ICP. Despite short-term effectiveness, cerebral vasoconstriction may eventually cause increasing ischemic brain injury, especially in vulnerable areas with previously compromised blood flow. Outcomes can worsen with its prolonged use. Therefore, hyperventilation is confined to brief intervals to urgently control sudden increases in ICP. When more permanent treatments are instituted (i.e., control of agitation, blood pressure regulation, or surgery), its use should be halted.

The relatively safe target level of PCO_2 is approximately 25–35 mm Hg; lower PCO_2 levels risk compromising cerebral blood perfusion with subsequent ischemia, which would eventually cause a seemingly paradoxic further increase in ICP. The usual approach is to increase respiratory rate but not tidal volume. Higher lung volumes increase intrathoracic pressure and total cerebral blood volume by compromising venous return from the brain to the heart.

OSMOTIC AGENTS AND DIURETICS

The osmotic agent mannitol (20–25% solution) has been the cornerstone of ICP management for decades and continues to be an effective and relatively safe treatment when used judiciously. It is usually administered rapidly over minutes (0.75–1.0 g/kg), with its initial effect usually occurring within 20 minutes and lasting approximately 6–8 hours. With repeated doses there is diminishing effectiveness and a shortening of the response duration over days. Depending on the clinical response and patient status, subsequent mannitol doses of 0.25–0.5 g/kg are administered every 4–6 hours. Concomitant measurement of serum osmolality, and sometimes ICP, is indicated. Repeated mannitol use requires extreme caution to avoid hypotension or a hyperosmolar state from too frequent or brisk diuresis. Using mannitol sparingly avoids the pitfalls of hypotension and electrolyte imbalance that can seriously undermine patient care. A staged approach in increasing the osmolarity initially to 295–300 mOsm/kg and then gradually to 310–320 mOsm/kg may be helpful. Osmolarities higher than 320 mOsm/kg are dangerous and add little to further control ICP. Standing orders for "maintenance" doses should be avoided; the clinical situation and osmolality should guide subsequent dosing. If the clinical examination, ICP and osmolarity are stable, no extra doses may be required. Serial measurement of renal function, electrolytes, and osmolarity are indicated every 4–6 hours. Potassium depletion is common, and frequent replacement is needed. Daily fluid balance and body weight measurements are essential to maintain the goal of a euvolemic hyperosmolar state. Only isotonic fluids should be used to replenish intravascular volume. Hypotonic fluids and free water should be avoided to avert recurrent brain edema.

Low doses of diuretics, such as furosemide (10–20 mg), may be used alone or with mannitol to enhance or hasten the response, especially when transient increase in intravascular volume, such as in congestive heart failure, may be problematic.

Hypertonic solutions have been used for more than 50 years in the treatment of ICP but, unlike mannitol, have only recently gained widespread use. Animal models and small human studies, mostly involving traumatic brain injury, show hypertonic solutions to have a more robust and longer effect in reducing ICP when compared to mannitol. They have the advantage of preserving CPP by repleting intravascular volume and enhancing microvascular circulation and well-being. Its effects on outcomes, however, have been variable and remain unestablished. There is no unified ICP protocol for hypertonic solution administration, with concentrations varying from 3% to 29.2% and given either as a bolus or as a continuous infusion to keep sodium levels about 145–155 mmol/L. Potential side effects include hypernatremia and electrolyte imbalance, non-anion gap acidosis, coagulopathies, and possibly renal failure.

BARBITURATE ANESTHESIA

The presumed mechanism for barbiturate anesthesia, another useful modality for controlling ICP, is its ability to reduce brain metabolic demand and therefore CBF. Evidence supporting its use is stronger for patients with head trauma than for those with nontraumatic injuries. It is difficult to use in a sustained fashion and its potentially serious adverse effects of hypotension and myocardial depression may offset its benefits in nontraumatic coma. Its use should be reserved for recalcitrant cases of increased ICP not responsive to conservative measures and osmotic agents in patients who are relatively hemodynamically stable. A short-acting barbiturate, pentobarbital, is used at a 1–3 mg/kg/hr drip after an initial loading dose of 3–10 mg/kg administered over at least 30 minutes followed by 5 mg/kg/hr for 3 hours. The maintenance dose is adjusted to obtain a burst suppression pattern on EEG, but this is not essential if other means of assessing ICP, such as a pressure bolt or intraventricular catheter, are available. Usually, adequate treatment occurs at barbiturate levels of approximately 30–50 mg/dL; higher levels may produce total electrocerebral silence and are not necessary. Blood pressure is maintained with pressor or inotropic infusion if needed.

OTHER AGENTS

Propofol infusion (1–3 mg/kg/hr) has some benefit in controlling increased ICP, but it must be used with caution because of its potential to cause hypotension, adrenal suppression, and increased risk of nosocomial infections. Halogenated inhalation anesthetics and ketamine are not recommended because of their direct dilatory effect on cerebral vasculature and CBF.

GENERAL MEASURES

In the care of patients with or at risk for increased ICP, several other modalities help prevent escalating ICP and improve outcome.

Head Position

If blood pressure is controlled and there is no threat of compromising CPP, head position should be kept upright at approximately 30° to aid brain venous outflow and reduce total brain blood volume. The head should be kept midline and not bent to the side, which may impede jugular venous drainage. If blood pressure is fluctuating or low, the patient should remain supine to prevent decreased CPP.

Blood Pressure

The parameters of blood pressure control in treating ICP remain hard to define. Cerebral autoregulation is absent in damaged or ischemic brain, and perfusion of these areas is directly related to systemic pressure. Relatively high systemic pressures may increase edema in areas of a disrupted blood–brain barrier, whereas low systemic pressures may compromise perfusion and cause further tissue ischemia. Cushing response, a reaction to increasing ICP, is a sympathetically mediated increase of systemic blood pressure with reflex bradycardia, which may play a protective role in preserving CPP (ICP minus mean arterial pressure). However, if untreated, it may eventually lead to increased tissue edema in damaged areas of the brain. Conversely, overaggressive treatment may exacerbate ischemia.

The principle of preserving CPP within the range of functioning cerebral autoregulation may be the best guide, as no definite directives exist. Because the range of cerebral autoregulation shifts upward with chronic hypertension, the parameters for each patient may vary. Ideally, arterial blood pressure should be kept near its premorbid range, determined if possible from previous documented measurements. If arterial pressure is low, then increasing it with isotonic fluids or mild pressor agents is indicated. In cases in which ICP is stable, systemic hypertension is treated independently. If both systemic pressure and ICP are increased in conjunction, then an attempt at reducing ICP (e.g., with mannitol) should be initiated first and blood pressure monitored closely for resolution of reflex hypertension. If there is no response within a few minutes, a gentle attempt to bring the systemic blood pressure down is made, preferably using agents with no cerebral vasodilatory effects, that is, diuretics, angiotensin-converting enzyme inhibitors, and β-sympathetic blockers. Reliance strictly on CPP alone may not always produce favorable outcomes, and following all parameters simultaneously may provide greater benefit.

When an ICP monitor is used, the goal is to preserve CBF above the level that ensures adequate cerebral oxygen metabolic needs while keeping CPP above 60 mm Hg and approximately 70 mm Hg and avoiding persistent or recurring ICP measurements of greater than 20 mm Hg.

Pathologic Stresses

Factors such as seizures and fever that may increase cerebral metabolic rate and blood flow require control. Seizures are emergently treated with benzodiazepines or short-acting barbiturates and for the long term with other anticonvulsants. Hypoxemia is avoided by monitoring blood oxygenation levels with O_2 saturation devices or repeated arterial blood gas samples. Hyperthermia requires prompt treatment with antipyretics and with antibiotics when an infectious cause is found. Because cerebral metabolic rate is directly proportional to temperature, some authorities have advocated hypothermia as a primary treatment for increased ICP. Although effective, its complications include cardiac arrhythmias, pancreatitis, infections, and rebound ICP during the rewarming process. Whether induced hypothermia improves neurologic outcome is still unknown and should not be used routinely or as a first-line treatment.

It is generally accepted that corticosteroids are not useful, and indeed may be detrimental, in most instances of sudden increase in ICP. Other than long-term control of tumor-associated edema, corticosteroids should not be used in the acute management of increased ICP.

Hemicraniectomy

In this surgical procedure, the lateral-coronal skull is removed and a dural flap is constructed without excision of necrotic brain tissue, permitting enlarging lobar lesions to expand outward without exerting pressure on deeper brainstem structures. Hemicraniectomy has been successfully used to control increased ICP when other measures have failed. Particularly used for large middle cerebral artery distribution strokes and traumatic brain injury, it is clearly effective in reducing mortality. Performing it as early as possible, at the first signs of deterioration, yields better results and may improve outcome. However, most survivors remain with significant disability, especially if they are older than 45 years. Hemicraniectomy for difficult-to-control ICP, regardless of the hemisphere involved, should not be done routinely. Careful consideration of residual functional abilities, life expectancy, patient wishes if known, and input from the family should all be considered.

BRAIN DEATH

Clinical Vignette

A 56-year-old man suddenly collapsed at home after experiencing severe chest pain. His wife called the emergency technicians, who found him pulseless and cyanotic. ECG demonstrated ventricular fibrillation, but he was successfully defibrillated. After an airway was established and 100% oxygen was given, he was transported to the ED. There, neurologic evaluation showed that he was unresponsive to any form of communication. His pupils were dilated and not reactive to light stimulation. Decerebrate posturing was noted to suctioning and to noxious stimulation. Bilateral Babinski signs were present. He eventually became flaccid, and cold caloric vestibular stimulation showed no ocular response. The next day, he developed generalized myoclonus and continued to require cardiac and full respiratory support. Three days later, there was no change in his neurologic status. An apnea test showed no respiratory response to induced hypercarbia. Although he was declared brain dead, his wife asked that further testing be performed to confirm the clinical diagnosis. An EEG demonstrated electrocerebral silence, and she agreed to have life support withdrawn.

This vignette is the classic example of a patient with prolonged cardiorespiratory arrest resulting in devastating diffuse cerebral ischemic damage. Until a precise determination of brain death is established, there are many medical and legal issues to address in caring for individuals who have no effective residual brain function despite cardiopulmonary function maintained with modern intensive care therapies.

In most medical communities, a person is considered dead once there is irreversible and total cessation of all brain function, regardless of a continuing functional circulatory system. The cause of brain damage must be clearly elucidated by history, examination, or medical tests before the diagnosis of brain death is entertained. Intoxicants, sedatives, and hypothermia may present similarly to brain death but are potentially reversible and must always be considered if the cause is not clear and well documented. In many countries, including the United States, "brain death" constitutes a legal definition of death, and all life support measures can be halted.

When caring for an individual, it is best to respect the family's wishes, religious or personal, regarding the timing of discontinuing life support. It is important to continue to explain the situation's finality and that circulatory collapse will invariably occur within hours to days of the onset of this clinical picture. The widespread difficulty in obtaining organs for an ever-growing list of patients awaiting transplant procedures makes it of paramount importance to broach the subject of organ donation as soon as possible as it is vital to harvest organs early. The physician who has an established relationship with the patient's family is perhaps the one best to initiate such discussion before involving the transplant team.

Brain Death Criteria

The criteria for brain death vary among states and countries. Usually the determination is clinical, with testing used only as an ancillary or confirmatory measure. The following are generally accepted principles of brain death determination:

1. A preceding coma of known irreversible cause must **not** be due to, or influenced by, CNS depressants, intoxicants, paralytic agents, hypothermia (less than 32°C/90°F), or endocrine or metabolic disturbances.
2. Cessation of all brain function must be documented as follows.
   a. There must be **no response to stimuli** in any way **other than** spinal **withdrawal** movements in the legs and arms. Spinal reflexes such as muscle stretch reflexes or extensor responses of the toes (Babinski signs) can be seen, but there must be no other spontaneous limb movements or posturing to painful stimuli, including decerebrate rigidity.
   b. **Brainstem reflexes must be absent**, including pupillary response to light (without mydriatic agents), oculocephalic reflexes by passive head turning or caloric stimulation, corneal reflexes, oropharyngeal reflexes (gag or swallowing), respiratory reflexes (spontaneous breaths or cough), and snout or jaw jerk reflex (Fig. 16-9).
   c. **Apnea test must be positive**, wherein the patient exhibits no evidence of respiratory effort or change in sinus

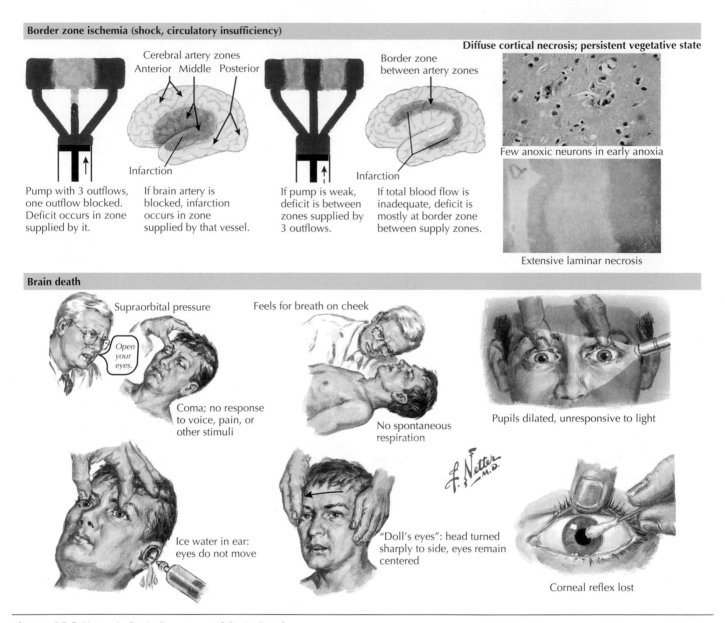

Figure 16-9 Hypoxic Brain Damage and Brain Death.

heart rate with induced hypercapnia. In this instance, the patient is ventilated with 100% O_2 for 15 minutes and then disconnected while an endotracheal catheter provides O_2 at 6 L/min. Apneic oxygenation is maintained for 10 minutes or until the PCO_2 is 55–60 mm Hg.

3. In the presence of a clear structural brain lesion without evidence of toxic or metabolic cause, neurologic reexamination should proceed 6 hours after the initial evaluation to confirm and document the findings. Repeat examination should be performed at 12 hours if the cause is uncertain or there is no evidence of irreversible severe structural brain damage.

4. When the clinical evaluation, apnea test, or both are unclear or unfeasible, confirmatory tests to document the absence of electrical or metabolic cerebral activity are conducted. CT or MRI scan may support the clinical examination.

a. A minimum 30-minute EEG isoelectric tracing (obtained with a "double" interelectrode distance bipolar montage) is sought. The first test is obtained no sooner than 8 hours after cardiac arrest and reconfirmed after 6 hours (American EEG Society Recommendations).

b. Documentation of cessation of cerebral circulation by conventional angiography, technetium isotope study, transcranial Doppler, or CT angiogram.

c. Absent auditory-evoked responses and short-latency somatosensory evoked responses may also be used to indicate absent brainstem function. However, these studies may be affected by peripheral lesions and are technically difficult to perform, especially in an intensive care unit setting, and their utility as a confirmatory test has been questioned.

Mitigating Factors

When a severe cerebral insult is suspected but brain death determination cannot be confirmed because of confounding issues, the utmost should be done to correct for these specific factors before brain death assessment can proceed. For example, hypothermia is treated with a warming blanket to bring and maintain core body temperature above 36.5°C. Fluid, and at times vasopressor agents, are administered for patients with systolic blood pressures lower than 90 mm Hg.

Patients with chronic hypercapnia secondary to lung disease such as chronic obstructive pulmonary disease have a higher respiratory center PCO_2 threshold, and a PCO_2 of approximately 60 mm Hg may not necessarily drive the chemoreceptors, even with a functioning brainstem. The CO_2 level may be allowed to climb to approximately 80 mm Hg, but such levels risk ensuing acidosis with direct cardiodepressor effects as well as arrhythmias and hypotension. Therefore, it is preferable in these instances to obtain confirmatory tests to bolster the diagnosis without risking untoward iatrogenic complications.

Although most centers in the United States uphold the general outline of the principles mentioned above, there are numerous variations and differences concerning how best to ensure diagnostic certainty. Most medical centers do not require confirmatory tests. The number of evaluations and the time span between them also differ. Many institutions require a brain death evaluation by two attending neurologists at different times and their presence at the apnea test. The specific brain death criteria and protocol for each medical center must be consulted before the evaluation is begun and a diagnosis is substantiated.

ADDITIONAL RESOURCES

Bullock R, Chestnut F, Clifton G, et al. Guidelines for the management of severe head injury. J Neurotrauma 2000;17:471-553.

Conrad GR, Sinha P. Scintigraphy as a confirmatory test of brain death. Semin Nucl Med 2003;33:312-323.

American Electroencephalographic Society. Guideline three: minimum technical standards for EEG recording in suspected cerebral death. J Clin Neurophysiol 1994;11:10-13.

Wijdicks EFM, Hijdra A, Young GB, et al. Practice Parameter: Prediction of outcome in comatose survivors after cardiopulmonary resuscitation (an evidence-based review): Report of the Quality Standards Subcommittee of the American Academy of Neurology. Neurology 2006;67;203-210. *A systematic review of the outcomes in coma after cardiopulmonary arrest identifying the factors that most reliably predict a poor prognosis.*

Hypothermia After Cardiac Arrest Study Group. Mild therapeutic hypothermia to improve the neurologic outcome after cardiac arrest. New England Journal of Medicine 2002;346(8):549-556.

Levy DE, Bates D, Corona JJ, et al. Prognosis in non-traumatic coma. Ann Intern Med 1981;94:293-301. *Landmark paper that details the examination of postanoxic coma and the various findings that predict outcomes.*

Muizelaar JP, Marmarou A, Ward JD, et al. Adverse effects of prolonged hyperventilation in patients with severe head injury: a randomized clinical trial. J Neurosurg 1991;75:731-739.

Piatt J, Schiff SJ. High dose barbiturate therapy in neurosurgery and intensive care. Neurosurgery 1984;15:427-444.

Presidents Commission on Guidelines for the Determination of Death. Neurology 1982;32:395.

Posner JB, Saper CB, Schiff ND, et al. The Diagnosis of Stupor and Coma. (Contemporary Neurology Series. 71). 4th ed. New York: Oxford University Press; 2007. *An expanded and exhaustive edition of the classic monogram on the pathophysiology of coma and its various etiologies. Detailed description of the associated vascular and anatomic pathology. It ends with a small section on the approach to the unconscious patient and treatment.*

Qureshi AI, Kirmani JF, Xavier AR, et al. Computed tomographic angiography for diagnosis of brain death. Neurology 2004;24;62:652-653.

Report of the Quality Standards Subcommittee of the American Academy of Neurology 1995;1-7.

Sazbon L, Zagreba F, Ronen J, et al. Course and outcome of patients in vegetative state of non-traumatic aetiology. J Neurol Neurosurg Psychiatry 1993;56:407-409.

Teasdale G, Jennet B. Assessment of coma and impaired consciousness: a practical scale. Lancet 1974;ii:81-84. *The first description of the Glasgow Coma Scale that has acquired widespread use and has subsequently been shown to be a reliable tool in predicting outcome in head trauma.*

The Multi-Society Task Force on PVS. Medical aspects of the persistent vegetative state: parts I and II. N Engl J Med 1994;330:1499-1508, 1572-1579.

Vahedi K, Hofmeijer J, Juettler E, et al; for the DECIMAL, DESTINY, and HAMLET investigators. Early decompressive surgery in malignant infarction of the middle cerebral artery: a pooled analysis of three randomized controlled trials. Lancet Neurol 2007;6:315–322. *Data pooled from three different studies showing that decompressive hemicraniectomy more than doubles the chance of survival from "malignant" middle cerebral artery stroke, and likely improves outcomes regardless of the side affected. However, most survivors are left with significant disability.*

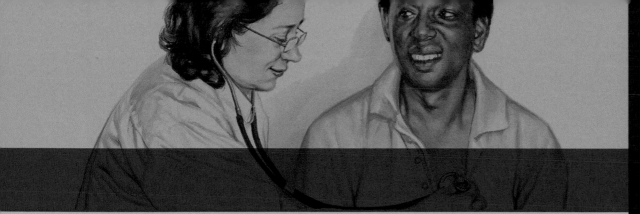

Cognitive and Behavioral Disorders

Delirium and Acute Encephalopathies

Yuval Zabar and Kenneth Lakritz

17

Clinical Vignette

A 62-year-old college professor was admitted to the hospital for elective hip replacement. Surgery was uncomplicated, but on the second postoperative day he was anxious, diaphoretic, and had a low-grade fever. A broad-spectrum antibiotic regimen was begun. That night, he began to hallucinate, insisting that strangers had come into his room. He hardly slept. The next morning he had a generalized convulsive seizure. A neurologic consultant noted agitation, disorientation, impaired recall, visual hallucinations, tremor, and tachycardia. The patient described his alcohol intake as "two per day," but his wife described his two drinks as tumblers of scotch and estimated his intake at a pint of whiskey daily. He had no history of liver disease, gastrointestinal bleeds, blackouts, withdrawal symptoms, solitary drinking, or occupational impairment.

He was treated with high-dose benzodiazepines, intravenous thiamine, intravenous fluids, and electrolyte replacement. His autonomic signs rapidly stabilized and no further seizures occurred. However he remained confused and agitated during the ensuing 2 weeks. Although he was carefully counseled about his alcohol abuse, and its inherent risks, he rejected the diagnosis of alcoholism, and refused follow-up treatment subsequent to his discharge.

Comment: This is a typical example of the understated abuser of alcoholic beverages. "Two a day" is a classic patient euphemism used to subconsciously or deliberately cover up their daily habit. The physician must always explore the precise meaning of such a statement vis-à-vis the actual amount of wine, beer, or spirits consumed. As in this instance, an observant and often concerned spouse is more frequently able to objectively report the actual degree of alcoholic consumption. A forewarned physician is much better able to critically observe the patient's in-hospital demeanor. At the slightest hint of cerebral and autonomic decompensation, so classic for early delirium tremens, appropriate therapies can be expeditiously initiated and a potentially fatal outcome prevented.

*D*elirium is a common, acquired neuropsychiatric disorder frequently encountered in clinical practice. Marked by cognitive and behavioral symptoms and a fluctuating course, delirium presents doctors and families with a host of challenges, from initial diagnosis and management, to ethical dilemmas surrounding informed consent, personal autonomy, and patient safety (Fig. 17.1). There is a lack of consensus regarding the definition and terminology pertaining to delirium. Terms such as "acute confusional state," "encephalopathy," and "change in mental status" are often used arbitrarily. As delirium often presents within the context of myriad medical and/or surgical conditions, it is often not appreciated to be a clinically independent entity. Nevertheless, delirium is associated with considerable morbidity and mortality, delaying or interfering with proper care as well as promoting great distress for nursing staff, physicians, and families.

DEFINITION

There are no universally accepted criteria for a diagnosis of delirium. The most often cited criteria are found in the DSM IV and include the following core features:

1. *Disturbance of consciousness*, with reduced ability to focus, sustain, or shift attention.
2. *Change in cognition or perception* that is not accounted for by a preexisting, established, or evolving dementing disorders.
3. *Disturbance develops acutely* (hours to days) and often fluctuates during the course of a day.
4. *Concomitant presence of another clinically active medical condition.* Evidence from the history, exam, or laboratory data indicates this disturbance is caused by substance intoxication, or medication side effects.

Additional clinical features of delirium may include:
a. *Psychomotor changes* such as hyperactivity, (or much less commonly hypoactivity), hypersympathetic activity, and disruption of circadian rhythms.
b. *Variable emotional disturbances* with wide-ranging emotions, including fear, euphoria, or depression.

Some clinicians reserve the term "delirium" to confusional states associated with agitated behavior, hallucinations, and delusions. The term "confusional state" might be applied preferentially to describe cases where cognitive disturbance predominates over psychiatric features. Although this distinction is academically enticing, it has no proven clinical utility. For the purposes of this text, the term *delirium* encompasses all variations of acute change in mental status.

EPIDEMIOLOGY

Nearly 30% of all patients aged 65 years or older will experience some degree of delirium during hospitalization. The risk varies from 10% to >50% depending on comorbidities, severity of illness, and hospital setting. For example, as much as 70% of intensive care patients experience delirium. Delirium prolongs hospitalization, rehabilitation, and promotes functional decline and risk of institutionalization. Mortality associated with delirium is high according to pooled data from several studies.

The prevalence of delirium in the nonacute setting is quite elusive. The Canadian Study of Health and Aging estimates a prevalence of <0.5% in a cohort of Canadians aged 65 years or older residing outside of the acute care setting. However, when nondemented subjects developed delirium, their 5-year survival was quite low. This suggests that the appearance of delirium per se may be a harbinger of serious illness in this cohort.

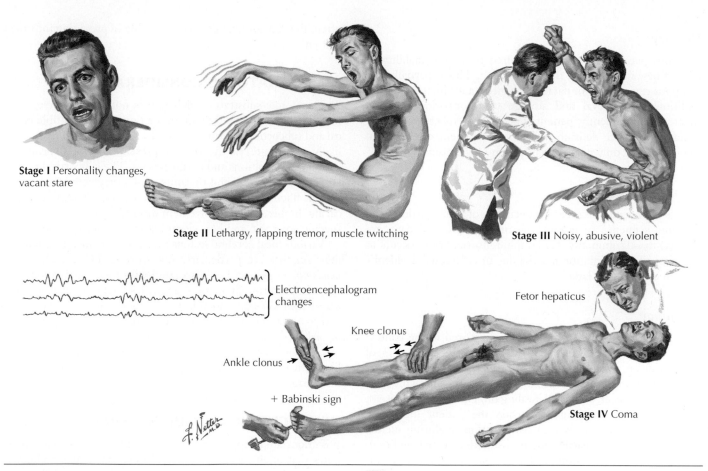

Stage I Personality changes, vacant stare

Stage II Lethargy, flapping tremor, muscle twitching

Stage III Noisy, abusive, violent

Electroencephalogram changes

Fetor hepaticus

Knee clonus

Ankle clonus

+ Babinski sign

Stage IV Coma

Figure 17-1 Delirium.

In contrast, the incidence of delirium within the hospitalized patient population ranges from 10% to 20% overall, and increases in direct relationship to increasing age. About 25% of hospitalized senior citizens, more than age 70 years, experience some degree of delirium. This age-related increased prevalence of delirium is more common in the setting wherein an underlying brain disease is present. In some instances, this may not have been previously identified, such as in the individual with occult Alzheimer disease. Sensory impairment (including poor hearing and vision) heightens the potential for delirium to develop in our senior citizens.

Despite such a potential prevalence, some studies suggest that delirium is neither detected nor documented in up to 66% of these patients. Precipitants of delirium include polypharmacy, infection, metabolic disturbance, malnutrition, and dehydration. Other inciting clinical settings often include intensive care setting, immobility (particularly when using restraints), frequent room changes, absence of a clock or a watch, and lack of reading glasses.

Another very high risk group for developing delirium is the patient who is in palliative care settings wherein close to half of these patients will be witnessed to have these mental status changes. Delirium is also common as a postoperative complication, occurring in up to 52% of these patients, and again preferentially in elderly individuals. Certain procedures are associated with a greater risk, such as coronary bypass and emergency hip surgery. The specific type of anesthesia does not influence risk. However, a low preoperative hematocrit (<30%) may increase the risk of postoperative delirium. Severe postoperative pain also increases the propensity for delirium. However, proper pain management may provide an excellent reduction in severity and duration of the delirium per se. Paradoxically, the initiation of opioid therapy may also precipitate delirium. Thus, it is essential to attempt to find a balance between pain control and opioid intoxication.

DIAGNOSIS

Attention and Vigilance

These patients are prototypically inattentive and distractible. They demonstrate difficulty maintaining focus and directing their attention to particular stimuli in the environment. Consequently, the patient cannot coherently follow a conversation or train of thought. Responses seem random and provided in a trivial fashion. Digit span testing is a sensitive way to assess impaired attention. The examiner lists five digits and asks the patient to repeat them in the same sequence. Then, the examiner lists three digits and asks the patient to repeat them in reverse sequence. Patients with normal attention and concentration should be able to do this accurately.

Memory

Delirious patients often have impaired recall and inability to acquire new information, that is, learning. This is partially due to a poor registration of data with concomitant inattentiveness. Additionally, retrieval and storage of information are also affected. Consequently, patients may be very repetitive or may confabulate. Once delirium resolves, the patient often has no recollection or only partial recollection of the event.

Disorientation

This is universally present. Appreciation of time relationships, the time sequence of events, the time of day, and date, are affected most commonly. Geographic disorientation occurs as well. Impaired orientation may be due to perceptual misidentification as discussed later.

Language

Typically, language function is relatively spared in the context of an episode of delirium. In some cases, the mechanics of articulation are disrupted, causing slurred speech, such as occurs in many cases of intoxication. Paraphasic errors with word substitution may occur, and word-finding difficulty may be present. Intrusion errors are common, when the patient introduces seemingly random words into conversation or during mental status exam. This is usually due to distractibility or inability to shift attention to new stimuli. These types of errors are manifestations of impaired attentional control rather than impaired language processing.

Misperception and Misidentification

Delusions and hallucinations occur commonly in the setting of delirium. Visual hallucinations are more common than other sensory misperceptions, although tactile, olfactory, and auditory hallucinations do occur. Delusional misidentification may also occur. Reduplicative paramnesia is the transposition of the current environment to another place. For example, patients may not recognize they are in a hospital bed but rather in their home, with doctors and nurses doing a home visit. *Capgras syndrome* is the belief that people in proximity to the patient, especially those who are most familiar, are replaced by exact duplicates. In contrast, the *Fregoli syndrome* is the belief that everyone the patient encounters is the same person in disguise. There are many variations of delusional misidentification, and these are often associated with paranoia, anxiety, and agitation.

Impaired Reasoning, Insight

Performance of tasks such as *identifying similarities and differences* between objects or *interpretation of proverbs* are useful means for assessing a patient's *abstract reasoning*. Typically, the delirious patient cannot produce and maintain the control of attention and recall to express a logical, coherent response. There may be *perseveration* or very concrete processing limiting normal comprehension and insight into the patient's condition. The *capacity for decision making is compromised* under such circumstances, and often, the delirious patient is not capable of providing informed consent.

NEUROANATOMIC CONSIDERATIONS

The anatomic substrate of delirium is not well understood; it most likely is composed of an interaction within multiple cortical and subcortical neuronal networks. Certain neuronal systems likely contribute to the overall presentation of delirium in various combinations and permutations. The subcortical reticular activating system and thalamic nuclei may contribute to the various fluctuations in level of consciousness, whereas the cortical and limbic system involvement most likely contributes to the specific cognitive and behavioral features at presentation.

Various focal cerebral lesions may produce differing states of delirium that are particularly noteworthy. These include the *nondominant parietal lobe*, associated with misidentification syndromes; posterior circulation territories, including *thalamus and mesial temporal lobes*, notable for various amnestic syndromes; and *frontal lobe* syndromes, characterized by differing attention disorders, executive dysfunction, or akinetic mutism. The delirious patient may exhibit a variety of these symptoms at once, likely fluctuating in severity over the course of a single episode of delirium.

NEUROCHEMICAL FOUNDATIONS

It is important to appreciate the important neurochemistry attributes that often accompany the delirious state. Acute administration of *benzodiazepines* may lead to not only sedation but also a disoriented and inattentive state. Chronically, these medications may produce short-term memory impairment as well. *Dopaminergic* pharmacotherapeutic agents may produce acute confusional states characterized by visual hallucinations and agitation. *Anticholinergic* therapies typically lead to a delirious state with prominent amnestic features. These various neuropharmacologic agents, each having a potential to lead to delirium, also offer a possible means to elucidate some of the neuroanatomic localizations responsible for the various features of delirium. Of particular importance is the observation that senior citizens are much more prone to experiencing these various neurotoxic side effects. Whenever one evaluates a delirious older individual, it is important to carefully review the patient's medication list for not only valid prescriptions per se but over-the-counter drugs and various dietary supplements.

EVALUATION

The bedside assessment of a delirious patient must include evaluation of a multiplicity of mental functions, including attention, orientation, short-term memory, abstract thinking, cognitive speed, and perception. Use of the digit span test, serial three subtractions, or listing months of the year backwards, provide very useful means for evaluation. When assessing patients' attention and concentration abilities at the bedside, their orientation to time and place must be assessed. Patients need to be able to estimate how long they've been in the hospital and the reason for their hospitalization, as well maintain their ability to readily identify familiar people. Healthy individuals are able to

Table 17-1 Clinical Differences Between Delirium and Dementia

	Delirium	Dementia
Onset	Acute to subacute	Subacute to chronic
Level of consciousness	Impaired, fluctuates	Unaffected until late stages
Cognition	Poor attention, disorientation	Poor memory; attention and orientation affected later
Motor behavior	Variably increased or reduced	Usually normal
Psychotic features	Common and prominent	Less common and usually less prominent

register three words and recall them spontaneously after 5 minutes. Normal persons are able to provide definitions of common words and interpret common proverbs. Asking about the similarities and differences between various items is another useful way to assess abstract reasoning. A mentally alert and healthy patient is able to easily produce a list of 12 animals within a 1-minute time frame. And, lastly, normal individuals are able to easily describe their immediate surroundings or look at a photograph in an organized fashion and then recall the details to their examiner.

Various disorders need to be considered in the differential diagnosis of the delirious patient. In order to *differentiate delirium from dementia*, there are some very simple means (Table 17-1). These include the following:

1. *Acute changes* are typical of delirium in contrast to the chronic time course characteristic of dementia.
2. *Clouding of consciousness* is also typical of delirium.
3. *Hyperactive sympathetic autonomic responses* are frequently apparent in the delirious patient.
4. *Aphasia* per se is more common in the demented patient.

Delirium also needs to be *differentiated from an acute psychosis* where, in contrast to the delirious individual, the psychotic patient maintains his or her:

1. memory and
2. orientation.

However, manic patients may mimic delirium as they often present with insomnia, agitation, delusions, even confusion. In such instances, ancillary studies such as electroencephalography (EEG) may prove useful. The psychotic patient typically has a normal EEG, whereas the delirious patient often has widespread slowing of brainwave activity.

TREATMENT

Management of delirium may be divided into two major categories. This includes (1) treatment of the precipitating mechanism leading to the delirium and (2) management of the problem behaviors associated with delirium.

The underlying cause of delirium is often readily identified; specific treatment is directed at the predisposing medical condition. Once this is defined, and therapy initiated, the delirium gradually resolves; however, it is not uncommon for the delirium to have an incomplete resolution during the initial treatment of the primary inciting mechanism. Thus, it may take days or weeks before patients return to their baseline mental status, well after they are discharged from hospital. Very specific interventions are required in some individuals presenting with delirium, as illustrated below.

In most cases of delirium, the specific treatment largely addresses the underlying medical precipitants of delirium. Sedative medications are largely used to address problem behaviors that disrupt the delivery of care and place patient and staff at risk. Neuroleptics and atypical neuroleptics are often used for this purpose. These medications must be prescribed judiciously to avoid side effects, which paradoxically may include toxic delirium and increased risk of falls. One also needs to be careful to gain a history of the patient's predelirious state to ascertain whether there were earlier signs of a dementing illness. If such is not recognized, these interventions are particularly worrisome. For example, those patients with previously unrecognized *dementia with Lewy bodies* (DLB) may be predisposed to a medication hypersensitivity. This is particularly the case with neuroleptics.

The various mental fluctuations found in DLB patients often mimic delirium as manifested by agitation and psychotic features. Even very low doses of neuroleptic medication in these patients can induce a severe parkinsonian syndrome or *neuroleptic malignant syndrome*.

Benzodiazepines may be used for their sedating and anxiolytic effects.

A paradoxical delirium and agitation may occur in many otherwise nonneurologically impaired, elderly patients. In some settings, benzodiazepines may exacerbate an underlying cognitive impairment with its increased risk of patient falling. Trazodone is sometimes helpful in reducing anxiety and helping to induce sleep. Any use of chemical restraints, to overcome problematic behavior, must be discontinued as quickly as possible.

Nonpharmacologic interventions are very important. The patient's eyeglasses and hearing aids need to be readily available. The hospital room must include a prominent clock in the patient's room, an easily readable calendar, consistent care providers with limited changes in personnel, and proper lighting. Frequent reorientation, one-to-one monitoring, and a structured environment to avoid environmental triggers of agitation may reduce the need for chemical and physical restraint in many cases.

Alcohol Withdrawal

These patients present with an agitated delirium characterized by early signs of hyperactive sympathetic activity. Large doses of benzodiazepines must be rapidly administered to prevent progression to *delirium tremens*. This is a severe form of alcohol withdrawal associated with a potentially high mortality if treatment is not expeditiously and vigorously pursued. These patients are often very tremulous and frequently have visual hallucinations that can be very frightening. For example, the agitated patient may report a feeling that snakes are crawling on them.

No degree of personal reassurance can help these patients. Rather they require very significant doses of benzodiazepines to gain control of the altered mental status in order to return to a nondelirious state. A subsequent medication taper can then be initiated.

Wernicke Encephalopathy

This is an acute neurologic emergency resulting from thiamine deficiency, commonly seen in malnourished patients such as alcoholics. This is manifested by confusion that is classically associated with significant ophthalmoplegia, with diplopia and nystagmus, and ataxia. These patients may acutely develop these symptoms during a period of just a few days. In other settings, Wernicke encephalopathy has a subacute presentation developing over a matter of weeks. The patient's delirium is characterized by disorientation, inattention, drowsiness, and indifference to surroundings. Conversation is sparse and tangential. Superimposed signs of alcohol withdrawal are seen in 15% of these patients.

Treatment of Wernicke encephalopathy is a neurologic emergency. This requires the immediate administration of large doses of thiamine, 100 mg intravenously in 0.5 NSS (but no glucose initially), in order to reverse the symptoms and prevent progression of pathology. This therapeutic protocol is a standard one provided in emergency rooms for most patients presenting with an acute confusional state. The subsequent intravenous fluid must contain glucose to avoid gray matter necrosis and permanent brain damage. To prevent Wernicke encephalopathy from developing in malnourished patients, thiamine and other B vitamins must be routinely administered as supplements to replenish body stores, especially when glucose is given intravenously. Without such supplementation the carbohydrates per se will paradoxically precipitate depletion of any thiamine stores and thus precipitate Wernicke encephalopathy. Progressive stupor, coma, and death develop if the condition is left untreated. In this setting, an autopsy will demonstrate symmetric necrosis of brainstem tegmentum nuclei, superior cerebellar vermis, and mammillary bodies, resembling lesions produced by disorders of pyruvate metabolism.

Portal-Systemic Encephalopathy

This is a progressive delirium resulting from hyperammonemia in patients with underlying liver failure. The mental changes progress in stages, initially manifested by confusion, sometimes with agitation, and then progressing to a sleep-like coma and eventual death. During the early stages, the patient also often exhibits *asterixis*; this is recognized by having patients extend their arms and wrists. The affected individual has motor impersistence, and is unable to maintain the wrists in a stable posture; rather, the hyperextended hands jerk back and forth, something known as a flap, or in the setting of the patient being an alcoholic this is known as a *liver flap*.

Treatment of portal encephalopathy requires reduction of arterial ammonia levels. This is often achieved by administering large doses of lactulose and sometimes antibiotics, such as neomycin, directed at changing the gastrointestinal track flora. Patients with advanced liver disease must maintain low protein diets to avoid high nitrogen load leading to elevated production of ammonia by gut flora.

SUMMARY

Delirium is a serious complication for many hospitalized patients; its presence must be identified early on, as well as its associated systemic precipitants, in order to provide a timely therapy that will reduce the patient's morbidity and mortality. EEG is a useful ancillary diagnostic study, especially in cases where acute psychiatric illness is a possibility. Here the EEG is typically normal. Nonpharmacologic interventions provide a safe means of reducing problem behaviors. The use of medications to reduce agitation must be done with specific goals in mind and in a limited fashion. In every instance, the patient's dignity must be respected as well as his family counseled and guided throughout the course of delirium. This helps to facilitate proper decision making on the patient's behalf.

ADDITIONAL READINGS

Andrew MK, Freter SH, Rockwood K. Prevalence and outcomes of delirium in community and non-acute care settings in people without dementia: a report from the Canadian Study of Health and Aging. BMC Medicine 2006;4:15.

Brown TM, Boyle MF. ABC of psychological medicine: delirium. BMJ 21 Sept 2002;325:644-647.

Francis J, Young GB. Diagnosis of delirium and confusional states. www.uptodate.com; 2009.

Johnson MH. Assessing confused patients. J Neurol Neurosurg Psychiatry 2001;71(Suppl. 1):i7-i12.

Meagher DJ. Delirium: optimising management. BMJ 20 January 2001;322:144-149.

Dementia: Mild Cognitive Impairment, Alzheimer Disease, Lewy Body Dementia, Frontotemporal Lobar Dementia, Vascular Dementia

Yuval Zabar

18

The diagnosis and management of dementia in older adults presents major challenges to the clinician and to society at large. The age-related increase in prevalence of dementia combined with increasing life expectancy is expected to result in a worldwide epidemic within the next few decades. Many of the diseases underlying dementia are definitively diagnosed only at autopsy, including the most common cause of dementia, namely Alzheimer disease (AD). Additionally, many neurodegenerative dementias develop without producing symptoms for many years, so-called "preclinical" disease. Consequently, many patients move through an early phase of illness that does not meet standard diagnostic criteria for dementia. This intermediate clinical phase is called mild cognitive impairment (MCI), reflecting the presence of significant cognitive decline minus the expected loss of function typical of dementia. As our clinical acumen improves and as public awareness of dementia increases, the number of MCI cases is likely to rise as well. With this in mind, this chapter reviews the definition of dementia and MCI and discusses the commonest causes of dementia.

Standardized diagnostic criteria for dementia in epidemiologic studies reveal three groups of patients, namely, those who meet the diagnostic criteria of dementia, those who are normal, and those who cannot be classified as normal or demented. The third group of patients represents individuals with isolated cognitive deficits (usually memory) or individuals without disability related to their cognitive deficits. This group of patients includes individuals with MCI.

MILD COGNITIVE IMPAIRMENT

Longitudinal follow-up of these patients reveals a substantially increased risk of cognitive decline and eventual "conversion" to dementia. This risk is estimated to be between 12% and 15% per year. The sensitivity and specificity of screening tools for dementia and MCI vary greatly. The more sensitive diagnostic instruments usually require more time to administer. Consequently, they are not helpful for routine screening. Current brief cognitive screening instruments, including the Mini Mental State Exam (MMSE) or the 7-Minute Screen, are more useful for detecting dementia than MCI when used in populations with elevated prevalence rates of dementia particularly in the elderly. Other brief, more focused cognitive screening tools such as the Clock Drawing Test or the Time and Change Test may offer additional sensitivity in screening for dementia.

The utility of these tests in detecting MCI is less reliable. Indeed, most patients with MCI score within the normal range on the MMSE. Interview-based dementia assessments, such as the Clinical Dementia Rating scale (CDR), provide a more sensitive means for reliable detection of MCI but may require considerably more time to administer. Another brief screening tool, the Montreal Cognitive Assessment Test (www.mocatest. org), may provide greater sensitivity in detecting MCI. The definitive diagnosis of MCI requires formal neuropsychological assessment. However, neuropsychological test batteries take several hours to administer and interpret. Therefore, they are not practical as screening tools. In the hands of an experienced neuropsychologist, formal neuropsychological tests provide the most sensitive means of detecting cognitive impairment. They may also provide greater specificity in identifying the underlying cause, although there may be significant variability among neuropsychologists' interpretations.

Neuropsychological batteries can differentiate MCI subtypes depending upon the predominant cognitive domain(s) involved. *Amnestic MCI* involves deficits in short-term memory localizable to mesial temporal structures. Neuropathologically, this subtype of MCI is most often associated with AD. *Nonamnestic MCI* includes patients with isolated non-memory related cognitive deficits, such as aphasia, apraxia, executive dysfunction, or agnosia. The neuropathology associated with non-amnestic MCI is more variable, but includes AD as well. Although detection of MCI is relatively easy, treatment of MCI remains controversial. In the largest randomized clinical trial to date, Donepezil was shown to delay "conversion" of amnestic MCI to AD better than placebo or vitamin E over 18 months' duration. Very disappointingly after 3 years of follow-up there was no difference in the rate of "conversion" nor in the severity of cognitive impairment.

DEMENTIA

The most common feature of dementia is impairment in short- and long-term memory, with additional impairment in at least one of the following: abstract thinking, impaired judgment, other disturbances of higher cognitive function, or personality change. The disturbance causes disability in usual social, occupational, or personal function. Of course, any 2 cognitive domains may be involved, and memory loss is not essential for every type of dementia. The diagnosis of dementia is not made if these symptoms occur in delirium (DSM IIIR).

Although this standard definition is adequate for diagnosis of dementia, it is limited in scope. Defined in this way, the diagnosis of dementia requires disability secondary to cognitive losses. However, an 80-year-old retired businessman with progressive deficits in multiple cognitive domains, but functioning independently, may not be considered "disabled" and, therefore, his condition does not technically meet the diagnostic criteria for dementia. Further refinements of diagnostic criteria, aimed at identifying the underlying neuropathologic disease process, require presence of more specific cognitive deficits for diagnosis. For example, the National Institute of Neurologic, Communicative Disorders and Stroke-AD and Related Disorders Association Work Group (NINCDS-ADRDA) criteria for a diagnosis of probable AD require deficits in short-term memory plus at least one additional cognitive domain. In this context, a 55-year-old businessman who can no longer work because of isolated short-term memory impairment also would not technically meet diagnostic criteria for dementia, despite having a disabling cognitive problem. Such cases should be monitored for future decline. Formal neuropsychological assessment must be considered in such cases to assess for more subtle deficits that standard bedside examination often misses. Additional diagnostic criteria may be applied to diagnose the underlying disease process once dementia is identified. In the future, there may be additional studies to improve the accuracy of diagnosis, such as CSF protein analysis for amyloid and tau proteins, and brain PET imaging.

Various comorbidities should be assessed to address potentially treatable factors contributing to cognitive impairment. Depression is particularly important because it commonly coexists with dementia in the elderly. Often depression may be a harbinger of impending dementia in many cases of late life onset of depression. Validated depression assessment instruments, such as Geriatric Depression Scale–Short Form or the Hamilton Depression scale, may facilitate office screening for depression.

Certain nutritional, endocrinologic, or infectious processes must also be considered in the evaluation of the demented patient. Vitamin B_{12} (cobalamin) deficiency is common in the elderly, although a specific causative relationship with dementia is not known. On rare occasions, vitamin B_{12} deficiency is associated with cognitive impairment that may reverse with vitamin supplementation. Hypothyroidism is also common in the elderly, and it is associated with impaired performance on cognitive tests. Although there is no well-established association with dementia, coincident hypothyroidism may impact dementia severity. The incidence and prevalence of tertiary syphilis in the United States is now virtually zero. Routine screening for syphilis as a cause of dementia in the elderly, therefore, is no longer recommended in most U.S. population groups.

The increasing recognition of possible biomarkers for various dementing diseases may also improve diagnostic accuracy. These include various cerebrospinal fluid protein assays, such as protein 14-3-3 in prion disease, and amyloid and tau proteins in AD. Imaging modalities such as fluorodeoxyglucose (FDG)–positron emission tomography (PET) scans, or ligand-based PET scans (detecting beta amyloid deposition in AD) may reveal the molecular changes in the brains of living dementia patients. However, the newer assays and brain imaging techniques still do not provide a definitive diagnosis of dementia, and are not utilized routinely. The definitive diagnosis of most dementing illnesses requires pathological confirmation. Today, diagnosis of dementia, therefore, remains largely clinical.

Dementia Management

The treatment of dementia requires pharmacologic and non-pharmacologic approaches. We will review general treatment strategies here. The target of treatment typically falls into one or more of three interdependent factors, namely (1) cognition, (2) behavior, and (3) functional capacity. Treatment of one factor may negatively impact the other factors. The literature on dementia treatments is too expansive for full review here. More detailed discussion of specific dementia treatment strategies follows in subsequent sections.

It imperative to recognize and treat dementia as early as possible, with a goal to maximize and preserve quality of life for both patient and caregiver. Treatment of cognitive impairment involves intervention either to reverse, slow, or delay progression of cognitive decline. For the most part, currently available pharmacologic agents prove valuable only in delaying decline, perhaps preventing more severe disability and behavior problems. Behavior problems range from disturbances of mood to psychotic symptoms, apathy to agitation, anxiety, and stereotypic, purposeless, rituals. Treatment of behavioral disturbance must address the behavior that proves disabling for the patient or the caregiver. In many cases, nonpharmacologic approaches may suffice. This may include diverting the patient's attention, changing the subject of conversation, comforting the patient affectionately, or occupying the patient with a task. Environmental manipulation, caregiver support, and day programs all provide structure and routine for the patient with behavior problems as well as his or her caregiver. In cases where such interventions prove less effective for behavior management, or safety is compromised by aberrant behavior, pharmacologic treatments should be used. The chosen medication should address the primary aspect of behavior aberration, such as antidepressants for low mood and vegetative symptoms, mood stabilizers for emotional lability, or antipsychotics for psychotic symptoms and combativeness. Prevention of functional decline requires comprehensive management of both cognitive and behavioral disturbances as well as provision of support and education to the caregiver. Routine follow-up of patients with their primary caregiver is essential to maximize quality of life for all involved.

Dementia and Driving

One of the most difficult aspects of counseling dementia patients and families relates to safety of operating a motor vehicle. Driving safety in AD is well studied and there is clear evidence that relative risk of crashes for drivers with AD, from mild to severe stages of dementia, is greater than accepted societal standards. Drivers with MCI seem to have risk for crashes similar to teenage drivers. Several studies link driving risk with dementia severity utilizing the Clinical Dementia Rating (CDR) scale. The CDR is an informant-based scale that includes direct assessment of the patient as well as information given by a knowledgeable informant. The CDR scores increase from 0 (normal) to 0.5 (possible dementia) to 1.0–3.0 (mild, moderate, severe dementia). Most clinicians do not routinely use this scale in their everyday practice and, therefore, translating the scale scores into everyday terms may be difficult. For practical purposes, the CDR score of 0.5 loosely translates into MCI, whereas a CDR score of 1.0 or greater translates to dementia. There may be exceptions to these findings, and further research is required to find more specific patterns of cognitive impairment that lead to driving risk. Risk of driving in non-Alzheimer dementia is relatively unstudied. It is safe to assume, however, that driving risk is increased in this population as well.

ALZHEIMER DISEASE

Clinical Vignette

A 75-year-old man became lost driving to his daughter's house; he was subsequently referred for cognitive evaluation. He is a retired accountant, college graduate, and competitive bridge player. The patient has no specific complaints, stating he came to the doctor's appointment because of family members' concerns about increasing short-term memory loss. He expresses frustration with family members' "overblown concerns," but he acknowledges occasionally forgetting people's names and trouble finding words during conversation. He excuses his recent driving error, stating "it could happen to anyone."

His wife paints a direful picture. She reports the patient's mentation is declining progressively. Two to three years earlier he began forgetting friends' and neighbors' names. Subsequently, he became increasingly repetitive and easily frustrated when she would try reminding him of recent conversation. About 1 year earlier, he made mistakes with the bills and bounced several checks, prompting her to take over the checkbook. He gave up playing bridge and reading. He spends increasing amounts of time sitting in front of his computer but does not seem to be accomplishing anything. When she tries to get him to go out to visit friends or family, he refuses and, occasionally, becomes angry with her. The patient recalls becoming angry but cannot recall the details of the events. She is concerned he may be mismanaging his medications because of recent changes in blood sugar levels. When he misplaces things, such as his wallet, he accuses her of taking it. He is reluctant to let her supervise his medications. Within the past 6 months, while driving he has had trouble finding his way around town.

On examination, he appears well. His mood is good and his affect is appropriate. He is fully awake and alert. He scores 18/30 on the MMSE, losing points on orientation items, all three memory items, and on serial seven subtractions. Additionally, he could not copy the intersecting pentagon figure. There was no evidence of apraxia or agnosia. His remaining neurologic examination was completely normal.

Brain MRI showed mild, diffuse atrophy, bilateral periventricular/subcortical white matter "microvascular" changes, and two chronic lacunar strokes in the right striatum and cerebellar hemisphere. Thyroid, vitamin B$_{12}$, folate, and rapid plasma reagin (RPR) studies were normal. Hemoglobin A1C was elevated.

Initially donepezil was prescribed and memantine added 6 months later. His MMSE scores remained relatively stable over the next 3 years. He never resumed bridge playing but he is more engaged and outgoing during this time. His wife enrolls him in a day program 4 days per week. There is a gradual decline in daily activities and, 4 years later, his MMSE score is 12/30. He now requires assistance with personal hygiene and with dressing. He continue to decline slowly until entering a nursing home approximately 10 years after disease onset.

Epidemiology

Alzheimer disease is the most common cause of dementia in adults, accounting for approximately 5 million cases of dementia in the United States of America. Age-specific disease incidence increases exponentially with advancing age; the risk of development of AD doubles every 5 years, beginning at 65 years of age. AD affects approximately 50% of the population aged 85 years and older. Given the growing elderly population in developed countries, projections of future AD prevalence show a fourfold increase through 2050. Because dementia is a major factor in health care costs, morbidity, and mortality, the high prevalence of AD places enormous burdens on the health care system. In many cases, diagnosis is delayed until an advanced stage, at which point caregiver stress is already high and treatment options are limited. Of the 5 million prevalent cases, only 3 million are diagnosed and only one third of diagnosed cases receive treatment. Of those that receive treatment, the percentage receiving adequate doses and follow-up is unknown. It is very important for clinicians to understand the natural history of AD, recognize early warning signs, implement appropriate screening and diagnostic tools, prescribe appropriate treatment, and follow patients regularly.

Pathogenesis

There is pronounced gross cerebral atrophy clearly evident on both imaging studies and post mortem. Typically, the dementia of AD preferentially affects the frontal, temporal, and parietal cortex. This is particularly evident in the temporoparietal and frontal association areas as well as the olfactory cortex. In contrast, other primary sensory cortical areas are unaffected. Additionally, the limbic system as well as subcortical nuclei as well as the nucleus basalis of Meynert are preferentially affected. Microscopically, there is clear loss of both neurons and neuropil. The classic findings include senile plaques and neurofibrillary tangles (Figs. 18-1 and 18-2). The white matter sometimes demonstrates a secondary demyelination.

β-AMYLOID

Alzheimer disease is a neurodegenerative disorder thought to result from deposition of the protein β-amyloid in the brain. β-Amyloid is formed by processing of the amyloid precursor protein (APP), a protein that may help regulate synaptic integrity and function, possibly by regulating excitotoxic activity of glutamate. APP is encoded on chromosome 21. It is processed

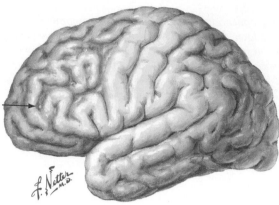

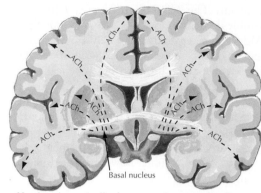

Regional atrophy of brain with narrowed gyri and widened sulci (arrow), but precentral and postcentral, inferior frontal, angular, supramarginal, and some occipital gyri fairly well preserved. Association cortex mostly involved.

Basal nucleus

Section of brain schematically demonstrating postulated normal transport of acetylcholine (ACh) from basal nucleus of Meynert (substantia innominata) to cortical gray matter

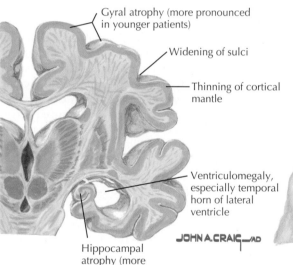

Gyral atrophy (more pronounced in younger patients)

Widening of sulci

Thinning of cortical mantle

Ventriculomegaly, especially temporal horn of lateral ventricle

Hippocampal atrophy (more pronounced in older patients)

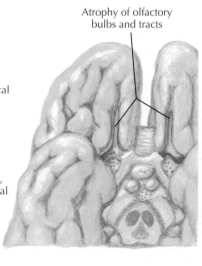

Atrophy of olfactory bulbs and tracts

JOHN A. CRAIG—AD

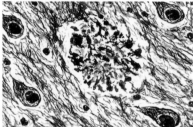

Senile plaque (center) made up of argyrophil fibers around core of pink-staining amyloid (Bodian preparation). Neurons decreased in number, with characteristic tangles in cytoplasm.

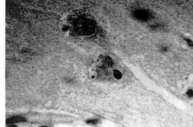

Section of hippocampus showing granulovacuolar inclusions and loss of pyramidal cells

Figure 18-1 Alzheimer Disease: Pathology.

at the cell membrane by secretase enzymes, called α-, β-, and γ-secretases. Two known membrane-bound proteins, called presenilins, comprise the active domains of the membrane-bound γ-secretase protein: presenilin 1 and presenilin 2 are encoded on chromosomes 14 and 1, respectively. Numerous genetic mutations of the presenilin and APP genes are known to cause familial, early-onset cases of AD. The familial forms of AD account for fewer than 5% of all AD cases. The known mutations account for approximately 50% of familial AD. In all cases, the genetic mutation leads to an overproduction of β-amyloid that may be the first step in the subsequent cascade of neurodegeneration.

β-Amyloid is a short fragment of the APP, typically 40–42 amino acids in length, which accumulates outside the cell during APP processing (Figs. 18-3 and 18-4). The tertiary structure of the 42–amino acid fragment is a β-pleated sheet that renders it insoluble. Consequently, it accumulates slowly, over many years,

in the extracellular space and within synapses. In vitro studies confirm that β-amyloid is toxic to surrounding synapses and neurons, causing synaptic membrane destruction and eventual cell death. Transgenic mouse models show a clear association between accumulation of β-amyloid fragments, formation of amyloid plaques, and development of cognitive impairment.

In vivo, β-amyloid fragments coalesce to form *"diffuse"* or *immature plaques*, best seen with silver-staining techniques. Diffuse plaques, however, are not sufficient to produce dementia; many nondemented elderly patients have substantial depositions of diffuse plaques throughout the cortex, a condition termed pathologic aging. It is when these plaques mature into *"senile"* or *neuritic plaques* that dementia becomes more likely (Fig. 18-5, top). Senile plaques consist of other substances in addition to β-amyloid, including synaptic proteins, inflammatory proteins, neuritic threads, activated glial cells, and other components. Unlike diffuse plaques, senile plaques are

In neocortex, primary involvement of association areas (especially temporoparietal and frontal) with relative sparing of primary sensory cortices (except olfactory) and motor cortices

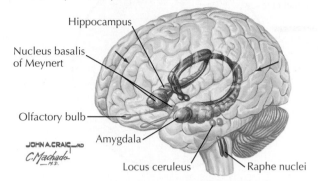

Pathologic involvement of limbic system and subcortical nuclei projecting to cortex

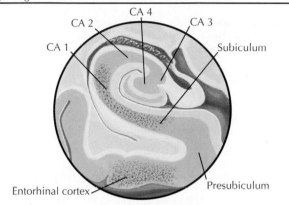

In hippocampus, neurofibrillary tangles, neuronal loss, and senile plaques primarily located in layer CA1, subiculum, and entorhinal cortex

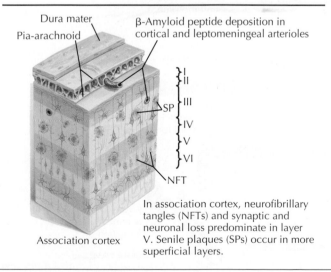

In association cortex, neurofibrillary tangles (NFTs) and synaptic and neuronal loss predominate in layer V. Senile plaques (SPs) occur in more superficial layers.

Figure 18-2 Distribution of Pathology in Alzheimer Disease.

composed of a central core of β-amyloid surrounded by a myriad of proteins and cellular debris. Senile plaques are distributed diffusely in the cortex, typically starting in the hippocampus and the basal forebrain. Senile plaque formation correlates with increasing loss of synapses, which correlates with the earliest clinical sign, namely, short-term memory loss. The anatomic

pattern of progression gradually spreads to neocortical and sub-cortical gray matter of the temporal, parietal, frontal, and, eventually, occipital cortex. Subcortical nuclei become involved relatively late in the process.

NEUROFIBRILLARY TANGLES

The second pathologic hallmark of AD is the neurofibrillary tangle (Fig. 18-5, bottom). These lesions develop and conform to an anatomic pattern that correlates with the clinical syndrome; the number and distribution of tangles are directly related to the severity and clinical features of the dementia. Neurofibrillary tangles form intracellularly, consisting of a *microtubule-associated protein, tau,* which has a vital role in the maintenance of neuronal cytoskeleton structure and function. Tau is hyperphosphorylated in AD, causing it to dissociate from the cytoskeleton and accumulate, forming a paired helical filament protein structure. The cytoskeleton is compromised structurally and functionally, disrupting normal cell function. The most commonly used pathologic criteria for definitive AD diagnosis at autopsy require the presence of senile plaques and neurofibrillary tangles. Other lesions, such as Hirano bodies, are also seen in AD but have little diagnostic specificity.

NEUROTRANSMITTERS

In addition to neuronal and synaptic loss, there is a gradual loss of various neurotransmitters. *Acetylcholine* synthesis is the earliest and most prominently affected. Most acetylcholinergic neurons arise within the *nucleus basalis of Meynert* in the basal forebrain (see Fig. 18-2). This nucleus is affected relatively early in the process; acetylcholine levels within the brain and spinal fluid of patients with AD quickly decline with disease progression. This observation supported the cholinergic hypothesis—that acetylcholine depletion results in the cognitive decline observed in patients with AD—eventually leading to the first symptomatic treatment of AD.

Risk Factors

Epidemiologic studies identify several potential risk factors for AD. The most consistent risk factors include advanced age, family history (especially in first-degree relatives), and ApoE genotype. Other risk factors include hypertension, stroke, and fasting homocysteine levels (Fig. 18-6). Because vascular risk factors are modifiable, they may affect risk reduction and treatment for patients with AD and those at risk for development of AD.

1. *Advanced age* is the single consistently identified risk factor for AD across numerous all-international studies. AD incidence and prevalence increase with advancing age, leading to the hypothesis that AD would develop in all individuals if they lived long enough. The true incidence in persons older than age 85 years is difficult to ascertain because of sharp decline in life expectancy. However, there are many instances of nondemented elders where no pathologic evidence of AD is found at autopsy, including in centenarians. Therefore, dementia is not considered a "normal" part of aging.

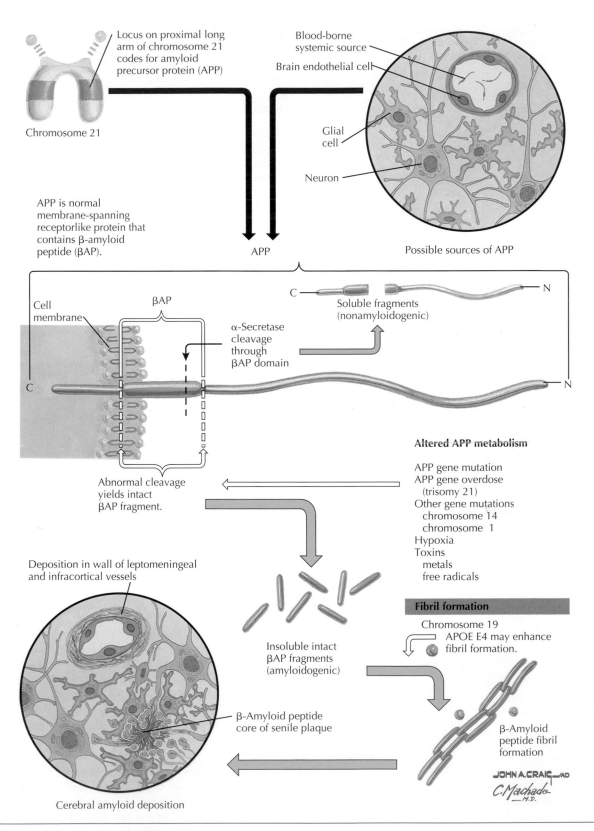

Locus on proximal long arm of chromosome 21 codes for amyloid precursor protein (APP)

Chromosome 21

Blood-borne systemic source

Brain endothelial cell

Glial cell

Neuron

Possible sources of APP

APP is normal membrane-spanning receptorlike protein that contains β-amyloid peptide (βAP).

APP

Cell membrane

βAP

Soluble fragments (nonamyloidogenic)

C

N

α-Secretase cleavage through βAP domain

C

N

Abnormal cleavage yields intact βAP fragment.

Altered APP metabolism

APP gene mutation
APP gene overdose (trisomy 21)
Other gene mutations
chromosome 14
chromosome 1
Hypoxia
Toxins
metals
free radicals

Deposition in wall of leptomeningeal and infracortical vessels

Insoluble intact βAP fragments (amyloidogenic)

Fibril formation

Chromosome 19
APOE E4 may enhance fibril formation.

β-Amyloid peptide core of senile plaque

β-Amyloid peptide fibril formation

Cerebral amyloid deposition

JOHN A. CRAIG—MD
C. Machado M.D.

Figure 18-3 Amyloidogenesis in Alzheimer Disease.

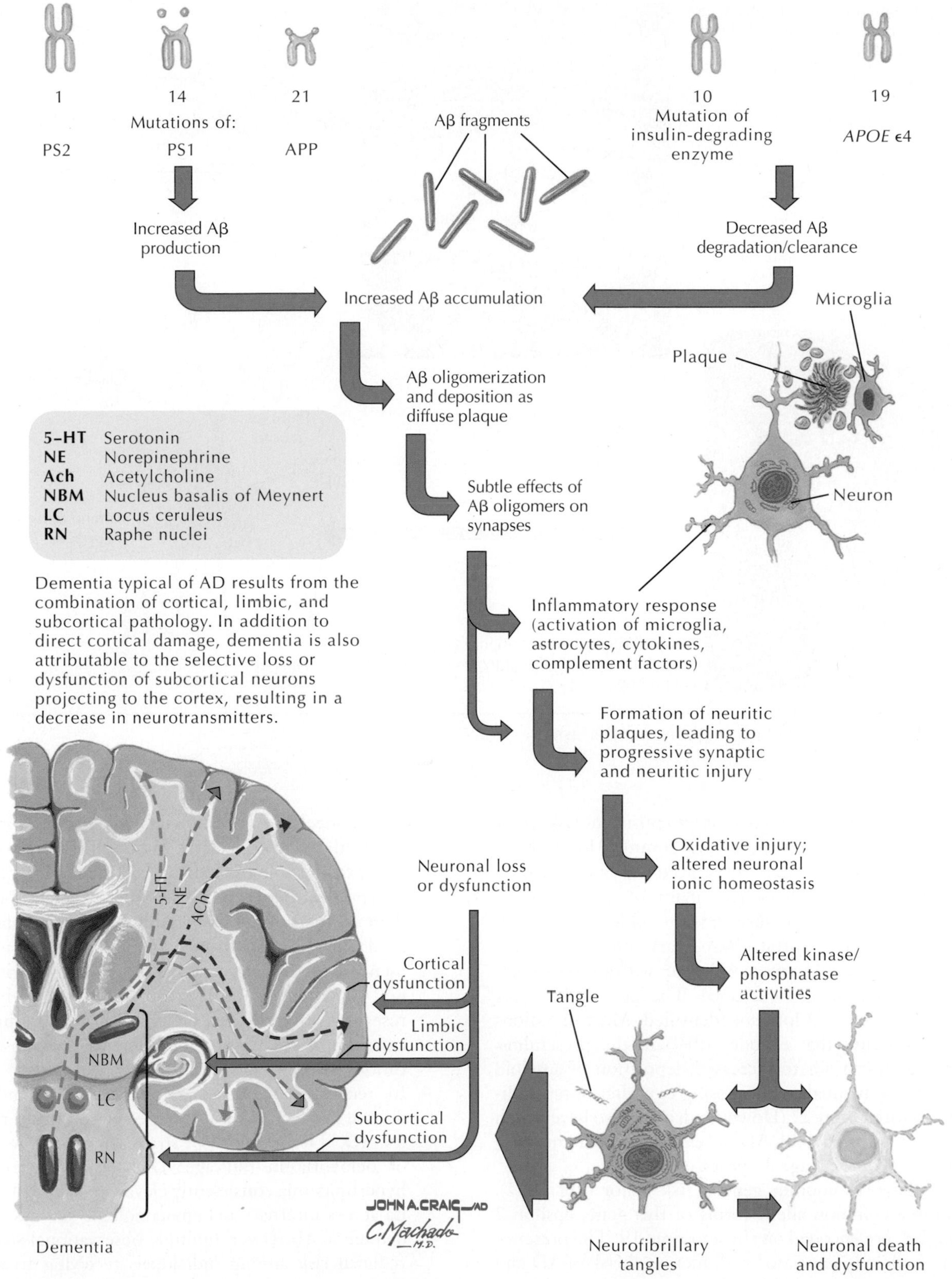
1
14
21
10
19
Mutations of:
PS2
PS1
APP
Aβ fragments
Mutation of insulin-degrading enzyme
APOE ϵ4
Increased Aβ production
Decreased Aβ degradation/clearance
Increased Aβ accumulation
Microglia
Plaque
Aβ oligomerization and deposition as diffuse plaque
5-HT Serotonin
NE Norepinephrine
Ach Acetylcholine
NBM Nucleus basalis of Meynert
LC Locus ceruleus
RN Raphe nuclei
Subtle effects of Aβ oligomers on synapses
Neuron
Dementia typical of AD results from the combination of cortical, limbic, and subcortical pathology. In addition to direct cortical damage, dementia is also attributable to the selective loss or dysfunction of subcortical neurons projecting to the cortex, resulting in a decrease in neurotransmitters.
Inflammatory response (activation of microglia, astrocytes, cytokines, complement factors)
Formation of neuritic plaques, leading to progressive synaptic and neuritic injury
5-HT
NE
ACh
Neuronal loss or dysfunction
Oxidative injury; altered neuronal ionic homeostasis
Cortical dysfunction
Limbic dysfunction
Altered kinase/ phosphatase activities
Tangle
NBM
LC
RN
Subcortical dysfunction
JOHN A.CRAIG—AD
C.Machado —M.D.
Dementia
Neurofibrillary tangles
Neuronal death and dysfunction

Figure 18-4 Amyloid Cascade Hypothesis in Alzheimer Disease.

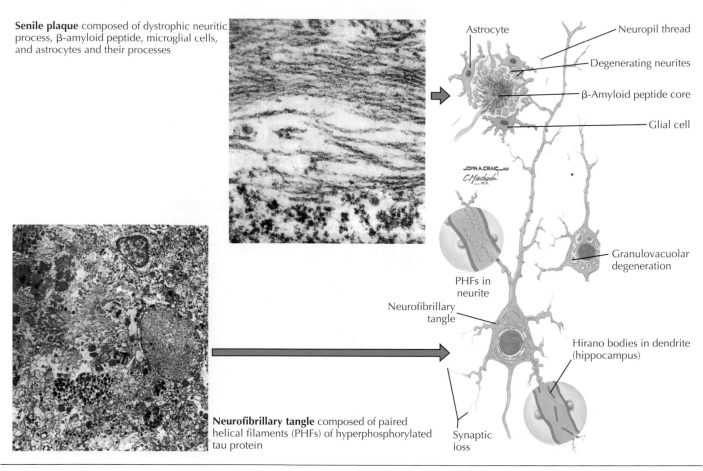

Senile plaque composed of dystrophic neuritic process, β-amyloid peptide, microglial cells, and astrocytes and their processes

Astrocyte

Neuropil thread

Degenerating neurites

β-Amyloid peptide core

Glial cell

JOHN A. CRAIG
C. Machado

PHFs in neurite

Granulovacuolar degeneration

Neurofibrillary tangle

Hirano bodies in dendrite (hippocampus)

Neurofibrillary tangle composed of paired helical filaments (PHFs) of hyperphosphorylated tau protein

Synaptic loss

Figure 18-5 Microscopic Pathology in Alzheimer Disease.

2. *Family history* of dementia is another consistent risk factor in many studies; however, the most common form of AD occurs sporadically. Establishing accurate family history of dementia is difficult because many of these patients' relatives may not have survived into older ages where dementia risk is greatest. Rare, early-onset, presenile (before age 65 years) forms of AD occur with an autosomal-dominant pattern of inheritance. The genetic basis for many hereditary AD forms is identified. Most mutations affect the genes that encode APP and the presenilins. Each mutation leads to increased deposition of amyloid in affected individuals, predisposing to earlier onset. Individuals with trisomy 21 (Down syndrome) also have a high deposition of β-amyloid. AD develops in all patients with Down syndrome by age 35 years.

3. *ApoE genotype* is another genetic risk factor (Fig. 18-7). The three common allelic forms of this gene, epsilon 2 through 4, are encoded on chromosome 19. The presence of an e4 allele is associated with increased risk of AD and younger age at onset. This risk is greatly increased in e4 homozygotes. Conversely, the e2 allele appears to impart a protective, risk-lowering effect, as replicated in numerous international, population-based studies. The association between the ApoE e4 allele and AD seems to be disease specific. There is no clear association between e4 and other neurodegenerative or amyloid-based diseases.

The mechanism underlying this increased risk associated with the Apo e4 allele is not well understood but may relate to the role of ApoE in cell membrane repair. Phenotypically, the e4 cases have greater amyloid deposition than do the non-e4 cases. Although ApoE genotyping is available, it is not a diagnostic test for AD, nor is it recommended for routine testing. Most patients with AD are non-e4 carriers. ApoE genotyping is largely used in research, primarily as a biological marker to differentiate cases. Some studies suggest differential response to medications in cases stratified by ApoE genotypes.

4. In recent years, cerebrovascular disease and vascular disease risk factors have emerged as significant risk factors for AD. The presence of stroke increases the likelihood of dementia in old age. Diabetes, hypertension, and hyperlipidemia consistently elevate relative risk of dementia across international epidemiologic surveys of AD and dementia. Moreover, multiple observational studies show reduced risk among individuals receiving treatment for these conditions. This connection between AD and cerebrovascular disease may provide an important focus for premorbid dementia prevention. It is unknown whether secondary stroke prevention reduces the likelihood of dementia or its rate of progression. Nevertheless, assessment of stroke risk factors may become increasingly important for the management of dementia patients.

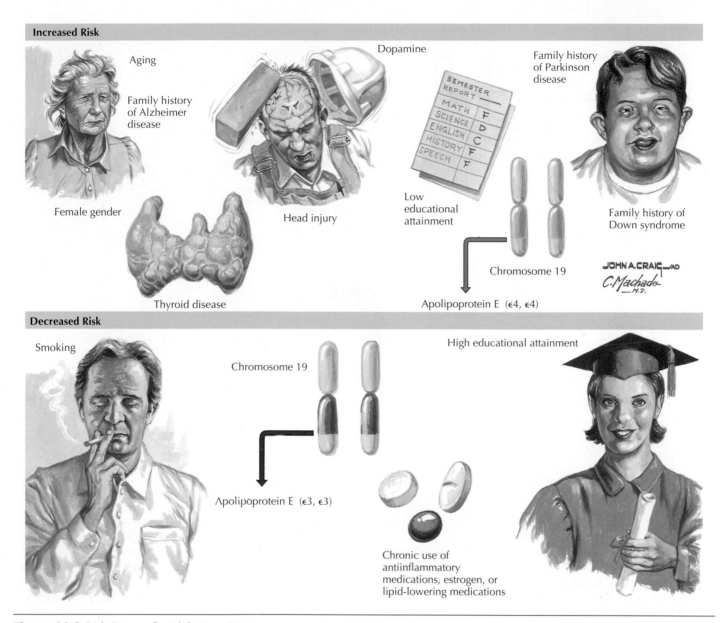

Increased Risk

Aging

Family history of Alzheimer disease

Female gender

Thyroid disease

Dopamine

Head injury

SEMESTER REPORT
MATH	F
SCIENCE	D
ENGLISH	C
HISTORY	F
SPEECH	F

Low educational attainment

Chromosome 19

Apolipoprotein E (ε4, ε4)

Family history of Parkinson disease

Family history of Down syndrome

JOHN A. CRAIG—AD
C. Machado M.D.

Decreased Risk

Smoking

Chromosome 19

Apolipoprotein E (ε3, ε3)

Chronic use of antiinflammatory medications, estrogen, or lipid-lowering medications

High educational attainment

Figure 18-6 Risk Factors for Alzheimer Disease.

Clinical Presentation

The early signs of AD may be subtle (Fig. 18-8). In the initial stages of AD, memory losses can be clinically distinguished from normal aging, although formal memory testing is often required to confirm suspicion of early dementia. The early signs of Alzheimer begin insidiously, progress slowly, and are often covered up by patients. Detection may be challenging even for close family members. The physician may observe changes in patient's pattern of behavior, such as missing appointments or poor compliance with medications. It is important to discuss such issues openly with family members given the patient often cannot recall examples of memory problems. Indeed, it is common for patients to have limited insight into their deficit, and for family members to initiate an evaluation for memory loss. In these early stages, patients maintain their social graces. It is not uncommon during mental status testing to discover the significant cognitive problems concealed by a patient's friendly

and sociable affect. "Very pleasant" patients sometimes fool even seasoned geriatricians. The Alzheimer's Association lists 10 key warning signs of AD.

Commonly, AD begins with short-term memory loss, although atypical presentations sometimes develop. Often, patients have increasing forgetfulness of words and names, relying more on lists, calendars, and family members for reminders. Disorganization of appointments, bills, and medications becomes commonplace. Family members often notice increasing repetitiveness, patients asking the same question or repeating the same conversation minutes after it was completed. Patients may forget to convey telephone messages or turn off the stove, or lose track of where they place things. Moreover, their ability to recall these incidents is impaired. They "forget that they forget." Affected individuals may become suspicious of others, thinking that misplaced items were stolen, for example.

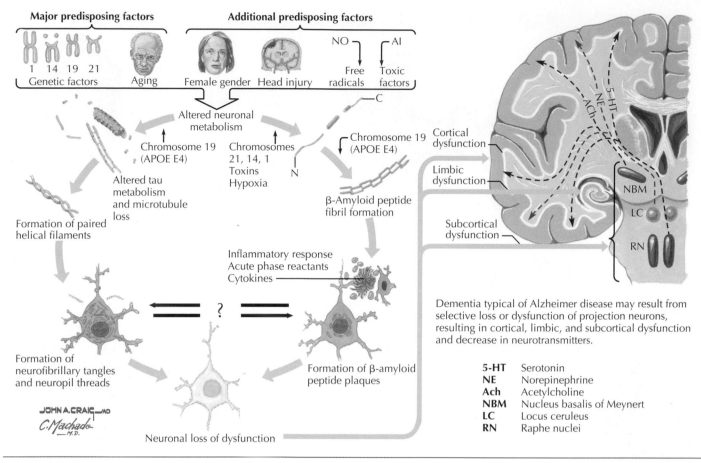

Figure 18-7 Possible Factors in Development and Progression of Alzheimer Disease.

Language function gradually declines. Word-finding and name-finding difficulties are common even in very early stages. Naming impairment and gradual loss of comprehension, expression, or both are universal. The perception of the temporal sequence of events is affected and disorientation eventually becomes pervasive. Geographic orientation declines, first affecting patients' ability to navigate in unfamiliar environments and later within their homes. Visuospatial skills decline and construction deficits may occur early.

Behavior and personality in patients with AD are often affected; combativeness, irritability, frustration, and anxiety become extremely common. Many patients seek medical attention only when family members are alarmed by behavioral changes, rather than because of their earlier progressive memory loss. Psychotic features may become prominent. Some patients also develop delusional thoughts and hallucinations, most commonly visual or auditory in nature. These may be benign, understated, hidden, or frightening and may lead to severe agitation. Family members may not speak freely in the patient's presence about these symptoms.

As cognitive and behavioral changes appear, the patients' ability to maintain personal independence declines. Altered activities that may occur early include medication mismanagement, financial disorganization, burnt pots on the stove, and driving errors. Eventually patients require assistance with activities of daily living: personal hygiene/bathing, eating, dressing, and toileting. Often, by this stage, patients exhibit signs

of Parkinsonism characterized by midline rigidity, symmetric bradykinesia and hypokinesia, stooped posture, and shuffling stride. The risk of falling increases. Seizures occur in up to 20% of cases. Myoclonic jerks are increasingly noted in advanced stages.

Later stages of AD are characterized by loss of bladder and then bowel control, failure to recognize family members, and eventually severe akinesia, requiring total nursing care. The most common cause of death is aspiration pneumonia. On average, AD has a duration of approximately 8 years. However, this varies substantially. Some patients live 20 years or more. Nursing care marks an important end point for many patients and their caregivers. The most common causes for nursing home placement include behavioral problems, immobility, and incontinence.

The Alzheimer's Association provides a staging system to allow doctors and caregivers a frame of reference when discussing the patient's level of impairment and possible future progression. It is important to emphasize that not every patient will follow through these stages in the same way or at the same rate.

Differential Diagnosis

The *absence of motor deficits* early in AD differentiates it from most other dementias. Other dementias lacking motor signs include amnestic syndrome (Korsakoff encephalopathy), Pick disease, vascular dementia, and HIV dementia complex.

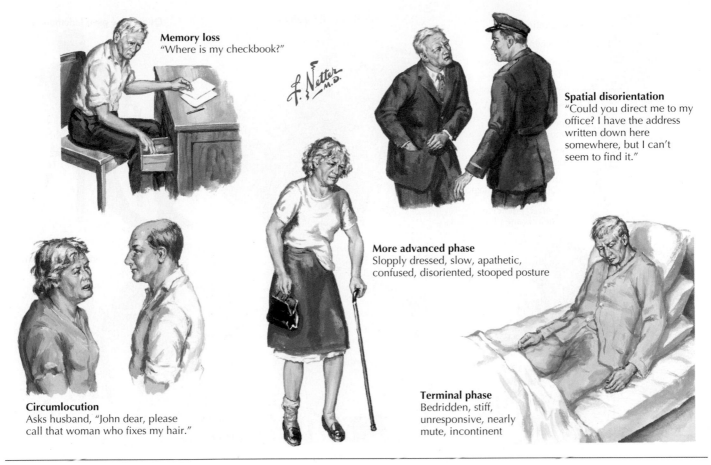

Memory loss
"Where is my checkbook?"

Spatial disorientation
"Could you direct me to my office? I have the address written down here somewhere, but I can't seem to find it."

More advanced phase
Slopply dressed, slow, apathetic, confused, disoriented, stooped posture

Circumlocution
Asks husband, "John dear, please call that woman who fixes my hair."

Terminal phase
Bedridden, stiff, unresponsive, nearly mute, incontinent

Figure 18-8 Alzheimer Disease: Clinical Manifestations, Progressive Phases.

Depression can also produce dementia-like symptoms without motor deficits. Poor concentration and short-term memory impairment result from lack of effort, disinterest, or distractibility. "Pseudo dementia" due to depression is usually not progressive, and functional loss is often disproportionately severe relative to cognitive impairment (Fig. 18-9).

Reversible causes of dementia without motor signs include toxic and metabolic causes of chronic delirium. Chronic use of medication with anticholinergic side effects (e.g., antihistamines and tricyclic antidepressants) is a possible cause of chronic delirium that may mimic AD. β-Blockers, digoxin, H_2 blockers, and various antibiotics may also contribute to chronic delirium. Chronic mass effect, caused by a slow-growing tumor (Fig. 18-9), may also produce reversible cognitive impairment.

Dementia *with motor deficits* includes a longer list of possibilities. Thyroid disease, vitamin B_{12} deficiency, and tertiary neurosyphilis are often considered; however, these conditions rarely cause dementia and usually present with characteristic metabolic or sensorimotor symptoms.

Normal pressure hydrocephalus is a relatively uncommon condition that late in its course may be characterized by a significant dementia (see Fig. 32-2). Typically, these individuals present with a broad-based magnetic gait as if their feet were partially glued to the ground. Eventually these patients may become unwittingly incontinent, unaware of their loss of sphincter control as the dementing process evolves. Although

these patients most often have no identifiable cause on occasion, they have previously sustained a subarachnoid hemorrhage or meningitis leading to poor cerebrospinal fluid (CSF) reabsorption. This leads to the characteristic hydrocephalus without an associated loss of cortical mantel. A CSF shunt may lead to a remarkable improvement.

The presence of spastic hemiparesis or dysarthria raises suspicion of cerebrovascular disease. Parkinsonism is associated with Parkinson disease (PD) and dementia with Lewy bodies. Progressive ataxia occurs with multisystem atrophy. Chorea characterizes Huntington disease. As AD progresses to late stages, parkinsonism often becomes evident, making clinical differentiation from other parkinsonian diseases more difficult. AD may also coexist with cerebrovascular or Lewy body pathology to produce dementia with motor signs.

Dementia may be further characterized by cortical and subcortical cognitive features, which also helps differentiate between different dementing diseases. Subcortical features include slower mental processing, slow retrieval of information, and often significant extrapyramidal motor signs, including bradykinesia or adventitious movements.

Diagnosis

The subjective complaint of memory impairment is not useful for dementia screening because it is a common complaint in

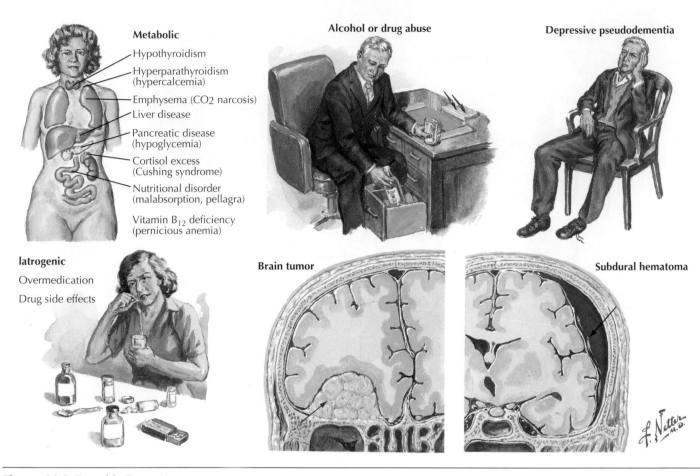

Metabolic
- Hypothyroidism
- Hyperparathyroidism (hypercalcemia)
- Emphysema (CO_2 narcosis)
- Liver disease
- Pancreatic disease (hypoglycemia)
- Cortisol excess (Cushing syndrome)
- Nutritional disorder (malabsorption, pellagra)
- Vitamin B_{12} deficiency (pernicious anemia)

Alcohol or drug abuse

Depressive pseudodementia

Iatrogenic
Overmedication
Drug side effects

Brain tumor

Subdural hematoma

Figure 18-9 Treatable Dementias.

older adults. Prospective evaluation of individuals aged 65 years who have complaints of memory loss show that dementia develops in fewer than 9% within a 5-year follow-up. However, dementia develops during a 5-year prospective follow-up in 50% of patients aged 85 years who had no complaints of memory loss at baseline. Consequently, clinicians must be proactive, particularly with patients aged 85 years or older, and screen for cognitive impairment.

Proper clinical assessment requires a detailed history, preferably provided by a trustworthy, knowledgeable informant particularly a spouse or child. The history should describe the cognitive decline, in temporal sequence, from earliest suggestion of cognitive impairment to most recent events. Examination in early stages may reveal no neurologic deficits other than cognitive impairment. In later stages, or in patients with coexisting neuropathology, such as stroke, there may be motor deficits or other focal CNS findings on physical examination.

MENTAL STATUS EXAM

The mental status examination (see Chapter 2) should assess all major cognitive domains, including *M*emory, *A*ttention, *L*anguage, *C*onstruction, *O*rientation, *P*raxis, and *E*xecutive function (MALCOPE). Standardized global measures of cognitive function such as the MMSE are of limited diagnostic value. The widely used MMSE is relatively insensitive to the milder stages of AD. Other tests, such as the Montreal Cognitive Assessment

test, include test items more suited to detecting earlier stages of cognitive impairment allowing improved sensitivity for detecting MCI. Another measure, the Alzheimer Disease 8 (AD8) is an informant-based tool that may shorten screening considerably. It must be emphasized that such instruments are not diagnostic tests, and interpretation of results must take into consideration level of education, native language, and physical or sensory impairment that might affect performance.

Impaired recording of information characterizes the memory loss of early AD. The inability to record information occurs when patients cannot recall information even with practice and when given hints or cues. Additional early cognitive deficits in AD include *dysnomia, reduced verbal fluency (especially in word categories), orientation to time,* and *construction impairment.* Having the patient list as many category words as possible within 1 minute provides a test of *verbal fluency.* For example, patients try to list animals, or words beginning with the letter *s.*

Clock drawing is useful when testing *construction and executive function* (Fig. 18-10). Patients draw a clock indicating 1:45, for example, on a blank sheet of paper. Their performance is observed from beginning to end, including the shape and size, number order and placement, hand size and placement, etc. The strategy (or lack thereof) used to draw the clock manifests itself readily, indicating impaired executive function in following a set of rules, or organizing and executing a multistep task. When patients finish, they should try copying a clock that the examiner

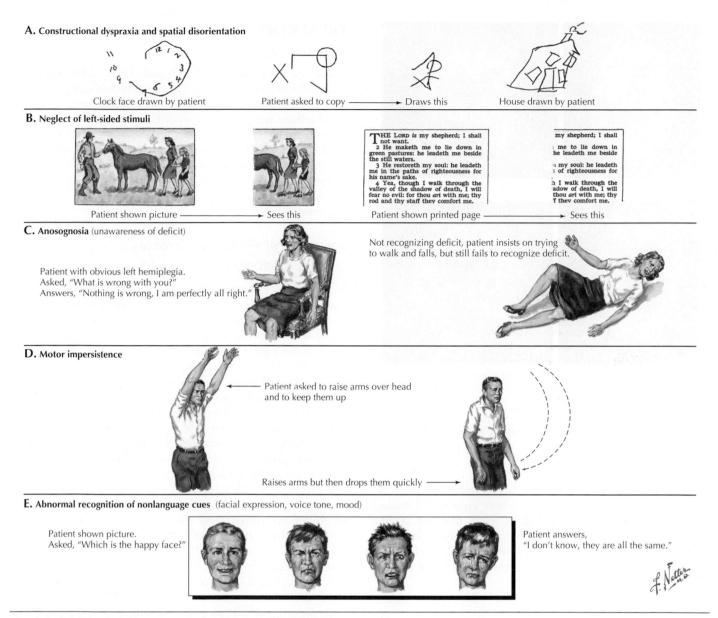

A. Constructional dyspraxia and spatial disorientation

Clock face drawn by patient

Patient asked to copy ⟶ Draws this

House drawn by patient

B. Neglect of left-sided stimuli

Patient shown picture ⟶ Sees this

Patient shown printed page ⟶ Sees this

C. Anosognosia (unawareness of deficit)

Patient with obvious left hemiplegia.
Asked, "What is wrong with you?"
Answers, "Nothing is wrong, I am perfectly all right."

Not recognizing deficit, patient insists on trying to walk and falls, but still fails to recognize deficit.

D. Motor impersistence

Patient asked to raise arms over head and to keep them up

Raises arms but then drops them quickly ⟶

E. Abnormal recognition of nonlanguage cues (facial expression, voice tone, mood)

Patient shown picture.
Asked, "Which is the happy face?"

Patient answers, "I don't know, they are all the same."

Figure 18-10 Nondominant Hemisphere Cortical Dysfunction.

draws in front of them. The numbers 12, 6, 3, and 9 are placed first, and the hands drawn accurately. If *construction problems* exist, patients have difficulty with the copy task as well as with the command task. If the copy is good, construction problems may not be a factor in cognitive impairment. There are many standardized, brief mental status tests like these available to clinicians. Routine use of such tests allows for longitudinal assessment and staging of dementia severity.

ADDITIONAL TESTING

Brain Imaging

All patients with evidence of cognitive impairment should undergo structural brain imaging with MRI or when not available, CT. This may show findings of non-AD-related changes such as stroke, subdural hematoma, tumor, or hydrocephalus (Fig. 18-9).

Quantitative or volumetric imaging may provide more accurate assessment of regional atrophy and provide better imaging resolution of AD-related changes. These modalities are not yet ready for routine clinical use. Functional imaging, such as FDG-PET and single photon emission computed tomography (SPECT) scans, may also be considered. FDG-PET scanning may be useful in differentiating AD from frontotemporal dementia (FTD) and could be considered in select cases as a diagnostic tool. The role of PET in MCI remains controversial, although PET imaging detects the changes of AD very early in the course. Eventually, PET scanning may provide a way to predict decline in MCI. Most recently, PET scanning using biomarkers for β-amyloid have allowed researchers to image the presence and distribution of amyloid plaque in AD patients. SPECT scans do not provide a significant improvement in detecting AD beyond routine assessment and are not recommended.

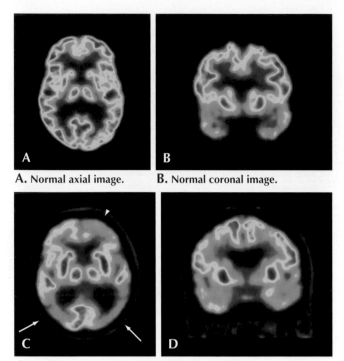

A. Normal axial image.

B. Normal coronal image.

C. and D. Reduced activity within temporal and parietal lobes (arrows) and early decreased activity in left frontal lobe consistent with advancing disease (arrowhead).

Figure 18-11 FDG-PET Typical Pattern for Alzheimer Disease.

CSF Biomarkers

Decreased β-amyloid and increase tau/phosphotau concentrations in spinal fluid may be detected very early in the disease. The sensitivity and specificity of these assays, however, is not a proven improvement over routine noninvasive, diagnostic approaches. More research into these tests is needed before they can be recommended for routine assessment of AD in most patients.

Blood Tests

There is no standard test panel to diagnose AD. Traditionally, levels of vitamin B_{12}, folate, TSH, and often serum RPR are measured. These tests may reveal a reversible cause of cognitive impairment that may contribute to overall dementia severity. The routine screening for syphilis is no longer recommended given the virtual absence of tertiary cases in the United States. Fasting homocysteine levels have been linked to increased risk of AD. The effect of decreasing homocysteine on the disease course of patients diagnosed with AD is unknown. However, premorbid reduction of homocysteine levels may decrease the risk of development of AD.

Genetic Tests

Apolipoprotein E genotyping is not diagnostic of AD. Moreover, ApoE genotyping should not be used routinely in family members because there is no specific genetic counseling to offer. The presence of an ApoE e4 genotype may only heighten anxiety unnecessarily.

TREATMENT

Treatment of MCI

There are currently no Food and Drug Administration–approved therapies for MCI. Several studies of currently available AD medications in MCI have shown mixed results. Prescriptions for patients with MCI may not be covered by insurance. The largest of these studies suggested limited benefit for donepezil in MCI for all study participants. It is noteworthy that the effect of donepezil was more pronounced and long-lived in patients with the ApoE e4 allele. The risks and benefits should be discussed carefully with MCI patients before initiating treatment.

Treatment of Alzheimer Disease

GENERAL APPROACH

Much of the management of the patient with AD revolves around family interactions. Caregivers should provide patients with a comforting and respectful living environment. As their cognitive abilities slip away, it is important to provide a setting that preserves patient dignity. AD patients particularly benefit from a structured simple approach to daily life, maintaining a routine of social and physical activities (Fig. 18-12).

MCI patients and those with very *early AD* and their caregivers should be counseled regarding driving risk as compared with cognitively healthy elder drivers. It is recommended that a driving performance evaluation be carried out. Even if felt to be safe, these patients should be reassessed on a regular basis, as progression of the disease will unequivocally require them to stop driving at a later stage of their illness.

Once an Alzheimer diagnosis is confirmed, it is imperative to protect the patient, and the public, from potential motor vehicle accidents. It is emphasized that the family and the treating physician assume responsibility for restricting the patient with AD from driving.

The assignment of simple daily chores where the individual can feel productive such as setting the table, folding clothes from the drier, or sweeping the sidewalk is recommended. Use of scheduled bathroom breaks or providing diapers keep the incontinent patient from the embarrassment of having soiled clothes that are socially obvious. Helping these individuals with simple activities of daily living such as dressing or feeding is eventually required. It is very important for the patient to have an easily seen identification bracelet. These patients have a tendency to "sun down," becoming easily confused in the dark; a simple bedlight can be very helpful for preventing this problem. Have the patient flip through an old photo album to comfort them with familiar, pleasant memories of their younger years, their childhood home, their parents.

As they become increasingly confused, it is typical for Alzheimer's patients to be more easily agitated; reassurance by relatives is often the best treatment. At times, simple anxiolytic medications, such as the SSRIs, may be useful. Eventually, a number of Alzheimer patients require long-term care to protect their family from the increasingly demanding nursing support that will eventually totally consume them emotionally and physically. The family should be reassured that the patient's cognitive decline prevents them from harboring any resentment

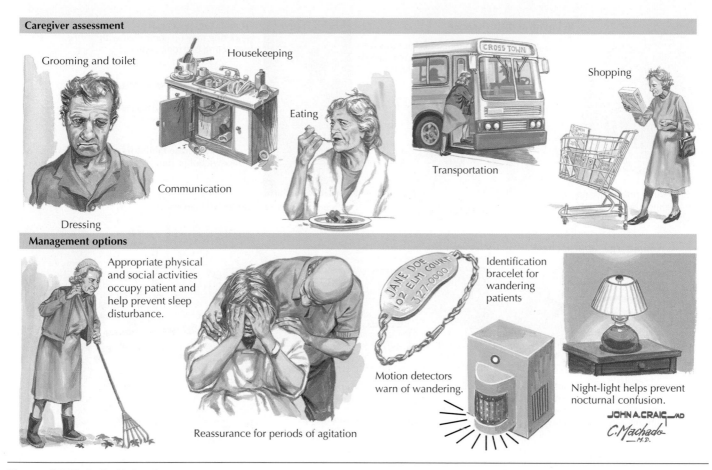

Figure 18-12 Daily Living Assessment.

for such a placement, otherwise their feelings of guilt may be overwhelming. This is a most challenging and sad experience for any family; their physicians and caregivers need to be very proactive and supportive.

CHOLINESTERASE INHIBITORS

The various agents available include donepezil, rivastigmine, and galantamine. Several studies show these medications reduce the decline on standardized tests better than placebo when used for 6–12 months, but do not slow the degenerative process. These drugs may provide some benefit if taken consistently over time. When initiating therapy patients need to increase the dose gradually. Additionally, the eventual maximum required doses of these medications is not predictable. **Cholinesterase inhibitors** are generally utilized in patients with mild to moderate AD (Fig. 18-13).

If these medications are stopped, patients may experience decline to the severity level that they would have reached without the medication. In such cases, restarting the medication may not regain lost ground. These medications are primarily effective at maximal doses. Rivastigmine is most effective at 4.5 or 6 mg twice daily. Recently, rivastigmine became available in transdermal patch form, significantly reducing the rate of side effects. Donepezil is only mildly effective at 5 mg/day, but greater benefit occurs with 10 mg/day doses. Similarly, galantamine should always be titrated to 12 mg twice daily to

maximize benefit. Galantamine is available in an extended-release formulation to allow for once-daily dosing. If patients do not tolerate these drugs at lower doses, it is prudent to try a different agent. It is unusual for patients to be unable to tolerate at least one of these three drugs. Typical adverse effects that may cause discontinuation include cholinergic effects, especially vomiting and persistent loose stools.

MEMANTINE

Memantine is an *N*-methyl-D-aspartate (NMDA) receptor antagonist that is approved for patients with moderate to severe AD. The involvement of glutamate-mediated neurotoxicity in the pathogenesis of AD is a hypothesis that is gaining increased acceptance. The keystone underlying this proposal is the assumption that glutamate receptors, in particular of the NMDA type, are overactivated in a tonic rather than a phasic manner in AD. Such continuous, mild, chronic activation may lead to neuronal damage/death. Memantine may improve memory by restoring homeostasis in the glutamatergic system—too little activation is bad, too much is even worse. Furthermore, memantine shows promise when used in combination with cholinesterase inhibitors. Memantine is primarily used as a supplemental medication in moderate to severe stages of AD. Clinical trials demonstrated that in combination with donepezil, there is improved stability of cognitive performance for 6–12 months compared to donepezil or memantine alone.

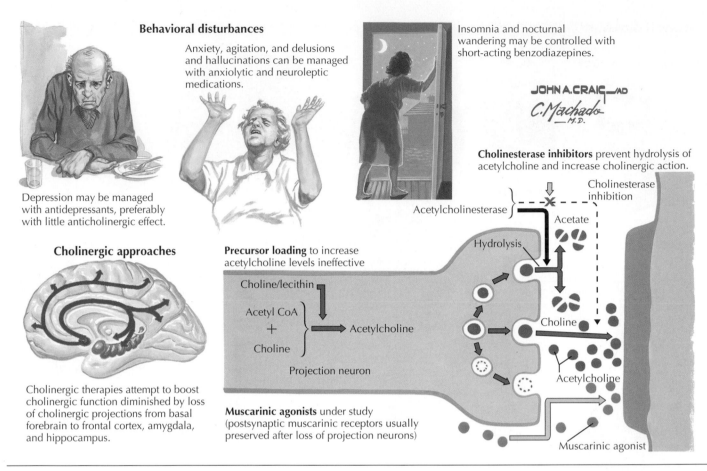

Behavioral disturbances

Anxiety, agitation, and delusions and hallucinations can be managed with anxiolytic and neuroleptic medications.

Insomnia and nocturnal wandering may be controlled with short-acting benzodiazepines.

JOHN A.CRAIG—AD
C.Machado
—M.D.

Cholinesterase inhibitors prevent hydrolysis of acetylcholine and increase cholinergic action.

Depression may be managed with antidepressants, preferably with little anticholinergic effect.

Acetylcholinesterase

Cholinesterase inhibition

Acetate

Hydrolysis

Cholinergic approaches

Cholinergic therapies attempt to boost cholinergic function diminished by loss of cholinergic projections from basal forebrain to frontal cortex, amygdala, and hippocampus.

Precursor loading to increase acetylcholine levels ineffective

Choline/lecithin

Acetyl CoA + Choline

Acetylcholine

Projection neuron

Muscarinic agonists under study (postsynaptic muscarinic receptors usually preserved after loss of projection neurons)

Choline

Acetylcholine

Muscarinic agonist

Figure 18-13 Pharmacologic Management.

The current pharmacologic treatment of AD is purely symptomatic. Long-term benefits of these medications may include a delay in need for nursing home placement. For example, using donepezil for 9–12 months may delay nursing home placement by approximately 20 months. However, functional decline continues and reasonable expectations for the effects of these medications must be emphasized to patients and their families. These treatments are associated with reduced behavioral problems and may reduce the need for sedatives in some patients. Determination of medication efficacy is challenging. When the maximum dosage is reached, annual follow-up examination is beneficial.

Repeated standardized mental status examinations are helpful. For example, the average rate of decline on the MMSE in AD is approximately 3 points per year. When a patient shows less than 3 points of decline, the medication may be helping. This method approximates the same measurements used in clinical trials of AD to assess medication efficacy. Such tests, in combination with the caregivers' subjective impressions, can help determine whether to continue or change medications.

Other potential therapies do not have unequivocal evidence to support their use. **Ginkgo biloba** may be useful with various unspecified (mixed) dementia, but efficacy data are lacking. Ginkgo showed no benefit versus placebo for treatment of AD in a large NIH-sponsored clinical trial. There is no reproduced clinical study to support utilization of anti-inflammatories (shown to lower the risk of AD in epidemiologic studies) or antioxidants. Estrogen treatment is not effective in the treatment of AD, and postmenopausal estrogen replacement in midlife may increase risk of dementia.

AD treatments of the future will likely focus on preventive strategies, including cerebrovascular risk factors in premorbid individuals at risk. For patients already demonstrating overt AD, there is increasing interest in disease-modifying therapies. Most noteworthy are a group of drugs that reduce accumulation of β-amyloid in the brain. These include a range of agents from γ-secretase inhibitors to monoclonal antibodies against amyloid.

DEMENTIA WITH LEWY BODIES

Clinical Vignette

A 78-year-old man is referred for evaluation of intermittent confusion. During the past 3 years, he had developed depression with prominent psychotic features requiring two psychiatric hospitalizations. The patient was initially very depressed and withdrawn. A trial of fluoxetine led to some disorientation and anxiety. When his hallucinations became persistently threatening, and his family could no longer distract his attention, he was switched to quetiapine. Initially, he had a poor response to low doses; gradual increases in dosage led to severe drowsiness and stiff gait. His first inpatient stay was related to increasing agitation at home because of vivid hallucinations characterized by a sensation of intruders coming into his home. During this hospitalization, he was treated with risperidone. Although his psychotic symptoms seemed to improve, he developed severe stiffness and a shuffling gait, prone to falling. Despite such he remained on this drug for nearly a year.

Once the medication was discontinued, the patient became more alert and his gait improved. However, he never returned to baseline, remaining slower than his baseline. Moreover, he appeared more forgetful, needing frequent reminders and prompts to complete tasks. Some days he seemed intoxicated, confused, disoriented, lethargic, and withdrawn. On other days, he appeared brighter, more alert, and competent. Subsequently, his psychotic symptoms returned; this led to his second psychiatric hospitalization. Formal mental status testing demonstrated significant impairment of both memory and visuospatial processing. A second trial of low-dose risperidone subdued the patient once again, but his mobility deteriorated to the point of needing a wheelchair.

During neurologic assessment, his wife revealed he had experienced severe nightmares over the past 10 years, causing him to yell, punch, and kick in his sleep. This forced his wife to sleep in another room. He fell out of bed a number of times. The patient never recalled these events. His exam was notable for an MMSE score of 22/30 and moderate symmetrical extrapyramidal motor signs, including, retropulsion, bradykinesia, and rigidity. There was no significant tremor. He did not initiate conversation and his affect was generally flat. Brain MRI showed diffuse atrophy and minimal microvascular changes. There were no metabolic signs of toxic/metabolic encephalopathy. Electroencephalography (EEG) revealed bitemporal slowing without epileptiform discharges or rhythmic abnormality.

Treatment with rivastigmine, a cholinesterase inhibitor, led to significant reduction in confusion and hallucinations. He was then taken off risperidone and remained psychiatrically stable for over a year. Although his Parkinsonism persisted, he no longer needed an assistive device to get around. Attempts at treatment with levodopa failed due to confusion and recurrent hallucinations. This patient's neurologic status slowly declined, with occasional bouts of agitated confusion. After a 5-year period nursing home placement was necessitated.

Pathogenesis

Lewy bodies (LBs), originally described at the turn of the 20th century in the substantia nigra of patients with PD, also occur in widespread areas of the cortex and other subcortical nuclei in many cases of Parkinsonism with dementia. Neurodegenerative changes with LB formation were first linked with dementia in the 1960s. Early case descriptions noted LBs distributed diffusely within the cerebral cortex and brainstem and were termed *diffuse Lewy body disease*. Subsequent neuropathologic studies found a surprisingly high frequency of LB pathology in the brains of patients with AD. These cases commonly show coexisting AD lesions and LBs and were classified as LB variant of AD.

In general, "variant" cases demonstrated relatively less AD pathology (especially NFTs) than pure AD cases matched for clinical dementia severity. Reports of Lewy neurites located in the CA2 region of the hippocampus suggest that dementia with Lewy bodies (DLB) is a unique neurodegenerative cause of dementia, independent of AD pathology. Interestingly, LBs are also found in the brains of patients with hereditary AD, suggesting a possible pathophysiologic link between these disorders. And LBs are occasionally found in the brains of nondemented elders. Few familial cases of DLB are described, and there are no known mutations associated with hereditary DLB.

A definitive pathologic diagnosis of DLB requires only the presence of cortical LB pathology, regardless of coexisting AD pathology. Many of these cases also fulfill pathologic criteria for a definitive diagnosis of AD and clinical criteria for a diagnosis of probable or possible AD. Consequently, controversy surrounds this diagnosis, and no agreement exists on a single-disease classification of cases with concomitant LB and AD pathology. Dementia autopsy series suggest that DLB is the second most common cause of elderly dementia after AD. Clinical epidemiologic studies are lacking.

Lewy bodies are intracytoplasmic inclusion bodies. They are the hallmark histopathologic lesions of primary PD where these occur within neurons of the substantia nigra and other brainstem nuclei. A spherical shape and eosinophilic staining properties characterize LBs morphologically (Fig. 18-14). The center stains densely, and a pale halo surrounds it. In cases of PD with dementia, LBs occur in cortical neurons and other gray matter regions. Cortical LBs are characterized by irregular shapes and do not have the characteristic pale halo seen with PD. Hence, cortical LBs can easily be missed with routine neuropathologic staining techniques. Moreover, LBs do not stain with silver-based stains often used to identify neuropathologic lesions in AD. A synaptic protein called *alpha synuclein* is the major LB component. Specific immunohistochemical stains for α-synuclein greatly improve LB detection throughout the brain. *Ubiquitin* staining also detects these lesions well. The function of α-synuclein is not completely understood. It may have a role in regulating presynaptic, nerve-terminal vesicular function. Mutations in the α-synuclein gene produce a mixed phenotype within members of affected kindred. Symptoms are predominantly PD-like, with cases of dementia occurring less frequently. α-Synuclein appears to be the main pathologic substrate in multiple systems atrophy (MSA) as well.

Clinical Presentation and Differential Diagnosis

DLB patients characteristically have cognitive decline, behavioral change, and motor dysfunction. The most crucial component for this clinical diagnosis is dementia, although the initial manifestations of DLB may be characteristically motor or behavioral impairment. A critical clinical feature of DLB is fluctuating mental status, which may be dramatic, ranging from relatively lucid to severe confusion. Episode duration and frequency vary greatly, lasting minutes, days, or weeks. Awareness and arousal levels may vary and include periodic somnolence and unresponsiveness. Transient neurologic symptoms (i.e., dysarthria, dizziness, or unexplained falls) may occur. Such episodes

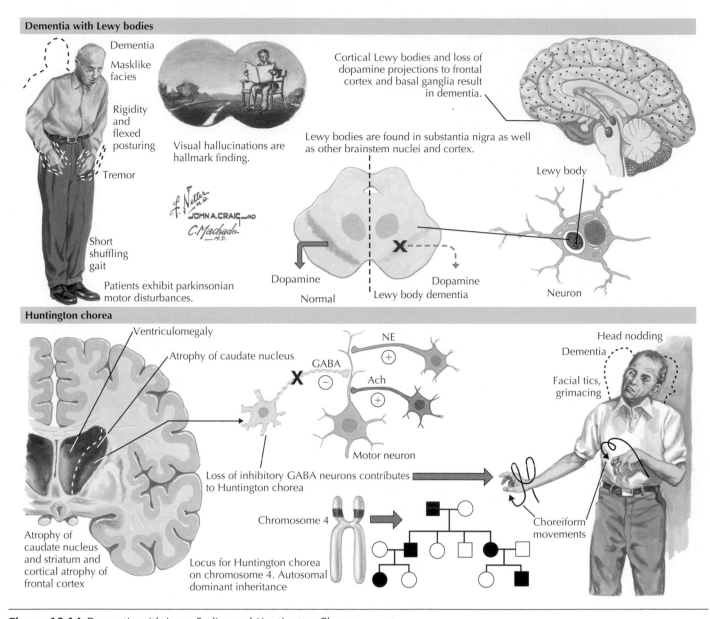

Figure 18-14 Dementia with Lewy Bodies and Huntington Chorea.

may suggest complex partial seizures, delirium, or transient ischemic attacks. Although patients with AD have "good and bad days," the fluctuations of patients with DLB are more pronounced. Clinical assessments may vary significantly from visit to visit. Caregivers often become stressed by the unpredictability of symptoms.

The cognitive impairment in DLB may be similar to that in AD, although there are some important differences. The memory loss in DLB tends to be less severe than in AD; however, retrieval deficits are more pronounced than encoding deficits. Therefore, patients with DLB have a greater problem retrieving previously learned information and show a greater benefit with cueing than do patients with AD. In AD, encoding difficulty predominates, and consequently, patients do not benefit as much from practice or from cueing. In DLB, visuospatial and construction skills may be impaired earlier than in AD. Patients

with DLB may present with geographic disorientation in familiar neighborhoods or even in their own homes while their memory is mildly impaired. Executive function is also impaired significantly earlier in DLB than in AD, manifested as impaired problem solving, inability to complete tasks, and marked disorganization of daily activities. Formal neuropsychological tests help to differentiate AD from DLB, particularly in early disease stages.

Prominent psychotic features, including hallucinations and delusions, also develop in patients with DLB, although such symptoms are not typically seen early in the disease course. In DLB, psychosis can be an early and severely disabling feature, sometimes heralding the onset of dementia. Recurrent vivid and detailed visual hallucinations are particularly prevalent in DLB. The emotional response to these hallucinations ranges from relative indifference to severe agitation and combativeness.

Table 18-1 Comparison of DLB and AD Manifestations

Manifestation	DLB	AD
Memory loss	Less pronounced, poor retrieval	Characteristic, poor encoding
Visuospatial and construction skills	Severely impaired early	Mildly impaired early
Executive function	Impaired earlier	Impaired later
Fluctuating mental status	Pronounced	Less pronounced
Psychotic features	Can be prominent early	Not typical early
Delusions	Bizarre, unrelated to impaired cognitive function	Often related to memory loss
Depression and anxiety	Common	Common
Parkinsonism	Within 1–2 years of dementia	Later in disease course

AD, Alzheimer disease; DLB, dementia with Lewy bodies.

Agitation typically occurs when the patient has little insight or the hallucinations are perceived as threatening. Hallucinations having other sensory (i.e., nonvisual) also occur but are less specific for DLB. Delusions are frequently bizarre, complex, and unrelated to cognitive impairment. In contrast, delusions in patients with AD often occur from misinterpretation secondary to forgetfulness. For example, patients with AD may become suspicious of others when they cannot find things they misplaced. Other behavioral problems such as depression and anxiety also occur frequently but are not unique to DLB (Table 18-1).

Motor signs of DLB include all the typical features of PD; however, here the bradykinesia and rigidity are more characteristic, whereas tremor is relatively uncommon. Signs tend to be distributed more symmetrically and axially than they are in PD. Unexplained falls occur early and often in patients with DLB, unlike postural instability in PD, which tends to mark more advanced disease. Response to dopaminergic medications is limited or absent with DLB, although they may exacerbate hallucinations. Parkinsonism is also seen in advanced AD and in frontotemporal dementia. When Parkinsonism occurs within 1–2 years of dementia, either before or after the onset of cognitive decline, DLB is a prime consideration in the differential diagnosis.

Diagnosis

The clinical evaluation for DLB is similar to that for AD. Formal neuropsychological tests can be useful early in the course to differentiate DLB from AD or other dementing illnesses. There are no specific findings on blood or spinal fluid analysis. Brain MRI and CT do not reveal any specific abnormalities. Volumetric MRI studies suggest there is relative sparing of hippocampal volumes in DLB cases. EEG shows nonspecific abnormalities, including focal or diffuse brain wave slowing. PET imaging may be helpful in the future, particularly in highlighting affected dopaminergic systems.

Treatment

Cholinergic CNS deficits occur in DLB as they do in AD. Some studies suggest that DLB is associated with greater cholinergic deficit than is AD. In theory, cholinesterase inhibitors—donepezil, rivastigmine, and galantamine—should be effective, and small, controlled clinical trials show that these medications have a favorable effect on cognitive outcome measures in DLB. The duration of drug benefit is not established but may be similar to that in AD. Cholinesterase inhibitors offer only symptomatic benefits, having no known effect on the degenerative process. Therefore, patients can delay cognitive progression for a limited amount of time only. It is not clear when these drugs truly lose their efficacy. As in AD, drug discontinuation, especially after several years of treatment, may result in rapid cognitive and functional decline. These drugs may reduce the extent and severity of cognitive fluctuations and behavioral problems throughout the disease course.

When psychotic features are disabling, use of atypical neuroleptic agents is common, similar to their efficacy in cases of PD with psychotic features. The efficacy of these drugs for DLB has not been studied in controlled clinical trials. As atypical neuroleptics produce fewer extrapyramidal adverse effects than "typical" neuroleptics, this must be an important consideration when treating DLB patients. However these atypical neuroleptics are associated with increased morbidity and mortality in nursing home patients. Their use in the elderly population with dementia, therefore, requires careful assessment of risk and benefit and close monitoring if used at all.

Additionally, patients with DLB often exhibit sensitivity to various centrally acting drugs, most prominently to neuroleptic medications, and may become completely incapacitated by severe akinesia, dystonia, or delirium. The incidence of neuroleptic malignant syndrome in DLB is unknown. Good clinical judgment and conservative dosing strategies should be used in every case. The treatment of psychotic features in DLB is one of the most challenging management issues. If at all possible, neuroleptic medication should be avoided.

Often, psychotic symptoms distress caregivers more than patients, but this should not prompt immediate initiation of such medications. Recently, use of cholinesterase inhibitors, such as rivastigmine, was shown to reduce hallucinations in patients with DLB. Therefore, cholinesterase inhibitors remain the first line of treatment in DLB, including cases with prominent psychotic features. Treatment of motor symptoms is based largely on anecdotal reports. Dopaminergic drugs may be tried with caution in selected cases; however, psychosis may be exacerbated, and efficacy is often minimal.

As in AD, caregiver counseling about the disease course and realistic treatment expectations is paramount for successful monitoring, intervention, and improved quality of life. The most common causes for nursing home placement in the demented population include psychosis with behavioral problems and parkinsonism. Patients with DLB are therefore at high risk for early nursing home placement. As in AD, use of cholinesterase inhibitors may help to delay nursing home placement.

mistaken for depression, and treatment with antidepressants is typically not effective.

c. *Stereotypic behavior* includes repetitive, ritualistic, and idiosyncratic behaviors. These individuals require a rigid daily routine, becoming agitated when their routine is interrupted. They may repeat, perseverate, the same story verbatim and with the same prosodic inflection numerous times during a single clinic visit. This is akin to "listening to a broken record." They evidence mental inflexibility and difficulty shifting mindset. Ritualistic behaviors, picking lint from the floor, rearranging the silverware drawer, rewriting a letter, etc., have a compulsive quality absent the anxiety associated with obsessive-compulsive disorder. The clinical features often overlap during the course of illness.

Patients may present with predominant apathetic features only to later develop increasingly disinhibited or stereotypic behavior or both. As symptoms progress, most patients experience akinesia, progressive rigidity, mutism, and incontinence, requiring total nursing care. Features of disinhibition are associated with degeneration within the orbital frontal and adjacent temporal lobes. Apathetic features correlate with degenerative changes within the dorsolateral frontal lobes. Stereotypic behavior type seems to correlate with more widespread involvement of frontal and temporal lobes, although greater emphasis may exist in the region of the cingulate gyrus.

Cognitive function may be relatively spared initially, so that mental status examination may be notable only for distractibility, inattentiveness, or perseveration rather than clear impairment of memory or constructional apraxia. One of the more striking cognitive features of bvFTD is executive dysfunction seen on sorting and sequencing tasks, loss of verbal fluency, and impairment in general problem-solving skills.

FRONTOTEMPORAL LOBAR DEGENERATION WITH MOTOR NEURON DISEASE

Frontotemporal lobar degeneration with motor neuron disease presents most often in men younger than age 65 years. Characteristic FTD typically precedes onset of motor neuron symptoms, and disinhibited-type behaviors predominate. The motor neuron component leads to a more rapid decline and death in these cases. Consequently, akinesia and mutism are not often seen. The duration of illness is typically 2–3 years. A family history of disease is only occasionally found.

PRIMARY PROGRESSIVE APHASIA

Primary progressive aphasia (PPA) presents in fluent and nonfluent subtypes. In both conditions, progressive aphasia is the predominant clinical feature, often remaining the only feature throughout the illness. Typically women, patients with fluent PPA usually present between the ages of 50 and 65 years. Illness duration ranges from 3 to 15 years. There is gradual loss of comprehension and naming, with relatively less impairment in reading and writing. Behavioral features include mental rigidity, stereotypic behaviors, self-centeredness, and disregard for personal safety. Many patients are easily agitated. Memory,

calculations, and constructional skills are relatively spared, whereas visual agnosia and prosopagnosia may occur relatively early.

Semantic Dementia may present as a fluent progressive aphasia and visual agnosia. Nonfluent PPA patients typically present at the same ages. Men and women are affected equally. Illness duration is between 4 and 12 years. There is overall good comprehension, with impaired verbal expression. Patients have effortful, agrammatic, stuttering speech, with impaired repetition and word retrieval. Reading and writing are also affected, but less so than speech. These individuals are aware of their impairment and become frustrated and depressed easily. Behavioral problems develop later in the disease and may include any FTD symptoms. Nevertheless, the focal characteristic of PPA clinically differentiates it from classic FTD.

Diagnosis

Brain MRI, important for excluding other mechanisms for frontal lobe syndromes such as tumor or infection, may demonstrate atrophy predominating within frontal and temporal lobes in neurodegenerative disease. Brain imaging may show focal lobar or asymmetric atrophy in PPA cases. EMG in cases of FTD/MND may be diagnostic. Brain SPECT may show deficits in a similar distribution, although it does not have a sensitivity that provides a definitive diagnosis. Brain FDG-PET scans are useful in distinguishing FTLD from AD. EEG is normal, especially early in the disease course. Blood work and CSF studies are not helpful. Formal neuropsychological tests are helpful in localizing deficits in cortical function.

Treatment

Treatment of FTD is supportive. There is no proven benefit to using the cholinesterase inhibitors, commonly used in AD. Caregiver education and reduction of caregiver stress are essential in successful management of agitation and other behavioral problems. When patients become aggressive and combative, caregivers tend to oppose their behavior. Distraction and redirection are more effective than verbal instruction in these instances.

Limited use of sedatives is recommended to avoid overmedication. Paradoxically, benzodiazepines may exacerbate agitation in some patients. SSRIs may reduce anxiety and restlessness. Other drugs, including mood stabilizers, and atypical anxiolytics (e.g., trazodone, buspirone), sometimes help with problematic behavior when used as monotherapy or in combination. There are few randomized clinical trials of classic and atypical neuroleptics in FTD, but they may be necessary in cases of aggressive or violent behavior.

VASCULAR COGNITIVE IMPAIRMENT

Clinical Vignette

A 67-year-old man with a history of hypertension and coronary artery disease, who had lived alone since his wife's death 3 years previously, came to the clinic at his daughter's insistence because he had become increasingly complacent and inactive. The daughter noted that he had stopped fixing his own meals and might not eat unless she brought something to him. He tended to eat junk food and sweets. She was unsure whether he was taking his antihypertensive medications regularly. He had neglected housework and the yard, stopped balancing his checkbook, and decreased participation in social activities.

The patient reported dizziness, and gradually worsening unsteady gait. Although he had not fallen, he felt off balance especially when turning. He also reported urinary frequency and occasional incontinence. He denied depression but was not particularly happy. He gave up previous interests because they were "too much to keep track of."

Five years previously, the patient had experienced a stroke causing transient weakness on the right side but no residual deficit. Approximately 1 year previously, he had stayed in the hospital for a transient ischemic attack characterized by transient right-sided weakness and dysarthria. Brain MRI showed extensive subcortical and periventricular white matter changes and numerous microvascular infarcts in the basal ganglia.

On exam, his affect was flat; he was slow to respond. Mental status examination results showed impaired motor sequencing, executive dysfunction, and memory impairment. He could not spell world backward. He was able to register four words but recalled only one of four spontaneously. With cueing, he recalled all four items. He could not draw a clock to command but copied a clock, drawn by the examiner, well. He had evidence of a wide-based, spastic gait, with bilateral Babinski signs. Stride and arm-swing amplitudes were reduced. Muscle stretch reflexes were brisk throughout. His blood pressure was 160/86 mm Hg. Repeated MRI demonstrated progressive subcortical and periventricular microvascular changes. Blood test results revealed normal cell counts, a normal B_{12} level, and a normal TSH level. Serum RPR was nonreactive. The fasting serum homocysteine level was slightly increased, at 17 mol/L.

Pathogenesis

The association between cerebrovascular disease and dementia has been recognized for many years. Some authors propose using the term *vascular cognitive impairment* (VCI) to describe the contribution of cerebrovascular disease to various dementia syndromes. This applies whether the dementia is primarily related to cerebrovascular disease or mixed with another dementing disorder. Indeed in the early and mid-20th century, cerebrovascular disease was postulated to be the specific etiology for senile dementia. It was not until the 1960s, that AD was recognized to be the most common pathophysiologic mechanism for the majority of individuals who have dementia. In subsequent decades, the concept of VCI underwent several revisions. Given the wide array of clinical syndromes possible with stroke, VCI presentation varies considerably. The heterogeneity of stroke complicates one's ability to specifically define VCI as a single clinical entity with specific diagnostic criteria. Autopsy series show cerebrovascular disease coexisting with AD, and influencing clinical dementia, in approximately 20% of dementia cases.

Vascular cognitive impairment occurs when multiple cerebral infarcts or hemorrhages cause enough neuronal or axonal loss to impair cognitive function. The core pathologic VCI syndromes include (1) *lacunar disease* (penetrator-vessel disease), (2) *multi-infarct* dementia (MID; medium- and large-vessel disease), (3) *strategic single-infarct* dementia (thalamus, angular gyrus, e.g.), and (4) *Binswanger* dementia. These conditions are not mutually exclusive; there are many instances wherein the patient has a mixture of small-vessel and medium-vessel infarcts. Furthermore, age-related microvascular disease, frequently defined by brain MRI scans of elderly patients, may also contribute to the onset, progression, and symptoms of old-age dementia.

Epidemiology

The risk of VCI increases with age just as the risk of stroke increases with age. Most epidemiologic studies of dementia do not differentiate among AD, cerebrovascular, and mixed dementia. The prevalence of a pure vascular cause of dementia in autopsy studies is probably less than 10% of old-age dementia cases. However, the prevalence of VCI may be much greater. There is often a prevalence of patients with mixed dementia, including the effects of both vascular and neurodegenerative disorders; this in fact may be much higher than current estimates. In general, diagnostic criteria for VCI lack sufficient sensitivity and specificity to recognize cases of VCI reliably. Many patients may also have other dementia types, like AD, DLB, or normal pressure hydrocephalus. Interestingly, cerebrovascular disease is extremely common and shares several risk factors for AD. These include hypertension, diabetes, and hyperlipidemia. Recent investigations also suggest a link between AD and metabolic syndrome. Stroke is identified more commonly in AD patients than in age-matched controls. It is, therefore, reasonable to suspect that cerebrovascular disease contributes significantly to old-age dementia.

Clinical Presentation and Differential Diagnosis

The potential for prevention of VCI highlights the importance of recognizing and treating the various vascular causes that may predispose to or contribute to dementia. Standard criteria for diagnosing vascular dementia are difficult to define given the variable nature of cognitive deficits following stroke, mainly depending upon the anatomical location of the stroke. The most common dementia is AD, typically characterized by short-term memory loss in the early stages. While vascular dementia may present in this way, it is not necessarily the "cardinal" feature of VCI. The cognitive consequence of stroke may include executive dysfunction, neglect, or aphasia. Additionally, the degree of cerebrovascular disease progression varies greatly. Residual symptoms following acute stroke may seem to initially but incompletely improve and then later on contribute to eventual cognitive dysfunction in the setting of mixed dementen. Moreover, there is now considerable evidence that stroke increases the risk of AD. "Silent" lacunar infarcts are particularly associated with increased risk of AD.

Almost all standard diagnostic criteria for VCI require imaging studies demonstrating evidence of stroke (Fig. 18-16).

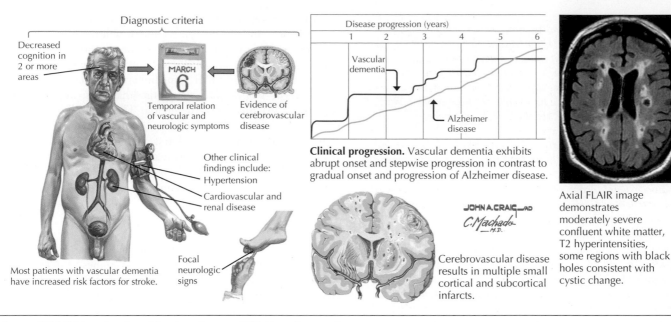

Figure 18-16 Vascular Cognitive Impairment (VCI)-Type Dementia.

However, there is no specific characteristic appearance on imaging studies that provide a diagnosis of VCI per se. The absence of specific cerebrovascular lesions of course mitigates this diagnosis. MRI is more sensitive than CT in showing subcortical and periventricular white matter changes consistent with small-vessel disease, and smaller infarcts. Therefore, a VCI diagnosis requires recognition of various syndromic features to correlate with findings on imaging studies.

Clinical presentation is arbitrarily divided into large-vessel and small-vessel disease, which are not mutually exclusive clinically. Large-vessel disease tends to affect large vascular territories, producing well-known clinical syndromes. For example, frontal lobe involvement may produce aphasia, apraxia, disinhibition, or apathy. Mesial temporal involvement produces amnesia, angular gyrus lesions lead to constructional apraxia, and parietal lesions produce alexia or apraxia.

The clinical syndrome of MID typically proceeds in a stepwise fashion with clear-cut stroke events leading to successive, cumulative impairment of various cognitive domains. Small-vessel disease typically eventuates in subcortical infarcts. These are sometimes localized within strategic locations, such as the thalamus or basal ganglia, and involve white matter tracts such as frontosubcortical and thalamocortical tracts.

Moreover, small-vessel pathology is often seen in the context of "normal" aging, where the smallest branches become increasingly tortuous, producing twists and loops along paths deep in the brain. Morphologic changes are amplified by hypertension and diabetes. This results in diffuse myelin loss within deep vascular territories such as periventricular and subcortical white matter regions. The clinical correlates of small-vessel disease may include executive dysfunction, apathy, inattentiveness, and personality changes typical of frontal lobe syndromes as occur with hydrocephalus and frontotemporal dementia (see Fig. 18-15). Involvement of specific circuits correlates with recognized clinical manifestations.

Dorsolateral prefrontal circuit dysfunction correlates with executive dysfunction, decreased verbal fluency, poor performance on sequencing tasks, impersistence, set shifting, and perseveration. *Subcortical orbitofrontal* circuits are associated with disinhibition, manic behavior, and compulsive behavior. *Medial frontal* circuits produce apathy, psychomotor retardation, and mood lability.

Binswanger Disease

This is the clinical representation of VCI dementia resulting from small-vessel disease. Characteristically, patients are aged between 50 and 70 years; more than 80% have a history of hypertension, diabetes, or both. Initial symptoms vary but often include behavioral changes such as depression, emotional lability, or abulia. Gait disturbances are characterized by lower extremity parkinsonism, ataxia, or spasticity. Dysarthria and other focal motor signs may be present. Urinary incontinence is common. Patients often have histories of dizziness or syncope. Progressive executive dysfunction, slow mental processing, and memory impairment affecting information retrieval rather than encoding characterize cognitive impairment.

Binswanger disease follows a clinical course having intermittent progression, often without clear stroke-like events. Typically, this follows a 3- to 10-year course. Pathologically, one finds numerous subcortical and periventricular infarcts that spare cortical u-fibers. When patients present with the clinical picture typical for Binswanger disease but do not have hypertension or diabetes, a diagnosis of cerebral autosomal-dominant arteriopathy with subcortical infarcts and leukoariosis (CADASIL) should be considered. It is one of the few hereditary causes of VCI.

In the elderly, the possibility of mixed dementia exists when patients exhibit clinical features of AD and VCI. Imaging studies reveal evidence of infarct, widespread microvascular disease, or both. Silent brain infarction, especially in the basal ganglia and thalamic regions, and significant ischemic white matter changes enhance the clinical presentation and progression of AD. In addition, various vascular risk factors, such as hypertension, hypercholesterolemia, and hyperhomocysteinemia (levels 14 mmol/L), also increase the risk of AD. Brains with mixed pathologies, matched for dementia severity, reveal fewer AD lesions compared with pure AD cases. Clearly the specific clinical presentation is influenced by cerebrovascular disease in these cases. Finally, the risk of developing poststroke dementia increases with advancing age, recurrent stroke, and larger periventricular white matter lesions on MRI. Hypoxic and ischemic stroke complications, such as pneumonia or seizure, also increase the risk of poststroke dementia.

Prevention and Treatment

Primary prevention must be pursued aggressively. When at-risk patients are identified, treatment of arterial hypertension, cardiac disease, lipid abnormality, and diabetes are important in reducing dementia risk. Secondary prevention, that is, treatment when cerebrovascular disease is initially recognized, begins with appropriate acute management of stroke and its complications. Prevention of stroke recurrence by appropriate antiplatelet or anticoagulant therapy and addressing primary risk factors are also very important. Use of calcium channel blockers in the treatment of hypertension may be more effective in dementia prevention than other antihypertensive medications. Dietary supplementation with folic acid and vitamins B_6 and B_{12} may help to reduce the levels of homocysteine, a possible contributory precursor to VCI. The role of "neuroprotective agents" in prevention of poststroke dementia is unknown.

To date, evidence-based controlled trials have not yet identified any pharmacologic agents for treatment of ischemic vascular (multiinfarct) dementia. However, when dementia develops, cholinesterase inhibitors may be helpful. As in AD, titration of these medications to maximum doses is recommended; their long-term efficacy in VCI is unknown. The efficacy of cholinesterase inhibitor treatment may be greater in cases of mixed dementia. However, acetylcholine deficits may be significant in VCI as well as in AD. Subcortical vascular disease often interrupts major cholinergic pathways from the basal forebrain to widespread regions of the cerebral cortex. Deficits of CSF acetylcholine levels are found in VCI cases when compared with healthy controls. As in all dementia cases, caregiver education and support are essential to long-term success and quality of patient life.

ADDITIONAL RESOURCES

ALZHEIMER DISEASE

Alzheimer's Association. www.alz.org.

Cummings JL. Alzheimer's disease. N Engl J Med 2004 Jul 1;351(1):56-67. Review.

Dubinsky RM, Stein AC, Lyons K. Practice parameter: Risk of driving and Alzheimer's disease (an evidence-based review): Report of the Quality Standards Subcommittee of the American Academy of Neurology. Neurology. 2000 Jun;54:2205-2211.

Klafki HW, Staufenbiel M, Kornhuber J, Wiltfang J. Therapeutic approaches to Alzheimer's disease. Brain 2006 Nov;129(Pt.11):2840-2855. Epub 2006 Oct 3. Review.

Knopman DS, Dekosky ST, Cummings JL, et al. The American Academy of Neurology. Practice Parameter: Diagnosis of Dementia (an evidence-based review—Report of the Quality Standards Subcommittee of the American Academy of Neurology). Neurology 2001;56:1143-1153.

Lesser JM, Hughes S. Psychosis-related disturbances. Psychosis, agitation, and disinhibition in Alzheimer's disease: definitions and treatment options. Geriatrics 2006 Dec;61(12):14-20. Review.

Raina P, Santaguida P, Ismaila A, et al. Effectiveness of cholinesterase inhibitors and memantine for treating dementia: evidence review for a clinical practice guideline. Ann Intern Med 2008 Mar 4;148(5):379-397. Review.

Small BJ, Gagnon E, Robinson B. Early identification of cognitive deficits: preclinical Alzheimer's disease and mild cognitive impairment. Geriatrics 2007 Apr;62(4):19-23. Review.

DEMENTIA WITH LEWY BODIES

Fantini ML, Ferini-Strambi L, Montplaisir J. Idiopathic REM sleep behavior disorder: toward a better nosologic definition. Neurology 2005 Mar 8;64(5):780-786. Review.

Huey ED, Putnam KT, Grafman J. A systematic review of neurotransmitter deficits and treatments in frontotemporal dementia. Neurology 2006 Jan 10;66(1):17-22. Review.

McKeith IG, Dickson DW, Lowe J, Consortium on DLB. Diagnosis and management of dementia with Lewy bodies: third report of the DLB Consortium. Neurology 2005 Dec 27;65(12):1863-1872. Review. Erratum in: Neurology. 2005.

Murphy J, Henry R, Lomen-Hoerth C. Establishing subtypes of the continuum of frontal lobe impairment in amyotrophic lateral sclerosis. Arch Neurol 2007;64:330-334. Review.

Sleegers K, Kumar-Singh S, Cruts M, Van Broeckhoven C. Molecular pathogenesis of frontotemporal lobar degeneration: basic science seminar in neurology. Arch Neurol 2008 Jun;65(6):700-704. Review.

van der Zee J, Sleegers K, Van Broeckhoven C. Invited article: the Alzheimer disease–frontotemporal lobar degeneration spectrum. Neurology 2008 Oct 7;71:1191-1197. Review.

FRONTOTEMPORAL DEMENTIA

Josephs KA. Frontotemporal dementia and related disorders: deciphering the enigma. Annals of Neurology 2008;64:4-14.

VASCULAR DEMENTIA

Bronge L, Wahlund LO. White matter changes in dementia: does radiology matter? Br J Radiol 2007 Dec;80(Spec No 2):S115-S120. Review.

Farlow MR. Use of antidementia agents in vascular dementia: beyond Alzheimer disease. Mayo Clin Proc 2006 Oct;81(10):1350-1358. Review.

Knopman DS. Cerebrovascular disease and dementia. Br J Radiol 2007 Dec;80(Spec No 2):S121-S127. Review.

Papademetriou V. Hypertension and cognitive function. Blood pressure regulation and cognitive function: a review of the literature. Geriatrics 2005 Jan;60(1):20-22, 24. Review.

Viswanathan A, Rocca WA, Tzourio C. Vascular risk factors and dementia: how to move forward? Neurology 2009 Jan 27;72(4):368-374. Review.

Transmissible Spongiform Encephalopathy (Creutzfeldt–Jakob Disease)

Yuval Zabar

19

Clinical Vignette

A 56-year-old man noted increasing clumsiness while writing. A tremor developed in his right hand, and he soon noted slurred speech over 2–3 weeks. Initial neurologic evaluation demonstrated an action tremor in the right hand and some reduction in fine dexterity. Brain magnetic resonance imaging (MRI) and electroencephalography (EEG) results were normal. During the next 2 months, the patient's wife believed that her husband became increasingly confused, as illustrated by his calling her by his sister's name. He had trouble initiating and maintaining sleep. His driving became erratic and dangerous. He was pulled over for driving too slowly and his license was revoked. On follow-up examination, 4 months later, he was disoriented. He spoke slowly and gave inappropriate responses. His dysarthria was more pronounced.

The results of repeated MRI and EEG were normal, as were cerebrospinal fluid (CSF) study results, including protein 14-3-3. Over the next 6 months, the patient's cognitive and motor function declined precipitously. His gait became progressively ataxic, and he fell numerous times. He lost proper use of his hands and legs, requiring assistance with eating, dressing, and bathing. Occasionally, his limbs would jerk suddenly, and he appeared startled and anxious. Speech output became largely unintelligible and palilalic. He would shout occasionally but mostly stayed quiet and passive.

Repeated EEG showed generalized slowing and intermittent periodic sharp waves, approximately 1 per second. Another MRI now demonstrated bright lesions on T2-weighted and flair imaging. Right frontal lobe biopsy showed vacuolar encephalopathy consistent with a transmissible spongiform encephalopathy (TSE). The final stages were characterized by increasing stupor and aspiration pneumonia. The patient died 14 months after onset. Autopsy confirmed the diagnosis.

EPIDEMIOLOGY

Transmissible spongiform encephalopathy includes rare, subacute, universally fatal neurodegenerative diseases affecting humans and animals. Clinical presentation and distribution of pathologic lesions vary widely, complicating classification of these diseases. Classification focuses on pathogenic mechanisms rather than clinical and pathologic features. Currently, human TSE is classified into three categories: sporadic, familial, and infectious. Most animal TSE cases fall into the infectious category, including scrapie (sheep); bovine spongiform encephalopathy (BSE), also known as mad cow disease (cattle); and chronic wasting disease (deer and elk). The sporadic form of human TSE, Creutzfeldt–Jakob disease (CJD), accounts for 85% of cases of this disorder. Sporadic fatal insomnia cases are also described. The inherited form of human TSE, accounting for 15% of cases, includes familial CJD, fatal familial insomnia, Gerstmann–Straussler–Scheinker disease, and other less well defined clinical syndromes.

The human epidemic forms of TSE, comprising less than 1% of cases, include iatrogenic cases of CJD (exposure via dural grafts, infected surgical instruments, and growth hormone injections), kuru (cannibalism), and variant CJD (vCJD; via ingestion of beef contaminated with BSE). In theory, transfusion of any blood product from an affected patient may pose a risk. To date, only a handful of vCJD cases are attributed to transmission from blood transfusion, much fewer than might be expected given the number of blood transfusions worldwide. There seems to be increased risk of CJD among venison eaters, although this is difficult to confirm. The incidence of human TSE is approximately 1.5/1 million people per year. This rate has remained stable over several decades.

The appearance of symptoms after exposure to "infected" tissue varies widely, and incubation periods lasting several decades are described. One hundred sixty-three vCJD cases have been reported in Europe since 1996. These occurred predominantly in the United Kingdom, where most cases of BSE occurred. No instances of vCJD originated in the United States. Given the potentially long incubation period (several years) of vCJD, all cases of TSE are reported and monitored by several European surveillance centers. A similar laboratory, the National Prion Diseases Pathology Surveillance Center, operates in the United States.

PATHOGENESIS

The histopathologic hallmarks of TSE include severe neuronal loss, spongiform vacuolization, and astrocytosis. There is no associated inflammatory response, and some disease forms have an accumulation of amyloid plaques. However, TSE amyloid differs from β-amyloid typically found in Alzheimer disease. The agent responsible for TSE is a "proteinaceous infectious particle," termed prion protein (PrPC). This is a normally occurring cell-surface glycoprotein, encoded on chromosome 20, which is highly conserved in mammals. Its normal function is not well defined, but it may have importance in response to oxidative stress.

All three TSE forms are thought to result from conversion of PrPC into PrPSc, also known as scrapie protein. PrPSc is a self-replicating and infectious agent lacking nucleic acid. The mechanisms by which PrPSc leads to neurodegeneration remain largely unknown. It is questionable whether the prion is the sole pathogenic mechanism of TSE. The disease can be experimentally transmitted between various animals, with some variability, by inoculation of infected nervous tissue. However, inoculation with pure PrPSc has not led to transmission of disease. Therefore, PrPSc alone does not account for horizontal transmission.

More than 20 pathogenetic mutations of the prion gene are identified, accounting for 15% of inherited human TSE. Mutations of the PrP gene predispose mutant PrP to transform into the PrPSc tertiary structure. A difference in just 1 amino acid can drastically affect the disease phenotype. With infectious TSE, PrPSc enters the central nervous system (CNS) via ingestion or iatrogenically and precipitates the conversion of PrPC into PrPSc. In sporadic cases, the conversion may occur via rare stochastic (random) changes of the normal protein. Individual susceptibility to conversion of PrPC also may be determined by genetic polymorphisms, some of which are identified and associated with varying phenotypic expression.

For example, patients who are homozygous for methionine at residue 129 tend to present with cognitive loss, aphasia, myoclonus, or insomnia and tend not to have plaque-like lesions at autopsy. Patients who are homozygous for valine at residue 129 present primarily with cognitive loss or insomnia but not aphasia or myoclonus, and all have plaquelike lesions at autopsy. Moreover, individuals who are homozygous for methionine at residue 129 are more susceptible to vCJD than individuals with other polymorphisms at the same residue.

CLINICAL PRESENTATION

Initial symptoms depend on the brain region involved. Cognitive impairment is often the first sign and may be recognized by attentive patients who note subtle changes in their intellectual capacities that are sometimes difficult for the examining physician to detect. Intellectual impairment may affect any cognitive domain. Behavioral and personality disturbances such as impulsivity, disinhibition, or apathy often occur. Progressive dementia eventually develops in all individuals, often with significant psychiatric and behavioral disturbance. A variety of motor signs and symptoms often develop, typically extrapyramidal features, and sometimes precede onset of cognitive deficits. Cerebellar ataxia develops in some patients and at times may be the presenting feature. Myoclonus develops in others; some also have a very hyperactive startle response. At times, these features do not occur until relatively late in the clinical course. Progressive parkinsonism, weakness with neurogenic muscle atrophy, and bulbar dysfunction also may occur. Motor signs may be unilateral or asymmetric, reflecting focal or multifocal disease, respectively. As symptoms progress, a multifocal pattern emerges with global cognitive impairment, severe loss of motor control, and marked behavioral changes.

Terminal TSE stages are characterized by progressive stupor, leading to coma and aspiration. Sporadic CJD cases usually present between the fifth and eighth decades of life, but vCJD occurs in younger adults and teenagers. The mean survival time for patients with sporadic disease is approximately 6 months; most expire within 12 months. Inherited forms of the disease and vCJD have younger onset ages and more protracted courses than do sporadic cases.

DIAGNOSIS

The results of routine laboratory studies are normal. Identification of pathogenic mutations in hereditary cases is available via rapid screening tests that can be performed on non-CNS tissue, including peripheral blood. Sporadic disease remains a diagnostic challenge. A family of proteins called 14-3-3 is increased in the CSF of affected patients. Although initially reported to have greater than 90% sensitivity and specificity for TSE, it is likely overestimated because 14-3-3 proteins are essentially markers for any acute to subacute brain neuronal damage. Nevertheless, CSF assays for protein 14-3-3 are useful when TSE is suspected. Noting that false positives do occur, *positive results must not be considered diagnostic of TSE.*

Brain MRI is now very useful in TSE diagnosis. In some cases of vCJD, bright lesions on T2-weighted and fluid-attenuated inversion recovery (FLAIR) imaging occur within the pulvinar, the so-called pulvinar sign. In CJD, focal hyperintense lesions may be found in the basal ganglia on T2-weighted images or multifocally within the cortex on diffusion-weighted images (Fig. 19-1). Diffusion-weighted MRI imaging has shown more than 90% sensitivity and specificity in some series, although the timing of MRI imaging along the course of illness is important. Repeated imaging may be required to detect typical changes. MRI abnormalities are also of supportive diagnostic value, similar to 14-3-3, but are not diagnostic of TSE. EEG may demonstrate 0.5- to 1-Hz periodic sharp waves focally or diffusely at some stage of the disease, particularly when there is clinical cerebral cortical dysfunction but certainly not all CJD individuals such as those presenting with cerebellar or striatal dysfunction. Nonspecific EEG slowing is more common but less specific than periodic sharp waves.

Brain biopsy needs to be considered in every case, particularly when the results of other studies are negative; however, brain biopsy per se is also susceptible to sampling error. This study will often differentiate CJD from other neurodegenerative disease and, more importantly, may help exclude potentially treatable conditions, such as CNS vasculitis. Frontal lobe and cerebellar biopsies can be particularly successful. In suspected vCJD, biopsy of lymphoid tissue such as the tonsils proves very reliable. CSF samples and brain tissue need to be sent to the National Surveillance Center for analysis and monitoring. Autopsy evaluation must be discussed with the family in advance of death because it is essential in confirming the diagnosis. Confirmation of a CJD diagnosis allows epidemiologic surveillance of disease activity as well as providing families a definitive conclusion to their previously unresolved tragic experience with a loved one.

TREATMENT

No anti-PrPSc prion therapies are available. Treatment is supportive. For individuals presenting primarily with cerebellar or striatal forms of these disorders, whose intellect may be maintained, it is important to include them in discussion of

Creutzfeldt-Jakob Disease

Demented patitent exhibiting myoclonus

Section from putamen showing extensive loss of neurons and spongiform brain tissue. Spinal cord usually shows similar loss of motor neurons.

EEG showing characteristic diffuse periodic wave pattern

Early Cortical Involvement

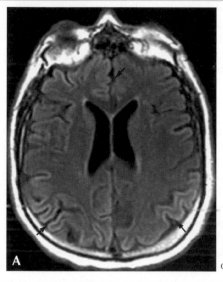

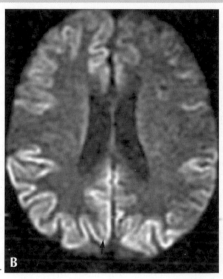

(**A**) FLAIR image shows increased intensity in frontal and parietal cortical gray matter. (**B**) Diffusion mimics the subtle restriction of diffusion in similar cortical regions.

Figure 19-1 Transmissible Spongiform Encephalopathy.

end-of-life issues. Hospice care is strongly encouraged where available.

In the absence of a definitive diagnostic test, frequent examinations and repeated testing including EEG, diffusion MRI, and CSF protein 14-3-3 assays are required. The means of preventing TSE transmission must be clearly defined. This requires significant regulatory and legislative measures to ensure appropriate standards in the meat packing industry, as well as a public education effort. Consistent case ascertainment including brain biopsies and autopsies, and reporting to the National Prion Disease Pathology Surveillance Center are imperative for the development of diagnostic and preventive strategies.

ADDITIONAL RESOURCES

Appleby BS, Appleby KK, Crain BJ, et al. Characteristics of established and proposed sporadic Creutzfeldt-Jakob disease variants. Arch Neurol 2009:208-215.

Brandel JP, Heath CA, Head MW, et al. Variant Creutzfeldt-Jakob disease in France and the United Kingdom: Evidence for the same agent strain. Ann Neurol 2009 Mar;65(3):233-235.

Brown P. Transmissible spongiform encephalopathy in the 21st century: neuroscience for the clinical neurologist. Neurology 2008 Feb 26;70(9):713-722. Review.

Collins SJ, Sanchez-Juan P, Masters CL, et al. Determinants of diagnostic investigation sensitivities across the clinical spectrum of sporadic Creutzfeldt-Jakob disease. Brain 2006;129:2278-2287.

Glatzel M, Stoeck K, Seeger H, et al. Human prion diseases; molecular and clinical aspects. Arch Neurol 2005;62:545-552. Review.

Goudsmit J. Obituary: Daniel Carleton Gajdusek (1923-2008). Nature 2009 Jan 22;457(7228):394.

Josephs KA, Ahlskog JE, Parisi JE, et al. Rapidly progressive neurodegenerative dementias. Arch Neurol 2009;66:201-207.

Kovacs GG, Budka H. Prion diseases: from protein to cell pathology. The American Journal of Pathology 2008;172(3):555-565.

Shiga Y, Miyazawa K, Sato S, et al. Diffusion weighted MRI abnormalities as an early diagnostic marker for Creutzfeldt-Jakob disease. Neurology 2004;63:443-449.

Ward HJ, Everington D, Cousens SN, et al. Risk factors for sporadic Creutzfeldt-Jakob disease. Ann Neurol 2008 Mar;63(3):347-354.

Warren JD, Schott JM, Fox NC, et al. Brain biopsy in dementia. Brain 2005 Sep;128:2016-2025. Review.

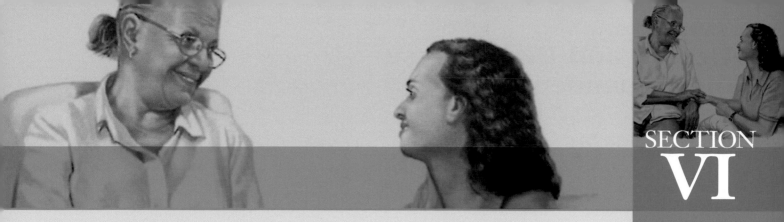

SECTION
VI

Psychiatric Disorders

SUBSTANCE DEPENDENCE

20   Alcohol and Drug Abuse and Dependence

PERSONALITY DISORDERS

21   Attention-Deficit/Hyperactivity Disorder
22   Obsessive-Compulsive Disorder
23   Borderline Personality Disorder
24   Panic Disorder
25   Posttraumatic Stress Disorder
26   Somatization Disorder
27   Eating Disorders

MOOD DISORDERS

28   Dysthymia
29   Major Depression
30   Bipolar Disorder

PSYCHOTIC DISORDERS

31   Schizophrenia

Alcohol and Drug Abuse and Dependence

Kenneth Lakritz and Yuval Zabar

20

Most physicians are intimately familiar with the protean manifestations of alcohol abuse and dependence (Fig. 20-1) and its characteristic clinical signs (Fig. 20-2). Incidence rates vary widely between cultural groups (alcoholism is almost unheard of in traditional Muslim communities), but lifetime rates of 5–10% are the rule in North America and Europe. Therefore, physicians who state that they *never see alcoholism* may not be recognizing the diagnosis. Patient denial significantly contributes to overlooking this potential diagnosis. This denial has several sources. Admitting to a problem with alcohol or other drugs may be humiliating for patients. Furthermore, alcohol use, even at dangerous levels, is a culturally embedded and approved, often pleasurable part of social life.

The rubric of drug and alcohol abuse subsumes dozens of syndromes, but a few useful generalizations can be offered. Most drugs have safe and unsafe uses. Physicians routinely employ opiates, sedative-hypnotics, psycho stimulants, and dissociative anesthetics, all of which have abuse and addiction potential. Even over-the-counter drugs, including anticholinergics, pseudoephedrine, and dextromethorphan, can be abused. Conversely, illegal or widely abused substances such as cannabinoids and nicotine have or are likely to have future medical uses.

Potentially *abusable drugs cause dopamine release* directly or indirectly in several forebrain structures. Beyond this, what makes a drug dangerous are the dosage, route of administration, and social context. High doses, routes of administration that rapidly deliver drug to the brain, and their ingestion beyond a stable social or religious context all predispose to initial abuse and eventual addiction. These factors rather than, for example, the pharmacology of cocaine per se, explain why the Peruvian practice of chewing coca leaves is safe; however, in contrast, smoking freebase cocaine is extremely harmful as is sometimes evidenced in many Western societies.

ETIOLOGY

Liability to alcohol abuse and dependence, especially early-onset abuse, runs in families, but the mechanism of inheritance is not understood. Findings of a link between alcoholism and a particular dopamine DR-2 receptor allele remain controversial. Some Asian populations are relatively protected from alcoholism because they possess a variant form of the enzyme alcohol dehydrogenase and metabolize alcohol poorly. This causes them to become flushed and nauseated with minimal doses. Conversely, young adults with a high alcohol tolerance, evaluated on measures of incoordination or subjectively, are at increased risk for later alcoholism. Young adults often assume they are not getting into difficulties with drinking because of their tolerance. Physicians must convince them that this is wrong.

Alcohol is a central nervous system (CNS) depressant with cross-tolerance to benzodiazepines, barbiturates, and some other sedatives. It is distinguished within this group by its ease of manufacture, legal status, wide availability, rapid absorption, and exceptionally low therapeutic index. The lethal dose of alcohol is only a few times the intoxicating dose; one bottle of whiskey can be lethal to an individual who has not acquired tolerance. The dose at which tissue damage occurs is lower in this setting and falls within the range of commonly ingested doses. In most adults, chemical signs of hepatic injury are detectable after consumption of three or more drinks within 24 hours. Alcohol is a potent fetal teratogen with no threshold dose; it is absolutely contraindicated in pregnancy.

CLINICAL PRESENTATION

Acute alcohol intoxication at moderate doses causes disinhibition and incoordination. Even at socially acceptable doses, it impairs driving and is implicated in approximately half of all highway accidents and deaths. Alcohol is linked to a similar proportion of sexual assaults.

Patients with most major psychiatric illnesses have increased rates of alcohol abuse. Alcohol interacts with psychiatric illnesses and treatments. Many patients use alcohol to treat mood disorders, anxiety, or insomnia, but it is not a safe or effective treatment for any medical disorder. The toxicity and short duration of action of alcohol make it useless as an anxiolytic, and it disrupts sleep architecture and decreases sleep efficiency. The combination of alcohol abuse and depression is especially lethal. Alcohol use makes patients who are depressed more depressed and interferes with antidepressant response. Drinkers who are depressed experience an approximately 10-fold increase in suicide rate compared with nondrinkers who are depressed.

Alcohol has direct toxic effects on multiple tissues, including the central nervous system, liver, the pancreas, and the heart. Patients may present with acute or chronic hepatitis, cirrhosis, esophageal varices, cardiomyopathy, and dementia. Acute withdrawal syndromes occur occasionally, leading to delirium tremens, Wernicke encephalopathy, and Korsakoff psychosis, as illustrated in Chapter 17.

Wernicke syndrome, an acute neurologic emergency resulting from acute thiamine and other B-vitamin depletion, is seen almost exclusively in alcoholics. It is initially manifested by gait ataxia, and subsequently oculomotor abnormalities and delirium, developing during a period of days to weeks and presents with confusion, ophthalmoplegia with diplopia and nystagmus, and ataxia. The delirium is characterized by disorientation, inattention, drowsiness, and indifference to surroundings. Conversation is sparse and tangential. Signs of alcohol withdrawal are seen in 15% of patients. Treatment of Wernicke syndrome requires immediate administration of large doses of thiamine, 100 mg intravenous (IV) in a non–glucose containing solution.

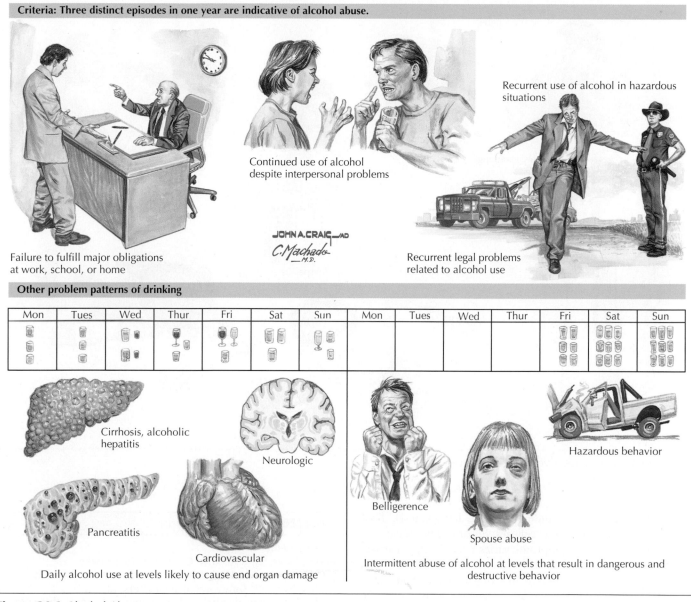

Figure 20-1 Alcohol Abuse.

This reverses the symptoms and prevents progression of pathology. This treatment is routinely provided in emergency departments for most patients presenting with an acute confusional state. Progressive stupor, coma, and death develop if the condition is left untreated. Thiamine and other B vitamins should be given to malnourished patients as supplements to replenish body stores.

Autopsy reveals symmetric necrosis of brainstem tegmentum nuclei, superior cerebellar vermis, and mammillary bodies. These findings resemble lesions produced by disorders of pyruvate metabolism.

Korsakoff psychosis is likely to develop without immediate repletion of thiamine in Wernicke syndrome patients. This disorder is mostly confined to alcoholics, with the only exception being individuals having bilateral hippocampal damage, typically from vertebral basilar infarction. This condition is a nonprogressive devastating irretrievable disorder of memory, affecting both new learning (anterograde amnesia) and past memory (retrograde amnesia). The patient cannot make new memories because of poor encoding, which is similar to the memory impairment of Alzheimer disease. The retrograde amnesia may extend back many years, rendering the patient "stuck in time." Recollection of past events is usually disorganized and erratic, sometimes suggesting deliberate confabulation. Additional cognitive impairment includes poor sequencing, arithmetic, and construction performance.

Hepatic encephalopathy occurs in stages. Patients with liver failure experience confusion, with decreased psychomotor activity associated with increasing serum levels of NH_3. Occasionally, hyperactivity and agitation occur. During this time, patients often exhibit asterixis, which is not a sign specific to hepatic encephalopathy because it can occur in many other metabolic disturbances, such as uremic encephalopathy. Progressive stages of drowsiness, stupor, and coma follow. Significant motor

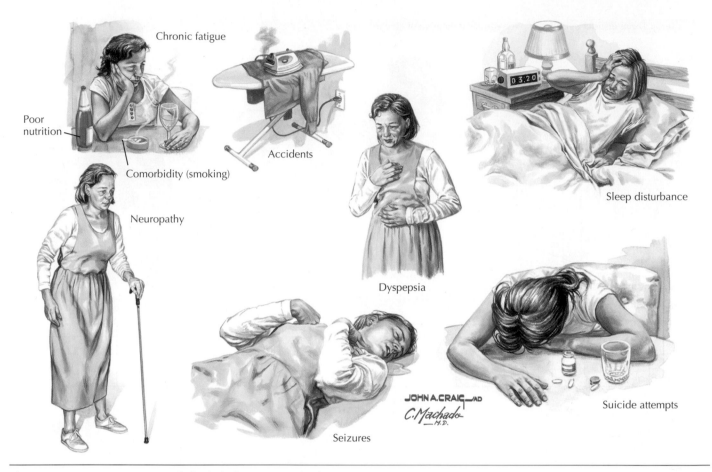

Figure 20-2 Signs Suggestive of Alcohol Abuse.

abnormality develops, including rigidity, bradykinesia, brisk reflexes, and extensor plantar reflexes. Seizures may occur.

The progression of symptoms varies considerably, particularly after treatment begins. However, left untreated, coma may persist and lead to death in up to 50% of patients. In some cases, a chronic disorder of cognition and behavior occurs, with pyramidal and extrapyramidal dysfunction lasting months or years. This condition is seen in patients with repetitive bouts of hepatic encephalopathy. EEG shows generalized slowing of background rhythm with prominent triphasic waves. The purpose of treatment is to attempt to decrease NH_3 levels by reducing dietary protein, acidifying colonic contents with lactulose, and, occasionally, suppressing urease-producing colonic bacteria with antibiotics.

DIAGNOSIS

To avoid missing the diagnosis of alcohol abuse or dependence, physicians must maintain a high index of suspicion directed at eliciting classic historic signs of *impending alcohol abuse* (Fig. 20-2). Similarly, asking about features suggestive of early *alcohol dependence* is equally important during what needs to be routine screening for alcoholism in any patient (Fig. 20-3). Asking about average levels and patterns of alcohol use should be part of every examination. Because patients underestimate their consumption, a useful rule of thumb is to double the amount reported

---

Box 20-1 CAGE Questionnaire

Ask patients whether:
They have felt a need to **C**ut down their intake
Others have **A**nnoyed them by criticizing their drinking
They have felt **G**uilty about their drinking
They have ever needed an **E**ye-opener (a morning drink) to calm their nerves or treat a hangover

---

by the patient. Patients also need to be questioned about binge drinking, withdrawal signs, blackouts, and excessive tolerance. The four-question CAGE questionnaire is a good screening instrument (Box 20-1). One positive answer to a CAGE question is cause for concern; two positive answers corresponds to a 50% risk of alcoholism.

Any individual who has had even one *driving while intoxicated* (DWI) drunk-driving conviction can be safely assumed to have a problem with alcohol, as can the occasional patient who presents in an intoxicated state for his appointment. In the latter case, the physician must take whatever steps are immediately necessary to prevent this patient from driving away from the medical office.

When diagnostic uncertainty persists, interviewing family or friends is often decisive; typically, they present a more accurate picture of the patient's drinking habits. Laboratory test results

Three or more incidences during 1 year indicate pattern of physical dependence

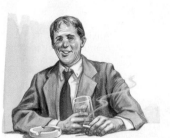

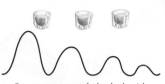

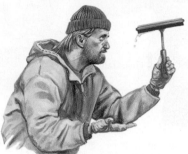

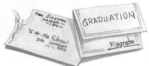

Increasing amounts of alcohol needed to achieve effect (tolerance)

Same amount of alcohol with decreasing effect

Great deal of time and effort spent on obtaining alcohol

Avoiding important social, occupational, or recreational events because of alcohol use

JOHN A. CRAIG—MD
C. Machado—M.D.

Typical withdrawal symptoms

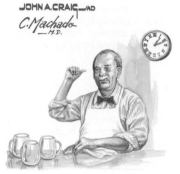

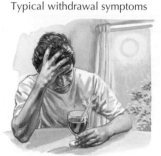

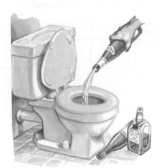

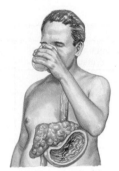

Drinking more or for longer periods

Similar substance used to avoid withdrawal symptoms

Persistent desire or unsuccessful efforts to curb abuse

Continued use of alcohol despite exacerbation of health problems

Figure 20-3 Alcohol Dependence.

that reveal increased GGTP or transaminase levels, mild macrocytic anemia, or both can add confirmatory evidence. Asking the patient to stop drinking for 6 months is helpful as both a diagnostic and a therapeutic maneuver. Heavy drinkers who achieve a few months of sobriety may feel so much better that they stay sober, and patients who refuse clearly have very serious trouble.

TREATMENT

Withdrawal from alcohol and *other cross-tolerant sedative hypnotics* (barbiturates, benzodiazepines, methaqualone, etc.) is potentially hazardous (Figs. 20-4 to 20-6). This can lead to *agitated delirium and seizures*. In contrast, most *other pharmacologic withdrawals* are characterized by *dysphoria* but are not medically dangerous; nevertheless, withdrawal from cocaine and amphetamines can lead to a profound depression.

Addicted patients must remove themselves from environments wherein these drugs are available and their use is encouraged or tolerated. Twelve-Step organizations like Alcoholics Anonymous and other self-help groups are extremely valuable in overcoming denial of illness and in providing patients a culture of sobriety and social support. The absolute treatment *goal* is total current and future *abstinence*. Although therapies incorporating a return to controlled use have been repeatedly proposed, these approaches are always unsuccessful.

Pharmacologic treatments for addiction are improving but are still adjunctive to psychotherapeutic and behavioral interventions. Long-term replacement of illicit opiates with methadone or buprenorphine is effective, as is the temporary use of nicotine administered by patch, gum, or inhalation to help smokers quit. The use of bupropion modestly increases the success rate of quitting cigarettes. Varenicline, a nicotine receptor partial agonist, works even better, but possibly at the cost of precipitating mood disturbances.

Disulfiram (Antabuse) is the oldest specific medicine to be prescribed to prevent use of alcohol. Unexpectedly, disulfiram also has been found to have some utility for therapy of cocaine abuse. By inhibiting a critical hepatic enzyme in the metabolic degradation of alcohol, disulfiram induces an unpleasant and potentially dangerous reaction to this therapy, whenever the reforming addict returns to alcohol ingestion. Disulfiram works best in highly motivated but intermittently impulsive binge drinkers. However, this therapeutic approach is not only potentially hazardous but totally dependent on patient motivation. It is easy for an alcoholic to simply choose to stop using the medicine.

Two other medications are approved for the treatment of alcoholism: *Naltrexone* is an opiate antagonist that also reduces alcohol intake, presumably by diminishing the rewarding effects of alcohol. *Acamprosate* is thought to subtly diminish protracted withdrawal systems by modulating glutamatergic activity. To

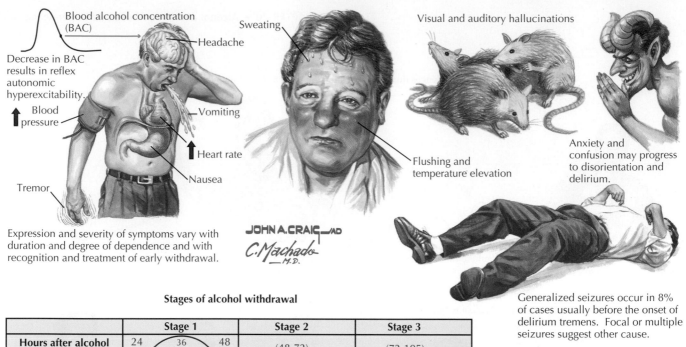

Stages of alcohol withdrawal

	Stage 1			Stage 2	Stage 3
Hours after alcohol consumption	24	36 (peak)	48	(48-72)	(72-105)
Symptoms	Mild-to-moderate anxiety, tremor, nausea, vomiting, sweating, elevation of heart rate and blood pressure, sleep disturbance, hallucinations, illusions, seizures			Aggravated forms of stage 1 symptoms with severe tremors, agitation, and hallucinations	Acute organic psychosis (delirium), confusion, and disorientation with severe autonomic symptoms

Stage 1 withdrawal usually self-limited. Only small percentage of cases progress to stages 2 and 3. Progression prevented by prompt and adequate treatment.

Figure 20-4 Alcohol Withdrawal.

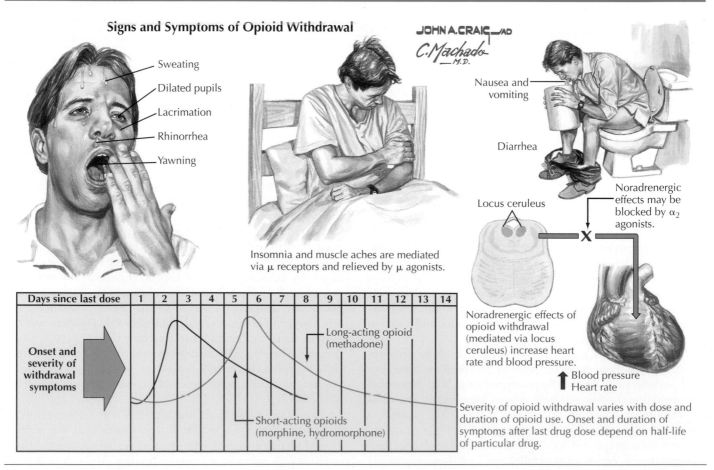

Figure 20-5 Opioid Withdrawal.

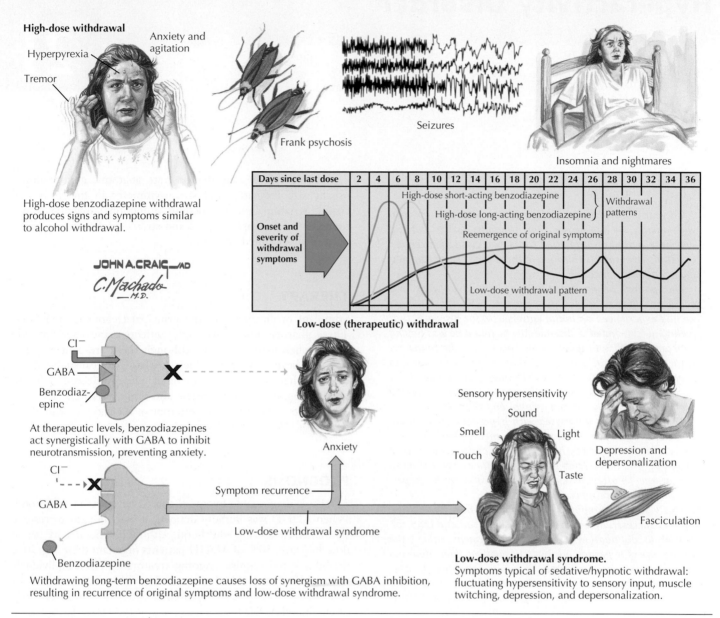

High-dose withdrawal

Hyperpyrexia

Anxiety and agitation

Tremor

High-dose benzodiazepine withdrawal produces signs and symptoms similar to alcohol withdrawal.

JOHN A.CRAIG—MD
C.Machado—M.D.

Frank psychosis

Seizures

Insomnia and nightmares

Days since last dose	2	4	6	8	10	12	14	16	18	20	22	24	26	28	30	32	34	36

Onset and severity of withdrawal symptoms

High-dose short-acting benzodiazepine

High-dose long-acting benzodiazepine } Withdrawal patterns

Reemergence of original symptoms

Low-dose withdrawal pattern

Low-dose (therapeutic) withdrawal

Cl⁻

GABA

Benzodiaz-epine

At therapeutic levels, benzodiazepines act synergistically with GABA to inhibit neurotransmission, preventing anxiety.

Cl⁻

GABA

Benzodiazepine

Withdrawing long-term benzodiazepine causes loss of synergism with GABA inhibition, resulting in recurrence of original symptoms and low-dose withdrawal syndrome.

Anxiety

Symptom recurrence

Low-dose withdrawal syndrome

Sensory hypersensitivity

Sound

Smell   Light

Touch

Taste

Depression and depersonalization

Fasciculation

Low-dose withdrawal syndrome.
Symptoms typical of sedative/hypnotic withdrawal: fluctuating hypersensitivity to sensory input, muscle twitching, depression, and depersonalization.

Figure 20-6 Benzodiazepine Withdrawal.

date, there are no accepted pharmacologic treatments for cocaine and other types of stimulant dependence. The most promising agents (topiramate, vigabatrin, etc.) increase GABA activity. Cocaine vaccines are also under investigation.

Liability to alcoholism, especially early-onset alcoholism, is *partially inherited,* as may be the case with other addictions. Physiologic and epidemiologic evidence suggest that the adolescent brain is especially vulnerable to addiction, particularly to nicotine; few smoking habits begin after age 18. Persons with psychiatric illnesses, especially *bipolar disorder, ADHD, and personality disorders,* are at heightened risk for drug abuse and dependence. ADHD is diagnosable by age 8 and never starts in adulthood.

Some psychiatrists believe that many addicts are in fact "self-medicating" an underlying psychiatric disorder—this idea remains controversial. However, "dual diagnosis" patients are the rule rather than the exception. These individuals need simultaneous treatment for both addiction and psychiatric illness.

ADDITIONAL RESOURCES

Hays JT. Efficacy and safety of varenicline for smoking cessation. Am J Med 2008 Apr;121(4 Suppl. 1):S32-S42.

Johnson BA, et al. Topiramate for treating alcohol dependence: a randomized controlled trial. JAMA 2007 Oct 10;298(14):1641-1651.

Karila L, et al. New treatments for cocaine dependence: a focused review. Int J Neuropsychopharmacol 2008 May;11(3):425-438.

Khantzian EJ. The self-medication hypothesis of substance use disorders: a reconsideration and recent applications. Harv Rev Psychiatry 1997 Jan-Feb;4(5):231-244.

Krupitsky EM. Antiglutamatergic strategies for ethanol detoxification: comparison with placebo and diazepam. Alcohol 2007 Apr;31(4):604-611.

Spanagel R, Kiefer F. Drugs for relapse prevention of alcoholism: ten years of progress. Trends Pharmacol Sci 2008 Mar;29(3):109-115.

Attention-Deficit/ Hyperactivity Disorder

Kenneth Lakritz

Clinical Vignette

A 26-year-old draftsman consulted a psychiatrist for help with anxiety. He had begun a job 3 months earlier and had just been placed on probation for slowness and inattention to detail. This was his third job in three years since completing vocational education.

This patient acknowledged falling behind at work, but could not offer an explanation for this behavior. Although he had experienced an initial enthusiasm for his work, that feeling quickly faded. Subsequently, he found he was having substantial difficulty maintaining focus when he found his work to be "boring." He agreed that he had a tendency to procrastinate, noting that despite having adequate funds he was behind on his taxes and mortgage. His wife reported that he sporadically abused alcohol and cocaine.

At age 8, he was diagnosed with hyperactive-type attention deficit disorder. Treatment with methylphenidate was successful. Subsequently he maintained adequate academic progress. The methylphenidate prescription was discontinued at age 18 after his high school graduation; his hyperactivity had not reappeared.

This vignette exemplifies an individual whose hyperactivity was successfully treated during childhood and later tolerated discontinuation of stimulant treatment without the recurrence of hyperactivity, but whose other associated cognitive impairments persisted. In adults, attentional disorders can present as apparent laziness, lack of focus, and procrastination. This patient needs a retrial of his ADHD medication.

CLINICAL PRESENTATION

Attention-deficit/hyperactivity disorder (ADHD) is a common, well-characterized, and very treatable neuropsychiatric disorder surrounded by social and political controversy.

This occurs in 3–9% of school-age children; it has a definite genetic predisposition. Although some researchers find a higher prevalence of ADHD in boys than girls, other investigators dispute this, claiming that the sex disparity is an artifact of the more manifest behavioral disturbance and hyperactivity in boys (Fig. 21-1).

The core symptoms necessary for the diagnosis of ADHD are (1) *distractibility* and (2) *difficulty sustaining attention*. Hyperactivity is not necessarily part of the clinical picture of ADHD. Affected children are at increased risk for school failure, antisocial personality disorder, and substance abuse.

Imaging studies may demonstrate anatomic abnormalities, usually size reduction and size asymmetry in the prefrontal cortex, striatum, and cerebellum. Functional imaging sometimes shows decreased frontal and striatal perfusion, especially on tests of sustained attention.

THERAPY

Stimulant medications are the principal treatment modalities. These pharmaceuticals are highly effective and have few side effects when used correctly. Although there are concerns that these medications promote illicit drug use, clinical studies demonstrate that appropriate treatment actually decreases future risk of drug abuse. Atomoxetine and other noradrenergic antidepressants are a reasonable alternative for patients who abuse or cannot tolerate stimulants.

PROGNOSIS

ADHD is diagnosable by age 8 and never starts in adulthood. When ADHD was initially defined, it was thought to resolve spontaneously during adulthood. Although hyperactivity per se does improve, 50% of ADHD patients maintain their cognitive disabilities and require ongoing treatment. These individuals need to be distinguished from adults with new complaints of restlessness, boredom, or impaired attention and no past history of childhood ADHD.

ADHD must also be distinguished from childhood mania. Both groups of patients are hyperactive and inattentive, but manic children are also irritable and usually overtalkative. This distinction can be difficult, in part because there is a comorbidity between the disorders; that is, most patients with childhood-onset bipolar disorder also have ADHD. These children's mood symptoms should be treated first with mood stabilizers. A stimulant can then be added later on as necessary.

Significant objections are expressed to the current approaches for diagnosis and treatment of ADHD. These stem from its high prevalence and the fear that children are being inappropriately drugged, rather than having their educational needs carefully defined and subsequently met. In reality, ADHD is both overdiagnosed and underdiagnosed: some children are inappropriately treated, but many others are missed. Although improper use of medication can occur, individual assessment and medical treatment are not mutually exclusive. The failure to diagnose and treat ADHD is as undesirable as overtreatment.

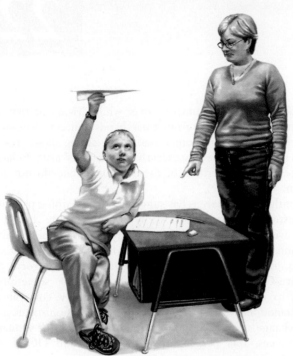

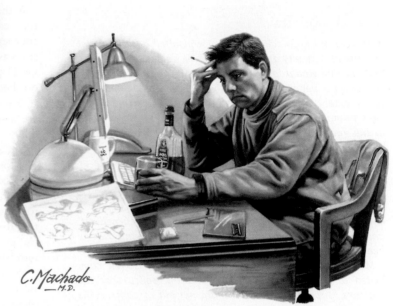

Attention-deficit disorder is a highly treatable neuropsychiatric disorder, common in school-age children, especially boys. Affected children are at increased risk for academic failure.

Hyperactivity improves or resolves spontaneously in adulthood, but 50% of patients maintain their cognitive disabilities. Substance abuse and antisocial personality disorder are commonly associated with ADHD.

Figure 21-1 Attention-Deficit Disorder.

ADDITIONAL RESOURCES

Barkley R. Attention-Deficit Hyperactivity Disorder. 3rd ed. A Handbook for Diagnosis and Treatment. New York, NY: Guilford; 2005.

Bush G, Valera EM, Seidman LJ. Functional neuroimaging of attention-deficit/hyperactivity disorder: a review and suggested future directions. Biol Psychiatry 2005 Jun 1;57(11):1273-1284.

Ellison-Wright I, Ellison-Wright Z, Bullmore E. Structural brain change in Attention Deficit Hyperactivity Disorder identified by meta-analysis. BMC Psychiatry 2008 Jun 30;8:51.

Faraone SV, Wilens TE. Effect of stimulant medications for attention-deficit/hyperactivity disorder on later substance use and the potential for stimulant misuse, abuse, and diversion. J Clin Psychiatry 2007;68(Suppl. 11):15-22.

Garrett A, Penniman L, Epstein JN, et al. Neuroanatomical abnormalities in adolescents with attention-deficit/hyperactivity disorder. J Am Acad Child Adolesc Psychiatry 2008 Nov;47(11):1321-1328.

Hallowell EM, Ratey JJ. Driven to Distraction: Recognizing and Coping With Attention Deficit Disorder from Childhood through Adulthood. New York, NY: Touchstone; 1995.

Obsessive-Compulsive Disorder

22

Kenneth Lakritz

Clinical Vignette

A 36-year-old high school teacher consulted a psychiatrist because of difficulty driving to work. He had a long-standing fear that he would lose control of his car and accidentally run down a pedestrian. Recently, this fear had intensified to the extent that he had to stop driving and examine his car's bumpers for signs of blood whenever he hit a bump in the road. It was taking him more than 2 hours each morning to make a 20-minute commute. On further questioning, the patient also admitted to fear that a knife or fork would accidentally slip from his hand while he ate dinner, and that he would inadvertently stab someone. He also had to check the appliances and faucets four times before leaving home to ensure they had been turned off, and he had a 1-hour ritual of washing and shaving that he needed to perform in strict order every morning.

Much to the patient's dismay, the psychiatrist felt compelled to warn both his family and the police that the patient's "suppressed anger" might get out of control. His family, however, was well aware of the patient's habits and fears, and declared that they were not frightened. Likewise, the police dismissed the case after finding no criminal history and no imminent threat.

Despite his time-wasting habits and rituals, the patient had a successful career. He was well liked by friends and family, who worked around his "eccentricities." His symptoms gradually diminished with combined treatment (provided by a second psychiatrist) with a serotonergic antidepressant and a behavioral program of exposure and response prevention.

*P*atients with obsessive-compulsive disorder (OCD) complain of unwelcome, intrusive, and repetitive thoughts or urge to act in ways they find meaningless or inappropriate. The thoughts or urges are "ego-dystonic"—they are perceived as unreasonable and seemingly imposed upon the patient. Someone who hoards newspapers and bits of string, or spends hours every day polishing a new car, but does so happily, does not have OCD, however odd the behavior. People with OCD are tormented by their thoughts and behaviors, usually struggling with them for years before seeking help.

CLINICAL PRESENTATION

OCD patients usually fit into one of a few categories. Some clean obsessively and worry about germs or contamination (Fig. 22-1). Others repeatedly check that they've turned off their appliances or locked their doors. Some are obsessed with symmetry or arranging their possessions in exactly the right order. Another group hoards what most would call "junk." Often, OCD patients are troubled by thoughts of violence; they may

fear that they will run someone over while driving or that as they eat a knife will slip from their hands and cut someone. Inexperienced clinicians sometimes err by seeing these obsessions as real threats, thereby exacerbating patients' fears. In fact, OCD patients are terrified of these thoughts and do not act on them.

Recently, factor analysis has suggested that hoarding patients are a distinct subtype, and possibly even a separate disorder. They have a different pattern of neuropsychological impairment, and they respond less well to medication.

Most diagnostic classifications employ a category of Obsessive-Compulsive Personality Disorder, or something similar, to describe individuals who are highly controlled, formal, emotionally distant, parsimonious, perfectionistic, resistant to change, and intolerant of ambiguity. Despite the similarity in names, this personality constellation and OCD are unrelated.

Several other disorders of impulse control seem superficially related to OCD. Pathologic gamblers and "sex addicts" seem obsessed and compulsive, as do sufferers from trichotillomania, the compulsion to pull out body hairs. However, these apparently similar patients share neither the unique pathophysiology of OCD described below nor the same pattern of response to treatment.

Patients with OCD typically have either no structural brain abnormalities or subtle loss of frontal tissue. In contrast, functional brain imaging (positron emission tomography or functional magnetic resonance) reliably shows excess metabolic activity in caudate and frontal regions; although OCD is a clinical syndrome, it can, in principle, be detected by brain scan! (This pattern is not required to diagnose OCD but the association is robust.) They typically exhibit minor difficulties on tests of executive function and less frequently disorders of short-term memory.

TREATMENT

OCD patients share a unique pattern of response to medications. They improve when given serotonin reuptake inhibitor antidepressants. However, at the clinical level, OCD does not respond as well to serotonergic antidepressants as does depression per se. Typically, higher doses of medication are required to treat OCD, the response is slower, and full remissions with medication alone are uncommon. In contrast, the antidepressants that block reuptake of norepinephrine, and that are as effective for treating depression as the serotonergic antidepressants, are ineffective for OCD. Curiously, a canine model for OCD, the Acral Paw Lick Syndrome, shows the same pattern of medication response. For patients with only a partial response, the addition of a low-dose neuroleptic medication is often helpful. Patients who are refractory to all other treatments and severely impaired by their illness are candidates for Deep Brain Stimulation or other neurosurgical interventions.

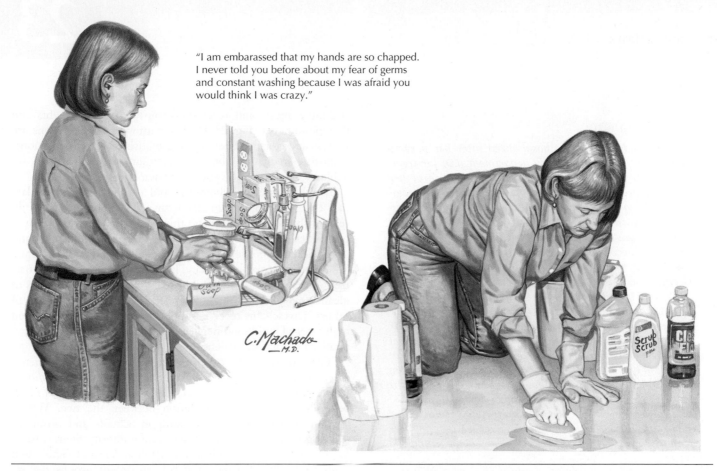

"I am embarassed that my hands are so chapped. I never told you before about my fear of germs and constant washing because I was afraid you would think I was crazy."

Figure 22-1 Obsessive-Compulsive Disorder.

Some form of behavioral therapy is almost always also required. The most effective of these is exposure and response prevention. If a patient has a compulsion to wash his hands, the quickest way to cure him is to get dirt on his hands and prevent him from washing them. Naturally, patients need support and encouragement to try this method. When patients improve, their functional imaging abnormalities resolve. This response is independent of whether their primary treatment modality was a specific medication or primary behavioral therapy.

Some cases of childhood-onset OCD, especially those with abrupt onset or associated movement disorders, are caused by *Streptococcal* infections. There is subsequent reactivity of anti-streptococcal antibodies within the basal ganglia. A combination of antibiotic treatment and plasmapheresis, to remove the antibodies, are helpful to these children.

ADDITIONAL RESOURCES

An SK, Mataix-Cols D, Lawrence NS, et al. To discard or not to discard: the neural basis of hoarding symptoms in obsessive-compulsive disorder. Mol Psychiatry 2008 Jan 8.

Burdick A, Goodman WK, Foote KD. Deep brain stimulation for refractory obsessive-compulsive disorder. Front Biosci 2009 Jan 1;14:1880-1890.

Clark DA. Cognitive Behavioral Therapy for OCD. New York, NY: Guilford; 2004.

Olley A, Malhi G, Sachdev P. Memory and executive functioning in obsessive-compulsive disorder: a selective review. J Affect Disord 2007 Dec;104(1-3):15-23.

Rapoport JL. The Boy Who Couldn't Stop Washing: The Experience and Treatment of Obsessive compulsive disorder. New York, NY: Signet; 1997.

Swedo SE, Swedo SE, Leonard HL, et al. Pediatric Autoimmune neuropsychiatric disorders associated with streptococcal infections: clinical description of the first 50 cases. Am J Psych 1998;155:264-271.

Borderline Personality Disorder

Kenneth Lakritz

23

Clinical Vignette

A 23-year-old woman was hospitalized after her parents brought her to the emergency department (ED) for treatment of an overdose of acetaminophen. Because of her history of drug abuse, her parents had refused to underwrite a spring-break vacation and the patient took the overdose to "punish" her parents The ingestion was minor and the patient was initially calm and friendly, but when ED staff expressed uncertainty about sending her home, the patient flew into a rage, accused staff of conspiring with her parents, and tried to bite a nurse.

This was her fifth psychiatric hospitalization in 3 years; all but one had been preceded by a suicide gesture or attempt. She lived with her parents and sporadically took adult education courses with a vague ambition to direct films. Despite high intelligence, she had failed three tries at college; in one instance, she had been dismissed for selling drugs. Although she had seen four respected therapists, she derided them as "only being in it for the money."

Her arms showed multiple burn marks, and she admitted to burning herself with cigarettes "to relieve tension." Her dentition was poor, and she acknowledged binge eating and purging.

Once admitted, she quickly established an alliance with a psychotic male patient and announced plans to move in with him when she was discharged. She was angry and sarcastic with some staff members but pleasant with others, leading to disagreements over her treatment and disposition.

Psychoanalysts of the 1920s and 1930s described patients who appeared superficially healthy but could not be psychoanalyzed because of their inability to establish a stable therapeutic relationship. These patients tended to have tumultuous life histories, poor social and vocational adjustment, and occasional brief regressions to psychosis. They were called "ambulatory schizophrenics," "pseudoneurotic schizophrenics," or "borderline schizophrenics." The term *borderline personality disorder* is now the accepted terminology.

CLINICAL PRESENTATION

In the 1950s, one subtype of *borderline patient* was isolated. These individuals had a persistent odd or flat affect, mild but stable thought disorder, and a family history of schizophrenia. Such patients suffer from a *forme fruste* of schizophrenia, and are now diagnosed with *schizotypal personality disorder*. The remaining borderline patients, those with *DSM borderline personality* disorder, are described as "the stably unstable." They have rapid and overwhelming mood fluctuations, are often strikingly angry, and react disastrously to minor slights and disappointments (Fig. 23-1). Their interpersonal relations are intense and stormy. They fail to establish consistent vocational identities, frequently abuse drugs, injure themselves, and are liable to brief psychotic episodes when stressed.

Developmental psychologists and psychoanalysts speculate that this syndrome originates with a disordered parent–child relationship in the second and third year of life. Either because of parental inconsistency or the child's innate mood lability and aggression, the borderline child is unable to integrate disparate experiences of parental love and hostility into a stable, "internalized" parent, leaving the child oscillating between extremes of idealization with devaluation in self-image and perception of others. This scheme receives support from the well-documented high rates of childhood neglect and sexual abuse found in hospitalized borderline patients.

These patients rely on two primitive psychological defense mechanisms: splitting and projective identification. *Splitting* is the tendency to see self and others as either all good or all bad, often with rapid fluctuation between the two. Within a confined environment as found in schools and hospitals, splitting often occurs among staff and authority figures; some are idealized, whereas others are hated and feared. This often leads to conflict between the two treatment groups per se, causing the patient's therapists to enact the patient's conflict among themselves.

Projective identification is the unconscious process of assuming that another person has an undesirable trait or attitude and then acting in such a way as to evoke those traits. Therapists of borderline patients may find themselves overwhelmed with rage or contempt for their patient and will be tempted to act on these feelings.

THERAPY

Borderline patients are exhausting to treat, because of their frequent crises, their simultaneous neediness and hostility, and their difficulty in establishing stable relationships. *Dialectical Behavioral Therapy* is demonstrating great promise. This is a comprehensive system of treatment with extensive institutional support for patients. Here therapists provide a persistent emphasis on diminishing unacceptable behavior as well as suicidal thinking.

No clear medication guidelines are available and none are likely to emerge, given the probable biological heterogeneity of this disorder. On the whole, though, second-generation antipsychotic medications have the most research support. Low-dose lithium and other mood stabilizers sometimes help. In contrast, benzodiazepines may not only disinhibit borderline patients but are apt to be abused. Whatever treatment is proposed, it is important to first rule out active substance abuse and bipolar disorder, two conditions with specific treatments that may mimic borderline personality disorder.

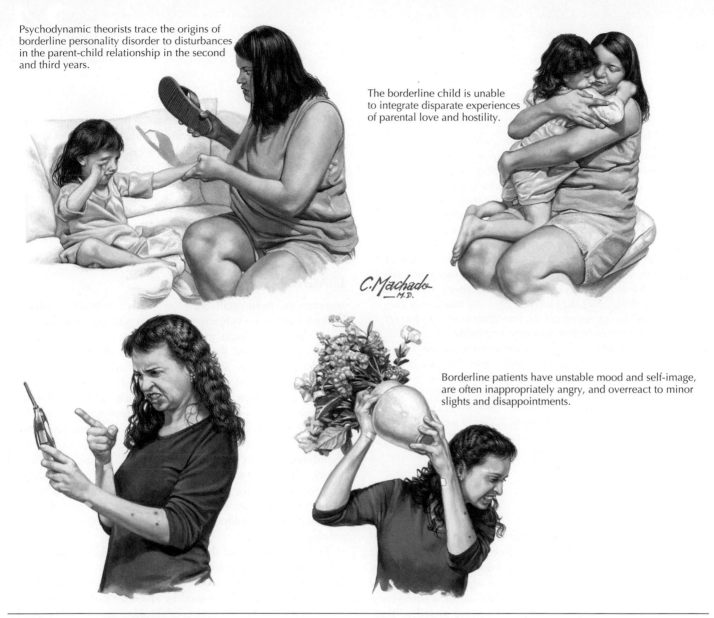

Psychodynamic theorists trace the origins of borderline personality disorder to disturbances in the parent-child relationship in the second and third years.

The borderline child is unable to integrate disparate experiences of parental love and hostility.

Borderline patients have unstable mood and self-image, are often inappropriately angry, and overreact to minor slights and disappointments.

Figure 23-1 Borderline Personality Disorder.

ADDITIONAL RESOURCES

Abraham PF, Calabrese JR. Evidence-based pharmacologic treatment of borderline personality disorder: A shift from SSRIs to anticonvulsants and atypical antipsychotics? J Affect Disord 2008 Feb 25.

Gunderson JG, Hoffman, PD, editors. Understanding and Treating Borderline Personality Disorder: A Guide for Professional and Families. Washington, D.C: American Psychiatric Association Press; 2005.

Linehan, M. Cognitive-Behavioral Treatment of Borderline Personality Disorder. New York, NY: Guilford; 1993.

Panic Disorder

Kenneth Lakritz

Clinical Vignette

A 33-year-old woman was referred to a psychiatric clinic after presenting to a hospital emergency department (ED) on four consecutive nights, complaining of chest pain, dyspnea, and faintness. Each time a careful cardiac and pulmonary examination was unremarkable, and the patient was sent home with a benzodiazepine prescription and reassurance from the ED staff that she was not ill.

She reported similar attacks since childhood, but not as frequently as recently. She felt a desperate need to have help available if an attack occurred and rarely left home unaccompanied. This lady worried that she would lose consciousness during an attack or lose control of her bowels but admitted that neither had ever happened.

Recently she had given up both driving and air travel. She worked at an undemanding job near home. Her lack of any substantive social life was something that significantly troubled her, but despite such she felt helpless to socialize any more. Caffeine made her feel "wired," and she presented the psychiatrist with a long list of medications to which she was "allergic." She acknowledged occasional excess alcohol consumption in order to lessen her anxiety.

*E*mergency department (ED) staff frequently encounter and diagnose patients with panic disorder. These individuals experience unpredictable and sudden bouts of intense anxiety and frightening physical symptoms, leading them to fear they are having a heart attack, stroke, or other medical emergency. This vignette is a classic illustration of a panic disorder. Typically, these patients require a combination of anxiolytic pharmacologic agents and behavioral psychotherapy.

CLINICAL PRESENTATION

Patients with panic disorder are invariably focused on the details of their bodily sensations and tend to reach catastrophic conclusions based on minor aches, palpitations, and shortness of breath (Fig. 24-1). They may present repeatedly in the ED with dyspnea, chest pain, tachycardia, and faintness. Extremity numbness or paresthesia suggest that patients are vasoconstricted from hyperventilation-induced respiratory alkalosis. Typically, patients are not reassured by a negative examination and may present again a few days later with the same complaints. Between episodes they may feel entirely well, but more commonly remain anxious and vigilant for signs of the next attack.

Many individuals with panic attacks develop *agoraphobia*. (Probably all agoraphobic patients have had panic attacks.) Agoraphobia is not—as the word would suggest—a fear of open spaces but a fear of being isolated from help and support. Agoraphobic patients avoid novel places and circumstances and may also avoid driving on familiar highways, fearing isolation in a traffic jam. Eventually, patients may become so fearful that they cannot leave home without accompaniment or at all. The presence of *panic* or intense anxiety in mood-disordered patients is a well-established *risk factor for suicide*. It is controversial as to whether panic disorder unassociated with depression, per se, heightens the risk for suicide.

DIAGNOSIS

Intravenous lactic acid infusion, which mimics respiratory acidosis but has no subjective effects in normal controls, reproduces the panic attacks in many patients. This and other evidence has suggested the "suffocation alarm" theory of panic disorder that asserts affected individuals are overly sensitive to minor changes in blood pH and PCO_2. Hence severe asthma, chronic obstructive pulmonary disorder, and a pulmonary embolus are some of the respiratory disorders that must be excluded in panicky patients. Other considerations include cardiac arrhythmias, myocardial infarction, ingestion of sympathomimetics (particularly cocaine), excess caffeine, alcohol and sedative-hypnotic withdrawal, hypoglycemia, partial complex seizures, and, rarely, pheochromocytoma or carcinoid tumors. Some of these diagnostic possibilities are eliminated by the chronicity of the illness; for example, no one survives daily pulmonary emboli.

Patients with panic disorder are more likely than most to smoke cigarettes. The suffocation alarm theory suggests that the high concentration of carbon dioxide in smoke and the chronic pulmonary dysfunction caused by smoking might both trigger panic attacks. In fact, initiation of smoking seems to precede the onset of panic attacks in most patients.

TREATMENT

Psychotherapeutic approaches to panic disorder include patient education about the syndrome's medically benign natural history and remediation of patients' catastrophic thinking and overgeneralizations. For some this is sufficient, although most phobic patients also need a course of graded exposure to feared situations.

Many patients also require pharmacologic management. Benzodiazepines abort panic attacks quickly and can be used as needed if attacks are infrequent. Most antidepressant medications (possibly excepting bupropion) have antipanic efficacy; they are the first choice for extended treatment. Anxious patients are sensitive to the initial activating or anxiogenic effects of antidepressants and need to begin with lower than usual doses. MAO inhibitors may work when other antidepressants are ineffective. However caution is needed with MAO inhibitors because of their potential for serious side effects (see Chapter 29).

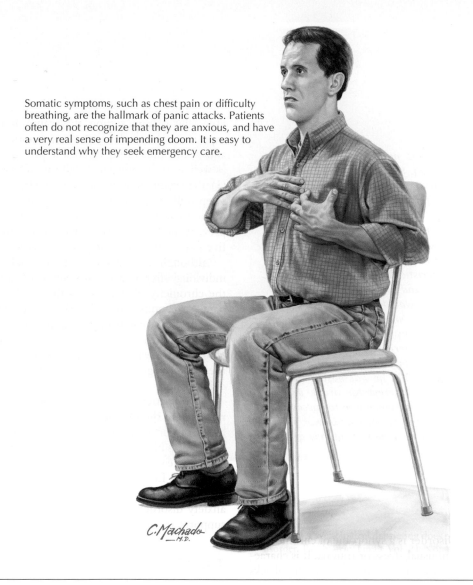

Somatic symptoms, such as chest pain or difficulty breathing, are the hallmark of panic attacks. Patients often do not recognize that they are anxious, and have a very real sense of impending doom. It is easy to understand why they seek emergency care.

Figure 24-1 Panic Disorder.

ADDITIONAL RESOURCES

Barlow D. Anxiety and Its Disorders: The Nature and Treatment of Anxiety and Panic. New York, NY: Guilford; 2002.

Breslau N, Klein DF. Smoking and panic attacks: an epidemiologic investigation. Arch Gen Psychiatry 1999 Dec;56(12):1141-1147.

Marks I. Living With Fear: Understanding and Coping with Anxiety. New York, NY: McGraw-Hill; 2005.

Preter M, Klein DF. Panic, suffocation false alarms, separation anxiety and endogenous opioids. Prog Neuropsychopharmacol Biol Psychiatry 2008 Apr 1,32(3):603-612.

Sareen J, et al. Anxiety disorders and risk for suicidal ideation and suicide attempts: a population-based longitudinal study of adults. Arch Gen Psychiatry 2005 Nov;62(11):1249-1257.

Somatization Disorder

Kenneth Lakritz

26

Clinical Vignette

At age 35 years, Barbara W. already had a 15-year career as a medical patient. When she consulted a new rheumatologist for unexplained fatigue, arthralgias, and muscle tenderness, a thorough examination revealed only an overweight, deconditioned, angry, and sullen woman demanding nonspecific relief from her suffering. She was dependent on an oral opiate and a benzodiazepine, which she simultaneously insisted were ineffective and necessary for her continued functioning. She also consumed startling quantities of nonsteroidal anti-inflammatory drugs and over-the-counter hypnotics.

A careful review revealed that she had seen at least 15 physicians in the past 5 years, had been hospitalized at four different institutions, and had undergone an appendectomy, two subsequent exploratory laparotomies for unexplained abdominal pain, and numerous steroid injections of her knees, shoulders, and lower back. She was an avid consumer of medical literature and believed herself to be suffering from fibromyalgia, chronic fatigue syndrome, multiple chemical sensitivities, sick building syndrome, chronic lyme disease, and mercury poisoning. When gently confronted about the absence of clinical findings and her lengthy history of unresponsiveness to medical intervention, she accused the rheumatologist of labeling her "a mental patient" and left angrily.

Somatization disorder, sometimes referred to as Briquet syndrome or hysteria, is a dramatic and severely disabling illness. Its diagnostic criteria require extensive unexplained physical symptoms, including pain in at least four different sites, two gastrointestinal complaints, one sexual symptom, and one pseudo-neurologic symptom such as fainting or paraparesis. Fortunately, few patients meet this exacting standard, but somatization disorder should be understood as just the most severe of a family of somatoform disorders. These include *conversion disorder* (one or more unexplained neurologic or general medical symptom), *hypochondriasis* (excessive preoccupation and worry about illness), *pain disorder* (unexplained pain), and *body dysmorphic disorder* (preoccupation with imagined or exaggerated physical defects). When all forms of unexplained medical symptoms are lumped together, they are surprisingly common; one study found them in more than 30% of patients presenting to neurology clinics.

CLINICAL PRESENTATION

Somatization and other somatoform disorders are hard to diagnose. By definition, *they are disorders of exclusion*, and a full medical workup always precedes the diagnosis. This step is complicated by the common presence of real physical illnesses in somatizing patients. Moreover, and confusingly, some real illnesses predispose to somatization.

Second, somatoform disorders must be distinguished from *deliberately feigned illness (malingering)* and the *intentional production of physical symptoms (factitious disorder)*. This distinction is notoriously tricky, especially in cases where insurance settlements and disability awards are at stake. There are two other disorders, namely fibromyalgia and chronic fatigue syndrome, that need consideration within the somatoform rubric as to date no specific organic definition process has been uncovered.

Fibromyalgia (see Fig. 28-1) is a common clinical syndrome typically found among women. It is characterized by complaints of widespread, migratory body pain, particularly myalgias and arthralgias (Fig. 26-1). These individuals frequently experience various combinations of psychological symptomatology, including an incapacitating fatigue, anxiety, depression, and poor sleeping. Often such patients are obsessed with finding a specific organic disorder as an explanation. In the neurologic clinic, one may see individuals who are convinced that they have a peripheral neuropathy, radiculopathies, or even complex regional pain syndromes. Because there is some clinical overlap with various neurologic and rheumatologic disorders, it is sometimes difficult to make a differential diagnosis in these patients between an organic versus somatoform disorder. As there is no specific neurologic testing modality that allows one to assign a formal pathophysiologic mechanism in these individuals, and the most detailed evaluations, including electromyography and muscle biopsy are normal, many neurologists conclude that these patients have a somatoform process. However, the neurologist must always maintain an open mind as each patient is evaluated.

Chronic fatigue syndrome is another commonly observed clinical entity that is also typically referred to the neurologist. Frequently these persons will relate the onset of their symptoms to a recent infectious illness such as Lyme disease of a viral disorder. These individuals are often convinced that they have a more serious illness such as amyotrophic lateral sclerosis (ALS) or multiple sclerosis. It is relatively easy to exclude the former with a careful clinical neurologic examination and electromyography. Multiple sclerosis (MS) offers a little more of a challenge as early on, the often diagnostic magnetic resonance imaging is sometimes normal. Careful clinical follow-up is necessary here to reassure physician and patient alike. Early-onset Parkinson disease is another important organic consideration that must also be considered in this setting.

TREATMENT

Somatization disorder and other somatoform disorders are rarely cured but they can be well managed. Somatizers need a primary doctor and should have regularly scheduled doctor visits, regardless of the level of their distress—if they get to see their doctor only when symptomatic, they get more

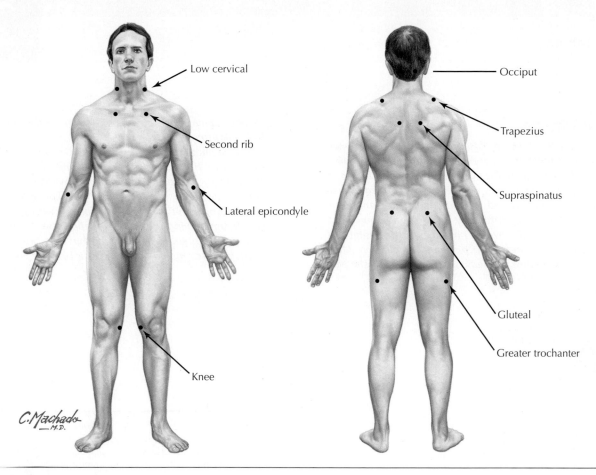

Figure 26-1 Fibromyalgia Tender Points.

symptomatic. These individuals need to be protected from both medical and surgical overtreatment and from quackery. Paradoxically, and most importantly, these patients always need close medical attention—as ALS, MS, and Parkinson disease are easily overlooked in somatizers and, despite their preoccupation with illness, these patients often neglect their health, especially by becoming physically inactive.

Somatizing patients benefit from psychiatric treatment. They are often concrete in their thinking and *alexithymic*—deficient in verbal access to their emotional state. These deficits are a suitable target for psychotherapy. But the biggest barrier to such treatment (apart from failing to diagnose the problem) is finding a way to tell the patient that he or she has a psychiatric disorder. Perhaps the best way to do so is to tell the patient that

he or she has a chronic medical illness of unknown etiology whose symptoms are exacerbated by stress. This is both tactful and true.

ADDITIONAL RESOURCES

Allen LA, Woolfolk RL, Escobar JI, et al. Cognitive-behavioral therapy for somatization disorder: a randomized controlled trial. Arch. Intern. Med 2006;166(14):1512–1518.

Andrade C, Singh NM, Bhakta SG. Simultaneous true seizures and pseudoseizures. J Clin Psychiatry 2006 Apr;67(4):673.

Eames P. Hysteria following brain injury. Journal of Neurology, Neurosurgery, and Psychiatry 1992;55:1046-1053.

Kroenke K. Efficacy of treatment for somatoform disorders: a review of randomized controlled trials. Psychosom Med 2007 Dec;69(9): 881-888.

Eating Disorders

27

Kenneth Lakritz

Clinical Vignette

Ellen W. had gained 15 pounds during her freshman year at college and felt out of control. She began a strict diet, limiting her intake to 1000 calories daily. She also began to run every day. By summer's end she had returned to her baseline weight but decided to continue her diet and exercise regime. She was continually hungry and sometimes binged, but she soon discovered how to induce vomiting and settled into a regular pattern of bingeing and purging. After another year, she came to medical attention when she was brought—against her objections—to an emergency room after collapsing while running.

On examination she was cachectic, hypotensive, and bradycardic. Her teeth were eroded and she had parotid enlargement. Laboratory studies revealed microcytic anemia, metabolic alkalosis, and hypokalemia. She was admitted and eventually required forced feeding to correct her life-threatening nutritional deficiencies. Throughout her hospitalization, she insisted that she was well but slightly overweight and needed to lose 10 more pounds. Five

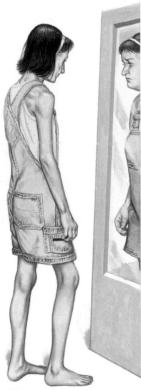

"No matter what anyone says, I am too fat!"

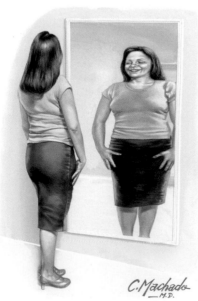

Two Forms	Restrictive anorexia nervosa. Bulimia nervosa; binge eating
Common Findings	Body image distortion @ ages 14-18; women > men Amenorrhea at least 3 months, and often precedes Weight loss >15% of ideal body weight Preserved secondary sex characteristics
Psychiatric Associated Disorders	Affective Anxiety OCD Personality Substance abuse
Differential Diagnosis	Adrenal insufficiency Inflammatory bowel and other GI disease Diabetes mellitus recent onset CNS posterior fossa lesions Primary depression
Endocrine Findings	Serum cortisol and growth hormone increased Serum LH & FSH low Insulin-like growth factor IGF-I low

Figure 27-1 Eating Disorders.

years later, she participated in regular individual and family psychotherapy. She had stopped bingeing and had negotiated a slightly less rigorous diet with her therapists, but she continued to monitor her caloric intake and weight every day.

Ellen W. suffers from anorexia nervosa, one of the two main eating disorders described in Diagnostic and Statistical Manual of Mental Disorders–Fourth Edition *(the other is bulimia). Anorexia nervosa is characterized by distorted body image, an unwillingness to maintain normal weight, emaciation, amenorrhea, and severely disordered eating habits. Anorexia nervosa is one of the deadliest of psychiatric disorders—a recent estimate is that 6% of anorectics die from their illness.*

ANOREXIA

Anorexia and other eating disorders are primarily diseases of young women. Its cause is unknown, but anorectic patients typically display high levels of anxiety and perfectionism, and twin studies suggest comorbidity with major depression and a substantial inherited risk (Fig. 27-1). However, unlike many other psychiatric illnesses, the prevalence of anorexia varies among different cultures; pressure to conform to cultural standards of thinness may play an important role in initiating the disorder.

The best treatment for anorexia is unclear, but there is general agreement that no progress can be made until the patient is restored to a safe weight. Zinc supplementation may be particularly important. Patients usually receive intensive individual and sometimes family psychotherapy. No medication is clearly effective.

BULIMIA

Bulimia, the other major eating disorder, is characterized by recurrent episodes of excessive food intake and loss of control, preoccupation with weight and body image, and inappropriate compensatory behaviors to control weight, such as fasting, excessive exercise, induced vomiting, and ingestion of laxatives and diuretics. Unlike anorectics, bulimic patients are usually obese or of normal weight.

Bulimia is less deadly than anorexia but much more common. The prevalence is especially high in settings where thinness is demanded, such as modeling, professional dance, and some athletics. There is a high rate of comorbidity with depression.

Bulimia is responsive to psychotherapy that includes education in healthy eating and weight management and a cognitive approach that addresses the all-or-none thinking that leads to binges.

Most antidepressant medications are at least partially effective in treating bulimia (the exception is bupropion, which is contraindicated in eating disorder patients because of a heightened risk of seizures). Selective serotonin reuptake inhibitors are considered first-line treatment. The anticonvulsant topiramate also appears to have a clinically useful antibingeing effect.

ADDITIONAL RESOURCES

Birmingham CL, Gritzner S. How does zinc supplementation benefit anorexia nervosa? Eating and Weight Disorders 2006;11(4):e109-e111.

Garner DM, Garfinkel PE. Socio-cultural factors in the development of anorexia nervosa. Psychol Med 1980;10(4):647-656.

Hay PJ, Bacaltchuk J. Psychotherapy for bulimia nervosa and binging. Cochrane Database Syst Rev 2003;(1):CD000562.

Herzog DB, Greenwood DN, Dorer DJ, et al. Mortality in eating disorders: A descriptive study. International Journal of Eating Disorders 2000;28(1):20–26.

Hudson JI, Hiripi E, Pope HG Jr, et al. The prevalence and correlates of eating disorders in the National Comorbidity Survey Replication. Biol Psychiatry 2007 Feb 1;61(3):348-358.

Lindberg L, Hjern A. Risk factors for anorexia nervosa: a national cohort study. International Journal of Eating Disorders 2003;34(4):397-408.

Toro J, Salamero M, Martinez E. Assessment of sociocultural influences on the aesthetic body shape model in anorexia nervosa. Acta Psychiatrica Scandinavica 1994;89(3):147-151.

Walsh BT, Roose SP, Glassman AH, et al. Bulimia and depression. Psychosomatic Medicine 1985;47(2):123–131.

Wonderlich SA, Lilenfeld LR, Riso LP, et al. Personality and anorexia nervosa. Int J Eat Disord 2005;37(Suppl.):S68-S71.

Dysthymia

Kenneth Lakritz

28

Clinical Vignette

A 47-year-old woman was referred to psychiatry by her internist who was caring for her chronic fatigue and diffuse achiness. He was uncertain of her diagnosis and wondered if the patient was depressed. Although the patient resented this referral, she agreed to a single consultation. This lady was experiencing inadequate and poor-quality sleep, impaired concentration, migratory chest pain, and migraine headaches. Utilizing the web, she had sought out a "Lyme specialist" and subsequently received antibiotic treatment for "chronic Lyme disease." However, her symptoms continued unabated despite this treatment.

Although she had been clearly depressed on two occasions, at age 19 years after her father's death and at age 26 years after the birth of her first child, she denied current feelings of sadness, guilt, or hopelessness. She described herself as overworked, justifiably pessimistic, socially isolated, and burdened with an unappreciative and unsympathetic husband. She wondered whether she had chronic fatigue syndrome, fibromyalgia, or multiple chemical

Some of the common complaints of dysthymic patients may include:

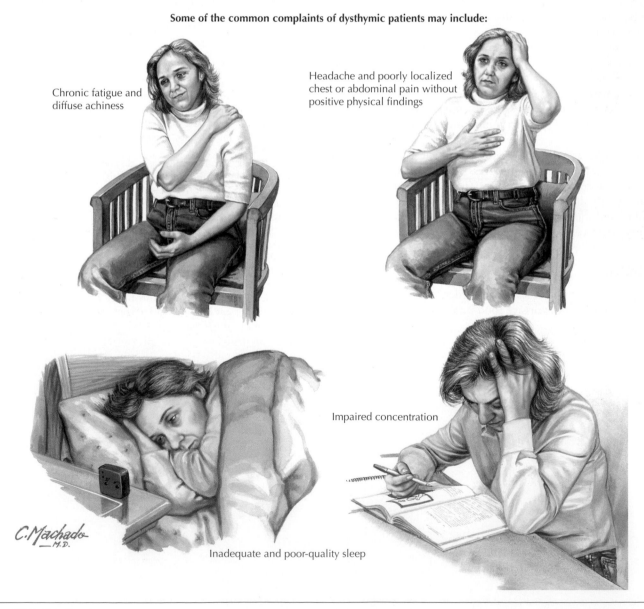

Chronic fatigue and diffuse achiness

Headache and poorly localized chest or abdominal pain without positive physical findings

Impaired concentration

Inadequate and poor-quality sleep

Figure 28-1 Dysthymia.

sensitivities, but she had no obvious delusions about her health. An extensive medical workup had revealed an iron deficiency anemia and hypothyroidism; however, their treatment was not helpful in resolving her many symptoms. An overnight sleep study was unremarkable, excluding sleep apnea as a potential mechanism. As this woman was generally sedentary, her physician recommended aerobic exercise, but she felt too tired to try it.

She reluctantly acknowledged that her pessimism and low mood might be contributing to her problems. She agreed to a trial of cognitive–behavioral therapy, which she found helpful especially as it induced her to exercise more and change jobs. She also convinced her husband to start marriage counseling.

CLINICAL PRESENTATION

Mood disorders are extremely common and diverse in their presentation and clinical course. Previously called "minor depression" and "subsyndromal depression," dysthymia is among the most common and easily overlooked.

Dysthymic patients have fewer and less-intense depressive symptoms than patients with major depression. To establish the diagnosis, the *Diagnostic and Statistical Manual of Mental Disorders–Fourth Edition* (DSM-IV) requires at least a 2-year course of predominantly depressed mood, while noting that chronic low mood may be such a fixture of the patient's life as to be unrecognized by the patient. Two other symptoms must also be present from a list, including sleep disturbance, appetite disturbance, fatigue, hopelessness, low self-esteem, and impaired concentration (Fig. 28-1). Dysthymia usually has an early and insidious onset and a chronic course. Family history of mood disorder is common.

Because of its restriction to overt and easily observable signs and symptoms, DSM-IV does not recognize the existence of a *depressive personality disorder*. However, patients who are characterologically prone to depression but not classically presenting with active symptoms of a mood disorder are extremely common. These individuals have an underlying conception (misconception) of themselves as defective or inadequate and are prone to feelings of guilt and shame. They overlap partially with patients suffering from dysthymia per se.

Although dysthymic patients do not meet the criteria for a diagnosis of major depression, dysthymia is not a benign illness. As a chronic disease, it causes immense suffering and loss of human potential. Dysthymic patients do less well than they should at school, work, and in personal relations. They overuse medical resources and substances, both legal and illegal. They are at high risk for the development of more severe affective disorders; one of the commonest is double depression, a pattern of repeated major depressive episodes with partial recovery to a state of dysthymia.

Most physician practices include a number of patients with poorly characterized pain or other vague but persistent physical complaints. Even after excluding appropriate and specific medical diagnoses, hypochondriasis, malingering, and delusional disorder, certain puzzling cases remain unclassified or specifically diagnosed per se. These are best understood as disguised presentations of dysthymia. Neurologists, rheumatologists, and gastroenterologists are frequently sought out by these relatively common dysthymic patients. Both the patients and the clinicians are usually frustrated and resentful of one another.

TREATMENT

Patients with dysthymia deserve careful evaluation and intensive treatment. They often respond well to specific counseling techniques such as cognitive–behavioral therapy or interpersonal therapy. Often a combination of psychotherapy and antidepressant medication produces the best outcome.

ADDITIONAL RESOURCES

Gureje O. The relation between multiple pains and mental disorders: results from the World Mental Health Surveys. Pain 2008 Mar;135(1-2): 82-91.

Ratey J, Johnson C. Shadow Syndromes: The Mild Forms of Major Mental Disorders That Sabotage Us. New York, NY: Pantheon; 1997.

Shedler J, Westen D. Refining personality disorder diagnosis: Integrating science and practice. American J Psych 2004;161:1350-1365.

Subodh BNJ, Avasthi A, Chakrabarti S. Psychosocial impact of dysthymia: A study among married patients. J Affect Disord. 2008;109:199-204.

Major Depression

Kenneth Lakritz

29

Clinical Vignette

A 69-year-old man was brought to the emergency room by his daughter for evaluation of weight loss, seeming inability to sleep, frequent periods of overwhelming anhedonism, and crying. The patient admitted that his appetite was poor, but was convinced he was losing weight because his bowels were being "eaten away" by cancer. He described himself as a useless individual whose productive life was over; he had become a burden to his family. Additionally he was experiencing intense anxiety, poorly localized back pain, difficulty concentrating, and insomnia. Ten years earlier he had been hospitalized for a depressive episode following a suicide attempt by overdose.

This vignette provides a classic picture of severe depression (Fig. 29-1). This is the most common serious psychiatric disorder; practicing physicians encounter it very frequently in many different guises. Depression is a very significant illness; it ranks second only to cardiovascular disease in overall morbidity and economic loss. Up to 20% of individuals within a general population will have at least one major depressive episode during their lifetime. Women have a higher incidence of depression between menarche and menopause, with an especially high risk postpartum. When depression affects men, the long-term risk of suicide is more common.

Depression usually begins in adolescence or early adulthood. It is a chronic illness with a propensity for recurrence. One common clinical pattern, called "double depression," is characterized by repeated episodes of depression (Fig. 29-2) with eventual remission to a milder "dysthymic" state (Chapter 28). Familial clustering is apparent, although specific genes have not been identified. Depression beginning after age 60 years is probably a different disorder. It is less often associated with a significant family history but is associated with cerebrovascular disease and periventricular white matter abnormalities.

CLINICAL PRESENTATION

Major depression predominantly presents with a 2-plus-week history of a sad or anxious mood; impaired energy and concentration; anhedonia (loss of pleasure from normally enjoyable experiences); insomnia, often with early morning wakening; loss of appetite; feelings of worthlessness or guilt; and recurrent thoughts of death or suicide. The presence of predominant diurnal mood fluctuation—feeling worse in the morning—is almost pathognomonic of depression. It is not uncommon to find disturbed sleep architecture with shortened rapid eye movement latency. Many patients have subtle endocrine disturbances, especially hypercortisolism that is not clinically apparent.

One of the major medical concerns vis-à-vis any severely depressed patient is that suicide ideation and very definite

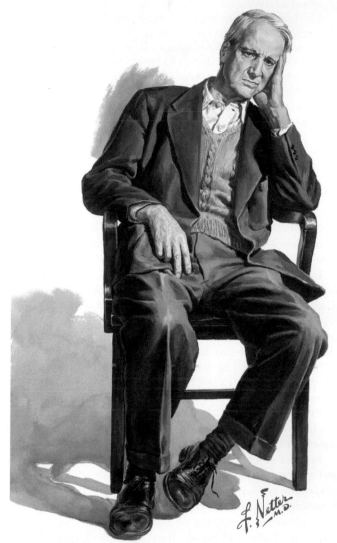

"I've lost interest in everything. It's even an effort to get out of bed in the morning. I don't want to go anywhere, see anybody, or do anything. It's all closing in on me."

Figure 29-1 Major Depression in Seniors.

attempts of the same are a common occurrence (Fig. 29-3). Although overt suicide attempts are notoriously difficult to predict, physicians must maintain a heightened sense of alertness to assessing suicide risk. One must always stand by to offer help and intervention per se when necessary, especially with the patient having significant suicidal risk factors. These include being a male, intense anxiety or agitation, social isolation, advanced age, history of previous suicide attempts, psychosis, and known alcohol abuse.

Certain medical conditions may provoke or mimic major depression. These most commonly include hypothyroidism, alcohol abuse, or need for corticosteroid therapy such as in the

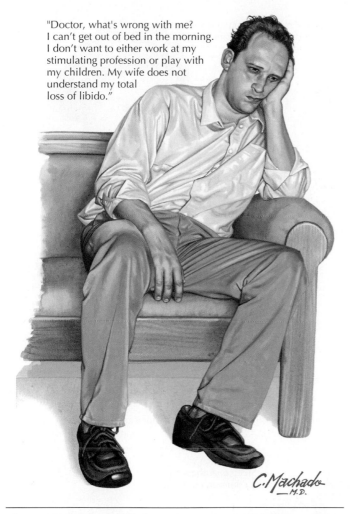

"Doctor, what's wrong with me? I can't get out of bed in the morning. I don't want to either work at my stimulating profession or play with my children. My wife does not understand my total loss of libido."

C. Machado
—M.D.

Figure 29-2 Severe Pathologic Depression in Otherwise Healthy, Vigorous Patient.

patient with myasthenia gravis. Depressed alcoholics and drug abusers are very unlikely to maintain a recovery from depression unless they maintain their sobriety.

Psychotic depression may develop in those individuals who are the most severely depressed at presentation. This is typically characterized by delusions that are "affect consonant," for example, delusions of poverty, moral depravity, or life-threatening illness. Bowel delusions are the most common of the various physical complaints that the depressed patient may express their inappropriate concern. The recognition of psychotic thinking in the depressed patient has very definite therapeutic consequences. This is particularly important because this subgroup of patients with depression fails to respond to standard antidepressant medications. There are two primary therapeutic options for psychotically depressed patients: (1) electroconvulsive therapy or (2) a combination of antidepressant and antipsychotic medication.

A primary bipolar disorder may underlie or be masked per se in at least 10% of individuals presenting with what appears on first pass to be unipolar depression. One single episode of mania will establish the bipolar diagnosis. A heightened level of suspicion for the presence of underlying bipolar disorder is necessary for anyone raised in a family with history of bipolar

disorder, having experienced a childhood onset of depressive illness, or a poor therapeutic response. Similarly, if the patient experiences a sudden response to initiation of antidepressant medication, that is, "switching," rather than following the usual delayed therapeutic response, a bipolar disorder requires further consideration. Efforts should be made to limit the exposure of patients with known or suspected bipolar disorder to the usual antidepressant medications (Chapter 30).

TREATMENT

Treatment of major depression combines specific pharmacologic medications with psychotherapy; the two are synergistic. Psychodynamic theorists divide depression as "anaclitic" or "introjective." Anaclitic patients feel ineffective and reliant on others for support. They get depressed when they feel abandoned, and respond well to supportive psychotherapy. Introjective patients set excessively high demands for themselves, are harshly self-critical, and feel guilty and worthless when they do not meet their own expectations. Both groups have characteristically distorted thinking even when well; they are overly passive, feel powerless, and evaluate problems in all-or-none terms. Cognitive therapies that target these patterns are the best-validated psychotherapeutic interventions.

The most useful information source for medical management of depression is the ongoing STAR*D study. This is a large multicenter, NIMH-funded trial dedicated to medication switching and augmentation strategies. Most antidepressant medications are equally effective, producing significant improvement in 60–70% of patients and full remission in 30–40%.

Selective serotonin reuptake inhibitors (SSRIs) are the preferred pharmacologic agents for initial treatment as they have milder side effects. Furthermore, the SSRIs are less lethal when taken as an overdose in comparison with the earlier developed tricyclic antidepressants. However, there is some controversy present as to whether SSRIs are as effective as tricyclics in severely depressed patients.

Although monoamine oxidase inhibitors (MAOIs) are often very effective for control of depression, unfortunately these pharmacologic agents have a unique potential for precipitating a hypertensive crisis and tachycardia. This occurs when norepinephrine is displaced from storage vesicles if patients are exposed to tyramine-containing foods. Tyramine is an amine that is typically produced by decarboxylation of the amino acid tyrosine during fermentation of various food products. These include Chianti and vermouth wines, aged cheeses, certain fruits such as eggplant, avocados, figs, grapes and prunes, as well as very high quantities of chocolate. A similar response may occur when MAOIs are given to patients already taking various other medications, particularly meperidine and SSRIs. A transdermal MAOI patch (containing selegiline) is now available. It causes fewer side effects but is very expensive.

Patients who have only a partial response to pharmacologic treatment may sometimes respond to various other therapeutic maneuvers. These include a switch to a different class of antidepressant, addition of a second antidepressant, or of an augmenting agent such as lithium and triiodothyronine (T3). Atypical antipsychotic agents and certain stimulants are also promising.

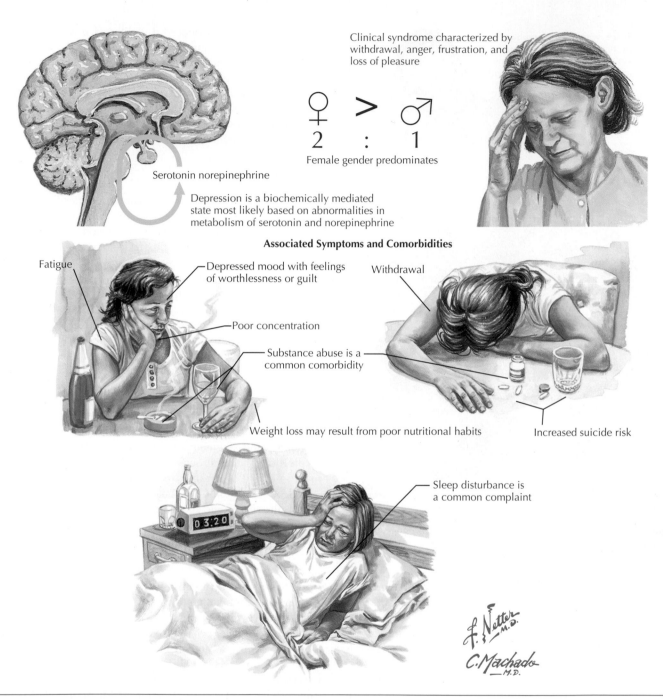

Clinical syndrome characterized by withdrawal, anger, frustration, and loss of pleasure

♀ > ♂
2 : 1
Female gender predominates

Serotonin norepinephrine

Depression is a biochemically mediated state most likely based on abnormalities in metabolism of serotonin and norepinephrine

Associated Symptoms and Comorbidities

Fatigue

Depressed mood with feelings of worthlessness or guilt

Withdrawal

Poor concentration

Substance abuse is a common comorbidity

Weight loss may result from poor nutritional habits

Increased suicide risk

Sleep disturbance is a common complaint

Figure 29-3 Major Depression.

Additionally, a combination of cognitive behavioral therapy as developed by Beck has proven to be a very useful additive therapeutic modality for some patients.

Electroconvulsive therapy (ECT) is a very important treatment modality for depression. It is indicated for severely depressed individuals who fail medication trials. It has more than a 90% response rate in well-selected populations. ECT is also the first-line treatment for psychotic depression, intense suicidal ideation, and the otherwise medically ill patients. Public misunderstanding may have led to its being underutilized. Unilateral electrode placement has significantly diminished the occurrence of post-ECT confusion. Today the concomitant employment of modern anesthetic agents has significantly decreased the frequency of other complications such as spinal compression fractures.

It is most important to recognize that depression is usually a chronic illness. Therefore a maintenance and prophylactic treatment protocol should be considered at time of diagnosis for each patient. Active treatment for first episodes should last at least six months, preferably one year. After three episodes, indefinite lifelong prophylaxis with full-dose antidepressant medication is indicated.

FUTURE DIRECTIONS

Because the treatment of depression remains somewhat unsatisfactory in certain cases, novel and experimental treatments abound. Patients who get depressed in the winter (seasonal affective disorder) often respond to bright light therapy, although standard antidepressant treatment is also effective. Vagus nerve stimulation, as used in certain cases of difficult-to-control epilepsy, is now approved by the Food and Drug Administration for refractory depression. However, definite controversy as to its effectiveness continues.

Hypericum, extract of St. John's Wort, is widely employed in Europe as a first-line treatment of depression, but controlled U.S. studies have been disappointing. S-adenosyl-methionine (SAM-E), a methyl donor, is an effective antidepressant with a benign side effect profile. However, a full dose is costly. Inositol, a sugar involved in second message signaling also has some experimental support and a favorable side effect profile. In a recent study, intravenous ketamine, an N-methyl-D-aspartic acid receptor antagonist, produced rapid and sustained improvement in depression.

Transcranial magnetic stimulation has been proposed as a more benign alternative to ECT, but it is less effective. Recently, stimulation of the anterior cingulated by implanted electrodes succeeded in a small study of desperately ill patients. Larger studies are under way.

ADDITIONAL RESOURCES

Beck AT, Rush AJ, Shaw BF, et al. Cognitive Therapy of Depression. New York, NY: Guilford Press; 1987.

Blatt SJ. Experiences of Depression: Theoretical, Clinical and Research Perspectives. Washington D.C.: American Psychological Association; 2004.

Maeng S, Zarate CA Jr. The role of glutamate in mood disorders: results from the ketamine in major depression study and the presumed cellular mechanism underlying its antidepressant effects. Curr Psychiatry Rep 2007 Dec;9(6):467-474.

Mayberg HS. Defining the neural circuitry of depression: toward a new nosology with therapeutic implications. Biol. Psychiatry 2007 Mar 15;61(6):729-730.

Mischoulon D. Update and critique of natural remedies as antidepressant treatments. Psychiatr Clin North Am 2007 Mar;30(1):51-68.

Solomon, A. The Noonday Demon: an Atlas of Depression. Scribner: 2002.

Warden D, Rush AJ, Trivedi MH, et al. The STAR*D Project results: a comprehensive review of findings. Curr Psychiatry Rep 2007 Dec;9(6):449-459.

Bipolar Disorder

Kenneth Lakritz

30

Clinical Vignette

An 18-year-old woman, currently a first-year college student, was admitted to an inpatient psychiatric unit after a deliberate overdose with acetaminophen. She complained of sadness and anxiety "for as long as I can remember," but in the preceding 3 months she had suffered from feeling of hopelessness, severe anhedonia, extreme fatigue, and hypersomnia. Her family history was positive for depression in three of five first-degree relatives and manic-depressive psychosis in her maternal grandmother.

   Treatment with a selective serotonin reuptake inhibitor (SSRI) was initiated, and the patient participated in individual and group psychotherapy. After 1 week, she announced that her energy had returned and that her need for sleep had decreased dramatically. She told staff that she was "cured," and developed a plan to move to Los Angeles with a fellow patient; they were both going to become movie stars. When she was prevented from leaving, she became agitated and threw chairs at the nursing staff, accusing them of a plot to keep her from succeeding. Despite this, she promised to buy everyone she knew a new car as soon as she left the hospital.

This vignette provides an example of a patient initially presenting with depression, and in a seeming clinical paradox, becoming manic after initiation of antidepressant therapy. This "switch" from depression may be the first indication that the patient has an underlying bipolar disorder. The presence of a strong family history of similar psychiatric illness is typical.

Typically mania has a unique presentation. The patient is often colorfully dressed and wearing too much jewelry, is excessively cheerful, overly familiar, brimming with schemes and ideas, and does not stop talking (Fig. 30-1). One of the surest sign of mania is the physician feeling the need to interrupt the patient. In the extreme, manic patients lose touch with reality; they may declare themselves an emperor, suddenly relocate to another state, or flirt dangerously with strangers. These patients often become irritable and sometimes aggressive. They may stop sleeping. In contrast to schizophrenic patients, who seem odd and distant, manic patients are often humorous, and frequently engaging.

Almost all manic patients eventually have serious depressions. (In contrast to unipolar depression, unipolar mania is uncommon.) With time, episodes of bipolar illness become more frequent, more autonomous—less clearly tied to external stresses—and more difficult to treat. Patients are at high risk for repeated hospitalizations, suicide, and drug and alcohol abuse.

CLINICAL PRESENTATION

Bipolar disease typically has its onset in the teens or twenties; however, on occasion a childhood onset may occur. The child who develops depression has a 50% chance of eventually becoming bipolar. There is no sexual predisposition.

Although classic clinical mania is hard to miss, it is an uncommon initial presentation. Early on bipolar disorder is often misdiagnosed. In most studies, the time from initial presentation to correct diagnosis is over 5 years. There are several reasons for this high rate of misdiagnosis:

1. Patients most often seek treatment when they are depressed. They may not yet have suffered a manic episode or, if they have, may not have recognized it as a problem.
2. Previous "high episodes" may have been either relatively mild or of "hypomanic" intensity, and not easily recognized as beyond the realm of normal behavior. A life history characterized by depressive episodes and mild or subsyndromal periods of elevated mood is known as Bipolar-2 Disorder. In fact, this variant may actually be the commonest variant of bipolar disorder. This form of bipolar disorder is thought to carry a high risk for development of substance abuse.
3. Although mania and depression seem to be polar opposites: happy/sad, accelerated/slowed, etc., the two states are more alike than different at a neurobiologic level. Patients often present with simultaneous features of mania (Fig. 30-2) and depression. In these atypical mood states, variously described as mixed states, dysphoric mania, or agitated depression, affected individuals present a confusing mix of symptoms. These patients are excited and restless but also sad or irritable, rapidly oscillating between elation and sadness. Most likely, such atypical states are actually more common than classic, euphoric mania.

A careful history is the essential diagnostic key in bipolar disorder as the very complex presentations may initially mask the primary psychiatric nature of this affliction. Patients' reluctance to see or acknowledge their own mania mandates that the physician take the time to inquire for more details from observant, reliable family members, friends or colleagues, and prior health care professionals.

As bipolar disorder is the most genetically determined of all major psychiatric illnesses, many of these patients have at least one affected relative. Conversely, anyone with a first-degree bipolar relative has at least a 10% chance of developing bipolar disorder. When individuals with this background present with a complaint of depression or alcohol abuse, suspicion of bipolar disorder must be high.

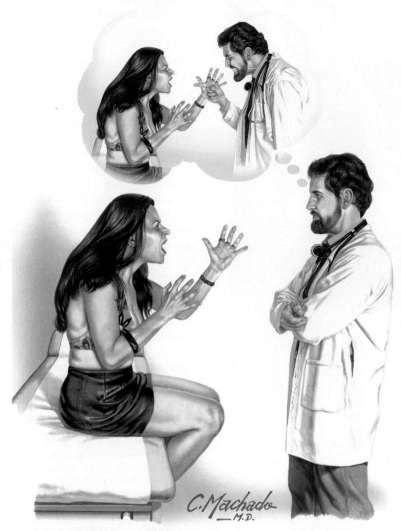

Patients with personality disorders often provoke intense and hostile feelings in their caregivers

Figure 30-1 Personality Disorders.

TREATMENT

Mood-stabilizing medications provide the primary treatment modality. Because of its natural history, once the diagnosis is established, bipolar patients must be treated indefinitely.

Lithium is effective for both the manic and depressed phases as well as for long-term prophylaxis. This medication is the first specific treatment for this disorder. Currently it continues to be the only medication clearly shown to reduce suicide rates in bipolar disorder. Because lithium has a narrow therapeutic index and many annoying side effects, frequent blood-level monitoring is required. One needs to also monitor renal and thyroid function.

Anticonvulsants are more effective than lithium in mixed or atypical cases, and especially for patients with "rapid cycling"—more than four episodes of illness per year. Valproic acid and carbamazepine are demonstrably effective; other anticonvulsants may also be effective. Atypical antipsychotics also have

mood-stabilizing properties. When these usual medications are ineffective, clozapine is sometimes helpful, although considered to be the last medication that should be tried.

The treatment of bipolar depression is especially challenging. Most patients with bipolar disorder experience depressive symptoms a significant larger proportion of their lifetime than those who demonstrate mania. Unfortunately antidepressants, per se, typically promote mood instability, often leading to rapid mood *cycling*. Any antidepressant can cause this switch to mania. Counterintuitively, there is little or no evidence that long-term use of antidepressant medications improves the outcome of bipolar depression. Nevertheless judicious use of antidepressants is often necessary, as most mood stabilizers have only weak antidepressant effects. Lamotrigine is the one anticonvulsant that may be specifically effective for bipolar depression. Another atypical antipsychotic, quetiapine, is now approved by the Food and Drug Administration for bipolar depression.

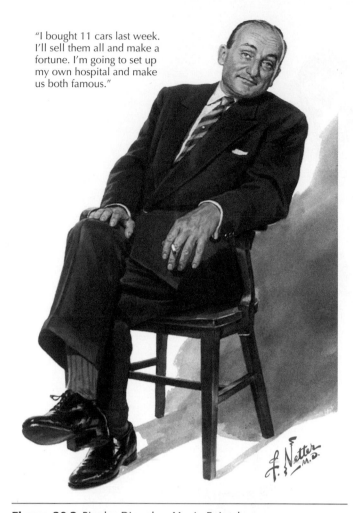

"I bought 11 cars last week. I'll sell them all and make a fortune. I'm going to set up my own hospital and make us both famous."

Figure 30-2 Bipolar Disorder: Manic Episode.

Electroconvulsive therapy is highly effective in both phases of bipolar disorder.

There is a paradoxical interplay between thyroid hormone activity in patients with bipolar disorder. In contrast to healthy individuals, supraphysiologic doses of thyroid hormone often help stabilize mood in these patients. Conversely, subclinical hypothyroidism is associated with rapid cycling. It is always important to test for such when lithium-treated patients are not responding well.

Therapeutic noncompliance almost universally occurs as most *successfully treated* bipolar patients eventually miss their high moods. Therefore, to avoid such remissions, a very strong interpersonal and educational relationship must be maintained between the psychiatrist, patient, and the family. Each individual who has a strong bond with a bipolar patient must learn to recognize and report early signs of relapse. Many authorities consider sleep loss to be the "final common pathway" to severe decompensation. The occurrence of insomnia in bipolar patients requires aggressive treatment.

Bipolar disorder appears to be less common in populations that consume large quantities of fatty fish. The typical Western diet is deficient. The fatty acids found in these fish—omega-3 unsaturated fatty acids—appear to play an important role in the secondary messenger systems activated by amine neurotransmitters. (Lithium is thought to affect the same pathways.) Dietary augmentation with omega-3 fatty acids appears to decrease relapse rates among bipolar patients. Because these dietary supplements appear harmless, and are known to benefit cardiovascular health, they can be widely recommended.

ADDITIONAL RESOURCES

Goodwin FK, Jamison KR. Manic-Depressive Illness. 2nd ed. New York, NY: Oxford Univ. Pr.; 2007.

Jamison KR. An Unquiet Mind: A Memoir of Moods and Madness. New York, NY: Vintage; 1997.

Goldberg JF, Perlis RH, Ghaemi SN, et al. Adjunctive antidepressant use and symptomatic recovery among bipolar depressed patients with concomitant manic symptoms: findings from the STEP-BD. Am J Psychiatry 2007 Sep;164(9):1348-1355.

Nierenberg AA, Ostacher MJ, Calabrese JR, et al. Treatment-resistant bipolar depression: a STEP-BD equipoise randomized effectiveness trial of antidepressant augmentation with lamotrigine, inositol, or risperidone. Am J Psychiatry 2006 Feb;163(2):210-216.

Owen C, Rees AM, Parker G. The role of fatty acids in the development and treatment of mood disorders. Curr Opin Psychiatry 2008 Jan;21(1): 19-24.

Wilens TE, Biederman J, Adamson JJ, et al. Further evidence of an association between adolescent bipolar disorder with smoking and substance use disorders: A controlled study. Drug Alcohol Depend 2008 Mar 14.

31

Schizophrenia

Kenneth Lakritz

Clinical Vignette

This 22-year-old electrician was brought to the emergency room after frequently confronting his parents, friends, and supervisors about being pursued by extraterrestrial aliens. With increasing frequency, he became obsessed with the idea of developing a barrier to electronic emissions that were "emanating from outer space." He was frightened that these signals were attempting to control his entire life by gaining control of his own body, and subsequently turn him into a baboon. When his parents attempted to be helpful, he found a lawyer and took them to court for persecuting him and invading his privacy.

Up until this time, he had been in perfect health with no outward signs of a thought disorder. He had never required any psychiatric treatment. He had done well in school, served in the armed forces for 4 years, where he learned to be an electrician and received an honorable discharge. Soon after arriving home and starting a civilian job, his parents recognized that a major personality change had occurred. This was characterized by both his paranoia and his withdrawal from most interpersonal relationships, spending almost all of his free time secluded in his room.

Psychiatric examination demonstrated him to be exceedingly tense and fearful. He stated that he was developing a computer system for his personal use that is to prevent alien communications from interfering with his daily activities. Further delusional thoughts were articulated, including his being concerned about a biologic invasion, voices telling him to do scary things, and feelings of being controlled by outside forces that are invading his own brain. Physical examination, cranial MRI, and routine laboratory testing, including drug screen, were unremarkable.

He was involuntarily hospitalized. An atypical antipsychotic drug helped to significantly improve his anxiety. Although this medication did not significantly impact on the presence and frequency of his delusional thinking, these thoughts seemed to be less bothersome to him. However, he was no longer capable of continuing in school and he withdrew from a formal educational environment to spend all of his time at home with his parents.

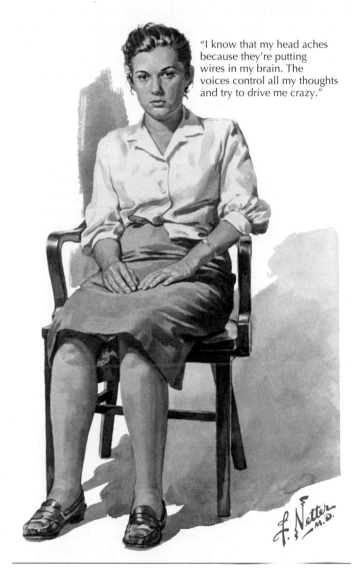

"I know that my head aches because they're putting wires in my brain. The voices control all my thoughts and try to drive me crazy."

Figure 31-1 Schizophrenic Disorder.

More than 120 years ago, Emil Kraepelin delineated schizophrenia as a global impairment of psychic functioning. It is distinguished from the affective psychoses by its unremitting course. Schizophrenia typically first occurs in late adolescence or early adulthood; this distinguishes it from the dementias. Sufferers, often initially odd or unsociable, eventually become progressively more isolated and eccentric, commonly failing to care for themselves and sometimes creating a public nuisance. It is quite uncommon for schizophrenia to first appear in midlife. However, when it does occur at this time in life, it overwhelmingly affects women, usually presenting with prominent paranoid symptoms.

During their initial evaluation, these patients overtly express their hallucinations—usually of commanding voices, disordered thinking, and delusional beliefs (Fig. 31-1). When untreated, schizophrenia patients exhibit declining cognitive function, especially early on during their first decade of the illness. Remissions and long-term improvement are eventually possible. Nevertheless, only a minority of schizophrenic patients achieve functional recovery. Most individuals are chronically disabled, accounting for a large proportion of nursing home and some prison populations. Sadly, one of the major consequences of schizophrenia is their very high suicide rate that approaches 10%.

Schizophrenia affects 0.5–1% of the population; a milder form of the illness, schizotypal personality disorder, is even more common. The pathophysiology continues to be elusive.

Familial clustering is obvious, but even identical twins have only ~50% disease concordance, excluding purely genetic explanations. More than 20 candidate genes are identified. Twin studies have refuted theories about defective parenting and "schizophrenogenic mothers." There are weak associations with winter birth, maternal malnutrition, and prenatal viral exposures, suggesting a stress-diathesis model, combining genetic vulnerability with early environmental insults. Immigrants, especially those who must learn a new language, are at increased risk. Schizophrenia is strongly associated with increased paternal but not maternal age, indicating that new germ-line mutations or epigenetic defects are involved in up to 25% of cases.

CLINICAL PRESENTATION

Schizophrenic symptoms can be categorized into three large clusters, with only weak associations between the clusters: positive symptoms, negative symptoms, and cognitive disturbance.

The schizophrenic delusions and hallucinations are *positive* symptoms, which are often more bizarre and illogical than compared with individuals having an affective psychosis. Many experts consider certain "first-rank" symptoms—delusions of passivity or outside control, thoughts being withdrawn from the patient's brain, thoughts being broadcast by the patient to others, for example—as pathognomonic for schizophrenia. Others maintain that only the long-term course of the illness reveals the diagnosis.

Negative symptoms are equally important components of the schizophrenic profile. These typically include emotional flatness, social withdrawal, and lack of initiative and self-care (Fig. 31-1). Additionally, the schizophrenic patient usually demonstrates a *cognitive* disturbance, with deficits in many areas of reasoning, such as working memory and abstract reasoning.

Schizophrenic patients have more than the expected number of neurologic "soft signs." Specific findings include abnormalities of smooth eye movement pursuit, auditory evoked potentials, and olfactory deficits. At least 50% of schizophrenic patients have gross central nervous system pathology visible on magnetic resonance imaging (MRI), including ventricular enlargement and decreased temporal and frontal lobe volume. Cerebellar abnormalities are also common. Ventricular enlargement appears to correlate with negative symptoms and treatment resistance. The underlying mechanisms explaining brain volume changes in schizophrenia are not yet understood, but the psychosis per se might be related to these changes. Five-year follow-ups on patients with first-episode schizophrenia who underwent brain MRI at inclusion and after 5 years demonstrated an association between longer duration of psychosis, larger gray matter volume decrease, and larger ventricular volume increase. These findings strongly suggest that psychosis contributes to brain volume reductions found in schizophrenia.

TREATMENT

Therapy of schizophrenic patients is challenging. Part of the difficulty is that patients are often strikingly unaware that they are ill. Because of this, they frequently stop their medications or drop out of treatment. Until neuroleptic medications were introduced in 1953, no effective biological treatments existed. The *classic neuroleptic agents* that work by blocking dopamine D_2 receptors are often *effective* against *positive symptoms*, but do *not help* and may exacerbate *negative* symptoms.

The first of the atypical neuroleptics, clozapine, was studied as early as the 1960s but was not introduced in the United States for more than 25 years because of its bone marrow toxicity—1% of patients develop potentially fatal agranulocytosis, and clozapine can only be prescribed when there is a mandatory monitoring of hematopoietic functions with regularly scheduled blood counts. Clozapine also causes seizures, metabolic syndrome, and weight gain at higher doses. Despite these problems, clozapine is clearly superior in efficacy to all other currently available antipsychotic drugs. Subsequent atypical or second-generation neuroleptics were developed to mimic clozapine's mechanism of action—thought to depend on weak D_2 antagonism combined with antagonism to the serotonin 5-HT2 receptor—without its inherent toxicity. The newer drugs are all, in varying degrees, less toxic, but none are quite as effective either.

Our current treatments are largely based on the idea that schizophrenia is a disorder of excess dopamine. This idea has some clinical support; dopaminergic drugs can cause or exacerbate psychosis, and antidopaminergic drugs treat psychosis. However, there is little direct evidence for this theory and no one believes that it comprises the entire story.

More recent research has focused on glutamate, especially on the NMDA receptor—in part because NMDA receptor antagonists such as phencyclidine precipitate psychosis. NMDA receptor agonists, such as the antituberculosis drug cycloserine, have been minimally effective. Recently, treatment with *N*-acetyl-cysteine, which is thought to act through glutamatergic mechanisms, has been promising.

Schizophrenic patients respond poorly to stress. Those living in rural or less industrialized settings tend to have better outcomes. Episodes of relapse correlate with "expressed emotion," a measure of interpersonal turbulence, in patients' households. Psychotherapy and educational measures focus on preventing these and other stressors.

ADDITIONAL RESOURCES

Amador X, David A. Insight and Psychosis: Awareness of Illness in Schizophrenia and Related Disorders. New York, NY: Oxford Univ. Pr.; 2004.

Cahn W, Rais M, Stigter FP, et al. Psychosis and brain volume changes during the first five years of schizophrenia. Eur Neuropsychopharmacol 2008 Dec 2. Epub ahead of print.

Kubicki M, Westin CF, Maier SE, et al. Uncinate fasciculus findings in schizophrenia: a magnetic resonance diffusion tensor imaging study. Am J Psychiatry 2002 May;159(5):813-820.

Lavoie S. Glutathione precursor, *N*-acetyl-cysteine, improves mismatch negativity in schizophrenia patients. Neuropsychopharmacology 2007 Nov 14.

Marom S. Expressed emotion: relevance to rehospitalization in schizophrenia over 7 years. Schizophr Bull 2005 Jul;31(3):751-758.

Sipos A. Paternal age and schizophrenia: a population based cohort study. BMJ 2004 Nov 6;329.

Straub RE, Weinberger DR. Schizophrenia genes—famine to feast. Biol Psychiatry 2006 Jul 15;60(2):81-83.

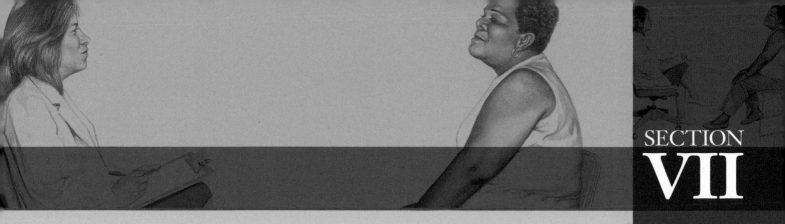

SECTION
VII

Gait and Movement Disorders

GAIT DISORDERS

HYPERKINETIC MOVEMENT DISORDERS

MISCELLANEOUS MOVEMENT DISORDERS AND THERAPY

Gait Disorders

Julie Leegwater-Kim

32

Clinical Vignette

A 70-year-old woman presented with a 2-year history of gait slowness and unsteadiness. Over that time, she experienced several falls, usually falling backwards. She began using a cane 1 year ago. She has noticed difficulty getting out of chairs or out of the car. Her husband described her walking as if "her feet are glued to the floor." In addition to her gait difficulties, she noted increased urinary urgency and had one episode of urinary incontinence. She also described being more forgetful.

Neurologic exam was notable for a slow, shuffled, broad-based gait with shortened stride length and heel strike, and en bloc turning. Arm swing was intact. When the patient was quickly pulled backward, she demonstrated marked postural instability and retropulsion. She could not arise from a chair without using her arms to push herself up. Cognitive testing was notable for limited object recall, one third objects at 5 minutes, as well as associated evidence of executive dysfunction.

The patient underwent testing, including a brain magnetic resonance imaging (MRI), which revealed an enlarged ventricular system out of proportion to the degree of brain atrophy. A large-volume lumbar puncture was performed, and the patient was noted to have marked improvement in her gait and balance afterwards. A ventriculoperitoneal shunt was placed, and the patient's gait improved to normal. She also experienced mild improvement in her urinary function. Her cognitive functioning was relatively unchanged.

*G*ait disorders are a common presentation of neurologic disease, and their prevalence increases with age. It is estimated that 15% of the population aged 60 years experiences gait abnormalities, whereas 82% of the population aged 85 years or older has a gait disorder. Approximately 40–50% of nursing home residents have walking difficulties and suffer from frequent falls. Gait disorder is associated with morbidity, particularly falls and loss of independence.

ANATOMY AND PATHOPHYSIOLOGY

Normal gait requires the integration and coordination of the central and peripheral nervous systems and the musculoskeletal system. Gait consists of two key components: (1) locomotion, the generation and maintenance of rhythmic stepping, and (2) equilibrium, the ability to keep the body upright and maintain balance. In quadripedal animals, locomotion is mainly dependent on spinal pattern generators, which produce rhythmic stepping movements. In contrast, locomotion in primates can be elicited by electrical stimulation of brainstem areas, including the posterior subthalamus, dorsal and ventral portions of the

caudal pons, and the mesencephalic tegmentum. The latter includes the pedunculopontine nucleus (PPN), a group of cholinergic neurons that receives input from the basal ganglia and motor cortex and projects to the spinal cord and reticular nuclei. Although the exact function of the PPN is not clear, it is uniquely situated to modulate the influence of the basal ganglia on locomotion and balance. Higher cortical centers are also important in the maintenance of gait and balance. The frontal cortex is implicated in the control, coordination, and planning of automatic and voluntary movements. In addition, the posterior parietal cortex is involved in the perception of body position and posture.

ETIOLOGY AND CLASSIFICATION

Because gait is dependent on the proper functioning and integration of different aspects of the nervous system, a variety of lesions in the central and/or peripheral nervous systems can produce walking difficulties. In a recent series of 120 patients presenting to an outpatient neurology clinic with gait disorder in which patients with hemiparesis, known Parkinson disease (PD), neuroleptic exposure, and orthopedic deformity were excluded, the distribution of etiologies were as follows: myelopathy (17%), sensory deficits (17%), multiple infarcts (15%), parkinsonism (12%), hydrocephalus (7%), cerebellar dysfunction (7%), psychogenic (3%) and toxic/metabolic causes (3%).

Gait disorders can be classified in a number of ways: etiologically (Table 32-1), anatomically (Table 32-2), and clinically (Table 32-3; Fig. 32-1). Perhaps the most useful approach to understanding gait disorders is a clinicoanatomic one. According to this method, gait disorders can be divided into roughly three anatomic categories: cortical, subcortical, and peripheral. A variety of well-defined clinical gait syndromes can be described under each anatomic rubric.

CORTICAL GAIT DISORDERS

Frontal Gait

Bilateral frontal lobe dysfunction and/or disconnection between cortical and subcortical motor areas (i.e., basal ganglia, brainstem, cerebellum) leads to a distinctive gait, variously known as magnetic gait, "marche a petits pas," lower-body parkinsonism, and frontal apraxia of gait. It is characterized by a combination of gait initiation failure, impaired walking and disequilibrium. The patient exhibits a wider than normal gait base, reduced stride length and heel strike, and shuffling steps (Fig. 32-2). There is often a pronounced hesitation to the initiation of the gait. Such patients frequently exhibit retropulsion, something that often leads to falls backwards. Paradoxically, there is usually preservation of other types of leg movements, that is, pedaling or bicycling in the recumbent position (hence the term *apraxia of gait*).

Table 32-1 Gait Disorders—Etiological Classification

Myelopathy
- Cervical spondylosis
- Vitamin B_{12} deficiency
- Demyelinating diseases (e.g., multiple sclerosis)
- Infectious diseases (e.g., human T-lymphotropic virus type 1 infection)

Parkinsonism
- Parkinson disease
- Atypical parkinsonism
  - Progressive supranuclear palsy
  - Corticobasal ganglionic degeneration
  - Dementia with Lewy body disease
- Secondary parkinsonism
  - Neuroleptic-induced parkinsonism

Multiple infarcts/small vessel disease
- Stroke
- Vasculitis
- Mitochondrial disease

Hydrocephalus
- Communicating
  - Normal pressure hydrocephalus
- Non-communicating

Cerebellar disease
- Toxic-metabolic
  - Alcohol-induced cerebellar degeneration
  - Medications (e.g., phenytoin)
  - Thiamine deficiency
- Heredodegenerative disorders
  - Spinocerebellar ataxias
  - Fragile X-tremor-ataxia syndrome
- Infectious/postinfectious diseases
- Paraneoplastic disorders
- Celiac sprue

Sensory Deficits
- Peripheral neuropathy (e.g., diabetic neuropathy)
- Dorsal root ganglionopathy (e.g., Sjögren syndrome)
- Posterior column lesions (e.g., tabes dorsalis)
- Vestibular disorders
- Visual disorders

Table 32-2 Gait Disorders—Anatomic Classification

Frontal/cortical
Subcortical-hypokinetic
Subcortical-hyperkinetic
Pyramidal
Cerebellar
Vestibular
Neuropathic
Myopathic
Orthopedic

Table 32-3 Clinical Gait Syndromes: Specific Examples

Gait Type	Clinical Features	Associated Findings
Frontal gait	Wide based Shortened stride length Reduced heel strike Start and turn hesitation Retropulsion	Frontal-release signs Cognitive impairment Behavioral changes Urinary disturbance
Cautious gait	Mildly wide-based Shortened stride Improvement with assistive device	Anxiety Fear of falling Fear of open spaces
Psychogenic gait	Bizarre, inconsistent movements Lurching and knee-bucking but rare falls Distractibility/ entrainment of movements	Abrupt onset/ resolution Positive psychiatric features Secondary gain Wide fluctuations over short time periods

freezing of gait (see hypokinetic-rigid gait) as well. Associated signs of frontal gait disorder include frontal release signs, behavioral changes, and executive dysfunction.

The most common cause of frontal gait is cerebrovascular disease (small vessel ischemic changes or infarcts) affecting the basal ganglia and/or periventricular white matter. Normal-pressure hydrocephalus (NPH) is another and very important etiology, particularly because it is potentially remediable. NPH is characterized by the clinical triad of frontal gait disorder, urinary incontinence, and dementia. Imaging of the brain demonstrates hydrocephalus (Fig. 32-2). Diagnostic workup includes large-volume lumbar puncture, which reveals improvement of gait hours to days after removal of CSF. Treatment involves placement of a ventriculoperitoneal shunt.

Cautious Gait

This is a very common disorder, especially among senior citizens who are beginning to show signs of being elderly. It is also seen among individuals made more cautious than usual after having experienced an unexpected or seemingly unprovoked fall. These patients assume a stance and gait pattern that *mimics walking on ice*. The base is widened and steps are slow, with reduced stride length. Turning is *en bloc* and the arms are abducted. This relatively common gait significantly improves with minimal support, i.e., the assistance of a companion, a cane, or a walker. There is usually associated anxiety and fear of falling. Cautious gait can improve with physical therapy and an assistive device. However, on occasion a patient presenting with a cautious gait may be offering a precursor of a more specific and serious gait disorder that may soon show itself.

Psychogenic Gait

This is also termed *hysterical gait disorder* or *astasia-abasia*. It is a most unusual gait to witness as it is not congruent with the

Frontal gait, on initial clinical assessment, can resemble parkinsonian gait, although there is generally only involvement of the lower body (hence the term *lower-body parkinsonism*). Features that can help differentiate frontal gait from typical parkinsonian gait are more erect posture, wide base, lack of tremor, and preserved arm swing. Patients can sometimes develop

Cerebellar Gait Disorders

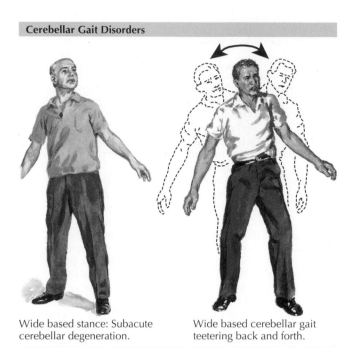

Wide based stance: Subacute cerebellar degeneration.

Wide based cerebellar gait teetering back and forth.

Spastic Gait	Peripheral Neuropathic Gait

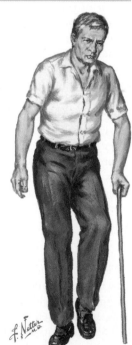

Cerebral, subcortical, or myelopathic lesons. Stroke, MS, or tumor at multiple sites: frontal lobe, internal capsule, pontine, or brainstem and cervical spinal cord, particularly spinal stenosis.

Painful burning feet with numbness and tingling. Foot drop.

Figure 32-1 Neuropathic Gait Disorders.

features of any known organic gait disorder. The gait is marked by bizarre, consistently inconsistent, and distractible movements. Some movements may be dramatic and lurching but subjects rarely fall. There are often significant clinical fluctuations over time. The diagnosis of psychogenic gait disorder

relies on the exclusion of organic etiologies but also on the presence of positive signs such as abrupt onset or resolution of symptoms/signs, false or giveway weakness, entrainability and distractibility of movements, somatization, la belle indifference affect, and psychiatric history and symptoms. Treatment is challenging, but a combination of intensive physical therapy and various psychiatric treatments including cognitive therapy may be beneficial.

One needs to be extremely cautious in arriving at such a diagnosis as is attested to by the following case history.

Clinical Vignette

A 28-year-old woman with depression had recently been evaluated by a psychiatrist; she began treatment using amitriptyline. Within a few weeks she appeared somewhat unsteady to others, who noted that she occasionally was bumping into furniture. Her internist stopped the antidepressant medication and scheduled a neurology consult. She reported to the neurologist that she was feeling significantly improved since the medication had been stopped. She still had a slightly abnormal poorly defined gait that suggested a primary emotional quality to the neurologist. Nevertheless, he wished to pursue this with imaging studies, but she failed to keep the appointment. Unbeknownst to the neurologist, she instead returned to see her psychiatrist; her depression worsened and noting her prior sensitivity to the amitriptyline, he elected to hospitalize her for electroconvulsive therapy (ECT).

After a few ECT treatments, she began to complain about problems with coordination of her left arm and leg. Her psychiatrist did not consult the neurologist but made an assumption that her new difficulties were psychogenic. He continued the daily ECT explaining her deteriorating neurologic status as a post-ECT effect. The patient's family demanded a recheck by the neurologist.

Unfortunately, he found that she had significant vertical nystagmus, left-hand finger to nose ataxia, and a spastic hemiparetic gait with brisk muscle stretch reflexes and a Babinski sign on the left. Imaging studies demonstrated a fourth-ventricle tumor. At surgery, this proved to be a malignant ependymoma with severe brainstem compression. She never awakened from the surgery.

Comment: One always needs to be very circumspect in evaluating any neurologic problem. Gait disorders are particularly prone to misinterpretation. Modern imaging studies generally prevent the unfortunate outcome experienced by this young woman.

SUBCORTICAL GAIT DISORDERS

Spastic Gait

This represents a pyramidal gait disorder, originating in the motor cortex or corticospinal tracts. Unilateral disease leads to a spastic hemiparetic gait characterized by stiff legged extension and circumduction of the affected leg (Fig. 32-1, middle row) and flexion of the ipsilateral upper limb. In the case of bilateral involvement, the patient exhibits adduction and scissoring of the

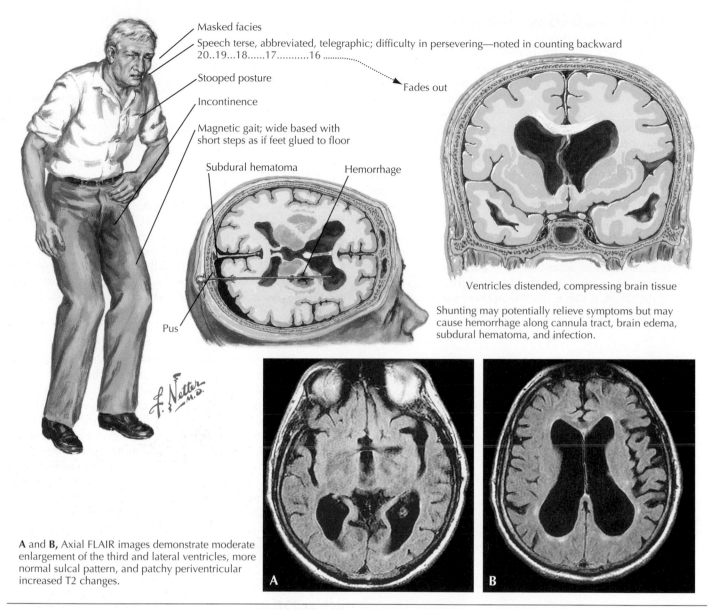

Masked facies

Speech terse, abbreviated, telegraphic; difficulty in persevering—noted in counting backward
20..19...18......17..........16 ....

Fades out

Stooped posture

Incontinence

Magnetic gait; wide based with short steps as if feet glued to floor

Subdural hematoma

Hemorrhage

Pus

Ventricles distended, compressing brain tissue

Shunting may potentially relieve symptoms but may cause hemorrhage along cannula tract, brain edema, subdural hematoma, and infection.

A and B, Axial FLAIR images demonstrate moderate enlargement of the third and lateral ventricles, more normal sulcal pattern, and patchy periventricular increased T2 changes.

A

B

Figure 32-2 Normal-Pressure Hydrocephalus: Gait and Other Clinical Characteristics.

legs. Associated findings include leg weakness, hyperreflexia, and extensor plantar responses. Causes of hemiparetic gait include stroke, demyelinating lesion, mass, or trauma. Paraparetic gait can be caused by cerebral palsy, primary lateral sclerosis, and spinal cord lesions. Botulinum toxin and oral medications such as baclofen and tizanidine can be beneficial.

Ataxic Gait

The gait has a lurching or veering quality, imitating a "drunken gait" that is marked by a widened base of support and irregular stepping. These patients also exhibit increased truncal instability that is exacerbated with standing with one's feet together or tandem walking. Ataxic gait disorders signal cerebellar dysfunction (Fig. 32-1 top row). On examination, other signs of cerebellar disease can be elicited: dysmetria, dysdiadochokinesia, nystagmus, hypermetric saccades, and scanning dysarthria.

Causes are myriad: (Table 32-4, Table 32-5) toxic/metabolic disorders (i.e. acute or chronic alcoholism), neurodegenerative diseases such as the spinocerebellar ataxias, paraneoplastic disease, and ischemic (Fig. 32-3) or demyelinating disorders affecting the cerebellum or its connections. Pharmacologic treatments to date have been unsuccessful. Physical therapy is the main treatment available.

Hypokinetic-Rigid Gait

This is also known as akinetic-rigid gait or parkinsonian gait and is seen in any of the various parkinsonian syndromes. The gait is characterized by flexed posture, reduced arm swing and stride length, shuffled steps, turning en bloc, and postural instability. Patients frequently exhibit festination, an acceleration of gait in which the steps get shorter and faster as the patient attempts to keep pace with his or her displaced center of gravity. Associated parkinsonian features may include bradykinesia, tremor, cogwheel rigidity, and freezing of gait (FOG). FOG refers to motor blocks in which the subject is unable to initiate and maintain locomotion.

Common etiologies of hypokinetic-rigid gait include neurodegenerative disorders such as idiopathic PD and atypical parkinsonian syndromes, that is, progressive supranuclear palsy (PSP) and corticobasal ganglionic degeneration (Fig. 32-4). One distinguishing feature between PD and other causes of parkinsonism is that the former is characterized by a normal or narrow base and the latter exhibits a broad-based gait. In addition, PD tends to start unilaterally versus the bilaterality seen with the atypical syndromes. Furthermore, the presence of a tremor is usually typical of idiopathic AD.

Patients with hypokinetic-rigid gaits should be given a trial of carbidopa/levodopa. A robust response to this medication supports a diagnosis of idiopathic PD. Patients with atypical parkinsonism may also benefit from carbidopa/levodopa; however, the effect, if any, is often temporary parkinsonian.

Table 32-4 Cerebellum: Acquired Disorders

Cerebral vascular disease
Toxic (alcohol, phenytoin, and other prescription drugs)
Tumors
Abscesses
Demyelinating, i.e., multiple sclerosis, progressive multifocal leukoencephalopathy
Viral
Prion disease
Metabolic diseases: hypothyroidism, thiamine deficiency, vitamin E deficiency, hyperpyruvic acidemia of childhood, Leigh syndrome, Refsum disease
Paraneoplastic

Hyperkinetic Gait

Hyperkinesias are excessive movements. Because many hyperkinesias represent abnormal movements, they are often termed dyskinesias. Hyperkinesias include chorea (random, brief movements that flow from one body part to another), dystonia (abnormal sustained involuntary movements), and myoclonus (rapid, involuntary, jerk-like movements). Patients with hyperkinesias often display distinctive gait patterns.

Choreic Gait

Choreic gait has a stuttering or dance-like quality that reflects superimposed choreic and choreoathetotic movements. Stride length and cadence are irregular and random. The base is variable. Steps often deviate from the direction of travel, giving the gait a somewhat ataxic quality. Choreic gait can be seen in patients with Huntington disease and in patients with PD who experience medication-induced dyskinesias.

Dystonic Gait

These patients demonstrate lower extremity and/or trunk dystonia. When the dystonia involves the foot, the gait is usually characterized by foot inversion. In the early stages of dystonia, the gait pattern is task-specific. For example, a patient with foot dystonia may exhibit dystonic gait when walking forwards but may walk backwards or run normally. In our clinic we evaluated a middle-aged patient who could only move forward emulating a cross country skiing gliding movement yet moved backward with impunity. In addition, dystonias can be temporarily improved with sensory tricks (i.e., placing hands in pockets, putting the hand on the back or hip). Isolated foot/leg dystonia can be due to early idiopathic PD, corticobasal ganglionic degeneration, or idiopathic torsion dystonia. Dystonia affecting the trunk can lead to retrocollis, anterocollis, Pisa syndrome (lateral flexion of the trunk), camptocormia, and opisthotonus. Causes of truncal dystonia include neurodegenerative disorders such as PSP (retrocollis) and multiple-system atrophy (Pisa syndrome, anterocollis), tardive syndromes (opisthotonus,

Table 32-5 Cerebellum: Degenerative and Hereditary Disorders: Some Examples

Name	Age at Onset (yr)	Symptoms/Findings	Mode of Inheritance	Pathology
Cortical cerebellar atrophy of Holmes	40	Ataxia, tremor, dysarthria	Familial and sporadic	Vermis
Multiple system atrophy— cerebellar type	50's	Ataxia Parkinsonism Autonomic dysfunction	Sporadic	Cerebellum Pons
Spinocerebellar ataxia type 3 (SCA3, Machado-Joseph disease)	Adolescence–late adulthood	Ataxia, parkinsonism Neuropathy Ophthalmoplegia Dystonia	Autosomal dominant Variable expression	Dentate nucleus Spinocerebellar tracts Pons Substantia nigra
Ataxia telangiectasia	1–2	Ataxia Chorea Oculomotor apraxia Oculomotor telangiectasis	Autosomal recessive	Cerebellum Posterior columns Peripheral nerves

Acute gait ataxia, sometimes truncal ataxia, vomiting, headache, dysarthria, with occasional hiccups and tinnitus

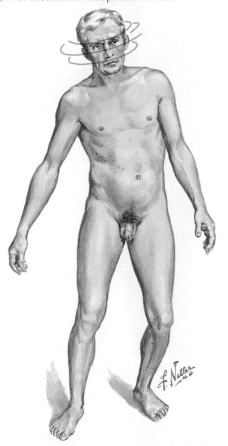

Acute gait disorder secondary to intracerebellar hemorrhage

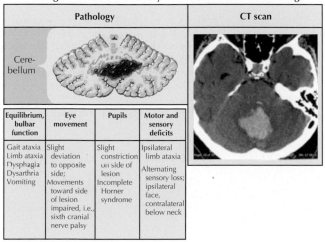

Pathology			CT scan
Cerebellum			
Equilibrium, bulbar function	Eye movement	Pupils	Motor and sensory deficits
Gait ataxia Limb ataxia Dysphagia Dysarthria Vomiting	Slight deviation to opposite side; Movements toward side of lesion impaired, i.e., sixth cranial nerve palsy	Slight constriction on side of lesion Incomplete Horner syndrome	Ipsilateral limb ataxia Alternating sensory loss; ipsilateral face, contralateral below neck

Figure 32-3 Vertebrobasilar Stroke: Gait and Other Clinical Findings.

retrocollis), and genetic disorders such as DYT-1 dystonia (generalized dystonia). Because dystonic gaits can appear unusual, be task-specific, and temporarily improve with sensory tricks, they are sometimes mistaken for psychogenic gaits. Treatments for dystonia include baclofen, trihexyphenidyl, and botulinum toxin. In severe cases, deep brain stimulation can be beneficial.

Myoclonic Gait

This is characterized by a bouncing gait and stance. This is due to the effects of positive myoclonus (quick jerk-like movements) and negative myoclonus (sudden give in muscle tone). Negative myoclonus while walking can lead to drop attacks. The classic example of myoclonic gait is posthypoxic (Lance-Adams) myoclonus. Other causes include neurodegenerative disorders, myoclonic epilepsies, myoclonic ataxia syndromes, and myoclonus-dystonia. A variety of pharmacologic agents may improve myoclonus and include clonazepam, piracetam, levetiracetam, and valproic acid. Posthypoxic myoclonus is exquisitely sensitive to alcohol. Sodium oxybate has recently been studied as a treatment for alcohol-responsive myoclonus.

PERIPHERAL GAIT DISORDERS

Sensory Gait

These patients have a loss of proprioceptive input from the legs; they tend to walk with a wide base and reduced stride length. Arms are usually held in abduction. Gait unsteadiness is markedly worsened when visual input is reduced, that is, in the dark or closing the eyes. Lesions of the large-fiber sensory afferent nerves including peripheral neuropathies, dorsal root lesions, sensory ganglionopathies, and posterior column damage account for the typical sensory gait disorders (Fig. 32-1, bottom row).

Steppage Gait

This gait disorder results from distal anterolateral leg muscle group weakness. Weakness of foot dorsiflexors causes foot drop, and patients compensate by adopting a high-stepping gait with excessive flexion of the hips and knees. When the foot touches down, the toe or anterolateral portion of the foot touches first. These patients cannot walk on their heels because of the weakness in the dorsiflexors of the feet and toes. Associated signs include distal muscle atrophy, reduced or absent ankle reflexes, and often sensory loss. The most common cause of steppage gait is peripheral neuropathy (Fig. 32-1, bottom row).

Waddling Gait

As its name implies, this is characterized by the swinging of the hip and trunk from side to side. The base is widened and lumbar hyperlordosis can develop. This type of gait arises from weakness affecting the proximal muscles of the leg and pelvic girdle muscles. Patients also have difficulty arising from a seated position and ascending stairs. Etiologies of waddling gait include myopathies, muscular dystrophies, neuromuscular transmission defects, particularly the Lambert-Eaton myasthenic syndrome, and on occasion a proximal peripheral nerve disorder such as chronic inflammatory demyelinating polyneuropathy.

Antalgic Gait

This classic gait is associated with orthopedic disorders such as arthritis. The gait is slow, limping, and painful (antalgic).

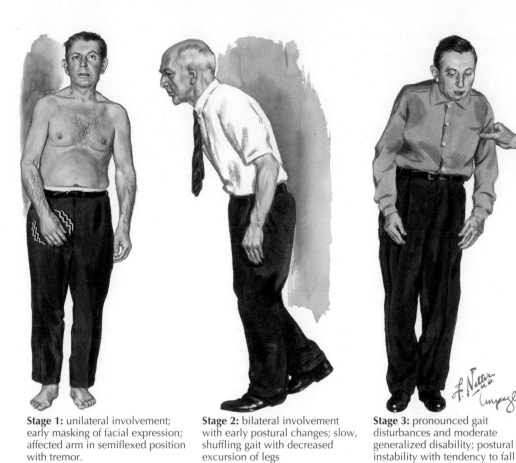

Stage 1: unilateral involvement; early masking of facial expression; affected arm in semiflexed position with tremor.

Stage 2: bilateral involvement with early postural changes; slow, shuffling gait with decreased excursion of legs

Stage 3: pronounced gait disturbances and moderate generalized disability; postural instability with tendency to fall

Figure 32-4 Parkinson Disease; Gait findings: Evolution of Disease Process.

Patients avoid weight-bearing on the affected leg, and there is limited range of movement of the leg and hip.

ADDITIONAL RESOURCES

Jankovic J, Nutt JG, Sudarsky L. Classification, diagnosis, and etiology of gait disorders. Adv Neurol 2001;87:119-133.

Nutt, JG. Classification of gait and balance disorders. Adv Neurol 2001;87:135-141.

Nutt JG, Marsden CD, Thompson PD. Human walking and higher level gait disorders, particularly in the elderly. Neurology 1993;43:268-279.

Ruzicka E, Jankovic JJ. Disorders of gait. In: Jankovic JJ, Tolosa E, editors. Parkinson's disease and movement disorders. Philadelphia, PA: Lippincott, Williams and Wilkins; 2002. p. 409-429.

Snijders AH, van de Waarenburg BP, Giladi N, et al. Neurological gait disorders in elderly people: clinical approach and classification. Lancet Neurol 2007;6:63-74.

Sudarsky L. Gait disorders: prevalence, morbidity, and etiology. Adv Neurol 2001;87:111-117.

Parkinson Disease

33

Diana Apetauerova

Clinical Vignette

This 54-year-old lady, a very dedicated high school art teacher, jammed her finger while playing basketball. Although the discomfort cleared rapidly, she continued to "favor" that hand. Her husband soon noted that her arm swing was absent on that side, telling her she carried the arm flexed "like Napoleon." Soon she lost the normal range of motion of that limb; eventually this arm became stiff, and she had increasingly limited motion at the shoulder. This led to her seeking chiropractic help; here she received manipulation, acupuncture, and heat. About 2 years after onset, she began to drag her right foot while walking. Subsequently, her art work became more limited, taking increasingly more time to do simple things such as coloring a boat. Her handwriting became more difficult as her hand began to shake and the figures increasingly small the longer she tried to write.

Neurologic examination demonstrated moderate masking of her face, a positive Myerson's sign, a mild 6-Hz rest tremor of her right hand, cogwheel rigidity of that wrist and elbow, diminished right arm swing, and a mild tendency to petit-pas gait. Extraocular muscle function was full, with no limitation of vertical gaze. Although a diagnosis of Parkinson disease (PD) was made here, initially she did not agree to take medication. Her tremor became much more pronounced at rest, particularly noticeable to her students. Activities of daily living were increasingly limited, such as getting dressed, going up and down stairs, and getting out of chairs. She had no problems with her left extremities.

Head computed tomographic (CT) scan was normal. No other investigations were indicated, as the diagnosis of PD is primarily a clinical one. Because of her moderately significant functional impairment, levodopa/carbidopa was initiated. Within 4 weeks, she demonstrated marked improvement. She was able to move faster, and her fine motor activities and tremor were significantly improved. This allowed her to return to a more vigorous approach to her celebrated teaching style. This excellent response made it most likely that idiopathic PD was the diagnosis.

In 1817, James Parkinson made the seminal observations on this disorder defining a specific neurodegenerative illness characterized by bradykinesia, resting tremor, cogwheel rigidity, and postural reflex impairment. Parkinson disease (PD) has a relatively stereotyped clinical presentation that now bears the name of this early 19th-century physician. PD is one of the most common neurologic disorders worldwide. It affects at least 1,500,000 persons within the United States. Its incidence typically peaks in the sixth decade; however, one can see classic clinical cases with onset as early as the fourth decade. On occasion, medication-induced Parkinson disease may also occur in early middle-aged individuals. In contrast, PD sometimes presents well into the late eighth or even the ninth decade. Usually the patient's clinical status progresses from a relatively modest limitation at diagnosis to an ever-increasing disability over 10 to 20 years in many but not all patients. The primary neuropathologic features are loss of pigmented dopaminergic neurons mainly in the substantia nigra (SN) and the presence of Lewy bodies—eosinophilic, cytoplasmic inclusions found within the pigmented neurons (Fig. 33-1). These neurons' primary projection is to the striatum, for example, the putamen and caudate. Dopamine is released primarily from these striatal cells. From here dopamine neurotransmission sequentially is directed through the globus pallidus, the subthalamic nucleus, to the thalamus per se, and then to the primary motor cortex (Figs. 33-2 and 33-3).

ETIOLOGY

Despite intensive research, the precise etiology of PD remains elusive. One conceptualization is that an unknown environmental toxin acts on genetically susceptible individuals to cause PD. The principal link between PD and an environmental toxin is the chemical MPTP (1-methyl-4-phenyl-1,2,3,6-tetrahydropyridine). This chemical was initially used by drug abusers in hopes of mimicking in the laboratory a synthetic narcotic-like substance. When ingested by humans, this narcotic model serendipitously led to a clinical entity that directly mimicked PD. As MPTP interferes with the function of nerve cell mitochondria, investigators next conjectured that chemicals impairing mitochondrial DNA may be one major pathophysiologic mechanism underlying human PD. It is here that evidence exists for a disturbance in oxidative phosphorylation, particularly reduced activity of complex I of the mitochondrial electron transport chain. Additionally, there are increased levels of free iron that may enhance toxic free radical formation.

Fifteen percent of Parkinson patients have a family history of PD; a small percentage of these individuals have at least three affected generations. It is unknown whether the clinical picture results from a defective gene per se, a shared environmental insult, or both. Currently there are several causative genes identified that are specific to young-onset PD. Although these well-identified PD genes are pathogenic in only a very small minority of individuals, their biochemical signatures are providing extraordinary insight into the molecular pathology of this disease. The currently identified genes are listed in Table 33-1.

GENES FOR PARKINSON DISEASE

Alpha-Synuclein

Alpha-synuclein (AS) is a ubiquitous neuronal protein of unknown function that may have a role in synaptic vesicle transport or recycling. Overexpression of AS in animal models leads to dose-dependent neurodegeneration, with dopaminergic cells

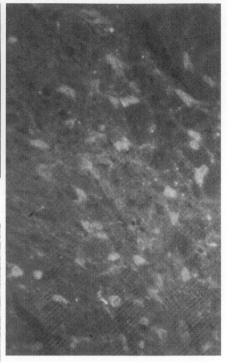

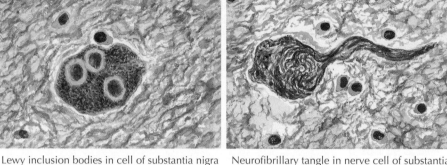

Normal: section through cerebral peduncles and substantia nigra

Parkinson disease: substantia nigra depigmented

Lewy inclusion bodies in cell of substantia nigra in Parkinson disease; may also appear in locus ceruleus and tegmentum, cranial motor nerve nuclei, and peripheral autonomic ganglia

Neurofibrillary tangle in nerve cell of substantia nigra as seen in postencephalitic parkinsonism, progressive supranuclear palsy, and parkinsonism-dementia complex

Section of substantia nigra of normal animal: treatment of section with formaldehyde vapor causes formation of polymers with monoamines (dopa and norepinephrine) that fluoresce to bright green under ultraviolet light

Figure 33-1 Neuropathology of Parkinson Disease.

in the substantia nigra being particularly susceptible. PARK 4 was identified as being a triplication of the normal AS gene, resulting in elevated protein levels and development of early-onset PD. In addition, AS promoter variants have been associated with increased risk for PD. Alpha-synuclein mutants are implicated for PD in several European families.

The discovery that mutant AS could cause PD quickly led to the discovery that AS also served as the principal component of Lewy bodies. These are proteinaceous cytoplasmic inclusions specifically found in the brains of PD patients; however, even today, the exact role of Lewy bodies is still unknown (see Fig. 33-1). The confirmation that triplication of the AS gene and the subsequent elevated protein levels (in the CSF) could cause PD has greatly strengthened the hypothesis that accumulation of protein is a fundamental event in the pathogenesis of PD.

Parkin

Parkin is an ubiquitin ligase, whose job is to add ubiquitins to proteins destined for degradation by the proteasome. Mutation of parkin impairs its ligation function, leading to protein accumulation within the cell. Homozygous mutation of parkin leads to early-onset PD, also called autosomal recessive juvenile PD (ARJP). Although classified as a recessive disorder, there is some evidence that haploinsufficiency may also occur, increasing susceptibility to disease in older patients. Parkin mutation is the single most common genetic cause of PD. In one European

study, this was identified in 40% of individuals with PD onset before age 40 years.

Other Proteins

UCHL1 is another member of the ubiquitin proteasome system (UPS). Ubiquitin carboxyterminal hydrolase L1 is involved in the metabolism of ubiquitins. *PINK1* is a recently identified mitochondrial protein kinase whose mutation may increase susceptibility to oxidative stress and apoptosis. *DJ-1* is a protein of unknown function.

These various genetic findings suggest that a critical step in the pathogenesis of PD is dysfunction of the UPS. Supporting this conclusion is evidence that specific inhibitors of the UPS cause the neuropathologic and motor abnormalities of parkinsonism in animal models. The precise pathophysiologic dysfunction that leads to dopaminergic cell death is still not certain. Possible mechanisms include a toxic gain of function of accumulated protein, mitochondrial impairment, and increased oxidative stress. These three mechanisms may also, in the face of other insults, act independently or interdependently to provoke dopaminergic cell death.

PATHOLOGY/PATHOPHYSIOLOGY

The pathologic sites responsible for the parkinsonian disorders reside in a group of brain gray matter structures known as the

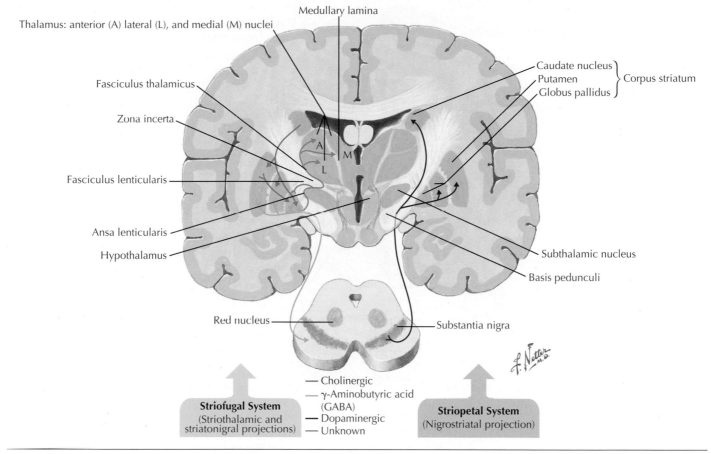

Thalamus: anterior (A) lateral (L), and medial (M) nuclei

Medullary lamina

Fasciculus thalamicus

Zona incerta

Fasciculus lenticularis

Ansa lenticularis

Hypothalamus

Red nucleus

Caudate nucleus
Putamen
Globus pallidus
} Corpus striatum

Subthalamic nucleus

Basis pedunculi

Substantia nigra

— Cholinergic
— γ-Aminobutyric acid (GABA)
— Dopaminergic
— Unknown

Striofugal System
(Striothalamic and striatonigral projections)

Striopetal System
(Nigrostriatal projection)

Figure 33-2 Parkinson Disease—Anatomy with Biochemical Pathways.

extrapyramidal system or basal ganglia (Fig. 33-2). These include striatum (caudate nucleus and putamen), globus pallidus interna and externa, subthalamic nucleus, substantia nigra pars reticulate and pars compacta, and the ventral nuclei of the thalamus.

Degeneration of the substantia nigra (SN) pars compacta is the pathologic hallmark of PD (Figs. 33-2 and 33-4). Neurons within the SN per se synthesize the neurotransmitter dopamine. These cells contain a dark pigment called neuromelanin. Parkinson symptoms develop when approximately 60% of these cells die. Concomitantly, direct inspection of the SN in PD demonstrates an abnormal pallor when compared with that characteristically seen with the normal hyperpigmented melanin-containing cells.

Direct dopaminergic projections from the SN influence motor processing within the basal ganglia by facilitating movement execution and concomitantly helping to suppress certain unwanted motor activity. When intra-SN dopaminergic neuron cell death occurs within the SN, the number of specific dopamine nerve terminals in the striatum decreases. These findings are associated with the classic PD clinical findings of rigidity and akinesia. In addition, basal ganglia function appears to extend beyond simple motor control concepts. The cortico-striato-pallido-thalamo-cortical circuit comprises several distinct and segregated loops, each having a different motor agonistic function. Within each loop are parallel pathways having antagonistic effects on this circuit outflow. The loss of

dopamine provokes a less active direct pathway and a more active indirect pathway. Disinhibition of the major output nuclei and increased inhibition of the thalamocortical system result in the classic pill rolling tremor.

The *direct pathway* arises from neurons that connect the striatum with the output nuclei, including the globus pallidum internum (Gpi) and substantia nigra pars reticularis (SNr). Direct pathway neurons contain GABA, the inhibitory neurotransmitter, and substance P (a neuropeptide that functions both as a neurotransmitter and neuromodulator), and *express the excitatory D1 dopamine receptor.* Direct pathway neurons receive glutamatergic projections from the cortex to the striatum. They also send GABAergic projections from SNr/Gpi to the ventral anterior and ventral lateral thalamic nuclei, completing the loop by sending glutamatergic fibers back to the cortex. The direct striatopallidal influence inhibits the Gpi neurons. These neurons inhibit the thalamic outflow to the cortex. The *net effect* of direct pathway activity is *excitatory* by stimulating cortical activity.

The *indirect pathway* includes intermediate synapses within the globus pallidum externum (Gpe) and subthalamic nucleus (STN). Neurons within this pathway contain enkephalins and express the inhibitory D₂ dopamine receptor. This pathway consists of three glutamatergic and three GABAergic-type neurons. Glutamatergic neurons in the cortex project to the striatum; striatal GABAergic neurons project to the Gpe. From Gpe, a second set of GABAergic neurons projects to a second set of glutamatergic neurons in the STN that project to the Gpi/SNr.

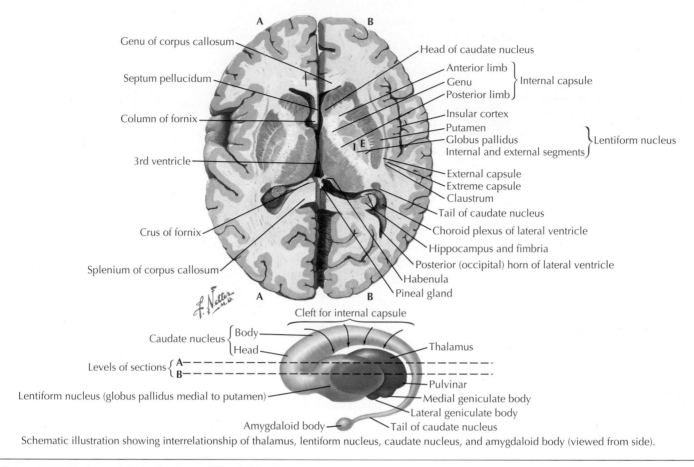

Genu of corpus callosum

Septum pellucidum

Column of fornix

3rd ventricle

Crus of fornix

Splenium of corpus callosum

Head of caudate nucleus

Anterior limb
Genu } Internal capsule
Posterior limb

Insular cortex
Putamen
Globus pallidus } Lentiform nucleus
Internal and external segments

External capsule
Extreme capsule
Claustrum
Tail of caudate nucleus
Choroid plexus of lateral ventricle
Hippocampus and fimbria
Posterior (occipital) horn of lateral ventricle
Habenula
Pineal gland

Cleft for internal capsule

Caudate nucleus { Body
Head }

Levels of sections { A
B }

Lentiform nucleus (globus pallidus medial to putamen)

Amygdaloid body

Thalamus

Pulvinar
Medial geniculate body
Lateral geniculate body
Tail of caudate nucleus

Schematic illustration showing interrelationship of thalamus, lentiform nucleus, caudate nucleus, and amygdaloid body (viewed from side).

Figure 33-3 Horizontal Brain Sections of Basal Ganglia.

Table 33-1 Genetic Causes of Parkinson Disease

Locus	Protein or Location	Inheritance	Ethnic Population
PARK 1	alpha-synuclein mutation	AD	Italian, Greek, German
PARK 2	Parkin	mainly AR	Global
PARK 3	2p13	AD, reduced penetrance	N. European kindred
PARK 4	alpha-synuclein triplication	AD, reduced penetrance	Iowa kindred
PARK 5	UCHL1	AD	German kindred
PARK 6	PINK1	AR	Italian
PARK 7	DJ-1	AR	Dutch
PARK 8	12p11.2-q13.1 LRRK2	AD, reduced penetrance	Japanese
PARK 10		Unclear	Icelandic
PARK 13	HtrA2	Unclear	German

The neurons from Gpi/SNr send GABAergic neurons to the thalamus. The final thalamocortical projection is glutamatergic. By contrast, increased indirect pathway activity excites the Gpi neurons, ultimately inhibiting cortical activity.

Decreased dopaminergic neurons in PD affects the direct pathway by reducing activity at Gpi and SNr leading to increased inhibitory output of Gpi and SNr. In the indirect pathway, dopamine deficiency in PD disinhibits striatopallidal neurons synapsing in Gpe, reducing activity in the inhibitory pallidosubthalamic neurons. Dopamine loss increases the striatal activity via the projections to GABAergic neurons that increase actions on the Gpe. Furthermore, dopamine loss causes a disinhibition of the STN through the indirect pathway.

CLINICAL PRESENTATION

The four *primary signs* of PD are bradykinesia, tremor, rigidity, and gait disturbance (Fig. 33-5). The primary criteria for a diagnosis of PD require that the patient's neurologic examination demonstrate at least two of these four features. There are certain additional features very suggestive of idiopathic PD. These include an asymmetric or unilateral onset and a clear response to levodopa treatment. Importantly from the point of differential diagnosis, neither of these features occurs in some of the atypical parkinsonism syndromes.

Bradykinesia, the most disabling PD symptom, is a decreased ability to initiate movement (akinesia is the extreme manifestation). This may affect multiple functions, particularly fine motor tasks such as buttoning a shirt or handwriting, the latter becoming micrographic. Other individuals may present with a masked facies nonemotional, bland, and expressionless, which later on becomes associated with decreased blink frequency, muted speech, and slowed swallowing. Typically, the gait is shuffling with decreased arm swing, stooped posture, and en bloc turning,

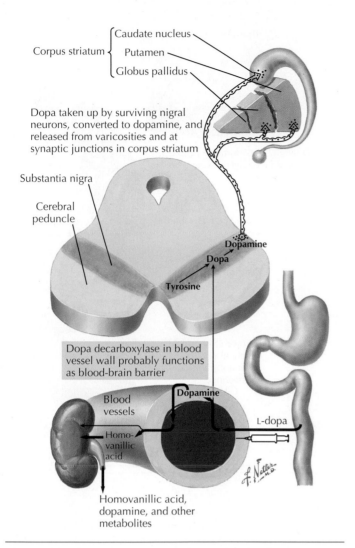

Corpus striatum {
Caudate nucleus
Putamen
Globus pallidus

Dopa taken up by surviving nigral neurons, converted to dopamine, and released from varicosities and at synaptic junctions in corpus striatum

Substantia nigra

Cerebral peduncle

Dopamine

Dopa

Tyrosine

Dopa decarboxylase in blood vessel wall probably functions as blood-brain barrier

Dopamine

Blood vessels

Homo-vanillic acid

L-dopa

Homovanillic acid, dopamine, and other metabolites

Figure 33-4 Parkinsonism—Hypothesized Role of Dopa.

The *Myerson's sign*, or glabellar tap sign, is elicited by having the patient look straight ahead while the examiner gently taps with her or his index finger tip between the medial ends of the eyebrows. Normally the patient blinks for the first few taps and then such is inhibited. In contrast, the PD patient persistently blinks as long as the tapping is maintained and thus a positive test.

Rigidity is a resistance to passive movement throughout the entire range of motion occurring in flexor and extensor muscles. This contrasts with spasticity, wherein there is an initial marked resistance to passive movement and then a sudden release, for example, *clasp-knife* phenomena. The classic cogwheel quality (stop-and-go effect) is from a tremor superimposed on the altered muscle tone. Very early on, patients are often concerned about stiffness, "weakness," or fatigue. Initially, the patient will just note a limitation in their daily activities or exercise capacity—unable to hike as long a distance, inability to get to the ball when playing tennis, or simply walking from the car to the store. When more pronounced, these bradykinetic symptoms may represent the combination of bradykinesia with rigidity.

Tremor occurs in 75% of patients. Typically, it is prominent at rest, having a frequency of 3–7 Hz. Although this tremor

usually does not significantly interfere with activities of daily living (ADLs), such as eating or writing, the patient finds it very embarrassing. PD patients frequently sit in the physician's office placing the affected hand out of sight down by their side or underneath a jacket. Sometimes they will actually hold the tremulous hand with the unaffected opposite hand. One should look for the tremor to be "uncovered" when asking the patient to walk; not only is the arm swing lost but a minor pill rolling tremor may become amplified as the hand comes away from the body and the patient is no longer able to cover it. Occasionally a PD tremor has a significant postural or action component complicating distinction from the more benign essential tremor.

Gait disturbance, postural instability, or both usually present at later stages of PD characterized by a change in the center of gravity typified by falling forward (propulsion) or backward (retropulsion) and a festinating (shuffling, slowly propulsive) petit pas (small steps) gait. When these symptoms are found early in PD, evaluation for other causes of parkinsonism, including progressive supranuclear palsy (PSP) and multiple system atrophy (MSA), is required.

Typically PD progresses in stages (Fig. 33-5). There are two commonly utilized rating scales to measure the degree of disability that these patients manifest: (1) UPDRS (Unified Parkinson Disease Rating Scale) and (2) Hoehn and Yahr (H&Y) scale (Box 33-1).

Two other less common symptoms, namely, *seborrheic dermatitis* and *hyposmia* (diminished sense of smell), although not diagnostic per se, may prove to be diagnostically helpful early on in the course of PD. This is especially true when these symptoms are seen in association with one primary PD criteria such as decreased arm swing. The recognition of either the seborrhea or a limited sense of smell may lead the astute clinician to an appropriate PD diagnosis even early in the disease course. Later in its course, certain *secondary features often occur*. Patients may experience difficulties with sleep initiation and maintenance. This *sleep disturbance* can occur secondary to the presence of an early morning dystonia or tremor, restless leg syndrome, or rapid eye movement (REM) behavior disorder. About 30% of PD patients also experience periodic leg movement of sleep.

Box 33-1 Parkinson Disease Rating Scales

Hoehn and Yahr

Stage I: unilateral disease
Stage II: bilateral disease with preservation of postural reflexes
Stage III: bilateral disease with impaired postural reflexes but preserved ability to ambulate independently
Stage IV: severe disease requiring considerable assistance
Stage V: end-stage disease, bed or chair confined

United Parkinson Disease Rating Scale (UPDRS)

Four major subsets
  Cognitive
  Activities of daily living
  Motor examination
  Complications of treatment
Scale 0–4 (0 = *normal*, 4 = *most severe*)

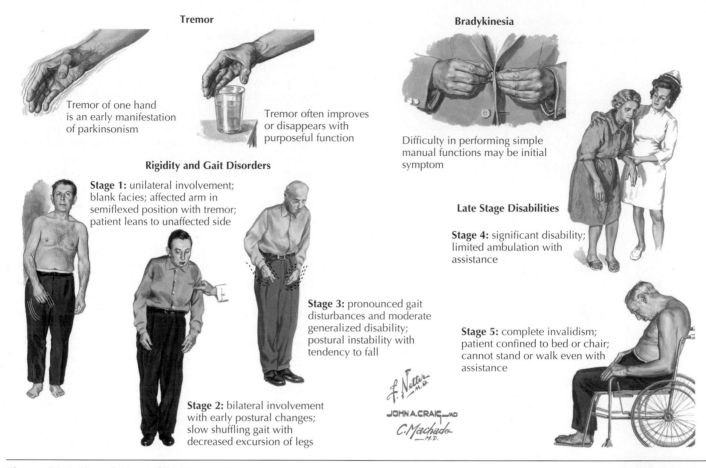

Tremor

Tremor of one hand is an early manifestation of parkinsonism

Tremor often improves or disappears with purposeful function

Bradykinesia

Difficulty in performing simple manual functions may be initial symptom

Rigidity and Gait Disorders

Stage 1: unilateral involvement; blank facies; affected arm in semiflexed position with tremor; patient leans to unaffected side

Stage 2: bilateral involvement with early postural changes; slow shuffling gait with decreased excursion of legs

Stage 3: pronounced gait disturbances and moderate generalized disability; postural instability with tendency to fall

Late Stage Disabilities

Stage 4: significant disability; limited ambulation with assistance

Stage 5: complete invalidism; patient confined to bed or chair; cannot stand or walk even with assistance

Figure 33-5 Clinical Signs of Parkinson Disease.

Autonomic dysfunction is seen commonly in PD. It is manifested as orthostatic hypotension, impaired gastrointestinal motility, urinary bladder dysfunction, disorders in thermoregulation, and sexual dysfunction.

Dysphagia is usually present later on in the PD patient. This relates to the development of oropharyngeal and esophageal motility disorders.

Psychiatric and cognitive symptomatology also frequently accompany or even precede the diagnosis of PD in some patients: about 40% suffer a major *depression* that may precede the diagnosis of the movement disorder; *anxiety* also occurs in up to 40% of patients. Later on in PD, *hallucinations* (visual, most likely nonthreatening), psychosis, and vivid nocturnal dreams are common. *Cognitive dysfunction* is typically a later manifestation. Clinically, it has the characteristics of a subcortical dementia (Chapter 18).

The clinical course or temporal profile of PD is quite variable. However, it usually progresses slowly and inexorably (Fig. 33-5). Typically, the illness begins unilaterally with focal tremor or difficulty using one limb. Eventually, the symptoms become more generalized and occur on the contralateral side, interfering with activities of daily living. Several secondary signs of parkinsonism also develop as previously noted.

Early on, the neurologic clinician must maintain a level of alertness for the presence of certain other clinical characteristics

that serve as "red flags" suggesting other non-Parkinson movement disorders. These are known as the "Parkinson plus" syndromes, including progressive supranuclear palsy (PSP), corticobasal degeneration (CBD), and multiple-system atrophy (MSA) (see Box 33-3).

If possible, it is useful to exclude these early in the disease course as they may change the treatment and prognosis. These are considered in detail in Chapter 34.

DIFFERENTIAL DIAGNOSES

When Parkinson-like findings are found in the face of other identifiable neurologic disorders, a primary diagnosis of PD should not be entertained. These include stroke, head injury, neuroleptic exposure, hydrocephalus, encephalitis, or brain tumor. The vast majority of PD patients present with at least two of the following classic findings, namely, bradykinesia; rigidity; tremor; and a petit pas, festinating gait disorder. When one only sees a single example of these physical changes, the patient may have early PD especially if associated with either seborrhea or anosmia. A certain set of clinical findings, such as the presence of supranuclear gaze palsy, must make one immediately consider other nontreatable movement disorders that are easily confused early on in these illnesses with PD (Box 33-2).

Box 33-2 Exclusion Criteria for Diagnosis of Parkinson Disease

Parkinsonism due to identifiable causes, such as stroke, head injury, encephalitis, neuroleptic exposure, hydrocephalus, or brain tumor
Supranuclear gaze palsy
Cerebellar signs
Autonomic insufficiency, early and severe, particularly orthostatic hypotension
Medication resistance, poor response to large doses of levodopa
Sustained remissions
Oculogyric crises

Box 33-3 Differential Diagnoses of Parkinson Disease

1. Essential tremor
2. Secondary parkinsonism
   a. Dopamine-blocking agents
   b. Vascular parkinsonism
   c. Normal-pressure hydrocephalus
   d. Infectious or postinfectious
   e. Toxic
   f. Metabolic
3. Atypical ("Parkinson plus"):
   a. PSP (Progressive supranuclear palsy)
   b. CBD (Corticobasal degeneration)
   c. MSA (Multisystem atrophy)
   d. DLBD (Dementia Lewy body disease)
4. Familial
5. Normal-pressure hydrocephalus
6. Other degenerative causes of parkinsonism

Table 33-2 Medications Causing Secondary Parkinsonism

Generic	Trade Name
Acetophenazine	Tindal
Amoxapine	Asendin
Chlorpromazine	Thorazine
Fluphenazine	Permitil, Prolixin
Haloperidol	Haldol
Loxapine	Loxitane, Daxolin
Mesoridazine	Serentil
Metoclopramide	Reglan
Molindone	Lidone, Moban
Perphenazine	Trilafon or Triavil
Piperacetazine	Quide
Prochlorperazine	Compazine, Combid
Promazine	Sparine
Promethazine	Phenergan
Thiethylperazine	Torecan
Thioridazine	Mellaril
Thiothixene	Navane
Trifluoperazine	Stelazine
Triflupromazine	Vesprin
Trimeprazine	Temaril

Otherwise, there is a relatively limited set of conditions to consider in the evaluation of such individuals (Box 33-3). These include essential tremor, secondary, atypical and familial parkinsonism, and other rare causes of parkinsonism.

Essential Tremor

Patients with essential tremor exhibit tremor only and do not have other parkinsonian signs. These individuals also do not respond to therapy with dopaminergic medications. Typically, an essential tremor is an action tremor and slower in frequency (4–8 Hz) than the PD resting (6 Hz) pill rolling tremor. Essential tremor occurs 20 times more frequently than PD; many such patients seek medical opinion because they are concerned they have the PD "shaking palsy" that will eventually incapacitate them. This does not predispose to PD; however, it may overlap some and cause early clinical confusion when it is accompanied by some minor normal signs of aging such as cog wheeling and bradykinesia. A small drink of an alcoholic beverage may clarify the diagnostic issue as essential tremors are commonly greatly inhibited by some ethanol derivative. Time also usually allows the PD differential to be confirmed as essential tremors do not typically progress to become associated with other motor limitations on the ADLs.

Secondary Causes of Parkinsonism

MEDICATIONS

Dopamine receptor-blocking agents used in psychiatry and for gastrointestinal symptoms are the most common drugs causing parkinsonism (Table 33-2). In the hospital, one may see patients who have newly developed parkinsonism after a relatively short course of symptomatic gastrointestinal medications such as metoclopramide. Of patients taking neuroleptic agents on a long-term basis, ~15% develop parkinsonism. Recovery following withdrawal of the offending agent may take weeks to months. If antiparkinsonian medication is required in these patients, anticholinergics are the drugs of choice.

INFECTIOUS DISEASES

It is very rare for one to need consider a secondary infectious mechanism to be responsible for a patient with parkinsonism. AIDS, cryptococcal meningoencephalitis, cysticercosis, fungal abscesses in the striata, herpes simplex encephalitis, Japanese B encephalitis, malaria, mycoplasma infection, postvaccinal parkinsonism, prion diseases (Creutzfeldt-Jakob disease), St. Louis encephalitis, subacute sclerosing panencephalitis, syphilis, tuberculosis, and Whipple disease may each lead to an encephalitis that presents with significant striatal involvement. Tremor rarely occurs in these syndromes. However, the infectious symptoms predominate, and the central nervous system involvement often demonstrates signs of a more widespread pathologic process affecting other neurologic systems.

Postencephalitic parkinsonism (PeP), also known as von Economo disease, encephalitis lethargica, or sleeping sickness, occurred in a pandemic in Europe and North America from 1916 to 1927. The precise infectious agent is still not identified. Typically, parkinsonism symptoms occurred immediately after the acute infectious process; however, in some patients prominent symptoms were not evident for up to 20 years. Clinically, patients had parkinsonism with other distinctive features: behavioral and mental disturbances in the acute illness, changes in sleep patterns, and ocular motor dysfunction, particularly oculogyric crisis (i.e., spasms of conjugate eye muscles, deviating eyes upward, downward, or to one side for minutes or hours). Levodopa was not as well tolerated as in idiopathic PD; high doses of anticholinergic medications were better tolerated. Today PeP is primarily a disorder of historic interest.

TOXINS

Rare forms of parkinsonism may also be related to various toxic chemical exposures. In 1976, the substance MPTP was inadvertently produced in an attempt to home manufacture an illicit narcotic analog of meperidine, namely, MPPP. Self-administration led to an acute Parkinson syndrome in this home-grown chemist. A few years later, a series of acute PD cases appeared in young Californians. These were also secondary to similar self-injection of illicitly manufactured "designer drugs," again being related to an MPTP formulation. This chemical is highly toxic to substantia nigra neurons; therefore, it has since been employed as a research means to produce animal models mimicking PD. The symptoms of MPTP parkinsonism respond well to levodopa.

The globus pallidus is another target for chemical toxins with the potential to produce parkinsonism. These include carbon monoxide, cyanide, and manganese. Manganese toxicity is seen in miners and industrial workers

METABOLIC CONDITIONS

Hypothyroidism, easily identified and treatable, is a metabolic condition that can cause some symptoms, particularly slowness of gait, mimicking parkinsonism. Other rare conditions include acquired chronic hepatocerebral degeneration leading to rigidity in hemochromatosis, ceroid lipofuscinosis, folate deficiency, Niemann-Pick type C disease, and postanoxic parkinsonism.

OTHER RARE SOMETIMES TREATABLE CAUSES

When parkinsonism develops before age 40 years, Wilson's disease must be considered in the differential diagnosis, requiring tests for copper metabolism and slit-lamp examination. Other forms of hepatolenticular degeneration also require consideration.

NORMAL-PRESSURE HYDROCEPHALUS

This must also be considered in the PD differential diagnosis. Normal-pressure hydrocephalus also typically presents with a gait disorder; however, it is somewhat different than that of idiopathic PD (see Chapter 32, Fig. 32-2). Typically slowness of gait is the initial symptom; characteristically this is a "magnetic" mildly wide-based finding likened to walking in cement. Cognitive decline may appear earlier in this syndrome than in PD, and "unwitting incontinence" may follow. It is important to recognize this relatively uncommon disorder early on as it is eminently treatable.

Table 33-3 Degenerative Causes of Parkinsonism

Alpha-synuclein Deposition	Tau Deposition	Polyglutamine Tract Deposition
Parkinson disease	Progressive supranuclear palsy	Juvenile Huntington's disease
Multiple-system atrophy	Corticobasal ganglionic degeneration	Autosomal dominant cerebellar ataxia (SCA-3)
	Parkinsonism dementia complex of Guam	Dentato-rubro-pallido-luyusian atrophy
	Postencephalitic Parkinson syndrome	Sporadic neuronal intranuclear inclusion disease
	Frontotemporal dementia with parkinsonism linked to chromosome 17	
	Posttraumatic parkinsonism	

SCA indicates spinocerebellar atrophy.

OTHER DISORDERS

Characterized by a poor levodopa response, *arteriosclerotic parkinsonism* (i.e., lower body parkinsonism) is the PD variant most likely to be associated with head CT or MRI abnormalities. They are primarily visible as periventricular white matter changes. Mass lesions, such as tumors, are exceedingly rare causes of parkinsonism. Multiple head trauma, as seen in boxers, can cause parkinsonism. Degenerative diseases causing parkinsonism are best classified by the type of abnormal degree of neurochemical deposition (Table 33-3).

Atypical Parkinsonism

Atypical parkinsonian syndromes or "Parkinson plus syndrome" (Chapter 34) are chronic, progressive neurodegenerative disorders, characterized by rapidly evolving parkinsonism in association with other signs of neurologic dysfunction not found within the spectrum of idiopathic Parkinson disease (PD) (Box 33-2). The presence of atypical signs on examination, sometimes called "red flags" (supranuclear gaze palsy, corticospinal pathway involvement, cerebellar signs, early autonomic dysfunction or dementia) with rapidly progressive course and minimal response to dopaminergic medications should trigger the clinician to look for atypical parkinsonism such as PSP, CBD, MSA or DLBD.

Familial Parkinsonism

A well-defined genetic component is present in a minority of PD patients even though most individuals developing classical parkinsonism have no specific etiology identified. Mutations in five causative genes (Table 33-1) together account for 2–3% of all patients with classical parkinsonism. These include alpha-synuclein (SNCA), parkin, PTEN-induced kinase 1 (PINK1),

DJ-1, and leucine-rich repeat kinase 2 (LRRK2). These patients are often clinically indistinguishable from others with idiopathic PD. Although the individual clinical course cannot be predicted, overall, many cases of genetic PD will progress more slowly and respond better to treatment than patients without mutations. Genetic testing frequently yields inconclusive results, is expensive, and does not have a current indication in the vast majority of PD patients. DNA testing is rarely indicated in suspected PD patients. It may be occasionally useful for diagnostic purposes but only after careful consideration in selected cases at specialty centers.

DIAGNOSTIC EVALUATION

Key diagnostic elements are the presence of two of the four cardinal signs: bradykinesia, tremor, rigidity, and gait problems (Fig. 33-5). However, it is unusual for a patient to present initially with the full-blown disease, and characteristic signs may not be present. Frequently, the patient may first become aware of a nonspecific fatigue in previously well-performed activities of daily living primarily affecting motor function. They may note a diminished reserve for distance demands. Clinical reexamination in several-month intervals is often needed to confirm a diagnosis of PD. Signs of another degenerative process sometimes become evident, interdicting the earlier diagnostic suspicion.

Although approaches to a specific preclinical detection of PD are constantly being investigated, a practical, inexpensive, sensitive, screening test is not available. Use of CT and MRI sometimes helps to distinguish idiopathic PD from other forms of parkinsonism. This is particularly relevant when the clinical findings are purely unilateral. Imaging studies may show atherosclerotic brain disease or normal-pressure hydrocephalus and rarely demonstrate a structural lesion. MRI sometimes shows signs typical for multiple-system atrophy (putaminal atrophy, hot cross bun sign, a hyperintense putaminal rim, and infratentorial signal changes).

One of the most specific diagnostic tools available today is a positive clinical response to a therapeutic trial of Parkinson medications. This is especially relevant with levodopa, particularly in the patient with unilateral symptoms, including bradykinesia, rigidity, and petit pas gait.

Once a specific PD diagnosis is confirmed, it is useful to qualitatively measure (Box 33-1) the disease severity. This allows the treating physician to establish a pretreatment clinical baseline. This will serve as a reference for future comparisons.

TREATMENT

PD treatment remains symptomatic; there is no neuroprotective therapy available to prevent ongoing evolution of this neurodegenerative disorder. Patient management requires careful consideration of the patient's symptoms and signs, stage of disease, degree of functional disability, and levels of activity and daily productivity. Treatment can be divided into (1) nonpharmacologic, (2) pharmacologic, and (3) surgical. Most patients with idiopathic PD have a significant therapeutic response to levodopa. The complete absence of a clinical response to a dose of 25/100 mg of carbidopa/levodopa 6–10 times a day strongly

---

Box 33-4 Pharmacologic Therapy for Parkinson Disease

1. Dopaminergic
   A. Levodopa
   B. Dopamine agonist
2. Anticholinergics
3. MAO inhibitors
4. COMT inhibitors
5. Amantadine

COMT, Catechol-O-methyltransferase; MAOI, monoamine oxidase inhibitor.

---

suggests that the original diagnosis was incorrect and should prompt a search for other causes of parkinsonism.

Pharmacologic therapy for PD consists of five types of medication (Box 33-4). There is no simple approach to treating PD; guidelines depend on functional impairment and response to therapy.

The treatment of PD can be divided into therapy of early and later stages (with motor fluctuations and dyskinesia). For patients requiring initiation of symptomatic therapy, there are three primary options: levodopa, dopaminergic agonists, or MAO-B inhibitors (level A, class I and class II evidence). Levodopa (LD) provides superior motor benefit but is associated with a higher risk of dyskinesia and motor complications. Dopaminergic agonists (DAs) result in fewer motor complications (wearing off, dyskinesia, on–off motor fluctuations) than levodopa treatment after 2.5 years of follow-up. However primary DA therapy is associated with more frequent adverse events, including hallucinations, somnolence, and edema, than levodopa therapy. The choice of either LD or DA, when initiating therapy, depends on the relative impact of improving motor disability (better with levodopa) compared with the lessening of motor complications (better with dopamine agonists) for each individual patient with PD (level A, class I and II evidence). For patients with PD in whom carbidopa/levodopa treatment is being instituted, either an immediate-release or sustained-release preparation may be considered (level B, class II evidence).

An important principle for early treatment of PD is that the introduction and use of medication must be tailored to the patient's individual needs. An arbitrary age of 70 years has been used as a guide to develop strategies for treatment initiation, although there must always be an emphasis on each individual patient's characteristics. As a general rule, for patients younger than age 70 years and having no cognitive dysfunction, the choice of initial drug may lie between MAO-B inhibitor and a dopamine agonist. Carbidopa/levodopa is started in Parkinson patients aged 70 years and older who have a significant motor disability, such as bradykinesia, rigidity, tremor, or gait problems. Senior citizens with PD may also be considered for MAO-B inhibitor or DA if they are cognitively intact and lack any significant comorbidity.

As PD progresses, the provision of effective symptom control becomes more challenging, and additional drugs may need to be added. For later stages of the disease, American Academy of Neurology guidelines suggest starting Entacapone, a COMT inhibitor, and rasagiline, an MAO inhibitor, as first choice to reduce off time (level A). DAs (pramipexole, ropinirole) and tolcapone should be considered to reduce off time as a second choice (level B). Tolcapone (hepatotoxicity) and pergolide (valvular fibrosis) should be used with caution and require monitoring. Apomorphine, cabergoline, and selegiline may be considered to reduce off time as third choice (level C). Amantadine may be considered to reduce dyskinesia (level C). DBS STN may be considered to improve motor fluctuation and reduce off time, dyskinesia and medication usage (level C). Sustained release carbidopa/levodopa and bromocriptine may be disregarded to reduce off time (level C).

Dopaminergic

LEVODOPA

Levodopa (LD) with carbidopa is the most commonly used, most potent antiparkinsonian medication and is equally beneficial for all symptoms. Levodopa is the immediate natural precursor of dopamine and is converted to dopamine by the enzyme aromatic amino acid decarboxylase (AAAD) (Fig. 33-6). Initially, levodopa was associated with a high rate of side effects, particularly nausea and vomiting, because of its ability to stimulate peripheral, non–central nervous system dopamine receptors. The addition of the decarboxylase inhibitor carbidopa decreased the incidence of the peripheral side effect, permitted more levodopa to cross the blood–brain barrier, and consequently allowed a reduction of the total levodopa dose. Carbidopa-levodopa is available in immediate-release form as tablets (Sinemet) or sublingual pills (Parcopa) and controlled-release formulations (Sinemet CR).

Early side effects, including nausea and orthostatic hypotension, are more easily managed than the late motor complications. Late side effects include involuntary movements, motor fluctuations, vivid dreams and nightmares, confusion, and psychosis, typically hallucinations and delusions, mania, or paranoia. In the geriatric population, particularly those individuals beginning to demonstrate early cognitive limitations, these levodopa side effects are more likely to occur. Treatment of these side effects also presents significant challenges as at times the commonly utilized antipsychotic drugs may worsen the parkinsonism per se.

With increasing duration of usage, there is a slower or delayed response to levodopa's therapeutic effect. LD also appears to have a shorter duration of action, a "wearing off" between doses. The patient's classic PD symptoms that had so nicely disappeared early in the course of treatment become prominent once again. Painful muscle spasms occur in some patients.

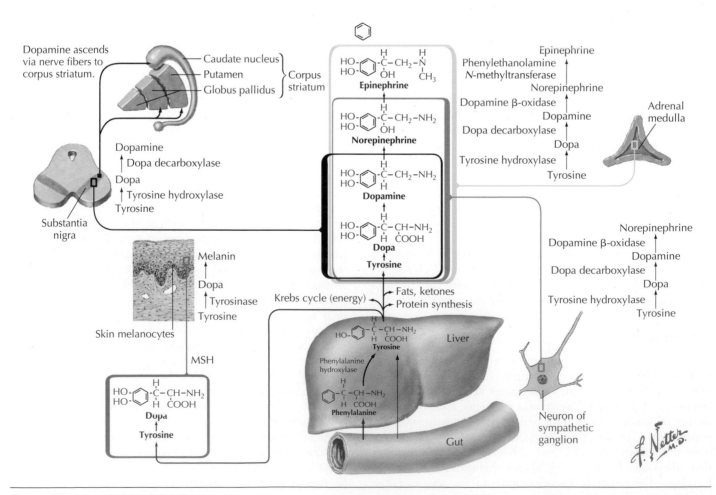

Figure 33-6 Catecholamine Synthesis.

Two of the most disabling long-term LD therapeutic side effects are the appearance of a variety of dyskinesias and motor fluctuations developing in a modest number of PD individuals. These involuntary movements are often choreiform; they can be particularly disabling, affecting various body parts; at times these rather bizarre postures may also be emotionally painful. The treatment of these complications is most difficult. Amantadine and the DAs are sometimes helpful adjuncts.

DOPAMINERGIC AGONISTS

DAs directly stimulate dopaminergic receptors. They are particularly indicated for monotherapy in younger patients, who are more prone to the early development of levodopa-related clinical fluctuations and who require long-term treatment. At least two general classes of dopamine agonists exist: one coupled to adenylate cyclases (D_1) and the other not so linked (D_2). Most effective antiparkinsonian dopamine agonists stimulate predominantly D_2 receptors.

DAs are used mainly early in the illness because they reduce the need for levodopa. Although not as effective as levodopa, DAs often provide satisfactory relief of mild symptoms. In those instances when severe symptoms interfere with the patient's social or occupational activities, early symptomatic treatment with carbidopa-levodopa, later combined with a DA, may be necessary. Commonly utilized preparations include pramipexole, ropinirole, bromocriptine, and pergolide (Box 33-5). Pergolide had been recently taken off the market because of potential heart valvular damage. Impulse control disorders or dysfunctional behaviors are problems that have been increasingly recognized with dopaminergic agonists but that occur much less commonly with levodopa. These disorders include hypersexuality, compulsive gambling, meaningless and repetitive activities (punding), hypomanic states, and addictive overuse of levodopa.

Anticholinergic

Anticholinergic agents are the oldest drug class used for PD. They act as muscarinic receptor blockers by penetrating the CNS to antagonize acetylcholine transmission by striatal interneurons. Anticholinergics are most effective for tremor, but because of their innate side effects these medications must be used with significant caution in the elderly. Usually used as monotherapy or an adjunct to dopaminergic therapy, the most commonly used anticholinergic agents include benztropine, procyclidine, and trihexyphenidyl.

Side effects, resulting from both peripheral and central cholinergic blockade, include dry mouth, narrow-angle glaucoma, constipation, urinary retention, memory impairment, and confusion with hallucinations.

COMT Inhibitors

Inhibition of the enzyme catechol-O-methyltransferase (COMT) blocks dopamine metabolism. COMT inhibitors prolong levodopa's benefits by extending the life span of the dopamine to which it is converted. There are two major COMT inhibitors. Entacapone is generally used adjunctively to levodopa. Tolcapone can cause severe hepatotoxicity, requires regular laboratory monitoring, and thus is used less frequently.

Monoamine Oxidase B Inhibitors

Selegiline is a selective inhibitor of monoamine oxidase B. Its primary mechanism of action is blockade of central dopamine metabolism. It is available as a swallowed pill (Eldepryl and generics) and as an orally disintegrating tablet (Zelapar ODT). It may improve response to levodopa, especially in patients with mild dose-related fluctuations. Selegiline has been studied as a neuroprotective agent because it can block free radical formation from the oxidative metabolism of dopamine. A large prospective, double-blind, placebo-controlled multicenter study (DATATOP) found that it delayed the progression of parkinsonian signs in previously untreated patients by 9 months. However, no persistent, long-term benefit in slowing PD progression has been demonstrated.

Rasagiline is a newer MAO-B inhibitor also available as Azilect. It received Food and Drug Administration approval for the treatment of signs and symptoms of Parkinson disease as initial monotherapy and as adjunct therapy to levodopa. As monotherapy, it may reduce parkinsonian disability. As adjunctive therapy, it may reduce off time and increase dyskinesia-free on time. Side effects include insomnia, hallucinations, and orthostatic hypotension.

Amantadine

Amantadine is an antiviral agent that was serendipitously found to have an antiparkinsonian effect. Its mechanism of action, thought to include blocking an N-methyl-D-aspartate receptor,

---

> **Box 33-5** Advantages and Disadvantages of Dopamine Agonists
>
> **Advantages**
> Some antiparkinson effect
> Reduced incidence of levodopa-related adverse events (dyskinesia and motor fluctuations)
> Selective stimulation of dopamine receptor subtypes and longer duration of action
> Levodopa-sparing effect
>
> **Disadvantages**
> Limited antiparkinson efficacy, always require levodopa adjunctive therapy
> Specific side effects (nausea, vomiting, postural hypotension, drowsiness, constipation, psychiatric reactions—hallucinations, confusion)
> Does not completely prevent development of levodopa-related adverse events. Once patients have developed dyskinesias, dopamine agonists exacerbate them further
> Do not treat all features of Parkinson disease, such as freezing, postural instability, autonomic dysfunction, dementia
> Unable to prevent disease progression

is controversial. Amantadine has a mild beneficial effect on tremor, bradykinesia, and rigidity. It is the only antiparkinsonian medication that can decrease the severity of levodopa-induced dyskinesias. Common side effects include livedo reticularis and lower extremity edema.

Future Directions

Because PD is more common with increasing age, its prevalence is expected to triple over the next 50 years because of the increased number of aging individuals in the westernized population. The most promising research is focused on the function and anatomy of the motor system, ways of controlling neurodegeneration, location of possible environmental factors, identification of a gene causing PD, and new medical and surgical therapies.

Animal models are used for studying methods for delivering dopamine to critical brain areas by implanting tiny dopamine-containing particles into brain regions affected by the disease. Such implants could partially ameliorate the movement problems exhibited by these animals. Also under investigation are implantable pumps that can produce a continuous supply of levodopa and help prevent fluctuations. Another promising method involves implanting capsules containing dopamine-producing cells into the brain. Neural grafting, or transplantation of nerve cells, is a proposed technique. Animal models show that damaged nerve cells can regenerate after fetal brain tissue from the SN is implanted. Other therapeutic attempts are directed to replace the lost dopamine-producing neurons with healthy, fetal neurons, and thereby improve movement and response to medications. A promising approach is the use of genetically engineered cells (e.g., modified skin cells grown in tissue culture) that could have the same beneficial effects. Skin cells would be much easier to harvest, and patients could serve as their own donors.

ADDITIONAL RESOURCES

Bonuccelli U, Ceravolo R. The safety of dopamine agonists in the treatment of Parkinson's disease. Expert Opin Drug Saf 2008 Mar;7(2):111-127.

Ho BL, Lieu AS, Hsu CY. Hemiparkinsonism secondary to an infiltrative astrocytoma. Neurologist 2008 Jul;14(4):258-261.

LeWitt PA. Levodopa for the treatment of Parkinson's disease. N Engl J Med 2008;359:2468-2476. *An excellent overall discussion of the current status of first-line medical therapy.*

McGoon DC. The Parkinson's Handbook. New York: WW Norton; 1990. *(An inspiring personal account of how a world-famed cardiothoracic surgeon discovered and dealt with his own PD that began during the height of his career. A very insightful commentary of value to both treating physician and patient alike.)*

Shapira AHV. Treatment options in the modern management of Parkinson's disease. Archives of Neurology Aug 2007;64(8):1083-1087.

The following Practice Parameter Guidelines from the American Academy of Neurology published in Neurology provide state-of-the-art reviews:

April 2006, Movement Disorders, Diagnosis and Prognosis of New Onset Parkinson Disease, Wendy Edlund at wedlund@aan.com. Endorsed by the National Parkinson Foundation and the Parkinson's Disease Foundation. Abstract Objective: To define key issues in the diagnosis of Parkinson's disease (PD), to define features influencing progression

April 2006, Movement Disorders, Initiation of Treatment for Parkinson's Disease. Practice Parameter: Initiation of Treatment for Parkinson's Disease (An Evidence-Based Review) Report of the Quality Standards Subcommittee of the American Academy of Neurology. J. M. Miyasaki, MD, W. Martin, MD, O. Suchowersky, MD, W. J. Weiner, MD.

April 2006, Movement Disorders, Evaluation Treatment of Depression, Psychosis and Dementia in Parkinson Disease, Endorsed by the National Parkinson Foundation and the Parkinson's Disease Foundation. Abstract Objective: To make evidence-based treatment recommendations for patients with Parkinson's disease (PD) with dementia, depression, and psychosis

April 2006, Movement Disorders, Treatment of Parkinson Disease with Motor Fluctuations and Dyskinesia.

Baltim A, Clinical Practice Parkinson Foundation and the Parkinson's Disease Foundation. Abstract Objective: evidence-based treatment recommendations for the medical and surgical treatment of Parkinson's disease. Methods: committee including movement.

Atypical Parkinsonian Syndromes

Diana Apetauerova

34

*A*typical parkinsonian syndromes previously called *Parkinson-plus syndromes*, are chronic, progressive neurodegenerative disorders, characterized by rapidly evolving parkinsonism in association with other signs of neurologic dysfunction beyond the spectrum of idiopathic Parkinson disease (PD). These include early postural instability, supranuclear gaze palsy, early autonomic failure, and pyramidal, cerebellar, or cortical signs. The most common disorders (Table 34-1) are progressive supranuclear palsy (PSP), corticobasal degeneration (CBD), and multiple-system atrophy (MSA). Unlike idiopathic PD, these uncommon syndromes have poor or transient responses to dopaminergic therapy and consequently a worse prognosis. These disorders are classified as *tauopathies* and *synucleinopathies* based on the accumulation of the abnormal proteins tau or alpha-synuclein within neurons and glial cells having various anatomic distribution within certain brain areas.

Tau is found in a hyperphosphorylated form in both PSP and CBD. In normal human brains, tau functions as a microtubule-binding protein as well as a stabilizer of the neuronal cytoskeleton. In diseased brain, tau is found in glial cells and neurons, where it produces a special cluster of fibrils called neurofibrillary tangle (NFT). Generally, there are six isoforms of tau made by alternative splicing from the tau gene. Tau also accumulates in the less common tauopathy, frontotemporal dementia with parkinsonism (FTPD). This is linked to chromosome 17 (FTPD-17).

Alpha-synuclein is a highly soluble synaptic protein found in the normal human brain. Typically, in MSA it accumulates as insoluble aggregates within white matter oligodendrocytes as glial cytoplasmic inclusions (GCIs).

There are no effective therapies for these syndromes. Therapeutic trials with free radical scavengers and better understanding of the abnormal proteins' roles within the brain may help improve understanding of these uncommon disorders.

PROGRESSIVE SUPRANUCLEAR PALSY

Clinical Vignette

A 71-year-old woman presented with poor balance starting 2 years ago. She would describe multiple episodes where she would suddenly fall backwards. She also recently noted visual blurring especially when she would be reading or going down the stairs. Frequently, she noted her eyes would be closed and she had difficulties opening them. Occasionally while drinking, she would spontaneously cough or choke; her speech became softer and slurred.

Neurologic examination demonstrated her to have a blank staring appearance, and dysarthric speech. She also demonstrated a vertical more than horizontal supranuclear gaze palsy; however, her vertical eye movements were

preserved with oculocephalic reflex maneuvers. Blepharospasm, prominent axial rigidity, and mild bradykinesia in all four extremities with minimal cogwheel rigidity and brisk muscle stretch reflexes were also identified. She was able to stand up slowly and walked with erect posture, stiff gait, and bilateral decreased arm swing. She had no postural reflexes and during pull test, she fell backwards easily.

PSP is a sporadic tauopathy that has a progressive clinical course characterized by parkinsonism with supranuclear gaze palsy (Fig. 34-1), early postural instability, falls, bradykinesia, and dysarthria as well illustrated in this vignette. PSP typically does not respond to dopaminergic therapy. Its prognosis is poor, with a median survival of 5–7 years. PSP's etiology, like that of CBD, is unknown. A genetic susceptibility may be invoked; however, to date, only the H1 MAPT haplotype has been consistently associated with a risk of developing progressive supranuclear palsy

PATHOPHYSIOLOGY

PSP is primarily a subcortical neurodegenerative tauopathy in contrast to both CBD and FTPD-17 having involvement of the cerebral cortex. Macroscopically, depigmentation is observable within the substantia nigra (SN) and locus coeruleus (LC), as well as atrophy of the pons, midbrain, and globus pallidum (Fig. 34-2). Microscopically, the most affected regions are brainstem nuclei III, IV, IX, and X, the red nucleus, LC, SN, globus pallidus, and cerebellar dentate nucleus. Tau protein accumulates within neurons as neurofibrillary tangle (NFT) and in glia as spherical neuropil threads.

CLINICAL PRESENTATION

PSP typically occurs between the sixth and seventh decades. Onset before age 40 years is rare. Prevalence varies between 1 and 6.4/100,000. PSP is sporadic in most individuals, but rarely an autosomal dominant inheritance is suggested.

Patients usually present with gait instability and tendency to unexpectedly fall backwards; in contrast, neither of these symptoms occurs early on in Parkinson disease. The parkinsonism of PSP is typically axial and symmetric, unlike the asymmetric often single limb presentation of PD. Most patients with PSP carry an erect posture in contrast to the flexed PD stance (see Fig. 34-1). Often they lack the typical PD tremor. Dystonia is a common finding particularly early on affecting limbs, neck dystonia, or even as blepharospasm.

The hallmark of PSP is the classic and characteristic finding of limited vertical eye movements; eventually a horizontal supranuclear gaze palsy may also become evident. In this clinical setting, the patient usually does not recognize the loss of eye

Table 34-1 Atypical Parkinsonian Syndromes

Syndrome	Abnormal	Clinical Features	Age at Onset (yr)	Genetic	Pathology	Therapy
PSP	Tau	Gait disorder, falls Abnormal eye movements Akinetic-rigid asymmetric parkinsonism Cortical signs Dystonia Action/postural tremor Myoclonus	55–70	Sporadic? Familial	Atrophy of BG and brainstem regions Normal cerebral cortex Globose, NFT	Poor response to dopaminergic medication Botulinum toxin for blepharospasm Supportive therapy
CBD	Tau	Alien limb phenomenon Symmetric axially predominant parkinsonism Dysarthria and dysphagia Frontal lobe abnormalities Cognitive impairment	60	Sporadic	Atrophy in FP cortex Tau-positive neurons in cortex Swollen and achromatic neurons (ballooned neurons)	Poor response to dopaminergic medication Botulinum toxin for blepharospasm Supportive therapy
FTDP-17	Tau	Highly variable: behavioral disturbance Cognitive impairment Motor disturbance (later in the disease) Positive family history	50	Autosomal dominant	Atrophy in FT cortex, BG, SN, LC Neuronal loss Argentophilic neuronal inclusions	Poor response to dopaminergic therapy
MSA	Alpha-synuclein	Parkinsonism Cerebellar signs Autonomic features Pyramidal features	60	Sporadic	Glial and neuronal cytoplasmic inclusions Absence of Lewy bodies	Poor or marginal response to dopaminergic therapy Fludrocortisone or midodrine for orthostatic hypotension

BG, Basal ganglia; CBD, corticobasal degeneration; FP, frontoparietal; FT, frontotemporal; FTDP-17, frontotemporal dementia with parkinsonism linked to chromosome 17; LC, locus ceruleus; MSA, multiple system atrophy; NFT, neurofibrillary tangle; PSP, progressive supranuclear palsy.

movement per se but rather perceives these limitations as blurry vision particularly manifested by difficulties with routine activities such as reading or walking down the stairs. Dysarthria and dysphagia are also commonly experienced early in the disease course. Cognitive dysfunction is a later development for most PSP patients.

DIAGNOSIS

PSP and other atypical parkinsonian syndromes including CBD, MSA, and dementia with Lewy bodies are often misdiagnosed as PD or as cerebrovascular disease (atherosclerotic parkinsonism). The most important diagnostic clues are (1) the results of a careful clinical evaluation and (2) a poor response to dopaminergic therapy.

Computed tomography (CT) and magnetic resonance imaging (MRI) (Fig. 34-3) often demonstrate generalized or brainstem (dorsal midbrain) atrophy. The combination of atrophy of the midbrain tegmentum with relative sparing of the basis pontis resembles "a lateral view of a standing penguin (especially, the king penguin), with a small head and big body" on a midsagittal MRI scan. Previously, appearance of the midbrain tegmentum was stated to resemble the head of a

hummingbird. Whether the penguin or hummingbird sign will take flight remains to be seen, but the implication of both studies is the same: the midbrain in PSP is atrophic and MRI can be helpful to verify the clinical diagnosis.

There are no more specific diagnostic studies available. Metabolic positron emission tomographic (PET) studies have demonstrated global reduction in cerebral metabolism; ^{18}F-fluorodopa PET uptake studies revealed reduced caudate and putamen uptake. Single photon emission computed tomography (SPECT) revealed bifrontal hypometabolism.

TREATMENT

There are no effective specific therapies available for the PSP patient. Although some of these individuals with slowness, stiffness, and balance problems initially may respond to antiparkinsonian therapies such as levodopa, or levodopa combined with anticholinergic agents, this effect is usually limited and at best a temporary one. Visual limitations, dysarthria, and dysphagia are usually unresponsive to any pharmacologic intervention.

Antidepressant drugs have had modest success in PSP; fluoxetine, amitriptyline, and imipramine are the most commonly

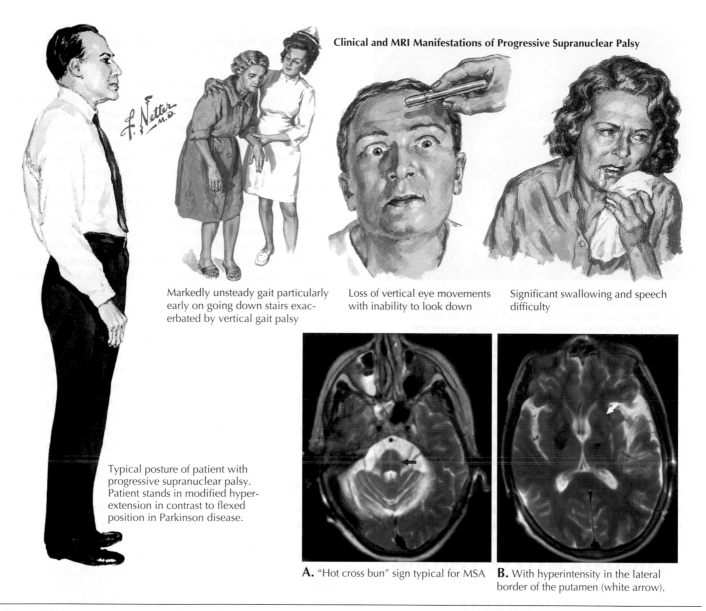

Clinical and MRI Manifestations of Progressive Supranuclear Palsy

Markedly unsteady gait particularly early on going down stairs exacerbated by vertical gait palsy

Loss of vertical eye movements with inability to look down

Significant swallowing and speech difficulty

Typical posture of patient with progressive supranuclear palsy. Patient stands in modified hyperextension in contrast to flexed position in Parkinson disease.

A. "Hot cross bun" sign typical for MSA

B. With hyperintensity in the lateral border of the putamen (white arrow).

Figure 34-1 Progressive Supranuclear Palsy.

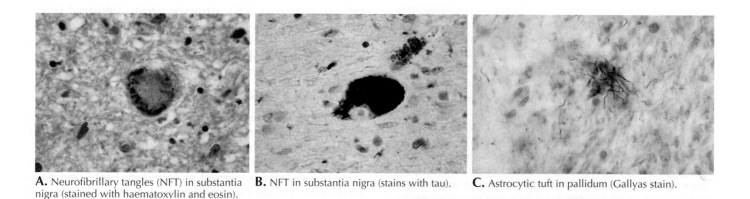

A. Neurofibrillary tangles (NFT) in substantia nigra (stained with haematoxylin and eosin).

B. NFT in substantia nigra (stains with tau).

C. Astrocytic tuft in pallidum (Gallyas stain).

Figure 34-2 Pathology of Progressive Supranuclear Palsy.

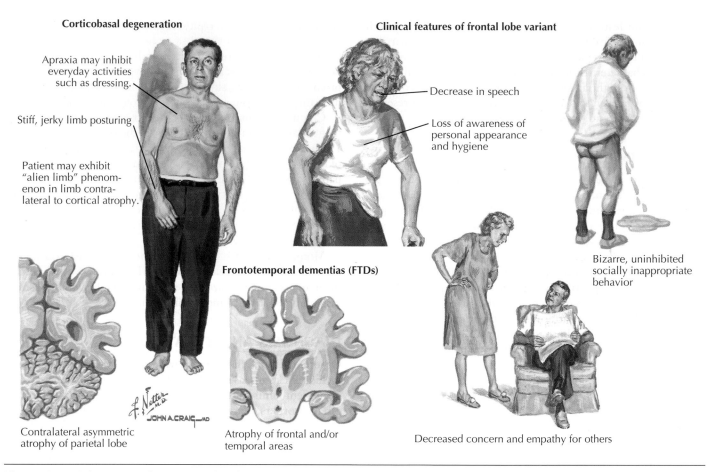

Corticobasal degeneration

Apraxia may inhibit everyday activities such as dressing.

Stiff, jerky limb posturing

Patient may exhibit "alien limb" phenomenon in limb contralateral to cortical atrophy.

Clinical features of frontal lobe variant

Decrease in speech

Loss of awareness of personal appearance and hygiene

Bizarre, uninhibited socially inappropriate behavior

Frontotemporal dementias (FTDs)

Contralateral asymmetric atrophy of parietal lobe

Atrophy of frontal and/or temporal areas

Decreased concern and empathy for others

Figure 34-4 Other Tauopathies. Corticobasal Degeneration and Frontotemporal Dementia.

His examination was notable for hypophonic speech, stridor, square wave jerks seen during eye movement exam, orofacial dyskinesia, and antecollis. He had asymmetric akinetic rigid syndrome with more involvement of the right-sided extremities with brisker muscle stretch reflexes and the presence of a right Babinski sign. Bilateral right greater than left, finger-to-nose-to-finger and heel-to-shin ataxia was identified, right more prominent than left. He was unable to ambulate independently and required two people to support him. His gait was characterized by a wide base with significant slowness, bilateral loss of arm swing, and poor postural stability. MRI demonstrated lateral putamen and pontine cruciate patterns of T2 hyperintensity (Fig. 34-5). He had abnormal autonomic testing.

MSA is a sporadic, degenerative CNS disease classified as a *synucleinopathy*. It presents with a combination of extrapyramidal, pyramidal, cerebellar, and autonomic symptoms and signs. Its clinical manifestations may change as it evolves.

MSA comprises three clinical conditions previously classified as (1) striatonigral degeneration (SND) with predominant parkinsonism and a *poor response to levodopa*; (2) Shy-Drager syndrome (SDS), parkinsonism or cerebellar syndrome, or both

with predominant *autonomic* dysfunction; and (3) sporadic *olivopontocerebellar atrophy* (OPCA) with predominant cerebellar dysfunction. MSA is a specific condition with a specific pathology, regardless of previous SND, SDS, or OPCA labels. It is characterized by oligodendroglial cytoplasmic inclusions that stain for alpha-synuclein. The etiology of MSA is unknown.

PATHOPHYSIOLOGY

Macroscopically, *neuronal loss and gliosis* are primarily seen in many subcortical areas such as the SN, LC, putamen, globus pallidus, inferior olive nucleus, pons, cerebellar cortex, autonomic nuclei of the brainstem, and intermediolateral columns of the spinal cord. *Glial cytoplasmic inclusions* (GCIs) are major microscopic findings that are characteristic of, but not specific for, MSA. These GCIs represent the accumulation of the protein alpha-synuclein within previously normal oligodendrocytes. These inclusions are distributed selectively within the basal ganglia, motor cortex, reticular formation, middle cerebellar peduncle, and the cerebellar white matter.

CLINICAL PRESENTATION

MSA affects a slightly younger age group than PD, with peak onset in the sixth decade. The clinical syndromes corresponding

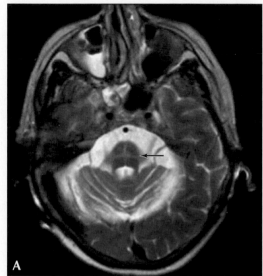

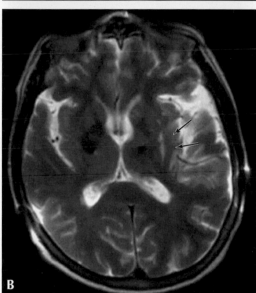

Typical brain MRI in MSA patient showing "hot cross bun" sign in the pons (arrow in A) and putaminal hyperintensity (arrows in B) .

Figure 34-5 Diagnosis of Multiple-System Atrophy.

to the previously named SND, OPCA, and SDS are parkinsonism, cerebellar dysfunction, and autonomic failure. Any one of these subcategories may be clinically predominant but still fall within the clinical spectrum of MSA.

The parkinsonism of SND tends to be more symmetric, rest tremor is less common, and postural instability develops earlier than in classic PD. Early stages, however, can be identical to the presentation of idiopathic PD. Similarly, an initial positive response to levodopa as well as negative fluctuations and dyskinesias may occur. Clinical "red flags" that should alert the clinician to a diagnosis of possible MSA include orthostatic hypotension, urinary retention or incontinence, ataxia, unexpected falls, stimulus-sensitive myoclonus, antecollis, slurred speech, stridor, and corticospinal tract signs.

MSA is a chronically progressive disorder characterized by the gradual onset of symptoms. Patients who present initially with extrapyramidal features commonly progress to develop autonomic disturbances, cerebellar disorders, or both. Conversely, patients whose first symptoms are cerebellar dysfunction often later develop extrapyramidal or autonomic disorders or both.

DIAGNOSIS

Distinguishing MSA from idiopathic PD and PSP is often challenging early in the illness. Some features such as autonomic dysfunction, poor or marginal response to levodopa with early clinical fluctuations, and dyskinesia can help to differentiate MSA from early PD. Autonomic failure is common in MSA and rare in early PD, whereas dementia and psychiatric features are more common in PD.

Cerebellar atrophy can be demonstrated even with brain CT scans. Characteristic MRI abnormalities include hypointensity on T1 or hyperintensities on T2 in the lateral border of the putamen or putaminal atrophy. Cerebellar and pontine atrophy with the *hot cross bun* sign (see Fig. 34-5) in the pons are seen; however, MRI is not specific and is often normal.

Other tests used in diagnosis of MSA include autonomic testing, external anal or urethral sphincter electromyography (EMG), and dopamine transporter scan.

TREATMENT

Only symptomatic therapy is available. Parkinsonism is treated with levodopa despite its inconsistent efficacy. Orthostatic hypotension may respond to conservative measures such as raising the head of the bed, binding stockings, and liberal salt intake. Medications such as fludrocortisone or midodrine are commonly required. Urinary dysfunction can be treated with antispasmodics such as oxybutynin and self-catheterization. Typical disease duration is 3–10 years. Breathing problems such as aspiration and cardiopulmonary arrest are common causes of death.

ADDITIONAL RESOURCES

Buee L, Delacourte A. Comparative biochemistry of tau in progressive supranuclear palsy, corticobasal degeneration, FTDP-17 and Pick's Disease. Brain Pathology 1999;9:681-693.

Dickson DW, Rademakers R, Hutton ML. Progressive supranuclear palsy: pathology and genetics. Brain Pathol 2007 Jan;17(1):74-82.

Frank S, Clavaquera F, Tolnay M. Tauopathy models and human neuropathology: similarities and differences. Acta Neuropathol 2008 Jan; 115(1):39053. Epub 2007 Sep 5.

Gibb RG, Luthert PJ, Marsden CD. Corticobasal degeneration. Brain 1989;112:1171-1192.

Gilman S. Multiple system atrophy. In: Jankovic J, Tolosa E, editors. Parkinson's Disease and Movement Disorders. Lippincott Williams & Wilkins; 1998. p. 245-295.

Gilman S, et al. Second consensus statement on the diagnosis of multiple system atrophy. Neurology 2008 Aug 26;71(9):670-676.

Houghton DJ, Litvan I. Unraveling progressive supranuclear palsy: from the bedside back to the bench. Parkinsonism Relat Disord 2007;13(Suppl. 3):S34106.

Litvan I, Cummings JL, Mega M. Neuropsychiatric features of corticobasal degeneration. J Neurol Nneurosurg Psychiatry 1998;65:717-721.

Melquist S, Craig DW, Huentelman MJ, et al. Identification of a novel risk locus for progressive supranuclear palsy by a pooled genomewide scan of 500,288 single-nucleotide polymorphisms. Am J Hum Genet 2007 Apr;80(4):769-778.

Oba H, et al. New and reliable MRI diagnosis for progressive supranuclear palsy. Neurology, 2005 Jun 28;64(12):2050-2055.

Rebeiz JJ, Edwin MD, Kolodny H, et al. Corticodentatonigral degeneration with neuronal achromasia. Arch Neurol 1986;(18):20-34.

Savoiardo M, Grisoli M, Girotti F. Magnetic resonance imaging in CBD, related atypical Parkinsonian disorders, and dementias. In: Litvan I, Goetz CH, Lang A, editors. Advances in Neurology, 82. Corticobasal Degeneration and Related Disorders. Lippincott Williams & Wilkins; 2000. p. 197-208.

Seppi K, Schocke MF, Wenning GK, et al. How to diagnose MSA early: the role of magnetic resonance imaging. J Neural Transm 2005 Dec;112(12):1625-1634. Epub 2005 Jul 6.

Wadia PM, Lang AE. The many faces of corticobasal degeneration. Parkinsonism Relat Disord 2007;13(Suppl. 3):S336-S340. Review.

Wenning GK, Stefanova N, Jellinger KA, et al. Multiple system atrophy: a primary oligodendrogliopathy. Ann Neurol 2008 Sep;64(3):239-243. Review.

Tremors

35

E. Prather Palmer and H. Royden Jones, Jr.

Clinical Vignette

A 31-year-old woman had the spontaneous onset of a relatively mild horizontal ("no-no") head tremor. She had no family history of neurologic disorders. This tremor was initially inconsequential but it gradually increased in severity. Turning her head to the right seemed to increase the tremor, whereas turning her head to the left decreased the tremor. Mild finger pressure on her left chin dampened the tremor and the involuntary movements of her head. Beta blockers, primidone, and alcohol had little effect. Eighteen months later, driving had become difficult because her head tended to turn involuntarily. Attempts to hold her head in the neutral position as well as stress markedly increased the tremor, leading to neck discomfort. Over time, the involuntary movements were continuously present. Neurologic examination demonstrated right sternocleidomastoid muscle hypertrophy. A trial of anticholinergic medication increased the tremor and precipitated a psychotic reaction. Eventually, the patient was treated with botulinum toxin in the right sternocleidomastoid muscle and some of the left paracervical muscles. This treatment controlled the involuntary movements and dampened the involuntary tremor.

Tremors are involuntary, rhythmic, and stereotyped oscillatory movements of a body part. These are the most prevalent movement disorders and are usually distinguishable from other abnormal involuntary movements by their rhythmic quality, with concomitant involvement of agonist and antagonist muscle groups. They result from alternating or irregularly synchronous contractions of reciprocally innervated skeletal muscles.

The precise pathogenesis for a tremor is unclear. With neurophysiologic testing, reciprocal bursts of electromyographic (EMG) activity occurring in agonist and antagonist muscles are separated by relative silence. Simultaneous EMG bursts in agonist–antagonist muscle pairs are not characteristic of tremors; the recorded pattern of any tremor can vary over a short period (i.e., co-contraction of the muscles, alternation of contraction, or contraction of the antigravity muscles alone). More complex relations between the agonist and antagonist muscles also occur. Hence, no universal method exists for definitively rating, measuring, or classifying tremors. Clinical examination is still the most important step in tremor evaluation.

PHYSIOLOGIC TREMOR

This is normally present in healthy individuals and is related to a number of factors. Physiologic tremor typically has an 8- to 12-Hz frequency in young adults and decreases to 6–7 Hz in the senior population (Table 35-1).

Peripheral components include muscle mass and stiffness, long and short loop reflexes, grouped motor neuron firing rates, and the inertia of muscles and other structures. The primary component of a physiologic tremor, the central generator, contributes weak 8- to 12-Hz low-amplitude movement not affected by inertial loading or physical manipulation. Other components, including the heartbeat (cardioballistics), may also contribute. This normal tremor is best seen by holding an arm straight in front of the body and placing a sheet of paper across the outstretched fingers.

The most common tremor is referred to as an enhanced physiologic tremor (EPT). It may result when motor units become discharged in groups. Typically this type of tremor becomes enhanced during muscular fatigue, fear, excitement, or emotional distress. It may occur in various medical conditions, for example, thyrotoxicosis, pheochromocytoma, catecholamine intake, methylxanthine use, drug withdrawal, and alcohol intoxication. Beta receptor agonists enhance physiologic tremor, and β-receptor blockade or $β_2$ receptor antagonists effectively decrease it. Early on, essential tremors (ETs) are difficult to separate from exaggerated physiologic tremors.

PATHOPHYSIOLOGY

The etiology of many tremors is unknown. Although Parkinson disease (PD) lesions predominate in the substantia nigra, experimental animal lesions within the substantia nigra do not cause tremor, and not all patients with lesions at this level have a tremor. Moreover, a tremor develops in only half of patients poisoned with the analog of meperidine (MPTP) that preferentially destroys part of the substantia nigra and classically leads to a mimic of PD. However, even with MPTP, the tremors are not the typical resting pill rolling ones of PD tremor; these have more of an action or postural component. In contrast, ventromedial tegmentum lesions made in a monkey midbrain do produce a resting-type tremor. Pathologic tremors such as ET, dystonic tremor, and the PD tremors are thought to have multiple central generators, resulting in variable frequencies of approximately 1–26 Hz (see Table 35-1).

PATHOLOGIC TREMOR

The most useful classification of pathologic tremors is based on their clinical features, especially anatomic distribution (proximal or distal, body part involved), symmetry, and the conditions that best activate them (Table 35-2). *Rest tremors* occur when a body part is completely supported against gravity (Fig. 35-1). *Action tremors* occurring during voluntary muscular contraction are further classified as (1) postural (occur in a body part maintained in position against gravity), (2) kinetic (occur during voluntary movement), or (3) isometric (occur within a muscle contracting against a stationary object).

Essential Tremor

This tremor is neither "essential" (an inherent characteristic of the individual) nor "benign." It is an acquired tremor that usually worsens with age and may eventually significantly interfere with normal activities. This type of action tremor has a lower frequency (4–8 Hz) than do physiologic tremors (7–12 Hz). It often occurs in isolation unrelated to any other neurologic disability. Approximately 50% of these patients have a positive family history, usually involving an autosomal dominant trait with virtually complete penetrance. These are referred to as *familial or hereditary tremor*. If the ET occurs late in life, it may be called a *senile tremor*. Although the familial forms tend to begin earlier, they rarely occur during infancy or after the sixth decade.

Table 35-1 Approximate Frequencies of Tremors

Frequency Range, Hz	Tremor Type
1–5	Holmes cerebellar tremor
2–10	Multiple sclerosis
2–12	Drug-induced tremor
2–12	Neuropathic tremor
3–10	Parkinsonian tremor
3–10	Task- and position-specific tremor
3–12	Dystonic tremor
4–10	Psychogenic tremor
4–8	Essential tremor
7–12	Physiologic and enhanced physiologic tremor
16–25	Orthostatic tremor

Adapted from Bain PG. The management of tremor. J Neurol Neurosurg Psychiatry. 2002;72(Suppl. 1):i3-i16.

ET is 20 times more frequent (prevalence, 0.2–33%) than PD. Many adult patients with ET tremors initially fear they have PD, and although classically it has not been thought that ET is an indication that PD will develop, more recent evidence demonstrates a small link between ET and PD. Similarly a postural tremor may appear years before the onset of other extrapyramidal symptoms of PD. Common genes or similar pathologic findings may underlie the development of both ET and PT and later PD. Functional neuroimaging studies demonstrate a dopaminergic deficit in some ET patients. Additionally, autopsy studies support such a relationship as some ET individuals have classic Lewy's body pathology in their brains similar to that present in PD.

Typically ETs are mild, symmetric postural tremors of the upper limbs, accentuated by voluntary movements. They commonly consist of pronation–supination and extension–flexion movements, and in severe or advanced cases, they may have a resting or kinetic component. They may spread to the head, face, lips, voice, jaw, tongue, chin, or occasionally the legs.

Head tremors may be horizontal ("no-no") or vertical ("yes-yes"). Although ET is a monosymptomatic illness, abnormalities in tandem gait are seen in nearly 50% of patients. Mild parkinsonian features (i.e., rest tremor, cogwheeling, and breakdown in rapid alternating movements) may also be present. As with classic ET, patients with the head tremor variation also have a somewhat greater incidence of PD. Additionally some instances of "no-no" head tremor may be a forme fruste later leading to spasmodic torticollis (dystonia) as per the vignette.

Treatment is not indicated for mild tremors that do not interfere with patients' quality of life. However, when the ET begins to interfere with the patient's daily activities, various therapeutic options are available. Although most patients

Table 35-2 Classification of Tremors

Type of Tremor	Clinical Features	Common Examples
Postural	A posture is maintained against gravity	Physiologic tremor Essential tremor Drug-induced tremor
Kinetic	With voluntary movements	Parkinson disease Cerebellar lesions (intention tremor) Writing tremor Holmes tremor
Isometric	With voluntary muscle contraction against a rigid, stationary object	Orthostatic tremor
Orthostatic tremor	Tremor of lower limbs on standing and remits on walking or sitting	Orthostatic tremor Head trauma Neuropathic tremor
Dystonic tremor	Tremor in body part affected by dystonia	Spasmodic torticollis
Resting tremor	Limb fully supported against gravity; improves with voluntary movement	Parkinson disease
Psychogenic tremor	Acute onset, inconsistent, fatigues, decreases amplitude with distraction	Somatoform disorders Malingering Depression
Asterixis	Arrhythmic lapses of sustained postures	Toxic and metabolic encephalopathies

Rest tremor

Usually called parkinsonian tremor, occurs in a limb that is not voluntarily activated. It is suppressed with voluntary movement. It may appear as "pill rolling."

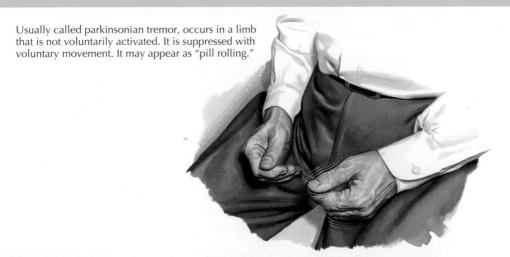

Action tremor (example: essential tremor)

Typically bilateral, this movement disorder is the most common. It may be accentuated with goal-directed movement of the limbs. Essential tremor affects the hands and facial musculature (in this order of prevalence). Most common presentation is the association of hand tremor and tremor in cranial musculature. Although considered benign, it can become incapacitating.

In the severe forms the patient may not be able to perform essential daily activities, such as drinking from a cup or dressing

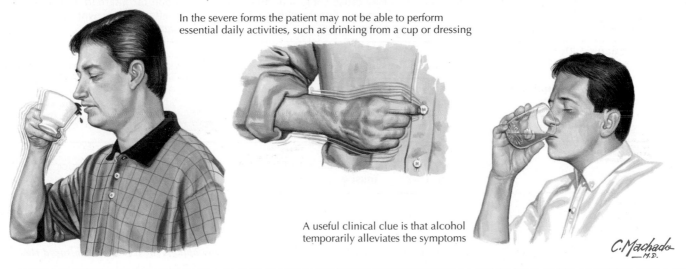

A useful clinical clue is that alcohol temporarily alleviates the symptoms

C. Machado
—M.D.

Figure 35-1 Tremor.

experience a reasonable response to beta adrenergic antagonists, such as propranolol, its side effects of bronchospasm, impotence, and sleep alterations are sometimes limiting. Other beta blockers may have a lower incidence of such side effects. The majority of ET patients experience a dramatic reduction in tremor after alcohol intake. Sometimes this response is helpful in making a differential diagnosis between ET and some variants of PD. Alcohol reduces the cerebellar overactivity that is demonstrated on PET scans of ET patients. However, over time, increasing amounts of alcohol are needed to produce this effect. Alcoholism is a potential outcome. Occasionally, treatment of ET can be very frustrating (Table 35-3). In the rare instance when the patient is very significantly incapacitated, surgical intervention (thalamotomy and deep brain stimulation) is effective.

Clinical Vignette

A 13-year-old boy was evaluated for a long-standing hand tremor that was accentuated by stress and physical activity, particularly having an essential quality. He had a grandmother with a head tremor and a grandfather with PD. Neurologic examination demonstrated intermittent bilateral action tremor of his hands most pronounced by finger-to-nose testing. His muscle stretch reflexes were hypoactive and he evidenced bilateral pes cavus. He refused an EMG. A trial of propranolol was considered. He returned 2 years later while attending vocational high school where he was studying welding. His tremor had increased and now involved his lower extremities and his head. He now had minimal distal weakness and sensory loss.

Table 35-3 Pharmacologic Options for Essential Tremor

Drug	Dosage	Precautions	Comment
Beta Blocker*			
Propranolol	30–240 mg/day	Avoid in patients with asthma, bradycardia, heart failure, or diabetes; may cause memory difficulties and confusion in the elderly	50% patients may benefit, and benefits may extend beyond 1 year, but escalation of the dose may be needed. Best tolerated by the young.
Metoprolol (Lopressor, Toprol)	50–200 mg/day	As above	Alternative to propranolol
Anticonvulsants*§			
Primidone*§ (Mysoline)	50–1000 mg/day	May cause ataxia, flulike symptoms, and drowsiness	Effective in up to 50% of patients; may be effective in patients who are unresponsive to beta blockers
Gabapentin†§ (Neurontin)	100–2400 mg/day	May cause mild drowsiness, headache, and abdominal discomfort	Studies show inconsistent improvement, well tolerated
Topiramate* (Topamax)	25–300 mg/day	May cause weight loss, paresthesiae, lethargy, or memory difficulties	Need to start with low doses and increase slowly
Benzodiazepines†			
Clonazepam (Klonopin)	0.25–4 mg/day	May cause confusion, drowsiness, ataxia, hypotension, and apnea	Good for intermittent use; loss of effectiveness with long-term use
Diazepam (Valium)	1–10 mg/day	Same as above	Same as above
Calcium Channel Blockers‡			
Nimodipine (Nimotop)	30–80 mg/day	May cause hypotension	Option if other drugs unsuccessful
Carbonic Anhydrase Inhibitors‡			
Methazolamide (Glauc Tabs, Neptazane)	100–200 mg/day	May cause paresthesiae, abdominal discomfort, and drowsiness	Adverse effects limit usefulness—may help with voice and head tremors
Botulinum Toxin‡			
Botox	Varies with injected muscles	Causes weakness of injected muscles	May be useful for voice or head tremors

*First-line drugs.
†Second-line drugs.
‡Drugs that may be helpful if others fail.
§Drugs better tolerated by the elderly.
Adapted from iHart after Evidente VGH. Understanding essential tremor: differential diagnosis and options for treatment. Postgrad Med. 200;108:138-149.

DNA testing was negative for Charcot–Marie–Tooth (CMT) polyneuropathy. Nerve conduction studies demonstrated multifocal demyelinating motor and sensory conduction slowing typical for an acquired chronic inflammatory demyelinating polyneuropathy (CIDP). Cerebrospinal fluid protein was 107 mg/dL. Treatment with intravenous immunoglobulin led to clinical improvement. Serendipitously, his Mom had an EMG that had some findings similar to his. Further DNA testing was carried out and demonstrated X-linked CMT polyneuropathy associated with 13-basepair deletion in the coding region of connexin-32.

Comment: Although this is a very uncommon clinical scenario, this patient's clinical presentation emphasizes the need to take a broad perspective when evaluating a patient with an ET as it can be mimicked by either acquired or hereditary demyelinating polyneuropathies.

Resting Tremor

PD and sometimes its variant are typified by a resting tremor (Chapters 33 and 34). The classic "pill-rolling" PD tremor has both a flexion–extension, abduction–adduction, of the fingers or hand and a pronation–supination component of the hand and forearm. This is typically unilateral at its first appearance and may remain asymmetric for a significant time. It is slowly progressive. Although this primarily affects the hand, it sometimes can include the feet, mandible, and lips. This PD tremor is somewhat suppressed by anticholinergic drugs and, less consistently but occasionally impressively so, by levodopa and other dopamine agonist drugs. On occasion, one sees patients with monosymptomatic resting tremors unassociated with other parkinsonian features. In contrast to PD per se, these isolated tremors are often refractory to treatment; however, sometimes other features of PD do respond to treatment eventually a number of years later.

Table 35-4 Essential Tremor Versus Parkinson Tremor

Characteristic	Essential Tremor	Parkinson Tremor
Type	Action/postural	Resting, "pill rolling"
Frequency	4–10 Hz	3–5 Hz
Age at onset	All ages	Middle age or elderly
Family history	First-degree relative often	None affected
Body part	Hands, head, voice	Hands, legs
Symmetry	Usually symmetric onset	Asymmetric onset, slowly
Course	Stable or slowly progressive	Progressive proximal as it generalizes to both sides
Other symptoms	Usually monosymptomatic	Rigidity, bradykinesia, flexed posture, balance problems
Origin	Olivocerebellar and other midbrain circuitry	Multiple generators within corticobasal ganglia and corticocerebellar circuitry
Other	Often transmitted as autosomal dominant, classically diminished by alcohol	May exhibit many types of tremors, including a postural one at the wrist at 5–8 Hz that may be difficult to distinguish from an essential tremor

With the increased understanding of the pathogenesis and treatment of PD, many patients mistakenly assume that most tremors are related to it. The physician must be able to differentiate the more common, postural ET from the serious resting tremor of PD (Table 35-4).

Orthostatic and Action Tremor

Clinical Vignette

A 72-year-old man had experienced difficulty playing golf during the past 6 months. When he would step to the tee standing still to get ready to hit the ball, his legs became increasingly tremulous. Although he could walk all 18 holes without difficulty, he was eventually unable to maintain his balance when he tried to stand still to make his shots. To compensate, he assumed an ever-widening posture, but this gradually became less helpful. Similarly, he had routinely begun to sit down when he urinated. Neurologic examination demonstrated an alert, pleasant man with normal facial expression. He arose from his chair without difficulty, walking with a normal gait, including a good arm swing. However, when he stopped and tried to stand still, he stood with an abnormally wide base and would soon develop an 18- to 20-Hz tremor involving both legs. It became necessary for him to hold on to someone to keep from falling. While seated, he had no rest tremor. He had no cogwheeling or rigidity, and his neurologic examination was otherwise normal.

Various medications were tried, including primidone, but no effective remedies were found.

Orthostatic tremor (OT) is a rare and often misdiagnosed problem of late middle age affecting the legs. It is typically precipitated by weight bearing and is characterized by a 16- to 25-Hz tremor. Isometric limb muscle contraction, the critical generation factor, induces the tremor. No other tremors have a frequency greater than 16 Hz. Often, if patients cannot sit down or resume walking, they become distressed and sometimes fall. The tremor classically abates in the non–weight-bearing setting

when the patient sits or begins to walk. Thirty percent of OT individuals also have an ET of the leg. In contrast to OT, this does not attenuate with walking.

The differential diagnosis of OT is a very limited one; the possibilities include aqueduct stenosis, pontine lesions, head trauma, and chronic inflammatory demyelinating neuropathy (CIDP). Brain MRI is important to exclude most of these. If this is normal, an EMG is indicated to exclude CIDP. Treatment is frequently problematic. Gabapentin may be helpful for OT. Treatment with topiramate, benzodiazepines, or valproic acid is sometimes of limited help. The nature of OT is commonly poorly understood by family and friends. They may need reassurance as to the nonpsychiatric nature of the patient's symptoms especially when he or she appears so normal in all other aspects. Patient anxiety is often a result; it may also require treatment (Table 35-5).

Ataxic Intention Tremor (AIT)

These are classified as either action or kinetic tremor. Their clinical characteristics have similarities to the tremor of cerebellar disorders and thus make this a separate clinical entity. The tremor is not intentional but occurs primarily during the demanding phase of active volitional movement. AIT is not apparent when the limbs are at rest and during the beginning of a voluntary movement. As an action is initiated and continues, fine motor adjustments are demanded (e.g., finger-to-nose task). In the instance of AIT, 2- to 4-Hz side-to-side oscillations eventually interrupt the movement and may continue for several beats after the target has been reached. Ataxic intention tremor always occurs in combination with cerebellar ataxia and may seriously interfere with performance of many skilled acts.

Another more violent form of an intention tremor, Holmes tremor, is associated with cerebellar ataxia, wherein slight lifting of the arms or maintenance of a static posture (e.g., arms abducted at the shoulders) results in a wide-range, rhythmic, 2- to 5-Hz "wing-beating" movement, often sufficiently forceful to throw patients off balance. The lesion is usually in the midbrain near the red nucleus (the tremor was formally called a rubral tremor). There is no treatment for these tremors. In severe cases, surgery (usually a thalamotomy) may help.

Table 35-5 Other Action-Type Tremors

Type	Description
Isolated chin tremors	Familial syndrome with onset in infancy or childhood; often intermittent and stress-induced
Dystonic tremor	A postural or kinetic tremor in an extremity or body part by dystonia; may at times be more obvious than the dystonic movement it accompanies.
Isolated voice tremor	May be a variant of essential tremor or dystonic tremor accompanying focal dystonia of the vocal cords (spasmodic dystonia)
Alcohol withdrawal tremor	An action/postural tremor is a prominent feature of the alcohol withdrawal syndrome; after recovery from the withdrawal state, some individuals have a persistent essential-type tremor; withdrawal of other sedative-type drugs (barbiturates, benzodiazepines) after prolonged use may also produce the same type of tremor
Task-specific tremors	May occur primarily during the performance of specific tasks or postures; primary writing tremor is the most common, but similar task-specific tremors have been described in typists, musicians, and sportsmen
Neuropathic tremor	Irregular, asymmetric, usually distal tremor, with frequencies of 3–12 Hz; may occur at rest, with posture with movement, and is associated with peripheral nerve disease; usually subsides with successful treatment of the underlying neuropathy or with beta blockers

Palatal Tremor (Palatal Myoclonus)

These rare tremors are rapid, rhythmic, and involuntary movements of the soft palate. Previously considered to be a form of myoclonus (hence the term *palatal myoclonus* or *palatal nystagmus*), palatal tremor has two forms: essential and symptomatic. *Essential palatal tremor* has no pathologic basis. It is associated with rhythmic activation of the tensor veli palatini, often recognized by the patient noting an audible click that ceases with sleep. MRI demonstrates no specific abnormalities in essential palatal tremor.

Symptomatic palatal tremor is often associated with a pendular vertical nystagmus, oscillopsia, and cerebellar signs. It is not inhibited by sleep. Unlike essential palatal tremor, this involves the levator veli palatini muscles. Symptomatic palatal tremor is associated with vascular disorders, multiple sclerosis, encephalitis, trauma, and neurodegenerative diseases. MRI demonstrates tegmental lesions as well as unilateral or bilateral inferior olivary nucleus enlargement.

Asterixis

This is typified by a series of arrhythmic interruptions in a sustained posture (i.e., sustained muscular contractions) with an intermittent lapse in postural muscle tone. The latter is associated with EMG silence for a period of 35–300 milliseconds. During this silence, gravity or the inherent elasticity of muscles produces the movement. Asterixis, therefore, differs physiologically from tremors and myoclonus. It is easily demonstrated by asking patients to hold their arms outstretched with hands dorsiflexed and fingers extended. Flexion hand movements may occur several times each minute. Asterixis can be produced by persistent contraction of any muscle group. Classically, this is precipitated by a sustained dorsiflexion of the wrists or less commonly protrusion of the tongue. It can occur in normal persons in the neck and arms with drowsiness.

Asterixis typifies the clinical picture of hepatic or uremic encephalopathy. Sometimes it is found in other metabolic and toxic states, including those iatrogenically induced by various medications such as phenytoin and other anticonvulsants.

Unilateral asterixis is rarely found with contralateral thalamic or brainstem lesions. Treatment with clonazepam, sodium valproate, tetrabenazine, and haloperidol is sometimes helpful.

Drug-Induced (Iatrogenic) Tremor

Many pharmacologic agents can induce tremors, depending on the individual and the underlying illness. Some drugs, such as lithium, can cause several types of tremor, depending on the dose or treatment duration. The most common drug-induced tremor is an enhanced physiologic tremor related to sympathomimetics or antidepressants (especially the tricyclics and serotonin reuptake inhibitors). Although specific predisposing risk factors are not well defined, patients with an ET, older patients, and women are thought to have a higher risk for drug-induced tremors.

A parkinsonian-like resting tremor may occur after ingestion of neuroleptic, antidopaminergic drugs (including dopamine-depleting drugs). Unlike the tremor of PD, the resting, pharmacologically induced tremor is initially bilateral and symmetric. An intention tremor may occur with lithium intoxication or chronic alcoholism. A tardive tremor is associated with long-term neuroleptic use. The anticonvulsants phenytoin and sodium valproate can cause various action tremors. An action tremor resembling an enhanced physiologic tremor is also produced by medications such as calcium channel blockers, amiodarone, theophylline, adrenaline, amphetamine, lithium, caffeine, cocaine, marijuana, and drug or alcohol withdrawal (Table 35-6).

Psychogenic Tremor

Unusual nonclassifiable tremors sometimes present as manifestations of underlying psychiatric disorders, particularly in patients with somatoform disturbances, malingering, or depression. Clinical presentations vary and are usually bizarre consistently inconsistent combinations of resting, postural, or intention tremors. Diagnosis of psychogenic tremor is often one of exclusion. It is frequently difficult to be certain of such a diagnosis

Table 35-6 Drug-Induced Tremors

Drug	Type of Tremor
Alcohol withdrawal	Postural, intention
Drug withdrawal	Postural
Insulin (by inducing hypoglycemia)	Postural
CNS acting	
Neuroleptics	Resting, postural
Reserpine	Resting, postural
Metoclopramide	Resting, postural
Antidepressants	Resting
Lithium	Resting, postural, intention
Cocaine	Postural
Alcohol	Postural, intention
Sympathomimetics	
Bronchodilators (β_2 agonist)	Postural, intention
Theophylline	Postural
Caffeine	Postural
Dopamine	Postural
Lithium	Postural
Thyroxine	Postural, action
Methylxanthines	Postural
Miscellaneous	Postural, action
Steroids	Postural, resting, intention
Valproate: Phenytoin	Postural, action
Antiarrhythmics (amiodarone)	Postural, action
	Postural
Antidopaminergic drugs (e.g., metoclopramide)	Postural, rest
	Postural
Mexiletine: Thyroid hormone	Postural
	Postural, intention
Cytostatics (vincristine, cytosine)	
Immunosuppressants	
Cyclosporine	Postural

early on. This is best confirmed by a tincture of time when no organic mechanism develops and psychotherapy leads to remission.

There are certain recognized diagnostic criteria for psychogenic tremor. These include an acute onset and spontaneous remission, distraction leading to a decrease in the tremor, variation of frequency and amplitude during movements; history of somatization, coactivation of antagonist muscles either during passive flexion or extension, and lack of responsiveness to acceptable treatment, placebo, or both. Rare patients present with whole-body shakes. Here, the tremor may cease spontaneously or during examination when the movements exhaust the patient. More difficult cases involve predominately extremity tremors, often without finger involvement. The prognosis in psychogenic tremors is poor without prompt recognition and treatment.

ADDITIONAL RESOURCES

Bain PG. The management of tremor. J Neurol Neurosurg, Psychiatry 2002;72(Suppl. 1):i3-i16.

Rodrigues JP, Edwards DJ, Walters SE, et al. Blinded placebo crossover study of gabapentin in primary orthostatic tremor. Mov Disord 2006 Jul;21(7):900-905.

Roze E, Coêlho-Braga MC, Gayraud D, et al. Head tremor in Parkinson's disease. Mov Disord 2006 Aug;21(8):1245-1248.

Stoessl AJ. Radionuclide scanning to diagnose Parkinson disease: is it cost-effective? Nat Clin Pract Neurol 2009 Jan;5(1):10-11. Epub 2008 Dec 9. *A recent study concluded that 123I-2β-carbomethoxy-3β-(4-iodophenyl)-n-(3-fluoropropyl)nortropane single-photon emission computed tomography (123I-FP-CIT SPECT) is helpful when there is difficulty making the differential diagnosis between essential tremor and Parkinson's disease.*

Tan EK, Lee SS, Fook-Chong S, et al. Evidence of increased odds of essential tremor in Parkinson's disease. Mov Disord 2008;23:993-997.

Zesiewicz TA, Hauser RA. Phenomenology and treatment of tremor disorders. Neurol Clin 2001;19:651-680.

Chorea

Diana Apetauerova

36

Clinical Vignette

John is a 56-year-old-right-handed architect who developed tick-like movements in his body within the past 3–4 years and was now "fidgety" all the time. His wife reported intellectual changes in her husband; he seemed withdrawn and forgetful, was occasionally inappropriate in his behavior, had difficulties with his job, and had to retire early due to inability to "concentrate." He had no other past medical history. He was adopted and there was no health information about his parents. Tourette syndrome was diagnosed by his primary care physician.

When seen in movement disorders clinic, he was unable to sit still. He had constant grimacing in his face, motor impersistence in his tongue, and piano-like playing movements in his hands. Brief, jerky choreiform movements were present in his trunk and extremities. His gait appeared very disorganized and unsteady. He had bradykinesia predominantly with testing of his hands. His demeanor was jovial and he had no signs of depression. The movements were not under any voluntary control and he had no urge to do them.

Because of the combination of cognitive decline and generalized chorea, Huntington disease was suspected. His genetic testing revealed 45 CAG repeats in the HD gene. He was treated with low doses of haloperidol 1 mg daily with substantial improvement in chorea. Recently, an addition of tetrabenazine was initiated, with further improvement of involuntary movements. However, his intellectual and behavioral decline continued.

Chorea (from Latin *choreus*, dance) is an abnormal involuntary movement usually distal in location, brief, nonrhythmic, abrupt, and irregular, that seems to flow from one body part to another. The movements are random, unpredictable in timing, direction, and distribution. Chorea can be partially suppressed; some patients can incorporate these into semipurposeful movements called *parakinesia*. Motor impersistence, the inability to maintain a sustained contraction, is a typical feature of chorea.

Athetosis and **ballism** are sometimes confused with chorea. *Athetosis* is a slow, writhing, continuous set of involuntary movements, usually affecting limbs distally, but it can involve the axial musculature (neck, face, and tongue). If athetosis becomes faster, it sometimes blends with chorea, that is, *choreoathetosis*. *Ballism* is large-amplitude, involuntary movements affecting the proximal limbs, causing flinging and flailing limb movements.

Patients with chorea are often initially unaware of these involuntary movements. The chorea is often first interpreted by observers as fidgetiness. The patients are usually frustrated by their own incoordination or clumsiness.

ETIOLOGY

Chorea results from disruption of the basal ganglia's modulation of thalamocortical motor pathways. Multiple pathophysiologic mechanisms may be implicated. These include neuronal degeneration in selective regions, neurotransmitter receptor blockade, other metabolic factors within the basal ganglia, and exceedingly rarely a structural lesion. Chorea is classified into inherited, primarily Huntington disease (HD), immunologic Sydenham chorea, drug-related, structural, and various miscellaneous etiologies (Table 36-1).

PATHOPHYSIOLOGY

The putamen, globus pallidus, and subthalamic nuclei are the key pathologic sites related to the development of chorea. Normal movement patterns depend on the presence of a critical physiologic balance between the direct and indirect motor pathways. Healthy individuals have an *excitatory glutamate pathway*, arising from within the subthalamic nucleus, that excites the globus pallidus interior and the substantia nigra. Concomitantly, these areas then signal the *GABA inhibitory pathway* within the thalamus. In a simplified model, the excitatory action of the subthalamic nucleus is reduced or lost, leading to a disinhibition of the pallidothalamic pathway.

The major neurodegenerative pathology in HD occurs within the caudate nuclei and the putamen (striatum). These changes primarily affect *medium-sized "spiny" neurons* that secrete the inhibitory neurotransmitter GABA. These neurons project from the striatum into the globus pallidus and substantia nigra. Selective loss of these specialized cells theoretically result in decreased thalamic inhibition, that is, leading to an increased activity. Consequently, such an inhibitory cell depletion causes an increased output to the cerebral cortex. The resultant motor activity leads to the disorganized, excessive (hyperkinetic) movement patterns of chorea. Concomitantly, HD patients also have a prominent associated temporal and frontal lobe cerebral cortex neuronal degeneration.

With Sydenham chorea, various streptococcal proteins or antigens (streptococcal M proteins) induce the body's production of antineuronal IgG antibodies. These antibodies cross-react against the body's own cells that provide the neuronal antigens within the basal ganglia, such as the caudate nuclei and subthalamic nucleus.

CLINICAL PRESENTATION

The spectrum of clinical findings in chorea varies, presenting in isolation or with other involuntary movements. At the simplest level, chorea appears as semipurposeful movements resembling fidgetiness. This is exemplified by the flitting movements of the fingers, wrists, toes, and ankles so characteristic of HD. The movements can be focal, as in tardive dyskinesia, where they are

Table 36-1 Causes of Chorea

Type of Chorea	
Inherited	Huntington disease
	Neuroacanthocytosis
	Wilson disease
	Benign hereditary chorea
	Olivopontocerebellar atrophy
	Ataxia telangiectasia
	Idiopathic torsion dystonia
	Tic disorder
	Myoclonic epilepsy
	Dentatorubropallidoluysian degeneration
	Gerstmann–Sträussler–Scheinker syndrome
Metabolic	Amino acid disorders (glutaric academia)
	Leigh disease
	Lesch–Nyhan disease
	Lipid disorders (gangliosidoses)
	Mitochondrial myopathy
	Nonketotic hyperglycemia
	Disorders of calcium, magnesium, or glucose
Immunologic	Sydenham chorea
	Systemic lupus erythematosus
	Antiphospholipid antibody syndrome
	Chorea gravidarum
	Reaction to immunization
Drug related	Tardive dyskinesia (neuroleptics, serotonin reuptake inhibitors, others)
	Withdrawal emergent syndrome
	Sympathomimetics
	Cocaine
	Anticonvulsants
	Contraceptives
	Lithium
	Tricyclic antidepressants
	Levodopa
	Amantadine
	Dopamine agonist
	Theophylline and β-adrenergic agents
	Ethanol
	Carbon monoxide
	Gasoline inhalation
Structural	Cerebrovascular disease
	Multiple sclerosis
	Traumatic brain injury
	Anoxic encephalopathy
	Pseudochoreoathetosis (spinal cord injury, peripheral nerve injury)
	Delayed onset following perinatal injury
Miscellaneous	Encephalitis (herpes simplex, HIV, Lyme disease)
	Endocrine dysfunction (e.g., hyperthyroidism)
	Metabolic disturbance (e.g., hypocalcemia, hyperglycemia, hypoglycemia)
	Kernicterus
	Nutritional (e.g., B_{12} deficiency)
	Postpump chorea (cardiac bypass)
	Normal maturation

more repetitive and stereotypical. They may present as lip pouting or pursing, cheek puffing, lateral or forward jaw movements, or tongue rolling or protruding.

Asymmetric chorea, such as hemichorea, primarily affects the limbs on one side of the body. Sometimes, chorea affects only specific functional muscle groups, such as respiratory chorea. When there is a more diffuse basal ganglia dysfunction, chorea is often accompanied by parkinsonism, tics, and dystonia. Later, chorea can interfere with activities of daily living; for example, limb chorea can cause falls and interfere with dressing and eating. Chorea of the face, jaw, larynx, and respiratory muscles may eventually limit verbal communication.

On neurologic examination, there is altered finger-to-nose testing. Rapid alternating movements are executed with a jerky and interrupted performance. When patients with significant chorea grasp an examiner's fingers, a squeezing motion called *milkmaid's grip* is sometimes noted. This is a sign of motor impersistence. As with other adventitious movements, seen with the various movement disorders, chorea is frequently aggravated while walking. Various oculomotor abnormalities may be observed. These include slow and hypometric saccades and saccadic pursuit, convergence paresis, and gaze impersistence. Parkinsonian features, particularly bradykinesia and dystonia, are sometimes evidenced with more advanced disease.

Huntington Disease

This hereditary, progressive neurodegenerative disorder is the most common cause of chorea. The classic signs of HD include the development of chorea, neurobehavioral changes, and gradual dementia (Fig. 36-1). Symptoms typically become evident during the fourth or fifth decade of life, although onset varies from early childhood to late adulthood. HD symptoms vary among patients in range and severity, as well as by age at onset, and in rate of clinical progression. An early onset is associated with increased severity and more rapid progression. For example, adult-onset HD typically lasts approximately 15–20 years, whereas the course of juvenile HD tends to last approximately 8–10 years.

The initial clinical presentation may be either neurologic or psychiatric. Characteristic early presentations include the gradual onset of subtle personality changes, forgetfulness, clumsiness, and development of choreiform, fidgeting movement of the fingers or toes. Neurobehavioral changes include both emotional and behavioral disturbance. Patients present with increased irritability, suspiciousness, impulsiveness, lack of self-control, and anhedonia. Sometimes anxiety, depression, mania, obsessive–compulsive behaviors, and agitation are seen early in the disease. Later, a severe distortion in thinking and occasionally hallucinations, such as the perception of sounds, sights, or other sensations without external stimuli, may develop. The juvenile form of HD more often presents with dystonia, rigidity, or cerebella ataxia than chorea per se.

Cognitive decline is characterized by progressive dementia or gradual impairment of the mental processes involved in comprehension, reasoning, judgment, and memory. Typical early signs include forgetfulness, inattention, increased difficulty in concentrating, and various forms of disinhibition manifested by emotional outbursts, financial irresponsibility, or sexual

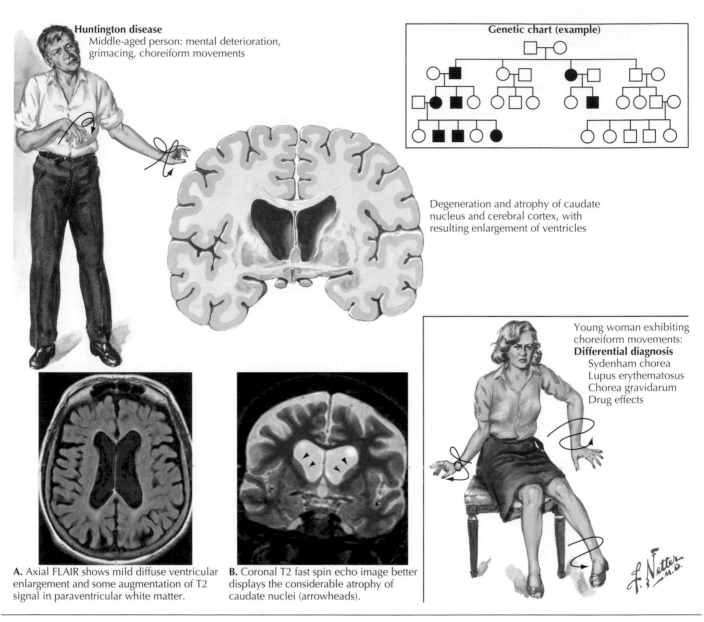

Huntington disease
Middle-aged person: mental deterioration, grimacing, choreiform movements

Genetic chart (example)

Degeneration and atrophy of caudate nucleus and cerebral cortex, with resulting enlargement of ventricles

Young woman exhibiting choreiform movements:
Differential diagnosis
Sydenham chorea
Lupus erythematosus
Chorea gravidarum
Drug effects

A. Axial FLAIR shows mild diffuse ventricular enlargement and some augmentation of T2 signal in paraventricular white matter.

B. Coronal T2 fast spin echo image better displays the considerable atrophy of caudate nuclei (arrowheads).

Figure 36-1 Chorea.

promiscuity. Communication difficulties develop, including problems expressing thoughts in words, initiating conversations, or comprehending others' words and responding appropriately.

Motor disturbances are characterized by the gradual onset of clumsiness, balance difficulties, and fidgeting movements. Early chorea may be limited to the fingers and toes, later extending to the arms, legs, face, and trunk. Eventually, chorea tends to become widespread or generalized. Parkinsonism and dystonia are sometimes seen later in the disease. Many patients with HD develop a distinctive manner of walking that may be unsteady, disjointed, lurching, and dance-like. Eventually, postural instability, dysphagia, and dysarthria appear.

Later disease stages are characterized by severe dementia and progressive motor dysfunction; patients usually become unable to walk, have poor dietary intake, become unable to care for themselves, and eventually cease to talk, leading to a persistent

vegetative state. Life-threatening complications may result from serious falls, sometimes even leading to subdural hematomas, poor nutrition, infection, choking, aspiration pneumonia, or heart failure.

Sydenham Chorea

This is the other well-recognized form of chorea. It is related to an autoimmune response to infection with group A beta-hemolytic streptococci leading to acute rheumatic fever (ARF). This is now very uncommon in economically developed countries with the widespread availability of antibiotics for *Streptococcus* A infection. The initial illness is usually characterized by pharyngitis, followed within approximately 1–5 weeks by the sudden onset of ARF. Chorea primarily occurs in patients between the ages of 5 and 15 years. It usually does not present until 1–6 months after the initial sore throat. Sydenham chorea

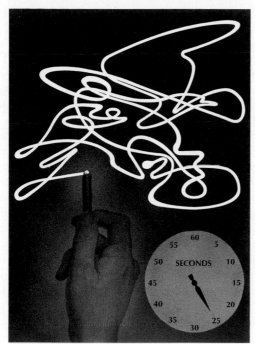

Sydenham chorea: spontaneous uncoordinated movements demonstrated by electric penlight held in patient's hand

Figure 36-2 Choreiform Movements.

---

may occur as an isolated condition or subsequent to other characteristic features of ARF. Initially, these children often are described as unusually restless, aggressive, or "excessively emotional." The distribution of chorea is usually generalized, and these movements consist of relatively fast or rapid, irregular, uncontrollable, jerky motions that disappear with sleep and may increase with stress, fatigue, and excitement (Fig. 36-2). Occasionally, the choreiform movements are so severe that they have a ballistic character. Some children also evidence emotional and behavioral disturbances.

Typically, in a significant majority of children, Sydenham chorea is a self-limited condition, resolving spontaneously within an average duration of 9 months to 2 years. However, sometimes residual signs of chorea and behavioral abnormalities fluctuate over a year or more. In approximately 20% of patients, Sydenham chorea may recur, usually within approximately 2 years of the initial occurrence. Recurrences are also reported during pregnancy and in association with certain medications in women who had ARF during childhood.

DIFFERENTIAL DIAGNOSES

Diagnostic considerations in a patient presenting with chorea is a broad one (Table 36-1). HD, the most common cause of chorea, is usually easily diagnosed when an adult has the typical triad of chorea, dementia, and family history. Several neurodegenerative disorders, some also having expanded trinucleotide repeats, are phenocopies of HD. These include spinocerebellar atrophy (SCA2, SCA3) and dentatorubral-pallidoluysian atrophy

Box 36-1 Initial Laboratory and Imaging Investigation of Chorea

Thyroid hormone assay
Electrolyte panel
Complete blood count (look for acanthocytes)
Antinuclear antibody test (SLE)
Antistreptolysin-O antibody test
Urine toxicological screen for illicit drugs
Brain MRI*/PET
Huntington disease gene testing

*MRI, magnetic resonance imaging; PET, positron emission tomography; SLE, systemic lupus erythematosus

(DRPLA). Additionally, there are some other HD-like diseases (HDL1, HDL2, HDL3) that may present with an HD-like phenotype. Sydenham chorea has an earlier onset, lacks the characteristic mental disturbances, and is usually self-limiting. Chorea with mental dysfunction may also occur as a manifestation of systemic lupus erythematosus (SLE). These patients usually have a more acute onset, with more localized chorea, and the characteristic SLE clinical and serologic abnormalities. There is a prior history of recurrent vascular thromboses or spontaneous abortions and disappearance after therapy with prednisone.

Involuntary movements occurring in psychiatric patients receiving long-term treatment with neuroleptic agents occasionally pose a diagnostic problem when they present with tardive dyskinesia (TD). Usually repetitive, these TD movements contrast with the nonrepetitive and flowing nature of chorea. Patients with TD usually have a predominant oral–lingual–buccal dyskinesia. Unlike in those with HD, these patients' gait is usually normal. Similar mental dysfunction occurs with some of the dementing disorders, particularly Alzheimer or Pick disease where language is more involved. Myoclonus is more typical than chorea with dementia, especially with spongiform encephalopathies, for example, Creutzfeldt–Jakob disease. Very rarely, a structural basal ganglia lesion, particularly an infarction or hemorrhage or an associated polycythemia rubra vera, leads to an acute focal chorea, or hemiballismus.

If the onset of chorea occurs during childhood, other inheritable disorders including the leukodystrophies and gangliosidosis require differentiation. *Neuroacanthocytosis* is another hereditary movement disorder also manifested by mild chorea, tics, parkinsonism, and dystonia. Laboratory findings include increased serum creatine phosphokinase and red cell acanthocytes. In all age groups, possible reactions to drugs or toxins must always be investigated.

DIAGNOSTIC EVALUATION

Huntington Disease

The evaluation of patients with chorea includes detailed family history and tests to exclude other possible pathophysiology (Box 36-1). Genetic testing is the most accurate test for HD. The mutation that is responsible for the disease consists of an unstable enlargement of the CAG repeat sequence. The gene is located at 4p16.3 and encodes for a protein called huntingtin.

Genetic testing is available for presymptomatic individuals at risk for HD; it requires careful pretest and posttest counseling to guard against suicidal risk in individuals who request the study and find out they have the illness. Other investigations are less important, but magnetic resonance imaging (MRI) or computed tomography (CT) are commonly performed. Head MRI is preferable to CT for better delineation of the affected subcortical tissue. Atrophy of the caudate nucleus may be demonstrated. Positron emission tomography (PET) typically demonstrates glucose hypometabolism within the striatum.

Sydenham Chorea

Diagnosis primarily relies on the recognition of acute chorea in a child or adolescent who recently had a Streptococcal pharyngitis. The combination fulfills the criteria for a diagnosis of ARF. Other manifestations of ARF are not mandatory for the diagnosis. Tests for acute-phase reactions are less helpful because of the latency between the early infection and the onset of the movement disorder. These include an erythrocyte sedimentation rate, C-reactive protein, and a leukocytosis. Supporting evidence of preceding streptococcal infections include positive throat culture for group A *Streptococcus*, increased antistreptolysin-O titer, or other antistreptococcal antibodies. Brain CT usually fails to display abnormalities. Head MRI is often normal but occasionally shows reversible hyperintensity in the basal ganglia. PET and SPECT demonstrate reversible striatal hypermetabolism.

Chorea Gravidarum

A chorea of any etiology beginning during a pregnancy is referred to as chorea gravidarum (CG). This is most common in younger woman, having an average age of 22 years. CG is frequently associated with eclampsia. At least 35% of CG individuals have a prior history of acute rheumatic fever (RF) with associated Sydenham chorea. CG is now quite uncommon, probably attributable to a decline in the incidence of RF with the more widespread use of antibiotics. It is postulated that estrogen and progesterone may sensitize dopaminergic receptors, inducing chorea in an individual with preexisting basal ganglia pathology.

TREATMENT

Readily reversible causes of chorea need to be excluded before considering pharmacologic intervention. Therapy depends on the severity of symptoms; mild chorea does not usually require any treatment. Chorea is treated with either dopamine-blocking or dopamine-depleting medications. Dopamine antagonists haloperidol and pimozide are the drugs of choice. Benzodiazepine drugs are another possible therapeutic modality offering a nonspecific means to suppress chorea. With severe chorea, dopamine-depleting agents such as reserpine or tetrabenazine are sometimes considered.

The overall treatment of Huntington disease patients requires an integrated, multidisciplinary approach, including symptomatic and supportive medical management; psychosocial support; physical, occupational, or speech therapy; and genetic counseling. Often more specific additional supportive services are helpful for individual patients and their families. There is no specific treatment available that slows, alters, or reverses the progression of HD. Tetrabenazine is a dopaminergic depleting medication that effectively lessens chorea; it was recently approved for treatment of HD patients.

Sydenham chorea is usually not a disabling disorder; however, the more severely affected patients with more severe chorea, requiring short-time treatment, may respond to dopamine antagonists or valproic acid. Severely affected patients may improve with immunosuppressants, plasmapheresis, or intravenous immunoglobulin. Drug treatment should be withdrawn after a short period because remission invariably occurs. Penicillin prophylaxis for ARF is advisable.

Prognosis depends on the cause of chorea. Drug-induced chorea is usually transient. Patients with a past history of rheumatic chorea are more susceptible to developing chorea during pregnancy or drug-induced chorea, for example, from phenytoin or oral contraceptives.

FUTURE DIRECTIONS

Current research is directed at better definition of the genetics, pathophysiology, symptoms, and progression of HD vis-à-vis the definition of new pharmacologic agents. Neuroprotection is the preservation of neuronal structure, function, and viability, and neuroprotective therapy is thus targeted at the underlying pathology of HD, rather than at its specific symptoms. Thus ultimately the development of disease-modifying neuroprotective therapies that can delay or even prevent the clinical presentation of HD is the ideal for those individuals who are at genetic risk. Preclinical discovery research in HD is identifying numerous distinct targets, along with options for modulating them. Some of these are now proceeding into large-scale efficacy studies in early symptomatic HD subjects. Cell models also offer a very important means to study early, direct effects of mutant huntingtin mRNA changes to identify groups of genes that could play a role in the early pathology of Huntington disease. In the meantime, alternative therapeutic agents that can slow progression for those who are already clinically affected with HD will be very welcome.

ADDITIONAL RESOURCES

Adam OR, Jankovic J. Symptomatic treatment of Huntington disease. Neurotherapeutics 2008 Apr;5(2):181-197.

Fahn S, Jankovic J. Huntington's Disease. Principles and Practice of Movement Disorders. Churchill Livingstone Elsevier 2007;369-392.

Hersch SM, Rosas HD. Neuroprotection for Huntington's disease: ready, set, slow. Neurotherapeutics 2008 Apr;5(2):226-236.

Huntington Study Group. Tetrabenazine as antichorea therapy in Huntington disease: a randomized controlled trial. Neurology 2006 Feb 14;66(3):366-372.

Jankovic J, Beach J. Long-term effects of tetrabenazine in hyperkinetic movement disorders. Neurology 1997;48:358-362.

O'Brien CH. Chorea. In: Jankovic J, Tolosa E, editors. Parkinson's Disease and Movement Disorders. Baltimore, MD: Williams & Wilkins; 1998. p. 357-364.

Wilson Disease

Isabel A. Zacharias and H. Royden Jones, Jr.

37

Clinical Vignette

Approximately 1 year ago, an 18-year-old woman began to have peculiar tremors of her arms and hands as well as difficulty with her speech becoming soft and slurred. This followed an insidiously progressive course to the point of being embarrassing when she was so poorly understood that family and colleagues sometimes found comprehension quite difficult as she started college. Concomitantly, she became irritable and had variable mood swings, at times leading to profound depression. On other occasions, she was belligerent. Within months, she took a medical leave of absence from school.

After initially being thought to be suffering from academic stress leading to profound somatization, she was referred to another neurologist. In addition to a poorly defined rather gross tremor of her arms and hands, a mildly masked bradykinetic facies and dysarthric speech were recognized. Ophthalmic examination demonstrated a gold/brown-pigmented ring at the limbus of his cornea. This was clearly visible with her blue irises. This proved to be a classic Kayser–Fleischer ring. She was mildly jaundiced.

Laboratory investigation demonstrated mildly abnormal general liver function tests (LFTs). Serologies were negative for hepatitis A, B, and C. Her serum ceruloplasmin level was low, and a 24-hour urine copper excretion level was increased. Magnetic resonance imaging (MRI) demonstrated variable degrees of cerebral cortical, brainstem, and cerebellar atrophy. Signal abnormalities were also noted in her putamen, caudate, midbrain, and pons. There was characteristic T2-W globus pallidal hypointensity with T1-W striatal hyperintensity.

Wilson disease (WD) was diagnosed, and she was started on penicillamine. Within 6 weeks, increased bradykinesia, rigidity, and mutism developed. However, these symptoms gradually cleared over the next 6 months. Twelve months later, the patient's speech had returned to normal, and her behavior had improved, although she still showed some depressive symptoms. Zinc acetate was started as a long-term therapy.

HISTORY

WD is a rare hereditary disorder of copper metabolism, biochemically characterized by abnormal accumulation of this essential trace metal in both the liver and the brain, leading respectively to cirrhosis and neuronal degeneration. WD has an autosomal recessive inheritance with a prevalence of approximately 1 case in 30,000 live births and a carrier rate of 1 in 90. Clinical presentations are quite variable. These include primarily neurologic, neuropsychiatric, or hepatic disturbances; less common are acute hemolytic crisis, arthralgias, nephrolithiasis, and cardiac arrhythmias.

This association between cirrhosis and progressive lenticular degeneration was first described by Kinnier Wilson in 1912. Subsequently excess copper deposits were demonstrated in both the liver and basal ganglia in a patient dying of WD. The finding of reduced serum ceruloplasmin level was recognized a few years later. Treatment was initially attempted using dimercaptopropanol (British Anti-Lewisite [BAL]) in 1951; the much more effective penicillamine treatment was introduced 5 years later. WD thus became the first inherited metabolic disorder with specific treatments. More recently, orthotopic liver transplantation performed for patients with WD has cured the disease in some instances, thus revolutionizing its treatment.

GENETICS

The genetic defect of WD is the ATP7B gene located on the long arm of chromosome 13. ATP7B binds copper and transports it across cellular membranes using ATP as an energy source. In WD, this defect leads to reduced copper binding to apoceruloplasmin, which normally forms ceruloplasmin. It also leads to decreased secretion of copper into the bile ducts. DNA analysis from patients with WD shows more than 100 mutations, thus complicating the opportunity for DNA diagnosis. Similarly, it is difficult to make a correlation between the various mutations and specific clinical features. Only a few patients are homozygous for the same mutation. The most frequently observed point mutation, H1069Q, results from the substitution of a histidine to a glutamine. This is present in nearly 30% of Wilson patients of European descent.

HEPATIC COPPER METABOLISM

Copper facilitates electron transfer in critical metabolic pathways involving cellular respiration, iron homeostasis, pigment formation, neurotransmitter production, peptide biosynthesis, connective tissue biosynthesis, and antioxidant defense. Within the brain, copper is found in particularly high concentrations in catecholamine-containing neurons. It is a component of the dopamine β-hydroxylase enzyme complex.

Copper balance is maintained entirely by gastrointestinal absorption and biliary excretion; urinary copper excretion cannot adequately compensate for reduced biliary excretion. Approximately 60% of dietary copper is absorbed in the proximal small intestine, most of which enters hepatoportal circulation, where it is rapidly taken up by hepatocytes. These cells regulate copper homeostasis by excretion of copper into the bile. This system is dependent on the degree of copper concentration as sensed by the ATP7B receptor that is located on the trans-Golgi network and the cytoplasmic vesicular compartment near the canalicular membrane. The absence or decreased function of ATP7B results in dysfunction of biliary copper excretion and consequently leads to copper accumulation within the liver.

Ceruloplasmin is a protein synthesized by hepatocytes and is the major carrier of copper in the bloodstream. Copper is thought to be incorporated into this protein via the ATP7B pathway. In WD, absent or diminished function of the ATP7B leads to reduced binding of ceruloplasmin to copper, thereby lowering circulating levels of ceruloplasmin.

Excess copper accumulation results in generation of free radicals, lipid peroxidation of membranes and DNA, and inhibition of protein synthesis leading to hepatocellular injury and necrosis. Release of free copper, from injured hepatocytes, into circulation is thought to be responsible for causing extrahepatic deposition of copper in the brain, kidneys, eyes, and joints.

CLINICAL PRESENTATION

WD patients have quite variable clinical presentations. Because WD is such an extremely rare disorder, and lacks a precise, stereotyped clinical presentation, these patients are often not diagnosed until long after the onset of their symptomatology. As with the above vignette, there are legendary recitals of individuals being told, not once but a number of times, that they are not organically ill and that a psychiatric evaluation is in order, only to later visit a dedicated physician who takes a careful history and closely examines the patient, often recognizing the classic and diagnostic Kayser–Fleischer (KF) ring and thus making the WD diagnosis.

One might suspect that as the liver is the primary site of both the abnormal copper storage, as well the specific genetic defect, the earliest signs of WD will be identified as having a hepatic origin. However, hepatic involvement is often clinically and laboratory-wise a subtle disorder because the copper accumulates very slowly. Eventually, subclinical cirrhosis develops. Concomitantly, as hepatocytic injury ensues, copper is released into the systemic circulation and subsequently is deposited within various other organs.

The subcortical nervous system is particularly sensitive to the free-ranging excess copper. Approximately 60% of WD patients present with a neurologic disorder (Box 37-1). Often they do not present until young adulthood with a variety of neurologic manifestations, including dysarthria, tremor, dysphagia, bradykinesia, and behavioral disturbance. *Speech manifestations* vary from rapid articulation to hypophonia and dysarthria. Any young adult patient who develops unexplained speech impairment needs to be evaluated for WD.

A *variety of tremors* are seen; these range from subtle in the outstretched fingers to severe, coarse, proximal tremors of the arms and legs that are totally different from those in Parkinson disease (PD). The reduced facial expression, bradykinesia, and tremors are sometimes confused with PD but such of course is only seen with rare exception in the WD age group. Upper extremity coarse tremors are quite common. Typically these adventitious movements are posturally dependent. Such tremors are especially prominent when the arms are elevated and flexed at the elbow, giving the appearance of "wing beating" or "chest beating."

Dystonia, hypertonicity, and choreoathetosis are common symptoms. Tremor and *dystonia* occur with equal frequency and sometimes coexist. The dystonia is more typically generalized, involving the extremities, neck (torticollis), and face (grimacing)

Box 37-1 Clinical Consideration for Diagnosis of Wilson Disease

Primary

Speech impairment that is progressive and unexplained
Extrapyramidal dysfunction that is progressive and unexplained
  1. Tremor of the arm, unusual course, positional, extreme = wing beating etc.
  2. Dystonia
  3. Bradykinesia to rigidity
Psychiatric disturbances of new onset in patients younger than 30 years, especially if associated with dysarthria, extrapyramidal dysfunction, or cognitive impairment
Chronic, unexplained liver disease
Acute hepatitis, especially if prolonged, recurrent, or associated with hemolysis
Siblings of patients with Wilson disease

Secondary

Hemolytic anemia
Fanconi syndrome with aminoaciduria and nephrolithiasis
Arthritis or arthralgias with early onset

---

but may be focal, involving a hand. Ultimately, patients may become severely rigid, with a pseudobulbar palsy. Usually, there is no evidence of cranial nerve, cerebellar, peripheral nerve, or skeletal muscle involvement.

Psychiatric disturbances are the presenting feature in at least a quarter of WD patients. However, there is no characteristic behavioral syndrome. Usually, the progressive change in personality develops in an insidious fashion. Irritability and aggression are typical; affective changes include depression and emotional lability. Cognitive changes, anxiety, catatonia, and psychosis are uncommon. A transient psychosis may be uncovered during treatment.

Ophthalmologic manifestations are not only common in WD but also are often crucial to a specific diagnosis. The classic and best-known finding is the dull, yellow-brown pigment at the limbus of the cornea. These are known as KF rings. They (Fig. 37-1) are most dense at the upper and lower poles of the cornea. These result from copper deposition in the Descemet membrane at the limbus of the cornea. KF rings are present in nearly all patients with WD who present primarily with neurologic or psychiatric symptoms. However, the uninitiated physician must maintain a level of clinical suspicion, or the actual identification of these KF rings may be missed on casual examination. This is particularly noticeable in the majority of patients as brown irises are the most common, providing a means for the copper deposition to inconspicuously blend into the human landscape. It is here that our ophthalmologic colleagues provide a major diagnostic keystone. Slit-lamp examination is often absolutely necessary for detection and verification. Early on KF rings are often absent in the asymptomatic individuals and in up to 50% of persons having a hepatic presentation. Other abnormal ophthalmologic signs include reduced saccadic velocity, interruption of smooth pursuit by saccadic intrusions, and sunflower cataracts (15–20% of patients).

Primary hepatic dysfunction is manifested in the early teens to the early 20s, although it may present in earlier childhood or

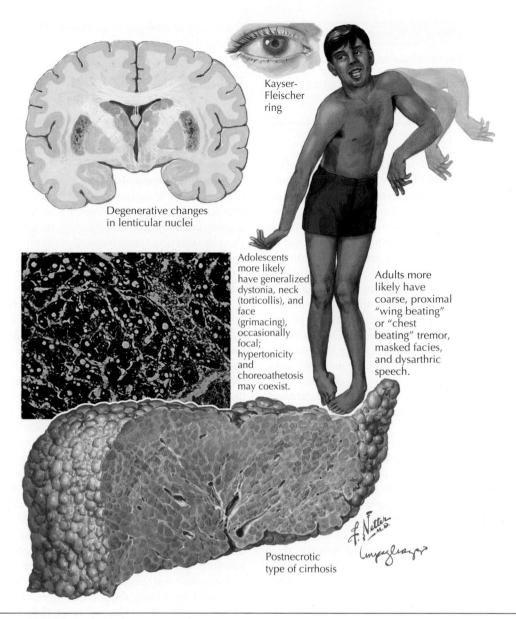

Kayser-Fleischer ring

Degenerative changes in lenticular nuclei

Adolescents more likely have generalized dystonia, neck (torticollis), and face (grimacing), occasionally focal; hypertonicity and choreoathetosis may coexist.

Adults more likely have coarse, proximal "wing beating" or "chest beating" tremor, masked facies, and dysarthric speech.

Postnecrotic type of cirrhosis

Figure 37-1 Wilson Disease.

late adulthood. This is the most common initial manifestation in childhood, with patients presenting at an average age of 10–13 years, a decade or more earlier than those who present with neuropsychiatric disorders. Symptoms of hepatocellular disease vary from a mild increase of serum transaminases in asymptomatic individuals to chronic hepatitis, portal hypertension, and cirrhosis. In earlier-stage disease, the immunohistochemical stains for copper may be negative because hepatocytic copper is diffusely distributed within the cytoplasm. When WD is unrecognized, fibrosis progresses and eventually cirrhosis develops. Rarely, WD patients can present with a fulminant hepatic failure associated with hemolytic anemia secondary to the acute release of copper into the circulation. Liver biopsy at these stages demonstrates a marked necrosis. In these patients, the alkaline phosphatase level is usually low. Hepatocellular carcinoma is a rare complication of WD.

DIAGNOSIS

Early diagnosis of WD is crucial to effective treatment and potential for a cure. This most depends on astute clinical collation in reference to the sometimes vague signs and symptoms (Box 37-1 and Fig. 37-1). This diagnosis should always be considered in patients between 10 and 40 years old who have unexplained dysarthria or tremor or psychiatric or hepatic disease. Devastating neurologic and hepatic deterioration may be prevented with early diagnosis and treatment.

Slit-lamp examination is required for any patient suspected of having WD. Although present in nearly every patient with neurologic involvement, KF rings may be absent in those who primarily present with hepatic involvement. Furthermore KF rings are not pathognomonic for WD. These are rarely seen in other chronic, severe liver diseases, such as primary biliary cirrhosis.

Box 37-2 Laboratory Testing in Wilson Disease

Slit-lamp examination for Kayser–Fleischer rings
Ceruloplasmin plasma levels reduced
24-hour urinary copper increased (in patients not using penicillamine)
Liver biopsy with measurement of liver copper

Ceruloplasmin levels are reduced in patients with WD, often with levels below 20 mg/dL (Box 37-2). A serum ceruloplasmin value less than 20 mg/dL and concomitant slit-lamp definition of a KF ring are diagnostic of WD. In acute liver damage, ceruloplasmin levels may be normal because it is an acute-phase reactant; therefore, a low ceruloplasmin concentration is not an absolute diagnostic test; this may also be seen in hypoproteinemic states.

Daily urinary copper excretion is elevated in WD patients. Its measurement provides a means to monitor the effectiveness of therapy. An elevated non-ceruloplasmin component of plasma copper is increased, filtered by the glomerulus, and incompletely reabsorbed by the renal tubules, causing urinary excretion of copper. The increased renal copper excretion does not adequately compensate for the reduced biliary copper excretion. Measurement of 24-hour copper excretion is a standardized and reliable diagnostic test and is often greater than 100 μg (Box 37-2).

Plasma copper concentration is not a useful or diagnostic laboratory parameter. Total plasma copper (ceruloplasmin bound plus non-ceruloplasmin bound) may be reduced, normal, or increased in WD. However *serum free copper levels* are elevated in WD patients. This is usually greater than 25 μg/dL. Aminotransferase levels of hepatic enzymes are usually mildly or moderately elevated.

Quantitative liver tissue copper concentrations greater than 250 μg/g of liver tissue are found in homozygous WD patients. Although heterozygotes for WD have elevated hepatic liver copper levels, these are not above the gold standard diagnostic level of 250 μg/g. Elevated liver copper levels can also be seen in patients with other causes of liver disease, including primary biliary cirrhosis and primary sclerosing cholangitis. Normal hepatic copper levels can also be found in patients with WD.

MRI is abnormal in most WD patients, mirroring the underlying basal ganglia pathology of both gliosis and neuronal loss with a concomitant significant increase in copper concentration. There are a wide variety of relatively symmetric MRI abnormalities resulting from combinations of edema, necrosis, cystic changes, and gliosis. These typically involve the striatum (caudate and putamen), globus pallidus, thalamus, and midbrain. Fluid-attenuated inversion recovery (FLAIR) pulse with diffusion-weighted imaging (DWI) and T2WI MRI modalities demonstrate hyperintense lesions but these are isointense to hypointense with T1WI. There is a tendency to confuse some of these images with multiple sclerosis (MS); however, WD white matter lesions are usually larger than those seen in MS. Furthermore, WD lesions do not directly come in contact with the ventricular ependymal something that is so common with MS. In general, brain MRI correlates with the presence or absence of neurologic impairment. The changes may improve with chelation therapy.

TREATMENT AND PROGNOSIS

The primary therapeutic goal in WD is to restore hepatic homeostasis by systemic chelation therapy or orthotopic liver transplantation. *Chelation therapies* include D-penicillamine and trientine. These agents bind copper in the plasma and organs, promote urinary copper excretion, and prevent copper accumulation in presymptomatic individuals. This therapeutic regime is indicated for symptomatic WD patients who have either neuropsychiatric or hepatic presentations. Clinical improvement is accompanied by marked decrease in hepatic copper content, thereby reversing symptoms and preventing progression of liver disease. KF rings will disappear with either medical or surgical treatment. If the rings return, it suggests noncompliance to medical therapy.

Penicillamine has multiple side effects, including fever, skin rash, thrombocytopenia, nephrotic syndrome, recurrent nephrolithiasis, and acute arthritis seen in up to 20% of patients. Late immune complex–mediated nephropathy, systemic lupus erythematosus, Goodpasture syndrome, oral ulcers, pseudoxanthoma, and autoimmune-mediated myasthenia gravis (MG) may develop.

The most significant adverse effect of penicillamine treatment is the paradoxical worsening or new appearance of neurologic deficits. Estimated to occur in up to 50% of patients, the mechanism is thought to be deposition of mobilized liver copper within the basal ganglia. After 4–6 months of treatment, lower doses are effective for maintenance therapy.

Triethylamine tetramine (trientine) is effective for treating penicillamine-intolerant patients and is also approved for initial, first-line WD therapy. Although less toxic, triethylamine tetramine also has a significant toxicity spectrum including autoimmune MG as well and requires similar monitoring.

Compliance to penicillamine and trientine is best monitored by recording urinary copper excretion. During the early phase of therapy, this should exceed more than 1000 μg/day. Eventually this decreases to 250–500 μg/day even with continuous use of chelation therapy after 4–6 months. Levels less than 250 μg/day suggest noncompliance with therapy.

Zinc salts are also used as an alternative to penicillamine or trientine-intolerant WD patients, as well as for safe and effective maintenance therapy. Zinc salts block intestinal absorption of dietary copper and also stimulate endogenous production of chelators in the liver. These often have a delayed onset of action; therefore, chelation therapy is preferred. Twenty-four-hour urinary copper excretion of patients taking zinc is not typically elevated because zinc prevents the intestinal absorption of copper rather than an increase in urinary copper excretion. Elevated urinary copper levels in these patients suggest noncompliance.

Orthotopic liver transplantation now provides another important treatment option for WD patients, particularly when they are compromised by significant cirrhosis or fulminant liver failure. After liver transplantation, there is no need to continue long-term therapy because the diseased liver (and therefore abnormal copper-transporting protein within the liver) is removed and replaced with a healthy liver. Transplantation may reduce neurologic symptoms in some patients.

Prognosis for compliant patients with WD is excellent, even if cirrhosis is present at time of initiating therapy. Rapid progressive liver failure due to WD carries a poor prognosis, unless liver transplantation is performed. Neurologic and psychiatric impairment are preventable if therapy is instituted in the early stages of disease. Therefore, early diagnostic recognition of WD is a very important challenge to every neurologic, psychiatric, or gastroenterologic physician. Not all patients improve to the same extent, and death may occur from neurologic (e.g., dysphagia) or hepatic complications.

ADDITIONAL RESOURCES

Ala A, Walker AP, Ashkan K, et al. Wilson's disease. Lancet 2007;369:397-408. *Excellent overview.*

Glazebrook AJ. Wilson's disease. Edinb Med J 1945;52:83-87. *Another historical milestone.*

Merle U, Schaefer M, Ferenci P, et al. Outcome of Wilson's disease: a cohort study Clinical presentation, diagnosis and long-term outlook. Gut 2007;56;115-120; *An overview.*

Pabón V, Dumortier J, Gincul R, et al. Long-term results of liver transplantation for Wilson's disease. Gastroenterol Clin Biol 2008 Apr;32(4): 378-381.

Pfeiffer RF. Wilson's Disease. Semin Neurol 2007 Apr;27(2):123-132. *A state-of-the-art neurologic review.*

Scheinberg IH, Gitlin D. Deficiency of ceruloplasmin in patients with hepatolenticular degeneration (Wilson's disease). Science 1952;116: 484.

Scheinberg IH, Jaffe ME, Sternlieb I. The use of trientine in preventing the effects of interrupting penicillamine therapy in Wilson's disease. N Engl J Med 1987;317:209-213.

Sinha S, Taly AB, Ravishankar S, et al. Wilson's disease: cranial MRI observations and clinical correlation. Neuroradiology 2006;48:613-621.

Steindl P, Ferenci P, Dienes HP, et al. Wilson's disease in patients presenting with liver disease—a diagnostic challenge. Gastroenterology 1997;113: 212.

Walshe JM. Wilson's disease; new oral therapy. Lancet 1956;267(6906): 25-26.

Wilson SAK. Progressive lenticular degeneration: a familial nervous disease associated with cirrhosis of the liver. Brain 1912;34:20-509. *The classic clinical definition.*

Myoclonus

Diana Apetauerova

38

Clinical Vignette

A 73-year-old right-handed man with history of coronary artery disease, myocardial infarction, peripheral vascular disease, and hypertension presented with cardiac arrest followed by resuscitation with subsequent development of anoxic brain injury. He was seen by a neurologist in the intensive care unit (ICU) setting 1 week after cardiac arrest. His family was very concerned about constant "jerkiness" of his body. Those movements seemed to worsen when people were touching the patient, which affected all four extremities as well as his trunk. He appeared very uncomfortable because of these jerks.

Neurologic examination demonstrated an elderly man who was intubated without any sedation. He was restless, inconsistently able to open his eyes to verbal commands, and followed very simple yes-and-no questions. His examination was notable for multiple, irregular, large-amplitude, brief shocklike jerks of the trunk, arms, and legs. These movements occurred randomly and many of them were stimulus sensitive. His magnetic resonance image (MRI) was unremarkable and electroencephalography (EEG) showed multifocal spike discharges. A diagnosis of postanoxic generalized myoclonus (Lance–Adams syndrome) was made and the patient was started on sodium valproate, which significantly diminished those movements.

M yoclonus is characterized by sudden, abrupt, brief, involuntary, jerk-like contractions of a single muscle or muscle group. They are related to involuntary muscle contractions (positive myoclonus) or sudden inhibition of voluntary muscular contraction, with lapses of sustained posture (negative myoclonus or asterixis). Myoclonus may affect any bodily region, multiple bodily regions, or the entire body, interfering with normal movements and posture.

There are various classifications of myoclonus; these include (1) etiology (Table 38-1), (2) affected body region (focal, segmental, multifocal, or generalized forms), (3) the presence or absence of specific provocative factors, and (4) specific site of nervous system origin of the abnormal neuronal discharges (Table 38-2). Spontaneous myoclonus has no clinically identifiable mechanism. Reflex myoclonus occurs in response to specific external sensory stimuli. Voluntary movement or attempts to perform specific movements induce action or intention myoclonus.

A neurophysiologic classification links the myoclonus to the anatomic origin for the abnormal neuronal discharge within the central nervous system (CNS). Cortical myoclonus arises from the cerebral cortex and is considered epileptic, often being associated with other seizure types. Subcortical myoclonus usually arises from the brainstem. Spinal myoclonus originates within the spinal cord. Clinically, differentiation is often impossible, but electromyography may help.

Another classification, based on etiology, categorizes myoclonus into physiologic or pathologic forms. Common examples of "normal," nonpathologic, physiologic myoclonus include hiccups or "sleep starts" occurring as one drifts into sleep. In pathologic myoclonus, the brief muscle jerks may occur infrequently or repeatedly. Examples include essential myoclonus, myoclonic epilepsy, and secondary myoclonus. Postanoxic encephalopathy and spongiform encephalopathy, that is, Creutzfeldt–Jakob disease, are the best-known examples of pathologic myoclonus. Additional rare forms include (1) palatal myoclonus, (2) periodic limb movements of sleep, and (3) psychogenic myoclonus. Although pathologic myoclonus is always a sign of CNS dysfunction, its pathophysiologic mechanism often remains enigmatic. Myoclonus may be an important clinical indicator in determining the proper diagnosis. It is also sometimes a nonspecific feature within more widespread neurologic abnormalities.

PATHOPHYSIOLOGY

The pathophysiologic mechanism leading to myoclonus is not well understood, thus complicating anatomic correlation. Cortical myoclonus is possibly a disorder of decreased cortical inhibition, although the reason for the reduced inhibition is unknown. Its frequent association with seizure disorders suggests a common pathophysiologic mechanism for myoclonus and some forms of epilepsy. Mechanisms for subcortical and spinal myoclonus are even less well appreciated.

CLINICAL PRESENTATION

Physiologic Nonpathologic Myoclonus

Shocklike contractions of the arms or legs during sleep or as individuals drift off to sleep are a common form of physiologic myoclonus, sometimes described as *physiologic sleep myoclonus*.

Pathologic Myoclonus

It is essential to distinguish the various forms of presumed pathologic myoclonus (Table 38-1).

Essential myoclonus is an isolated neurologic finding that has no association with seizures, dementia, or ataxia. It is nonprogressive, usually multifocal in distribution, typically induced by voluntary movements (action myoclonus), and usually responds to alcohol (Fig. 38-1).

Although often familial, essential myoclonus can occur sporadically. Familial essential myoclonus appears to be an autosomal dominant trait with reduced penetrance and variable expressivity. Symptoms typically begin before the age of 20 years. Essential myoclonus often occurs in association with other movement disorders, particularly tremor and dystonia.

Table 38-1 Etiologies of Pathologic Myoclonus

Type of Myoclonus	Etiologies
Essential	Autosomal dominant trait with reduced penetrance and variable expressivity
Myoclonic epilepsy	Juvenile myoclonic epilepsy, benign myoclonus of infancy
Secondary	Brain trauma, infection, inflammation (encephalitis, Creutzfeldt–Jakob disease), tumors (neoplasms), or cerebral hypoxia due to temporary lack of oxygen (i.e., posthypoxic myoclonus or Lance–Adams syndrome)
Spinal	Spinal cord trauma, infection, inflammation, or lesions may produce segmental myoclonus
Inborn biochemical errors	Inborn errors of metabolism (lysosomal storage diseases: Tay–Sachs disease, Sandhoff disease, sialidosis)
Infectious	Creutzfeldt–Jakob disease
	Subacute sclerosing panencephalitis (SSPE)
	Whipple disease (facial myoclonus—oculofacial masticatory monorhythmia)
Neuroimmunologic	Stiffman variant: Encephalomyelitis with rigidity
Neurodegenerative	Parkinsonism, Huntington disease, Alzheimer disease, Lafora disease, corticobasal degeneration, progressive supranuclear palsy, or olivopontocerebellar atrophy
Metabolic	Metabolic conditions, such as kidney, liver, or respiratory failure, hypokalemia, hyperglycemia, etc.
Mitochondrial	Mitochondrial encephalomyopathy, particularly MERFF syndrome (myoclonus epilepsy with ragged-red fibers), or other progressive myoclonic encephalopathies, including those characterized by epilepsy and dementia (e.g., Lafora disease) or epilepsy and ataxia (e.g., Unverricht–Lundborg disease)
Medications: Drug-induced myoclonus	Serotonin receptor inhibitors: serotonin syndrome; toxic levels of anticonvulsants, levodopa, and certain antipsychotic agents (tardive myoclonus)
Toxins	Exposure to toxic agents, such as bismuth or other metals

Table 38-2 Classification of Myoclonus

Classification Bases	Classifications
Affected body part	Focal
	Segmental
	Multifocal
	Generalized
Provoking symptom	Spontaneous
	Reflex
	Action
Neurophysiology	Cortical
	Subcortical
	Spinal
Etiology	Physiological
	Essential
	Myoclonic epilepsy
	Secondary
Additional forms	Palatal myoclonus
	Periodic limb movements of sleep
	Psychogenic myoclonus

Various forms of epilepsy may be accompanied by myoclonus. For example, in forms of idiopathic epilepsy, such as juvenile myoclonic epilepsy and benign myoclonus of infancy, myoclonus may be a primary finding.

Any underlying disease process or cause of CNS dysfunction may lead to secondary myoclonus (Fig. 38-1).

Additional Forms of Myoclonus

Palatal myoclonus has rapid, rhythmic jerking of muscle of one or both sides of the soft palate. It is more appropriately classified as a form of tremor despite continued use of the term *palatal myoclonus*.

Periodic limb movements of sleep differ from physiologic sleep myoclonus in that they typically consist of repeated, stereotypic, upward extension of the great toe and foot, possibly followed by flexion of the hip, knee, or ankle. These usually involve both legs, tend to occur in repeated episodes lasting a few minutes to several hours, and occur during non-REM sleep. An association with restless legs syndrome is common.

In psychogenic myoclonus, symptoms have a mental or emotional basis rather than an organic origin. In most patients, the condition worsens with stress or anxiety. The myoclonus can be segmental or generalized.

DIFFERENTIAL DIAGNOSIS

Myoclonus must be differentiated from other movement disorders, including tics, tremors, ataxia, and chorea. When the jerks are single or repetitive but arrhythmic, a tic diagnosis should be considered. A history of an urge associated with tics is helpful in the diagnosis. In contrast, organic myoclonus is usually briefer and less coordinated or patterned than tics.

Rhythmic forms of myoclonus may be confused with tremors. The pattern of myoclonus is more repetitive, abrupt-onset, square-wave movements, unlike the smoother sinusoidal activity of tremor. Rhythmic myoclonus usually ranges from 1 to 4 Hz, differing from faster tremor frequencies.

Myoclonus, particularly action (intention) myoclonus, is often confused with cerebellar ataxia. Myoclonic jerking occurs during voluntary motor activity, especially when patients attempt to perform a fine motor task, such as reaching for a target.

DIAGNOSTIC EVALUATION

A diagnosis of myoclonus is based on a thorough clinical assessment, evaluation of the nature of the myoclonus (e.g.,

Essential Myoclonus

Usually multifocal in distribution, often familial, typically induced by voluntary movements causing a single jerk of the extremity (action myoclonus). Symptoms begin before age 20 and frequently occur associated with tremor, dystonia, and other movement disorders.

Commonly, essential myoclonus responds to ingestion of alcohol.

Lance-Adams Syndrome

Prolonged hypoxia may result in posthypoxic myoclonus, which is usually stimulus sensitive.

A variety of stimuli such as noise, light, and touch can provoke this type of myoclonus in multiple areas of the body.

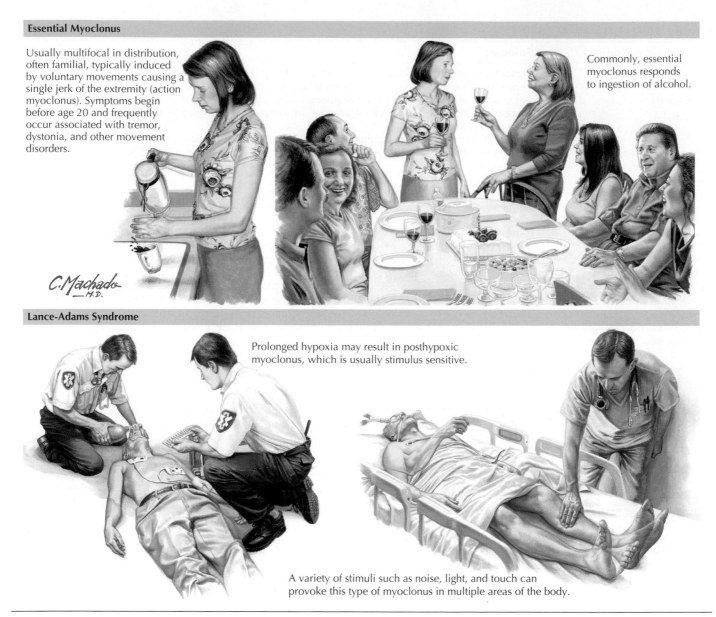

Figure 38-1 Myoclonus (Essential and Posthypoxic).

electrophysiologic characteristics), bodily distribution, provocative factors, and a careful family history. Examination and observation of patients with myoclonus are important diagnostic steps. However, patients with myoclonus can have entirely normal examination results, particularly with physiologic and essential myoclonus. When myoclonus is present during examination, characterization of its rhythm, repetitiveness, onset, and frequency is important. Because myoclonus may occur with other movement disorders, it is important to look for evidence of dystonia, tremor, ataxia, or spasticity.

The clinical distribution of the myoclonus is also helpful. Focal myoclonus is more commonly associated with CNS lesions. Segmental involvement may suggest brainstem or spinal cord lesions. Multifocal or generalized myoclonus suggests a more diffuse disorder, as seen in diffuse postanoxic insults. This particularly involves the reticular substance of the brainstem. Precipitating factors are important for stimulus-sensitive

myoclonus. Therefore, somesthetic sensory input testing is needed. It is important to determine whether the myoclonus occurs spontaneously and whether symptoms improve or worsen with voluntary activity.

During testing for negative myoclonus (asterixis), patients are asked to extend their arms with the wrists back or to perform another movement that requires holding the limb against gravity. In this way, a sudden loss of muscle contraction causes the hand or the arm to fall downward.

Specialized testing can be used to determine the site of the abnormal neuronal discharge within the CNS (e.g., cerebral cortex, brainstem, or spinal cord) and establish the underlying cause. These studies typically primarily include EEG, and less commonly electromyography, or somatosensory evoked potential testing. Neuroimaging studies such as MRI or computed tomography can on rare occasions demonstrate structural lesions. Other specialized diagnostic tests may help to exclude particular conditions such as hereditary, metabolic, mitochondrial, infectious, vascular, neoplastic, toxic, or neurodegenerative processes.

TREATMENT AND PROGNOSIS

The treatment of myoclonus varies depending on the type. If a specific cause is found, myoclonus usually resolves with effective treatment of the underlying disease. A good example is juvenile myoclonic epilepsy. This usually responds to valproate and may require lifelong treatment. Less specific symptomatic therapy typically includes medications to reduce the severity of the myoclonus, such as benzodiazepines. Cortical myoclonus may respond to valproate, piracetam, levetiracetam, or lamotrigine. Myoclonus from a hypoxic event may respond to 5-hydroxytryptophan, and this may help in other causes. Carbamazepine may worsen myoclonus and should be avoided.

Prognosis depends on the form of myoclonus. Generally, although myoclonus is not a life-threatening condition, it may be secondary to serious, debilitating fatal diseases such as individuals with Creutzfeldt–Jakob disease. Postanoxic myoclonus is another disorder that is associated with an extremely poor prognosis in the post–cardiac arrest individual.

Researchers are attempting to clarify the genetic and molecular aspects of myoclonus. Newer physiologic techniques, such as magnetoencephalography, are being used to study cortical activity in cortical reflex myoclonus.

ADDITIONAL RESOURCES

Caviness JN. Myoclonus. Parkinsonism & related disorders 2007;13(Suppl. 3):S375-S384.

Gordon MF. Toxin and drug-induced myoclonus. Adv Neurol 2002;89:49-76.

Hallet M. Neurophysiology of brainstem myoclonus. Adv Neurol 2002;89:99-102.

Obeso JA. Therapy of myoclonus. Clin Neurosci 1995-1996;3:253-257.

Rubboli G, Tassinari CA. Negative Myoclonus. An overview of its clinical features, pathophysiological mechanism, and management. Nerurophysiol Clin 2006 Sep-Dec;36(5-6):337-343. Epub 2007 Jan 23.

Shafiq M, Lang AE. Myoclonus in parkinsonian disorders. Adv Neurol 2002;89:77-83.

Watts RL, Koller WC, editors. Movement Disorders: Neurologic Principles and Practice. New York, NY: McGraw-Hill Companies, Inc; 1997.

Tic Disorders

39

Julie Leegwater-Kim

Clinical Vignette

A 12-year-old boy presented to the neurology clinic with approximately 1 year of excessive eye blinking. He was accompanied by his parents. He was a full-term infant and reached all developmental milestones appropriately. School-work has been average; he frequently loses pencils and articles of clothing. He also has difficulty finishing his home-work. During the past year, his parents have noted increased frequency of eye blinking. The patient is aware of the blink-ing and has been told by his classmates that he "squints" and "makes funny faces." He is embarrassed by the move-ments. His neurologic exam was notable for eye blinking, sniffing, nose wrinkling, and contraction of the platysma. He was able to suppress the movements volitionally. He was prescribed clonidine. After 8 weeks, he returned to the office with his parents. He reported lessening of his tics. His parents felt he was performing better at school.

PHENOMENOLOGY AND CLASSIFICATION

Tics are sudden, relatively quick, stereotyped movements (motor tics) or sounds (phonic tics) which are repeated at irregular intervals. Tics are often preceded by a premonitory urge or inner sensory stimulus, and can be suppressed at will. They are, therefore, referred to as semivoluntary, or unvoluntary, movements.

Tics are categorized as simple or complex (Box 39-1). Simple motor tics involve only one group of muscles and are character-ized by quick, jerk-like movements. Usually they are abrupt in onset and brief (*clonic tics*) but they can also be slower and sustained (*dystonic tics*). Examples of *simple motor tics* include eye blinking, nose twitching, and shoulder shrugging. Simple phonic tics include sniffing, throat clearing, and grunting. *Complex motor tics* are sequenced and coordinated movements that can resemble gestures or fragments of normal behavior, e.g., kicking, jumping, and, rarely, inappropriate behavior, e.g., showing the middle finger. Complex phonic tics have a semantic basis, including words, parts of words, and obscene words (coprolalia).

It is important to distinguish tics from other hyperkinetic movement disorders. For example, simple motor tics can resem-ble myoclonus. However, clonic tics are stereotyped, rather than random, are suppressible, and are typically accompanied by a premonitory sensation.

The most common tic disorder is *Tourette syndrome* (TS), which is characterized by motor and phonic tics. The Tourette Syndrome Classification Study Group has formulated diag-nostic criteria for TS that include the presence of both motor and phonic tics, though not necessarily concurrently; the presence of tics for at least 1 year; fluctuation in tic type, fre-quency, and severity; and onset before age 21 years. Tics of duration less than a year are classified as *transient tic disorder*. When only one category of chronic tics can be identified, the terms *chronic motor tic disorder* or *chronic vocal tic disorder* are used.

CAUSES OF TIC DISORDERS

Tic disorders can be primary or secondary (Box 39-2). Primary tic disorders are discussed in the previous section and include transient tic disorder, chronic motor tic disorder, chronic vocal tic disorder, and Tourette syndrome. Less commonly, tics can be secondary to other causes, including neurodegenerative ill-nesses (i.e., Huntington disease, neuroacanthocytosis), infection (i.e., viral encephalitis), global developmental syndromes (i.e., static encephalopathy, autism spectrum disorders), and drugs (i.e., amphetamines, lamotrigine). Secondary causes should always be considered in adult-onset tic disorders.

The pathogenesis of tic disorders is unknown but biochemi-cal, neuroimaging, and genetic data suggest an abnormality in the cortico-striato-thalamo-cortical circuits and their neu-rotransmitter systems. One hypothesis suggests that there is disinhibition of excitatory neurons in the thalamus resulting in hyperexcitability of the cortical motor areas. Dysfunction of dopamine neurotransmission has been implicated, with recent evidence suggesting excessive dopaminergic activity via abnormal presynaptic terminal function, dopamine hyperinner-vation, and/or dopamine receptor supersensitivity.

CLINICAL COURSE AND NATURAL HISTORY OF TOURETTE SYNDROME

In TS, symptoms typically begin in childhood, usually by age 7 years. Early in the course, tics frequently involve the face, head, and neck (Fig. 39-1). Vocal tics tend to start later (ages 8–15 years). The frequency and severity of tics fluctuate over time, with peak severity occurring at about 10 years of age. The anatomic locations and complexity of tics also tend to change over time. The vast majority of TS patients (85%) experience reduction in tics during and after adolescence. Tics can be exacerbated by stress, fatigue, CNS stimulants, and caffeine. Alleviation of tics can occur with focused mental and physical exercise, relaxation, and exposure to nicotine and cannabinoids.

Tic disorders are frequently associated with a wide range of neuropsychiatric disorders. Approximately 50% of patients with TS have obsessive–compulsive disorder (OCD), and 50% exhibit attention deficit hyperactivity disorder (ADHD). In addition, affective disorders, impulse control disorders, anxiety, and rage attacks can be seen in patients with TS.

THERAPIES

There are both nonpharmacologic and pharmacologic treatments for tics. It is important to recognize that the mere presence of tics does not necessarily imply a need to initiate pharmacologic treatment. One initially needs to determine the degree to which tics are interfering with functioning at school, at work, or at home and any disability associated with tics. In addition, comorbidities such as ADHD, OCD, and mood disorders need to be assessed. If tics are mild, educational and psychosocial interventions can be implemented for treatment of tics. If tics are more severe and disabling, medication treatment should be considered (Box 39-3).

The *alpha agonists* clonidine and guanfacine have moderate efficacy in treating tic disorders and are often considered as *first-line treatments* because of their relatively low side effect burden. In addition, they can be effective in treating concomitant ADHD.

Box 39-1 Tic Types—Examples

Simple Motor

Eye blinking
Nose twitching
Head jerking
Shoulder shrugging
Tensing of abdominal muscles

Simple Vocal

Sniffing
Grunting
Throat clearing
Screaming

Complex Motor

Touching
Throwing
Hitting
Jumping
Obscene gestures (copropraxia)

Complex Vocal

Repetition of words
Repetition of obscenities (coprolalia)
Repetition of parts of words (palilalia)
Repetition of another person's words (echolalia)

Box 39-2 Tic Disorders—Causes

Primary

Transient tic disorder
Chronic motor or vocal tic disorder
Tourette syndrome

Secondary

Infection
• Encephalitis
Neurodegenerative
• Pantothenate kinase–associated neurodegeneration
• Huntington disease
• Wilson disease
• Neuroacanthocytosis
Autoimmune
• Sydenham chorea
• Antiphospholipid antibody syndrome
Drug-induced
• Side effect: lamotrigine, carbamazepine, methylphenidate, cocaine
• Tardive syndrome: typical and atypical neuroleptics
Toxins
• Carbon monoxide
Developmental
• Mental retardation
• Autism spectrum disorders

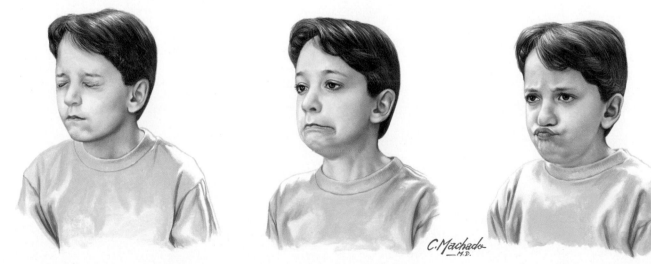

Tics involving the eyes, i.e., eye-blinking, are the most common tics in childhood-onset tic disorders. Patients with tic disorders frequently develop other motor tics of the head and neck, including grimacing and frowning.

Figure 39-1 Common Motor Tics.

Box 39-3 Pharmacologic Treatment for Tics

Alpha agonists: clonidine, guanfacine
Neuroleptics
  Atypical neuroleptics: risperidone, olanzapine, aripiprazole
  Typical neuroleptics: pimozide, haloperidol, fluphenazine
Benzodiazepine: clonazepam
Dopamine depletor: tetrabenazine
Dopamine agonists: pergolide, ropinirole
Botulinum toxin injections

Box 39-4 Proposed Criteria for Identification of Tourette Syndrome Candidates for Deep Brain Stimulation

Inclusion Criteria

- Age >25 years
- Chronic and severe tic disorder with severe functional impairment
- Failure of conventional medical therapy for tics
- Trial of behavioral treatment, if suitable
- Optimization of treatment of comorbid medical, neurologic and psychiatric disorders for >6 months
- Active involvement and compliance with psychological interventions to address psychosocial problems for >6 months

Exclusion Criteria

- Secondary tic disorder
- Severe medical, neurologic, psychiatric, or cognitive disorders
- Significant psychosocial factors that increase the risk of the procedure or complicate recovery period
- Unwillingness to be involved in ongoing treatment for psychosocial problems

---

Dopamine receptor–blocking drugs are the most potent drugs for treatment of tics. These drugs include both typical (haloperidol, fluphenazine, pimozide) and atypical (risperidone, olanzapine) neuroleptics. Although these drugs are often highly effective, they can cause numerous side effects, including sedation, weight gain, metabolic syndrome, and tardive dyskinesia. The atypical neuroleptics quetiapine and clozapine are associated with low risk of tardive syndrome but they tend to be less effective in treating tics.

Tetrabenazine, a *dopamine-depleting* agent, has also shown efficacy in treatment of tics. Common side effects include depression, apathy, parkinsonism, and sedation.

Other agents that have tic-suppressing effects include clonazepam, dopamine agonists (low-dose ropinirole and pergolide), and levetiracetam.

Botulinum toxin can be considered for simple motor tics, especially dystonic tics. Many patients who have had botulinum toxin treatment for tics report decrease in premonitory urges to tic.

The role of *deep brain stimulation* (DBS) in the treatment of tic disorders is being studied as a possible treatment for severe, disabling, medication-refractory tic disorders. A number of different anatomic locations are targeted, including the medial portion of the thalamus, the globus pallidus internus, the nucleus accumbens, and the anterior limb of the internal capsule. Inclusion and exclusion criteria to determine suitable TS candidates for DBS have been devised and are listed in Box 39-4. Further controlled trials of DBS in TS will need to be done to confirm the efficacy of DBS in TS and the optimal surgical target.

ADDITIONAL RESOURCES

Ackermans L, Temel Y, Visser-Vandewalle V. Deep brain stimulation in Tourette syndrome. Neurotherapeutics 2008;5:339-344.

Rampello L, Alvano A, Battaglia G, et al. Tic disorders: from pathophysiology to treatment. J Neurol 2006;253:1-15.

Shprecher D, Kurlan R. The management of tics. Mov Disord 2009; 24:15-24.

Clinical Vignette

A 22-year-old previously healthy woman developed slurred speech, difficulty walking, and hand tremors over the course of 1 month after a severe psychological trauma. She had mild neck pain and took cyclobenzaprine without benefit. She denied history of fever, head trauma, or exposure to dopamine receptor–blocking agents. There was no family history of neurologic disease. Exam revealed lower facial dystonia, including risus sardonicus and tongue dystonia, dysarthria, bradykinesia, mild cogwheel rigidity, mild rest and kinetic tremor, dystonic gait, and loss of postural reflexes. After several weeks, her symptoms plateaued. Trial of carbidopa/levodopa was ineffective. She reported slight benefit on high doses of trihexyphenidyl.

Workup included blood glucose, creatinine, electrolytes, complete blood count, liver function tests, thyroid-stimulating hormone, erythrocyte sedimentation rate, antinuclear antibodies test, vitamin B_{12}, ceruloplasmin, and 24-hour urine copper, all of which were within normal limits. Slit-lamp exam was negative for Kayser–Fleischer rings. Spinocerebellar ataxia genetic testing was negative. Brain magnetic resonance imaging was unremarkable. Electroencephalography and electromyography were unremarkable. ATP1A3 genetic sequencing revealed a mutation.

Dystonia is a hyperkinetic movement disorder characterized by involuntary, sustained muscle contractions that frequently cause twisting and repetitive movements or abnormal postures. Dystonic movements are patterned, meaning they repeatedly involve the same group of muscles. There is simultaneous contraction of agonist and antagonist muscles. In general, the duration of dystonic muscle contractions is longer than other hyperkinesias (i.e., chorea), though sometimes the movements can be rapid enough to resemble repetitive myoclonic jerking. One of the characteristic features of dystonia is that it is often temporarily diminished by tactile sensory tricks (gestes antagonistes). For example, a patient with cervical dystonia may be able to reduce dystonic movements by placing a hand on the chin or the side of the face. Patients with orobuccolingual dystonia often experience improvement by touching the lips or placing an object, such as a toothpick, in the mouth. In some patients, simply thinking about performing the sensory trick diminishes dystonia. The efficacy of sensory tricks can be exploited in the development of therapies. For example, some patients with lower cranial dystonia may benefit from wearing a mouthguard.

The initial presentation of dystonia is usually focal (affecting one body part) and task-specific—the dystonia occurs with a particular action. For example, a subject with foot dystonia may initially note dystonia when walking forward, but not walking backward or running. In the majority of patients, the dystonia remains focal without spreading to other parts of the body. If dystonia spreads, it tends to involve contiguous body parts and becomes a segmental dystonia. In more severe cases, the dystonia can become generalized. As a rule, the younger the age at onset, the more likely the dystonia is to spread. Recent data have also suggested that in the primary dystonias there is a caudal-to-rostral anatomic gradient in the site of onset as a function of age.

As dystonia progresses, it emerges with other actions of the affected body part, therefore becoming less task-specific. For example, the patient with foot dystonia may experience it when walking forwards and backwards, running, or tapping the foot. Further progression can lead to "overflow dystonia," in which movement of a distant body part elicits the dystonia. As dystonia worsens, it can occur at rest. In the most severe cases of dystonia, contractures may develop.

Dystonia is frequently worsened by fatigue and stress and diminished with relaxation and sleep. Pain is generally uncommon in dystonia except for cervical dystonia, in which ~75% of patients report pain.

CLASSIFICATION OF DYSTONIA

There are several recognized classification schemes for dystonia: (1) age at onset, (2) anatomic distribution, and (3) etiology.

Age at Onset

Early-onset dystonia is defined as dystonia developing at or before the age of 26 years and late onset is defined as dystonia developing after age 26 years. Age at onset is an important factor determining prognosis in patients with dystonia, with earlier age at onset correlating with increased likelihood of spread of dystonia to other body parts. In general, young-onset dystonia tends to begin in a limb and become generalized whereas adult-onset dystonia tends to be craniocervical and remain focal or become segmental.

Anatomic Distribution

The topographic characteristics of dystonia are useful in defining the severity of the dystonia and guiding treatment. Focal dystonia affects a single body part. Virtually any part of the body can be involved in dystonia and many types of focal dystonia have specific names: blepharospasm (dystonic eye closure), spasmodic torticollis (rotational cervical dystonia), and writer's cramp (focal hand dystonia). When dystonia involves two or more contiguous body parts/regions, it is referred to as segmental dystonia. Multifocal dystonia refers to the involvement of two or more noncontiguous body parts. Generalized dystonia represents a combination of crural dystonia (one or both legs plus trunk) and any other area of the body. In hemidystonia, as its name implies, dystonia affects one half of the body. Hemidystonia suggests a symptomatic (secondary), rather than primary, dystonia.

Etiology

The growth in our understanding of the genetics of dystonia has contributed significantly to the etiologic classification of dystonia. There are essentially two broad categories: primary and secondary.

PRIMARY DYSTONIA

Primary dystonias are characterized by pure dystonia (with the exception that tremor can be present) and they may be sporadic or familial. Most primary dystonias are sporadic with onset in adulthood and a focal or segmental presentation. The most common focal dystonia presenting to movement disorders clinics is cervical dystonia (Fig. 40-1). After cervical dystonia, the most common focal dystonias are blepharospasm, spasmodic dysphonia, oromandibular dystonia, and hand dystonia.

A minority of primary dystonias have an identified genetic etiology (Box 40-1). Perhaps the best studied of the primary dystonias is DYT1 dystonia, or Oppenheim's dystonia, a generalized torsion dystonia that usually begins in childhood affecting the limbs first. DYT1 dystonia is caused by a deletion in the DYT1 gene, which encodes for the *torsin A* protein. The disease

is inherited in an autosomal dominant fashion and has 30–40% penetrance. Phenotype can vary widely within an affected family. The DYT1 mutation is estimated to account for 90% of limbonset dystonia cases in the Ashkenazi Jewish population and 50–70% of cases in the non-Jewish population. A number of

---

Box 40-1 Dystonia Classification Schemes

- Age at Onset
  - Young-onset: ≤26
  - Late-onset: >26
- Anatomic Distribution
  - Focal—single body part
  - Segmental—two or more contiguous body parts
  - Multifocal—two or more noncontiguous body parts
  - Generalized—segmental crural dystonia plus one other body part
  - Hemidystonia—dystonia affecting one half of the body
- Etiologic
  - Primary (Idiopathic)
    - Familial
    - Sporadic
  - Secondary Dystonia
    - Heredodegenerative
    - Degenerative—sporadic
    - Dystonia-plus syndromes (inherited nondegenerative)
    - Drug-induced
    - Injury/trauma
    - Structural lesions
    - Psychogenic

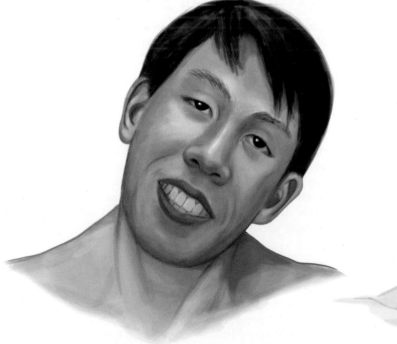

Young man with muscular torticollis. Head tilted to left with chin turned slightly to right because of contracture of left sternocleidomastoid muscle.

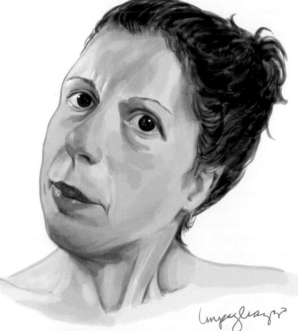

Untreated torticollis in middle-aged woman. Thick, fibrotic, tendon-like bands have replaced sternocleidomastoid muscle, making head appear tethered to clavicle. Two heads of left sternocleidomastoid muscle are prominent.

Figure 40-1 Cervical Dystonia.

Table 40-1 Genetic Dystonias

Dystonia	Etiologic type	Inheritance	Clinical Features	Chromosome Gene
DYT1	Primary	Autosomal dominant	Early onset (age <40 years) Limbs affected first	9q34 Torsin A
DYT2		Autosomal recessive	Early onset	Not mapped
DYT3	Secondary	X-linked recessive	Dystonia/parkinsonism (Lubag)	Xq13.1
DYT4		Autosomal dominant	Whispering dysphonia	Not mapped
DYT5	Secondary (dystonia-plus)	Autosomal dominant	Dopa-responsive dystonia (DRD) parkinsonism	14q22.1 GCH1
DYT6	Primary	Autosomal dominant	Childhood and adult onset Cranial and upper limb	8p
DYT7	Primary	Autosomal dominant	Adult onset Cervical dystonia	18p
DYT8		Autosomal dominant	Paroxysmal nonkinesigenic dyskinesia (PNKD)	2q33-35
DYT9		Autosomal dominant	Episodic chorea/ataxia spasticity	1p21
DYT10		Autosomal dominant	Paroxysmal kinesigenic choreoathetosis (PLD)	16
DYT11	Secondary (dystonia-plus)	Autosomal dominant	Myoclonus–dystonia (MD)	7q21 e-sarcoglycan 18p11
DYT12	Secondary (dystonia-plus)	Autosomal dominant	Rapid-onset dystonia–parkinsonism (RPD)	19q Na+/K+-ATPase
DYT13	Primary	Autosomal dominant	Adult onset Cervical–cranial dystonia	1p36.13-p36.32
DYT14		Autosomal dominant	DOPA-responsive dystonia (DRD)	14q13

other primary dystonias (DYT6, DYT7 and DYT13) have had their genetic loci mapped (Table 40-1).

SECONDARY DYSTONIA

Secondary dystonia encompasses a broad clinical category that includes inherited degenerative disorders, degenerative disorders of unknown etiology, acquired dystonias (i.e., drug-induced, structural lesions, trauma), and psychogenic dystonia. Patients with secondary dystonia frequently display associated clinical abnormalities including other movement disorders besides tremor (i.e., parkinsonism), dementia, spasticity, ataxia, weakness, reflex changes, eye movement abnormalities, or seizures. Other historical and clinical features that suggest secondary dystonia include history of trauma, perinatal anoxia, toxin or drug exposure, onset of dystonia at rest, and hemidystonia.

A number of heredodegenerative disorders may present with dystonia. **Autosomal dominant disorders** (Huntington disease, spinocerebellar ataxia type 3, neuroferritonopathy), autosomal recessive disorders (Wilson disease, pantothenate-kinase associated degeneration), X-linked recessive disorders (DYT3 or Lubag), and mitochondrial disorders (Leigh disease) have been described and are listed in Box 40-2.

Dystonia can also be seen in various neurodegenerative parkinsonian syndromes, including Parkinson disease, as well as the atypical parkinsonian syndromes including progressive supranuclear palsy and corticobasal ganglionic degeneration (CBD). Adult-onset focal foot or leg dystonia can be the initial presentation of Parkinson disease (PD). Patients with PD may also develop dystonia as an off-symptom or as part of levodopa-induced dyskinesias. A dystonic, apraxic limb is a hallmark of CBD.

Dystonia-plus syndromes are a rare group of inherited nondegenerative diseases that include dopa-responsive dystonia (DRD), myoclonus–dystonia (MD), and rapid-onset

Box 40-2 Heredodegenerative Disorders Causing Dystonia

- Autosomal dominant
  - Huntington disease
  - Spinocerebellar ataxias (SCA3)
  - Dentatorubro-pallidoluysian atrophy (DRPLA)
- Autosomal recessive
  - Wilson disease
  - Neuroacanthocytosis
  - Niemann–Pick type C
  - Glutaric aciduria
  - GM1 gangliosidosis
  - GM2 gangliosidosis
  - Metachromatic leukodystrophy
  - Homocystinuria
  - Friedreich ataxia
  - Pantothenate-kinase–associated neurodegeneration (PKAN)
  - Neuronal intranuclear hyaline inclusion disease (NIHID)
- X-linked dominant
  - Rett syndrome
- X-linked recessive
  - DYT3 (Lubag)
  - Deafness–dystonia syndrome
- Mitochondrial
  - Leigh disease
  - Leber disease

dystonia–parkinsonism (RDP). These diseases are considered neurochemical disorders because they are due to biochemical defects that are not associated with neuronal loss. Dystonia is associated with parkinsonism in DRD and RDP and with myoclonus in MD.

1. *Dopa-responsive dystonia (DRD)*, also called Segawa disease or DYT5, is characterized by the onset of progressive

dystonia and parkinsonism in midchildhood. Patients exhibit a diurnal variation in symptoms and the feet and legs are predominantly involved. The disease is inherited in an autosomal dominant pattern and is caused by genetic mutations in the GTP-cyclohydrolase I (GCHI) gene. GCHI is the rate-limiting enzyme in the synthesis of tetrahydrobiopterin, an essential cofactor for tyrosine hydroxylase. Patients respond dramatically to small doses of levodopa.

2. ***Rapid-onset dystonia–parkinsonism (RDP)*** is an autosomal dominant disorder characterized by young-onset dystonia and parkinsonism. The symptoms appear dramatically over days to weeks and can often emerge in the setting of a stressor. Bulbar symptoms are very common. Symptoms tend to plateau after weeks. Patients exhibit little if any response to levodopa. The gene for RDP has been identified as ATP1A3, which encodes an Na^+/K^+ ATPase.

Myoclonus-dystonia (MD) is an autosomal dominant disorder characterized by alcohol-responsive myoclonus and dystonia. Symptoms can emerge in childhood or in adulthood. Psychiatric disorders such as obsessive–compulsive disorder and alcohol abuse are frequently seen. This disorder has been associated with mutations in the epsilon sarcoglycan gene.

3. ***Iatrogenic dystonia*** can occur with exposure to dopamine receptor–blocking agents, levodopa, and selective serotonin reuptake inhibitors. Tardive dystonia may be focal, segmental, or generalized and often is characterized as retrocollis and opisthotonic posturing. Acute dystonia reactions may also develop in association with exposure to dopamine receptor–blocking agents.

A variety of lesions causing damage to the basal ganglia are associated with dystonia. These include perinatal hypoxia, stroke, head trauma, brain tumor, infection, and autoimmune disorders.

Psychogenic dystonia is perhaps the most diagnostically challenging type of secondary dystonia as illustrated by the record that many now-recognized organic dystonia patients were initially thought to have a primary psychiatric disorder. It is also important to recognize that a minority of patients with organic movement disorder may have a superimposed psychogenic movement disorder including dystonia. Features on history and exam that can suggest a psychogenic dystonia include abrupt onset, spontaneous remission, distractible or entrainable movements, variability and inconsistency of movements (i.e., non-patterned dystonic movements), false weakness or sensory complaints, multiple somatizations, the presence of secondary gain, and concomitant psychiatric disease.

PATHOPHYSIOLOGY

Although the genetics of a number of primary dystonias have been elucidated, the pathophysiology of dystonia remains unclear. Lesions in the basal ganglia, particularly the thalamus and putamen, point to these structures as having key roles in the development of dystonia. Models of basal ganglia circuitry suggest that there is an imbalance between direct and indirect pathways leading to reduced pallidal inhibition of the thalamus with subsequent overactivity of the premotor cortex. However, this hypothesis does not square with the finding that pallidotomy and deep brain stimulation of the globus pallidus internus can improve dystonia. A more complex pathophysiological model of dystonia is emerging that incorporates not only rate but pattern, synchronization, and somatosensory responsiveness of neuronal activity.

TREATMENT

Treatment of dystonia is determined by etiology and anatomic region(s) involved. All children and young adults presenting with dystonia should be given a trial of levodopa to rule out DRD.

The first-line treatment for cervical dystonia, blepharospasm, focal limb dystonia, and spasmodic dysphonia is botulinum toxin. Both serotypes A and B are available in the United States. Botulinum toxin and baclofen can be beneficial for oromandibular dystonia. In addition to medications, physical therapy is an important adjunct in the treatment of dystonia.

For patients with generalized dystonia, trihexyphenidyl at high doses (~90 mg per day) can provide some benefit. Baclofen may also be tried for generalized dystonia and can also be given at high doses. The benzodiazepines may provide adjunctive benefit. Variable results have been found for diphenhydramine, carbamazepine, dopamine agonists and dopamine antagonists. Tetrabenazine can be helpful, especially in tardive dystonia.

For medication-refractory dystonia, surgery can be considered. Peripheral denervation surgeries such as rhizotomy have produced variable results. More recently, deep brain stimulation (DBS) of the globus pallidus has been performed in patients with medication-refractory dystonia. In a recent prospective, double-blind, video-controlled study of patients with primary generalized dystonia (DYT1 and non-DYT1), DBS patients experienced ~50% improvement in motor and disability scores at 1 year. A follow-up study in this group of patients has shown a sustained improvement in both motor and quality of life at 3 years postsurgery. Case series have described benefit of DBS in the treatment of cervical dystonia. DBS also shows promise for treating tardive dystonia.

ADDITIONAL RESOURCES

Fahn S, Bressman SB, Marsden CD. Classification of dystonia. Adv Neurol 1998;78:1-10.

Fahn S, Jankovic J. Principles and practice of movement disorders. Churchill and Livingstone 2007.

Tarsy D, Simon DK. Dystonia. N Engl J Med 2006;355:818-829.

Vidailhet M, Vercueil L, Houeto JL, et al. Bilateral deep-brain stimulation of the globus pallidus in primary generalized dystonia. N Engl J Med 2005;352:459-467.

Vidailhet M, Vercueil L, Houeto JL, et al. Bilateral, pallidal, deep-brain stimulation in primary generalised dystonia: a prospective 3 year follow-up study. Lancet Neurol 2007;6:223-229.

Medication-Induced Movement Disorders

41

Diana Apetauerova

Clinical Vignette

A 57-year-old woman with history of chronic nausea and concomitant use of antiemetic medications presented for evaluation of slowness and tremor. She had been followed by a gastroenterologist for the past 3 years for her nausea. No specific mechanism was identified to explain her symptoms; treatment was initiated with various antinausea medications. Approximately 1.5 years ago, metoclopramide was initiated; it was continued daily. This led to significant improvement of her nausea. Her past medical history was not otherwise of note.

One year ago, she began to note that both hands were shaking and her dexterity diminished, particularly with her handwriting becoming smaller and progressively telescoping. Her family also noticed that she had developed facial masking, a shuffling gait, and a hunched posture. On occasion, her speech had an indistinct and low volume. There was no family history of Parkinson disease or other neurologic conditions. She denied any prior toxic exposure.

Neurologic examination revealed facial masking; hypophonic speech; mild perioral tremor; symmetric generalized bradykinesia and rigidity; a bilateral 5-Hz frequency postural as well as action hand tremor; and a slow, shuffling parkinsonian gait. The diagnosis of drug-induced parkinsonism was suspected. Metoclopramide was discontinued. She had complete resolution of her symptoms and was normal when seen 6 months later.

There are a large number of pharmaceutical agents with the potential to cause a movement disorder (Table 41-1). These medications primarily interfere with dopaminergic transmission within the basal ganglia (levodopa, dopamine agonists, dopamine receptor–blocking agents [DRBs]). Other classes of these movement disorder–inducing agents do not have as precisely defined biochemical mechanisms. These medications include central nervous system (CNS) stimulants, anticonvulsants, tricyclic antidepressants, and estrogens. From a clinical perspective, the medications most commonly responsible for iatrogenic movement disorders are the various neuroleptics and pharmacologic agents that block or stimulate dopamine receptors.

The clinical temporal profile of drug-induced movement disorders can be acute, subacute, or chronic. Acute syndromes include dystonia, choreoathetosis, akathisia, and tics. Subacute syndromes include drug-induced parkinsonism and tremor. Chronic syndromes include levodopa-induced dyskinesias in Parkinson disease and tardive dyskinesia (TD). There is no direct evidence of precise CNS pathology predisposing to the development of drug-induced movement disorders. Because no precise pathoanatomic correlation or model is known, a primary biochemical mechanism is therefore the likely responsible pathophysiologic mechanism here.

CLINICAL SYNDROMES

Neuroleptic Malignant Syndrome

Neuroleptic malignant syndrome (NMS) is a very unusual complication and is one of the most severe reactions to neuroleptic therapy. It has a relatively high incidence (0.5–1%) considering the very large numbers of patients taking neuroleptic medication. Symptoms typically occur shortly after institution of neuroleptic therapy or at time of initiating increased dosage. Young men are at higher risk than the general population. Pathogenesis is thought to involve both central and peripheral effects of dopamine receptor blockade.

Typically, NMS patients present with an acute onset of a severe movement disorder characterized by rigidity, tremor, and dystonia. There are often manifestations of very significant dysautonomic disturbances, including fever, diaphoresis, and cardiovascular/pulmonary dysfunction. Often the patients are stuporous, and a very intense concomitant myonecrosis usually accompanies the NMS; this leads to significant elevation of serum creatine kinase with its own innate risk of significant renal compromise. There is an associated leukocytosis. The fatality rate in NMS may reach as much as 20% because of the various associated complications, including dehydration, cardiac arrhythmias, pulmonary embolism, and renal failure. As soon as this clinical setting of NMS is recognized, it is very important to begin treatment. Medications that are frequently useful include levodopa, dopamine agonists, and the antispastic agent dantrolene.

Acute Dystonic Reactions

These very dramatic movement disorder syndromes usually develop within 5 days after initiation of various neuroleptic medications. This clinical picture typically presents very rapidly after initiation of the responsible therapeutic agent. The craniocervical region is the most commonly affected site. These patients are sometimes thought to have tetanus what with the facial spasms mimicking the classic trismus with risus sardonicus (Fig. 41-1).

Pathophysiologically, these disorders are related to a sudden imbalance between the striatal dopamine and cholinergic systems. Typically these disorders are diagnosed by their relatively acute resolution either spontaneously subsequent to drug withdrawal or more immediately by parenteral administration of an antihistamine, such as diphenhydramine, or sometimes anticholinergics.

Table 41-1 Types of Drug-Induced Movement Disorders and Responsible Medications

Syndrome	Responsible Medication	Syndrome	Responsible Medication
Postural tremor	Sympathomimetics	Chorea, including tardive and orofacial dyskinesia	Antipsychotics
	Levodopa		Metoclopramide
	Amphetamines		Levodopa
	Bronchodilators		Direct dopamine agonists
	Tricyclic antidepressants		Indirect dopamine agonists and other catecholaminergic drugs
	Lithium carbonate		Anticholinergics
	Caffeine		Antihistaminics
	Thyroid hormone		Oral contraceptives
	Sodium valproate		Phenytoin
	Antipsychotics		Carbamazepine
	Hypoglycemic agents		Ethosuximide
	Adrenocorticosteroids		Phenobarbital
	Alcohol withdrawal		Lithium carbonate
	Amiodarone		Methadone
	Cyclosporin A		Benzodiazepines
	Others		Monoamine oxidase inhibitors
Acute dystonic reactions	Antipsychotics		Tricyclic antidepressants
	Metoclopramide		Methyldopa
	Antimalarial agents		Digoxin
	Tetrabenazine		Alcohol withdrawal
	Diphenhydramine		Toluene sniffing
	Mefenamic acid		Flunarizine and cinnarizine
	Oxatomide	Dystonia, including tardive dystonia (excluding acute dystonic reactions)	Antipsychotics
	Flunarizine and cinnarizine		Metoclopramide
Akathisia	Antipsychotics		Levodopa
	Metoclopramide		Direct dopamine agonists
	Reserpine		Phenytoin
	Tetrabenazine		Carbamazepine
	Levodopa and dopamine agonists		Flunarizine and cinnarizine
	Flunarizine and cinnarizine	Neuroleptic malignant syndrome	Antipsychotics
	Ethosuximide		Tetrabenazine with α-methyl-*para*-tyrosine
	Methysergide		Antiparkinsonian drugs withdrawal
Parkinsonism	Antipsychotics	Tics	Levodopa
	Metoclopramide		Direct dopamine agonists
	Reserpine		Antipsychotics
	Tetrabenazine		Carbamazepine
	Methyldopa	Myoclonus	Levodopa
	Flunarizine and cinnarizine		Anticonvulsants
	Lithium		Tricyclic antidepressants
	Phenytoin		Antipsychotics
	Captopril	Asterixis	Anticonvulsants
	Alcohol withdrawal		Levodopa
	MPTP (1-methyl-4-phenyl-1,2,3,6-tetrahydropyridine)		Hepatotoxins
	Other toxins (manganese, carbon disulfide, cyanide)		Respiratory depressants
	Cytosine arabinoside		

Medication-Induced Parkinsonism

Various medications have the potential to interfere with the synthesis, storage, and release of dopamine, as well as the varied dopamine-blocking agents, and may precipitate an akinetic-rigid syndrome that is nearly indistinguishable from idiopathic Parkinson disease (Fig. 41-2). Substituted benzamides, particularly metoclopramide, used to treat gastrointestinal disorders, and calcium channel blockers particularly have the potential to produce a medication-induced parkinsonism. The basic pathophysiologic mechanism here is related to a predominant presynaptic effect on dopamine and serotonin neurons.

In contrast to Parkinson disease where the presentation often has a focal distribution, therapeutic medication-induced parkinsonism is often characterized by a symmetric bilateral presentation. Bradykinesia predominates over typical rigidity and resting tremor. When a tremor is present, it is usually postural instead of resting. Although drug-induced parkinsonism may persist long after withdrawal of the offending drug,

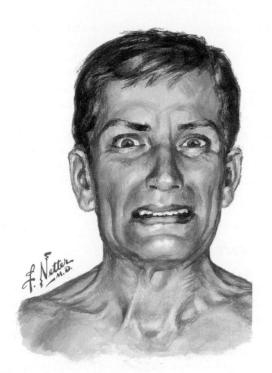

Spasm of jaw, facial, and neck muscles (trismus [lockjaw], risus sardonicus), and dysphagia are often early symptoms after variable incubation period.

Figure 41-1 Acute Dystonic Reaction.

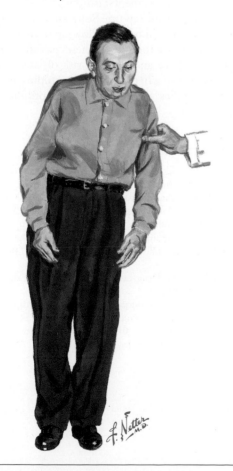

Figure 41-2 Medication-Induced Parkinsonism.

eventually most patients improve without further therapeutic interventions if use of the offending drug can be stopped.

Akathisia

This unusual disorder is typified by an inability to keep still; subjectively, it is often accompanied by feelings of restlessness, primarily resulting from the initiation of neuroleptic therapy. Akathisia is the most poorly understood, acute drug-induced syndrome; no neuroanatomic correlates explain it. Dose reduction or withdrawal of the offending drug is the most effective treatment. At times, introduction of other medications, such as propranolol and clonidine, can provide reasonable treatment. The pathophysiologic mechanisms are not well defined. It is known that these neuroleptics have little or no direct effect on β-adrenergic receptors.

Tardive Dyskinesia Syndromes

The prevalence of TD varies between 0.5% and 65%, making it the most feared complication of long-term neuroleptic therapy. These syndromes present after a latency period following initiation of these various inciting medications. They usually do not present until at least 3 months after—or, more commonly, 1 to 2 years after—the patient begins taking the responsible medication. The timing of presentation for these disorders can be varied during treatment per se, after dose reduction, or subsequent to medication withdrawal. Unfortunately, some of these syndromes are irreversible. Neuroleptics are the most common offending drugs, particularly because of dopamine receptor blocking (DRB).

Most commonly, TD clinically affects the orofacial region, in particular, various chewing movements, tongue protrusion, vermicular tongue motion, lip smacking, puckering, and pursing (Fig. 41-3A). TD patients also have hyperkinesias, including chorea (Fig. 41-3B), athetosis, dystonia, and tics affecting the limb and truncal regions, or paroxysms of rapid eye blinking. Various risk factors are thought to be operative, including female sex, older age, and duration and dosage of therapy. It may take months for TD to resolve if they are going to do so, and sadly this is not predictable.

The primary pathophysiology of TD is only partly appreciated. Currently it is thought that striatal dopamine receptors are chronically blocked by DRBs. Subsequently, these receptors develop a supersensitivity to small amounts of dopamine that would be too small to induce dyskinesia in an otherwise healthy individual. The persistence of TD after drug withdrawal also suggests that there is underactivity of GABA-mediated inhibition of the thalamocortical pathway and an excitotoxic DRB mechanism.

DIAGNOSIS

Careful clinical observation and review of the patient's medication history are the primary keys to the diagnosis of drug-induced movement disorders. When there is no well-defined pharmacologic predisposition defined, the possibility of other etiologic mechanisms must be considered to exclude hereditary or systemic illness. Extraordinarily rare structural basal ganglia

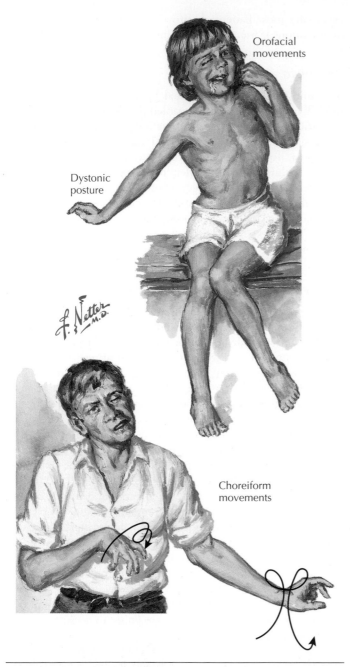

Orofacial
movements

Dystonic
posture

Choreiform
movements

Figure 41-3 Tardive Dyskinesia.

lesions require consideration and an MRI needs to be performed.

The differential diagnosis of TD is sometimes a difficult one, including idiopathic movement disorders such as psychotic patients having stereotypic behavior, Tourette syndrome, simple or complex motor tics, and possible dental problems. Other drug-induced dyskinesias deserve consideration, particularly with the acute dystonic reaction secondary to antiemetics such as chlorpromazine. Here intravenous diphenylhydramine can be both therapeutic and diagnostic. Inheritable disorders including Huntington disease, Wilson disease, and pantothenate kinase–associated neurodegeneration with brain iron accumulation type 1 disease also require consideration in the differential diagnosis. Some systemic illnesses are also associated with various dyskinesias; hyperthyroidism, hypoparathyroidism, hyperglycemia, chorea of pregnancy, Sydenham chorea, and inflammatory or space-occupying brain lesions rarely cause a pseudo-TD.

TREATMENT

No single therapeutic strategy is significantly effective for TD. The best methods are prevention and early recognition. Reduction or withdrawal of medication, when possible, is advisable. Drugs used in its treatment include dopamine-depleting agents (reserpine, tetrabenazine), benzodiazepines, GABA mimetics (valproate sodium and baclofen), and dopamine agonists in low doses. Use of antioxidants such as vitamin E has been proposed, but study results conflict.

PROGNOSIS

Medication-induced movement disorders have primarily been studied in individual case reports. Solid epidemiologic data are lacking. Of interest would be the follow-up of metoclopramide-induced PD as to whether once these patients are back to normal, they then have an increased risk of later development of this disorder. Prospective, multicenter studies are needed to elucidate the specifics of individual susceptibility for these syndromes.

ADDITIONAL RESOURCES

Esper CD, Factor SA. Failure of recognition of drug- induced parkinsonism in the elderly. Mov Disord 2008 Feb 15;23(3):401-404.

Gershanik OS. Drug-induced dyskinesia. In: Anodic J, Tolosa E, editors. Parkinson's disease and movement disorders. Baltimore, Md: Williams & Wilkins; 1998. p. 579-600.

Kiriakakis V, Bhatia K, Quinn NP, et al. The natural history of tardive dystonia: a long-term follow-up study of 107 cases. Brain 1998;121: 2053-2066.

Mena MA, de Yebenes JG. Drug-induced parkinsonism. Expert Opin Drug Saf 2006 Nov;5(6):759-771.

Pierre JM. Extrapyramidal symptoms with atypical antipsychotics; incidence, prevention and management. Drug Saf 2005;28(3):191-208.

Woerner MG, Alvir JMJ, Saltz BL, et al. Prospective study of tardive dyskinesia in the elderly: rates and risk factors. Am J Psychiatry 1998;155:1521-1528.

Psychogenic Movement Disorders

Diana Apetauerova

42

Clinical Vignette

A 35-year-old woman with a medical history of depression presented with intermittent head tremor. Several months ago while driving, with her seat belt on, and stopped at a traffic signal she had a motor vehicle accident (MVA) when her car was rear ended. She had no immediate overt injuries, but did complain of mild neck pain after that. Subsequently, just 3 weeks later, she first noted tremor. Her tremor was fairly persistent and did not improve after drinking alcoholic beverages or disappear at night. She "had to leave work" due to this tremor; she then filed formal litigation against the offending driver. Her family history included a younger brother with dystonic cerebral palsy. This patient used fluoxetine (Prozac) long-term for her depression.

This patient appeared very anxious; however, her general physical examination was unremarkable. Her neurologic examination demonstrated an intermittent shaking horizontal "no–no" head posture as well as "yes–yes" vertical tremor of her head. The tremor continually changed in frequency as well as amplitude; there was no consistent pattern evident; that is, it was consistently inconsistent. She had no dystonic posturing or hypertrophy of any neck muscles. Her tremor became very prominent while discussing the details of the MVA and completely disappeared when she was deliberately distracted. Similarly, the tremor was totally absent during other portions of the neurologic examination. However, her muscle strength testing also demonstrated consistently inconsistent "weakness" of the "give way" type typical of nonorganic secondary gain patients. The remainder of her examination was unremarkable. She did not have any tremor in other body parts, nor any cogwheeling, rigidity, or signs of dystonia. While ambulating, her head tremor again became very prominent.

Laboratory testing for Wilson disease, thyroid, vitamin B$_{12}$ level, head and neck magnetic resonance imaging (MRI), and magnetic resonance angiography were all normal. With her consistently inconsistent neurologic findings, a diagnosis of psychogenic tremor was suspected. Several treatment options including propranolol, anxiolytics, and antidepressants were tried without either objective or subjective improvement. Later, after undergoing psychotherapy, she experienced a sudden and complete remission of these symptoms.

Psychogenic, psychosomatic, hysterical, or functional movement disorders are conditions related to an underlying psychiatric illness with no evidence of any organic etiology. One has to be very cautious. There is a major inherent difficulty whenever one entertains a diagnosis of a psychogenic movement disorder as studies demonstrate that this is a too common and poorly documented diagnosis, in that up to 30% of patients diagnosed with *psychogenic disorders* eventually are found to have an organic neurologic illness. Because, with just a few exceptions, most movement disorders have no specific diagnostic laboratory or imaging study available, beyond clinical observation, there is a temptation by the uninitiated to label a patient hysterical when the clinician cannot arrive at a definitive organic diagnosis. An important diagnostic caveat is for the evaluating physician to not rush to judgment when the patient's findings do not initially fit a specific diagnostic set, such as pill-rolling rest tremor, cogwheel rigidity, masked facies, and en bloc walking as is typical of Parkinson disease. Astute clinicians often use a "tincture of time" to prospectively and carefully follow patients by repeated clinical evaluations. Here one monitors the individual patient for the gradual development of recognized classic signs of an evolving and well-recognized neurologic process. Barring the later clinical evolution of symptoms and findings into a more classic organic movement disorder, the clinician will gradually acquire information from the patient or family to become more comfortable with the importance of underlying psychogenic factors.

A variety of underlying psychiatric diagnoses are found in patients with psychogenic neurologic movement disorders; these include various somatoform and factitious disorders, malingering, depression, anxiety, and histrionic personality disorders. Although a specific psychiatric diagnosis cannot always be confirmed for these various abnormal and consistently inconsistent motor symptoms, despite the clinician's high suspicion of psychogenicity, an emotionally based diagnosis is not totally precluded. Often it is only time and a cautious diagnostic approach that will allow one to sort out the majority of these challenging patients' specific diagnosis. In young women, one has to be particularly careful to not overlook sexual abuse, particularly incest.

Psychogenic tremor, dystonia, myoclonus, chorea, and parkinsonism are the typical means for a functional movement disorder to present and are particularly common in women (Fig. 42-1). These patients usually have multiplicity and variability of symptoms superimposed on a significant psychiatric background. The neurologic findings do not fit a specific diagnostic set typical of the classic organic movement disorders. These factitious patients present with movements that are consistently inconsistent and are particularly liable to change or decrease during distraction. Frequently, patients with psychogenic movement disorders display uneconomic postures demonstrating a most exaggerated effort during examination that may also produce fatigue. They may demonstrate marked slowness when asked to perform certain tasks such as rapid alternating movements.

Therapeutically, psychogenic movement disorders often respond to placebo or suggestion.

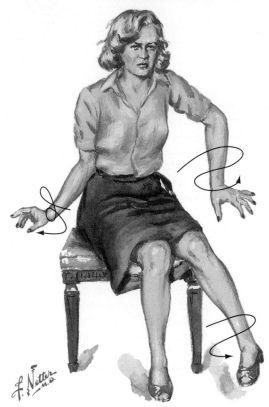

One must exclude organic disorders including pregnancy (chorea gravidarum), lupus erythematosus, medication- or drug-induced chorea, Sydenham chorea, and Wilson disease.

Figure 42-1 Psychogenic movement disorder, pseudochoreoathetosis.

ETIOLOGY

Because the etiologies of psychogenic movement disorders are unknown, no anatomic correlation can be made. It is totally conjectural as to whether any neurochemical interplay exists, or will later be recognized, between the effect of the presumed underlying psychiatric condition and the patient's clinical presentation.

CLINICAL PRESENTATIONS

Psychogenic Dystonia

Dystonia is an involuntary, sustained muscle contraction causing repetitive twisting and abnormal postures. Most patients with dystonia have no identified mechanism, although some have a genetic basis. Because no specific test for organic dystonia exists, the diagnosis of psychogenic dystonia is very difficult to initially confirm. There is a broad clinical presentation for the organic dystonias. And the neurologist must always take such into consideration, keeping an open mind before making a psychogenic diagnosis.

Patients with psychogenic dystonia may present with foot or leg involvement, a distribution that is relatively unlikely but not exclusive of an organic adult-onset idiopathic dystonia. An important clue to a diagnosis of a psychogenic dystonia is the presence of symptoms at rest; this often helps to differentiate such individuals from those with an action-specific organic dystonia.

Psychogenic Tremor

Tremors are rhythmic, bidirectional, oscillating movements resulting from contraction of agonist and antagonistic muscles. Tremors can be resting, postural, or action.

Psychogenic tremor usually varies in frequency and amplitude, is complex, occurs at rest, during various postures, and with various actions. Psychogenic tremor often has amplitudes unlike that of even midbrain tremor. It typically lessens with distraction.

Psychogenic Myoclonus

Myoclonus is defined as brief, shocklike movements caused by muscle contraction or lapses in posture. The frequency, amplitude, body distribution, symmetry, and course differ with various etiologies. Psychogenic myoclonus decreases in amplitude during distraction and often occurs at rest, in contrast to organic myoclonus, which decreases at rest.

Psychogenic Parkinsonism

Parkinsonism is a symptom complex consisting of resting tremor, rigidity, bradykinesia, and impaired postural reflexes. Psychogenic tremor varies in frequency and rhythmicity, remitting with distraction. Rigidity related to psychiatric problems consists of voluntary resistance without any evidence of cogwheeling. As with other psychogenic movement disorders, the symptoms of psychogenic parkinsonism lessen with distraction. Gait is atypical, with extreme or bizarre postural instability.

DIFFERENTIAL DIAGNOSES

Psychogenic movement disorders have certain common characteristics, such as acute onset, static course, spontaneous remissions, consistently inconsistent character of their movements in amplitude, frequency, distribution, and a selective disability. Furthermore, these psychiatrically affected individuals are unresponsiveness to appropriate medications, may sometimes respond to placebo, have their movements increase with attention, while these same adventitious movements decrease with distraction. A remission may occur with psychotherapy, once a specific psychopathology is diagnosed. The clinician strives to make a distinction between these psychogenic clinical presentations and those of organic movement disorders. It is very often a most challenging diagnostic algorithm and sometimes may take several years to confirm.

Certain factors support the possibility of a psychogenic movement disorder. This is particularly relevant when there is a patient history of multiple poorly defined, somatic complaints. Other supportive evidence for an emotional basis includes specific findings on neurologic examination. These include a nonanatomic sensory loss such as when one places a tuning fork on the forehead and the patient states he or she does not feel it when it is tilted to the left but does so when tilted to the right, while the examiner maintains the instrument's base in the precisely same anatomic spot for each testing. Similarly, a consistently inconsistent weakness and a seemingly deliberate slowness of movement are also typical of psychogenic movement disorders.

Questioning the individual or family to potentially uncover possible secondary gain are also important. This is especially true when one determines that there is a pending litigation or workman's compensation action. On some occasions, psychiatrically ill patients use a family member or friend with an organic movement disorder to serve as a subconscious model for their own adventitious movement or gait disorder. Thus, one may sometimes find a positive family history by meeting with and observing family members important in the individual's daily life. These encounters may provide a good means for establishing the true identity of the patient's problem. Such a meeting may be overwhelming when one identifies the precise model for the specific movement. Some patients are truly great actors!

DIAGNOSTIC EVALUATION

The diagnosis of psychogenic movement disorder usually requires both a neurologist and a psychiatrist as well as a direct meeting with family members. The initial step is a detailed clinical history and examination, review of current and previous medications, and subsequent exclusion of a true organic movement disorder. Diagnostic tests follow clinical assessment and may include brain MRI, serum ceruloplasmin and urine copper excretion, thyroid functions, and other tests based on clinical suspicion. The diagnostic evaluation may also include an appropriate trial of specific medications typically used for various organic movement disorders and tailored to the patient's clinical picture. After these steps are taken, and certain clinical suggestions of psychogenicity are defined, a diagnostic psychiatric evaluation is needed. However, the definition of a psychiatric illness still does not absolutely prove that the movement disorder has a psychogenic basis as patients with psychiatric disorders of course also develop organic neurologic diseases.

Thus, careful neurologic as well as psychiatric follow-up is often mandated. Wilson disease is a good example of patients presenting with seemingly bizarre movements that have led to psychiatric diagnosis early on. Careful attention to search for a Kayser–Fleischer ring when looking at the patient's iris and obtaining copper screening studies may occasionally uncover this important but very rare movement disorder. There is no more grateful patient.

TREATMENT AND PROGNOSIS

These patients present a therapeutic challenge equal to the diagnostic challenge that led to a proper diagnosis. Treatment of these individuals is often very difficult. No specific treatment protocols exist. Periodic neurologic follow-up with the same neurologist, in conjunction with psychotherapy, is often necessary to alleviate residual concerns that an organic illness is present. These visits will also provide reassurance to the patient and subsequently lead to a reduction or remission of the adventitious motor symptoms. Careful neurologic follow-up can be exceedingly reassuring for not only the patient but often the physician. It is not appropriate to make a psychogenic diagnosis without providing for careful follow-up. Ongoing psychotherapy and physical therapy are important, as is treatment of the underlying psychiatric conditions (antidepressants, anxiolytics, etc.). Finally, the use of placebo is debatable. Some physicians and patients interpret this as confrontational. Unfortunately, some patients resist accepting both the diagnosis and psychiatric treatment.

Prognosis depends on the psychodynamic specifics underlying the movement disorder. Generally good prognostic signs include acute onset, short duration of symptoms, healthy premorbid functioning, absence of coexisting organic and psychogenic disease, and presence of an identifiable stressor.

FUTURE DIRECTIONS

When specific laboratory tests, possibly neurochemical or autoimmune in type, become available for the diagnosis of organic movement disorders, psychogenic movement disorders will be easier to confirm. More research in the field of neurotransmitters, more specific brain studies, such as functional MRI, and genetic testing will eventually aid the understanding of this complex and difficult therapeutic problem. It is not out of the question that eventually some new previously misunderstood organic movement disorders will be identified in some of these individuals.

ADDITIONAL RESOURCES

Fahn S, Williams D. Psychogenic dystonia. Adv Neurol 1988;50: 431-455.

Halle M, Fahn S, Jankovic J, et al. Psychogenic Movement Disorders. Neurology and Neurosurgery. Baltimore, MD: Lippincott Williams & Wilkins; 2006.

Koller WC, Marjama J, Troster A. Psychogenic movement disorders. In: Jankovic J, Tolosa E, editors. Parkinson's Disease and Movement Disorders. Baltimore, MD: Williams & Wilkins; 1998. p. 859-868.

Surgical Treatments for Movement Disorders

43

Jeffrey E. Arle

Surgical therapies for certain movement disorders are important treatment modalities, particularly in medically refractory cases where the patient has become significantly disabled. Early on, thousands of surgically induced brain lesions were performed between 1950 and 1970 after a serendipitous surgical "mistake" led to loss of a classic Parkinson disease (PD) tremor in one patient. Very rapidly an initial enthusiasm developed for this therapeutic modality. However, the introduction of levodopa in 1966 led to a significant cessation in the development of more sophisticated surgical treatment for PD. Subsequently our understanding of the physiology of movement disorders and our ability to better assess baseline and outcome data in these patients have markedly improved since the initial historical period. Concomitantly, it became clear that medical management would not provide long-term resolution of the classic PD in many patients. Today PD primarily includes mostly the idiopathic subset in contrast to the combined idiopathic as well as the postencephalitic variants present when surgical therapeutic methodologies were in their infancy. Currently there are several operations performed for the rather few neurologic disorders that are treated effectively by surgery (Table 43-1). These include very specific intentional destructive lesions targeting specific basal ganglia sites as well as deep brain stimulation (DBS) within the basal ganglia and thalamus.

PATIENT SELECTION

Patients who are candidates for DBS are typically refractory to standard medical therapy that included multiple trials with varying dosages and combinations of pharmacotherapy. Once a diagnosis of PD is confirmed, expeditious medication trials are encouraged, in order that years of potential benefit from subsequent surgery are not lost if the patient eventually becomes a medication failure. Ideally the surgeon prefers to consider patients whose clinical severity has not progressed toward end stages where surgical intervention becomes less appropriate. However, in most centers, DBS and lesion placement for PD are performed as late as age 80 years. This is predicated on the patient still evidencing good results to preoperative neuropsychological testing that demonstrates no more than minimal signs of dementia. Similar criteria are applied when contemplating DBS treatment for tremor per se.

Dystonia, in contrast, typically involves children as young as ages 6–8 years. Although adequate genetic testing is helpful for diagnosis, many dystonia patients are DYT-1 negative. The presence or absence of genetic confirmation does not determine which child will benefit from DBS.

Decisions to pursue DBS for patients with variable clinical presentations, including severe essential tremor, PD, or dystonia, are clinical ones. Patients are initially selected from those who have failed various medication protocols. The neurosurgeon then considers the potential contribution of the invasive

procedure to the patient's overall quality of life as well as its potential acute and chronic side effects and thus its relative risk benefits.

GENERAL PROCEDURE

The operations are performed stereotactically, typically with the help of a frame affixed to the head of the patient (Fig. 43-1). This frame serves to create a space with x, y, and z coordinates that the head, and thus the brain, lies within. As such, any particular location within that space can be targeted using devices to place and hold a probe tip, recording electrode, or stimulating electrode at the desired coordinates. These systems are highly accurate, provided the surgeon is specifically trained and able to precisely focus the probe target within just 1 mm of an intended therapeutic site deep within the appropriate target brain structures including the basal ganglia, thalamus, or subthalamic brain structures. A system of stereotactic targeting software is used to define readily appreciated common brain structures as initial reference points. These systems typically use measurements based on the location of the anterior and posterior commissures.

During the intraoperative procedure, the patients are kept awake and monitored by a clinical neurophysiologist. As the probe is advanced, specific cell types are verified physiologically by having a clinical neurophysiologist make microelectrode recordings along the probe's trajectory toward the intended subcortical target. Cells in certain specific areas have reproducible physiologic signatures vis-à-vis their firing rates and patterns. The utilization of these physiologic markers helps validate the exact location of the electrode (see Fig. 43-1). There are major albeit relatively uncommon risks associated with these procedures, the most significant being a debilitating or fatal intracerebral hemorrhage; currently, these complications still occur in approximately 0.5–3% of cases.

OPERATIONS PERFORMED FOR MOVEMENT DISORDERS

Pallidotomy

The postero-ventro-lateral region of the globus pallidus pars interna (Gpi) was reexamined in the early 1990s when earlier studies of the 1960 decade were revived. "Lesions," that is, intended damage to brain parenchyma, are made in this area after an initial test lesion. In this setting, the probe is heated to a lower temperature for a shorter time period. This test allows the neurosurgeon to observe the development of any potentially adverse but usually totally reversible side effects of the intended procedure. Additionally, great care needs to be applied to avoid causing any part of this deliberately made lesion to damage the adjacent optic tract. Thousands of pallidotomies have been

Table 43-1 Summary of Current Best Procedures for Movement Disorders*

Disorder	Procedures
Essential (familial) tremor	Vim Thalamic DBS or Thalamotomy (unilateral)
Parkinson disease	DBS either to the STN or Gpi or Pallidotomy (unilateral)
Dystonia	Gpi DBS

*DBS, deep brain stimulation; Gpi, globus pallidus pars interna; STN, subthalamic nucleus; Vim, ventralis intermedius.

performed historically, and after a resurgence in the 1990s, subsequent emphasis has now shifted to stimulation procedures. In general, a unilateral pallidotomy provides very good results in the treatment of contralateral dyskinesia, rigidity, tremor, and bradykinesia. Unfortunately, however, prior attempts to perform bilateral pallidotomy lesions resulted in a high percentage of patients becoming cognitively impaired. Thus, it is now very rare to perform bilateral pallidotomies.

Thalamotomy

A unilateral thalamotomy provides very good results; it is a procedure that has been used since the mid-1950s. Although

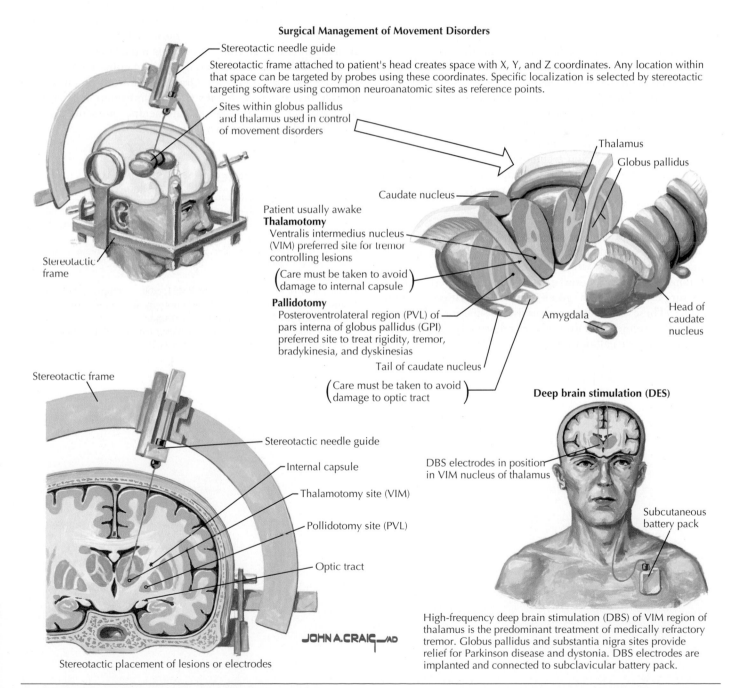

Surgical Management of Movement Disorders

Stereotactic needle guide

Stereotactic frame attached to patient's head creates space with X, Y, and Z coordinates. Any location within that space can be targeted by probes using these coordinates. Specific localization is selected by stereotactic targeting software using common neuroanatomic sites as reference points.

Sites within globus pallidus and thalamus used in control of movement disorders

Stereotactic frame

Thalamus

Globus pallidus

Caudate nucleus

Patient usually awake
Thalamotomy
Ventralis intermedius nucleus (VIM) preferred site for tremor controlling lesions

(Care must be taken to avoid damage to internal capsule)

Pallidotomy
Posteroventrolateral region (PVL) of pars interna of globus pallidus (GPI) preferred site to treat rigidity, tremor, bradykinesia, and dyskinesias

Amygdala

Head of caudate nucleus

Tail of caudate nucleus

(Care must be taken to avoid damage to optic tract)

Stereotactic frame

Stereotactic needle guide

Internal capsule

Thalamotomy site (VIM)

Pollidotomy site (PVL)

Optic tract

Stereotactic placement of lesions or electrodes

JOHN A. CRAIG—MD

Deep brain stimulation (DES)

DBS electrodes in position in VIM nucleus of thalamus

Subcutaneous battery pack

High-frequency deep brain stimulation (DBS) of VIM region of thalamus is the predominant treatment of medically refractory tremor. Globus pallidus and substantia nigra sites provide relief for Parkinson disease and dystonia. DBS electrodes are implanted and connected to subclavicular battery pack.

Figure 43-1 Surgical Management of Movement Disorders.

several regions of the thalamus may play a role in movement disorders and have effects if stimulated or lesioned, the ventralis intermedius (Vim) nucleus seems to have evolved as the best area to make tremor-controlling lesions. These lesions are generally produced in the same manner as pallidotomies. Great care must be taken to avoid therapeutic damage to the adjacent internal capsule lying immediately lateral to the targeted thalamic regions that manage sensory processing. Unfortunately, bilateral lesions in the thalamus are associated with dysarthria or poor cognitive outcomes just as with pallidotomies for movement disorder control. Thus, bilateral therapeutic thalamotomies are typically avoided similar to bilateral pallidotomies.

Deep Brain Stimulation

In the early 1990s, reports of the initial attempts to control tremor, utilizing high-frequency deep brain stimulation (DBS) of the thalamus's Vim region, began to surface. Interestingly, this new approach developed before the resurgence of interest in pallidotomy. This procedure has continued to gather a following among movement disorder experts. DBS is currently the predominant treatment for medically refractory tremor (typically benign essential tremor, but also tremor-predominant PD).

Subsequently stimulation techniques were then reported in both the globus pallidus (Gpi) and the subthalamic nucleus (STN) for other indications. DBS has now also been tried in several other areas of the brain, though most experience is with stimulation in the Gpi and STN for PD and dystonia. Excellent relief of major parkinsonian symptoms, including rigidity, bradykinesia, tremor, and akinesia, can be achieved using DBS in the majority of patients with true PD. More recent publications, providing longer-term follow-up perspectives comparing either sham surgical controls or good historical validation are now available. These demonstrate a persistent superior efficacy of DBS for PD, tremor, and dystonia over destructive lesions such as thalamotomy or pallidotomy.

In all instances when indicated, DBS four-contact electrodes may be placed bilaterally. This also includes settings where prior thalamotomies or pallidotomies have been unsuccessful. However, the stimulating electrodes need to be placed in a healthy area and not one previously lesioned. The electrodes are brought out through the brain and secured at the skull edge. A battery is placed in a small subcutaneous pocket just under the clavicle and tunneled to the electrode with a connecting wire (see Fig. 43-1).

Patients with dystonia are increasingly receiving DBS as a primary therapeutic modality. The consensus to date indicates that Gpi DBS is the best site to achieve therapeutic success. Although these results are especially applicable for genetically positive DYT-1 patients, similar encouraging results are also documented in individuals with secondary dystonias. Thus, Gpi DBS has the potential to relieve most dystonic posturing, particularly in any or all four limbs. This modality is also proving to be valuable wherein there is dystonia of either the neck musculature and speech muscles. Drawbacks for utilization of DBS include the somewhat higher risks for infection and the need to reprogram the stimulation parameters, often over several months in the postoperative period.

ADDITIONAL RESOURCES

Arle E, Shils JL. Essential neuromodulation. Oxford, Elsevier, 2011.

Krack P, Batir A, Van Blercom N, et al. Five-year follow-up of bilateral stimulation of the subthalamic nucleus in advanced Parkinson's disease. NEJM 2003;349:1925-1934.

Kupsch A, Benecke R, Muller J, et al. Pallidal deep-brain stimulation in primary generalized or segmental dystonia. NEJM 2006;355: 1978-1990.

Schuurman PR, Bosch DA, Bossuyt PMM, et al. A comparison of continuous thalamic stimulation and thalamotomy for suppression of severe tremor. NEJM 2000;342:461-468.

Yu H, Neimat JS; The treatment of movement disorders by deep brain stimulation. Neurotherapeutics 2008;5(1):26-36.

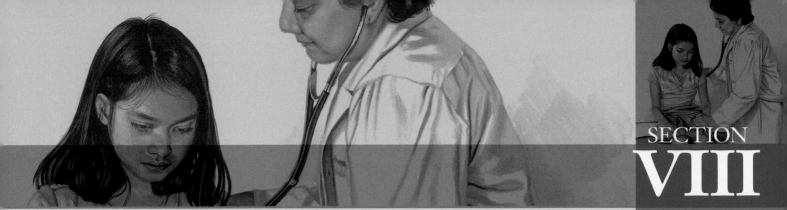

Spinal Cord Disorders

Anatomic Aspects of Spinal Cord Disorders

H. Royden Jones, Jr., Ann Camac, and Jose A. Gutrecht

44

*D*isorders of the spinal cord provide one of the best opportunities in clinical neurology to apply the basic science of neuroanatomy to the diagnosis and eventual management of patients having myelopathies. Detailed knowledge of spinal cord neuroanatomy is crucial to providing appropriate care to patients with the many various myelopathies as presented in the subsequent chapter (Chapter 45).

ANATOMIC CORRELATIONS
External Structure

The spinal cord has major functional and teleologic importance, yet it is almost paradoxical that its total mass represents just 2% of the entire central nervous system volume. The spinal canal dimensions are slightly larger, allowing the cord to move freely within the canal during neck and back flexion/extension as its perspective changes with movement. The spinal cord per se is a cylindrical elongated structure flattened dorsoventrally, having a length of 42–45 cm (Fig. 44-1). It lies within the vertebral canal extending from the atlas, continuous with the medulla through the foramen magnum, to the level of the 1st and 2nd lumbar vertebra. Here it tapers into the conus medullaris and terminates as the cauda equina (Fig. 44-1). In conditions such as meningitis, one *must not* place the spinal needle above the L3 vertebra in order not to specifically damage the underlying spinal cord. It is safe to enter the spinal canal distal to this level because the spinal nerves originating from the distal cord and forming the cauda equina, as nerve roots L2-S5, are anatomically arranged so that they are gently moved aside by the passage of the needle in contrast to the fixed spinal cord that may be easily pierced by the needle insertion and thus cause significant damage.

The cervical and lumbar enlargements of the spinal cord provide the nerve roots innervating, respectively, the upper and lower limbs. There are 31 pairs of spinal nerves, each having dorsal sensory and ventral motor roots that exit the cord (8 cervical, 12 thoracic, 5 lumbar, 5 sacral, 1 coccygeal). Although there are 7 cervical vertebrae, there are 8 cervical nerve roots (Fig. 44-2). The C1-7 roots exit above their respective vertebrae whereas C8 exits below the 7th cervical vertebra and all thoracic, lumbar, and sacral roots exit below their specific vertebrae.

Three protective membranes, the meninges including the dura mater, being the outer layer, then the arachnoid, and the most inner one, the pia, surround the cord (Fig. 44-2). Cerebrospinal fluid flows between the arachnoid and pia. Epidural fat is present in the epidural space between the spinal canal and dura mater. When clinical myelopathies develop, these various disorders are classically categorized as *intramedullary*, that is, intrinsic to the cord, or *extramedullary*, occurring secondary to disorders extrinsic to the cord. Extramedullary disorders are further subdivided into those with either an *intradural* extramedullary locus or a purely *extradural* site of pathology.

Internal Structure

White matter, consisting of myelinated fibers, surrounds the butterfly or H-shaped gray matter that contains cell bodies and their processes within the cord's center. These include both primary ascending sensory fibers and descending motor fibers. The sensory pathways are most superficial, while the motor fibers such as the corticospinal fibers are more deeply situated but still superficial and superior to the ventral horn containing the anterior horn cells that are the primary receptors for the corticospinal tract fibers. Longitudinal furrows on the cord's surface divide the white matter into columns or funiculi that are large bundles of nerve fibers having diverse functions. The anterior median fissure, posterior median, posterior intermediate, and the anterolateral sulci divide the dorsal or posterior, lateral, and anterior columns. The posterior columns are further divided into two fasciculi, gracilis medially (present at all spinal levels) and cuneatus laterally (T6 and above).

Specific Spinal Tracts

Ascending and descending tracts within the cord are interrupted at sites of cord damage (Figs. 44-3 to 44-5). The subsequent clinical sequelae develop based on the specific tracts that are affected.

ASCENDING SENSORY TRACTS (see Fig. 44-4)

Dorsal columns subserving *touch*, *pressure*, *position*, and *movement* sensations arise from dorsal root fibers and ascend posteriorly. Their fibers do not decussate (i.e., cross) until within the medulla. They then travel to the ventral posterolateral thalamic nuclei.

Lateral spinothalamic tracts arise from secondary *pain and temperature* neurons within the spinal cord, cross into the anterior commissure, and ascend in the lateral funiculus to the reticular formation and ventral posterolateral thalamic nuclei.

Anterior spinothalamic tracts arise from dorsal horn neurons within the spinal cord, cross in the anterior commissure, and ascend anterolaterally to the posterior thalamic and ventral posterolateral thalamic nuclei. The anterior spinothalamic tract provides *light touch* sensation.

Dorsal spinocerebellar tracts are uncrossed, ascending in the lateral funiculus to the cerebellar vermis. At subconscious levels, they provide fine coordination of posture and limb muscle movement.

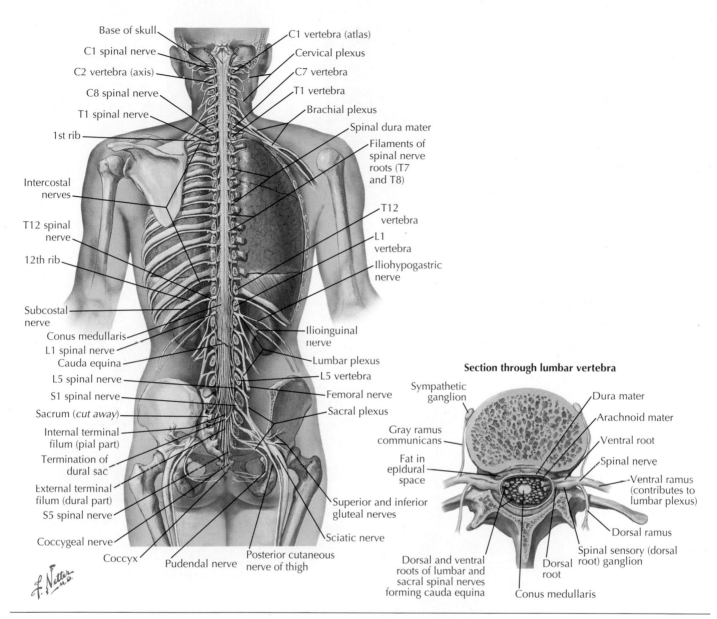

Figure 44-1 Spinal Cord and Vental Rami in Situ.

Anterior (ventral) spinocerebellar tracts are dedicated to lower extremity movement and posture, initially cross and then ascend the lateral funiculus to the cerebellum.

Cuneocerebellar tracts (not illustrated) contribute to upper extremity coordination and movement, are uncrossed, and ascend to the cerebellum.

DESCENDING MOTOR TRACTS

Corticospinal tracts are responsible for *voluntary, skilled movement*. They originate in the motor cortex (precentral and premotor areas 4 and 6), postcentral gyrus, and adjacent parietal cortex (see Fig. 44-5). These primary motor fibers descend via the corona radiata, posterior limb of internal capsule, pons, and into the medulla where most distally they then divide into three separate motor tracts (see Fig. 44-3). Up to 90% of these fibers descend in the lateral funiculus as the *lateral corticospinal tract.*

Most decussate within the distal medulla; the *uncrossed lateral corticospinal tract* is much smaller. The *anterior corticospinal tract* travels in the anterior funiculus, crossing within the cord.

Tectospinal, rubrospinal, and vestibulospinal tracts (see Fig. 44-3) originate in the superior colliculus, red nucleus, and the lateral vestibular nucleus, respectively. These tracts variously affect reflex postural movements, tone in flexor muscles, and facilitate antigravity and extensor muscles.

Spinal Gray Matter

The gray matter within the central cord from dorsal to ventral respectively includes the dorsal horn, the medial commissure, and the anterior horn. Various types of sensory fibers end in different layers of the dorsal horn. The high-threshold, very thin, and unmyelinated A delta and C fibers, conducting impulses from the nociceptors, end almost exclusively in the substantia

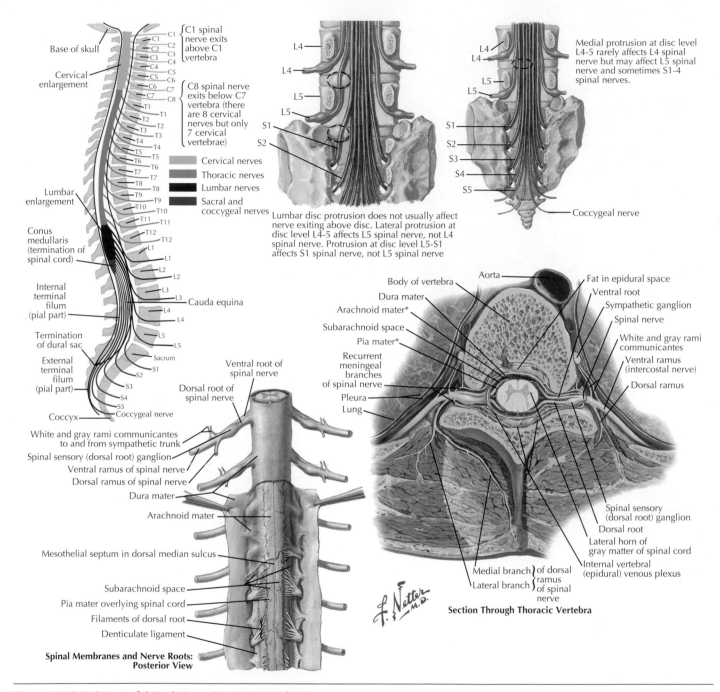

Figure 44-2 Relation of Spinal Nerve Roots to Vertebrae.

gelatinosa (lamina I and II). In contrast, nerves carrying the low-threshold mechanoreceptors subserving A beta fibers terminate in the deeper layers of the dorsal horn Rexed layers III-V. Lastly the largest, A alpha joint position sensory nerves end in the deepest layer VI of the dorsal horn (see Fig. 44-4).

Motor neurons are primarily contained within the anterior horn. The preponderant numbers of these somatic efferent neurons are primarily located within the cervical and lumbosacral enlargements (see Fig. 44-5). Here these provide the motor innervation for their respective extremities. In contrast, the ventral horn areas subsume a much smaller portion of the thoracic cord. Here the lateral horn of the gray matter becomes

preeminent, where it includes the **intermediolateral nucleus**. Here the preganglionic sympathetic neuron perikarya are located; similar neurons are also found within the brainstem (Fig. 44-6).

Vascular Supply

ARTERIAL

One anterior and two posterior spinal arteries course the length of the cord supplying the anterior two thirds and posterior one third of the cord, respectively (Fig. 44-7). Sulcal or central branches of the anterior spinal artery supply the central cord,

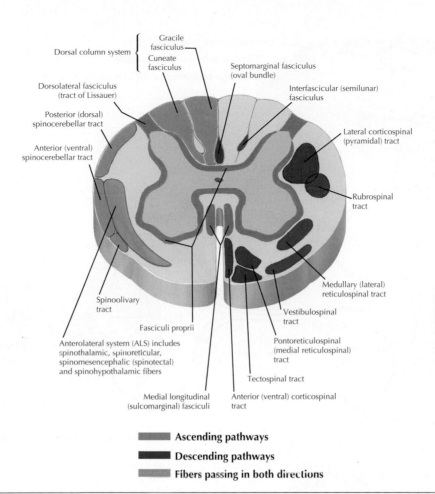

Figure 44-3 Principal Fiber Tracts of Spinal Cord.

whereas coronal or circumferential branches supply the ventral and lateral columns (Fig. 44-8).

Anterior spinal artery supplies the anterior horn, spinothalamic tract, and corticospinal tract.

Posterior spinal artery supplies the dorsal column, dorsal gray matter, and superficial dorsal aspect of lateral columns.

Vertebral artery medullary branches join the anterior and posterior spinal arteries to supply the cervical cord.

Aortic segmental arteries provide the supply for the remainder of the cord by branching into dural arteries that supply the dura and nerve root sleeve. *Radicular* branches supply the anterior and posterior nerve roots, and *medullary* branches join the anterior and posterior spinal arteries to supply the cord. Adamkiewicz's artery, at the lumbar enlargement, usually arises from the left side between T6 and L4. It provides the major arterial supply to the lower cord. The cord levels of C1–T2 and T9 caudally have excellent vascular supplies. In contrast, the T3–T8 arterial vasculature is more limited in number of vessels. Thus, this is usually considered a watershed area that is quite vulnerable to ischemic events.

Venous

The anteromedial cord (anterior horns and white matter) is drained by the central or sulcal veins into the anterior median spinal vein that extends the length of the cord. The anterolateral, peripheral, and dorsal cord capillary plexus drains into the radial veins. The radial veins subsequently drain into the coronal venous plexus on the spinal cord surface (Fig. 44-9). This plexus, with superficial spinal cord veins (anterior median, anterolateral, posterior median, posterior intermediate), drains into medullary veins. These are anatomically linked to the nerve roots traveling through the intervertebral foramen forming the epidural venous plexus. Subsequent drainage is to the inferior vena cava, azygous, and hemizygous veins.

PATHOANATOMY

Although a magnetic resonance image often expeditiously demonstrates the site and type of spinal cord abnormality, an appreciation of the anatomy and clinical temporal profile of the precise spinal cord disorder per se is fundamental to the care of every patient presenting with a myelopathy. Focal spinal cord lesions lead to degeneration of ascending tracts above the pathoanatomic site and descending tracts below the lesions. The key to localizing the site of spinal cord involvement is identifying the exact distribution of the various motor, reflex, and sensory deficits. These findings are the clinical expression of the site of pathology. Usually, but not always, a variable degree of motor dysfunction develops. All muscles subserved by the adjacent

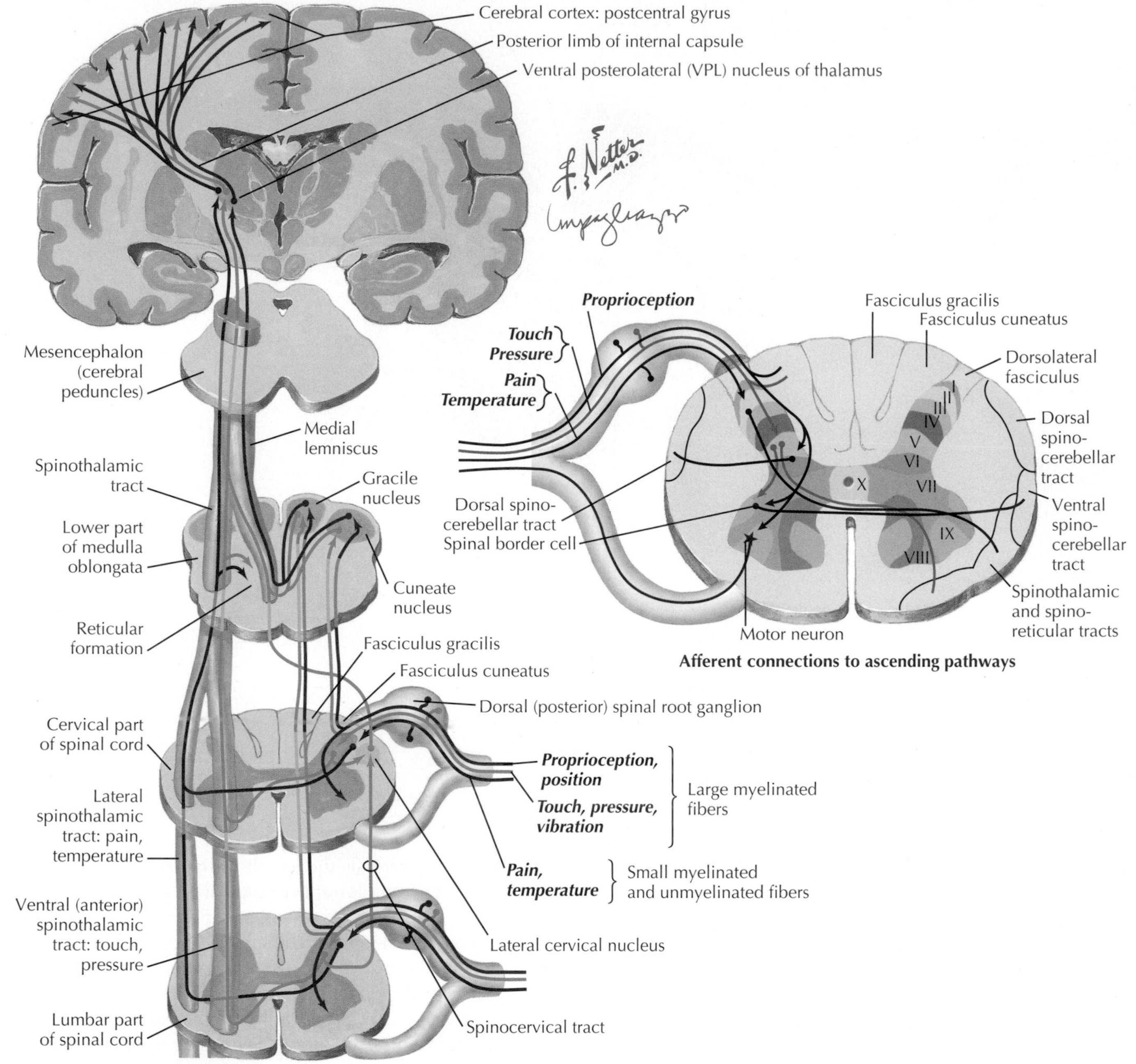

Cerebral cortex: postcentral gyrus
Posterior limb of internal capsule
Ventral posterolateral (VPL) nucleus of thalamus

Mesencephalon (cerebral peduncles)

Medial lemniscus

Spinothalamic tract

Gracile nucleus

Lower part of medulla oblongata

Reticular formation

Cuneate nucleus

Cervical part of spinal cord

Fasciculus gracilis
Fasciculus cuneatus

Dorsal (posterior) spinal root ganglion

Lateral spinothalamic tract: pain, temperature

Ventral (anterior) spinothalamic tract: touch, pressure

Lumbar part of spinal cord

Spinocervical tract

Lateral cervical nucleus

Proprioception, position
Touch, pressure, vibration } Large myelinated fibers

Pain, temperature } Small myelinated and unmyelinated fibers

Proprioception
Touch Pressure
Pain Temperature

Fasciculus gracilis
Fasciculus cuneatus
Dorsolateral fasciculus
Dorsal spinocerebellar tract
Ventral spinocerebellar tract
Spinothalamic and spinoreticular tracts

Dorsal spinocerebellar tract
Spinal border cell

Motor neuron

Afferent connections to ascending pathways

Figure 44-4 Spinal Cerebral Afferent Systems.

corticospinal tracts and/or the segmental anterior horn cells are affected respective to the spinal cord level (Fig. 44-10). Even though a patient is aware of subtle changes in performance, more indolent lesions are often not evident at first examination even by a skilled neurologist. This is particularly true with segmental lesions wherein one may have a subtle foot drop (L5) or weakness of intrinsic hand muscles (C8, T1).

Muscle stretch reflex examination can point to a precise site when there is loss of a specific reflex; for example, a diminished or absent triceps reflex pointing to a lesion at C7 or loss of the quadriceps (knee jerk) pointing to an L3, 4 lesion. Total loss of muscle stretch reflexes may occur with an acute spinal cord

lesion (spinal shock), such as a traumatic severance. Thus although loss of muscle stretch reflexes usually points to a peripheral nerve lesion such as the Guillain-Barré syndrome, one always needs to keep the possibility of an acute myelopathy. More traditionally, muscle stretch reflexes are increased with a central nervous system lesion; often Babinski signs and spinal clonus are also identified.

Lastly a very precise sensory evaluation is essential to the proper investigation of any potential myelopathy (Fig. 44-11). When the pathology affects the spinothalamic tract, assessment of pain and temperature sensation often provide the best evidence of a distinct *spinal level* of sensory loss. Often a *"cord level"*

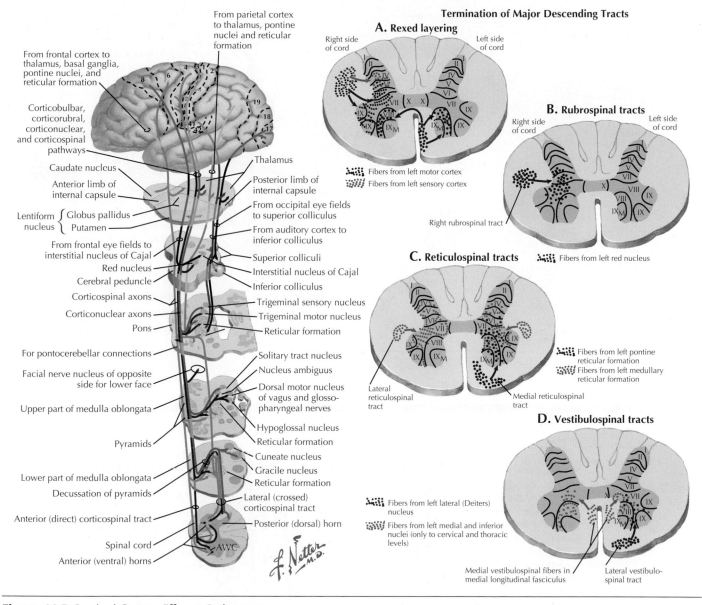

Figure 44-5 Cerebral Cortex: Efferent Pathways.

is a dramatic and distinct finding to elicit *if* one takes the time to do so. This can be elicited by using variable sensory modalities: a cold stimulus, such as the handle of a tuning fork; a safety pin; or just touching the skin (Fig. 44-12). Here the examiner takes one of these sensory tools and starting proximally or distally looks to see if there is a dramatic loss of appreciation if coming from the neck to the buttocks, or significant increased appreciation if one moves proximally in a reverse fashion. The patient's trunk must be examined both anteriorly and posteriorly. On occasion, one sees a patient in whom such was not performed at the initial evaluation and the precise anatomic localization not appreciated—thus a temporally important opportunity for treatment delayed or missed in its entirety. It is also vital to examine sensation in the extremities. Modalities such as position sense are best evaluated by moving the great toe or a finger subtly up or down and asking the patient to report its direction of movement from its prior position.

Utilizing the data obtained from these careful motor, sensory, and reflex examinations, one can make a very logical clinical judgment as to the type of lesion, that is, intramedullary, intradural extramedullary, and extradural extramedullary. There are some very classic patterns, as summarized in Figure 44-13.

INTRA-AXIAL SPINAL CORD PATHOLOGIES

Intramedullary Loci

Syringomyelia, or more rarely either an intramedullary cord tumor or a central hemorrhagic spinal necrosis present with a classic dissociated sensory syndrome. Classically these patients have a "cape loss" of pain and temperature modalities. That is, the patient may note loss of temperature and pain sensation limited to their hands, arms, and shoulders with preservation of

Sections through spinal cord at various levels

Dorsal lateral sulcus
Dorsal intermediate sulcus
Dorsal median sulcus
Lateral horn of gray matter (intermedio-lateral nucleus)
Gelatinous substance
White matter
Dorsal (posterior) horn
Gray matter
Commissure
Ventral (anterior) horn
Anterior white commissure
Ventral lateral sulcus
Ventral median fissure

C5
T2
L2
S2

Intermediolateral sympathetic column fiber tracts
Sympathetic trunk
Sympathetic trunk ganglion
Dorsal root
Thoracic part of spinal cord
Spinal ganglion
Spinal nerve to vessels and glands of skin
Ventral root
Recurrent meningeal branch (to spinal meninges and spinal perivascular plexuses)
White ramus communicans
Gray ramus communicans

Sympathetic fibers	Parasympathetic fibers	
—— preganglionic	—— preganglionic	—— Afferent fibers to spinal cord
- - - - postganglionic	- - - - postganglionic	—— Afferent fibers to brain stem

Figure 44-6 Spinal Cord Cross Sections: Fiber Tracts.

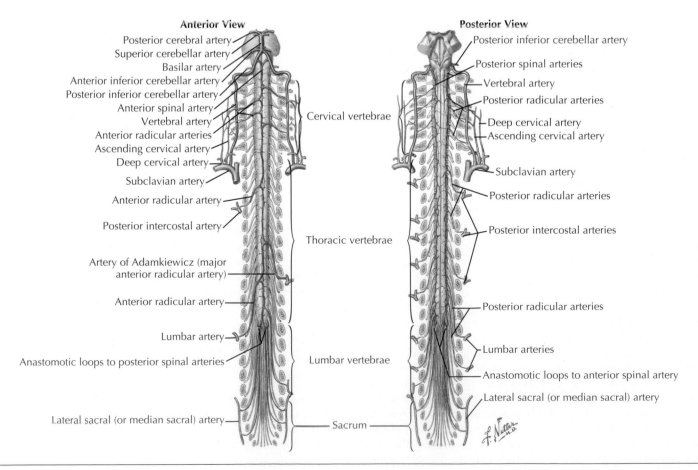

Anterior View

Posterior cerebral artery
Superior cerebellar artery
Basilar artery
Anterior inferior cerebellar artery
Posterior inferior cerebellar artery
Anterior spinal artery
Vertebral artery
Anterior radicular arteries
Ascending cervical artery
Deep cervical artery
Subclavian artery
Anterior radicular artery
Posterior intercostal artery
Artery of Adamkiewicz (major anterior radicular artery)
Anterior radicular artery
Lumbar artery
Anastomotic loops to posterior spinal arteries
Lateral sacral (or median sacral) artery

Cervical vertebrae
Thoracic vertebrae
Lumbar vertebrae
Sacrum

Posterior View

Posterior inferior cerebellar artery
Posterior spinal arteries
Vertebral artery
Posterior radicular arteries
Deep cervical artery
Ascending cervical artery
Subclavian artery
Posterior radicular arteries
Posterior intercostal arteries
Posterior radicular arteries
Lumbar arteries
Anastomotic loops to anterior spinal artery
Lateral sacral (or median sacral) artery

Figure 44-7 Arteries of Spinal Cord: Schema.

Section through Thoracic Spine

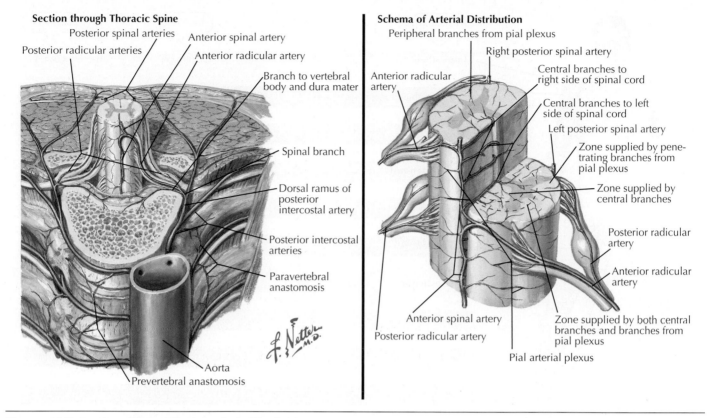

Posterior spinal arteries
Anterior spinal artery
Posterior radicular arteries
Anterior radicular artery
Branch to vertebral body and dura mater
Spinal branch
Dorsal ramus of posterior intercostal artery
Posterior intercostal arteries
Paravertebral anastomosis
Aorta
Prevertebral anastomosis

Schema of Arterial Distribution

Peripheral branches from pial plexus
Right posterior spinal artery
Central branches to right side of spinal cord
Anterior radicular artery
Central branches to left side of spinal cord
Left posterior spinal artery
Zone supplied by penetrating branches from pial plexus
Zone supplied by central branches
Posterior radicular artery
Anterior radicular artery
Anterior spinal artery
Posterior radicular artery
Zone supplied by both central branches and branches from pial plexus
Pial arterial plexus

Figure 44-8 Arteries of Spinal Cord: Intrinsic Distribution.

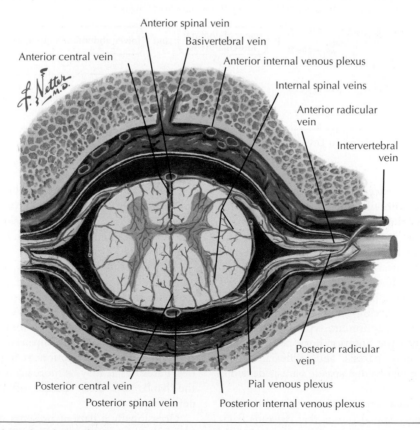

Anterior spinal vein
Basivertebral vein
Anterior central vein
Anterior internal venous plexus
Internal spinal veins
Anterior radicular vein
Intervertebral vein
Posterior radicular vein
Posterior central vein
Pial venous plexus
Posterior spinal vein
Posterior internal venous plexus

Figure 44-9 Veins of Spinal Cord and Vertebrae.

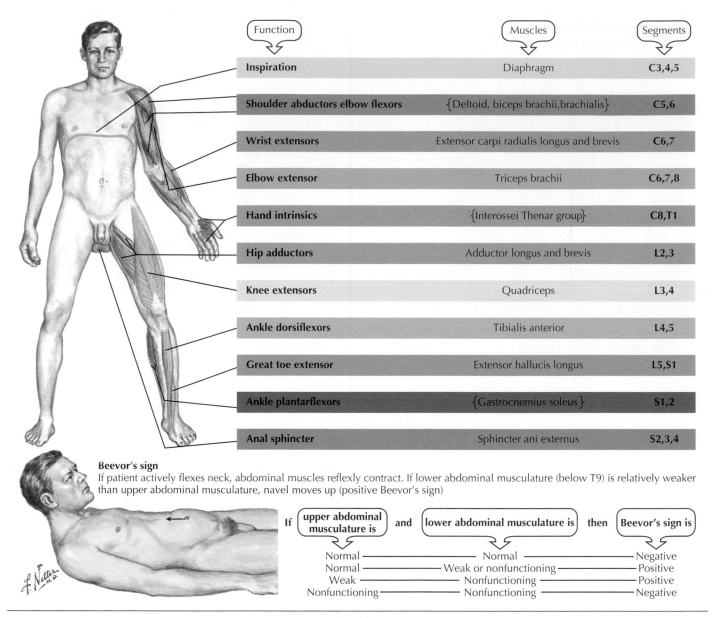

Function	Muscles	Segments
Inspiration	Diaphragm	**C3,4,5**
Shoulder abductors elbow flexors	{Deltoid, biceps brachii,brachialis}	**C5,6**
Wrist extensors	Extensor carpi radialis longus and brevis	**C6,7**
Elbow extensor	Triceps brachii	**C6,7,8**
Hand intrinsics	{Interossei Thenar group}	**C8,T1**
Hip adductors	Adductor longus and brevis	**L2,3**
Knee extensors	Quadriceps	**L3,4**
Ankle dorsiflexors	Tibialis anterior	**L4,5**
Great toe extensor	Extensor hallucis longus	**L5,S1**
Ankle plantarflexors	{Gastrocnemius soleus}	**S1,2**
Anal sphincter	Sphincter ani externus	**S2,3,4**

Beevor's sign
If patient actively flexes neck, abdominal muscles reflexly contract. If lower abdominal musculature (below T9) is relatively weaker than upper abdominal musculature, navel moves up (positive Beevor's sign)

If upper abdominal musculature is	and lower abdominal musculature is	then Beevor's sign is
Normal	Normal	Negative
Normal	Weak or nonfunctioning	Positive
Weak	Nonfunctioning	Positive
Nonfunctioning	Nonfunctioning	Negative

Figure 44-10 Motor Impairment Related to Level of Spinal Cord Injury.

same on the trunk and lower extremities. In this instance, the decussating pain and temperature fibers, such as C5-8 fibers, are damaged as they pass under the spinal cord's expanding central canal. Normally, these fibers join the ascending spinothalamic tracts from the legs and trunk to ascend to the brain (Fig. 44-14). Here temperature and pain sensation are intact distal to the site of the intramedullary lesion; thus there is a dissociation in the patient's ability to perceive these basic modalities proximally at the midcervical levels but preserving same below the affected areas. Light touch and proprioception are typically preserved. Extension of the lesion into the anterior horn cells leads to segmental neurogenic atrophy, paresis, and areflexia. As the corticospinal tracts become involved, a spastic paresis develops below the level of the syrinx.

Another form of dissociated sensory loss occurs in the rare instance of an intramedullary spinal tumor that expands from within destroying fiber tracts that are deep within the cord while it leaves intact the most peripheral portions of the spinothalamic tract carrying pain and temperature sensation from the S1-S5 regions, that is, the posterior thighs and buttocks. In this instance, when one examines the buttocks, a "saddle sparing" is present.

The posterior-lateral columns and often the adjacent corticospinal tracts may also be preferentially affected. Common examples include multiple sclerosis, vitamin B12 (cyanocobalamin) or copper deficiency, and HIV-associated vacuolar myelopathy. Here position and usually vibration modalities are primarily affected concomitant with impaired corticospinal tract function. Vibration and proprioception are impaired in the lower extremities. Paresthesiae may be more pronounced in the feet, although the hands are often earlier affected with cyanocobalamin deficiency.

Occasionally a patient presents with a primary intramedullary lesion that primarily affects the anterior spinal cord. The

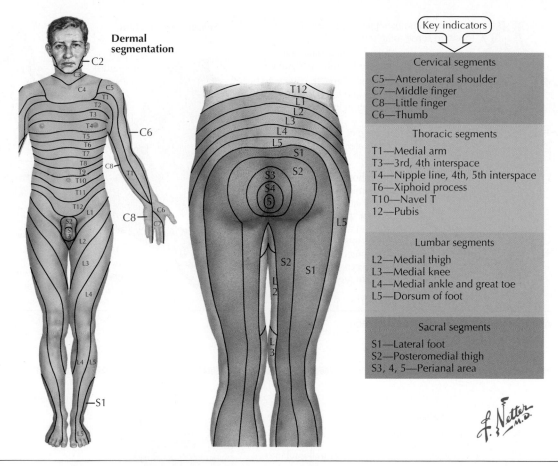

Dermal segmentation

Key indicators

Cervical segments

C5—Anterolateral shoulder
C7—Middle finger
C8—Little finger
C6—Thumb

Thoracic segments

T1—Medial arm
T3—3rd, 4th interspace
T4—Nipple line, 4th, 5th interspace
T6—Xiphoid process
T10—Navel T
12—Pubis

Lumbar segments

L2—Medial thigh
L3—Medial knee
L4—Medial ankle and great toe
L5—Dorsum of foot

Sacral segments

S1—Lateral foot
S2—Posteromedial thigh
S3, 4, 5—Perianal area

Figure 44-11 Sensory Impairment Related to Level of Spinal Cord Injury.

primary damage occurs within the spinal cord anatomy dependent on anterior spinal artery supply. In this instance, the patient experiences damage to the lateral spinothalamic and anterior and lateral spinothalamic tracts as well as the relevant anterior horn cells (see Fig. 44-12). Typically these patients become paraparetic or paraplegic, with a complete pain and temperature sensory loss below the level of the lesion. In essence, this is an anterior two thirds transverse spinal cord lesion. Therefore, these patients characteristically have preservation of proprioception modalities (position sense) as the posterior columns remain intact. Very rarely, weakness occurs in all four extremities when the cervical cord is infarcted; however, the abundance of collateral circulation at this level makes this an exceedingly rare clinical scenario. A posterior one-third myelopathy would be expected to lead to a sensory ataxia, spasticity, and hyperreflexia with preserved pain and temperature and corticospinal tract function; however, this clinical picture is extremely rare.

Intradural Extramedullary

Hemi-cord lesions: The *Brown-Sequard syndrome is a classic example*. The corticospinal tract subserves the ipsilateral extremities, as its decussation has previously occurred at the cervical medullary junction. Therefore, these patients have weakness appropriate to the side of the spinal lesion. In contrast, pain and temperature loss is confined to the contralateral

body as the fibers composing the spinothalamic tract have already decussated as it ascends within the cord. Thus, a left-sided lesion affects the right side's ability to perceive these modalities, whereas the motor loss is ipsilateral to the lesion site.

This combination of incongruous motor and sensory dysfunction is known as a *dissociated clinical pattern*. A good illustration is a 40-year-old woman who noted that her left leg was occasionally scuffing somewhat when she played tennis. Subsequently, she did not recognize having cut her right leg while shaving. Thus, she was developing a *hemicord Brown-Sequard syndrome* that proved to be at the thoracic spine level (Fig. 44-15).

As a lesion such as this increases in size, the other sensory modalities are sometimes affected ipsilateral to the spinal lesion. These include loss of position, that is, proprioceptive function. Sometimes vibration and touch modalities are also affected.

Extradural Extramedullary

Patients with this type of pathologic process may have either a diffuse or a solitary lesion. Many extradural processes are manifested by a widespread "seeding" representing an extension of some systemic process, including metastatic tumors, various parameningeal infections, or very rare granulomatous processes.

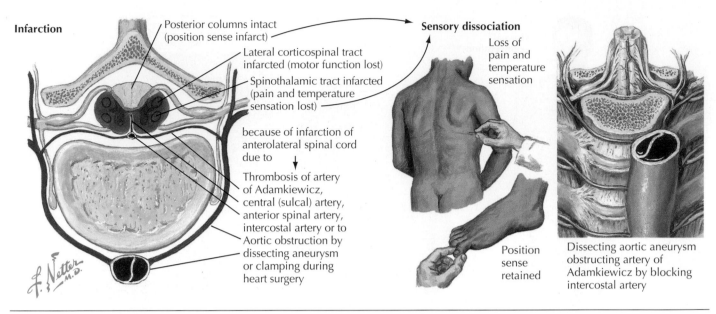

Infarction

Posterior columns intact
(position sense infarct)

Lateral corticospinal tract
infarcted (motor function lost)

Spinothalamic tract infarcted
(pain and temperature
sensation lost)

because of infarction of
anterolateral spinal cord
due to

Thrombosis of artery
of Adamkiewicz,
central (sulcal) artery,
anterior spinal artery,
intercostal artery or to
Aortic obstruction by
dissecting aneurysm
or clamping during
heart surgery

Sensory dissociation

Loss of
pain and
temperature
sensation

Position
sense
retained

Dissecting aortic aneurysm
obstructing artery of
Adamkiewicz by blocking
intercostal artery

Figure 44-12 Acute Spinal Cord Syndromes Pathology.

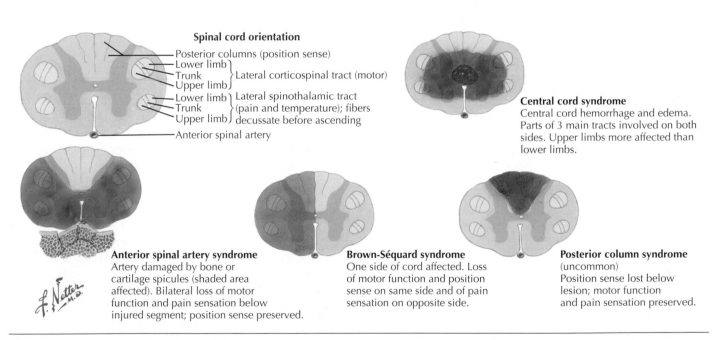

Spinal cord orientation

Posterior columns (position sense)

Lower limb ⎫
Trunk ⎬ Lateral corticospinal tract (motor)
Upper limb ⎭

Lower limb ⎫ Lateral spinothalamic tract
Trunk ⎬ (pain and temperature); fibers
Upper limb ⎭ decussate before ascending

Anterior spinal artery

Central cord syndrome
Central cord hemorrhage and edema.
Parts of 3 main tracts involved on both
sides. Upper limbs more affected than
lower limbs.

Anterior spinal artery syndrome
Artery damaged by bone or
cartilage spicules (shaded area
affected). Bilateral loss of motor
function and pain sensation below
injured segment; position sense preserved.

Brown-Séquard syndrome
One side of cord affected. Loss
of motor function and position
sense on same side and of pain
sensation on opposite side.

Posterior column syndrome
(uncommon)
Position sense lost below
lesion; motor function
and pain sensation preserved.

Figure 44-13 Incomplete Spinal Cord Syndromes.

Focal bony lesions, often from metastases, are the typical example of an extramedullary extradural lesion. These may present subacutely or relatively acutely from pathologic fracture dislocation and extension of the tumor leading to rapid cord compromise (Fig. 44-16). Characteristically, these patients experience pain secondary to involvement of the pain-sensitive meninges, its adjacent sensory nerve roots, or the concomitant bone as occurs with metastatic cancers. Therefore, pain is one of the hallmarks of many extradural extramedullary disorders. As the size of the lesion increases, direct pressure is applied to the adjacent spinal cord, or the primary vascular supply is compromised, predominantly affecting the anterior two thirds of the cord, or both. Often these lesions expand or displace cord tissue acutely, essentially leading to a pathophysiologic cord transection. Thus, the final clinical picture may mimic a traumatic myelopathy; it is therefore of paramount importance to expeditiously evaluate these patients in order to preserve cord function.

More chronically, a progressive cervical spondylosis will produce spinal stenosis leading to a gradual relatively symmetric

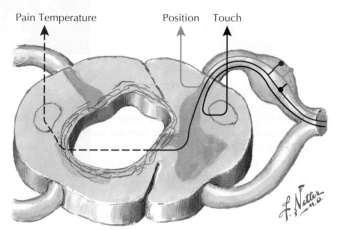

Pain Temperature   Position   Touch

Diagram demonstrating interruption of crossed pain and temperature fibers by syrinx; uncrossed light touch and proprioception fibers preserved

Figure 44-14 Syringomyelia.

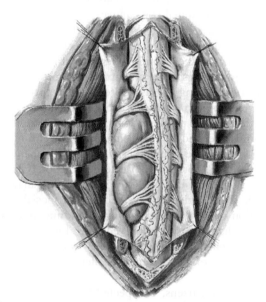

Intradural extramedullary tumor (meningioma) compressing spinal cord and deforming nerve roots

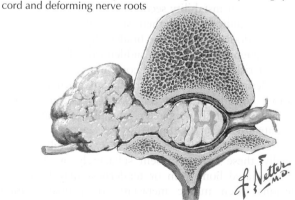

Dumbbell tumor (neurilemmoma) growing out along spinal nerve through intervertebral foramen (neurofibromas of von Recklinghausen disease may act similarly)

Figure 44-15 Intradural Extramedullary Tumors of Spinal Cord.

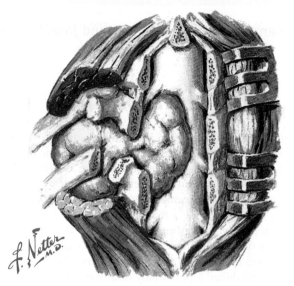

Lymphoma invading spinal canal via intervertebral foramen, compressing dura mater and spinal cord

Figure 44-16 Extradural Tumors.

cord compression. Typically, these patients evidence posterior column and corticospinal tract dysfunction. This is manifested by numbness in the feet and tendency to a spastic gait.

Transverse Myelopathy, Complete Spinal Cord Lesions

When one is faced with lesions extensively damaging the entire spinal cord, the resultant clinical picture is characterized by total interruption of all sensory and motor functions below the damaged level. An acute insult causes flaccid paralysis and areflexia secondary to "spinal shock"; subsequently, spasticity and hyperreflexia develop, as in more ingravescent lesions. These chronic lesions are associated with a slowly evolving weakness. If the anterior horn cells, ventral roots, or both are also involved, lower motor neuron signs, including fasciculations, atrophy, areflexia, and weakness, occur at the lesion level. An extensive cord insult is necessary to completely affect touch sensation as both the posterior columns and spinothalamic tracts provide touch. The demonstration of a sensory level, assessed by testing pain and temperature (spinothalamic tract), segmental paresthesiae, or radicular pain, often helps to localize the spinal cord level.

ADDITIONAL RESOURCES

Bradley WG, Daroff RB, Fenichel B, et al. Neurology in Clinical Practice. 5th ed. Philadelphia: Elsevier; 2008.

Brodal P. The Central Nervous System. 3rd ed. Oxford, UK: Oxford University Press; 2003.

Ropper A, Samuels M. Adams and Victor's Principles of Neurology. 9th ed. New York: McGraw-Hill; 2009.

Rowland LP, Pedley TA. Merritt's Neurology. 11th ed. Baltimore, MD: Lippincott, Williams, and Wilkins; 2010.

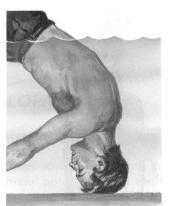

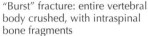

"Burst" fracture: entire vertebral body crushed, with intraspinal bone fragments

Mechanism: vertical blow on the head as in diving or surfing accident, being thrown from car, or football injury

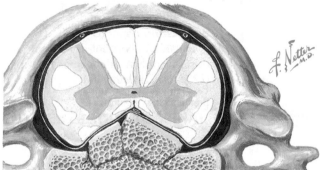

Dislocated bone fragments compressing spinal cord and spinal artery: blood supply to anterior two thirds of spinal cord is impaired

Figure 45-2 Trauma.

thoracic spine pain. During the next 2 days, his pain worsened even while lying in bed. Neither meperidine, a narcotic agent, nor a muscle relaxant relieved his pain and paraspinal muscle spasm. His difficulties rapidly worsened as he began to have trouble walking, lost sensation in his legs, and became unable to urinate.

Neurologic examination demonstrated an acutely ill febrile individual with a flaccid paraplegia, brisk muscle stretch reflexes at the knees, bilateral Babinski signs, loss of position sense in the feet and a cord level to both pin and temperature sensation at T6. There was percussion tenderness over his upper thoracic spinous processes. MRI demonstrated an extensive epidural collection extending from C6 to T10. Emergency laminectomy was performed, which demonstrated a purulent epidural abscess. Despite the emergent surgery, the patient was still significantly limited a few months later.

Epidural spinal abscess is a rare clinical process occurring in 2–20 cases per 100,000 hospital admissions. Its incidence appears to be increasing; these are usually seen in middle-aged adults, more often men. Despite its rarity, the potential for an epidural abscess to cause permanent paraplegia makes it one of the most urgent spinal cord emergencies (Fig. 45-6). Even though back

pain is such a ubiquitous and usually benign process, it is very important for any physician to consider the potential diagnosis of an epidural abscess in every patient presenting with acute and increasing back pain, especially when febrile. The epidural space in the posterior thoracic cord is the primary site for an epidural spinal abscess to develop. These may extend to the cervical cord and rarely into the lumbar spine. Experimental studies suggest that the mass effect of the abscess, leading to cord compression, is the important clinicopathologic mechanism.

Staphylococcus aureus is the predominant etiologic microorganism leading to epidural spinal abscesses. Usually a distant septic focus provides bacterial seeding via the bloodstream, for example, skin furuncles, dental abscesses, simple pharyngitis, or a recently infected traumatic site (see Fig. 45-6). Often there is a concomitant history of diabetes mellitus, alcoholism, drug abuse, or recent spinal or extraspinal trauma. Less commonly, epidural spinal abscesses develop subsequent to vertebral osteomyelitis, pulmonary or urinary infection, sepsis, or extremely rarely bacterial endocarditis. Invasive procedures, including epidural anesthesia, spinal surgery, vascular access lines, and paravertebral injections, also provide potential mechanisms for bacterial seeding. Corticosteroid therapy may contribute to immune suppression and the possibility of secondary nosocomial infections.

Percussion tenderness over the posterior spinal processes, as well as fever, are important diagnostic clues compatible with an epidural spinal abscess Some of these individuals also develop signs of meningeal irritation such as Kernig's sign. A rapidly developing combination of motor, sensory, and sphincter dysfunction then occurs. Often the patient becomes paraplegic and demonstrates a spinal cord sensory level. The differential diagnosis includes acute central disc, epidural metastasis often with acute pathologic fracture, and spontaneous or anticoagulation-induced hematoma.

An urgent MRI easily identifies the epidural abscess. Concomitantly, there may be a highly elevated C-reactive protein and erythrocyte sedimentation rate, often >70 mm/hour, with a modestly elevated WBC count. Emergency surgical decompression is the treatment of choice. Occasionally when no significant neurologic compromise exists, antibiotics are the primary treatment. However, careful follow-up is indicated as the patient's clinical picture may rapidly evolve with motor and sensory loss leading to need for another MRI and surgical intervention.

Prognosis depends entirely on the patient's expeditious presentation to a medical facility and the clinician's level of suspicion leading to relatively early diagnosis of the epidural spinal abscess. If treatment is not initiated until after the patient becomes paraplegic, prognosis is extremely guarded.

Spinal Epidural Hematoma

Fortunately a spinal epidural hematoma is a relatively rare lesion with an acute to subacute onset. Some of these occurrences are related to anticoagulation therapy, particularly warfarin or heparin. If an anticoagulated patient sustains back or neck trauma or develops symptoms mimicking an acute meningitis that in most circumstances requires an emergent spinal puncture, and the unwary clinician has not recognized that the patient is anticoagulated, performance of a lumbar puncture

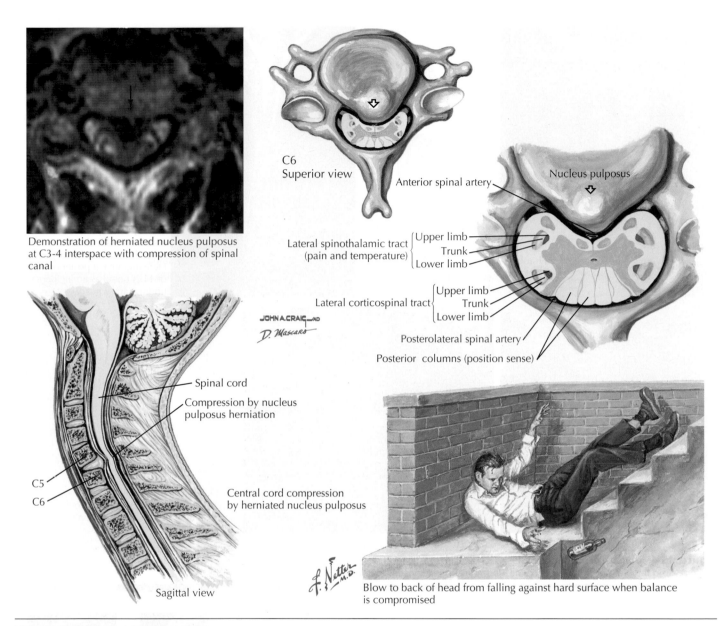

Demonstration of herniated nucleus pulposus at C3-4 interspace with compression of spinal canal

C6 Superior view

Anterior spinal artery

Nucleus pulposus

Lateral spinothalamic tract (pain and temperature) { Upper limb / Trunk / Lower limb

Lateral corticospinal tract { Upper limb / Trunk / Lower limb

Posterolateral spinal artery

Posterior columns (position sense)

Spinal cord

Compression by nucleus pulposus herniation

C5

C6

Central cord compression by herniated nucleus pulposus

Sagittal view

Blow to back of head from falling against hard surface when balance is compromised

Figure 45-3 Cervical Disc Herniation.

(LP) is very dangerous. The patient is at risk to develop an acutely evolving paraparesis/paraplegia within 12–24 hours. By the time the effects of the anticoagulation are reversed, surgical intervention may be too late to regain neurologic function; this is truly an iatrogenic lesion that is preventable by careful assessment of all patient medications prior to performing the LP.

Spontaneous spinal epidural hematomas are being defined more frequently with the more widespread use of MRI. Very occasionally, spinal epidural hematomas seem to occur spontaneously. However, it is suggested that antiplatelet agents such as acetylsalicylic (Aspirin) or clopidogrel (Plavix) therapy may be a contributory risk factor. These lesions may present with subacutely evolving thoracic or cervical spine pain, evolving weakness, and urinary retention. Surgical decompression is the usual means of therapy, and the prognosis may be better than with those for the patient taking major anticoagulants.

ACUTE INTRADURAL INTRAMEDULLARY SPINAL LESIONS

Myelitis Secondary to Multiple Sclerosis

Clinical Vignette

Right arm weakness acutely developed in a 30-year-old woman. In retrospect, she had noted some numbness in that arm for the past 3 months, and 16 months earlier she experienced blurred vision in her right eye, with intermittent dizziness. She also had experienced episodic momentary electric shock, lightning-like sensation radiating to her buttocks often precipitated by bending her neck. Hot weather was more uncomfortable for her as she reported worsening of these symptoms and nonspecific fatigue. She

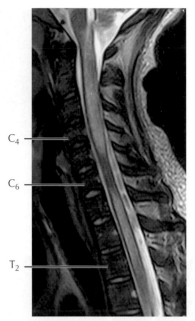

A. Transverse myelitis. Sagittal T2-weighted fast spin echo fat-saturated image demonstrates increased signal from the medulla to C5 with a short skip segment continuing from C7 into the upper thoracic spinal cord. The signal changes are accompanied by swelling within the spinal cord with long segment involvement more typical of transverse myelitis seen in neuromyelitis optica (Devic).

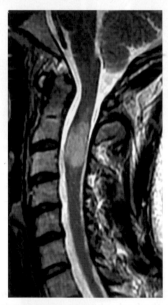

B. Acute cervical spinal cord multiple sclerosis. Sagittal T2-weighted fast spin echo image demonstrates increased signal involving the upper spinal cord in addition to expansion (arrows).

Figure 45-7 Myelitis Secondary to Neuromyelitis Optica (Devic) and Multiple Sclerosis.

had involvement of her right arm, implying extension into the right anterior horn. The presence of the subclinical brain MRI abnormalities, as well as the prolonged VERs, point to multiplicity of demyelinating lesions in time and space consistent with the diagnosis of MS (Table 45-1).

Table 45-1 Acute Intradural Intramedullary Myelopathies	
Inflammatory	
Transverse myelitis	Multiple sclerosis
	Neuromyelitis optica
	Systemic lupus erythematosus
	Sjögren syndrome
	Sarcoidosis
	Schistosomiasis
Vascular	Infarction
Anterior cord syndrome	
Infectious	HTLV-I
	HIV
	Syphilis
	Tuberculosis
	Other bacteria, viruses, fungi, and parasites, e.g., schistosomiasis
Trauma	Hematomyelia
Central cord syndrome	

Transverse Myelitis

Clinical Vignette

A 16-year-old boy suddenly began to walk with both knees in a flexed posture. Initially, his parents thought he was just joking. However, later that evening he began to experience knife-like pain in midback radiating around his ribs toward his epigastrium. The next morning, he awakened unable to get out of bed. He was unable to void. On neurologic examination he was paraplegic, his muscle stretch reflexes were absent, and his plantar response "ambiguous." Sensory exam suggested a T10 level for both pain and temperature modalities.

Pertinent laboratory findings included CSF findings with a protein 175 mg/dL, and 30 WBC with 90% lymphocytes. Nerve conductions demonstrated prolonged F waves but otherwise normal motor and sensory nerve conductions. The spinal cord had a focal demyelinating lesion with gadolinium enhancement involving most of its transverse diameter at T9–T11. Unfortunately a course of intravenous (IV) methylprednisolone was ineffective; he remained paraplegic, with a persistent dense sensory level and ongoing incontinence.

Very often, there is no underlying pathology identified with many transverse myelitis (TM) cases. Acute transverse myelitis most likely represents another type of autoimmune CNS disorder. A nonspecific "viral infection" may be the inciting mechanism or sometimes a bacterial infection, and rarely this may occur subsequent to immunization. Sometimes, a transverse myelitis is preceded by or associated with optic neuritis. This is known as neuromyelitis optica (NMO), an unusual autoimmune demyelinating disorder associated with a very specific serum autoantibody referred to as NMO-IgG (Fig. 45-7). This antibody binds to the CNS-dominant water channel, aquaporin 4; this is a structure that is normally present on astrocytes. The diagnostic criteria for neuromyelitis optica include optic neuritis, acute myelitis, and two of the following three: brain MRI not characteristic for multiple sclerosis, contiguous spinal cord MRI lesion extending over three or more vertebral segments, and NMO-IgG positive status.

Motor, sensory, and sphincter disturbances vary in degree if the process begins subacutely. However, with an acute onset, a lesion can rapidly develop, mimicking a traumatic lesion with paraplegia or quadriplegia, total sensory loss, and absence of bladder and rectal sphincter function as per the above vignette. A complete transverse myelitis interrupts all ascending tracts below the lesion, leading to a "sensory level" and concomitantly a flaccid paraplegia or tetraplegia depending on the lesion level as all descending tracts above the pathologic site, particularly the corticospinal tracts, are compromised. Over time, spasticity develops. Interruption of the anterior and lateral spinothalamic tracts and dorsal columns leads to the cord level. Pinprick or temperature sensation is the most easily localized, with loss 1–2 levels below the lesion site. Bladder and bowel functions are also impaired.

Differential diagnosis includes cord infarct, arteriovenous malformation, radiation myelopathy, metastatic or intrinsic tumors, and central cord compression for a spondylotic central disc. Very rarely, TM is part of an acute disseminated encephalomyelitis. Systemic lupus erythematosus (SLE), other types of vasculitis, sarcoidosis, Sjögren syndrome, antiphospholipid antibody syndrome, and *Schistosoma mansoni* parasitic infection are other predisposing mechanisms.

MRI with gadolinium is the procedure of choice to exclude compressive lesions, especially when history and exam suggest a specific level of spinal cord dysfunction (see Fig. 45-7). Brain lesions consistent with MS are demonstrated with MRI in approximately half of all TM patients. Transverse myelitis appears with T2 signal hyperintensity on MRI. The area of signal abnormality may be focal or extensive in cross section and length. Gadolinium enhancement is frequent. Cord swelling is present to variable degrees. Large cross-sectional area, multi-segment length, cord expansion, and peripheral enhancement are most consistent with a diagnosis of TM. In contrast, MS lesions tend to be smaller, usually involving only 1–2 segments, and are often multifocal. Total cross-sectional area and multi-segment length are uncommon in MS, although cord expansion and enhancement are frequent with larger acute inflammatory MS lesions. Gadolinium-enhanced brain MRI, and optical coherence tomography (OCT), even more than visual evoked potentials (Chapter 46), help determine the presence of multifocal demyelinating disease. Associated cerebral white matter lesions and oligoclonal bands in CSF increase the later probability of developing unequivocal MS. Oligoclonal bands, however, are nonspecific for multiple sclerosis and not always present in individuals with multiple sclerosis.

When evaluating a patient with TM for the presence of infection or systemic inflammatory disease, a lumbar puncture is indicated for CSF analysis (cell count, protein, oligoclonal bands, culture, glucose, and viral polymerase chain reactions [PCR]) and or viral titers, and serologies. Blood work required includes ESR, C-reactive protein, antinuclear antibodies, anti-DNA antibodies, SSA, SSB, anticardiolipin antibodies, lupus anticoagulant, complement, and angiotensin-converting enzyme. Viral and bacterial screen might include varicella zoster,

enterovirus, Coxsackie virus, Epstein-Barr virus, cytomegalovirus, herpes simplex, hepatitis, HIV, and Lyme titers.

Methylprednisolone, 1 g intravenously for 5–10 days, is indicated in all TM patients as occasional NMO patients respond to this therapy and/or plasma exchange. However, there is always a variable degree of response. The degree of recovery depends on the rapidity of development and severity of deficit. Unfortunately, most NMO patients may have significant optic nerve and spinal cord deficits and a tendency to have severe relapses. Intermittent or chronic immunosuppressive treatment is often indicated. Such a temporal profile also occurs with SLE, antiphospholipid antibody syndrome, and vascular malformations of the cord. In contrast, a relapsing and recurring transverse myelitis is rare when TM is not a manifestation of either NMO or MS.

Spinal Cord Infarction/Ischemic Myelopathy
ANTERIOR SPINAL ARTERY SYNDROME

Clinical Vignette

A vigorous 56-year-old state police officer was found to have an extensive thoracoabdominal aneurysm requiring heroic surgical repair with replacement of his entire descending aorta from its arch in the chest to the distal bifurcation within the abdomen. Although the primary surgical procedure appeared to be successful, when the patient awakened he was unable to move his legs or empty his bladder and he had numbness distal to T8–T10. Neurologic examination demonstrated the patient to be paraplegic but with preserved strength in his arms and upper body, loss of temperature and pain sensation, with a vague numbness from his upper abdomen to the tips of his toes, and preserved position and vibratory sensation.

Thoracic and cervical MRI performed within a few hours of his awakening was normal. This excluded a mass lesion potentially capable of being surgically treated but could not reveal an early spinal cord infarct. The patient's clinical course was otherwise stable. When there was no improvement in his neurologic status, he was transferred to a spinal rehabilitation unit.

The clinical picture of paralysis secondary to loss of corticospinal tract function and sensory change from impaired spinothalamic function, as well as infarction of the anterior horn cells, but with very preserved posterior column function, is classic for an anterior spinal artery distribution spinal cord infarction (Fig. 45-8). Onset of anterior spinal artery syndrome, although usually sudden, may occasionally be gradual over hours or days.

Because of the significant collateral circulation, spinal cord infarction is very much less common than cerebral ischemia; thus spinal cord infarction and transient ischemic attacks involving the spinal cord rarely occur. This diagnosis must be considered in patients who present with sudden onset of nontraumatic weakness, a sensory loss with a definable level to pain and temperature with preserved posterior column function, and bladder dysfunction. Paresthesia or radicular pain can occur at

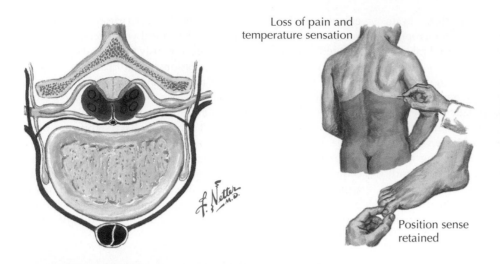

Loss of pain and temperature sensation

Position sense retained

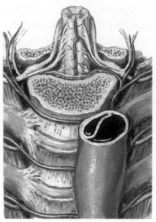

Dissecting aortic aneurysm obstructing artery of Adamkiewicz by blocking intercostal artery

A. Sagittal T2-weighted MR image showing slightly enlarged spinal cord with patchy increased T2 signal representing edema. **B.** Sagittal T1-weighted MR image with only minimal enhancement within the spinal cord.

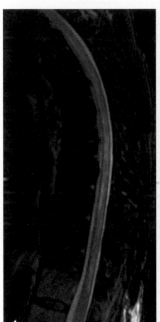

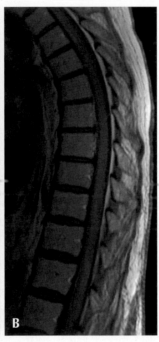

Figure 45-8 Spinal Cord Infarction.

the infarct level. Patients may develop either a bilateral flaccid paraplegia or quadriplegia depending on the site of cord occlusion. At the cervical level, the arms are flaccid and eventually atrophic because of anterior horn involvement, although the legs become spastic. Thoracic cord infarcts lead to a spastic paraplegia. Initial areflexia changes to hyperreflexia with the presence of Babinski signs.

Spinal cord infarction is typically secondary to inadequate arterial flow through the anterior spinal artery, which supplies the anterior funiculi, anterior horns, base of the dorsal horns, and anteromedial aspects of the lateral funiculi. Thus, the corticospinal and spinothalamic tracts are affected bilaterally. The upper to midthoracic spinal cord is poorly vascularized, and these watershed zones are more susceptible to infarction. Interruption of blood supply from the aorta to the intramedullary spinal vasculature can cause infarction. In contrast, a posterior spinal artery infarction is rare because of well-developed collaterals.

Spontaneous dissecting aneurysms of the descending thoracic or upper abdominal aorta can occlude the ostia of segmental spinal arteries; atherosclerosis of the aorta and its branches, and iatrogenic ischemia from recent aortic surgery are the usual pathophysiologic mechanisms predisposing to spinal cord infarction. Aortic surgical procedures may reduce vascular supply to the radicular and spinal arteries. Procedures such as thoracotomy and nephrectomy sometimes compromise intercostal or lumbar artery flow, which give rise to radicular arteries. The presence of concomitant chest or abdominal pain, limb ischemia, or loss of peripheral pulses suggests a possible aortic dissection.

Very rarely emboli or arteritis may be responsible for an intramedullary cord infarction. Emboli to the anterior spinal artery may be derived from atheromatous, septic, fibrocartilaginous, and air (decompression illness/caisson disease) sources. Vascular angiitis with subsequent thrombosis from primary CNS vasculitis, syphilis, tuberculosis, sarcoidosis, and schistosomiasis can all cause cord infarction.

Differential Diagnosis

Any condition that leads to a rapid onset of a partial transverse spinal cord lesion must be considered, including trauma, metastatic cancer, dural arteriovenous malformations, acute transverse myelitis, MS, and intramedullary tumors. Usually these lesions do not spare posterior column function, and thus position sense is affected in contrast to its presence with anterior spinal artery lesions. Spinal claudication alternatively presents as exercise-induced painless lower extremity weakness.

MRI can exclude these other lesions. Infarction appears isointense on T1 and eventually hyperintense on T2. When MRI is not available or contraindicated, a CT/myelogram can exclude cord compression, but provides less information regarding the spinal cord per se. Spinal fluid evaluation can help detect infection, demyelinating disease, and subarachnoid hemorrhage. In the acute setting, the potential concomitant diagnosis of a dissecting aortic aneurysm must be considered and appropriate body imaging pursued. If negative, studies to search for a cardiac source of embolism, vasculitis, hypercoagulable states, and aortic atherosclerosis are indicated.

Therapy

With the exception of an aortic dissection where surgery may be indicated to preserve life, treatment is supportive. Aneurysmal repair will not affect spinal cord damage. Underlying etiologic factors must be corrected, if possible, when discovered.

Prognosis

This depends on the level of anterior spinal artery occlusion, which determines whether the patient is paraplegic or quadriplegic. Once the infarction occurs recovery is rare, although it is possible. Less commonly, the arterial occlusion is farther from the cord, so the chance for collateral arterial supply is greater. Slow, gradual occlusion is offset by collateral development. Anatomic variations are also important; damage to a particular intercostal artery can be of variable importance. Hypoxia and low perfusion pressure aggravate damage caused by ischemia.

POSTERIOR SPINAL ARTERY SYNDROME

A rare spinal stroke, the posterior spinal artery syndrome presents with ataxia, loss of position, vibration, and fine tactile sensation and bladder and bowel disturbance. Well-developed arterial collaterals on the posterior cord account for the extreme rarity of this type of myelopathy.

CHRONIC MYELOPATHIES

EXTRADURAL MYELOPATHIES

Cervical Spondylosis

Clinical Vignette

An obese septuagenarian, with previously diagnosed diabetic polyneuropathy manifested by burning discomfort in his feet, presented with a 4- to 6-month history of increasing leg numbness. These new symptoms were totally different from the mild tingling and burning that had been chronically present for the past 10 years. He began to require a cane to maintain his equilibrium when walking. Although he initially tolerated the newer symptoms, he began to be concerned that he could not walk safely without relying on a walker. He sought further medical opinion. He previously had a myocardial infarction.

Neurologic examination demonstrated a broad-based, spastic gait, brisk muscle stretch reflexes, and bilateral Babinski signs. Pinprick and temperature sensation were reduced in a stocking-glove distribution in his legs. There was a question of a bilateral cord level to pin sensation at C-7. Position sense was absent at the toes, and vibratory sense lost at the ankles.

MRI revealed spinal stenosis and cord edema at C5–C6. He had severe spinal stenosis with multilevel spondylosis, disc protrusion, and end-plate osteophytes. After a 3-month period of observation, his gait difficulties increased. A cervical posterior laminectomy was performed. Subsequently, after a period of rehabilitation hospitalization, he gradually regained the ability to walk independently.

One needs to always carefully evaluate the patient with a chronic primary sensory polyneuropathy who begins to develop disproportionately increased gait difficulty. Cervical spinal stenosis is a common chronic disorder. As occurred in this instance, one may define a quite remediable condition.

Spondylosis, a normal aging process, is the most common cause of a cervical myelopathy (Figs. 45-9 and 45-10; Box 45-2). This results from disc degeneration followed by reactive osteophyte formation, fibrocartilaginous bars, spondylotic transverse bars, articular facet hypertrophy, and thickening of the ligamentum flavum causing spinal canal narrowing. Subsequently, gradual spinal cord compression may occur; it is particularly likely in patients having congenitally narrowed spinal canals. In its simplest form, a chronically herniated central nucleus pulposus in patients with congenital stenosis can produce a cervical myelopathy. Although many senior individuals have radiographic signs of cervical spondylosis, most are asymptomatic.

Box 45-2 Chronic Extradural Extramedullary Myelopathies

Spondylosis disc osteophyte complex with chronic disc protrusion
Arteriovenous malformation
Lymphoma
Miscellaneous disorders sometimes affecting spinal cord:
  Pott disease (tuberculosis)
  Paget disease
  Rheumatoid arthritis
Primary bone tumors with secondary invasion of the epidural space:
  Hemangioma, chondrosarcoma, osteogenic sarcoma
Lipoma

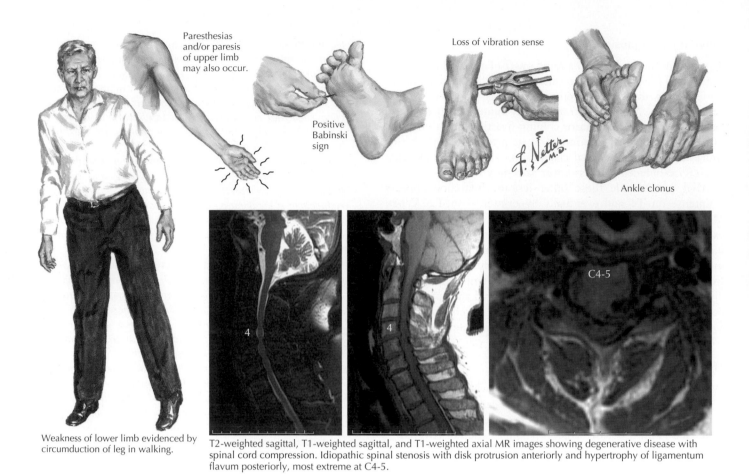

Paresthesias and/or paresis of upper limb may also occur.

Positive Babinski sign

Loss of vibration sense

Ankle clonus

Weakness of lower limb evidenced by circumduction of leg in walking.

T2-weighted sagittal, T1-weighted sagittal, and T1-weighted axial MR images showing degenerative disease with spinal cord compression. Idiopathic spinal stenosis with disk protrusion anteriorly and hypertrophy of ligamentum flavum posteriorly, most extreme at C4-5.

Figure 45-9 Cervical Spondylosis.

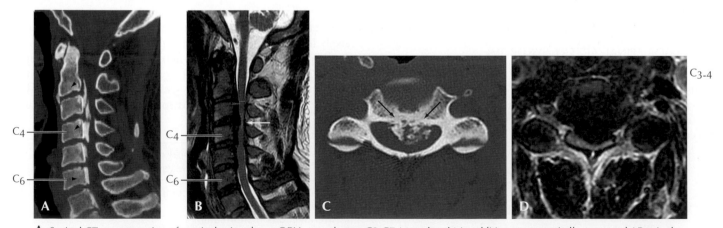

A. Sagittal CT reconstruction of cervical spine shows OPLL at each area C2-C7 (arrowheads) in addition to congenitally narrowed AP spinal canal dimensions. **B.** Sagittal T2-weighted fast spin echo image demonstrates similar findings with ossification demonstrated as signal void anterior to the compressed spinal cord. Note spinal cord edema at C3-C4 (arrow). **C.** Axial CT image with large ossification in anterior spinal canal (arrows). **D.** Axial T2-weighted fast spin echo fat-saturated image demonstrates severe spinal cord compression with edema most remarkable on the left.

Figure 45-10 Imaging of Ossification of Posterior Longitudinal Ligament (OPLL).

When a myelopathy develops, clinical findings can present acutely, subacutely, or over many years. Sometimes both a cervical myelopathy and adjacent radiculopathy may occur in the same spondylotic patient.

PATHOPHYSIOLOGY AND ETIOLOGY

Typically, the spinal canal is 17–18 mm in diameter between C3 and C7. A narrower cervical spinal canal may range from 9 to 15 mm; however, a compressive spondylitic myelopathy rarely occurs when the canal diameter is >13 mm. Cervical cord diameter ranges from 8.5 to 11.5 mm, averaging approximately 10 mm. Disc protrusion and other reactive and degenerative processes further reduce canal dimension. Direct cord compression, compromised blood supply to the cord or venous stasis, and other mechanical factors, such as rheumatoid arthritis, can in combination or independently cause irreversible damage.

Normally, the spinal cord moves cephalad and posteriorly within the canal during neck flexion and caudally and anteriorly during neck extension. If osteophytes, discs, and hypertrophied ligaments make contact with the cord, the cord sustains additive trauma, leading to development of a clinical myelopathy. The disc levels affected are C5–C6, C6–C7, and C3–C4, in order of their clinical frequency.

In this setting, the spinal cord may become pathologically, grossly flattened, distorted, or indented. Demyelination of the lateral columns occurs at the lesion site with consequent lateral column degeneration below the lesion. Concomitant dorsal column degeneration occurs at and above the damaged segment(s). There may also be damage and loss of nerve cells in gray matter. Ischemic changes, gliosis, demyelination, and even cavitation necrosis sometimes also result.

CLINICAL PRESENTATION

The patient may initially note a tendency for his foot to drag or scuff on rugs or curbs. Limb paresthesias are generally relatively mild dysesthesiae often mimicking a polyneuropathy. As this disorder evolves with more significant cervical cord involvement, an increasingly severe proprioceptive loss occurs, often leading to a sensory ataxia. Examination demonstrates mild asymmetric spasticity with upper motor neuron corticospinal tract findings including hyperreflexia, and Babinski signs primarily related to lateral cord compression. Diminished position and/or vibration sense are markers of posterior column pressure. Bowel and bladder disturbances are usually late findings. If there is concomitant ventral cord compression, the anterior horn cells within the gray matter may be damaged, characterized by muscle fasciculations, atrophy, and weakness appropriate to the affected nerve roots.

Neck pain varies. Lhermitte's sign may occur, characterized by recurrent lightning-like paresthesias traversing down the back with neck flexion. When the syndrome is purely spinal, a myelopathy without root signs or symptoms occurs. However, a radicular syndrome occasionally accompanies the myelopathy presenting with radicular pain, sensory or motor deficit, or both. This is localized to the area innervated by the specific nerve root.

The clinical course varies among patients. Although some individuals have a mild protracted insidious course, even over decades, others have subacute temporal profiles progressing over a few months to a relatively severe disability. Infrequently, these patients are prone to acute cord compression secondary to a fall, as the compromised spinal canal diameter makes it more likely that the cord will be contused with sudden hyperextension or flexion. This may even mimic a stroke, as noted in the initial vignette in this chapter. Here it is important to emphasize clinical evaluation for a cervical spinal sensory level as the important defining feature of an acute myelopathy.

Rarely, sudden neck hyperextension leads to a temporary "person in the barrel" syndrome. Here there is an acute compression of the anterior spinal cord. This transiently impairs the segmental anterior horn cells innervating the arm musculature. The clinical picture of isolated arm and hand weakness relates to the preserved lateral column corticospinal tract function; thus the legs are unaffected.

Clinical Vignette

A very unique scenario occurred in a 40-year-old man who, while skiing, noted that his ankles "vibrate" each time he "hit the bumps." This advanced skiing technique involves rapidly traversing through and over these mounds of snow (moguls) that routinely pile up on steep ski trails. The skier negotiates a field of moguls repetitively coming across these bumps, and then "jumps," making a 90-degree turn to land on his skies with significant force. Our patient had performed this action in an almost perfunctory fashion for a number of winters. However, he recently noted that each time he landed on the mogul his legs grossly vibrated, sometimes causing him to fall.

His examination demonstrated bilateral ankle clonus, and a left Babinski sign. The patient likened this feeling of clonus to his skiing experience. Cervical spinal cord MRI demonstrated disc extrusion primarily at the C5–C6 level along with abnormal intramedullary enhancement compatible with a severe spondylotic cervical myelopathy (see Figs. 45-9 and 45-10). In this instance, the patient's vivid description of a most unusual complaint ("mogul clonus") led to careful investigation and eventual surgery. Six months postoperatively, "skiing the bumps" no longer produced clonus. Most importantly, his risk of permanent spinal cord injury was greatly lessened if he were to subsequently sustain a severe fall.

Comment: Presumably, this patient's jumps onto the snowfield moguls, while skiing, dorsiflexed his feet abruptly enough to elicit a spontaneous clonus by a mechanism essentially similar to that used by a neurologist routinely checking for clonus. The force of his body coming down on the hard packed snow induced the "vibration," that is, mogul clonus. The basic pathophysiology identified by the MRI was a congenital, very tight cervical spinal stenosis.

DIAGNOSIS

MS, amyotrophic lateral sclerosis, vitamin B_{12} deficiency, human T cell leukemia/lymphotrophic virus type 1 (HTLV-I) myelopathy, adrenoleukodystrophy, syringomyelia, and spinal cord tumors need to be considered in the differential diagnosis of cervical spinal spondylosis with cord compression. The presence of hand or leg paresthesia, Lhermitte's sign, prominent neck pain, or significant sensory loss provides historic and examination evidence to distinguish cervical spondylosis with myelopathy from motor neuron disease/amyotrophic lateral sclerosis.

MRI is the diagnostic procedure of choice. It provides longitudinal segmental views of the cord, dural space, and relationships to bony and ligamentous structures. CT/myelogram is an alternative when MRI is contraindicated because of cardiac pacemakers or severe claustrophobia. CT can provide additional information about the bony structure regarding the foramen, facets, and uncovertebral joints. Electromyography/nerve conduction can help identify concomitant peripheral nerve disease or nerve root compression when the differential diagnosis includes a process in the peripheral motor sensory unit.

TREATMENT

Epidemiologic data regarding the natural history of cervical spondylosis are lacking. In patients with mild deficits from cervical myelopathy, it is unclear whether surgical decompression is superior to conservative management. Some patients remain stable or improve without treatment. For patients with evolving symptoms and deficits, surgical decompression is the treatment of choice to arrest progression of the myelopathy. Functional recovery may not occur if the deficit is already severe, possibly because of chronic ischemic cord damage from spinal artery compression.

Surgical approaches include the posterior approach, which allows for generous decompressive laminectomies, and the anterior approach, which enables operation on bars and spurs anterior to the cord and fusion when instability or subluxation is present. Discectomy, corpectomy, laminectomy, and laminoplasty are other surgical options.

Significant variations exist in the degree of postsurgical clinical improvement. Duration and severity of the myelopathy before surgery are key determinants for clinical outcome. Cord atrophy, irreversible signal change within the cord on T2-weighted MRI (gliosis rather than cord edema), superimposed trauma, and advanced age are negative prognostic factors. Maintaining spinal stability and treating anterior compression improve outcome.

Spinal Cord Arteriovenous Malformations

Clinical Vignette

During the past year, this very healthy 45-year-old neuropsychologist experienced intermittent lower extremity paresthesia and heaviness in her legs. On one occasion, she experienced the precipitous onset of severe difficulty walking. This lasted for a few hours, and then resolved. Two months later, she developed low back pain, constipation, and problems voiding. She had a second episode of inability to walk lasting for several hours.

On neurologic examination, her proximal leg muscles were significantly weak; distal leg and all muscles in her arms were normal. Pinprick sensation was reduced in a patchy distribution in both legs. Her gait was broad based and unsteady and she was unable to walk on her heels or toes. Muscle stretch reflexes were increased in both legs and a right Babinski sign was present.

MRI demonstrated a swollen conus with increased vasculature. A selective intercostal angiogram revealed a dural AVM with its feeder vessel nidus at T11 on the left, and not involving the artery of Adamkiewicz.

A T10–T11 laminectomy was performed to remove the AVM. Large arterialized vessels were found medial to the nerve roots filling the dorsal subarachnoid space. These epidural vessels and large feeders at T10–T11 were coagulated. The patient's strength improved postprocedure, returning to normal within 1 year. Bladder dysfunction was minimal. She has had excellent long-term follow-up examinations.

Comment: Spinal AVMs are a group of vascular disorders that can cause acute, subacute, or chronic spinal cord dysfunction. Dural AVMs present in later adulthood and may be acquired. The most common type is the **dural AVM** *(80–85%), although intradural AVMs, combination intradural and extradural AVMs, and cavernous angiomas (cavernous malformations) also occur. A high index of suspicion is needed so as not to miss the diagnosis in any patient with unexplained myelopathy. An associated venous hypertension or bleeding of these spinal AVMs leads to the intermittent and eventually progressive myelopathy. Complete spinal angiography with concomitant obliteration of the AVM is usually indicated.*

PATHOPHYSIOLOGY AND ETIOLOGY

Dural AVMs primarily occur in the mid to lower thoracic and lumbar spine. Many dural AVMs are AV fistulas that essentially have a single hole in an artery connected to a vein (Fig. 45-11). Radicular or dural branches from the segmental arteries supply the AVM, usually within the dura of an intervertebral foramen. The AVM nidus is typically a low-flow shunt drained by a single vein that joins the *coronal plexus* on the dorsal cord surface. The coronal plexus is arterialized by the AVM fistula and becomes dilated, coiled, and elongated. Blood flow through this vessel is slower than normal and thus leads to venous congestion with increased venous pressure that is transmitted intramedullarly, reducing the arteriovenous pressure gradient within the cord. Cord perfusion decreases, leading to prolonged ischemia/hypoxia and a progressive myelopathy. The effects of hypoxia that are initially reversible later lead to an irreversible degenerative cord necrosis. The corticospinal tracts, lateral white matter, and dorsal columns are especially vulnerable.

Intradural AVMs originate from intramedullary arteries arising from the anterior spinal artery. The nidus can be in the cord (intramedullary), in the pia on cord surface (extramedullary), or be a combination of intramedullary and extramedullary. These AVMs are high-pressure systems with rapid blood flow. These can contain arterial aneurysms that can spontaneously hemorrhage within the cord or into the subarachnoid space. Unlike dural AVMs, intradural AVMs occur throughout the length of the cord. These intradural AVMs affect younger

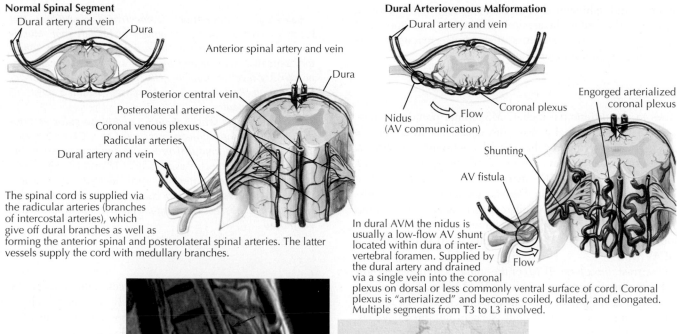

Normal Spinal Segment

Dural artery and vein

Dura

Anterior spinal artery and vein

Dura

Posterior central vein

Posterolateral arteries

Coronal venous plexus

Radicular arteries

Dural artery and vein

The spinal cord is supplied via the radicular arteries (branches of intercostal arteries), which give off dural branches as well as forming the anterior spinal and posterolateral spinal arteries. The latter vessels supply the cord with medullary branches.

Dural Arteriovenous Malformation

Dural artery and vein

Engorged arterialized coronal plexus

Coronal plexus

Nidus (AV communication)

Flow

Shunting

AV fistula

Flow

In dural AVM the nidus is usually a low-flow AV shunt located within dura of intervertebral foramen. Supplied by the dural artery and drained via a single vein into the coronal plexus on dorsal or less commonly ventral surface of cord. Coronal plexus is "arterialized" and becomes coiled, dilated, and elongated. Multiple segments from T3 to L3 involved.

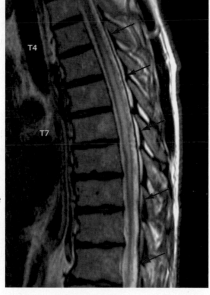

Sagittal T2 image shows increased T2 signal in the central cord representing edema and/or gliosis. Multiple signal voids behind the spinal cord are secondary to tortuous vessels from the malformation.

Spinal angiogram of radicular artery, left T6, with arteriovenous fistula filling multiple draining veins at the dural level. These join to form a complex medullary venous plexus.

Figure 45-11 Spinal Arteriovenous Malformations.

patients than do the dural lesions. These may be of congenital origin. Recurrent subarachnoid and intramedullary hemorrhage are the primary pathophysiologic mechanisms.

Cavernous angiomas or malformations are rare, isolated or multiple lesions, more common in the cerebral hemispheres than in the cord. These low-flow lesions can spontaneously hemorrhage and are best shown by MRI (spinal arteriography is normal).

CLINICAL PRESENTATION

Dural AVMs occur more commonly in men. Symptoms typically emerge after age 40, peaking at 50–70 years. The thoracolumbar (T6–L1) region is most frequently involved. Symptoms are gradual in onset and slowly progressive. Back or radicular pain is the most frequent presenting symptom. Patients often have a combination of upper and lower motor neuron findings

with spasticity, weakness, fasciculations, atrophy, hyperreflexia, hyporeflexia, and Babinski signs. A variable degree of leg weakness can progress from abnormal stance or gait to needing an assistive walking device to wheelchair or bed dependence. Sensory dysfunction is manifested by impaired joint position, vibration, pain, and temperature sensation. A discrete or vague sensory level may sometimes be identified. Various degrees of bladder, bowel, and sexual dysfunction develop. Very rarely auscultation over the spine demonstrating a bruit can help diagnose a high-flow AVM. Certain activities or postures may precipitate or exacerbate symptoms. Dural AVMs rarely hemorrhage.

Intradural AVMs affect men and women more evenly. They present at an early age, usually <40 years, sometimes during childhood. The AVM nidus is distributed evenly along the cord from the foramen magnum to the conus medullaris. Early clinical findings usually result from an intramedullary or subarachnoid hemorrhage. Patients usually develop progressive weakness, numbness, and sphincter dysfunction. Because the intradural AVM may be located in the cervical spinal cord, both upper and lower extremities are sometimes affected. Recurrent hemorrhages leads to clinical deterioration.

DIAGNOSIS

Entities in the differential include MS, spinal pseudoclaudication associated with spinal stenosis, disc disease, acute or chronic infection, tumor, syringomyelia, and subarachnoid hemorrhage. All these conditions can have acute or slowly progressive courses.

With *dural AVMs*, MRI demonstrates serpentine filling defects of reduced signal in the subarachnoid space corresponding to blood flow in the dilated, tortuous coronal venous plexus. Sometimes cord signal is increased from edema or venous congestion. Rarely an MRI will fail to demonstrate a dural AVM.

In contrast, *intradural AVMs* of the spinal cord may have low signal corresponding to an intradural AVM nidus. A target sign may be seen at the site of previous hemorrhage.

Myelography may demonstrate serpentine linear defects. However, this medium is less helpful in distinguishing intramedullary from extramedullary lesions. Selective spinal arteriography offers more precise information regarding AVM anatomy.

TREATMENT AND PROGNOSIS

Treatment depends on the location, size, source of arterial supply and site of the shunt. Surgical removal, endovascular embolization, or both are often helpful.

For *dural AVMs*, goals are to eliminate the dural nidus and interrupt the AV fistula between the nidus and coronal venous plexus, resolving the venous hypertension and congestion, subsequently improving the myelopathy. Elimination of the fistula/nidus at the intervertebral foramen can be curative. The dilated veins of the coronal plexus can remain; their removal can be damaging and unnecessary.

Intramedullary AVMs are often inoperable. Embolization can occlude feeding vessels and the nidus, reducing flow and allowing lesion thrombosis. Collateral spinal vascular supply is needed to prevent cord damage from the subsequent ischemia. If the treated vessels recanalize, reembolization may be required.

Early detection and treatment can improve gait disturbances, sometimes bladder dysfunction, and other myelopathy signs, especially if they are less severe. A previously progressive course can be arrested by surgery.

Epidural Lipomatosis

Clinical Vignette

A 64-year-old man, hospitalized for an acute myocardial infarction, was dyspneic, with worsening heart failure. He complained of weakness and inability to ambulate. Additional medical history included obstructive pulmonary disease and low back pain, for which he received chronic intermittent steroids, including epidural injections.

Neurologic examination demonstrated significant iliopsoas weakness and no movement of his left foot. Muscle stretch reflexes were brisk with a right Babinski sign. Vibratory sensation was absent in lower extremities. There was no sensory level to pinprick. His thoracic spine was tender to palpation. Rectal tone was decreased. Within 5 days, his legs became plegic.

The patient was febrile. Sputum and blood cultures grew pseudomonas. A pacemaker precluded MRI. CT/myelogram demonstrated an epidural process extending dorsally T4–T10, and severe stenosis especially at T8 and T9. The spinal cord was displaced anteriorly with marked compression. The patient was taken to surgery for decompression and possible abscess drainage. Epidural lipomatosis was diagnosed.

Epidural lipomatosis is defined as excess adipose tissue deposition posterior to the spinal cord. Rarely described in children, it occurs primarily in a thoracic (61%), sometimes lumbar (39%) distribution, but not within the cervical spine. Men are affected more than women with average age 44, range 18–64 years.

PATHOPHYSIOLOGY AND ETIOLOGY

Epidural fat accumulation leads to cord compression with corticospinal tract and dorsal column compromise. Venous thrombosis can be a significant part of the pathology.

Epidural lipomatosis is sometimes a rare consequence of therapeutic corticosteroids, that is, part of an iatrogenic Cushing syndrome. The correlation between duration and dosage of steroid treatment is unknown. It can occur with prednisone dosages ranging from 5 to 180 mg/day (average 30–100 mg/day). Epidural lipomatosis is also seen in patients who use steroid inhalers or have had epidural steroid injections. It can occur as early as 6 months or more than 10 years after initiation of steroid treatment.

Idiopathic epidural lipomatosis rarely occurs in obese patients who may or may not have concurrent hypercortisolism. An abundance of epidural fat and congenitally narrowed spinal canal are predisposing factors.

CLINICAL PRESENTATION

Weakness is the most frequent (72%) symptom and finding. Progressive paraparesis sometimes develops over months. Acute irreversible paraplegia rarely occurs. Other common complaints include low back pain (66%), radicular pain (50%), numbness/dysesthesias (50%), and changes in muscle stretch reflexes (50%). Lumbar radiculopathy, cauda equina syndrome, and neurogenic claudication are other possible manifestations.

DIAGNOSIS AND TREATMENT

Extraaxial tumors, epidural abscess, epidural hematoma, and other rare extrinsic compressive processes need consideration.

MRI is the study of choice, especially noting the unique signal characteristics of fat. When MRI cannot be performed,

CT/myelogram demonstrates complete block in 69% of patients.

Weight loss and discontinuation or reduction of the corticosteroid dose are the primary medical modalities. The choice of medical versus surgical management is based on the severity of the clinical picture, possibility for reversing the causative mechanism, and the potential for surgical complications. Sometimes a multilevel laminectomy with debulking of lipid tissue is required; however, this has high morbidity and mortality.

INTRADURAL EXTRAMEDULLARY SPINAL CORD LESIONS

Meningioma

> ### Clinical Vignette
>
> *A 43-year-old woman had a history of numbness and cold sensation in her right leg for several months. She did not perceive pain in her right leg while she cut it while shaving. She felt that her tennis game was slipping. Medical history was otherwise unremarkable.*
>
> *Initial neurologic exam was normal. At follow-up 6 weeks later, her exam demonstrated reduced light touch, pinprick and temperature sensation to a level of T12 on the right. Position and vibration senses were intact. Strength, gait, and reflexes were normal.*
>
> *MRI demonstrated a thoracic meningioma on the left at T5–T6 that was intradural and extramedullary. The spinal cord was markedly thinned. Surgical resection of the meningioma led to rapid and full recovery.*

Spinal cord meningiomas comprise at least 25% of primary spinal cord tumors although they are less common than intracranial meningiomas (Box 45-3). Most are intradural. They can be located ventrally, dorsally or laterally to the cord.

PATHOPHYSIOLOGY AND ETIOLOGY

Typically, corticospinal tract dysfunction is the most prominent feature of cord compression secondary to an intradural extramedullary tumor. As the tumor enlarges, spinothalamic tract and dorsal column compromise also become evident. Localized radicular pain sometimes occurs; this is secondary to mass effect on adjacent nerve roots by the meningioma.

Spinal cord meningiomas have the same histologic classification as intracranial meningiomas (Chapter 51) and can become densely calcific. Meningothelial (syncytial), psammomatous, transitional, and fibroblastic meningiomas are seen; meningotheliomatous meningiomas are the most frequent.

CLINICAL PRESENTATION

Almost any age group may present with a meningioma; individuals in their fourth to seventh decades are most vulnerable, particularly women. The thoracic cord is the most frequent site (~80% of cases); however, on occasion these occur in the high cervical cord at the foramen magnum. Meningiomas rarely occur at the lumbar level. Localized radicular pain may antedate other symptoms, as the nerve root is affected early on. Weakness, sensory loss, bladder and bowel dysfunction, and gait difficulty very gradually occur.

Spasticity, hyperreflexia, and Babinski signs ipsilateral to the lesion characterize the corticospinal tract involvement. Ipsilateral loss of proprioception may occur from pressure on the dorsal columns. When the spinothalamic tract is affected, contralateral pain and temperature loss are produced. When this is combined with corticospinal tract involvement, it is referred to as the Brown–Sequard syndrome indicating a hemi-cord lesion.

DIAGNOSIS

Intradural extramedullary spinal tumors include meningiomas, schwannomas, and neurofibromas. Ependymomas can affect the filum terminale or any part of the spinal cord. Other spinal cord tumor categories include extradural and intradural intramedullary lesions (Table 45-2). Additional diagnoses in the differential

---

Box 45-3 Chronic Intradural Extramedullary Myelopathies

Meningioma
Schwannoma
Neurofibroma
Arteriovenous malformation

Table 45-2 Chronic Intradural Intramedullary Myelopathies

Type	Examples
Congenital or acquired	Syringomyelia
	Hydromyelia
Genetic	Hereditary spastic paraparesis
	Friedreich ataxia
	Adrenomyeloneuropathy
Neurodegenerative	Amyotrophic lateral sclerosis
	Primary lateral sclerosis
Infectious	HTLV-I
	HIV
	Syphilis
	Tuberculosis
	Schistosomiasis
	Other bacteria, viruses, and fungi
Inflammatory	Multiple sclerosis
	Sjögren syndrome
	Sarcoidosis
	Systemic lupus erythematosus
Neoplasms	Ependymoma
	Astrocytoma
	Hemangioblastoma
	Metastasis
Vascular	Cavernous malformation
Nutritional deficiencies: Subacute combined degeneration	Vitamin B_{12} (cobalamin)
	Copper
Toxic	Lathyrism
	Konzo
	Radiation
	Intrathecal chemotherapy

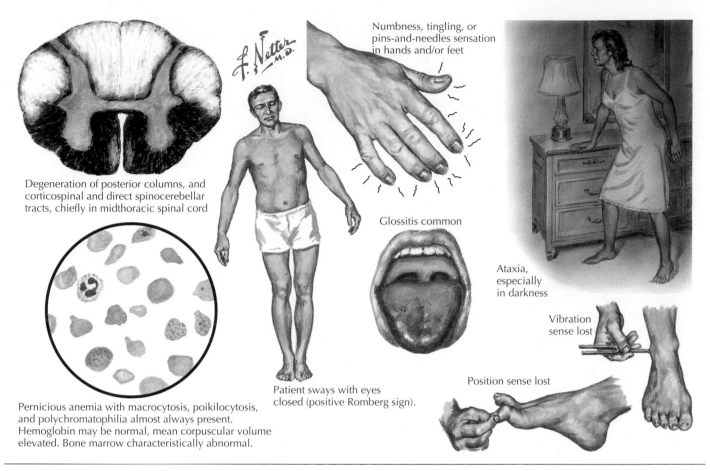

Degeneration of posterior columns, and corticospinal and direct spinocerebellar tracts, chiefly in midthoracic spinal cord

Numbness, tingling, or pins-and-needles sensation in hands and/or feet

Glossitis common

Ataxia, especially in darkness

Vibration sense lost

Position sense lost

Patient sways with eyes closed (positive Romberg sign).

Pernicious anemia with macrocytosis, poikilocytosis, and polychromatophilia almost always present. Hemoglobin may be normal, mean corpuscular volume elevated. Bone marrow characteristically abnormal.

Figure 45-12 Subacute Combined Degeneration.

are MS, spinal dural AVMs, vitamin B$_{12}$ deficiency, central disc herniation, and syringomyelia.

MRI provides an excellent means to diagnose intradural extramedullary lesions (Fig. 45-12). Meningiomas enhance homogeneously with gadolinium. Axial MRI helps to determine if the tumor is circumferential. When an initial MRI at the thoracic level is normal, further study needs to be performed to the foramen magnum. This is because what initially appears to be sensory localizing signs at the low thoracic level may actually be found due to a lesion situated higher in the canal. CT/ myelogram is also a valuable diagnostic tool that can demonstrate a partial or complete block and also assess for tumor calcification, but is primarily used when MRI cannot be performed. Plain spine films may demonstrate erosion of a pedicle or articular process by the meningioma and intraspinal calcification.

TREATMENT AND PROGNOSIS

Most meningiomas are benign, slow growing, and well circumscribed; the majority are successfully resected. Radiation therapy may be administered in cases of early recurrence or limited surgical resection.

Prognosis is often very good with improved motor, sensory, and sphincter function after surgical removal, particularly when the tumor is diagnosed at an early stage. Postoperative mortality

is low. The tumor recurs in only a minority of patients. Negative prognostic factors include elderly age, severe neurologic deficits, long duration of symptoms before diagnosis, subtotal tumor resection, and extradural extension.

INTRADURAL INTRAMEDULLARY SPINAL CORD LESIONS

Vitamin B$_{12}$ Deficiency

Clinical Vignette

A 72-year-old man presented with distal paresthesia, more pronounced in his hands than feet, an unsteady gait, and frequent falls, particularly when in the dark. This was especially limiting when in the shower and washing his face where he could no longer see to establish his place in space or at night when getting out of bed in the dark. His family noted some subtle memory loss of unclear duration.

On examination, he was oriented to self and place, but not to month or year. He registered three items at zero minutes, but recalled only one item at 5 minutes even when clues were provided. Visual acuity was poor. On motor exam, he had mild weakness in his legs, a broad-based, spastic, and ataxic gait. Romberg testing was very positive.

He had loss of position sense in toes, vibratory sense as high as his knees, and hyperesthesia to pin in his distal extremities. Two-point discrimination was very limited in his fingers. Babinski signs were present, although muscle stretch reflexes were normoactive. Hematocrit was 29%, with a mean corpuscular volume of 112. Vitamin B₁₂ level was 34 (normal >190). A diagnosis of pernicious anemia (PA) was made.

Vitamin B₁₂ replacement was vigorously initiated and within just 3–4 months he was immensely better, no longer falling or having any residual gait difficulties, particularly in the dark.

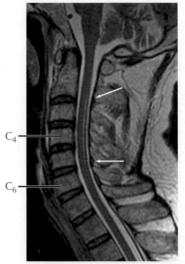

A. Vitamin B₁₂ deficiency

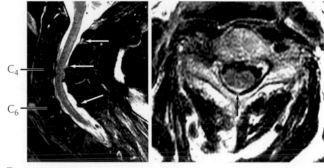

B. Copper deficiency

Figure 45-13 Nutritional Myelopathies.

Vitamin B₁₂, also known as cobalamin, deficiency causes both neurologic and hematologic difficulties. Myelopathy and peripheral neuropathy with a megaloblastic anemia are the cardinal features; rarely there is cognitive impairment. The degrees of neurologic and hematologic abnormalities do not always correlate. Although most patients present with the anemia, occasionally the neurologic symptomatology is the initial clinical presentation. This disorder characteristically affects both the posterior columns and the corticospinal tracts and thus the designation of *subacute combined degeneration*. Until the discovery of the role of intrinsic factor in the gastric absorption of this vitamin, this was eventually a progressively severe disorder leading to death.

PATHOPHYSIOLOGY AND ETIOLOGY

Vitamin B₁₂ deficiency is called "subacute combined degeneration of the spinal cord" or "combined system disease." White matter degeneration of the cord is the characteristic pathology; occasionally this also affects the brain. Symmetric loss of myelin, particularly in the posterior and lateral columns, exceeds the coexistent axonal damage. Typically the process begins in the posterior columns of the thoracic cord, spreading laterally, anteriorly, inferiorly, and superiorly. Although spinal cord involvement is the more significant clinical component, there is also a concomitant peripheral nerve involvement. The widespread availability of serum vitamin B₁₂ levels makes it relatively easy to make a diagnosis early on. Impaired vitamin B₁₂ absorption most commonly results from an autoimmune-mediated process resulting in the clinical picture of pernicious anemia (PA). Rarely B₁₂ deficiency is a component of a postgastrectomy syndrome, or a deficient diet (vegetarians) with secondary peripheral nerve damage.

CLINICAL PRESENTATION

Although most patients with PA do not have signs of neurologic compromise, some individuals occasionally present with what appears to be a primary neurologic syndrome and minimal or no hematologic abnormalities. Distal paresthesia, particularly in the hands, and gait ataxia are the typical presenting symptoms in patients with primary neurologic involvement (Fig. 45-13). Loss of vibratory sensation, abnormal joint position sense, sensory ataxia, and positive Romberg signs correlate with posterior column damage. Later appearance of lower extremity weakness and spasticity reflect the corticospinal tract damage.

Muscle stretch reflexes can be increased or decreased depending on whether the myelopathy or the peripheral neuropathy components predominate. Memory loss, confusion, paranoia, irritability, and hallucinations rarely develop.

DIAGNOSIS

Because hand paresthesia may be the initial symptom, an initial diagnosis of carpal tunnel syndrome (CTS) may be considered in some individuals. This contrasts with the peripheral neuropathy patient, in whom the initial symptoms occur in the feet. In the patient with PA, the hand symptoms likely reflect cervical spinal cord involvement and not a peripheral neuropathy per se. Another important differentiation from CTS is that these symptoms are persistent throughout the day and do not have either the typical nocturnal awakening or symptom exacerbation when driving an automobile.

HIV vacuolar myelopathy also requires diagnostic consideration because the posterolateral cord is the primarily affected site. The coexistence of a peripheral neuropathy and dementia may also be comorbid AIDS complications.

A megaloblastic anemia is an important clue to the diagnosis of vitamin B₁₂ deficiency. However, because some patients have few or no hematologic abnormalities, awareness of the pure neurologic clinical syndrome is important. Diagnosis is straightforward when vitamin B₁₂ levels are low. When B₁₂ levels are normal or only slightly abnormal, then elevation of methylmalonic acid and homocysteine are important indicators of cobalamin deficiency.

MRI images may demonstrate T2 accentuated posterior column changes (Fig. 45-13).

TREATMENT AND PROGNOSIS

In the early and moderate deficiency state, the administration of parenteral vitamin B_{12} (initially 1000 μg every 1–2 weeks and later monthly) can reverse the disorder. Oral supplementation is insufficient in the severely depleted patient. Hematologic abnormalities improve more rapidly than neurologic ones, although clinical changes can be dramatic over weeks to months.

Prognosis for neurologic recovery is best with early diagnosis. The course is progressive and can be fatal without treatment.

Copper Deficiency Myelopathy

Clinical Vignette

During the past 18 months, this 74-year-old man developed numbness that began distally in his legs and feet progressing up to his waist and within 6–8 months his hands and arms. A severe gait ataxia followed; it gradually worsened, eventually leading to him becoming wheelchair-bound. Neurologic examination demonstrated a "combined system" clinical picture with loss of proprioceptive sensation and corticospinal tract dysfunction manifested by severe spasticity. As this mimicked a patient having vitamin B_{12} deficiency, a therapeutic trial of intramuscular injections of B_{12} was tried but this was unsuccessful and led to our evaluation at Lahey Clinic.

His past medical history was notable for severe peptic ulcer disease occurring more than 30 years earlier. This led to a series of partial gastrectomies that over the ensuing few years formed a de facto total gastrectomy. Subsequently, he required long-term enteral nutrition via a feeding jejunostomy tube.

The neurologic examination demonstrated a "stocking/glove" sensory loss, particularly compromising vibratory and proprioceptive modalities, spasticity, a positive Romberg sign, and severe truncal, limb, and gait ataxia.

Laboratory studies demonstrated a normocytic anemia with a normal platelet count. Vitamin B_{12} level was 314 pg/dL (normal 200–1200 pg/dL). He had a severely decreased serum copper level of 4 g/dL (normal = 70–140 g/dL) and ceruloplasmin values of 6 mg/dL (normal = 14–28 mg/dL). A 24-hour urine study failed to detect any copper excretion. Cerebrospinal fluid (CSF) studies were normal. Dietary copper supplementation led to stabilization of his neurologic symptoms, but unfortunately no significant improvement occurred.

Comment: This patient's clinical picture was one that totally mimicked subacute combined degeneration. However, laboratory parameters did not support this. With his past history of severe gastric compromise, studies of his copper metabolism led to the appropriate diagnosis.

Copper is a trace metal that is an essential micronutrient necessary for both the neurologic and hematologic systems. Acquired copper deficiency in humans leads to a syndrome similar to the subacute combined degeneration of vitamin B_{12} deficiency.

PATHOPHYSIOLOGY AND ETIOLOGY

Copper deficiency is extremely rare because of its low daily nutritional requirements as well as its ubiquitous nature within the environment. Various seeds, grains, nuts, beans, shellfish, and liver are the primary dietary sources for copper consumption. A variety of clinical settings negatively affect copper stores, including malnutrition, nephrotic syndrome, excess zinc, and treatment with penicillamine or alkali agents. Additionally parenteral feeding with insufficient copper content, and the consequences of major gastrointestinal surgery leading to need for long-term enteral feedings into the proximal and midjejunum, are joint risks that predispose to the development of clinically defined copper deficiency.

Patients who take too much zinc (i.e., 15–30 times the normal daily requirements) with health fads, such as to protect against the common cold, are also prone to develop copper deficiency when hyperzincemia occurs, blocking copper absorption.

CLINICAL PRESENTATION

Acquired copper deficiency classically mimics the posterior column, corticospinal, and dorsal root ganglion dysfunction so typical of vitamin B_{12} deficiency. Symptoms include loss of proprioception and vibratory sensation, severe ataxia, as well as peripheral neuropathy. Examination demonstrates gait instability and severe sensory ataxia secondary to dorsal column dysfunction, and severe lower limb spasticity with brisk muscle stretch reflexes and positive Babinski signs.

DIAGNOSIS

Evaluation of serum copper, ceruloplasmin, and urinary copper excretion are the primary means to make this diagnosis. Zinc levels are normal or elevated in most patients. No laboratory findings are identified to suggest other mechanisms for a peripheral neuropathy and/or myelopathy.

Most patients who develop primary neurologic dysfunction have an associated anemia or leucopenia; however, some do not develop an anemia.

Spinal cord imaging sometimes demonstrates increased signal intensity within the posterior columns on T2-weighted MRI images.

TREATMENT

Although a few patients report that their paresthesia improved with parenteral administration of copper, the result was not sustained with oral repletion, despite restoring serum copper levels to normal in more than half of so identified patients. This therapeutic approach will prevent further progression of neurologic disability.

DEMOGRAPHICS AND PROGNOSIS

Although gastric surgery for peptic ulcer disease is rarely required in the era of treatment of *Helicobacter pylori* and use of proton-pump inhibitors, there is a very increased use of bariatric surgery. This procedure physiologically isolates the stomach, duodenum, and proximal jejunum—the preferred sites for copper absorption. Gastric bypass surgery is both a restrictive and a malabsorptive method for weight reduction and results in micronutrient deficiencies.

Today with the almost epidemic numbers of individuals having morbid obesity, and candidates for bariatric surgery, there are increasing numbers of patients at risk for copper deficiency. These patients require vitamin and mineral supplementation and periodic assessment. Furthermore, enteral feeding is increasingly being used.

Currently, in the absence of a prospective study, it is unclear how to best replete copper and to what levels. However, there is no doubt that there is a need for early recognition of copper deficiency and eventual therapy with oral or parenteral copper. With increasing awareness of the clinical manifestations of copper deficiency and by identifying those patients at risk, these individuals need to be treated earlier, in hopes of preventing permanent neurologic damage.

AIDS-Associated Vacuolar Myelopathy

This AIDS complication generally occurs relatively late during the course of HIV infection. Earlier onset of coexistent neurologic conditions including dementia and peripheral neuropathy may detract from the diagnosis. The incidence of a myelopathy among AIDS patients is unknown.

PATHOPHYSIOLOGY AND ETIOLOGY

The intramedullary white matter of the thoracic cord is the primary target site for the AIDS vacuolization to occur. This primarily involves the lateral and posterior white matter columns; the anterior and anterolateral columns are less affected. Wallerian degeneration of the posterior columns also occurs. Vacuolization increases over time, and more cord segments become involved, although the process is confined to white matter.

Etiology is unknown. Macrophage secretion of cytokines that damage the cord and a metabolic disorder of the B_{12}-dependent transmethylation pathway are among the theories postulated.

CLINICAL PRESENTATION

HIV-associated vacuolar myelopathy occurs in the later stages of this systemic illness. These patients usually present with slowly progressive leg weakness, spasticity, gait disorder, and painless sensory changes, including vibratory and position sense impairment and sensory ataxia. If paresthesia is present, these patients may also have a coexistent HIV peripheral neuropathy. On occasion, bladder and bowel dysfunction also develops. Impotence can occur in some men. The upper extremities are usually uninvolved or minimally so, as the thoracic cord is the primary pathologic site. Rarely, an acute transverse myelitis

occurs at the time of HIV seroconversion, but this is a different entity.

DIAGNOSIS

Intrinsic spinal cord disease and extramedullary compressive lesions are the main differential diagnostic considerations. Various other infectious myelopathies may also occur. These are sometimes opportunistic organisms such as cytomegalovirus, herpes simplex virus, varicella zoster, toxoplasmosis, tuberculosis, syphilis, and HTLV-I. What with the increased incidence of CNS lymphoma in HIV patients, this also needs to be thought of in these patients. And considering the propensity for HIV to involve the posterior columns, B_{12} deficiency is also part of the differential.

As there is no specific diagnostic set of clinical and laboratory findings, HIV vacuolar myelopathy becomes a diagnosis of exclusion. MRI of the spinal cord helps exclude a mass, focal enhancement, abnormal cord signal, cord enlargement, or atrophy. Focal cord enlargement suggests lymphoma or toxoplasmosis. The cord may often appear normal or mildly atrophic. Cord signal may or may not be increased.

The utilization of brain MRI augments the cord imaging. Serologies and CSF studies help exclude other causes of myelopathy. The CSF may have slight pleocytosis and protein elevation. Vacuolar myelopathy may be difficult to distinguish from HIV myelitis. Myelitis is less common and is usually seen concomitant with HIV encephalitis.

TREATMENT AND PROGNOSIS

Treatment is supportive. Anti-spasticity agents, treatment of sphincter dysfunction, and physical therapy are the mainstay therapies. Antiretroviral drugs can sometimes improve symptoms or slow myelopathy.

AIDS-associated vacuolar myelopathy is slowly progressive. Patients sometimes progress to wheelchair dependence and double incontinence.

Schistosomal (Bilharziasis) Myelopathy

There are more than 200 million persons worldwide who are infected with schistosomiasis. Three to five percent of patients acquiring this parasite primarily develop either a myeloradiculopathy secondary to inflammation of the spinal cord and the nerve roots or an acute cerebritis often mimicking a brain tumor. Neurologists in more temperate climates may not consider this disorder in the differential diagnosis of patients presenting with a myeloradiculopathy, myelopathy, or radiculopathy because of the schistosomiasis predominance in tropical climates. These areas include the Nile and Amazon river basins, Lake Victoria in East-Central Africa, the Caribbean, and the Middle East. Schistosomiasis is one of the most common etiologies for myelopathy in Brazil with its massive Amazon territorial drainage areas. Its incidence in endemic tropical areas is not well defined and it may be greatly underestimated. Initially *Schistosoma mansoni* resides within the inferior mesenteric venules eventually affecting Batson's plexus and then invading the spinal venous circulation.

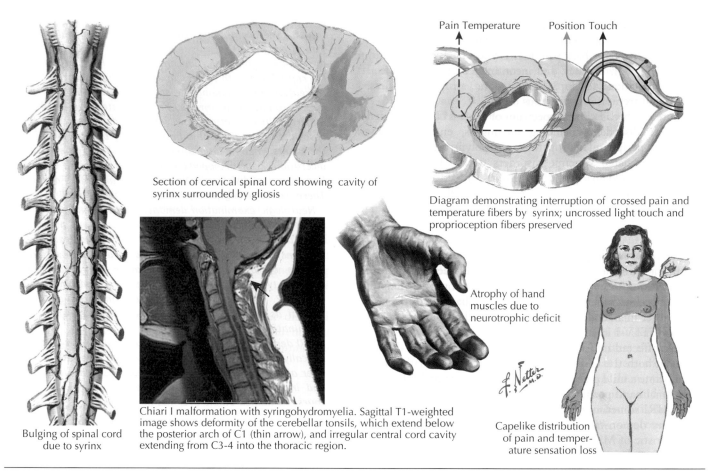

Section of cervical spinal cord showing cavity of syrinx surrounded by gliosis

Diagram demonstrating interruption of crossed pain and temperature fibers by syrinx; uncrossed light touch and proprioception fibers preserved

Pain Temperature   Position Touch

Atrophy of hand muscles due to neurotrophic deficit

Chiari I malformation with syringohydromyelia. Sagittal T1-weighted image shows deformity of the cerebellar tonsils, which extend below the posterior arch of C1 (thin arrow), and irregular central cord cavity extending from C3-4 into the thoracic region.

Bulging of spinal cord due to syrinx

Capelike distribution of pain and temperature sensation loss

Figure 45-14 Syringomyelia.

Although no specific pathophysiologic mechanism is recognized, the increased incidence of certain concomitant lesions, such as the *Arnold–Chiari malformation* (ACM), suggests a congenital origin. An ACM is characterized by the extension of cerebellar tonsils below the foramen magnum. These may occur in isolation, typically presenting with postural induced headaches and on examination down-beating nystagmus. Rarely a syrinx develops after spinal trauma, possibly by creation of a central hematomyelia. Intramedullary neoplasms such as ependymomas or astrocytomas may lead to central canal obstruction and the development of a secondary syrinx.

CLINICAL PRESENTATION

These patients often present with a history of unexplained finger skin ulcerations and an atrophic weak hand. On neurologic examination, the dissociated sensory loss, preferentially affecting pain and temperature modalities in a cape distribution at the cervical level, concomitant with distal upper extremity muscle weakness, atrophy, and fasciculations, are the classic clinical findings. Eventually with cavity enlargement, corticospinal and dorsal column function is affected.

The temporal profile of clinical progression varies from an insidiously evolving lesion to episodes of sudden worsening as noted in the prior vignette. Occasionally the loss of pain sensation leads to a *Charcot joint* in the shoulder or arm. In this setting, the patient suffers repeated trauma to the joint but does not experience pain. Thus the joint is subjected to repetitive trauma eventually damaging the joint. There are classic findings on radiographic inspection of the joint. Another unusual complication is the development of a severe cervical kyphoscoliosis secondary to anterior horn cell damage primarily affecting the paraspinal muscles.

DIAGNOSIS

The differential diagnosis is a broad one. Amyotrophic lateral sclerosis is often the first consideration because of the painless atrophied and weak hand. Other possibilities in the differential are ulnar or median neuropathies or both; a medial brachial plexus lesion, particularly a Pancoast tumor; and a primary intramedullary spinal cord tumor.

MRI is the diagnostic modality of choice. CT/myelography is also useful when MRI is contraindicated.

TREATMENT AND PROGNOSIS

Decompression of the frequently accompanying cerebellar tonsillar herniation of an associated Arnold–Chiari lesion may sometimes be sufficient. If this lesion is not present, sometimes a syringotomy is performed providing a communication to drain fluid from the self-contained central canal/syrinx to the subarachnoid space. Within two decades of diagnosis, approximately 50% of syringomyelia patients become wheelchair bound. Some of these individuals have a rapidly evolving course becoming quadriplegic within just 10 years. Factors explaining the disparity in clinical progression are not well appreciated, increasing the difficulty of counseling recently diagnosed patients with relatively mild compromise.

Hereditary Spastic Paraplegia

Clinical Vignette

A 25-year-old man who jogged short distances daily began to trip over pavement and uneven surfaces. His jogging became slower and more labored over the course of a year. Eventually, he completely stopped running. He noted that when he sat his child on his knee and wanted to balance him and emulate a pony ride, all he had to do was to push down on the sole of his foot and he could induce a continued up and down movement of his leg, in essence a self-induced self-sustaining clonus. On examination, he had a slightly broad based, spastic gait, hyperreflexia with pronounced ankle clonus, and bilateral Babinski signs. He was adopted and had no knowledge of family medical history. However, DNA testing demonstrated positive results with a mutation in the SPG4 gene encoding spastin.

Hereditary spastic paraplegia (HSP) is a genetically and clinically heterogeneous condition characterized by progressive spastic weakness of the lower extremities. Commonly, these patients notice gradual physical limitations, particularly affecting their walking. Sometimes patients note spontaneous clonus.

PATHOPHYSIOLOGY AND ETIOLOGY

Corticospinal tract and dorsal column involvement cause motor and sensory findings, respectively. Axonal degeneration of the distal ends of long axons in the spinal cord occurs.

The condition is genetically heterogeneous with autosomal dominant, autosomal recessive, and X-linked inheritance. Multiple genes and loci are defined; the SPG4 gene encodes spastin. Mutations in SPG4 account for ~40% of autosomal dominant HSP cases. This is the most common form of HSP and is linked to chromosome 2p. It is thought that spastin located within the cytoplasm interacts with microtubules. Another gene, SPG3, encodes atlastin. The genetic basis for this disease entity continues to expand as more kinds are identified and new loci and genes are discovered for other autosomal dominant, recessive, and X-linked forms.

CLINICAL PRESENTATION

Progressive lower extremity spasticity and weakness are the main clinical findings seen in HSP patients. Age of onset and the severity of symptoms may vary widely within a given family. The *pure or "uncomplicated"* form is the more common expression; this is characterized by spastic gait, increased muscle tone in the legs, quite exaggerated muscle stretch reflexes, and Babinski signs. The presence of self-induced clonus occasionally can

be annoying, although sometimes it can provide delight to a youngster in a fashion as noted in the above vignette. Vibratory sensation is sometimes mildly decreased. Occasional patients experience sphincter disturbances manifested by a spastic bladder with urgency and frequency.

The *complicated form* can include other neurologic and nonneurologic impairments: cognitive impairment, mental retardation, aphasia, dysarthria, dysphagia, optic disc pallor, nystagmus, cataracts, upper extremity weakness, motor neuronopathy, amyotrophy, cerebellar or cerebral atrophy, hydrocephalus, white matter changes, and thin corpus callosum. Additionally some patients experience bladder and bowel dysfunction as well as gastroesophageal reflux.

DIFFERENTIAL DIAGNOSIS

Important HSP differential diagnostic considerations include MS, primary lateral sclerosis, B_{12} deficiency, HTLV-I myelopathy, leukodystrophies, intrinsic or extrinsic cord tumor, syringomyelia, and dural AVMs.

A positive family history is one of the most important diagnostic clues for HSP. Genetic screening for the spastin (SPG4) or atlastin (SPG3) genes now provide a definitive diagnostic modality in a number of individuals with the classic clinical presentation. Other DNA studies will eventually become available. When these are negative, the C26:C22 long-chain fatty acid analysis for X-linked adrenoleukodystrophy needs consideration, especially when the mother may be the carrier.

Severe spinal atrophy is the typical HSP finding on MRI. However, this is a nonspecific finding as it can also be seen in other degenerative disorders such as adrenoleukodystrophy. More importantly, other causes of spastic paraparesis such as congenital spinal stenosis, syringomyelia, and spinal cord tumors are easily excluded by performing brain and spinal MRI. This study is especially important in the absence of an associated family history or positive DNA analysis for HSP.

TREATMENT

There is no specific treatment or gene therapy available to prevent, reverse, or modify the underlying disease process. Thus, the patient requires excellent supportive care, including gait and bladder training, and intensive physical therapy to keep the limbs limber in attempting to counterbalance the progressive spasticity. However, once their spasticity becomes significantly symptomatic with painful extensor spasms, the use of baclofen or even spinal cord stimulators may reduce or hopefully eliminate the patients' severe end-stage manifestations of HSP. Eventually, most of these individuals require ambulatory aids, including canes, walkers, and wheelchairs.

Friedreich Ataxia

Clinical Vignette

A 12-year-old girl presented with complaints of difficulty running and standing stationary and frequent stumbling. General exam demonstrated scoliosis and pes cavus. On

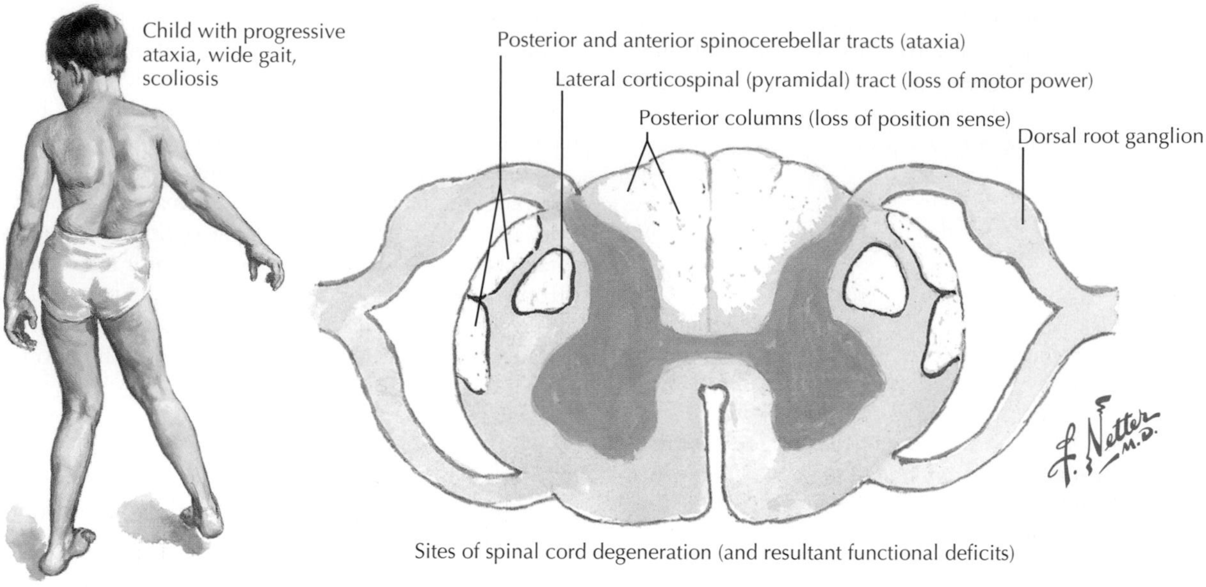

Child with progressive ataxia, wide gait, scoliosis

Posterior and anterior spinocerebellar tracts (ataxia)

Lateral corticospinal (pyramidal) tract (loss of motor power)

Posterior columns (loss of position sense)

Dorsal root ganglion

Sites of spinal cord degeneration (and resultant functional deficits)

Figure 45-15 Friedreich Ataxia.

neurologic exam, she had truncal and gait ataxia, positive Romberg, areflexia, and extensor plantar responses. Electromyography (EMG) demonstrated total absence of sensory nerve action potentials (SNAPs) but was otherwise normal. Cardiomegaly was present on chest radiography. An electrocardiogram demonstrated intermittent atrial fibrillation. A hyperexpansion of a GAA trinucleotide repeat was identified in the first intron of the frataxin gene on the long arm of chromosome 9. Because of the inherited abnormal code, a particular sequence of bases (GAA) is repeated too many times. Normally, the GAA sequence is repeated 7–22 times, but in people with Friedreich ataxia (FA) it can be repeated hundreds or even over a thousand times. This type of abnormality is called a triplet repeat expansion and has been implicated as the cause of several dominantly inherited diseases. FA is the first known recessive genetic disease that is caused by a triplet repeat expansion. Although ~98% of FA carriers have this particular genetic triplet repeat expansion, it is not found in all cases of the disease. A very small proportion of affected individuals have other gene coding defects responsible for causing disease.

The triplet repeat expansion apparently disrupts the normal assembly of amino acids into proteins, greatly reducing the amount of frataxin that is produced. Frataxin is found in the energy-producing parts of the cell called mitochondria. Research suggests that without a normal level of frataxin, certain cells in the body (especially brain, spinal cord, and muscle cells) cannot effectively produce energy and have a buildup of toxic byproducts leading to what is called "oxidative stress." This clue to the possible cause of FA came after scientists conducted studies using a yeast protein with a chemical structure similar to human frataxin. They found that the shortage of this protein in the yeast cell led to a toxic buildup of iron in the cell's mitochondria.

FA is an autosomal recessive neurodegenerative condition characterized by progressive ataxia. The disease affects the posterior columns, lateral corticospinal tracts, dorsal and ventral spinocerebellar tracts, dorsal roots and ganglia, and peripheral nerves, causing a combination sensory and cerebellar ataxia.

PATHOPHYSIOLOGY AND ETIOLOGY

The spinal cord atrophies secondary to a fiber loss in the corticospinal and spinocerebellar tracts. Neuronal loss also occurs in Clarke's column, the dorsal root ganglia, and especially the dentate nuclei (Fig. 45-15). Compensatory gliosis follows axonal degeneration and demyelination. The heart is affected, with myocardial muscle fibers replaced by myophages and fibroblasts.

A hyperexpansion of GAA triplet repeat in the first intron of the frataxin gene interferes with gene transcription, leading to deficiency of frataxin, a nuclear-encoded mitochondrial protein. This product depletion is responsible for FA in most patients. The larger the size of the expanded repeat, the greater the severity of the specific phenotype. Longer repeats are associated with earlier onset and more severe disease.

Frataxin plays a role in iron homeostasis. Its deficiency leads to increased mitochondrial iron accumulation, sensitivity to oxidative stress, and free radical–mediated cell death—particularly to neurons and cardiomyocytes.

CLINICAL PRESENTATION

A midchildhood or adolescent onset is typical, but FA may present from infancy far into adulthood. Gait ataxia is the earliest symptom. Affected individuals may stumble and have difficulty standing steadily or running. The ataxia is progressive. Hand clumsiness and dysarthria may occur months or years later. Vibration and position sense are also compromised early.

Areflexia results from peripheral nerve damage; however, in what initially seems to be a paradox, plantar responses are extensor, because of concomitant corticospinal tract damage. Nystagmus, tremor, athetoid, and choreiform movements and visual and hearing loss can also occur.

High arched feet and hammer toes may present at birth or later, or can be a forme fruste in individuals who do not develop full-blown disease. Scoliosis often develops later on. A very serious cardiomyopathy with potential for the development of various serious arrhythmias develops in most affected individuals.

DIAGNOSIS

This was formerly made on clinical grounds alone, in an older child between 8 and 15 years, who has developed a progressive ataxia, skeletal deformities, and cardiomyopathy. These cardinal features demonstrate varying degrees of scoliosis and cardiomyopathy. Genetic testing shows most affected individuals to have an abnormal gene located on chromosome 9 leading to a triplet repeat expansion. FA is a recessive genetic disease and the initial one to be identified as being caused by a triplet repeat expansion. A sequence of bases (GAA) is repeated many times more than normal. In healthy individuals, this GAA sequence is repeated 7–22 times. FA patients are often found to have hundreds or even over a thousand repeats. This classic genetic triplet repeat expansion occurs in 98% of FA carriers. Frataxin production is reduced; this interferes with intracellular energy production especially in the brain, spinal cord, and muscles.

Differential diagnosis includes MS, HSP, tabes dorsalis, ataxia telangiectasia, peroneal muscular atrophy, and olivopontocerebellar and spinocerebellar degeneration. Most of these diagnoses can be readily distinguished clinically.

TREATMENT AND PROGNOSIS

Affected individuals should maintain activity as long as possible. Balance training and muscle strengthening can be helpful. If bracing is inadequate, orthopedic surgery for scoliosis may be necessary. Regular orthopedic and cardiology follow-up is important. Scoliosis and cardiomyopathy treatment can prolong life. Over time, individuals may become wheelchair dependent or bed-bound. Death is usually secondary to cardiac arrhythmia, infection, or restrictive pulmonary disease.

Antioxidants to enhance respiratory chain function and free radical scavengers are being studied. Idebenone, a short-chain analogue of coenzyme Q10 with antioxidant properties, has been used to treat FA; however, to date there is still no effective therapy available.

ADDITIONAL RESOURCES

Anderson O. Myelitis. Current Opinions in Neurology 2000;13(3): 1311-1316.

Bhigjee AI, Madurai S, Bill PLA, et al. Spectrum of myelopathies in HIV seropositive South African patients. Neurology 2001;57:348-351. *In South Africa, the majority of HIV-seropositive patients presenting with a myelopathy have a treatable cause. Vacuolar myelopathy is rare. These features must be borne in mind when managing these patients.*

Bohlman HH. Cervical spondylosis and myelopathy. Instr Course Lect 1995;44:81-97.

Chan KF, Boey ML. Transverse myelopathy in SLE: clinical features and functional outcomes. Lupus 1996;5:294-299.

Clarke MJ, Patrick TA, White JB, et al. Spinal extradural arteriovenous malformations with parenchymal drainage: venous drainage variability and implications in clinical manifestations. Neurosurg Focus 2009 Jan;26(1):E5. *Although nontraumatic spinal arteriovenous malformations and fistulas restricted to the epidural space are rare, they can lead to significant neurologic morbidity. Careful diagnostic imaging is essential to their detection and the delineation of the pathologic anatomy. Aggressive endovascular and open operative treatment can provide arrest and reversal of neurologic deficits.*

de Seze J, Stojkovic T, Breteau G, et al. Acute myelopathies—clinical, laboratory and outcome profiles in 79 cases. Brain 2001;124:1509-1521.

Ferguson RJL, Caplan LR. Cervical spondylitic myelopathy. Neurologic Clinics 1985;3(2):373-382.

Fink JK. The hereditary spastic paraplegias: nine genes and counting. Archives of Neurology 2003;60(8):1045-1049.

Groen RJ. Non-operative treatment of spontaneous spinal epidural hematomas: a review of the literature and a comparison with operative cases. Acta Neurochir (Wien) 2004 Feb;146(2):103-110.

Harris MK, Hadi Maghzi A, Etemadifar M, et al. Acute demyelinating disorders of the central nervous system. Curr Treat Options Neurol 2009 Jan;11(1):55-63. *This paper summarizes clinical manifestations of these disorders, as well as treatment strategies. Currently, immunosuppression with corticosteroids for the acute events is the mainstay of treatment.*

Kerr DA, Ayetey H. Immunopathogenesis of acute transverse myelitis. Current Opinion in Neurology 2002;15:339-347.

Kovacs B, Lafferty TL, Brent LH DeHoratius RJ. Transverse myelopathy in systemic lupus erythematosus: an analysis of 14 cases and review of the literature. Annals of Rheum Dis 2000;59:120-124.

Kumar N, McEvoy K, Ahlskog JE. Myelopathy due to copper deficiency following gastrointestinal surgery. Arch Neurol 2003;60:1782-1785. *This paper is not only the first report on copper myelopathy but also the seminal one to date.*

Kumar N. Spinal cord, root, and plexus disorders. Continuum June 2008;14:1-271. *This is a brilliant overview of the subject.*

Lestini WF, Wiesel SW. The pathogenesis of cervical spondylosis. Clinical Orthopedics and Related Research 1989;239:69-93.

Levin MC, Jacobson S. HTLV-1 associated myelopathy/tropical spastic paraparesis (HAM/TSP): a chronic progressive neurologic disease associated with immunologically mediated damage to the central nervous system. Journal of Neuro-Virology 1997;3:126-140.

McArthur JC, Brew BJ, Nath A. Neurological complications of HIV infection. Lancet Neurol 2005 Sep;4(9):543-555.

Makinson A, Morales RJ, Basset D, et al. Diagnostic approaches to imported schistosomal myeloradiculopathy in travelers. Neurology 2008;71: 66-68.

Narvid J, Hetts SW, Larsen D, et al. Spinal dural arteriovenous fistulae: clinical features and long-term results. Neurosurgery 2008 Jan;62(1):159-166; discussion 166-7. *Sixty-three patients presenting symptoms were consistent with progressive myelopathy, and included lower extremity weakness (33 patients, 52%), parasthesias (19 patients, 30%), back pain (15 patients, 24%), and urinary symptoms (four patients, 6%). Thirty-nine patients underwent an initial endovascular embolization, with 27 requiring only this first procedure for complete obliteration. On the other hand, 24 patients underwent an initial surgical procedure, with 20 of them treated successfully with a single operation.*

Novy J, Carruzzo A, Maeder P, et al. Spinal cord ischemia: clinical and imaging patterns, pathogenesis, and outcomes in 27 patients. Arch Neurol 2006 Aug;63(8):1113-1120. *An excellent review based on 14 years' experience with 27 patients.*

Pandolfo M. Friedreich ataxia. Arch Neurol 2008 Oct;65(10):1296-1303.

Sellner J, Lüthi N, Schüpbach WM, et al. Diagnostic workup of patients with acute transverse myelitis: spectrum of clinical presentation, neuroimaging and laboratory findings. Spinal Cord 2008 Nov 18. [Epub ahead of print]

Thiele RH, Hage ZA, Surdell DL, et al. Spontaneous spinal epidural hematoma of unknown etiology: case report and literature review. Neurocrit Care 2008;9(2):242-246.

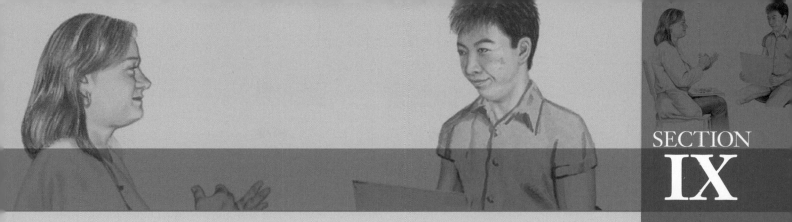

Multiple Sclerosis and Other Autoimmune CNS Demyelinating Disorders

Multiple Sclerosis

Mary Anne Muriello

46

Clinical Vignette

A 23-year-old woman suddenly noted pain behind her right eye; this discomfort was exacerbated whenever she moved her eyes horizontally or vertically. Within 2 days, she lost central vision in her right eye; she could not read with that eye alone; however, her left eye was normal. She was otherwise perfectly healthy.

Neurologic examination demonstrated her visual acuity as 20/200 OD and 20/30 OS; associated findings confined to her right eye included a slightly irregular, poorly reactive pupil, diminished color vision, and papilledema. A magnetic resonance image (MRI) of the brain demonstrated a few periventricular demyelinating lesions. Treatment was begun with daily intravenous methylprednisolone infusions for 10 days. Her vision returned to normal within a few weeks.

She was well for another 4 years until the sudden onset of an annoying swollen and numb feeling in her left leg and concomitant occurrence of an electric shock–like sensation that spread down her back whenever she bent her neck. Examination demonstrated brisk muscle stretch reflexes, left greater than right, a left Babinski sign, ipsilateral decreased position sense, and contralateral diminished temperature appreciation from her right foot to her high thoracic region. MRIs demonstrated demyelination within her left cervical-thoracic spinal cord junction, and concomitant increased T2 signal within the corpus callosal and periventricular cerebral white matter. Although she once again responded well to methylprednisolone, and despite beginning ongoing therapy with beta-interferon, this young woman continued to have occasional exacerbations with some degree of remission. Eventually, she developed a persistent gait ataxia; nevertheless, she has maintained a very successful professional career, is married, and has a 3-year-old child.

Comment: This is a classic example of a previously healthy young person, whose initial optic neuritis held a relatively poorer prognosis as her brain MRI at that time showed signs of "silent" central nervous system (CNS) demyelination. Today, with that initial combination of optic neuritis and MRI findings, a diagnosis of multiple sclerosis (MS) would be made and an "ABC" medication begun at the outset of her illness.

Multiple sclerosis is the most common central nervous system disorder to affect young and middle-aged adults. Because the disease process has such protean manifestations and a variable course, demyelinating disorders have a broad clinical spectrum, ranging from a single benign episode to one that is potentially fatal. Epidemiologic studies demonstrate that MS is more prevalent in northern latitudes, twice as common in women, and most often presents during the third and fourth decades. Caucasians are twice as likely as people of color to acquire MS in the United States and Canada. Interestingly, when MS develops among Asian populations, it predominantly affects the optic nerves and spinal cord with much less involvement of the brain in contrast to North American and European persons. Individuals born in a northern latitude, who are race- and age-matched, gain the innate diminished risk of equatorial region habitats if they move south before age 15 years. Other persons who also move from the north to the south, but do not do so until after age 15 years, maintain their innate higher risks. Although there are some yet to be precisely identified genetic predisposing factors for MS, these alone cannot account for the above-defined variabilities, as genetically comparable populations vary in MS prevalence depending on place of birth and age of migration.

GENETIC FACTORS

There is no well-defined typical genetic pattern defined on review of the natural heritability of MS. However occasional familial disease clusters do exist. The risk of MS in a first-degree relative of an affected individual (estimated at 1 in 500–1000) is approximately 20 times that in the general population. Of patients with MS, 10–15% have at least one affected first-degree relative, but the risk is not much different for parent–child relationships than for other relationships, thus negating typical dominant, recessive, or sex-linked inheritance. The risk of MS in first-degree relatives is never greater than 5%, except in monozygotic twins, where concordance rates are approximately 25%.

It is unlikely that any single gene is responsible for conferring susceptibility; therefore, a polygenic mode of transmission is assumed. Comparison of concordance rates between half-siblings reared together and those reared apart demonstrates no significant difference, suggesting that environment does not account for the slightly higher rate of MS in half-siblings of affected persons. Furthermore, it does not matter whether the shared biologic parent is the mother or the father. Thus, a mitochondrial inheritance pattern is most unlikely.

PATHOLOGY

With classic MS, the primary process is one of demyelination leading to loss of myelin from central nervous system (CNS) axons. Myelin loss (a nonspecific term) occurs concurrently with other pathologic processes that also affect the axons, glial elements, or vasculature. CNS oligodendrocytes are responsible for the elaboration of brain myelin. This is a predominantly lipid-based (70%) structure, with the remainder being protein based. One part, myelin basic protein, is particularly immunologically susceptible and experimentally encephalitogenic.

Inspection of the gross brain of an MS subject does not demonstrate any sign of abnormalities that would indicate the presence of the myriad histologic changes that are to be found on microscopic evaluation. However, the optic nerves, optic

Multiple Sclerosis: Central Nervous System Plaques

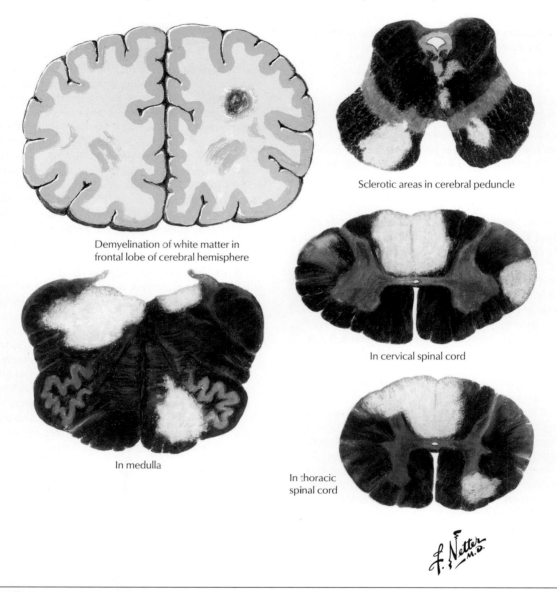

Demyelination of white matter in
frontal lobe of cerebral hemisphere

Sclerotic areas in cerebral peduncle

In cervical spinal cord

In medulla

In thoracic
spinal cord

Figure 46-1 Central Nervous System Pathology.

chiasm, and spinal cord may be atrophic to the native eye. Sometimes, areas of patchy demyelination are seen on the basis pontis surface, the cerebellar peduncles, and the surface of the medulla and floor of the fourth ventricle.

Coronal brain sections reveal changes similar to those noted on MRI, where variously sized MS plaques are apparent. Recently acquired lesions are pink and soft, whereas chronic MS lesions are gray, translucent, and firm (Fig. 46-1). It is often difficult to correlate the multiple lesions found at autopsy or by MRI throughout the neuraxis with a patient's history. Sometimes classic MS plaques exist in patients who were never clinically suspected of harboring it.

Microscopic analysis demonstrates that many plaques have no relation to specific nerve tracts. Often, the plaques have a perivenular and paraventricular distribution. Myelin loss from a nerve fiber is distinct and best defined by toluidine blue stains. Macrophage accumulation is a frequent accompaniment. Active plaques contain myelin debris. Severe loss of oligodendrocytes within MS plaques is associated with the concomitant nonspecific finding of hypertrophic astrocytes. Signs of leptomeningeal inflammation, not unlike that found in acute disseminated MS, may be evident.

There is also a very significant component of axonal and neuronal damage in multiple sclerosis. This is particularly relevant to the long-term outcome and eventual disability. One can find evidence of axonal injury early on in the disease process. This is found in areas of obvious demyelination as well as areas of white and gray matter that appear normal to gross inspection. It is proposed that an antigen-specific destructive component related to both T cells and autoantibodies as well as the effects of activated macrophages and microglia lead to very significant axonal damage in the pathogenesis of MS. Mitochondrial function may also be impaired as various cellular substrates further contribute to this pathologic component.

CLINICAL SUBTYPES

The natural history of MS varies with the subtype of disease. Functional consequences may relate to some degree of axonal loss occurring after demyelination.

Benign MS

Clinical Vignette

A 52-year-old woman with migraine headaches since childhood, tobacco use throughout her adult years, and a history of transverse myelitis at age 14 years with complete recovery was subsequently noted to have a normal neurologic examination. She remained well until 65 years of age when she had an acute episode of left hemisensory deficit. An MRI scan of the brain revealed an acute lacunar infarct in the right thalamus on diffusion-weighted imaging, a chronic lacunar infarct in the left basal ganglia, and 10 bright lesions on T2 and FLAIR images, several of which were linear to ovoid in shape, configured perpendicularly to the ventricular walls, none enhancing with contrast. MRI of the cervical spine showed mild myelomalacia at C5 to C7 without other abnormality. She quit smoking and recovered with very little sensory impairment throughout her left side and lived without further neurologic symptoms until the age of 72 years, when she died of lung cancer.

Comment: This patient experienced a single bout of transverse myelitis as an adolescent, often a harbinger of more generalized MS. Medical technology at that time did not afford a simple way to explore her central nervous system for occult signs of multiple sclerosis. Clinical signs of more diffuse disease never developed. However, approximately 50 years later, when the patient required an MRI for a question of stroke, clinically inactive, more widespread MS became evident. In fact there was more than one explanation for the periventricular white matter abnormalities on MRI, namely, microvascular disease and migraine headaches. However, taken in the context of her prior episode of transverse myelitis, and the number and configuration of her white matter lesions, a diagnosis of relatively benign MS is likely. Certainly, whatever the idiosyncrasies of her immune system are that protected her, thus preventing further expression of more diffuse signs of clinical multiple sclerosis over her lifetime, once unlocked, they might provide the key for better appreciating the pathophysiology of MS and therefore direct more specific therapeutic research intervention in the future.

Relapsing–Remitting MS

Clinical Vignette

A 47-year-old woman sustained lower back and neck injury and concussion at 25 years of age in a motor vehicle accident. She underwent a C2-3 fusion and L4-5 diskectomy at that time and made a good recovery. She delivered two healthy children when she was ages 28 and 30 years. Five months after the birth of the first child, she began to experience numbness in the left leg and urinary urgency, with occasional leakage of urine. She was felt to have a

recrudescence of her lumbar radicular symptoms and postpartum stress incontinence. Her primary care physician referred her for physical therapy, and her symptoms improved over the ensuing 2 months.

Just 1.5 years later, at age 32 years, she experienced increased difficulty lifting simple kitchen objects such as a milk carton and a frying pan and noted some numbness in her hands. She had increasing problems carrying her children, particularly placing them into their car seats. Her internist found Tinel signs at each wrist and thought she might have bilateral carpal tunnel syndrome; wrist splints were not helpful, and she remained relatively symptomatic. Over the years, she tried to remain active with her children, but increasingly found herself altering bicycle routes that they had once taken with ease as a family. She could not drink anything for 3 hours prior to going out on a bike ride to avoid urinary incontinence. Because she more commonly fatigued with any sustained walking, particularly during the warmer summer months, she curtailed her shopping.

Eventually she was referred to a neurologist after she developed a right foot drop, a subsequent series of falls, and then an exacerbation of her bladder symptoms. Examination demonstrated tandem ataxia, circumduction of her right leg, with diminished right arm swing, very brisk muscle stretch reflexes more on the right, sustained ankle clonus, bilateral Babinski signs, and markedly diminished vibration sense. Brain MRI revealed scattered bihemispheric periventricular and subcortical T2 and FLAIR hyperintensities without enhancement. MRI of the cervical and thoracic spine showed a stable C2-3 fusion, myelomalacia from T7 to T9 with patchy hyperintensity throughout this region, and an enhancing lesion at the conus. Cerebrospinal fluid examination demonstrated five oligoclonal bands without pleocytosis.

Comment: This is a relatively classic case of relapsing–remitting multiple sclerosis (RRMS) beginning subtly during the childbearing years. On occasions the onset may be more precipitous, almost mimicking a stroke; however, the clinical setting is with rare exceptions not quite as abrupt, and the findings do not replicate the damage one finds when a specific vessel is obstructed. Often, as in this instance, the symptoms are attributed to more benign entities such as various mononeuropathies, for example, the median nerve with her first visit to an internist, and to a peroneal lesion when the foot drop developed and she first visited an osteopath. Her limited exercise reserve, as exemplified by her diminished ability to walk or bike-ride any significant distance, could easily have been ascribed to fatigue, hysteria, or depression, something that commonly occurs during the first years of a demyelinating illness. This is particularly the case for a young woman who has recently taken on the new responsibility of caring for two babies. With time, the clinical setting clarifies itself.

Even the most skilled neurologist often had trouble confirming an MS diagnosis prior to the era of MRI. Today the brain MRI is sometimes normal or nonspecific early on, and it is not until one also obtains spinal imaging that the MS diagnosis is established. Lastly one needs to fastidiously maintain an objective approach to this type of patient, especially early on in the illness. It is important to be willing to reevaluate PRN and/or at a set interval. Corollary to this is that it is blatantly unfair to label the patient with new-onset symptoms as being histrionic when she has a normal neurologic examination and especially a normal brain MRI.

Secondary Progressive

Clinical Vignette

This now 50-year-old woman presented with a 29-year history of neurologic difficulties. She had reported having diplopia at age 21 years, making a good recovery. She was diagnosed with RRMS just 2 years later, after an episode of subacute right-sided weakness and cerebrospinal fluid (CSF) analysis demonstrating oligoclonal bands. She was treated with adrenocorticotropin hormone (ACTH). Although subsequently she required a right ankle–foot orthosis (AFO), she was able to return to an active life. In the early 1990s, she was prescribed subcutaneous interferon beta-1b that she tolerated poorly because of excessive injection-site reactions; she discontinued these within a few months. Subsequently she developed increasingly severe relapses every 1 to 2 years, each time undergoing treatment with intravenous (IV) methylprednisolone. She than began interferon beta-1a intramuscularly in the late 1990s when she visited a new neurologist because of increasing dependence on a cane and frequent bouts of urinary incontinence. Subsequently, mounting lower extremity weakness, spasticity, and fatigue evolved but she no longer experienced distinct flare-ups of her disease. It became increasingly difficult for her to keep up with the frequent travel that her work as an executive required.

Neurologic examination revealed an internuclear ophthalmoplegia (INO) and spastic paraparesis. Ultimately, the patient required an electric wheelchair to maintain mobility.

Comment: Typically, RRMS continues over many years, gradually leading to incremental decline in a range of neurologic functions resulting in varying degrees of neurologic disability. Eventually, the severity and discreteness of relapsing symptoms tend to wane, but dysfunction concomitantly becomes more insidious, resulting in secondary progressive MS (SSMS). Rarely, MS begins with a fulminant course followed by poor recovery, rapid progression, or both, ending in significant disability or death in a relatively short period after disease onset.

Primary Progressive

Clinical Vignette

A 45-year-old man who worked as a New York stockbroker had a gradual change in his commuting routine to and from work. For years, he would forego the subway for a brisk walk to the stock exchange after taking commuter rail from the suburbs. By the age of 40, he had universally taken to riding the train the entire distance. He attributed his "laziness" to aging and knee problems related to his high school basketball career. No longer could he keep himself out in front when bicycle-riding with his wife nor could he lift nearly the weight with his legs during his gym workouts

that he had earlier on. To his embarrassment, he tripped on the stairs when walking with a coworker and knocked out his two front teeth.

Neurologic examination demonstrated a spastic gait with mild circumduction of the right leg, mild weakness of the iliopsoas bilaterally, brisk muscle stretch reflexes in the legs, bilateral Babinski signs, and loss of vibration perception at the toes, ankles, and knees.

Comment: In approximately 15% of patients with MS, the clinical course is more chronically progressive from the outset, in contrast to the more typical history of remissions and exacerbations of relapsing–remitting disease. This clinical setting defines another group of patients, those with primary progressive MS (PPMS). Most of these individuals have clinical evidence of significant spinal cord disease but a paucity of intracranial findings. Typically, progressive gait dysfunction and spasticity characterize their clinical course. Unlike RRMS, this subtype exhibits a male predominance, older age of onset, and poor response to disease-modifying strategies.

Therefore, the MS clinical spectrum can range from a relatively asymptomatic disorder, after an initial few benign episodes of CNS or optic nerve disorder, to an acute life-threatening illness that may mimic a brain tumor.

DIFFERENTIAL DIAGNOSIS

Because MS can affect any area of the CNS from the optic nerves to the distal spinal cord, patients present with extremely varied manifestations occurring over a wide age range from midchildhood into the early sixth decade. Whenever one is confronted with an acute neurologic process primarily affecting the CNS in a previously healthy young person, the physician must always consider if this could be the initial presentation of MS. There is a very broad differential diagnosis predicated on the patient's initial symptomatology.

Ocular

Blurred vision, likely a manifestation of acute optic neuritis, is a very common initial symptoms of MS. This may have great variability in degree from gross total unilateral blindness to a subtle change in visual acuity. Vision changes may also be related to a poorly expressed diplopia secondary to an INO, one of the most common neuro-ophthalmologic manifestations of MS (Fig. 46-2). In the first instance, the differential diagnosis includes any process affecting the retina or cornea, and in the second, the diplopia may be related to a pseudo-INO, mimicking MS. This is typical of myasthenia gravis. Sometimes a true INO secondary to a stroke may occur in older hypertensive patients.

At times a subtle demyelinating lesion may be clinically uncovered by exposure to heat. For example, during a summer heat wave, or even just taking a shower, a patient may note relatively short-lived symptomatology, sometimes visual blurring or just a change in gait; this is known as Uhthoff syndrome. The symptoms are usually fleeting. These routinely disappear when the patient returns to more normal ambient temperatures.

The prognostic significance of an acute episode of optic neuritis (ON) has been the subject of numerous investigations. Today MRI provides an important means to put the ON event into a long term perspective. A recent ON study, with a median

Optic neuritis

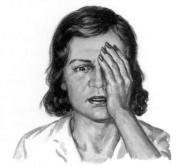

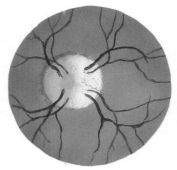

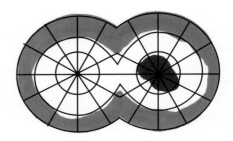

Sudden unilateral blindness, self-limited (usually 2 to 3 weeks). Patient covering one eye, suddenly realizes other eye is partially or totally blind.

Temporal pallor in optic disc, caused by delayed recovery of temporal side of optic (II) nerve

Visual fields reveal central scotoma due to acute retrobulbar neuritis

Internuclear ophthalmoplegia

(OD = right, OS = left)

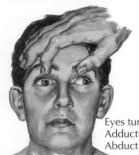

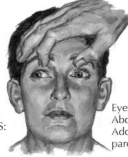

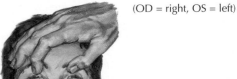

Eyes turned to left. OD: Adduction paralysis; OS: Abduction nystagmus

Eyes turned to right. OD: Abduction nystagmus; OS: Adduction lesser mild paresis

Convergence. Fully preserved adduction; both eyes have full medial movement

Figure 46-2 Multiple Sclerosis: Visual manifestations.

6 years' follow-up, demonstrated that slightly less than 50% of these patients had converted to *clinically definite MS* (CDMS). Most importantly, both the presence and the number of MRI-defined spinal cord lesions, and to a lesser extent gadolinium-enhancing lesions, as well as the number of infratentorial lesions at baseline were significant independent predictors of an even higher disability manifested as CDMS.

When temporally associated with a myelopathy, this clinical presentation is referred to as *Devic syndrome*, or *neuromyelitis optica* (NMO). This is a humorally mediated autoimmune demyelinating disorder that is immunologically distinct from MS. It is characterized by an autoantibody that recognizes aquaporin 4 (AQP4), a water channel expressed on astrocyte podocytes. NMO may sometimes have a poorer prognosis than MS although on occasion it is more acutely responsive to immunosuppression or chemotherapy. This Devic syndrome does not typically benefit from first-line long-term MS disease modifiers (Chapter 47).

Inner Ear or Cerebellum

A vague feeling of unsteadiness, dizziness, and sometimes a whirling vertigo with nausea are frequent symptoms of MS. Precise definition of exactly what patients mean by "dizzy" is essential. Frequently, patients are in fact reporting a sense of dysequilibrium likely representing cerebellar dysfunction and less commonly reflecting vestibular pathways. Such patients

typically demonstrate a broad-based gait, various signs of dysmetria, a tremor not seen in patients with a primary vestibular lesion, and often vertical nystagmus (Fig. 46-3).

The most common cause of true vertigo is either a primary vestibular neuronitis or the recurrent Ménière syndrome associated with hearing loss. These are both benign processes originating within the inner ear. However, one needs to always consider the possibility that the patient's dizziness/vertigo has a primary CNS basis. One very important differential diagnostic clue to the latter is the finding of vertical nystagmus on the neurologic examination. This is not found when a peripheral mechanism for vertigo is present. The clinical demonstration of vertical nystagmus in a patient with vertigo requires an MRI to look for primary CNS disease.

Although spontaneous downbeat nystagmus is often the hallmark of another specific central nervous system lesion, namely an Arnold-Chiari malformation, this may also occur in MS patients reporting feelings of dizziness.

Myelopathies

Sensations of tingling, tightness, pins and needles, and electric shocks are common MS symptoms. Relatively early in the disease course, some of these patients report an electric shock–like sensation that usually radiates down the back or arms, occurring spontaneously when the patient bends his or her neck. This is known as *Lhermitte's sign* (Fig. 46-4). This most

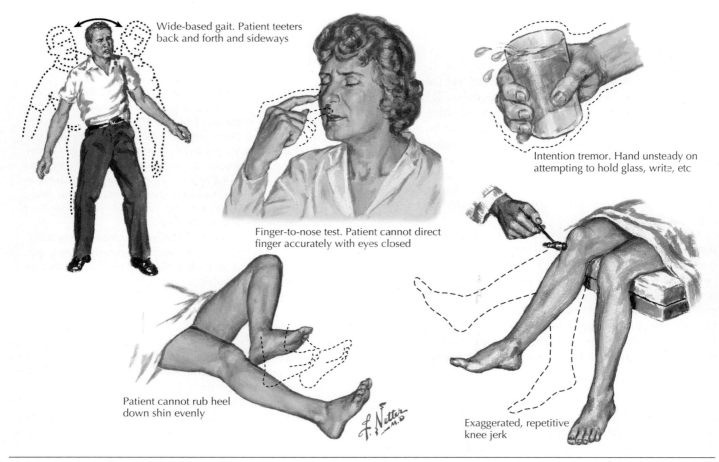

Wide-based gait. Patient teeters back and forth and sideways

Intention tremor. Hand unsteady on attempting to hold glass, write, etc

Finger-to-nose test. Patient cannot direct finger accurately with eyes closed

Patient cannot rub heel down shin evenly

Exaggerated, repetitive knee jerk

Figure 46-3 Multiple Sclerosis: Cerebellar and Brain Stem Manifestations.

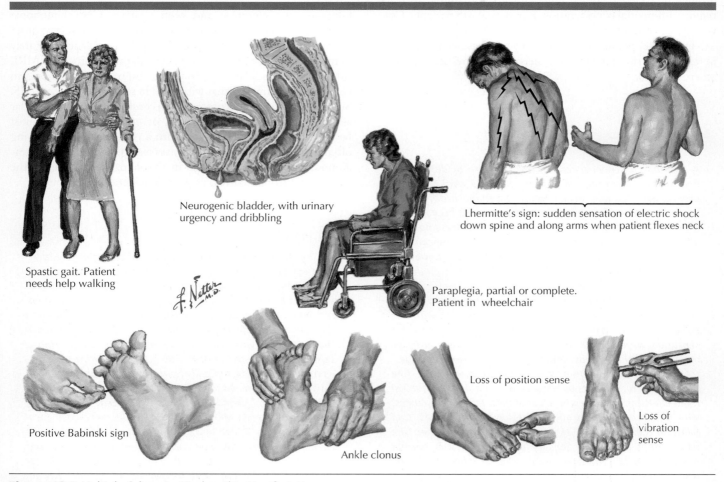

Spastic gait. Patient needs help walking

Neurogenic bladder, with urinary urgency and dribbling

Paraplegia, partial or complete. Patient in wheelchair

Lhermitte's sign: sudden sensation of electric shock down spine and along arms when patient flexes neck

Positive Babinski sign

Ankle clonus

Loss of position sense

Loss of vibration sense

Figure 46-4 Multiple Sclerosis: Myelopathic Manifestations.

commonly occurs with MS patients but often the patient does not report this per se. Rather the skilled examiner is trained to ask about such as it is pathognomonic and indicative of spinal posterior column dysfunction. *Lhermitte's sign* can be reported with almost any form of spinal cord disease, including spondylosis with significant cervical spinal stenosis, a space-occupying lesion, vitamin B_{12} (cobalamin) deficiency, or copper deficiency syndromes, especially in individuals who have had major gastrectomies or unusual diets, such as excess zinc that blocks copper absorption.

Other patients with MS frequently report a tight bandlike distribution of numbness. When circumferential or hemicircumferential, particularly in the midtrunk, the immediate concern is a possible transverse myelitis or primary spinal cord mass lesion. Sometimes patients describe a distribution suggestive of a polyneuropathy with bilateral symmetric numbness. On other occasions, numbness may occur acutely in the hand, compatible with mononeuropathy or stroke. Other myelopathies deserving consideration relate to tropical spastic paraparesis or AIDS.

Strokes and TIAs

Although MS is one of the most common neurologic disorders in young to middle-aged adults, stroke must always be considered. Carotid or vertebrobasilar dissection, paradoxical emboli, and CNS vasculitis are some of the more common stroke syndromes in younger adults. These may often mimic MS and require differential consideration in potential MS patients. Conversely, as technology has improved, the ability to recognize MS in an older population (aged >50 years) has become possible in cases that masquerade as microangiopathy secondary to atherosclerosis.

Clinical Vignette

A 58-year-old school teacher with a history of depression and sciatica noted the presence of left-sided weakness that progressed gradually over a year. She found it difficult to maneuver her left leg into a pair of pants and occasionally experienced buckling of the right leg when dressing. Her left-handed grasp of a pen was increasingly compromised and her handwriting was changing. Advancing fatigue was making it increasingly difficult for her to get through her work day. She began to experience difficulty driving due to stiffness and shaking of the right leg, and, eventually, she could not exit her car without lifting her right leg with her hands. This was associated with a band-like constriction sensation around her thorax and intermittent urinary incontinence that she attributed to child-bearing and age.

Neurologic examination demonstrated diminished fine coordinated movements of her dominant left hand, bilateral hand clumsiness, and right greater than left leg weakness, with increased tone distally in the lower extremities, and bilateral Babinski signs. Her gait was wide-based and she had a right foot drop. Sensory examination was normal except for mild symmetrically decreased vibration in the distal lower extremities.

MRI scan of the brain with and without contrast showed scattered focal areas of T2 and FLAIR hyperintensity in the periventricular white matter, some oriented perpendicularly to the ventricles. There was a single lesion in the anterior corpus callosum and one area of faint enhancement in the left cerebral peduncle. Diffusion-weighted imaging was normal. Thoracic spine MRI showed an enhancing lesion in the cord at T9. Visual evoked responses showed some delay on the right, and CSF analysis revealed four oligoclonal bands and negative Lyme testing.

In retrospect, the patient recalled a transient visual disturbance in the right eye at age 19 years that was construed as migraine. When questioned, she also recalled an occasional Lhermitte sign occurring as a young woman.

A wider diagnostic net needs to be cast in older patients who are considered to possibly have had a cryptogenic stroke who do not have underlying risk factors for stroke. As so well illustrated in this vignette, a careful history is once again the essence of neurologic diagnosis, especially knowledge of what are the best questions to ask. Diffusion-weighted imaging and MRI perfusion studies can be very helpful in distinguishing subacute ischemic lesions from demyelinating lesions.

Cerebral Mass Lesions

Gliomas, meningiomas, and even primary CNS lymphoma always require consideration in young patients with recent onset of focal neurologic dysfunction. Lymphomas particularly may mimic MS because of their periventricular distribution on MRI. Additionally, the relatively promising response of lymphoma to corticosteroids mimics that witnessed in some patients with MS. Similarly when patients present with cerebellar ataxia, cerebellar astrocytomas, hemangioblastomas, or other mass lesions must be excluded. When confronted with a patient with an evolving often asymmetric paraparesis, a mass lesion, particularly meningiomas, originating anywhere in the spinal axis, or even the parasagittal frontal cortex, require consideration.

Clinical Vignette

A 30-year-old woman, previously healthy, began to experience episodes of déjà vu and derealization. In her work as a bank teller, colleagues noted that she had distinct periodic slowness in her work and an occasional latency in responsiveness when dealing with customers. A friend suggested that she was suffering from anxiety, and she consulted a therapist who witnessed one of her spells. Suspecting a seizure disorder, the patient was referred to a neurologist, who found her to be diffusely hyperreflexic with a left Babinski sign, mildly increased tone in the lower extremities, and a jaw jerk. EEG demonstrated left temporal lobe slowing with sharp waves. MRI scan of the brain revealed a focal enhancing mass lesion in the left temporal lobe with modest edema and three tiny, non-enhancing white matter lesions located subcortically as well as in the periventricular regions. A glioblastoma multiforme was suspected; however,

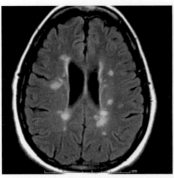
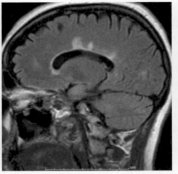
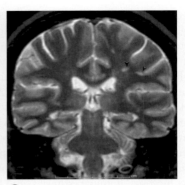

A. and **B.** Axial and sagittal FLAIR images with increased T2 signal within the corpus callosum and paraventricular white matter with extension into central white matter along vascular pathways.

C. Coronal T2, where the typical oval lesions are oriented along vascular pathways, typical of "Dawson fingers" (*arrowheads*).

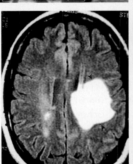
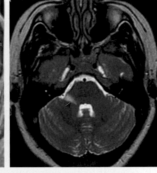

D. Coronal T1-weighted, fat-saturated, post–gadolinium-enhanced image shows enhancement and enlargement of the right optic nerve (*arrow*).

E. Cerebellar Peduncle: Axial T2 Brain MR: Multiple Sclerosis: Cleft-like right brachium pontis plaque (arrowhead).

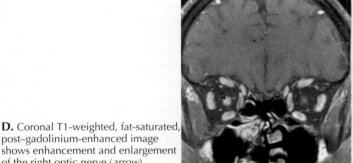
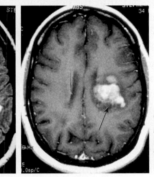

F. Fulminate MS 1: Tumefactive Multiple Sclerosis: Axial FLAIR Brain MR: Large demyelinating mass left frontoparietal periventricular white matter (arrowheads).

G. Fulminate MS Contrast: Tumefactive Multiple Sclerosis: Axial Postcontrast T2 Brain MR: Markedly enhancing large left frontoparietal periventricular white matter demyelinating mass (arrow).

Figure 46-5 Brain MRI in Multiple Sclerosis.

stereotactic biopsy showed demyelination with axonal sparing, sparse perivascular lymphocytic infiltration, and numerous periodic acid Schiff-positive macrophages.

The patient received a short course of IV methylprednisolone, and phenytoin therapy was initiated. Her episodes resolved and repeat MRI in 3 months showed near complete resolution of the mass-like region.

Occasionally an acute focal cerebral lesion may be the presenting sign of MS leading the clinician to suspect that the patient has a glioblastoma multiforme, the most malignant of brain tumors. Fortunately, stereotactic biopsy occasionally demonstrates a rare monofocal form of MS, monofocal acute inflammatory demyelination (MAID) (Fig. 46-5). This can mimic a primary brain tumor or abscess. It is a rare and unique demyelinating disorder that may herald, or be superimposed on, more typical MS or may be seemingly unassociated with MS. MAID usually affects the cerebral hemispheres, and its clinical and radiologic features suggest a brain tumor. In contrast, an acute myelitis or optic neuritis is a more common example of a monofocal demyelinating process. Patients with the "cerebral form" of demyelinating disease have symptoms atypical for MS, including an acute hemiplegia, hemisensory complaints, and visual field deficits. Less common symptoms include headaches, seizures, aphasia, an alteration in level of consciousness, and cognitive or psychiatric manifestations.

Rarely, patients with a similar acute clinical presentation have multifocal CNS lesions, diagnosed as acute disseminated encephalomyelitis (ADEM) (Chapter 47). ADEM usually has widespread or multifocal MRI abnormalities.

Spinal Dural Arteriovenous Malformations

Patients with MS typically experience evanescent or waxing and waning symptomatology. However, there are two different forms of vascular anomalies that sometimes present with a relapsing–remitting temporal profile mimicking MS. Firstly a spinal dural arteriovenous fistula must also be an important part of the differential diagnosis. Although the physician typically suspects MS whenever a patient experiences intermittent myelopathic symptoms, very precise inspection of the MRI is essential in order to define the possibility of an epidural vascular lesion. Once diagnosed, surgical treatment or an embolization procedure is performed to obliterate the abnormal cord vasculature. Secondly the very rare pontine cavernous hemangiomas require consideration in the differential of intermittent brainstem symptoms, including diplopia, hemiparesthesias, and bilateral Babinski signs. Here the MRI is again essential in reaching this diagnosis. These patients have a focal pontine lesion identified and there is no evidence of a diffuse, multifocal set of demyelinating abnormalities characteristic of MS.

Peripheral Neuropathy

In patients with MS, the "numbness" per se is commonly a feeling of tightness or pressure rather than the more classic tingling sensation of a peripheral nerve disorder. Individuals with MS frequently complain of a poorly defined, and often variable, multifocal numbness. This is typically not confined to a single nerve root or peripheral nerve distribution; it may occur with both a chronic and acute temporal profile. When this is a slowly evolving process, entities such as vitamin B_{12} deficiency, particularly when associated with a myelopathy manifested by Babinski signs, Lyme disease, HTLV-I, copper deficiency, or even the relatively unusual migrant sensory neuritis of Wartenberg, are part of the differential diagnosis. When both legs are involved in a relatively acute and symmetric fashion, with an evolving weakness, either the Guillain–Barré syndrome or a spinal mass lesion are common possibilities.

Neuromuscular Transmission Defects

Like MS, myasthenia gravis tends to occur in young women. It is characterized by combinations of intermittent visual difficulties, particularly diplopia often referred to by the patient as blurring, dysarthria, and fatigue, symptoms that also occur in MS. Lambert–Eaton myasthenic syndrome (LEMS), a presynaptic autoimmune, often paraneoplastic, disorder, also may cause intermittent weakness, bulbar signs, and fatigue (Chapter 70), mimicking the fatigue or nonspecific tiredness that are so commonly presenting signs of MS.

Myopathies

These disorders, often either mitochondrial myopathies or late-onset dystrophies of the oculopharyngeal type, present with an increased tendency to muscular fatigue. On neurologic examination, these patients frequently have both ptosis and limited extraocular muscle (EOM) function. However, as the EOM deficits are symmetric, most of these patients do not report any diplopia. Individuals with periodic paralysis have intermittent symptomatology; however, these events usually start in childhood and adolescence, are symmetric, are relatively short-lived, and rarely affect bulbar musculature.

Conversion Hysteria

All too often, patients eventually diagnosed with MS do not have any definitive findings on their initial neurologic examination. This often leads the initial and unsuspecting physician into a common and sad differential diagnostic error. One must take great care not to falsely apply diagnostic significance to various situational anxieties such as occupational stresses, marital discord, or financial worries as being emotional precipitants for ill-defined clinical presentations and suggest that the patient has a somatoform disorder (Chapter 26). Conversion hysteria must always be a diagnosis of exclusion. This relatively rare disorder frequently occurs in young adults, particularly women, within the setting of poorly articulated psychologic stress, sometimes related to sexual abuse such as incest.

These individuals invariably have normal examination results, although their subconscious attempts to demonstrate neurologic abnormalities often result in consistently inconsistent neurologic findings. These may often be a "give-way" weakness or very bizarre gait problems known as "astasia-abasia." Repeat clinical neurologic evaluations, MRI, evoked potentials (EPs), and CSF examinations are all warranted. This allows one to always give the patient the benefit of doubt, repeatedly searching for clues to a much more common organic disease. Most importantly, there is no illness more likely to lead the physician to this clinical conundrum than MS.

DIAGNOSTIC APPROACH

Although there are no specific criteria for making the diagnosis of MS, MRI is the most helpful diagnostic adjunct. When typical MRI findings are found in the presence of a classic history and physical findings, there is little need to resort to other testing modalities in most clinical settings.

Magnetic Resonance Imaging

The diagnosis of MS has become very well defined with MRI; a positive study provides the physician with a solid diagnostic base leading in most instances to an accurate MS diagnosis in upwards of 95% of patients. New lesions typically have uniform gadolinium enhancement, whereas a ringlike enhancement is compatible with reactivation of prior lesions. Acute-phase plaques appear as rounded areas of high-signal intensity on FLAIR and T2 sequences. Gadolinium enhancement on T1 sequences is secondary to inflammatory damage to the blood–brain barrier. Earlier-onset, but nonreactivated, lesions do not enhance at all. T2-weighted MRI has the highest degree of sensitivity and is particularly useful for demonstrating disease dissemination; however, this lacks somewhat in specificity. A primary value of T1-weighted gadolinium-enhanced imaging is that it provides an increased specificity by differentiating enhancing from nonenhancing lesions.

Classic MRI findings are typified by multiple well-demarcated ovoid plaques whose long axis are situated perpendicularly along callososeptal interfaces and demonstrate a perivenular extension within the corpus callosum (Dawson fingers). Furthermore, plaques have a propensity for the periventricular and subcortical white matter, middle cerebellar peduncle, pons, or medulla (see

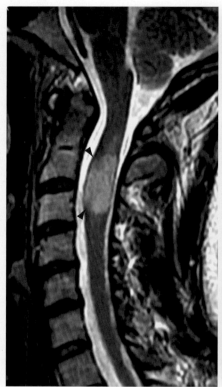

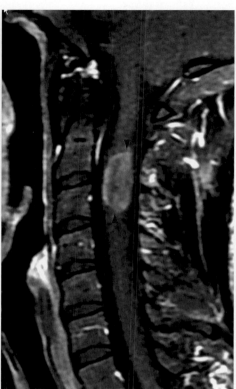

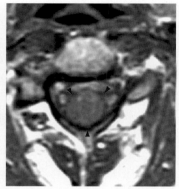

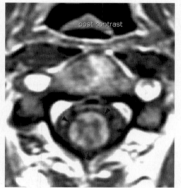

A. Sagittal T2 cervical MR (arrowheads).

B. Sagittal T1 post-gadolinium cervical MR: Large expansile hyperintense upper cervical cord plaque (arrowheads).

C. Axial precontrast T1 cervical MR: Markedly expanded cervical spinal cord (arrowheads).

D. Axial postcontrast T1 cervical MR: Expansile peripherally enhancing plaque (arrowheads).

Figure 46-6 Spinal Cord MRI in Multiple Sclerosis.

Fig. 46-5). Within the spinal cord per se, white matter lesions can involve any part of the many afferent or efferent tracts, particularly the dorsal columns. At times the lesion can be so large that it mimics an intramedullary tumor as characterized by a large expansile hyperintense upper cervical cord plaque as seen in Figure 46-6. MRI has unequivocally replaced CSF analysis, the oldest methodology, as well as various forms of evoked neurophysiologic potentials, as the primary diagnostic methodology.

Increasingly powerful magnets and techniques, able to resolve variations from the norm, that sometimes mimic MS but may not be pathologic, sometimes complicate interpretation of abnormalities. "Unidentified bright objects (UBOs)" are the classic imitators seen in those who smoke, have hypertension, migraine headaches, or Lyme disease, or are present for indeterminate reasons. Similarly, Virchow-Robin spaces, dilated CSF-filled vascular areas, may give high T2 signal intensity. However, these can be distinguished from demyelinated plaques of MS because they are not present with proton density images.

MRI of the spinal cord may be particularly useful in substantiating a diagnosis (see Fig. 46-6). In clinically suspicious cases with normal or equivocal brain MRI, spinal cord lesions can be compelling, even without symptoms referable to the spinal cord. Spinal cord lesions, however, are sometimes not as easily identified because of the constraints of motion artifact. The increased availability of 3-Tesla magnets in the coming

years will add further image refinement, particularly with primary spinal forms of MS.

There is a most interesting subset of patients who eventually prove to have MS but are first evaluated with symptoms that are seemingly nonspecific and definitely not classic for MS. They undergo MRI scanning primarily to assuage patient fears of a structural abnormality, such as a tumor or perhaps MS. In a serendipitous fashion, the study then uncovers unexpected white-matter demyelinating lesions compatible with MS. For the physician, these MR findings do not seem to collate with the patient's presenting symptoms. However, these observations need to be taken seriously. Such results are extending our definition of the initial clinical picture of multiple sclerosis and are making the neurologic clinician even more alert to the relative subtleties of this disorder early in its course.

Clinical Vignettes

A 27-year-old woman with a history of depression since early adolescence experienced painful spasm in her neck after her psychiatrist increased her dose of Zyprexa. An MRI of her cervical spine revealed an abnormality in the left dorsolateral spinal cord at C7. It was a nonenhancing lesion, bright on T2 and FLAIR image. Her torticollis resolved

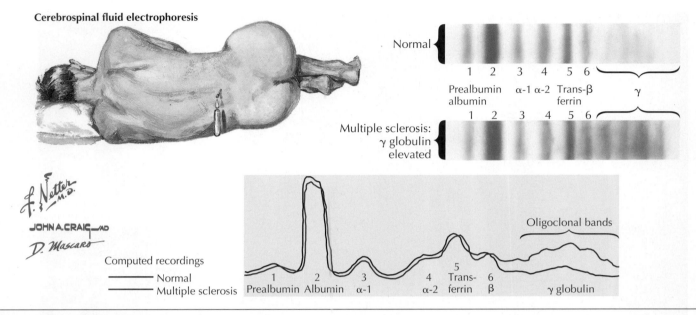

Cerebrospinal fluid electrophoresis

Figure 46-7 Diagnostic Tests—Spinal Fluid.

following reduction of her Zyprexa dosage. Brain MRI showed two lesions within the corpus callosum. Visual evoked response was significantly delayed on the right eye compatible with a lesion between the retina and the optic chiasm.

A 34-year-old landscaper was struck by the trunk of a tree that was felled by a coworker, failing to heed a warning to stand clear. He lost consciousness and was taken to a local emergency room. He had awakened and was noted to be fully alert and oriented. CT of the spine showed a T3 compression fracture. The day after his injury, he developed a severe headache. Magnetic resonance angiography of the head and neck revealed no dissection or any other vascular abnormality. Although brain MRI revealed no hemorrhages, there were 11 periventricular lesions seen on T2 and FLAIR images. Some of these were oriented perpendicularly to the ventricles, the largest of which, in the right frontal lobe, showed some cystic changes with low attenuation on T1 images and mild enhancement. CSF analysis demonstrated six oligoclonal bands and the presence of myelin basic protein. None of these findings could be related to his long history of ADH.

These two vignettes emphasize how MRI can serendipitously demonstrate findings of MS in the absence of active clinical symptoms, raising the question, "How early is too early to offer immunomodulatory therapy?" There is no consensus on the approach to such patients. How to identify patients with a potentially benign course versus those at risk for significant future disease with later disability remains unknown. MRI will be a keystone as this treatment algorithm is eventually defined. With the increasing evidence of the efficacy of the various ABC drugs in lessening long-term deficits, if these medications are begun when the diagnosis of MS is well defined, there is an increased tendency to begin active therapy once the diagnosis is ensured in patients such as these.

Cerebrospinal Fluid

Lumbar puncture for CSF is becoming superfluous when the diagnosis is established by history, examination, and unequivocal and very supportive MRI images. MRI is also very useful in excluding other diagnoses, particularly Lyme disease, sarcoidosis, lymphoma, or multi-infarcts secondary to a primary CNS vasculitis. However, when there is no definite MRI confirmation or collation of an MS diagnosis, a CSF examination can still be a very useful diagnostic procedure. When indicated, this procedure is typically performed by neurologists and neuroradiologists.

The typical CSF profile of a patient with MS is summarized in Figure 46-7. The white blood cell count is typically normal, with less than 6 mononuclear cells/mm³ being present; however, occasionally one may see MS patients with up to 50 lymphocytes per cubic millimeter. This usually does not exceed 25 cells/mm³. Lymphocyte counts greater than 100/mm³ must arouse suspicion of other inflammatory or even neoplastic processes. Given the expectation of subtle, if any, pleocytosis, it is paramount to strive for an atraumatic tap. The number of cells present may correlate with enhancing MRI lesions and thus with disease activity. However, there is no apparent correlation between cell count and T2 lesion burden. The CSF glucose level is normal, appropriate to the generally benign cell counts.

The CSF total protein is normal in 60% of MS cases; rarely is it greater than 70 mg/dL. Healthy individuals may have a CSF banding pattern similar to that found within a concomitant serum immunoglobulin electrophoresis. In contrast, if CSF bands outnumber serum bands, an abnormal CNS immune response is suggested. Whenever a few well-defined B-cell clones migrate to the CNS, these cells begin to produce distinct populations of immunoglobulins that separate into the bands seen on electrophoresis. CSF IgG is relatively increased when compared with albumin and with the IgG present in the serum of the same subject. This is related to changes in the permeability of the blood–brain barrier and IgG synthesis by plasma cells within the abnormal CNS. In healthy patients, there is no discrete CSF banding; instead, a diffuse single band represents a mixture of polyclonal immunoglobulins that do not segregate into distinct groups. An in-situ CNS hyperimmune response may be associated with oligoclonal band production. However, this is not specific for MS as it may occur with other CNS inflammatory or infectious diseases.

Myelin basic protein is a molecularly large component of myelin that can be detected in a degraded form by CSF immunoassay. Although its presence is thought to correlate with active demyelination, this is a relatively nonspecific finding. When detected, the level seems to be related to the amount and rate of myelin destruction. Thus, a relatively inactive instance of "smoldering" MS is not typically associated with the presence of myelin basic protein. In contrast, other pathologic processes that rapidly destroy large amounts of myelin (e.g., stroke) also produce high levels of CSF myelin basic protein.

Evoked Potentials

Neurophysiologic studies provide a means to objectively analyze the integrity of neuronal pathways in both the central and peripheral nervous systems. Prior to the availability of MRI, EPs were a useful modality to identify subclinical CNS disease. Testing is relatively easy to perform and requires minimal patient cooperation, particularly when testing the visual and, less commonly, auditory pathways. Today the primary value of EP testing occurs when a patient presents with a myelopathy and one is attempting to define the presence of multiple areas of clinical involvement in space and time to establish a diagnosis of MS. As some patients either forget or previously had a prior subclinical optic neuritis, visual evoked responses (VERs) may still be quite useful in this one instance. However, brainstem and somatosensory EPs are no longer of major diagnostic value when considering a diagnosis of MS.

With VERs, a peripheral stimulus, typically a reversing high-contrast checkerboard pattern, provides a means to study the integrity of the visual system. The response latencies can yield objective data regarding the ability of the nervous system to transmit impulses efficiently from the optic nerve to the occipital cortex. If there is a unilateral absence or delay, one can conclude that there is slowing in conduction between the retina and the optic chiasm (Fig. 46-8). This is typical for a unilateral optic neuritis. It is particularly helpful as even if the patient totally regains his or her vision, the remyelination is not perfect; thus a marker is left for future reference. When bilateral changes are present with the potentials delayed, attenuated, or blocked because of a prior instance of CNS demyelination, one cannot precisely localize the lesion to the optic nerve as the lesion could be any place in the visual pathway.

If a number of years later a patient develops a myelopathy, VER testing can provide an opportunity to define the previous presence of some damage to these pathways. The combination of an abnormal VER response and a myelopathy is almost unique for a diagnosis of MS.

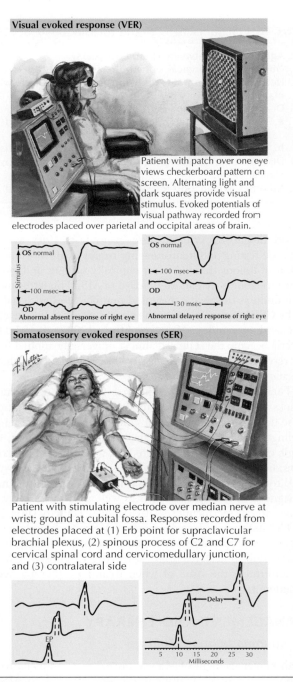

Visual evoked response (VER)

Patient with patch over one eye views checkerboard pattern on screen. Alternating light and dark squares provide visual stimulus. Evoked potentials of visual pathway recorded from electrodes placed over parietal and occipital areas of brain.

Abnormal absent response of right eye

Abnormal delayed response of right eye

Somatosensory evoked responses (SER)

Patient with stimulating electrode over median nerve at wrist; ground at cubital fossa. Responses recorded from electrodes placed at (1) Erb point for supraclavicular brachial plexus, (2) spinous process of C2 and C7 for cervical spinal cord and cervicomedullary junction, and (3) contralateral side

Figure 46-8 Tests—Evoked Responses.

Multiple Sclerosis Diagnostic Criteria

Although MRI provides a superb diagnostic testing modality, it always needs to be accompanied by an appropriate clinical setting to make an unequivocal diagnosis of MS. Clinicians utilize a set of consensus criteria that continually evolve as new technological advances become available. Clinical history and examination were the mainstays of diagnosis in 1965 when Schumacher et al. issued the first widely used criteria for MS; these required that five of six of the conditions shown in Box 46-1 be met before making a clinically definite diagnosis of multiple sclerosis.

Box 46-1 Schumacher Criteria for Diagnosis of MS

1. Age on onset between 10 and 50 years.
2. Objective neurological signs on exam.
3. Neurological symptoms and signs referable to CNS white matter.
4. Dissemination in time with
   a. Two or more attacks lasting at least 24 hours and separated by at least 1 month.
   b. Progression of signs and symptoms over 6 months.
5. Dissemination in space with respect to localization by clinical exam.
6. No other explanation for symptoms (always required).

Box 46-2 McDonald Criteria for Diagnosis of MS

1. Two or more attacks with objective clinical evidence of two or more clinical lesions is enough to make a diagnosis of MS.
2. Two or more clinical attacks:
   a. But only one clearly defined lesion on clinical examination,
   b. Fulfillment of additional criteria of dissemination in space may be evidenced by
      1. New MRI lesion.
      2. Combination of an MRI lesion plus positive CSF findings or another clinical attack at a new site.
3. Isolated clinical attack occurs; criteria for MS may be met if there are two or more lesions with evidence of dissemination in time by either
   a. New lesion by MRI or
   b. Second clinical attack
4. Clinically isolated syndrome with only one objective lesion PLUS, can make a diagnosis of MS with
   a. Dissemination in space demonstrated by second MRI lesion with positive CSF findings.
   b. Dissemination in time if demonstrated by
      1. MRI or
      2. Second clinical attack.
5. Insidious progression of disease can lead to a diagnosis of MS
   a. If disease has progressed for at least 1 year and
   b. Two of the following three conditions are met:
      1. positive brain MRI findings,
      2. positive spinal cord MRI findings (given more weight than previously), and
      3. positive CSF findings.

From Pohlman CH, Reingold SC, et al. Diagnostic criteria for multiple sclerosis: 2005 revisions to the "McDonald criteria". Ann Neurol 2005;58(6):840-846.

MS diagnostic criteria were revised in 1983 as evoked response testing and neuroimaging began to allow the identification of lesions that were not clinically evident and gave credence to laboratory data supportive of MS. The latter included CSF findings of specific increased number of oligoclonal bands in the CSF in comparison to the serum, elevated IgG levels, and increased IgG index. Most recently in 2001, the McDonald criteria became the standard almost universally applied in clinical research as well as to justify disease-modifying therapies specific for MS treatment.

These preserved the traditional requirement of multiple attacks of disease separated in time and space. Additionally, these new criteria provided for consideration of MRI and CSF findings when only one objective MRI lesion is found, only a single clinical attack has occurred, or when disease progression is insidious. The McDonald Diagnostic Criteria were revised in 2005 to incorporate the growing role of MR imaging for making a diagnosis of multiple sclerosis as well as to foster early treatment without sacrificing sensitivity and specificity (Box 46-2).

The ability to make a diagnosis of MS as early and accurately as possible is critical to patient care and to producing the most meaningful clinical research. Once the diagnosis of MS can be confirmed, the issue of when to initiate therapy becomes paramount.

MANAGEMENT AND THERAPY

Immunomodulatory Therapy

Medical management of MS was once limited to palliative care. Although symptom treatment remains integral to MS care, immunomodulatory therapies are changing treatment. Pharmacologic interventions modify the course of MS through the reduction of relapse rate and MRI lesion burden, both of which are likely to affect disease progression.

Five drugs are approved by the USFDA for treatment of RRMS: interferon beta-1b, intramuscular interferon beta-1a, glatiramer acetate, subcutaneous interferon beta-1a, and natalizumab infusion. *Subcutaneous interferon beta-1b* (8 million U every other day) became available early in the 1990s, followed by *intramuscular interferon beta-1a* (30 μg once weekly) later in that same decade. An alternative *form of subcutaneous interferon beta-1a* used in Europe became available in the United States in 2002 and is injected three times per week (22–44 μg), delivering a greater weekly dose of interferon beta-1a. Flulike symptoms, the most prominent adverse effect, occur in approximately 60% of those who use interferons, but these effects are mitigated over time and can be treated effectively with NSAIDs.

Glatiramer acetate (20 mg subcutaneously daily) became available in the United States in 1996 and is an unrelated compound of polypeptides that may have fewer potential adverse effects and perhaps more than one mechanism of action on the aberrant immune response. Some of its benefit may be realized later in the course of treatment than with the interferons.

In 2004, *natalizumab* was approved for use in the United States and the European Union. It was temporarily withdrawn by the manufacturer in February 2005 due to the occurrence of two cases of progressive multifocal leukoencephalopathy (PML) in MS patients treated with a combination of interferon beta 1-a and natalizumab. PML is a rare, progressive, and universally fatal central nervous system infection primarily occurring in immunodeficient individuals, particularly those with HIV-AIDS or very rarely those taking long-term immunosuppressive medications, particularly corticosteroids. PML is caused by the unmasked virulence of the fairly ubiquitous papillomavirus, JC virus.

In 2006, *natalizumab* returned to the market with more stringent guidelines for administration and solely as monotherapy for relapsing forms of MS. To date, however, additional cases of PML continue to accrue at a low incidence even with natalizumab monotherapy. Although the risk of evolving PML remains the greatest deterrent for many patients and clinicians, cases of liver toxicity and a questionable association with melanoma have since come to light. Thus far, there have been no controlled trials to adequately assess the efficacy of natalizumab for secondary progressive multiple sclerosis (SPMS).

Each of these agents reduces relapse rates and decreases the MRI burden of lesions within the central nervous system. Differences in trial design make effective drug-to-drug comparisons very difficult. To date, the reduction in relapse rate over 2 years hovers around 30–35% each for interferon therapies and for glatiramer acetate, whereas natalizumab was shown to reduce relapse rate over 1 year by as much as 68% when compared to placebo. Preexisting factors may influence the choice of therapy in treatment-naive patients. For example, a history of depression, suicidal ideation, or both, which may be adverse effects of the interferon drugs, may make glatiramer acetate the drug of choice in certain individuals. Some patients may be more compliant with one medication than another, depending upon individual tolerances for site reactions, flu-like symptoms, frequency of treatment, and impact upon lifestyle. Patients who cannot achieve compliance with intramuscular or subcutaneous injection may be able to tolerate monthly infusion with natalizumab.

Mechanisms of Immunomodulatory Therapies

Interferons and glatiramer acetate alter the mechanism of antigen presentation in MS. A host of immune mechanisms are stimulated by the presentation of a candidate antigen, perhaps an intrinsic myelin protein or a viral antigen cross-reacting with a native myelin protein. Myelin reactive T cells become activated and cross the blood–brain barrier, where they can initiate inflammation of myelin-rich white matter. Interferons do not actually enter the CNS and hence exert their effects external to it. Although, like interferons, glatiramer acetate does not itself cross the blood–brain barrier, it does affect activity within the CNS by increasing the production of neurotropic factors in the brain.

Natalizumab is a humanized recombinant monoclonal antibody that exerts its effect upon activated T cells by binding to the alpha 4 subunit of integrins expressed on the T-cell surface. This disables the transport of activated T cells across the blood–brain barrier by blocking their binding to endothelial adhesion molecules, thus dramatically reducing the elaboration of abnormally proliferating white blood cell populations and associated cytokines present within the CNS of the MS patient.

Neutralizing Antibodies

Although the long-term safety of available first-line immunomodulating therapies is unclear, each type seems to be relatively well tolerated. However, the interferons, glatiramer acetate, and natalizumab are not naturally occurring human proteins and, as such, are prone to inducing antibodies in human recipients. The propensity for antibody production depends on the agent, dose, and route of administration. Substantial controversy exists as to the impact of these antibodies on long-term effectiveness of immunomodulatory medications.

Drug-induced antibodies simply bind to the molecules of the active agent and may have no significant function. Neutralizing antibodies are a subset of these binding antibodies that might interfere with drug activity by a steric hindrance of drug binding to its receptor or via remote effects on drug activity through binding at distant sites.

Some agents are more "foreign" than others and have a higher likelihood of inducing antibodies. Glycosylation renders substances more soluble in suspension; without it, aggregates that may be immunogenic are likely to form. This may account for the higher incidence of neutralizing antibodies with the use of interferon beta-1b (30–35%) compared with interferon beta-1a (15%). The latter is glycosylated, has no amino acid substitutions, and looks almost exactly like naturally occurring IFN-β. Higher doses of the drug, more frequent exposures, and delivery via subcutaneous injection may affect antibody induction. Natalizumab therapy is associated with antibody production that persists for greater than 6 months in 6% of patients. Natalizumab antibodies present beyond 6 months of monthly treatments appear to neutralize the drug and negate its benefits completely; therefore, antibody testing for natalizumab has become routine under a carefully administered monitoring program (TOUCH program) required for patients who are treated with natalizumab and their prescribing physicians. True hypersensitivity reactions to natalizumab have occurred in 2–9% of patients administered the drug, and these patients are more inclined than those without reactions to evolve persistent antibodies.

Treatment of More Severe Multiple Sclerosis

The protocol for treating recalcitrant MS is not formulaic. Only two agents are approved by the USFDA for rapidly progressive MS: mitoxantrone and interferon beta-1b. *Mitoxantrone* (12 mg/m^2 IV given every 3 months to a cumulative maximum dose of 144 mg) is a chemotherapeutic agent used to treat other immune-mediated disorders. Usually considered a treatment of last resort after multiple treatment failures, its categorization is due to its potential toxicities, the most worrisome of which is cardiac toxicity.

Two trials offered some evidence that *interferon beta-1b* favorably impacts secondary progressive disease with respect to various outcome measures (progression of disability scores, relapse rate reduction, MRI activity), not all of which were significant in both studies. High-dose *interferon beta-1a* has also been investigated in secondary progressive disease; two studies demonstrated efficacy compared with placebo. Although heterogeneity of study populations and outcome measures make these studies difficult to compare, they offer some rationale for choosing a new therapy in patients who have advanced from relapsing–remitting disease to a more aggressive RRMS or secondary progressive disease, regardless of previous treatments. Multi-interferon therapy and interferon plus glatiramer acetate are being investigated. Despite multiple investigations focused on other treatment strategies, their efficacies have remained largely anecdotal.

Azathioprine, Cyclosporine, and Cyclophosphamide

The equivocal benefits of *azathioprine* (2–3 mg/kg daily) in MS are realized in decreasing relapse rates and MRI lesion burden.

Cyclosporine inhibits the production of lymphokines and seems to foster the expansion of certain populations of suppressor T cells. One cyclosporine and azathioprine comparison showed no differences between the two agents with respect to relapse frequency or expanded disability status scale, but therapy complications were more than twice as likely in the cyclosporine group as in the azathioprine group. Other studies of cyclosporine have been marred by high attrition in the treatment groups due to toxicities (renal failure, hypertension) that likely occur before any benefit is achieved. These observations have taken cyclosporine out of the usual arsenal of immunosuppressive therapy for the treatment of MS in many centers.

Cyclophosphamide is another immunosuppressive agent widely used to treat various neoplastic and autoimmune disorders. One study suggested some response based on expanded disability status scale scores to induction with booster infusions in patients younger than age 40 years. Toxicities include hemorrhagic cystitis, leukopenia, myocarditis, pulmonary interstitial fibrosis, malignancy, interstitial pulmonary fibrosis, and infertility. Mitoxantrone tends to be better tolerated, with fewer adverse effects, and has better evidence of efficacy in secondary progressive MS.

Methotrexate. Low-dose weekly oral methotrexate is not approved for use in MS but is used as an adjunct therapy in off-label use based on a limited number of studies in patients with MS and its efficacy in rheumatoid arthritis, another autoimmune disease. Methotrexate is a competitive inhibitor of dihydrofolate reductase and interferes with the production of reduced cofactors required for the synthesis of DNA and RNA. It seems to have both immunosuppressive and antiinflammatory effects and immunoregulatory action. Toxicities include pulmonary and liver fibrosis, cirrhosis, and bone marrow suppression.

Monthly Intravenous Methylprednisolone

In addition to its efficacy as acute therapy in relapses, cyclical infusions of 500–1000 mg IV glucocorticoids can be useful as a scheduled monthly or bimonthly treatment in patients whose frequent relapses signal a transition from RRMS to secondary progressive MS. This is generally a safe, well-tolerated approach for patients who have waning response to other conventional immunomodulators but are unwilling to undertake chemotherapeutic options.

Plasma Exchange

Plasmapheresis intervenes primarily at the level of humoral responses, thought to be less important in MS than cellular responses. There are no data supporting a significant treatment effect.

Intravenous Immunoglobulin

Limited data exist regarding IV immunoglobulin for MS. There are few long-term adverse effects but no evidence that it is more effective than other approved therapies for MS. Because MS is not a USFDA–approved indication for IV immunoglobulin, the expense of treatment is usually prohibitive.

Adjuvant Medical Problems and Treatments

Despite new therapies, for most people, MS eventually involves some adaptation in lifestyle. It may mean adopting a less frenetic pace with curtailed work hours, help with household management, less travel, napping, or avoidance of excessive heat. The demand for lifestyle modification can be one of the more frustrating aspects of MS.

Clinical Vignette

A 31-year-old ICU nurse had no explanation for her complaints of fatigue. She had long worked 36 hours per week in three 12-hour shifts with additional shifts in overtime, more often than not. She was not married, had no children, and had always made exercise a regular part of her routine. She was in the habit of running with her dog in the mornings and, while she used to find this invigorating and an energy booster for the coming day, she began to feel that she was really pushing herself to keep up with her usual activities on most days. By late morning, she would feel exhaustion setting in, even though she made it more of a point than ever to get plenty of sleep in her down time and began taking vitamin supplements.

She found herself cutting back on social activities, and her friends and colleagues saw the change and wondered whether she was depressed. Overall she had no history of mood disorder or any other perceived stressors, and had been happy with her life until she began to have significant physical and mental fatigue. From the neurologic perspective, she had no overt limb weakness, subjective sensory impairment, imbalance, visual difficulties, or pain. Similarly, there was nothing to suggest any underlying systemic disorder. However, the fatigue was taking over her life and she decided to seek further medical evaluation.

Her primary care physician found her thyroid function and B$_{12}$ levels normal; an ANA was positive with a speckled pattern. Consideration of an occult depression diagnosis led to a trial of an SSRI. However, she felt no better. Soon thereafter, she began to experience a vibrating sensation in her feet and a feeling of tightness in her upper thorax, as if she was wearing a bra that was too tight. She became convinced that either she was becoming a hypochondriac or her doctor was "missing something." When she voiced this concern, her physician made referrals to a rheumatologist, an endocrinologist, and a neurologist. The endocrinologist felt that she had mild vitamin D deficiency and recommended some additional supplementation to her multivitamin, but was otherwise unconcerned. The rheumatologist felt there was no evidence for systemic lupus erythematosus or any connective tissue disorder, apart from possible fibromyalgia.

Her neurologist elicited a history of urinary frequency with relatively little urine volume with each void. On examination, she found diminished vibratory perception in the patient's lower extremities up to the knees and diffuse hyperreflexia. A postvoid residual of 180 mL was measured by ultrasound. MRI revealed multifocal areas of chronic demyelination in the brain, cervical, and thoracic spinal cord.

Comment: This clinical scenario is not all that uncommon and emphasizes the importance of a careful neurologic evaluation in previously well-functioning young to middle-aged persons who begin to develop limitations in their abilities to perform their daily activities. One must be careful to not invoke the common diagnosis of chronic fatigue syndrome in such individuals until careful and often ongoing neurologic evaluations precisely exclude a diagnosis of MS.

RELATED MS MANAGEMENT PROBLEMS

Fatigue

Fatigue is often one of the most debilitating symptoms, particularly early on in MS. The primary "lassitude" of MS is an overwhelming sense of physical and mental exhaustion that has no identifiable cause but significantly interferes with normal activity. The majority of patients with MS rank it as their most disabling symptom affecting daily living. This eclipses bowel and bladder dysfunction, weakness, and balance problems. Although fatigue can be secondary to deconditioning, the advanced symptoms of MS that limit physical activity are not a prerequisite for fatigue. It has been associated with every stage of the disease, regardless of clinical subtype, and is often present in an apparently well-compensated individual who otherwise has little objective disability.

Persistent but ineffective neuronal firing of short-circuited neural pathways that do not affect movement in weak limbs, transmit cohesive visual impulses, or recruit the reflexes necessary to maintain balance may be a pathophysiologic correlate of primary MS fatigue. There is no specific link evident to provide objective measures of disease activity such as commonly used MS functional scales or MRI findings.

Additionally, some evidence exists of an association among MS-related fatigue, depression, and cognitive dysfunction. That this is true in patients without significant deficits and in patients who have not received a diagnosis suggests that the mental fatigue is not simply an epiphenomenon of a reactive depression. The fatigue of MS is likely a direct consequence of demyelination, inflammation, and axonal injury along shared neuronal networks that affect attention, depression, and cognitive dysfunction. Hypometabolism in the frontal cortex and basal ganglia resulting from this type of damage has been implicated in primary MS fatigue.

Sufficient rest is critical to managing fatigue in MS. Additionally some pharmacologic therapy is a useful adjunct to behavioral and lifestyle strategies. Despite the incomplete understanding of the pathophysiology of MS-related fatigue, clearly valuable pharmacotherapies mitigate a profoundly low energy level through modification of altered neurochemistry that results from damage to the CNS.

Wakefulness involves various arousal systems with complex circuits that project between the reticular activating system, limbic system, and frontal cortex. From the brainstem, monoamine-mediated pathways (dopamine, norepinephrine, serotonin, acetylcholine) ascend through the reticular activating system. Several useful agents operate along this pathway. The stimulant medications (methylphenidate, amphetamine salts, dextroamphetamine [Dexedrine], pemoline) affect this mesocorticolimbic system by enhancing global CNS activation but

may produce undesirable side effects such as dependence through stimulation of central "reward mechanisms" (governed by the nucleus accumbens in the striatum), insomnia, appetite suppression, and peripheral autonomic effects, including tachycardia, dysrhythmia, and hypertension. Amantadine enhances dopamine release and seems to have some benefit in improving central attention and processing speed. Modafinil, used to treat narcolepsy, is also helpful in treating MS fatigue by increasing activity in the frontal cortex via activation of histaminergic neurons arising from the hypothalamus.

Pain

Multiple sclerosis is usually regarded as a disease of progressive neurologic dysfunction without significant pain. However, pain is a common problem deserving appropriate attention. Years of gait disturbance, abnormal forces on joints, repetitive motion injuries, wheelchair confinement, disuse, and painful muscle spasms are all typical sources of pain in MS. A regular exercise program is essential to prevent additional disability from deconditioning.

NSAIDs, gabapentin, pregabalin, and tricyclic antidepressants are often useful. For pain, narcotic medications are probably best avoided because they are likely to exacerbate fatigue and cognitive dysfunction. Aqua therapy is an excellent form of exercise that does not put undue stress on joints and provides buoyant support for weak limbs, allowing patients to maximize range of motion. Yoga is helpful for relaxation and flexibility maintenance. Shiatsu massage therapy may help to prevent contractures, but deep muscle massage may be overzealous and increase rather than mitigate pain. Acupuncture may disrupt aberrant pain pathways.

Bladder Dysfunction

Bladder symptoms, one of the most vexing problems commonly experienced, significantly influence quality of life in 50–80% of patients with MS. The degree of impairment usually parallels the degree of other neurologic deficits. Bladder hygiene is compromised by increased spasticity, loss of strength, and diminished mobility. Although bladder dysfunction rarely leads to life-threatening infection or secondary renal failure, the resultant recurrent or chronic urinary tract infections can potentiate other MS symptoms and are a common trigger for significant exacerbations.

On rare instances, an acute pyelonephritis may develop with a high fever; this may lead to a temporary exacerbation of the underlying neurologic deficits. In a way, this mimics the Uhthoff phenomena. This emphasizes the need to look for evidence of an underlying infection in anyone with MS who has an acute exacerbation; appropriate antibiotics will not only clear the infection but also lead to the resolution of the MS exacerbation.

Control of urination depends on the complex coordination of reflexive and volitional activities that rely on the integrity of complex pathways that traverse the subcortical white matter, spinal cord tracts, and reflex spinal cord centers. Lateral and posterior cervical spinal tracts are among the most common sites of demyelination in MS and are critical for all aspects of coordinating voluntary voiding.

Bladder dysfunction in MS is managed both pharmacologically and with adaptations in toileting. The most common pharmacologic agents diminish bladder contraction. Typically this is an antispasmodic anticholinergic, oxybutynin chloride. Dosage is usually initiated at 5 mg, the maximum being 20 mg daily. These are generally more effective than attempts to improve bladder emptying with cholinergic agents. Alpha-adrenergic agents increase bladder outlet resistance and sometimes help to treat urinary incontinence. Emptying the hyporeflexic or areflexic bladder is best accomplished by clean, intermittent self-catheterization.

Sexual Dysfunction

Unfortunately this continues to be a problem of "don't ask, don't tell" type. The presence of societal inhibitions have greatly disappeared about discussing this important part of the human condition in healthy individuals as well illustrated by the magazine covers at any supermarket checkout lane. However, this is a subject that most practitioners are woefully undertrained to adequately discuss so that the patient may receive appropriate guidance and therapy. Certainly this is a very important quality-of-life issue for the MS population. Neurologists must be cognizant of its frequent occurrence in MS and need to always ask the patient about whether they have concerns about their sexual abilities, particularly as influenced by their illness. If so, it is important to refer them to an appropriate urologic/endocrinologic sexual dysfunctions clinic for further care.

Pregnancy

Pregnancy in women with MS seems to have no long-term effects on MS progression. It may have some protective value, because the incidence of exacerbations is actually lower during pregnancy. In the 6 to 12 months after pregnancy, the exacerbation rate is higher than expected. The decision to bear children should probably take into account the pre-pregnancy tempo of disease and whether a woman with MS feels physically capable of keeping up with the rigorous demands of raising children. Family support and financial resources are also factors.

Heat

High ambient temperatures and high levels of humidity are often associated with MS worsening and possibly even exacerbations just as with febrile illnesses as noted above. During summer months, especially within temperate countries, patients are advised to avoid the stress of overexposure to high ambient temperatures, especially during heat waves. Where possible, air conditioning, ceiling fans, or avoidance of strenuous activities may lessen the chances for causing deterioration in the overall status of patients with MS.

PROGNOSIS

Patients newly diagnosed with MS are relieved to know that it has a broadly based prognostic spectrum; some have a benign course, and others encounter a debilitating disease. Most patients have an experience between these extremes. Only 10% of patients have "benign" MS. Of MS patients, 85% begin with a relapsing–remitting course, and 90% of these eventually enter a secondary progressive phase; in the preponderance of patients with a diagnosis of MS, a long-term life-altering morbidity eventually develops. However, it is important to emphasize that the overall mortality is only a few years less than that of the general population.

There are exceptions wherein MS follows a relentlessly progressive course over relatively few years, leading to death much earlier than anticipated. If untreated, 20% of patients with MS are unable to walk without assistance 5 years after diagnosis. At 15 and 30 years after diagnosis, this increases to 50% and 80%, respectively.

ADDITIONAL RESOURCES

Comi G, Filippi M, Barkhof L, et al. Effect of early interferon treatment on conversion to definite multiple sclerosis: a randomized trial. Lancet 2001;357:1576-1582.

European Study Group on Interferon beta-1b in Secondary Progressive MS. Placebo-controlled multicentre randomized trial of interferon beta-1b in treatment of secondary progressive multiple sclerosis. Lancet 1998;352:1491-1497.

Fletcher SG, Castro-Borrero W, Remington G, et al. Sexual dysfunction in patients with multiple sclerosis: a multidisciplinary approach to evaluation and management. Nat Clin Pract Urol 2009;6:96-107. *An important review of particular importance to any MS patient with spinal cord dysfunction.*

Goodin DS, Cohen BA, O'Connor P, et al. Assessment: the use of natalizumab (Tysabri) for the treatment of multiple sclerosis (an evidence-based review). Neurology 2008;71:766-773.

Guo S, Bozkaya D, Ward A, et al. Treating relapsing multiple sclerosis with subcutaneous versus intramuscular interferon-beta-1a: modelling the clinical and economic implications. Pharmacoeconomics 2009;27(1):39-53. *This study provides a useful cost analysis comparing effectiveness of two of the most common preparations of interferon beta-a.*

Hartung HP. New cases of progressive multifocal leukoencephalopathy after treatment with natalizumab. Lancet Neurol 2009;8:28-31.

Kappos L, Pohlman CH, Freedman MS, et al. Treatment with interferon beta 1-b delays conversion to clinically definite and McDonald MS in patients with clinically isolated syndromes. Neurology 2006;67(7):1242-1249.

Kumar N, McEvoy K, Ahlskog JE. Myelopathy due to copper deficiency following gastrointestinal surgery. Arch Neurol 2003;60:1782-1785.

Lassmann H. Axonal and neuronal pathology in multiple sclerosis: What have we learnt from animal models. Exp Neurol 2009 Oct 17. [Epub ahead of print]. *A review of the increasingly recognized importance of axonal damage in the early pathophysiology of MS.*

Lovblad KO, Anzalone N, Dorfler A, et al. MR imaging in multiple sclerosis: review and recommendations for current practice. AJNR Am J Neuroradiol 2009 Dec 17. [Epub ahead of print]

Pohlman CH, O'Connor PW, et al. A randomized, placebo-controlled trial of natalizumab for relapsing remitting multiple sclerosis. N Engl J Med 2006;354(9):899-910.

Pohlman CH, Reingold SC, et al. Diagnostic criteria for multiple sclerosis: 2005 revisions to the "McDonald criteria." Ann Neurol 2005;58(6):840-846.

Swanton JK, Fernando KT, Dalton CM, et al. Early MRI in optic neuritis: The risk for disability. Neurology 2009;72:542-550. *This is an important prospective analysis of the risk of development of clinically active MS among a cohort of newly diagnosed optic neuritis patients.*

47

Other Autoimmune CNS Demyelinating Disorders

Mary Anne Muriello, Claudia J. Chaves, and H. Royden Jones, Jr.

There are three very rare acute demyelinating central nervous system disorders that are distinct from multiple sclerosis (MS). These initially appear de novo in previously healthy individuals. Although some instances may occur in isolation, and respond to very high dose immunosuppressive therapy, on other occasions their consequences can be devastating.

NEUROMYELITIS OPTICA / DEVIC DISEASE

Optic neuritis (ON) is very commonly the first clinical event experienced by patients who later develop full-blown multiple sclerosis. Approximately 50% of ON patients will demonstrate clinical evidence of MS within 5–6 years of onset. Rarely an occasional patient, presenting with what seems to be classic ON, very soon thereafter develops an acute and clinically severe myelopathy. The combination represents an entirely different nosologic and pathophysiologic entity from MS. This entity, known as neuromyelitis optica (NMO), is a syndrome that is both relapsing and much more rapidly disabling than occurs in the typical MS patient. For example, about half of NMO patients become wheel chair bound within 5 years and almost two thirds will be legally blind (no better than 20/200) within that same time frame. There is no chronic progressive stage as most often eventually occurs in classic multiple sclerosis. NMO also has a relatively high early mortality, something almost unheard of in MS. These relatively rare NMO deaths usually follow disease extension into the brainstem and/or upper cervical cord.

DIAGNOSIS

The diagnosis of NMO, rather than MS, in a patient with a history of ON (Fig. 47-1) and myelitis is largely dependent on documentation of longitudinally extensive spinal cord lesions (more than three spinal segments). Such extensive intramedullary spinal cord lesions are unique to NMO in contrast to the very short segment MRI findings in MS (Fig. 47-2).

A very specific NMO-IgG serum autoantibody is identified that binds to the central nervous system (CNS)–dominant water channel aquaporin-4, a structure that is normally present on astrocytes. This leads to the primary pathologic change, namely, loss of this aquaporin-4 water channel protein. This is occasionally associated with secondary demyelination. Hypothalamic and periventricular demyelination, the latter previously thought to be almost MS specific, are now also recognized to be associated with NMO-IgG/anti-AQP4 seropositivity. This particular distribution of lesions corresponds with the site of AQP4 expression within the brain. Preliminary experiments suggest that anti-AQP4 autoantibodies are pathogenic. This antibody has a high sensitivity and specificity for NMO being present in at least 75% of these cases; its presence now provides a specific diagnostic modality. This totally contrasts with MS, where there is nothing absolutely specific present to confirm that diagnosis.

PROGNOSIS

When one is confronted with a new case of ON, the testing for NMO-related *anti-AQP4 antibodies* is very important diagnostically as well as prognostically. In this setting, the finding of this specific seropositivity predicts poor future visual outcome, and possibly rapid onset of NMO. In the converse, the patient presenting with longitudinally extensive transverse myelitis (LETM) and who is found to be antibody positive for the NMO antibody has more than a 50% chance of developing ON or recurrent severe ON within just 1 year. This is an important designation as NMO has a much worse prognosis than MS per se because the antibody-positive NMO patient does not respond to the usual immunomodulatory treatments that are often initially effective for MS.

TREATMENT

In contrast to MS where beta-interferon is often the therapy of choice for prevention of disease relapses, a few immunosuppressant medications are the treatment of choice for both NMO and relapsing optic neuritis (RON). Previously, before specific

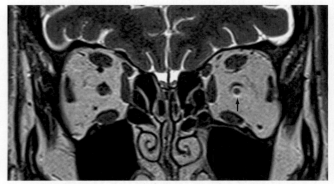

Coronal T2 fast spin echo with fat saturation demonstrates striking atrophy of left optic nerve resulting from previous optic neuritis (arrow).

Figure 47-1 Optic Nerve Atrophy.

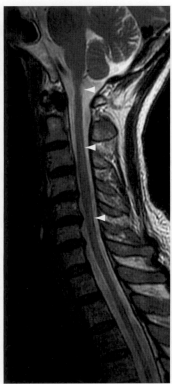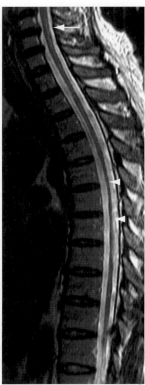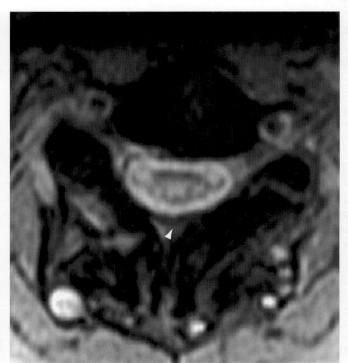

C. Axial T2 cervical MR: Extensive central and dorsal cervical plaque (arrowhead).

A. Sagittal T2 cervical MR: Moderate cervical spinal cord atrophy with multifocal (arrowheads) spinal cord plaques.

B. Sagittal T2 thoracic MR: Marked midthoracic spinal cord atrophy (arrowheads) with cervicothoracic junction plaque (arrow).

Figure 47-2 Neuromyelitis Optica.

antibody testing had been available for a precise NMO diagnosis, classic clinical cases sometimes responded to very high doses of daily intravenous methylprednisolone.

Recently treatment with rituximab, a monoclonal antibody against CD20⁺ B cells, appears to reduce the frequency of attacks for NMO. It also appears to potentially stabilize or even lessen disability. This proved effective by decreasing the number of relapses as well as improving or at least stabilizing disability in 80% of previously medically refractory NMO patients in one recent multiinstitution trial. However, this is not a panacea as this medication has been associated with serious infectious complications, including progressive multifocal leukoencephalopathy (PML) and even death in a few patients. Currently these concerns are limiting the adoption of rituximab as the drug of choice for NMO. Unfortunately, previous experience with other chronic immunosuppressive agents, including azathioprine, cyclophosphamide, cyclosporine, methotrexate, mitoxantrone, and mycophenolate mofetil have proved disappointing. NMO patients taking these various drugs are found to continue to have relapses and progression of their disease.

ACUTE DISSEMINATED ENCEPHALOMYELITIS

This clinical entity is an acute monophasic demyelinating CNS disorder characterized by multifocal white matter involvement.

Acute disseminated encephalomyelitis (ADEM) usually occurs without any recognized antecedent cause or within 6 weeks of an antigenic challenge after exanthems (measles, rubella, variola, varicella), vaccination (rabies, smallpox, and pertussis), or respiratory infections (mycoplasmal pneumonia, Epstein–Barr virus, and cytomegalovirus). An uncommon disease, it affects children more than adults.

CLINICAL PRESENTATION

A severe focal or multifocal encephalopathy associated with pyramidal, cerebellar and brainstem signs is typically evidenced. Seizures occur with 25% of patients. An association with bilateral optic neuritis and transverse myelitis is particularly suggestive of a demyelinating disease such as ADEM. These various presentations reflect the disseminated CNS involvement.

DIAGNOSTIC APPROACH

MRI is the primary diagnostic methodology. Commonly one sees multifocal asymmetric gadolinium-enhancing lesions throughout the brain and spinal cord (Fig. 47-3). Typically these lesions have varied imaging patterns, including nodular, gyral, amorphous, spotty, and ringlike shapes. ADEM patients typically have MRI abnormalities seen at the cortical gray and subcortical white matter interface. This contrasts significantly with

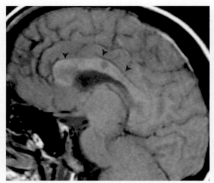

A. Sagittal T1-weighted image shows expanded corpus callosum with mixed signal characteristics (arrowheads).

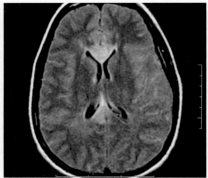

B. Axial FLAIR image demonstrates enlargement and increased T2 signal in corpus callosum.

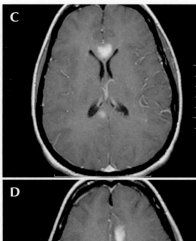

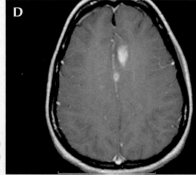

C. and D. Axial T1-weighted, gadolinium-enhanced scans with multiple enhancing lesions within corpus callosum and beyond.

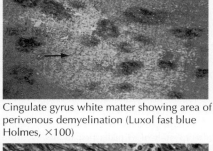

Cingulate gyrus white matter showing area of perivenous demyelination (Luxol fast blue Holmes, ×100)

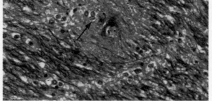

Cerebral white matter with scattered deep hemorrhages in pale, edematous areas (H and E stain, ×10)

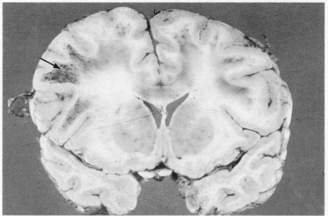

Coronal section of cerebral hemispheres at level of corpus striatum showing punctate hemorrhagic lesions in subcortical white matter

Figure 47-3 Acute Disseminated Encephalomyelitis.

MS, where the periventricular white matter is most commonly involved.

The cerebrospinal fluid (CSF) is abnormal in 70% of patients, showing a modest lymphocytosis, increased protein with 60% having oligoclonal bands, and normal glucose. Electroencephalography often shows diffuse slowing compatible with an encephalopathic process. Epileptiform spike discharges are unusual in ADEM.

DIFFERENTIAL DIAGNOSIS

This includes acute MS, various acute aseptic meningoencephalitides, vasculitides, and very rare metabolic leukoencephalopathies, such as Schilder disease or Leigh syndrome. Cerebral biopsy is often necessary to confirm an ADEM diagnosis, especially in adults and atypical cases. Perivenous mononuclear cell infiltration associated with demyelination within the cellular cuff is the typical finding in patients with ADEM (Fig. 47-2).

THERAPY AND PROGNOSIS

Methylprednisolone, in very high doses. is the treatment of choice as most patients with ADEM improve with this modality. However, if that fails, intravenous immunoglobulins, plasmapheresis, or cytotoxic drugs are given. Acute disseminated encephalomyelitis is usually associated with a good prognosis. Most patients sustain mild residual deficits or even achieve complete recovery.

ACUTE HEMORRHAGIC LEUKOENCEPHALOPATHY

Acute hemorrhagic leukoencephalopathy (AHL) is considered a hyperacute form of ADEM. As in ADEM, AHL is a monophasic disease. It is usually postinfectious, secondary to an autoimmune process directed against the CNS myelin. However, the clinical course of AHL is much more fulminant than that of ADEM and more frequently fatal.

CLINICAL PRESENTATION

Early symptoms of AHL include fever, headaches, and malaise. These rapidly progress to confusion, decreased level of consciousness (obtundation) and coma. Aphasia, hemiparesis, brainstem signs, and seizures are common focal signs.

DIAGNOSIS

Peripheral leukocytosis is often present in AHL, with WBC counts as high as $40,000/mm^3$. The lesions on MRI are usually larger and have more edema than in ADEM. Hemorrhages are frequently seen. The CSF usually demonstrates polymorphonuclear pleocytosis, increased protein, and a normal glucose level. Although AHL is associated with petechiae, the number of RBCs can vary from none to thousands. Increased levels of CSF gamma globulins may be present.

PATHOLOGY

The pathologic findings in AHL are unique and show widespread edema in the white matter, ball and ring hemorrhages, perivascular exudates, and perivenous foci of microglial proliferation (Fig. 47-2). Areas of demyelination are seen around the vessels.

TREATMENT

Early and aggressive treatment of AHL patients with high-dose corticosteroids is indicated and may occasionally lead to an improved clinical outcome.

ADDITIONAL RESOURCES

Cree B. Neuromyelitis Optica: Diagnosis, pathogenesis, and treatment. Current Neurology and Neuroscience Reports 2008;8:427-433. *Excellent overview of the immunologic aspects of this disorder.*

Dale RC. Acute disseminated encephalomyelitis. Semin Pediatr Infect Dis 2003;14:90-95.

Giovannoni G. To test or not to test NMO-IgG and optic neuritis. Neurology 2008;70:2192-2193. *A fine "state of the art" overview.*

Jacob A, Weinshenker BG, Violich BS, et al. Treatment of neuromyelitis optica with rituximab: retrospective analysis of 25 patients. Arch Neurol 2008;65:1443-1448.

Lennon VA, Wingerchuk DM, Kryzer TJ, et al. A serum autoantibody marker of neuromyelitis optica: distinction from multiple sclerosis. Lancet 2004;364:2106-2112. *The original report defining the presence of this specific antibody.*

Matiello M, Lennon VA, Jacob A, et al. NMO-IgG predicts the outcome of recurrent optic neuritis. Neurology 2008;70:2197-2200.

Roemer SF, Parisi JE, Lennon VA, et al. Pattern-specific loss of aquaporin-4 immunoreactivity distinguishes neuromyelitis optica from multiple sclerosis. Brain 2007;130:1194-1205.

Rust RS. Multiple sclerosis, acute disseminated encephalomyelitis, and related conditions. Semin Pediatr Neurol 2000;7:66-90.

Tenembaum S, Chamoles N, Fejerman N. Acute disseminated encephalomyelitis: a long-term follow-up study of 84 pediatric patients. Neurology 2002 Oct 22;59(8):1224-1231.

Waters P, Jarius S, Littleton E, Leite MI, Jacob S, Gray B, Geraldes R, Vale T, Jacob A, Palace J, Maxwell S, Beeson D, Vincent A. Aquaporin-4 antibodies in neuromyelitis optica and longitudinally extensive transverse myelitis. Arch Neurol 2008 Jul;65(7):913-919.

Wingerchuk DM, Lennon VA, Pittock SJ, Lucchinetti CF, Weinshenker BG. Revised diagnostic criteria for neuromyelitis optica. Neurology 2006;66:1485-1489.

Wingerchuk DM, Pittock SJ, Lucchinetti CF, Lennon VA, Weinshenker BG. A secondary progressive clinical course is uncommon in neuromyelitis optica. Neurology 2007;68:603-605.

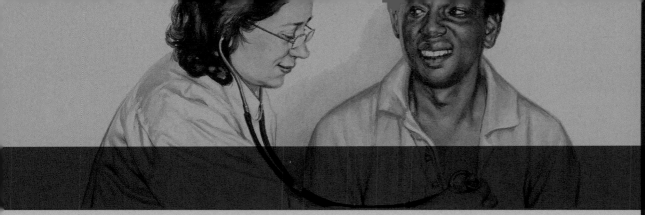

SECTION
X

Infectious Disease

Bacterial Diseases

Daniel P. McQuillen, Donald E. Craven, Robert A. Duncan, Winnie W. Ooi,
Robert Peck, Samuel E. Kalluvya, Johannes B. Kataraihya, and H. Royden Jones, Jr.

48

*B*acterial infections of the central nervous system can present as acute medical emergencies, exemplified by bacterial meningitis and spinal epidural abscess, or develop more insidiously, as occurs in brain and spinal tuberculosis. This chapter will first discuss the most common clinical syndromes of bacterial infections of the central nervous system followed by detailed discussion of specific pathogens that represent common clinical scenarios or difficult diagnostic entities.

COMMON SYNDROMES

BACTERIAL MENINGITIS

Clinical Vignette

A 19-year-old woman presented to the emergency department with confusion, lethargy, and neck stiffness. Her dorm mates reported that she had experienced upper respiratory symptoms for 3 or 4 days before presentation. She had no significant past medical history. On physical examination, her temperature was 37° C (98.6° F), her pulse was 100 beats/min, respirations were 20/min, and her blood pressure was 110/70 mm Hg. Although her neck was stiff, Kernig and Brudzinski signs were absent. The pharynx was slightly injected without exudate. Heart and lung examination results were normal. No rash was present. Neurologic examination revealed a slightly obtund, sleepy woman with otherwise intact mental status, intact cranial nerves, no motor or sensory deficits, and normal reflexes.

The patient's white blood cell (WBC) count was 22,900/ mm³, with a marked left shift, including 34% bands and 62% polymorphonuclear neutrophils (PMNs). Her platelet count was 120,000/mm³. Her electrolytes revealed a mild metabolic acidosis. A chest radiograph and brain computed tomography (CT) were normal.

Initial cerebrospinal (CSF) fluid examination was normal. However, she was admitted for observation. Very soon thereafter, she complained of increasingly severe headache and neck pain. On exam, she was definitely confused and now had a fever of 39.1° C (102.4° F). Repeat lumbar puncture demonstrated a cloudy CSF with 670 WBCs (90% PMNs), a glucose level of 1 mg/dL, and a protein level of 220 mg/ dL. Gram stain revealed rare gram-negative diplococci that on culture grew Neisseria meningitidis. Blood cultures also grew N. meningitidis. She was treated with 24 million U/ day intravenous (IV) penicillin G and recovered completely. Before discharge, she was given rifampin to eliminate nasopharyngeal carriage of N. meningitidis.

One of the most serious neurologic emergencies involves the evaluation and care of patients with bacterial meningitis. Usually, these individuals are vigorous and previously healthy when they suddenly develop a severe headache, fever, and stiff neck. Despite more than 50 years of experience with antibiotic therapies, bacterial meningitis remains a very lethal disease. Expedient diagnosis is essential to prevent such an outcome. In the preceding vignette, typical for meningococcal meningitis, despite the history and findings suggestive of a meningeal infection, the initial CSF examination was normal. Emergency physicians wisely admitted the patient for observation. When she experienced sudden deterioration, repeat CSF examination led to diagnosis and appropriate therapy. Any delay in diagnosis and therapy of bacterial meningitis can be irretrievable as death may occur soon after a clinical change unless appropriate antibiotic therapy is begun immediately.

Pathophysiology

Bacterial meningitis is defined as a microbial infection primarily involving the leptomeninges (Fig. 48-1). Typically, bacteria seed the leptomeninges via the bloodstream or from a contiguous site of infection, such as sinusitis, otitis media, or mastoiditis. Rarely a defect in the normal anatomic barriers, as with a perforating cranial or spinal injury or congenital dural defect, leads to a predisposition to recurrent bacterial meningitis.

The responsible microorganisms often differ between children and adult patients. Those commonly responsible for meningitis in adults include *Streptococcus pneumoniae*, *N. meningitidis*, and *Listeria monocytogenes*. *Haemophilus influenzae* still causes 20–50% of meningitis in developing countries, but in the United States, this rate has been reduced 90% with the *H. influenzae* type b vaccine. In neonates, *Escherichia coli* and group B β-hemolytic streptococci comprise most cases. *L. monocytogenes* particularly leads to meningitis in immunocompromised patients and rarely in the newborn. *N. meningitidis* infection often occurs with a primary sepsis, and a characteristic petechial and/or purpuric rash, or disseminated intravascular dissemination. Conditions predisposing to pneumococcal meningitis in adults include sickle cell disease as well as conditions predisposing to immune deficiencies, including alcoholism, cirrhosis, splenectomy, and HIV/AIDS.

Gram-negative bacilli (*E. coli*, *Proteus*, *Pseudomonas*, *Serratia*, *Klebsiella*, and *Citrobacter*) are rarely found in community-acquired meningitis but more commonly occur in association with head or spinal trauma or after neurosurgery. These organisms always need to be considered with the immunocompromised hosts. Meningitis due to *Staphylococcus aureus* may follow penetrating trauma, neurosurgery, or bacteremia. Coagulase-negative staphylococci (*Staphylococcus epidermidis*) or *S. aureus*

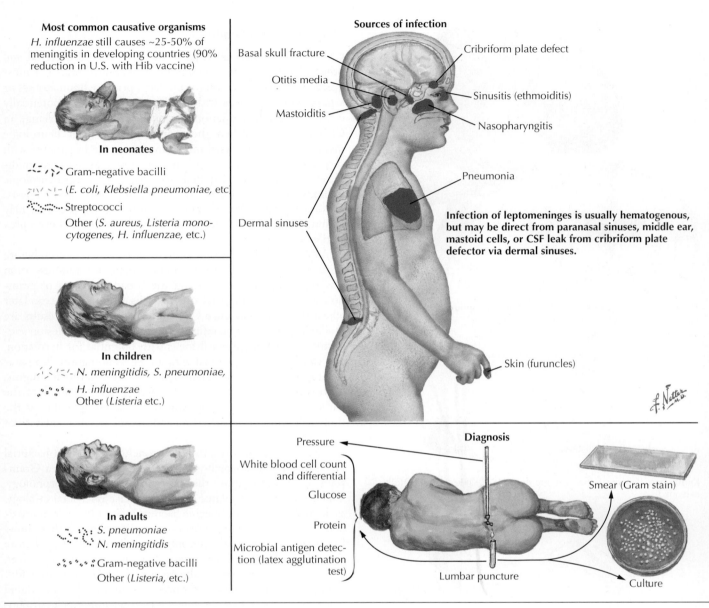

Most common causative organisms

H. influenzae still causes ~25-50% of meningitis in developing countries (90% reduction in U.S. with Hib vaccine)

In neonates

Gram-negative bacilli (*E. coli, Klebsiella pneumoniae*, etc)

Streptococci

Other (*S. aureus, Listeria monocytogenes, H. influenzae*, etc.)

In children

N. meningitidis, S. pneumoniae, H. influenzae
Other (*Listeria* etc.)

In adults

S. pneumoniae
N. meningitidis
Gram-negative bacilli
Other (*Listeria*, etc.)

Sources of infection

Basal skull fracture
Otitis media
Mastoiditis
Dermal sinuses
Cribriform plate defect
Sinusitis (ethmoiditis)
Nasopharyngitis
Pneumonia
Skin (furuncles)

Infection of leptomeninges is usually hematogenous, but may be direct from paranasal sinuses, middle ear, mastoid cells, or CSF leak from cribriform plate defector via dermal sinuses.

Diagnosis

Pressure
White blood cell count and differential
Glucose
Protein
Microbial antigen detection (latex agglutination test)
Lumbar puncture
Smear (Gram stain)
Culture

Figure 48-1 Bacterial Meningitis–I.

and other organisms are associated with infected ventricular shunts.

Clinical Presentation and Diagnosis

The onset of acute bacterial meningitis is rapid: hours to a day or so. Classic clinical findings include signs of an acute cerebral disorder, with lethargy, seizures, and agitation as well as specific signs of meningeal involvement manifested by severe neck stiffness, called *meningismus*, and fever that may not be immediately present. The patient rapidly becomes confused, sleepy, obtunded, and often comatose.

The examining physician needs to carefully search for signs of nuchal rigidity in any febrile patient who presents with a headache or any changes in level of alertness. Two clinical maneuvers are very important for identifying the presence of inflamed meningeal coverings involving the lumbosacral nerve

roots: the Kernig and Brudzinski signs (Fig. 48-2). The **Kernig sign** is elicited by flexing the patient's hip to a 90-degree angle and then attempting to passively straighten the leg at the knee; pain and tightness in the hamstring muscles prevent completion of this maneuver. This sign should be present bilaterally to support a diagnosis of meningitis. The **Brudzinski sign** is positive if the patient's hips and knees flex automatically when the examiner flexes the patient's neck while the patient is supine. Because host responsiveness to the infection varies, these signs of meningeal irritation are not invariably present, especially in debilitated and elderly patients and infants. When the clinical picture is typical of meningitis, it is also very important to exclude the concomitant presence of a focal parameningeal source such as a brain abscess. Further history, careful neurologic examination, and various imaging studies are essential (Figs. 48-3 and 48-4). Frequently there may be concomitant dermatologic findings present. A maculopapular or petechial/

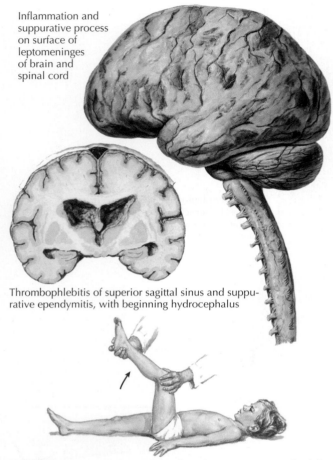

Inflammation and suppurative process on surface of leptomeninges of brain and spinal cord

Thrombophlebitis of superior sagittal sinus and suppurative ependymitis, with beginning hydrocephalus

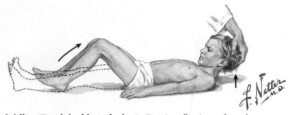

Kernig sign. Patient supine, with hip flexed 90°. Knee cannot be fully extended.

Neck rigidity (Brudzinski neck sign). Passive flexion of neck causes flexion of both legs and thighs.

Figure 48-2 Bacterial Meningitis–II.

purpuric rash usually indicates infection with *N. meningitidis* although an echovirus may mimic such. However, in these instances, the CSF findings are significantly different, usually with predominant lymphocytosis, normal CSF sugar, and negative Gram stain. The dermatologic findings of *N. meningitidis* are usually secondary to an underlying vasculitis; they are rarely related to concomitant coagulation defects or a combination of the two. Meningococcal infection more commonly has a rash that affects the trunk and extremities in contrast to the echovirus exanthem that usually involves the face and neck early in the infection. Purpuric lesions may also rarely be found in a fulminant pneumococcal bacteremia with meningitis as well as staphylococcal endocarditis, the latter primarily involving the finger pads.

Diagnostic Approach

CSF examination is essential to the diagnosis of bacterial and other microbial forms of meningitis. Generally, a brain CT must precede CSF examination to rule out a primary brain abscess or a parameningeal focus with significant mass effect, potentially causing cerebral herniation secondary to a sudden change in CSF dynamics. When there are signs of focal neurologic involvement or increased intracranial pressure in patients with suspected meningitis, a lumbar puncture may be contraindicated. These include papilledema, coma, and focal neurologic findings, such as dilated pupils, hemiparesis, and aphasia. Accompanying signs of increased intracranial pressure may include bradycardia, Cheyne–Stoke respirations, and even projectile vomiting.

As soon as diagnosis of meningitis is considered, even before proceeding with a CT scan and lumbar puncture, administration of empiric antibiotics covering the broad spectrum of gram-positive and gram-negative organisms is essential. One can later adjust the treatment once CSF culture examination results are available. If CT exam confirms that there is no mass lesion suggestive of a parameningeal focus with potential for herniation, one can then safely proceed with a CSF examination. If a parameningeal mass lesion is identified as a source of the meningitis, its treatment is paramount. The precise identification of the pathogenic bacteria, per se, will then become possible at the time of surgical decompression, and the spinal tap as such is not required.

CSF analysis provides the only conclusive proof of bacterial infection of the subarachnoid space. It must include a Gram-stained smear to define the offending organism morphology. The Gram stain correlates with the precise microbial etiology, as defined by the more specific bacteriologic culture, in approximately 80% of patients. This is a simple technique that allows for better selection of appropriate antibiotic therapy before definitive culture and sensitivity data are available. However, one does not need to await the results of the Gram stain before immediate initiation of appropriate antibiotic therapy. Rapid detection of microbial antigens by counterimmunoelectrophoresis or latex agglutination tests can aid diagnosis when CSF Gram stain and cultures are not diagnostic. Newer molecular diagnostic techniques are anticipated.

The initial CSF analysis needs to include measurement of the opening pressure, color (clear, turbid, or purulent), WBC count and differential, and levels of glucose and protein. Typically in bacterial meningitis, the CSF opening pressure is increased (>200 mm of CSF lying down and >35 mm Hg upright). The fluid is usually turbid or frankly purulent and contains predominantly (>90%) polymorphonuclear leukocytes. The CSF glucose level is very low, usually less than 50% of that found with measurement of concomitant serum glucose. A low glucose level (<40 mg/100 mL) is also found in some other types of microbial meningitides including *L. monocytogenes*, *Mycobacterium tuberculosis*, and *Cryptococcus neoformans*. Normal glucose levels are common in viral meningitis. Usually, CSF protein levels are increased, often greater than 100 mg/dL (reference range, <45 mg/dL). In patients with parameningeal foci, such as a brain or epidural spinal abscess, or with multiple septic emboli, CSF glucose may not be as low as with typical bacterial

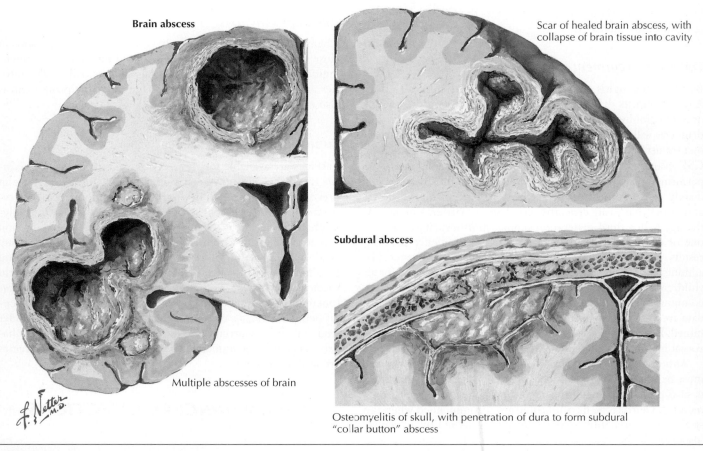

Brain abscess

Scar of healed brain abscess, with collapse of brain tissue into cavity

Subdural abscess

Multiple abscesses of brain

Osteomyelitis of skull, with penetration of dura to form subdural "collar button" abscess

Figure 48-3 Parameningeal Infections.

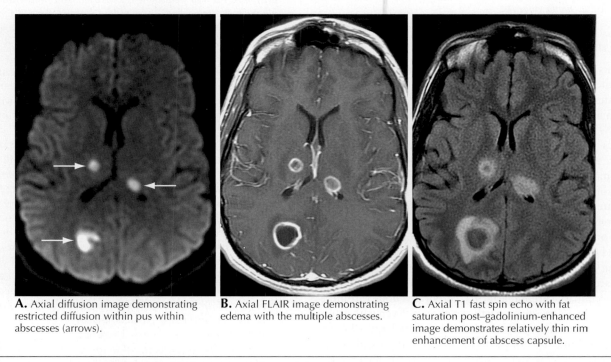

A. Axial diffusion image demonstrating restricted diffusion within pus within abscesses (arrows).

B. Axial FLAIR image demonstrating edema with the multiple abscesses.

C. Axial T1 fast spin echo with fat saturation post–gadolinium-enhanced image demonstrates relatively thin rim enhancement of abscess capsule.

Figure 48-4 Multiple brain abscesses in a 32-year-old with septicemia.

meningitis, even though in these instances the CSF protein level is significantly increased.

Optimum Treatment

Bacterial meningitis is an extremely life-threatening infection. Any delay in its diagnosis by not initially assessing the patient or not beginning therapy at the first consideration of this critical diagnosis will increase morbidity and mortality. Antibiotic treatment must be initiated as soon as possible, and later guided by CSF examination results. When CSF examination cannot be performed promptly, empiric therapy must be instituted immediately. Patients must receive at least 10 days of high-dose IV antibiotics that easily cross the blood–brain barrier. Empiric IV therapy with a third-generation cephalosporin, such as ceftriaxone or cefotaxime, plus vancomycin must commence pending results of the bacterial cultures. High-dose corticosteroids, administered before antibiotic therapy, are recommended for all children and should be seriously considered for adults with community-acquired meningitis. When culture and sensitivity data are available, a specific antimicrobial therapy can be determined. Penicillin G is recommended for documented meningococcal meningitis.

Antimicrobial therapy for meningitis caused by *S. pneumoniae* must be based on antibiotic sensitivity test results. If the strain is susceptible to penicillin, penicillin or ceftriaxone are recommended. Ceftriaxone or cefotaxime are recommended when the strain is not susceptible to penicillin and is susceptible to cephalosporins. If the strain is susceptible to neither cephalosporins nor penicillin, vancomycin must be added to a third-generation cephalosporin (cefotaxime or ceftriaxone). In patients older than age 50 years, empiric therapy with ampicillin must be added to vancomycin and a third-generation cephalosporin to provide coverage for *L. monocytogenes*.

Complications

Of patients with bacterial meningitis, approximately 15% experience acute and chronic complications, including various cranial nerve dysfunction, particularly those affecting extraocular function (cranial nerves [CNs] III, IV, and VI), CN-VII, and sometimes CN-VIII, although this is less common today with the antibiotics lacking specific ototoxicity or vestibular toxicity. However, permanent sensorineural hearing loss occurs occasionally, most commonly with pediatric meningococcal infections. Assorted cranial neuropathies are generally secondary to the exudate common with the more purulent forms of bacterial and tuberculous meningitis.

Focal or generalized seizures, various focal cerebral signs, coma, and acute cerebral edema occasionally occur. Findings mimicking a stroke, such as a hemiparesis, aphasia, and hemianopsia, are relatively infrequent; persistence of such findings suggests secondary cerebral arteritis, cerebral venous thrombosis, or rarely a mass lesion, especially an abscess. Even with astute and early diagnosis, mortality rates are still at least 10% for meningococcal and 30% for pneumococcal meningitis, although the latter has very significantly decreased in frequency with the recent introduction of a pneumococcal immunization. Whenever any diagnostic delay occurs leading to less than immediate treatment, mortality and morbidity are significantly higher.

Chemoprophylaxis

Chemoprophylaxis is particularly recommended for persons in close contact with patients who acquired meningococcal meningitis, especially in confined settings such as college dormitories and army barracks. Rifampin is preferred; ciprofloxacin is also effective.

Future Directions: Vaccines

Vaccines are available for three common organisms. *H. influenzae* type b protein-polysaccharide vaccine is highly effective in preventing meningitis in newborns and young infants. *N. meningitidis* (meningococcus) serogroups A, C, Y, and W135 polysaccharide vaccine is recommended for high-risk adults and contacts of persons with meningococcal disease. Although group B accounts for >50% of cases, its capsule is an autoantigen and thus not a suitable vaccine target; several recombinant protein vaccines are in late-stage clinical development. *S. pneumoniae* (pneumococcus), pneumococcal protein-polysaccharide heptavalent vaccine, is recommended for children and is under study in adults. Currently, 23-valent pneumococcal polysaccharide vaccine is recommended for adults. Several new vaccines are in development.

PARAMENINGEAL INFECTIONS

Clinical Vignette

A 76-year-old man presented with sinus headaches and underwent surgical drainage of the frontal sinuses. Postoperatively, he had headaches, seizures, and mild right-sided weakness, diagnosed as a mild CVA. He was discharged home, where he had some difficulty walking and speech was "not quite normal." He gradually worsened and 6 weeks after his surgery he could not hold anything in his right hand and became aphasic. He complained of some chills but no fever. On examination, he was awake and alert but globally aphasic, cranial nerves were intact, and gaze was conjugate. There was a right hemiparesis. WBC count was 9,700/mm³ with a normal differential. Brain CT demonstrated a hypointense left frontal lobe structural lesion with midline shift. Brain magnetic resonance imaging (MRI) demonstrated a multiloculated lesion with marked ring enhancement and surrounding edema extending through the frontal lobe and posteriorly toward the left parietal lobe (see Fig. 48-3). There was 1.5 mm midline shift. The lesion was aspirated using a stereotactic technique; Gram stain revealed many PMNs, many gram-positive cocci, and rare gram-negative rods. Culture grew Proteus mirabilis and Bacillus species. He was treated with 4 months of ceftriaxone and metronidazole with full resolution of speech and recovery of ambulation with the assistance of a walker.

Comment: Although parameningeal infections are relatively uncommon disorders, these lesions must always be considered in the differential diagnosis of any acute cerebral or spinal lesion (see Fig. 48-3). These processes may easily be unsuspected and thus unrecognized until it is too late to prevent permanent neurologic deficits. CT scanning is a very useful tool to exclude such predisposing lesions. Although these abscesses are easily considered within the setting of an overt infection, a precise microbial source is not always defined by the character of the clinical presentation. It is essential to always consider whether any acute spinal or cerebral lesion possibly has an infectious basis. This is particularly important in the setting of a chronic illness such as diabetes mellitus, something that often predisposes individuals to spinal epidural abscesses. The highest diagnostic and therapeutic priority is required in these settings. When identified, such processes are among the most urgent neurologic emergencies. These require immediate diagnostic and therapeutic attention. Even when appropriate diagnostic and therapeutic focus occurs, the patient's outcome may still be guarded, as in the preceding vignette in this chapter.

BRAIN ABSCESS

Clinical Vignette

A 26-year-old woman had the sudden onset of numbness in her right hand and face. This cleared within a few minutes only to recur on two more occasions within the next 48 hours. She then suddenly became aphasic with numbness and weakness of her right hand and face. Neurologic examination demonstrated a fluent aphasia, with a right central facial and hand weakness. Her muscle stretch reflexes were enhanced in her right arm associated with a right Babinski sign. She had a grade III/IV systolic murmur at the apex of her heart. Brain imaging demonstrated a left parietal temporal mass suggestive of a cerebritis or an abscess. Empirical antibiotics were begun. Within 36 hours, blood cultures demonstrated a gram-positive diplococcus. The antibiotics were adjusted appropriately. Within 48 hours, her condition had stabilized. Repeat imaging studies 1 week later showed improvement. Surgical decompression was considered early on; however, the antimicrobial therapy was sufficient. She gradually improved having an almost complete recovery. When her speech improved, she subsequently recalled having had a dental hygiene appointment a few weeks before the onset of her illness. Previously, she had not been aware of having a mitral valve lesion. She was instructed that she needed antimicrobial therapy prior to any dental or other medically invasive procedure in the future.

Brain abscess, which may be indolent or fulminant, results from direct extension of a contiguous focus, such as middle ear or sinus infections, congenital heart disease with a right-to-left shunt, or very rarely a pulmonary arteriovenous malformation having similar shunt mechanisms. Hematogenous spread may occur from distant infection sites in the head and neck, heart (infectious endocarditis), lung, or abdomen, or direct introduction of bacteria after penetrating head injuries. Brain abscess can occur after surgical procedures, as in the vignette on p. 408. The cardinal symptom of brain abscess is relentless and progressive headache, usually followed by focal neurologic manifestations. Only two thirds of patients have fever. Papilledema

and other signs of increased intracranial pressure may occasionally develop; however, the availability of imaging studies makes it more likely that the abscess will be identified prior to its obtaining significant enough mass to create increased intracranial pressure.

Most brain abscess cases are polymicrobial. Etiologic agents often include aerobic bacteria, such as streptococci, Enterobacteriaceae, and staphylococci. *Streptococcus milleri* normally resides in the oral cavity, appendix, and female genital tract and has a proclivity for abscess formation. Anaerobic microorganisms, such as *Bacteroides* and *Prevotella* species, are present in up to 40% of cases. Fungi are uncommon but increasingly recognized among immunosuppressed patients.

MRI is most helpful for making the initial diagnosis (Fig. 48-3). The characteristic appearance is a focal cerebral lesion with a hypodense center and a peripheral uniform ring enhancement subsequent to contrast material injection. Sometimes there is a concomitant area of surrounding edema. In these circumstances, if at all possible lumbar puncture should be avoided to prevent abscess herniation or rupture into the ventricular system.

Therapeutically, the abscess may be directly aspirated. Empiric medical therapy is started with a third- or fourth-generation cephalosporin or penicillin plus metronidazole, depending on the setting. Surgery may not be necessary if follow-up CT demonstrates decreased abscess size. Brain edema associated with acute brain abscess necessitates use of steroids and mannitol, as well as phenytoin, to prevent convulsions.

SUBDURAL ABSCESS

This is another form of life-threatening neurologic infection. It is typically characterized by a purulent collection within the potential space between the dura mater and arachnoid membrane (Fig. 48-3). An active paranasal sinusitis, particularly originating within the frontal sinuses or mastoid air cells, usually precedes extension of the infection into the subdural space. Occasionally, it is directly introduced through operative or traumatic wound sites.

Streptococci usually comprise 50% of cases; *S. aureus*, gram-negative bacteria, and anaerobic bacteria such as microaerophilic streptococci, *Bacteroides* species, and *Clostridium perfringens* are sometimes identified. Occasionally, polymicrobial infections occur.

Localized swelling, erythema, headache, or tenderness of the site overlying the primary infection may occur. As the illness progresses, the headache becomes generalized and severe, with a high fever, vomiting, and nuchal rigidity developing. Seizures, hemiparesis, visual field defects, and papilledema sometimes occur.

CSF contains 10 to 1000 WBCs; protein level is increased, and glucose level is normal in contrast to bacterial meningitis; this is a particularly important clue if imaging studies have not been previously obtained. CT or MRI demonstrates a low-absorption extracerebral mass. A thin, moderately dense margin may be visualized with the contrast medium (Fig. 48-3).

Treatment includes a combination of prompt surgical drainage and intensive antimicrobial therapy. The initial antibiotic choice requires intravenous third- or fourth-generation cephalosporin for aerobic bacteria and metronidazole for anaerobic bacteria. Prophylactic use of anticonvulsants and corticosteroids may also be required.

SPINAL EPIDURAL ABSCESS

Clinical Vignette

A 52-year-old diabetic man experienced a nonspecific upper respiratory tract syndrome typically thought of as influenza. Within just a few days, he developed increasingly severe midthoracic spine pain. He soon developed rigors, chills, and vomiting. His symptoms rapidly worsened over the subsequent 12–24 hours. He then suddenly noted numbness in both legs spreading up to his midback. He soon had trouble climbing stairs and after lying down to regain his strength was unable to arise from bed even with his wife's attempted help. He could not urinate. His family called the local emergency ambulance and had him taken to the hospital.

Neurologic examination demonstrated that he was paraplegic and had a T6 sensory level with marked loss of sensation below his nipple line. The patient required urinary catheterization. Spinal MRI demonstrated an epidural abscess extending between T4 and T10. Although an immediate neurosurgical decompression was carried out, unfortunately this patient had only partial resolution of his neurologic deficit.

Epidural spinal abscess patients typically present with fever and relatively severe back pain, sometimes with varying degrees of leg weakness. There are four clinical stages: (1) focal vertebral pain, (2) radicular pain corresponding to the dermatomal course of the specific involved nerve roots, (3) early signs of spinal cord compression such as paresthesias, weakness, or delayed ability to urinate, and (4) paralysis below the lesion level.

A purulent or granulomatous collection within the spinal epidural space may overlie or encircle the spinal cord, nerve roots, and nerves (Fig. 48-5). Although the infection is usually localized within three to four vertebral segments, it rarely extends the length of the spinal canal.

S. aureus is the most common organism leading to a spinal epidural abscess, but aerobic or anaerobic streptococci and gram-negative organisms are occasionally isolated. Mixed anaerobic and aerobic organisms are sometimes responsible. When no organism is isolated or if granulomas are identified, *M. tuberculosis* infection of the spine, for example, Pott disease, also requires consideration. A skin infection, especially a furuncle, is the most common focus for a hematogenous spread to the epidural space. An antecedent vertebral osteomyelitis with a prior hematogenous source is responsible for approximately 40% of spinal epidural abscess. Dental and upper respiratory tract infections are other common predisposing lesions.

Any patient presenting with back pain, fever, and localized tenderness or signs of cord compression requires immediate and complete spinal MRI. Surgical or CT-guided needle aspiration is necessary to define an accurate diagnosis and possible decompression. Blood cultures are recommended. Lumbar puncture

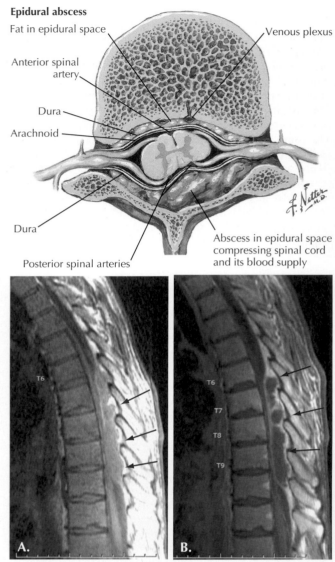

Epidural abscess

Fat in epidural space

Anterior spinal artery

Dura

Arachnoid

Dura

Posterior spinal arteries

Venous plexus

Abscess in epidural space compressing spinal cord and its blood supply

Epidural abscess. Sagittal T1-weighted images without (**A.**) and with (**B**) gadolinium enhancement demonstrate an extensive posterior epidural process from T6 to T11. Enhancement of the granulation tissue allows appreciation of nonenhancing focal pus collections.

Figure 48-5 Spinal Epidural Abscess.

should **not** be performed. Appropriate parenteral antibiotics are necessary for 3 to 4 weeks in uncomplicated cases and for up to 8 weeks or more if osteomyelitis is present.

SPECIFIC PATHOGENS

LYME DISEASE (BORRELIA BURGDORFERI)

Clinical Vignette

A 39-year-old woman presented with complaints of fatigue progressing over a month followed by aching in her back

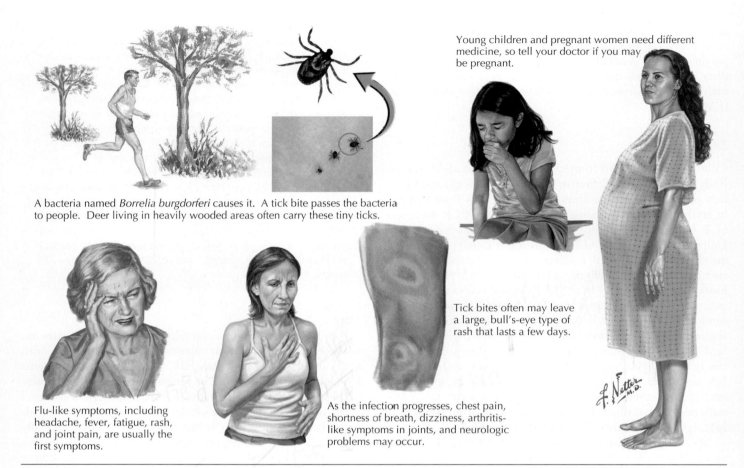

A bacteria named *Borrelia burgdorferi* causes it. A tick bite passes the bacteria to people. Deer living in heavily wooded areas often carry these tiny ticks.

Young children and pregnant women need different medicine, so tell your doctor if you may be pregnant.

Tick bites often may leave a large, bull's-eye type of rash that lasts a few days.

Flu-like symptoms, including headache, fever, fatigue, rash, and joint pain, are usually the first symptoms.

As the infection progresses, chest pain, shortness of breath, dizziness, arthritis-like symptoms in joints, and neurologic problems may occur.

Figure 48-6 Lyme Disease Clinical Settings.

behind her right shoulder for 2 weeks. She developed a severe headache with photophobia and nausea over the week before admission. On questioning, she remembered a bug bite followed by a 5-cm rash at about the time her fatigue began. At the time, she developed upper back and neck stiffness that she sought chiropractic treatment for. She was afebrile on examination, with no neck stiffness or neurologic deficits. A 5-cm oval area of erythema was noted near her left axilla. WBC was 6.58 and metabolic profile normal. CSF examination showed 129 WBC (89% lymphocytes, 3% neutrophils) and 363 RBC, glucose 48, and protein 54. CT scan of the brain was unremarkable. Serum Lyme Western blot testing was positive. A Lyme IgM was positive in the patient's CSF and Lyme polymerase chain reaction (PCR) was negative. She was treated with 1 month of ceftriaxone 2 g IV daily with complete resolution of symptoms.

Comment: Lyme disease, which is caused by the tick-borne spirochete Borrelia burgdorferi, is endemic in parts of the United States, particularly northeast Atlantic coastal areas from Maine to Maryland, the upper Midwest, including Minnesota and Wisconsin, as well as the northern Pacific including California and Oregon. Currently, about 15,000 cases per year are reported in the United States. It is also endemic in Europe and Asia in forested areas.

Clinical Presentation

In 80% of patients in the United States, Lyme disease presents with a slowly expanding skin lesion called erythema migrans that occurs at the site of the tick bite (Fig. 48-6). Influenza-like symptoms, such as malaise, fatigue, fever, headache, arthralgias, myalgias, and regional lymphadenopathy, frequently accompany the rash and are often the presenting manifestation of Lyme disease. Early localized infection is followed within days to weeks by a systemic dissemination that variously affects the nervous system, heart, or joints. Untreated, late or persistent Lyme infection ensues.

In the United States, 15% of untreated neuroborreliosis patients develop objective signs and symptoms of early disseminated infection. A variety of neurologic manifestations develop, including lymphocytic meningitis with episodic headache and mild neck stiffness, a subtle encephalitis with impaired memory, a cranial neuropathy (most commonly uni- or bilateral facial palsy, sometimes an optic neuropathy), cerebellar ataxia, myelitis, motor or sensory radiculoneuritis, or a mononeuritis multiplex.

Untreated, acute neurologic abnormalities usually improve or resolve within weeks or months. However 5% of untreated patients may develop a chronic neuroborreliosis with subtle cognitive changes. This is termed Lyme encephalopathy. Although the cerebrospinal fluid in these patients shows no inflammatory changes, intrathecal antibody production against *B. burgdorferi* is often demonstrated. Sometimes a chronic axonal polyneuropathy, generally presenting as spinal radicular pain or distal paresthesias, may develop. Diffuse involvement of proximal and distal nerve segments is found on electromyography (EMG).

Diagnosis

Culture of *B. burgdorferi* from specimens in Barboud–Stoenner–Kelly medium allows definitive microbiologic diagnosis, but is only possible early in the illness and usually only from biopsies of erythema migrans lesions. In late infection, PCR detection of *B. burgdorferi* is superior to culture from joint fluid. In the United States, diagnosis of Lyme disease is usually made based on characteristic clinical findings, history of exposure in an endemic area, and antibody response to *B. burgdorferi* by enzyme-linked immunosorbent assay (ELISA) and Western blotting interpreted according to Centers for Disease Control and Prevention (CDC) criteria. Serology is insensitive during the first several weeks of infection (only 20–30% positive and usually IgM alone), but by four weeks 70–80% are seropositive (generally IgM and IgG), even after antibiotic treatment. A positive IgM test alone after 1 month of illness is likely to represent a false-positive result. Patients with acute neuroborreliosis, especially meningitis, often demonstrate intrathecal production of IgM, IgG, or IgA antibody against *B. burgdorferi*.

MRI may demonstrate meningitic findings (Fig. 48-7a&b), as well as cranial nerve involvement. Intraparenchymal white matter changes in the corpus callosum as well as centrum semiovale mimicking multiple sclerosis may be seen. Active enhancement is a good marker of active disease (Fig. 48-7c–f).

Treatment

Evidence-based recommendations for Lyme disease have been developed by the Infectious Diseases Society of America. Early or localized disseminated infection can be successfully treated with 14–21 days of oral doxycycline. Children and pregnant women may be treated with amoxicillin. An advantage of doxycycline is efficacy against *Anaplasma phagocytophilum*, a possible coinfecting pathogen that causes human granulocytic ehrlichiosis. Cefuroxime axetil is a third alternative in those allergic to the first options. Patients with objective neurologic abnormalities can be treated with 14–28 days of intravenous ceftriaxone (cefotaxime and penicillin G are possible alternatives). Manifestations of acute neuroborreliosis usually resolve within weeks, but chronic neuroborreliosis generally resolves over a period of months. Objective evidence of relapse is rare after 4 weeks of therapy.

TUBERCULOSIS: BRAIN AND SPINE (*MYCOBACTERIUM TUBERCULOSIS*)

Clinical Vignette

A 51-year-old Vietnamese woman presented with 7 days of headache, vomiting, and episodic left facial and arm tingling numbness while visiting the United States. She reported diplopia, having fallen twice and fractured her nose. Some seizurelike activity was witnessed. The patient's temperature was equivocally febrile. On neurologic examination, she was confused and only intermittently fluent. She had bilateral sixth cranial nerve palsies and early papilledema. Her neck was stiff, and her lungs were clear.

A lumbar puncture revealed a CSF opening pressure of 500 mm CSF, protein of 218 mg/dL, glucose of 22 mg/dL (serum glucose level 137 mg/dL), an RBC count of 190/mm³, and a WBC count of 1390/mm³ (4% polymorphonuclear leukocytes, 94% lymphocytes). CSF acid-fast bacilli smear and PCR results were negative. Cranial CT and MRI results were normal. The patient was treated with isoniazid, rifampin, ethambutol, pyrazinamide, and methylprednisolone (Solu-Medrol). The CSF ultimately grew M. tuberculosis.

The incidence of CNS tuberculosis in the United States has markedly decreased; it most commonly occurs in foreign-born adults and those infected with HIV. Neurologically, it presents as a meningitis, mass lesion, or vertebral lesion. Because tuberculosis is still endemic in Southeast Asia, it must be considered in the differential diagnosis of patients immigrating from this area who present with a meningoencephalopathy, especially with cranial neuropathies; the vignette in this chapter is classic. It is important to make a clinical diagnosis and begin treatment while awaiting CSF culture results.

Tuberculous Meningitis

Tuberculous meningitis usually results from hematogenous meningeal seeding or contiguous spread from a tuberculoma or parameningeal granuloma, with subsequent rupture into the subarachnoid space (Fig. 48-8). Local foci of infection along the meninges, brain, or spinal cord, thought to be present from hematogenous seeding of the primary infection, also release bacilli directly into the subarachnoid space. Infection then spreads along the perivascular spaces into the brain. An intense inflammatory reaction at the brain base causes an occlusive arteritis, with small vessel thrombosis and resultant brain infarction. Direct cranial nerve compression and obstruction of CSF flow at the foramina of the fourth ventricle or at the basal cisterns may result in subarachnoid block and cerebral edema.

Tuberculous meningitis progresses rapidly, with headache, fever, meningismus, and cranial nerve deficits, especially sixth nerve palsy. Focal cerebral or cerebellar deficits are followed by altered sensorium and coma.

CSF examination is critical in establishing the diagnosis. Classically, the CSF glucose level is less than two thirds that of the serum glucose level; the CSF protein level is greater than 50 mg/dL; and the WBC count is increased, with a lymphocyte predominance. PCR analysis and culture are the most sensitive diagnostic tools. PCR can detect fewer than 10 organisms in clinical specimens compared with the 10,000 necessary for smear positivity. False-negative PCR results have been reported (sensitivity in acid-fast smear-negative cases varies from 40% to

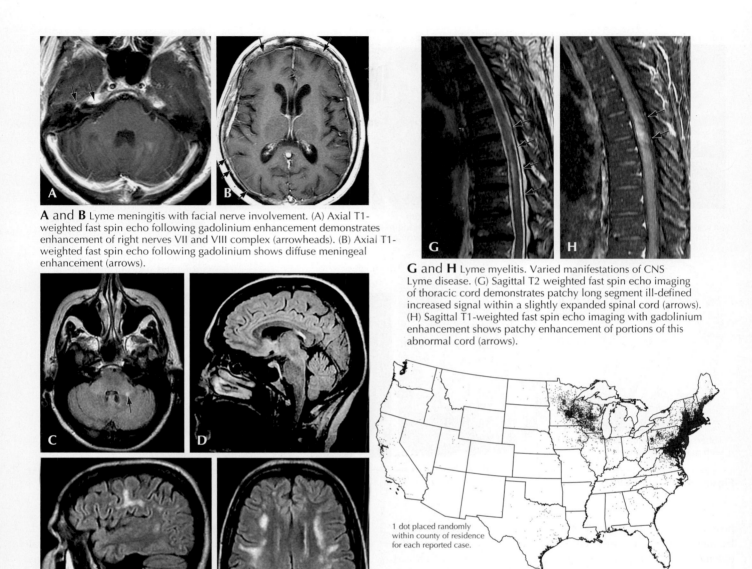

A and B Lyme meningitis with facial nerve involvement. (A) Axial T1-weighted fast spin echo following gadolinium enhancement demonstrates enhancement of right nerves VII and VIII complex (arrowheads). (B) Axial T1-weighted fast spin echo following gadolinium shows diffuse meningeal enhancement (arrows).

G and H Lyme myelitis. Varied manifestations of CNS Lyme disease. (G) Sagittal T2 weighted fast spin echo imaging of thoracic cord demonstrates patchy long segment ill-defined increased signal within a slightly expanded spinal cord (arrows). (H) Sagittal T1-weighted fast spin echo imaging with gadolinium enhancement shows patchy enhancement of portions of this abnormal cord (arrows).

1 dot placed randomly within county of residence for each reported case.

I Reported cases of Lyme Disease—United States, 2009. From the Centers for Disease Control and Prevention, Division of Vector-Borne Infectious Diseases. www.cdc. gov/ncidod/dvbid/lyme/ld_Incidence.htm

C–F Lyme CNS disease. Note primary demyelinating pattern as evidenced by the intraparenchymal brain lesions. Multiple FLAIR images demonstrate multiple regions of involvement, including left cerebellar peduncle (C), splenium of corpus callosum and posterior subfrontal region (D), and central white matter and subcortical involvement (E and F).

Figure 48-7 Lyme Disease.

77%). Unfortunately, acid-fast (Ziehl–Neelsen) smears are positive only 25% of the time, and more commonly with concentrated CSF specimens.

It is imperative to initiate therapy at the slightest suspicion of CNS tuberculosis as death may follow within a matter of weeks if this is present and left untreated. Because of worldwide increases in drug resistance, whenever there is a clinical suspicion of this diagnosis, therapy must be instituted immediately. Isoniazid, rifampin, ethambutol, and pyrazinamide are the medications of choice until diagnostic identification and sensitivity testing are available. Both isoniazid and pyrazinamide achieve CSF concentrations equaling those in blood, and rifampin crosses the blood–brain barrier adequately. Corticosteroids are added when cerebral edema, subarachnoid block, or both occur. Mortality is greatest at the extremes of age (20% at <5 years and 60% at >50 years) or if the illness has been present more than 2 months (80%). HIV infection does not seem to alter the clinical course or prognosis of tuberculous meningitis, although CNS mass lesions are more likely to occur in this setting.

Cerebral Tuberculomas

Cerebral tuberculomas are less common than tuberculous meningitis. These are often calcified and are usually located in the

TB with involvement of basal cisterns with vasculitis and ischemia

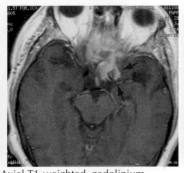

Midsagittal T2-weighted image shows increased T2 signal within ischemic frontal lobe.

Axial T1-weighted, gadolinium-enhanced image with enhancing mass at left basal cisterns and subfrontal region.

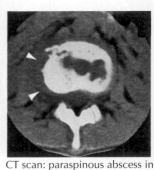

CT scan: paraspinous abscess in addition to bony destruction

X-ray film: destruction of disc space (arrow) and adjacent end plates of vertebrae

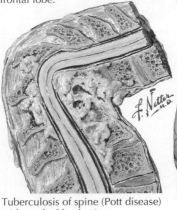

Tuberculosis of spine (Pott disease) with marked kyphosis

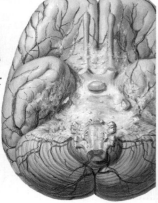

Tuberculous basilar meningitis

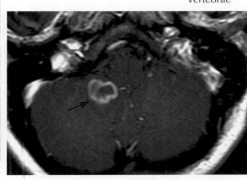

Tuberculoma. Axial T1-weighted fast spin echo post–gadolinium enhanced image demonstrates a rim enhancing inferior right cerebellar mass (arrow).

Figure 48-8 Tuberculosis.

posterior fossa, particularly the cerebellum. Although most frequently multiple, tuberculomas can be single. Contrast-enhanced MRI is generally considered the modality of choice in detecting and assessing CNS tuberculosis (Fig. 48-8). PCR and CSF culture or culture of biopsied lesional material confirms the diagnosis. Because standard medical therapy is usually successful if multidrug resistance is not identified, antituberculous therapy must be attempted before surgery is contemplated. Of course, if there are signs of impending herniation, immediate surgery is indicated.

Vertebral Tuberculosis (Pott Disease)

Clinical Vignette

A 30-year-old man who emigrated from India to the United States 2 years previously to take a job with a software company presented with complaints of back pain, fever, and leg numbness. His examination was normal. Tuberculin skin testing elicited an 18-mm reaction. Chest radiograph demonstrated an infiltrate in the posterior-apical segment of the right upper lobe. CT scan revealed a paraspinal abscess at the L5 level. Both the sputum and an aspirate of the abscess grew M. tuberculosis.

Skeletal joints most subject to trauma are primarily affected. The spine—typically the disc space and adjacent vertebral bodies, the epidural space, or both—is involved in approximately 50% of tuberculosis cases. Back pain and fever are often followed by progressive spinal cord compression from unrecognized epidural infection or fracture, collapse, or angulation of vertebral segments.

Standard spinal radiographs reveal disc space infection with spread to adjacent vertebrae (Fig. 48-8). MRI and/or CT myelography are the diagnostic procedures of choice. Bone biopsy or disc space aspiration is required for culture diagnosis before therapy.

A 9- to 12-month regimen of isoniazid and rifampin is appropriate. Prolongation of therapy is indicated for tuberculosis in sites that are slow to respond.

Future Directions

Reliable methods for rapid determination of *M. tuberculosis* drug susceptibility are needed. Multiple investigators have identified chromosomal mutations associated with drug resistance. Genotypic assays are highly specific but of variable sensitivity. Phenotypic susceptibility assays under development use mycobacteriophages to detect metabolically active mycobacteria grown in the presence of antituberculous drugs. Although these assays are not widely clinically available, they reduce turnaround time for results from 3 weeks to as little as 54–94 hours.

HANSEN DISEASE (LEPROSY—MYCOBACTERIUM LEPRAE)

Clinical Vignette

A 56-year-old woman from Cambodia was evaluated because she had been tripping on her left foot for 6 months. For the past month, she noticed difficulty gripping objects with her right hand and had associated elbow and median forearm pain.

Neurologic examination demonstrated weakness of finger abduction and adduction, mild clawing of the fourth and fifth digits, and sensory loss of the medial 1½ fingers, consistent with a right ulnar neuropathy affecting ulnar innervated structures in her right hand. Examination of the left leg revealed focal weakness of foot dorsiflexion and eversion with sensory loss on the lateral aspect of the left calf and the dorsum of the foot indicating a left common peroneal neuropathy. Both ulnar and peroneal nerves were thickened and palpable. Two subtle hypopigmented, anesthetic macules were found on her upper arm and trunk. Sensation was diminished on the ear pinna and tip of the nose.

EMG confirmed moderately severe right ulnar and left peroneal axonal neuropathies. Skin biopsy revealed noncaseating granulomas with lymphocytic infiltration and giant cells; acid-fast bacilli were seen on the modified Fite–Faraco stain. The diagnosis was tuberculoid leprosy; dapsone and rifampin were administered.

Hansen disease is a chronic infectious granulomatous disease of skin and peripheral nerves. The reader should understand that although leprosy has been the name of this disorder for many years, its use has led to unfortunate discrimination. Therefore Hansen disease, in recognition of the scientist who discovered the responsible mycobacterium, is now the preferred nomenclature. However, these names are still interchangeably used in some circles.

Worldwide, Hansen disease is one of the most common causes of neuropathy. Any patient from an area endemic for this disorder who has multiple mononeuropathies, particularly ulnar and peroneal, and has skin lesions, especially in superficial sensory areas that have cooler ambient temperatures, is most likely to have this disorder. The etiologic agent is *Mycobacterium leprae*, an acid-fast bacillus identified by Hansen in 1873. Today this occurs primarily in Asia, Africa, and Latin America. Subsequent to the World Health Organization redefining Hansen disease cases as only those under active treatment, and active case detection is now eliminated, the global registry of new cases has steadily declined since 2001, with 259,017 new cases reported in 2006. Active case detection is now relegated to the primary care physician. However, these bureaucratic finesses create a false sense of security. Thus, we feel that the actual numbers of patients with Hansen disease are grossly underestimated.

Bacteriology

The leprosy bacillus's genome demonstrates reductive evolution with extensive deletion and inactivation of genes and abundant pseudogenes; <50% of the genome contains functional genes. That may explain the unusually long generation time and the inability to culture *M. leprae* in artificial media.

Hansen disease is transmitted by respiratory droplets and direct skin contact during frequent, close exposure to untreated patients. Other routes of infection include contact with armadillos (a reservoir in Texas), infected soil, and rarely direct dermal implantation during procedures such as tattooing. The incubation period is usually 5–7 years. *M. leprae*/laminin-α_2 complexes bind to alpha/beta dystroglycan complexes expressed on Schwann cells and induce rapid demyelination by a contact-dependent mechanism. Myelinated Schwann cells are resistant to *M. leprae* invasion but undergo demyelination on bacterial attachment; Schwann cells proliferate and generate a nonmyelinated phenotype, where *M. leprae* multiply intracellularly in large numbers. The clinical development of leprosy depends on host immune responses and genetic factors. The disease spectrum varies widely from limited tuberculoid forms (where few bacilli can be demonstrated) to an extensive lepromatous (LL) form (where more than 10 million organisms per high power field can be seen on skin biopsies).

Clinical Presentation and Diagnosis

The three cardinal diagnostic criteria are anesthetic skin patches, thickened nerves, and acid-fast bacilli in skin smears (Fig. 48-9). The World Health Organization (WHO) recommends classification based on clinical criteria: *paucibacillary* if less than five skin lesions and/or one nerve is involved, or *multibacillary* if there are five or more skin lesions, more than two nerves involved, or both. This system determines the therapy type and duration for patients evaluated in the field where laboratory help is not available. The commonly used classification is based on the disease's clinical spectrum, extending from tuberculoid (TT) to borderline tuberculoid (BT), borderline (BB), borderline lepromatous (BL), and lepromatous (LL). Indeterminate leprosy, seen early in the infection, is diagnosed by the presence of a single or a few skin macules having variable sensory loss.

In tuberculoid (TT and BT) Hansen disease, preserved cell-mediated immunity prevents significant dissemination of the bacillus precluding more severe disease. Patients usually have asymmetrically distributed hypopigmented anesthetic lesions with erythematous margins and an associated asymmetric multifocal neuropathy (mononeuritis multiplex). Involved nerves are concomitantly enlarged, particularly the ulnar, posterior auricular, peroneal, and posterior tibial nerves. Skin or nerve biopsies demonstrate well-demarcated, noncaseating granulomas with many lymphocytes, Langhans giant cells. Acid-fast bacilli are infrequently seen, especially in tuberculoid leprosy. Nerve biopsies are infrequently needed to make this diagnosis.

Borderline (BB) leprosy stands between lepromatous and tuberculoid leprosy in severity and disease manifestation. Once patients receive treatment, they usually move toward the tuberculoid pole of the spectrum.

Lepromatous Hansen disease (LL and BL) is the most severe form, with unrestricted bacterial multiplication and hematogenous dissemination. The organisms have a predilection for multiplying in cooler body areas such as the superficial nerves, nose,

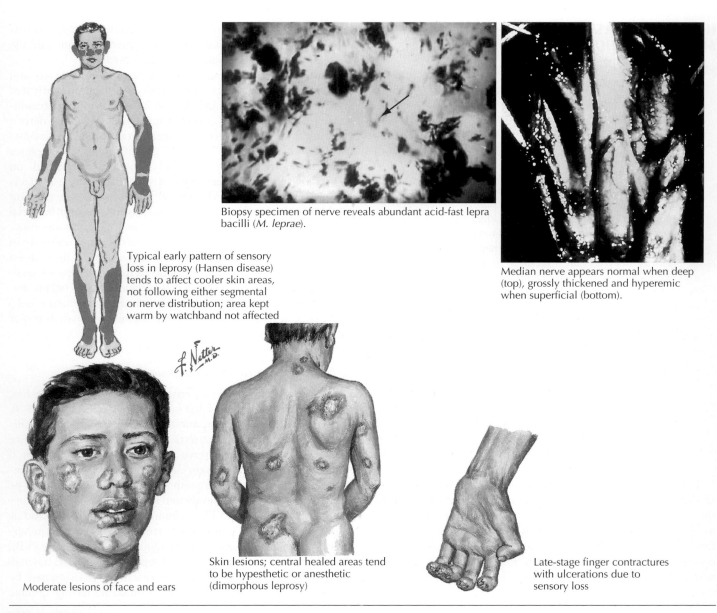

Biopsy specimen of nerve reveals abundant acid-fast lepra bacilli (*M. leprae*).

Typical early pattern of sensory loss in leprosy (Hansen disease) tends to affect cooler skin areas, not following either segmental or nerve distribution; area kept warm by watchband not affected

Median nerve appears normal when deep (top), grossly thickened and hyperemic when superficial (bottom).

Moderate lesions of face and ears

Skin lesions; central healed areas tend to be hypesthetic or anesthetic (dimorphous leprosy)

Late-stage finger contractures with ulcerations due to sensory loss

Figure 48-9 Leprosy.

earlobes, skin, testes, and eyes. Nerve involvement is symmetric and more extensive than in tuberculoid leprosy but more frequently involves the superficial cutaneous nerves. Large nerves are less frequently affected than in tuberculoid leprosy. Cutaneous lesions are skin-colored nodules or papules that coalesce to form extensive symmetric raised plaques or more diffuse infiltration of the skin. On the face, they result in leonine facies. Skin biopsies demonstrate vacuolated foam cells within the dermis containing large numbers of *M. leprae*, with few inflammatory cells, and rare granulomas.

The ulnar nerve is the most commonly affected peripheral nerve; when this is associated with median nerve involvement, the combination leads to clawing of the hand. Peroneal neuropathies are most common in the leg. At its extreme, patients with leprotic neuropathies develop auto-amputation of digits, recurrent nonhealing ulcers that often result in osteomyelitis, and nasal bridge collapse.

Erythema Nodosum Leprosum and Reversal Reactions

Leprosy can be complicated by different reactional states, namely, erythema nodosum leprosum (ENL) and reversal reactions. ENL is thought to be an immune complex–mediated process and is characterized by the development of crops of new, small tender subcutaneous nodules accompanied by fever, arthralgias or arthritis, adenopathy, and neuritis. Reversal reactions present as inflamed, indurated skin plaques with neuritis and represent an upgrading of the cell-mediated response in the patient's immunity to the infection. Both ENL and reversal reactions can occur before, during, and after the completion of antimycobacterial treatment for leprosy. Tumor necrosis factor–alpha and other proinflammatory and anti-inflammatory cytokines are considered key mediators in these reactional states.

Diagnostic Approach and Treatment

Other disorders that may present with similar skin lesions include sarcoidosis, leishmaniasis, lupus vulgaris, syphilis, yaws, and granuloma annulare. However, no other disease has hypopigmented anesthetic skin lesions. Hansen disease diagnosis depends on clinical findings and skin biopsy, a much less invasive procedure than nerve biopsy.

Multidrug treatment (MDT) with the antibiotic combination of rifampin, dapsone, and clofazimine is highly effective. The risk of recurrence is increased with higher bacterial loads and may not occur until 5–10 years after completion of treatment. Severe neural damage is the major complication of reactional states and responds to oral prednisone. Thalidomide, the preferred medication for severe ENL, has significant teratogenic potential. Additionally, thalidomide usage can be complicated by a dose-dependent sensory polyneuropathy; electrophysiologic studies have shown that monitoring sural sensory amplitude may help in the early diagnosis of an emerging sensory neuropathy. Management also includes injury prevention to anesthetized areas, hygiene maintenance, and reconstructive plastic surgery such as nasal reconstruction.

Future Directions

Multidrug treatment has resulted in a 90% reduction in disease prevalence. The global Hansen disease elimination campaigns of early disease detection, prevention of deformity, and completion of predefined treatment regimens are now replaced by the integration of detection and treatment of cases into the less than adequate primary care framework of endemic countries. The WHO definition of a case of leprosy includes only any patient who is on active MDT and therefore excludes the treatment of Type 1 and 11 reactions (that may occur for up to 10 years after effective MDT) with the ensuing deforming neuropathies. Although specific preventive vaccines are not available, bacille Calmette-Guerin (BCG) is variably effective. The successful mapping of the genome for the *M. leprae* bacterium and a better understanding of disease pathogenesis may result in more effective prevention and therapies.

The main drawback to treating this eminently curable disease is the limited resource availability in countries where Hansen disease is endemic. Although the decrease in prevalence rates due to MDT is admirable, this has also led to decreased funding of leprosy research and treatment programs. Greater provision of funds and medical expertise by the international community would help overcome this.

TETANUS (CLOSTRIDIUM TETANI)

Tetanus is caused by a potent neurotoxin, tetanospasmin, released by a gram-positive spore-forming obligate anaerobe, *Clostridium tetani*, that is typically found in occasional wound infections. This bacterial infection can be introduced at any site; contaminated wounds or retained foreign bodies are particularly dangerous. Although common in developing countries, tetanus very uncommonly occurs in North America mostly after the age of 60 years. Rarely, patients contract tetanus despite adequate immunization.

Tetanus results from the release of tetanospasmin into the bloodstream from a focus of infection by *C. tetani*; subsequently, it binds to the neuromuscular junction and then attaches to peripheral motor neuron nerve endings. It travels centrally up the nerve, in retrograde fashion (antidromically), to the anterior horn cells, where it enters adjacent spinal inhibitory interneurons, exerting its primary pathophysiologic effect by blocking inhibitory neurotransmitter release to the anterior horn cell. This leads to the classic muscular hypertonia and muscle spasms as agonist and antagonist muscles simultaneously contract as reciprocal inhibition is blocked (Fig. 48-10).

Clinical Presentation

Generalized Tetanus varies from mild to severe, depending on the incubation period, usually 2–14 days. It is occasionally delayed by weeks to months after the injury. A more severe clinical picture occurs when the incubation period is less than 8 days and the onset period is less than 48 hours.

In patients with partial or complete immunization, tetanus sometimes occurs as a mild form. It is often more severe in nonimmunized patients. Muscles close to the infection site are more severely affected initially. Typically trismus (lockjaw) and risus sardonicus (a spasmodic tetanic involuntary smile) are early and constant signs.

Subsequently shocklike painful spasms of all muscles are provoked by the slightest disturbance, including sight, sound, or touch, or occur spontaneously. Between the intermittent severe spasms, continuous muscle rigidity is often characterized by the clenched jaw, risus sardonicus, and a stiff back, neck, abdominal wall, and limbs, sometimes associated with laryngeal and respiratory muscle spasms that may cause airway obstruction.

Tetanus patients are fully conscious because this toxin does not affect cortical function or sensory nerves. They experience severe pain with every muscle contraction. The spasms become progressively severe in the first week after onset, gradually improving over 1–4 weeks. Sympathetic overactivity may occur with tachycardia, labile hypertension, and arrhythmias.

Focal Tetanus is an unusual manifestation, and is limited to muscles at the wound site. It is thought to occur when circulating antitoxin neutralizes the toxin, preventing systemic circulation of the toxin. However, this does not prevent the spread of the tetanus toxin regionally. Painful muscle spasms adjacent to the wound site may last a few weeks. Sometimes, focal tetanus proceeds to generalized tetanus. If generalization does not occur, there is eventually good recovery.

Diagnosis

Abdominal rigidity, generalized spasms, trismus, and risus sardonicus are highly characteristic clinical signs of tetanus. They may be mistaken for encephalitis, encephalomyelitis, meningitis, intracranial hemorrhage, or even stiff man syndrome. Normal CSF parameters and absence of an altered level of consciousness differentiate tetanus from primary CNS infections. Certain local conditions, including dental and peritonsillar abscesses, may also mimic tetanus. Hypocalcemic tetany is usually distinguished by carpopedal spasms and a positive Chvostek sign. Phenothiazine toxicity sometimes results in

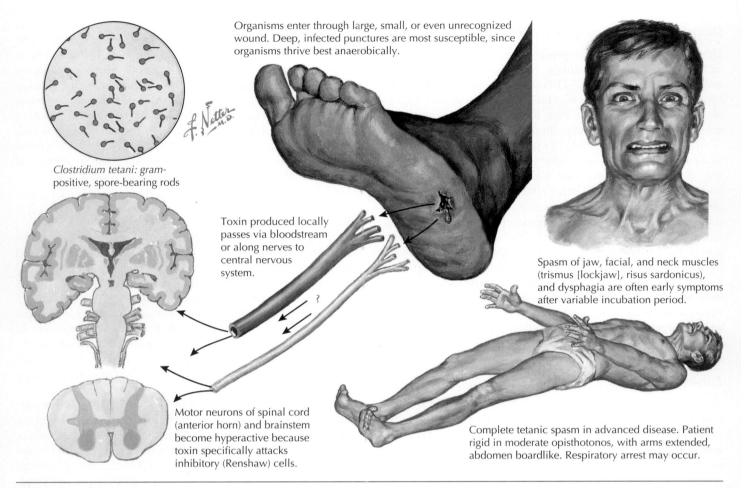

Organisms enter through large, small, or even unrecognized wound. Deep, infected punctures are most susceptible, since organisms thrive best anaerobically.

Clostridium tetani: gram-positive, spore-bearing rods

Toxin produced locally passes via bloodstream or along nerves to central nervous system.

Motor neurons of spinal cord (anterior horn) and brainstem become hyperactive because toxin specifically attacks inhibitory (Renshaw) cells.

Spasm of jaw, facial, and neck muscles (trismus [lockjaw], risus sardonicus), and dysphagia are often early symptoms after variable incubation period.

Complete tetanic spasm in advanced disease. Patient rigid in moderate opisthotonos, with arms extended, abdomen boardlike. Respiratory arrest may occur.

Figure 48-10 Tetanus.

dystonia and opisthotonus mimicking tetanus; prompt response to IV diphenhydramine helps to distinguish this medication-induced partial mimic of tetanus. Epileptic seizures and drug withdrawal reactions also occur in the differential diagnosis.

Fortunately, tetanus has a characteristic clinical picture, because *C. tetani* organisms are isolated from the wound in only one third of affected patients. There are no specific confirmatory blood studies or CSF analyses for tetanus. Sometimes EMG supports the diagnosis.

Treatment and Prognosis

Tetanus is entirely preventable with immunization. Treatment modalities include appropriate antibiotics and tetanus immunoglobulin, local wound care, control of spasms with muscle relaxants such as benzodiazepines and magnesium sulfate, anticonvulsants, ventilatory support, meticulous nursing care, and maintenance of adequate nutrition and hydration.

The incubation period and time to onset are important predictors of prognosis. If the incubation period is less than 8 days, the onset period is less than 48 hours, and reflex spasms have been present during more than 12– 24 hours, the prognosis is generally poor. With multimodality treatment, mortality from tetanus may be substantially reduced in the coming years throughout the world.

NEUROSYPHILIS (TREPONEMA PALLIDUM)

Clinical Vignette

A 27-year-old man was brought to the hospital by his friends who reported he had been "acting strange" before complaining of headache, nausea, and vomiting. He was afebrile and his examination was normal except for anisocoria, palsies of the right seventh and eighth cranial nerves, and a positive Romberg sign. CSF examination revealed 105 WBC (96% lymphocytes), protein 87, glucose 49. CSF VDRL (Venereal Disease Research Laboratory) was positive, as was serum rapid plasma reagin (RPR). HIV testing was negative. He was treated with 14 days of penicillin G 4 million units IV every 4 hours, with complete resolution of his symptoms.

Syphilis, or lues, is an uncommon disorder occurring primarily within the immune-compromised population, particularly in those with AIDS. *Treponema pallidum*, a spiral bacterium that is difficult to culture in the laboratory, causes syphilis. The diagnosis is made by spirochete identification in material from primary lesions using dark-field microscopy or serologic methods. CNS syphilis occurs in less than 20% of patients with primary infection. Typical of many patients with CNS lues, the diagnosis is made only by clinical signs, particularly the disparate pupillary responses to light and accommodation, along with often subtle findings of posterior spinal cord column and dorsal root ganglion involvement.

Untreated, *T. pallidum* causes chronic inflammation of CNS cellular and interstitial tissues, culminating in a granulomatous process, producing endarteritis and gummatous lesions. In the United States, syphilis occurs primarily in persons aged 20 to 39 years. Reported rates in men are one and a half times greater than those found in women. The incidence is highest in women aged 20–29 years and men aged 30–39 years.

Cases of primary and secondary syphilis in the United States increased 2% between 2000 and 2001 and 12% between 2001 and 2002. Increases were observed only in men; several outbreaks, associated with high rates of HIV coinfection and high-risk sexual behavior, were seen among men who had sex with men. From 2000 to 2002, the number of primary and secondary syphilis cases decreased 19% among women and 10% among African Americans. Poverty, inadequate health care access, and lack of education are associated with disproportionately high syphilis incidence in certain populations.

Clinical Presentation

There are five classic neurologic presentations: meningitis, meningovascular syphilis, tabes dorsalis, general paresis, and gumma.

Syphilitic meningitis develops early on after primary infection, usually coinciding with the secondary-stage syphilis rash. Common symptoms are nocturnal headache, malaise, stiff neck, fever, and cranial nerve palsies. CSF examination demonstrates increased lymphocyte count and total protein; serum RPR test results are usually positive.

Meningovascular syphilis is a more chronic disorder. Usually evident 20 or more years after initial exposure, it rarely occurs as early as 2 years after the primary untreated infection. Chronic inflammation produces brain or spinal cord infarction leading to cranial nerve palsies, cerebrovascular accidents, seizures, or paraplegia. Argyll Robertson pupils, which are small and irregular and accommodate to near vision but do not react to light or painful stimuli, are present.

Tabes dorsalis develops 10 to 20 years after primary infection, usually in persons aged 25–45 years. Both direct invasion by the spirochete and an immunologic reaction may occur, producing degenerative and sclerotic changes in the posterior nerve root fibers of the spinal cord, spinal ganglia cells, long fibers of the posterior columns of the spinal cord, optic nerves, and oculomotor nuclei. Symptoms may include lightning-like, very brief severe nerve root pains, gastric crisis, and spastic gait, failing vision, and urinary and sexual dysfunction. Optic nerves show progressive primary atrophy; Argyll Robertson pupils are small and irregular. Impaired vibration sense, ataxia, and a positive Romberg sign are present. Knee and ankle jerks are absent. In 54 patients with tabes dorsalis and positive serum VDRL, CSF VDRL and fluorescent treponemal antibody (FTA) test were positive in only 18% and 73%, respectively.

General paresis (dementia paralytica) occurs most commonly in patients older than age 40 years, from direct spirochete invasion of neural tissue causing neuronal degeneration, astrocytic proliferation, and meningitis (Fig. 48-11). Resultant degenerative and sclerotic changes produce a thickened dura mater, chronic subdural hematoma, cortical cell atrophy, and astrocyte proliferation. The frontal lobes are disproportionately affected. Progressive dementia occurs in 60% of patients, but headaches, insomnia, personality change, impaired judgment, disturbed emotional responses, slurred speech, and tremors can also develop. Argyll Robertson pupils are characteristic. RPR test results in blood and VDRL test results in CSF are positive in more than 90% of patients.

Gumma of the brain and spinal cord are rare. Symptoms are consistent with expanding CNS lesions.

Diagnosis and Treatment

Diagnosis is based on serologic tests with blood RPR and CSF VDRL tests for screening and FTA absorption test or microhemagglutination–*T. pallidum* test for specific confirmation. The CSF usually demonstrates a modest increase primarily in lymphocytic cells, with a moderate protein increase and normal glucose level.

Penicillin is the treatment for all forms of syphilis. Repeated therapeutic blood and CSF levels are necessary to effect a cure if the syphilis stage is treatable.

Future Directions

Although no large-scale randomized trial has compared azithromycin directly to benzathine penicillin, preliminary studies support the efficacy of azithromycin (a single oral dose of 1 or 2 g) in treatment of early-stage syphilis. Evidence does not yet support its use in late- or tertiary-stage disease. Additional data support the use of ceftriaxone in early-stage disease. Ceftriaxone (2 g intramuscular once daily for 10 days) produced similar CSF responses for treatment of neurosyphilis in HIV-infected individuals. In aggregate, the data do not establish the equivalence or superiority of these agents to standard penicillin regimens but support their use as alternatives when penicillin is not a therapeutic option. Concurrent HIV infection may modify the natural history of syphilis, but the overall response to standard therapy has been no different than in HIV-seronegative individuals.

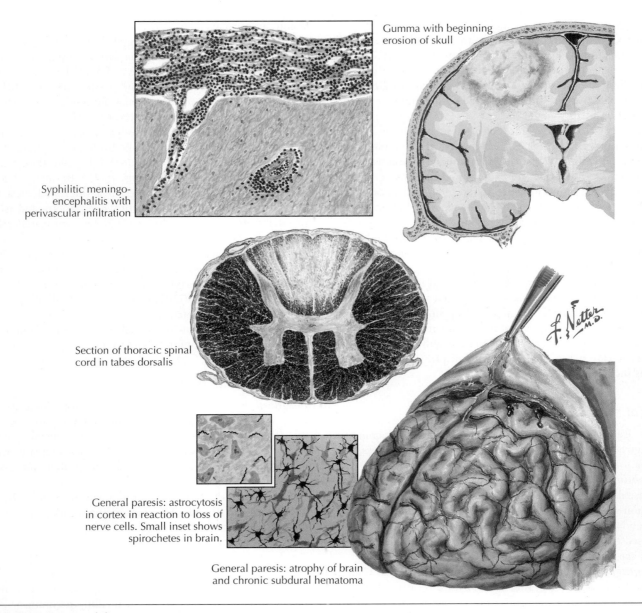

Gumma with beginning erosion of skull

Syphilitic meningo-encephalitis with perivascular infiltration

Section of thoracic spinal cord in tabes dorsalis

General paresis: astrocytosis in cortex in reaction to loss of nerve cells. Small inset shows spirochetes in brain.

General paresis: atrophy of brain and chronic subdural hematoma

Figure 48-11 Neurosyphilis.

EVIDENCE

Case records of the Massachusetts General Hospital. Weekly clinicopathological exercises. Case 12-2001: A 16-year-old boy with an altered mental status and muscle rigidity. N Engl J Med 2001;344:1232-1239. *Classic description of a case of tetanus*

Dariouche RO. Spinal epidural abscess. N Engl J Med 2006;355:2012-2020. *This review addresses the pathogenesis, clinical features, diagnosis, treatment, common diagnostic and therapeutic pitfalls, and outcome of bacterial spinal epidural abscess.*

Garcia-Monco JC. Central nervous system tuberculosis. Neurol Clin 1999;17:737-759. *Comprehensive review of diagnosis and treatment of central nervous system tuberculosis*

Heilpern KL, Lorber B. Focal intracranial infections. Infect Dis Clin North Am 1996;10:879-898. *Review of the diagnosis and management of focal intracranial infections including the use of MR imaging and MR angiography as well as early surgical intervention*

Steere AC. Lyme Disease. N Engl J Med 2001;345:115-25. *Comprehensive review of the many manifestations of Lyme disease*

Stoner BP. Current controversies in the management of adult syphilis. Clin Infect Dis 2007;44:S130-S146. *Review summarizing recent research on syphilis treatment efficacy and outcomes*

Tunkel AR, Hartman BJ, Kaplan SL et al. Practice guidelines for the management of bacterial meningitis. Clin Infect Dis 2004; 39:1267-84. *Evidence-based guidelines for the diagnosis, management, and treatment of bacterial meningitis developed by the Infectious Diseases Society of America*

van de Beek D, de Gans J, Tunkel AR, Wijdicks EF. Community-acquired bacterial meningitis in adults. N Engl J Med 2006;354:44-53. *This review summarizes the current concepts of the initial approach to the treatment of adults with bacterial meningitis, highlighting adjunctive dexamethasone therapy and focusing on the management of neurologic complications.*

ACKNOWLEDGMENT

We gratefully acknowledge the contributions of Samuel Kalluvya and J. B. Kataraihya of Weill Bugando Medical Center, Mwanza, Tanzania.

ADDITIONAL RESOURCES

Halperin JJ, Shapiro ED, Logigian E, et al. Practice parameter: treatment of nervous system Lyme disease (an evidence-based review). Neurology 2007;69:91-102.

Hildenbrand P, Craven DE, Jones R, Nemeskal P. Lyme Neuroborreliosis: manifestations of a rapidly emerging zoonosis. AJNR Am J Neuroradiol 4-3-2009. www.ajnr.org. doi 10.3174/ajnr.A1579 Evidence-based guidelines for the treatment of nervous system Lyme disease developed by the American Academy of Neurology.

Ooi WW, Moschella SL. Update on leprosy in immigrants in the United States: status in the year 2000. Clin Infect Dis 2001;32(6): 930-937.

Ooi WW, Srinivasan J. Leprosy and the peripheral nervous system: basic and clinical aspects. Muscle Nerve Muscle Nerve 2004 Oct;30(4): 393-409.

Practice Guidelines of the Infectious Diseases Society of America. Available at: http://www.idsociety.org/Content.aspx?id=9088. Accessed April 28, 2011. *Evidence-based statements developed to assist practitioners and patients in making decisions about appropriate health care for specific clinical circumstances. Guidelines for treatment of infections by organ system and organism may be found here.*

Sabin TD, Swift TR, Jacobson RR. Leprosy. In: Dyck PJ, Thomas PK, editors. Peripheral Neuropathy. Philadelphia: WB Saunders; 2005. p. 1354-1379.

Viral Diseases

Daniel P. McQuillen, Donald E. Craven, and H. Royden Jones, Jr.

49

HERPES SIMPLEX ENCEPHALITIS

Clinical Vignette

An independent 74-year-old man left a family wedding reception early because he did not feel well; he complained of mild nausea and general malaise. His daughter called the next day and when he did not answer the phone she went to his home to check on him, discovering him wandering in his backyard acutely confused. She convinced him to go to the emergency department, where he was found to be febrile with a temperature of 38.5° C (101.3° F). He soon became unresponsive to verbal stimuli, had conjugate right eye deviation, neck stiffness, and bilateral palmar grasps. He withdrew to noxious stimuli; plantar responses were flexor.

A noncontrast head computed tomography (CT) was unremarkable. Cerebrospinal fluid (CSF) examination demonstrated a WBC count of 45/mm³, predominantly lymphocytes, protein of 110 mg/dL, and a normal glucose level. Intravenous acyclovir 10 mg/kg every 8 hours was begun. A magnetic resonance image (MRI) of the brain demonstrated T2-weighted hyperintensity with edematous changes in the left insular cortex region of the inferior temporal lobe, the parahippocampal gyrus, and the hippocampus, extending into the subthalamic nucleus suggestive of herpes simplex virus (HSV) encephalitis. Electroencephalography (EEG) demonstrated periodic lateralized epileptiform discharges (PLEDs). This diagnosis was confirmed by HSV polymerase chain reaction (PCR) 4 days after symptom onset. The patient gradually improved and was treated with a 21-day course of acyclovir. After a short stay in a rehabilitation facility, he was discharged home.

Comment: This is a fine example of the rapidity with which herpes simplex encephalitis (HSE) will declare itself and the urgent need to consider the diagnosis in any acutely confused patient, initiating treatment based on clinical judgment alone without waiting for definitive diagnostic proof to become available. Unless this type of decision making takes place, the HSE will have caused irreversible cerebral damage, particularly involving the temporal lobes with their memory and language function modalities.

ETIOLOGY

A wide spectrum of viral agents may cause an infectious encephalitis. Diagnosis and management are dependent on identifying the precise causative agent. Only a few viruses are amenable to specific antiviral therapy. Therefore, prevention strategies are particularly important, especially for arthropod-borne viruses such as West Nile virus (WNV) and eastern equine encephalitis (EEE).

HSE is the most common acute encephalitis in the United States, with an annual incidence of 1 in 250,000 to 1 in 500,000. It affects all ages and both sexes equally, without significant seasonal variation. Early antiviral treatment significantly reduces mortality, but morbidity remains unacceptably high. Most cases of HSE are caused by oral herpes (herpes simplex virus [HSV] type 1); however, genital herpes (HSV-2) is more common among neonates with disseminated disease. HSE commonly develops as a recurrent infection but on occasion may occur during primary infection. Animal data verify the presence of retrograde virus transport into the brain via olfactory or trigeminal nerves. However, the human disease pathogenic pathways are not fully clarified. There is a predilection for HSE, once established, to lead to a hemorrhagic necrosis with inflammatory infiltrates and cells containing intranuclear inclusions.

CLINICAL PRESENTATION

The symptoms and signs of patients with subacute or acute focal encephalitis are generally rather nonspecific, with fever, headache, and altered consciousness being the most common. Focal manifestations often include seizures, typically complex partial in character because of the temporal lobe's predisposition to develop a herpes infection. It is common for these patients to also develop language difficulties, personality changes, hemiparesis, ataxia, cranial nerve defects, and papilledema (Fig. 49-1). The differential diagnosis includes stroke, brain tumors, other viral encephalitides, bacterial abscesses, tuberculosis, cryptococcal infections, and toxoplasmosis.

DIAGNOSIS

One of the major issues in diagnosis is for the examining clinician to put HSE into his or her diagnostic spectrum very early on in the temporal profile of the patient's illness. If this is not applied, a major therapeutic window allowing for successful treatment is sometimes lost. One of the saddest neurologic clinical scenarios is to evaluate a patient for confusion that has been present for the past 3–5 days and wrongly attributed to medication, or minor infection such as one involving the urinary or respiratory tracts. This is particularly liable to occur in a previously mentally vital senior citizen who develops a febrile illness with acute confusion and the change in mental status is presumed to be secondary to the fever per se, secondary nonspecific metabolic or toxic effects of empirical antibiotics, a stroke, or even "sundowning."

For patients with suspected encephalitis, the initial diagnostic studies must include a CT scan (to rule out a mass effect) and then immediate CSF examination. CT scan results are abnormal in 50% of cases early on and usually demonstrate localized edema, low-density lesions, mass effects, contrast enhancements, or hemorrhage. MRI and EEG may be subsequently

Possible route of transmission in herpes simplex encephalitis

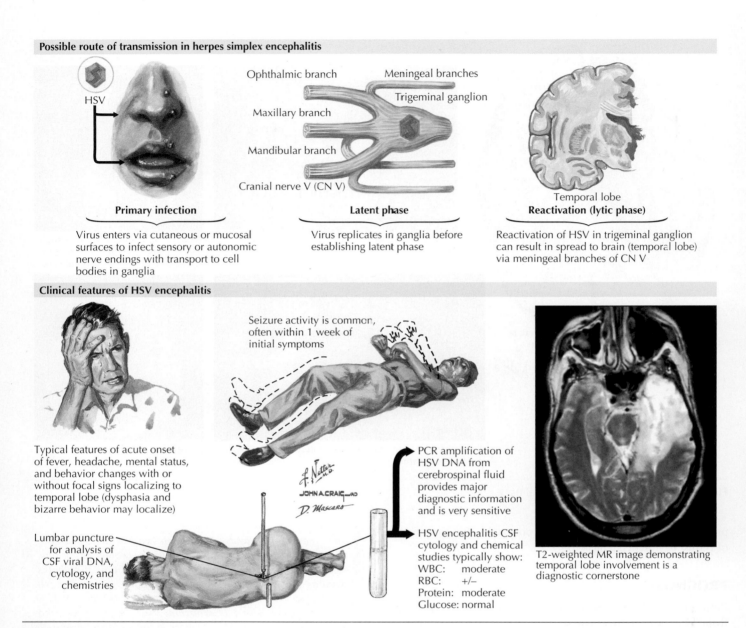

HSV

Primary infection

Ophthalmic branch

Maxillary branch

Mandibular branch

Cranial nerve V (CN V)

Meningeal branches

Trigeminal ganglion

Latent phase

Temporal lobe
Reactivation (lytic phase)

Virus enters via cutaneous or mucosal surfaces to infect sensory or autonomic nerve endings with transport to cell bodies in ganglia

Virus replicates in ganglia before establishing latent phase

Reactivation of HSV in trigeminal ganglion can result in spread to brain (temporal lobe) via meningeal branches of CN V

Clinical features of HSV encephalitis

Typical features of acute onset of fever, headache, mental status, and behavior changes with or without focal signs localizing to temporal lobe (dysphasia and bizarre behavior may localize)

Seizure activity is common, often within 1 week of initial symptoms

Lumbar puncture for analysis of CSF viral DNA, cytology, and chemistries

PCR amplification of HSV DNA from cerebrospinal fluid provides major diagnostic information and is very sensitive

HSV encephalitis CSF cytology and chemical studies typically show:
WBC: moderate
RBC: +/–
Protein: moderate
Glucose: normal

T2-weighted MR image demonstrating temporal lobe involvement is a diagnostic cornerstone

Figure 49-1 HSV Encephalitis.

obtained for further confirmation. These usually demonstrate major temporal lobe damage (Fig. 49-2); however, a normal study does not exclude an HSE diagnosis. If such does occur, it is often wise to repeat the study within a few days, particularly if the patient continues to be confused.

CSF findings are nonspecific, often including a lymphocytic pleocytosis with a slight protein increase. Abnormal CSF findings are found in 96% of biopsy-proven HSE cases. EEG may show repetitive spiked, sharp wave discharges and slow waves localized to the involved area often as PLEDs.

The accuracy of PCR testing for HSV-DNA to detect HSV-1 and -2 in CSF compares favorably with the previous use of brain biopsy. This methodology provides excellent sensitivity and specificity (90–98%). The viral sequence for HSV may be detected months after the acute episode and may be negative in early disease phases. PCR should not be used to monitor therapy success. No standardized commercial assay is available. Brain

biopsy was previously the gold standard for specificity, but it is rarely indicated now with the widespread availability of HSV PCR testing. If used, biopsy specimens are examined for both histopathologic changes and HSV antigens by immunofluorescence testing and appropriate culture techniques.

THERAPY

Immediate initiation of acyclovir is indicated the moment HSE is clinically suspected. This relatively benign medication has the greatest chance of efficacy if it can be initiated very early on in the patient's clinical course. The excellent outcome of the patient in the initial vignette in this chapter emphasizes the absolute importance for primary care and emergency medicine physicians to immediately consider HSE in individuals of any age who experience relatively acute changes in mental status. Unfortunately, if immediate therapy is not commenced at

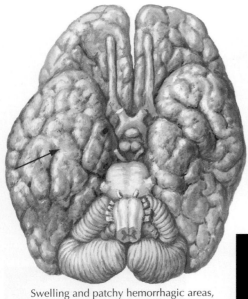

Swelling and patchy hemorrhagic areas, most marked in right temporal lobe

f. Netter
M.D.

Perivascular infiltration with mononuclear cells in disrupted brain tissue

Axial FLAIR image with extensive intracranial signal in right temporal lobe and medial left temporal lobe

Immunofluorescent staining shows presence of herpesvirus antigen in neurons

Diffusion with right temporal and insular changes

Figure 49-2 Herpes Simplex Encephalitis.

presentation, the outcome is usually poor, with minimal chance of return to independent living.

PROGNOSIS

Before the availability of intravenous (IV) acyclovir, mortality from HSE was approximately 70%. If one is able to initiate antiviral therapy within the first 24 hours of symptom onset, the prognosis is much better for long-term outlook if the patient is fully treated for 21 days. This approach has reduced both mortality and morbidity substantially. Overall, although morbidity remains high, with 60–70% of patients having significant neurologic deficits, the mortality is now 10–20%.

On rare occasions, a patient seemingly doing well with initial therapy has a relapse. Inadequate early dosing of the acyclovir is the usual cause. Thus, initial treatment regimens must include daily doses of 30 mg/kg intravenously usually in three separate aliquots of 10 mg/kg.

EASTERN EQUINE ENCEPHALITIS

Clinical Vignette

A 60-year-old New Hampshire man presented in mid-August with 2 weeks of headache followed by dizziness and unsteady gait, then nausea and vomiting. He walked his black Labrador retriever past a local pond in the woods every day, sustaining multiple mosquito bites. He had type II diabetes mellitus and history of a prior nephrectomy for renal cell carcinoma. At clinical presentation he was febrile, 38.3° C (101° F), somnolent but arousable, was vague answering questions, there were fine tremors in his hands, and muscle stretch reflexes were globally depressed.

Brain MRI revealed increased signal with mild mass effect in the left hippocampus. Spinal fluid examination demonstrated a WBC of 1,860/mm³ (81% polymorphonuclear neutrophils (PMNs), 11% lymphocytes, 8% monocytes), 26 red blood cells/mm³, protein 106 mg/dL, glucose 98 mg/dL (serum 209), and Gram stain negative. He had continued fevers with progressive gait ataxia, upper extremity weakness, and memory loss. Bacterial cultures and studies for Borrelia burgdorferi, Treponema pallidum, herpes simplex virus, and West Nile virus were negative. CSF IgM and plaque assay were positive for eastern equine encephalitis. He gradually recovered motor function over the next few months with supportive care and 1 year later he had minimal residual cognitive deficits.

EPIDEMIOLOGY

Eastern equine encephalitis virus is a member of the family Togaviridae, genus alphavirus, that is found in the eastern half of the United States. Eastern equine encephalitis (EEE) is a mosquito-borne viral disease. Here it causes disease in humans, horses, and some bird species. It generally takes from 3 to 10 days to develop symptoms of EEE after being bitten by an infected mosquito. An average of 5 human cases occur per year (approximately 220 confirmed cases in the United States between 1964 and 2004, most frequently in Florida, Georgia, Massachusetts, and New Jersey). EEE virus transmission is most common in and around freshwater hardwood swamps in the Atlantic and Gulf Coast states and the Great Lakes region. The main EEE virus transmission cycle is between birds and mosquitoes.

CLINICAL PRESENTATION AND TREATMENT

Most persons infected with EEE virus do not demonstrate a clearly discernible illness. In those individuals who do develop clinical illness, symptoms range from mild flu-like illness to a fulminating encephalitis eventually leading to coma and death. The mortality rate from EEE is approximately 33%, making it one of the most deadly mosquito-borne diseases in the United States.

DIAGNOSIS

Laboratory diagnosis of EEE virus infection is based on serology, especially IgM testing of serum and CSF, and neutralizing antibody testing of acute- and convalescent-phase serum. MRI is the most sensitive imaging modality for diagnosis of EEE (Fig. 49-3). The most commonly affected areas of the central nervous system (CNS) include the basal ganglia (unilateral or asymmetric, with occasional internal capsule involvement) and thalamic nuclei. Other areas include the brain stem (often the midbrain), periventricular white matter, and cortex (most often temporally). Affected areas appear as increased signal intensity on T2-weighted images.

THERAPY/PROGNOSIS

There is no specific treatment for EEE; optimal medical care includes intensive hospitalization and supportive care.

Approximately half of those persons who survive EEE will have mild to severe permanent neurologic damage, particularly involving cognitive impairment. Those older than age 50 and younger than age 15 years appear to be at greatest risk for developing severe EEE.

WEST NILE VIRUS

ETIOLOGY/EPIDEMIOLOGY

West Nile virus is a flavivirus usually found in Africa, West Asia, and the Middle East. The Middle Eastern strains are most closely related genetically to the St. Louis encephalitis virus found in the United States. There are many potential animal, ornithologic, and insect reservoirs including humans, horses, some other mammals, birds, and mosquitoes. The West Nile virus was not documented in the Western Hemisphere until 1999. In the temperate zones of the world, West Nile

encephalitis cases occur primarily in the late summer or early autumn. In southern climates, where temperatures are milder, WNV can be transmitted year-round.

CLINICAL PRESENTATION

West Nile fever is typically a mild disease characterized by flu-like symptoms that develop 3–15 days after the bite of an infected mosquito. West Nile fever usually lasts only a few days and does not seem to cause any long-term health effects. Mild fever, headache, body aches, occasional skin rash, and swollen glands are the most common symptoms.

However, there is a more severe disease spectrum that can manifest as encephalitis, meningitis, or meningoencephalitis. A poliomyelitis-like illness is also described, with an acute proximal and asymmetric flaccid paralysis, very occasionally occurring during recent outbreaks in the United States. Neurophysiologic, radiologic, and pathologic studies suggest that WNV has a proclivity to damage anterior horn cells within the spinal cord.

DIAGNOSIS

Diagnosis is made by serologic assays of blood and CSF.

THERAPY

Treatment is entirely supportive; there is no specific drug treatment or vaccine available. In the rare instances of a polio-like illness, the long-term outcome hinges on the degree and distribution of anterior horn cell damage.

HUMAN IMMUNODEFICIENCY VIRUS (HIV)

Clinical Vignette

A 31-year-old mother of a 13-month-old child presented to the emergency department with headache, vertigo, diplopia, and an unsteady gait. She had been treated with antibiotics for acute sinusitis during the preceding 8 days. Her neurologic examination demonstrated a lethargic, restless, febrile woman with meningismus, photophobia, horizontal nystagmus, and slight appendicular ataxia of her right arm and leg.

Brain CT demonstrated diminished absorption bilaterally in both thalami and to a lesser degree her internal capsules, midbrain, pons, and right posterior temporal lobe. There were signs of a primary maxillary and sphenoid sinusitis. Spinal tap demonstrated a CSF with moderate increased pressure of 275 mm/CSF, a cell count of 485 white blood cells (84% neutrophils), a protein concentration of 106 mg/mL, and glucose of 66 mg/dL. Intravenous antibiotics as well as acyclovir were begun. Gram stain and culture were negative initially and on a repeat study within less than 1 day.

During the first day of admission, she developed increased obtundation and intermittently varied automatisms. Bilateral flexor posturing and intermittent left-sided extensor

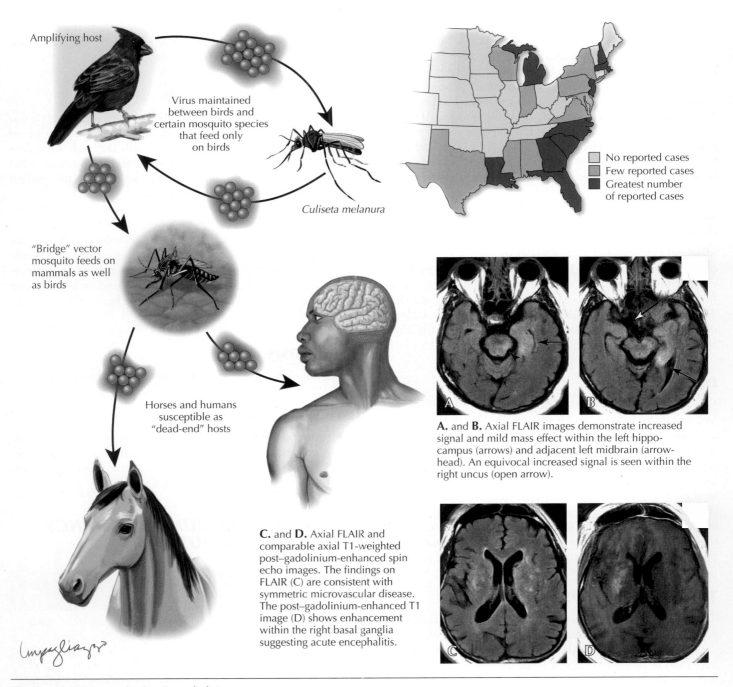

A. and **B.** Axial FLAIR images demonstrate increased signal and mild mass effect within the left hippocampus (arrows) and adjacent left midbrain (arrowhead). An equivocal increased signal is seen within the right uncus (open arrow).

C. and **D.** Axial FLAIR and comparable axial T1-weighted post–gadolinium-enhanced spin echo images. The findings on FLAIR (C) are consistent with symmetric microvascular disease. The post–gadolinium-enhanced T1 image (D) shows enhancement within the right basal ganglia suggesting acute encephalitis.

Figure 49-3 Eastern Equine Encephalitis.

posturing developed during her second day of hospitalization. Dexamethasone was administered every 6 hours. EEG demonstrated bilateral 3–5-Hz activity. Repeat imaging demonstrated extension of the low-density lesions into the basal ganglia and frontal lobe operculum. Temporal lobe biopsy was negative for HSV virus. Three days after admission, all spontaneous movements ceased; her pupils became dilated, fixed, and nonreactive; she was now areflexic and did not respond to any form of sensory stimulation. EEGs were electrically silent on two occasions over the next 24 hours. She died on the fifth hospital day.

A history of marked sexual promiscuity became available during her hospitalization. CSF culture was eventually positive for HIV although no serum or CSF antibodies to HIV were defined; all other cultures for various microbes were negative. Pathologically, there was an encephalopathic demyelinating process affecting cerebral white matter, the thalamus, and brain stem with acute neuronal damage. There was no associated vasculitis.

Comment: This case, seen at Lahey in the mid-1980s, added further support to the proposal that HIV is a primary neurotropic virus. Our experience emphasized the

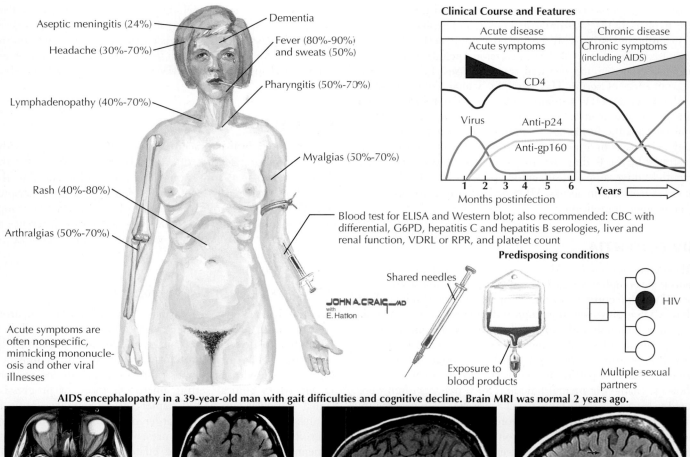

Aseptic meningitis (24%)

Dementia

Headache (30%-70%)

Fever (80%-90%) and sweats (50%)

Lymphadenopathy (40%-70%)

Pharyngitis (50%-70%)

Myalgias (50%-70%)

Rash (40%-80%)

Arthralgias (50%-70%)

Acute symptoms are often nonspecific, mimicking mononucleosis and other viral illnesses

Clinical Course and Features

Acute disease — Acute symptoms

Chronic disease — Chronic symptoms (including AIDS)

CD4

Virus — Anti-p24 — Anti-gp160

1 2 3 4 5 6
Months postinfection

Years

Blood test for ELISA and Western blot; also recommended: CBC with differential, G6PD, hepatitis C and hepatitis B serologies, liver and renal function, VDRL or RPR, and platelet count

Predisposing conditions

Shared needles

JOHN A. CRAIG—MD with E. Hatton

Exposure to blood products

HIV

Multiple sexual partners

AIDS encephalopathy in a 39-year-old man with gait difficulties and cognitive decline. Brain MRI was normal 2 years ago.

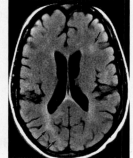

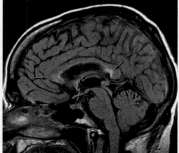

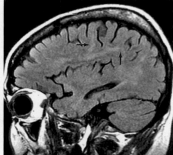

A. Axial T2 fast spin echo demonstrates ill-defined area of augmented T2 signal in upper left pons (arrow).

B. Axial FLAIR shows moderate sulcal and ventricular enlargement consistent with diffuse atrophy for age 39 in addition to paraventricular augmentation of T2 signal which in some regions extends to subcortical white matter and cortex (arrows).

C. Midsagittal FLAIR with ill-defined augmentation in both genu and splenium of corpus callosum (arrows).

D. FLAIR imaging more laterally again demonstrates paraventricular involvement extending to subcortical white matter (arrows).

Figure 49-4 Primary HIV Infection of the Nervous System.

importance of considering HIV in the differential diagnosis of any acute encephalitis even if the patient is HIV antibody negative. Here the initial antibody negativity supported the concept that this patient's encephalitis represented the primary phase of her HIV. Today when one wishes to consider an acute HIV infection in the setting of a negative HIV antibody one now has available an HIV viral load study. This will be positive, despite a negative HIV antibody study, if the patient has an active HIV infection. Thus, one will not need to depend on a viral culture to make the diagnosis as occurred with this patient. Such was not available at the time we evaluated this person.

PRIMARY NEUROLOGIC HIV INFECTION (PNHI)

Acute aseptic meningitis is the most common neurologic disorder to develop among individuals presenting with primary HIV infection (PNHI) (Fig. 49-4). Such patients present with headache, meningismus and sometimes myalgias, and arthralgias. As per the above vignette, on rare occasions, a meningoencephalitis, an encephalopathy, an acute disseminated encephalomyelitis, a myelopathy, a meningoradiculitis, and a peripheral neuropathy, particularly a Guillain–Barré syndrome may be seen as the presenting clinical picture of HIV. Other systemic symptoms and signs seen with acute HIV infection include fever, night sweats, weight loss, rash, fatigue, lymphadenopathy, oral ulcers, thrush, pharyngitis, gastrointestinal upset, and genital ulcers. As HIV antibody testing may be negative in PNHI, laboratory clues to the presence of seroconversion include leucopenia, thrombocytopenia, and elevated transaminases. In such cases, determination of serum HIV viral load may yield a positive result. A repeat HIV antibody study is often positive if the patient survives the initial neurologic illness. The primary infectious encephalitic forms have a significant morbidity and mortality perhaps as high as 50%. Its importance in adolescents is illustrated by the finding that in the United States, HIV is the seventh leading cause of death among patients aged 15–24 years. Once seroconversion occurs, AIDS patients are at risk for a host of neurologic complications.

HIV DEMENTIA

AIDS dementia complex (ADC) is the most important "primary" neurologic complication of HIV infection. It is almost universal for HIV-1 infection to occur within the cerebrospinal fluid when AIDS is previously unrecognized and thus untreated. This was quite common early on in the AIDS epidemic prior to the availability of specific highly active antiretroviral therapy (HAART) protocols. These individuals presented with a varied dementia that was particularly characterized by early- to mid-adult-age changes in mental function. Such patients often were noted to have a relatively rapid to subacute change in personality with prominent apathy, inattention, inability to form new memory, and language dysfunction. ADC individuals were unable to carry out the basic requirements of normal activities of daily living. Although a number of AIDS patients develop a variety of opportunistic brain infections, as per Chapter 51, at autopsy many proved to have a primary subacute demyelinating process with some mild cellular response, particularly characterized by clusters of foamy macrophages, microglial nodules, and multinucleated giant cells.

Once effective, combinations of HAART became available in the mid-1990s, the prevalence of ADC declined dramatically. Because the brain is a viral sanctuary, further therapeutic effort to deal with long-term HIV effect is of importance. The prevalence of HIV-associated neurocognitive disorders (HANDs) is high even in long-standing aviremic HIV-positive patients. However, from the practical viewpoint, HANDs does not usually have any daily functional repercussions. It is of concern, however, that as people with HIV live longer, the frequency of HIV-related neurologic impairment may be rising once again despite successful administration of life-prolonging HAART. There is little evidence that HAART per se leads to primary CNS toxicity. The benefits and risks of HAART in the preservation or enhancement of neurocognitive function in well, HIV-infected patients with more than 500 CD4+ cells/μL are unknown. Abnormal brain MRIs typified by both white matter (demyelination) and gray matter (atrophy) may be demonstrated in seemingly clinically asymptomatic persons living with HIV.

HIV PRIMARY CNS ANGIITIS

Central nervous system vascular involvement may develop in HIV infection. This is usually a result of associated opportunistic infections including bacterial, viral (Epstein–Barr virus, CMV, hepatitis B), fungal, or parasitic organisms. Very rarely, neoplastic disease, or toxic drug abuse may provide the mechanism for CNS angiitis in this setting. At autopsy, in some studies, perhaps a quarter of HIV-infected patients have cerebral infarcts.

HIV MYELOPATHY

Occasionally a primary vacuolar and inflammatory myelopathy is the presenting feature of AIDS. Its predisposition for the dorsal lateral spinal cord mimics the distribution and thus the clinical spectrum of B_{12} or copper deficiency syndromes (Chapter 45). There is no effective treatment for HIV-associated myelopathy. The introduction of HAART has made little difference to its natural history. Spinal cord pathology reveals vacuolization and inflammation.

HIV Anterior Horn Cell Myelopathy

Very rarely, one may see various forms of a motor neuron, anterior horn cell, disorder with HIV infection. This is attributed to direct HIV damage to the motor neurons by neurotoxic HIV viral proteins, cytokines and chemokines. Opportunistic viruses may also directly attack motor neurons in the AIDS clinical setting mirroring those of progressive spinal muscular atrophy (Chapter 67). This may result in an inexorably progressive disorder of upper and lower motor neurons. One most unusual presentation has been the rare patient presenting with severe bilateral arm and hand weakness unassociated with either bulbar and/or leg weakness or any corticospinal tract findings. This is referred to as a neurogenic "man-in-the-barrel" syndrome or brachial amyotrophic diplegia.

HIV PERIPHERAL NEUROPATHY

There are other HIV-related syndromes, primarily various polyneuropathies that mimic motor neuron disease. These include chronic inflammatory polyradiculoneuropathy, a multifocal motor neuropathy with anti-GM1 antibodies, or a primary axonal motor polyradiculoneuropathy.

The most common HIV-related polyneuropathy is a distal symmetric primary sensory polyneuropathy (DSP). This occurs in more than one third of infected patients but may occur in twice as many if asymptomatic patients are also considered. DSP patients develop slowly progressive symmetric numbness and burning sensations in their feet. The pathophysiologic mechanism underlying the development of HIV-associated DSP is not known. Possibilities include cytokine/HIV protein neurotoxicity or primary mitochondrial damage. In addition, several of the early nucleoside reverse transcriptase inhibitor (NRTI) drugs (zalcitabine [ddC], didanosine [ddI], and stavudine [d4T]) have been shown to produce a toxic neuropathy that resembles HIV peripheral neuropathy clinically and electrically. This neuropathy has been postulated to be due to mitochondrial toxicity of these agents, may be additive to HIC neuropathy, and has led these agents to be replaced by newer NRTIs in modern HAART regimens.

HIV MYOPATHY

Some AIDS patients develop proximal weakness and rarely rhabdomyolysis. Clinically these patients sometimes appear to have an inflammatory myopathy; some of these individuals may occasionally respond to corticosteroid therapy. At other times the HIV virus has been primarily implicated as the cause of this myopathy. One of the original therapies, zidovudine, was also thought to be primarily myotoxic although it is difficult to separate this from a primary viral mechanism.

SHINGLES (HERPES ZOSTER)

ETIOLOGY AND EPIDEMIOLOGY

Shingles is the most common neurologic disease. In America, it is estimated that 15% of our population will experience shingles during their lifetime. An aging population, increasing prevalence of immunosuppressed hosts from myriad causes, and widespread adoption of varicella vaccination in children are causing these rates to rise. Advancing age is the most significant risk factor for acute herpes zoster reactivation and development of the chronic neuropathic pain of postherpetic neuralgia (PHN).

The growing use of varicella vaccine reduces the rates of chickenpox in children. As a consequence, fewer adults have experienced viral exposure. Waning varicella-specific immunity in older adults leads to higher rates of shingles. The precise breach of immune surveillance that allows for varicella reactivation remains unknown. Although most cases affect healthy adults, 10% of all patients with lymphoma will develop shingles. In addition to treatment of acute symptoms, further diagnostic evaluation for an underlying carcinoma or lymphoma needs to be considered. Other patients at high risk for herpes zoster include organ-transplant recipients and those receiving corticosteroid therapy. Immunocompromised persons can experience recurrent, multifocal, protracted bouts of acute neuralgia.

PATHOPHYSIOLOGY

Focal reactivation of latent varicella-zoster virus (VZV) in sensory ganglia causes the distinctive rash known as shingles. This occurs in 2 discrete stages. VZV causes varicella (chickenpox) primarily during childhood. Once this disorder clears, this virus becomes inactive and remains latent within the peripheral nervous system sensory ganglia. Here it persists in the host for many years, with the potential to be reactivated later in life. Reactivation is associated with a declining, virus-specific, cell-mediated immune response. If this dormant virus does regain virulence it typically presents as shingles. In immunocompetent hosts, this is generally an isolated event although with an increasingly aging population some individuals may have more than one episode.

The dorsal root ganglion is the primary site of infection. The virus spreads transaxonally to the skin. Cellular-level examination reveals hemorrhagic inflammation extending from the sensory ganglion to its projections in the nerve, skin, and adjacent soft tissue. Virions also spread centrally into the spinal cord, causing an occult focal myelitis in the anterior horn cells.

The damage may also ascend into the CNS at the level of the dorsal columns and brainstem.

CLINICAL PRESENTATION

The clinical onset is often heralded by a few days of relatively severe localized pain or nonspecific discomfort in the affected area. The acute pain of shingles is characterized by burning discomfort associated with volleys of a severe lancinating sensation. At times, this is so uncomfortable that it may mimic an acute to subacute intra-abdominal or intrathoracic disorder such as an acute peptic ulcer or even a myocardial infarction. Nociceptive pain from soft tissue inflammation and itching may also be associated. Rarely, VZV produces pain without a rash (zoster sin herpete).

The eruption is unilateral and typically does not cross the midline. It overlaps adjacent dermatomes in 20% of cases. A vesicular skin rash, within a dermatomal distribution, forms the clinical signature of VZV reactivation in the dorsal root ganglion. Although any spinal segment or cranial nerve may be involved, the lower thoracic roots and the ophthalmic sensory ganglia are most commonly affected and thus a zoster rash is found frequently in these levels. Vesicles usually appear 72–96 hours later (Fig. 49-5). The lesions have an erythematous base

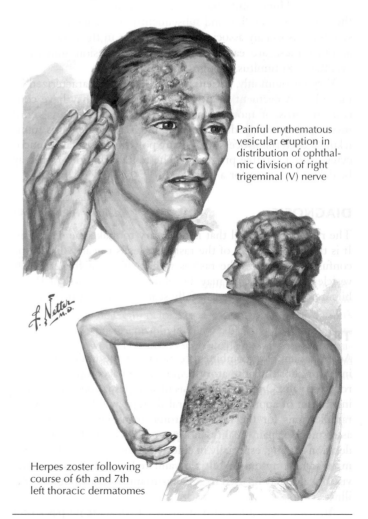

Painful erythematous vesicular eruption in distribution of ophthalmic division of right trigeminal (V) nerve

Herpes zoster following course of 6th and 7th left thoracic dermatomes

Figure 49-5 Herpes Zoster.

particularly refused immunizations, reported headache, fever, nausea, and general malaise 1 week after camping. Two days later, he felt better, but 48 hours after that, the general symptoms returned, with more headache, generalized muscle aching and pain, and some drowsiness. When weakness supervened a week after illness onset, he was brought to the emergency department.

The patient's temperature was 39.5° C (103.1° F), his pulse was 100 beats/min, and his blood pressure 130/70 mm Hg. He had a stiff neck, generalized muscle tenderness, asymmetric weakness (right arm and left leg more than elsewhere), preserved though hypoactive muscle stretch reflexes, flexor plantar responses, normal sensation, and intact cranial nerves.

His cough was weak, with a vital capacity of barely 1 L. His WBC count was 15,000/mm³ (40% lymphocytes). Lumbar puncture revealed somewhat cloudy fluid under increased pressure (220 mm Hg), 170/mm³ nucleated cells (60% polymorphonuclear leukocytes), 150 mg/dL protein, and 80 mg/dL glucose. Spinal MRI showed enhancement of the cord interiorly, especially the right cervical region.

Comment: this is a classic case of infantile poliomyelitis as one would have experienced prior to the widespread utilization of oral and parenteral polio vaccines. In this instance, the patient was at high risk of developing polio either from exposure to a baby recently immunized with live vaccines or the more remote setting here wherein this young man was inadvertently exposed to wild-type polio virus.

EPIDEMIOLOGY AND ETIOLOGY

Poliomyelitis is a word derived from the Greek polio (gray) and myelin (marrow), indicating the spinal cord. Spinal cord infection with poliomyelitis virus leads to the classic paralysis secondary to destruction of the anterior horn cells. The incidence of polio peaked in the United States in 1952 with more than 21,000 cases but rapidly decreased after introduction of effective killed parenteral Salk vaccines in 1954 and the live Sabin vaccine a few years later.

The last case of wild-virus polio acquired in the United States was in 1979, and the Global Polio Eradication Program dramatically reduced transmission elsewhere. Polio is eradicated from most of the world but still circulates in many developing countries, particularly in Africa and the Indian subcontinent, and to a lesser degree in Indonesia, a few remote parts of Russia, as well as China and the Arabian Peninsula. Travelers to areas where naturally occurring poliovirus still circulates need to be vaccinated as follows: persons who completed an adequate primary series during childhood should have a one-time booster dose of inactivated poliovirus vaccine (IPV); those who have not received a primary series should receive it although even a single dose prior to travel is of benefit.

Humans are the only known reservoir. Transmission occurs most frequently with an unapparent infection. An asymptomatic carrier state occurs only in those with immunodeficiency. Person-to-person spread occurs predominantly via the fecal–oral route. Infection typically peaks in summer in temperate climates, with no seasonality in the tropics. Poliovirus is highly infectious and may be present in stool up to 6 weeks; seroconversion in susceptible household contacts of children is nearly 100%, and that of adults is greater than 90%. Persons are most infectious from 7 to 10 days before and after symptom onset.

IPV, an inactive, killed vaccine, was licensed in 1955 and used until the early 1960s, when trivalent oral poliovirus vaccine (OPV), containing attenuated strains of all three serotypes of poliovirus in 10:1:3 ratios, largely replaced it. Enhanced potency trivalent poliovirus vaccine (IPV) was introduced in 1988. The viruses are grown in monkey kidney (Vero) cells and are inactivated with formaldehyde. An occasional live vaccine–associated case of paralytic polio continued to occur in infants after their first immunization at approximately 3 months of age until the CDC mandated in the late 1990s that initial vaccinations must be with the Salk IPV. Since then, no such incidents have been reported. Between 1980 and 1999, a total of 152 confirmed cases of paralytic polio occurred in the United States. Of these, 145 (95%) were vaccine-associated. For this reason, in 2000, the recommendation was made to use IPV exclusively in the United States. Vaccine-associated paralytic polio is thought to occur from a reversion or mutation of the vaccine virus to a more neurotropic form.

Live attenuated polioviruses replicate in the intestinal mucosa and lymphoid cells and draining lymph nodes. Vaccine viruses are excreted in stool for up to 6 weeks, with maximal shedding in the first 1–2 weeks after vaccination. IPV is highly effective in producing immunity (99% after three doses) and protection from paralytic poliomyelitis. IPV seems to produce less local gastrointestinal immunity than OPV. Thus, persons immunized with IPV could still become infected with wild-type poliovirus and shed it on return to the United States, with subsequent potential spread. Although most individuals in economically privileged countries are immunized, occasionally, an instance such as described in the vignette in this chapter is seen. Asymmetric weakness distribution and CSF findings help to differentiate it from Guillain–Barré syndrome.

PATHOGENESIS

Poliovirus is a member of the family Picornaviridae, enterovirus subgroup. Enteroviruses are transient inhabitants of the gastrointestinal tract and are stable at acid pH. Picornaviruses have an RNA genome; the three poliovirus serotypes (P1, P2, and P3) have minimal heterotypic immunity among them. The virus enters through the mouth and multiplies primarily at the implantation site in the pharynx and gastrointestinal tract; usually, it is present in the throat and stool before clinical onset (Fig. 49-7). Within 1 week of clinical onset, little virus exists in the throat, but it continues to be excreted in the stool for several weeks. The virus invades local lymphoid tissue, enters the bloodstream, and then may infect CNS cells. Viral replication in anterior horn and brainstem motor neuron cells results in cell destruction and paralysis.

CLINICAL PRESENTATION

The incubation period for poliomyelitis is usually 6–20 days, with a range of 3–35 days. Clinical response to poliovirus

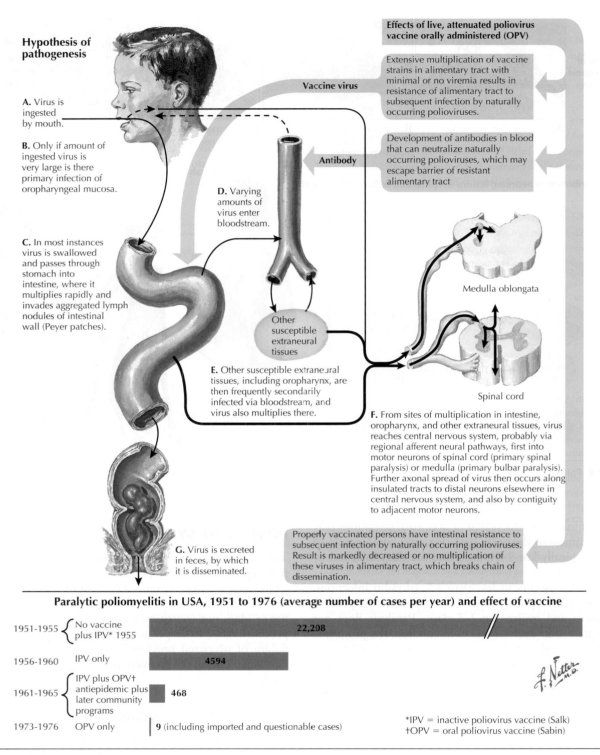

Hypothesis of pathogenesis

A. Virus is ingested by mouth.

B. Only if amount of ingested virus is very large is there primary infection of oropharyngeal mucosa.

C. In most instances virus is swallowed and passes through stomach into intestine, where it multiplies rapidly and invades aggregated lymph nodules of intestinal wall (Peyer patches).

D. Varying amounts of virus enter bloodstream.

E. Other susceptible extraneural tissues, including oropharynx, are then frequently secondarily infected via bloodstream, and virus also multiplies there.

Other susceptible extraneural tissues

F. From sites of multiplication in intestine, oropharynx, and other extraneural tissues, virus reaches central nervous system, probably via regional afferent neural pathways, first into motor neurons of spinal cord (primary spinal paralysis) or medulla (primary bulbar paralysis). Further axonal spread of virus then occurs along insulated tracts to distal neurons elsewhere in central nervous system, and also by contiguity to adjacent motor neurons.

G. Virus is excreted in feces, by which it is disseminated.

Vaccine virus

Antibody

Medulla oblongata

Spinal cord

Effects of live, attenuated poliovirus vaccine orally administered (OPV)

Extensive multiplication of vaccine strains in alimentary tract with minimal or no viremia results in resistance of alimentary tract to subsequent infection by naturally occurring polioviruses.

Development of antibodies in blood that can neutralize naturally occurring polioviruses, which may escape barrier of resistant alimentary tract

Properly vaccinated persons have intestinal resistance to subsequent infection by naturally occurring polioviruses. Result is markedly decreased or no multiplication of these viruses in alimentary tract, which breaks chain of dissemination.

Paralytic poliomyelitis in USA, 1951 to 1976 (average number of cases per year) and effect of vaccine

1951-1955	No vaccine plus IPV* 1955	22,208
1956-1960	IPV only	4594
1961-1965	IPV plus OPV† antiepidemic plus later community programs	468
1973-1976	OPV only	9 (including imported and questionable cases)

*IPV = inactive poliovirus vaccine (Salk)
†OPV = oral poliovirus vaccine (Sabin)

Figure 49-7 Poliomyelitis-I.

infection varies. Up to 95% of all polio infections are asymptomatic even though infected persons shed virus in stool and are contagious.

Abortive poliomyelitis occurs in 4–8% of infections. It causes a minor illness, without evidence of CNS infection. Complete recovery characteristically occurs within 1 week.

Upper respiratory infection (sore throat and fever), gastrointestinal disturbances (nausea, vomiting, abdominal pain, constipation, or rarely diarrhea), and influenza like illness can all occur and are indistinguishable from other enteric viral illnesses.

Nonparalytic aseptic meningitis, usually occurring several days after a prodrome similar to the minor illness, occurs in a small

Parasitic and Fungal Disorders and Neurosarcoidosis

Winnie W. Ooi, Daniel P. McQuillen, and H. Royden Jones, Jr.

50

*P*arasitic infections of the nervous system range from acute syndromes such as diffuse cerebritis in cerebral malaria to more chronic mass lesions causing seizure disorders such as neurocysticercosis. This chapter will focus on the most common parasites causing central nervous system infections.

CEREBRAL MALARIA

Clinical Vignette

A 45-year-old previously healthy, Indian male, working as an engineer in the United States returned from India in August after a 6-week stay visiting with his parents. One week after his return, he presented to the emergency ward with 4 days of fever to 102° F, headache, and diarrhea. His facies was flushed; he had mild confusion, severe lethargy, a moderately stiff neck, and a temperature of 39.4° C (103° F). A lumbar puncture demonstrated a normal cerebrospinal fluid (CSF). His peripheral WBC was 12,000/mm³, with a hemoglobin of 10 g and a platelet count of 40,000/mm³. His blood glucose level was 56 mg/dL. A peripheral blood smear demonstrated multiple intraerythrocytic ring forms consistent with the trophozoites of Plasmodium falciparum *with a parasite count of 3%.*

The patient was treated with intravenous artesunate, obtained from the Centers for Disease Control and Prevention (CDC), and doxycycline. He became afebrile, alert, and oriented after 3 days of intravenous therapy. His oral treatment regimen was completed after 7 days of doxycycline.

***Comment**: Malaria remains a major cause of morbidity and mortality in the developing world and the most important treatable cause of acute parasitic infection in travelers returning to their Westernized homelands. In the United States, 1564 imported cases were reported during 2006; 39% were attributable to P. falciparum. Immigrants who have recently visited with friends and relatives in their countries of origin often do not take antimalarial prophylaxis and are at higher risk of acquiring malaria.*

Malaria continues to have a global presence, primarily affecting individuals living in South and Central America, Africa, and Asia (Fig. 50-1). Close to a half billion individuals are affected annually with up to a million deaths each year. Previously endemic

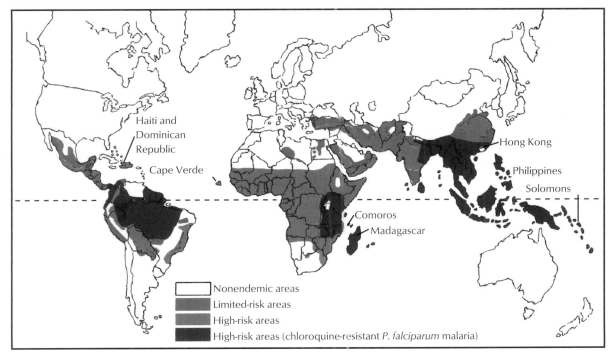

Figure 50-1 Geographic Distribution of Malaria.

in the United States, public health measures have greatly decreased its incidence here. However, at least a thousand cases are reported annually here and are primarily related to *P. falciparum* affecting travelers to endemic geographic areas.

EPIDEMIOLOGY

Malaria is caused by four common species of parasites: *P. falciparum*, *P. vivax*, *P. ovale*, and *P. malariae*. Each form is transmitted to the human from the bites of infected Anopheles mosquitoes. Erythrocytes infected with mature parasites of *P. falciparum* adhere to endothelial cells in the microvasculature of many organs, including the brain, and undergo a complex interplay with host factors, leading to the manifestations of cerebral malaria.

CLINICAL FEATURES

Cerebral malaria is the most life-threatening form, having an adult mortality rate of 20–50%; this is even worse in children. It is caused by *P. falciparum*, with rare exceptional instance of *P. vivax*. Its primary neurologic features range from irritability and confusion to seizures and coma. Early on there are usually several days of fever and other nonspecific symptoms indistinguishable from those of uncomplicated malaria. Patients may gradually develop coma or in contrast deteriorate suddenly and persistently after a generalized seizure. Grand mal convulsions occur in about half of adult patients. The seizures are often exacerbated by hypoglycemia and lactic acidosis metabolic features that often accompany severe malaria. Hypoglycemia is a common and important abnormality in patients with cerebral malaria and may not be suspected clinically because the symptoms (anxiety, restlessness, and tachycardia) are attributed to the infection itself.

DIAGNOSIS

If malaria is suspected, peripheral blood smears need to be examined every 8–24 hours by an experienced microscopist. In a patient with fever and abnormal mental status who was potentially exposed to malaria, antimalarial chemotherapy must be started immediately even if blood smears are repeatedly negative. Microscopic examination and culture of CSF is also essential in patients with cerebral malaria to exclude other treatable central nervous system (CNS) infections.

THERAPY

Increased drug resistance has led to combination therapy for malaria. The treatment of cerebral malaria consists of either intravenous quinidine or artesunate accompanied by doxycycline (Fig. 50-2). Intravenous quinidine has to be administered in an ICU setting with electrocardiographic monitoring, as it may lead to severe arrhythmias. Exchange transfusion should be strongly considered for persons with a parasite density of more than 5–10% or even with a lower level of parasitemia if the cerebral malaria is severe or other complications of the malaria occur, including non–volume overload pulmonary edema, or renal complications.

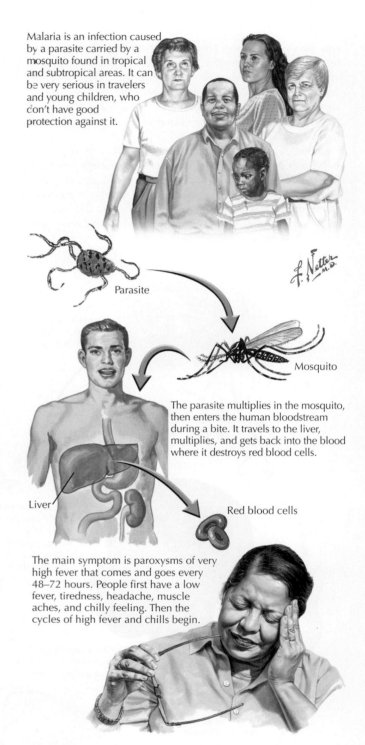

Figure 50-2 Treatment of Malaria.

AFRICAN TRYPANOSOMIASIS (SLEEPING SICKNESS)

Clinical Vignette

A 38-year-old West African woman, who migrated from her native country 4 months ago, was evaluated in an emergency department for a few weeks of bizarre behavior. In the preceding months, she noted modest weight loss and progressive failure to thrive. She was referred to an inpatient psychiatric service, where she became more lethargic. Her physical examination revealed a low-grade fever with a suspicion of hepatomegaly but was otherwise normal.

Laboratory tests demonstrated a white cell count of 6400/mm, hemoglobin 10 g, and normal platelets. Her liver function tests revealed a mild transaminitis. A careful exam of her peripheral blood smear showed a trypomastigote. HIV antibody was negative. The patient's basic CSF parameters were normal. However, both her indirect fluorescent antibody (IFA) and enzyme-linked immunosorbent assay (ELISA) to Trypanosoma gambiense in her CSF were positive. Treatment was started with melarsoprol but was stopped because of progressive encephalopathy. The patient's family signed her out of the hospital against medical advice and she was lost to follow-up.

Comment: With the world becoming "smaller," previously "exotic" infectious diseases may now be seen anywhere, including economically highly developed countries. Cultural issues also arise, as well illustrated here, where the family made a decision not to allow attempts at a second line of therapy such as intravenous eflornithine when the first medication trial was not successful.

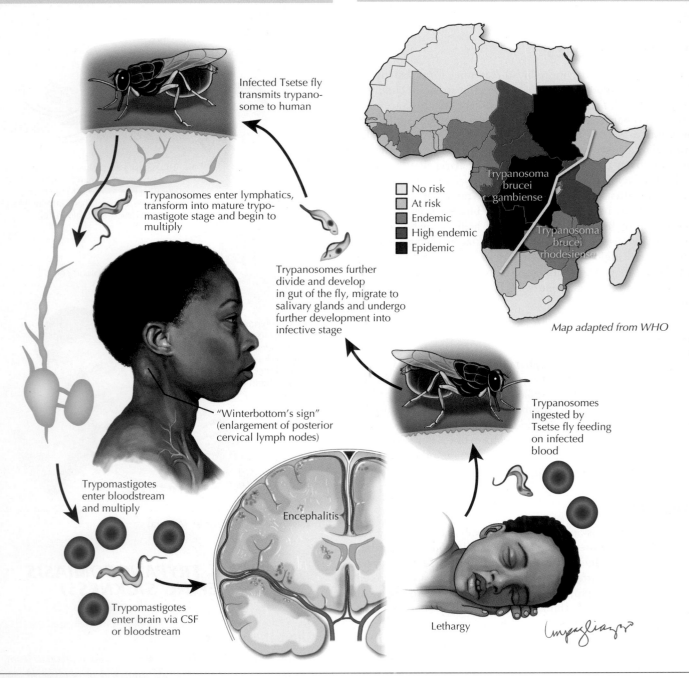

Figure 50-3 Trypanosomiasis (African Sleeping Sickness).

EPIDEMIOLOGY

After being brought under control for many years, ever since the 1970s, African trypanosomiasis has reemerged, as a new epidemic of enormous proportions. This disease is divided into two different forms, each characterized by meningoencephalitis when it reaches more advanced stages. Both are transmitted by the bites of infected tsetse flies.

CLINICAL FEATURES

West African sleeping sickness accounts for more than 90% of reported cases of sleeping sickness and causes a chronic infection primarily occurring in west and central Africa. It is caused by *Trypanosoma brucei gambiense*. Individuals can be infected for months or even years without experiencing any major symptoms or signs. Initially, the systemic disease presents with fever, fatigue, weight loss, cervical lymphadenopathy and hepatosplenomegaly.

Once the neurologic manifestations emerge, the patient often has developed an advanced stage of central nervous system (CNS) infection. Personality changes are common; patients are frequently mistaken as having psychiatric disorders, as in this case. In the early phases of CNS disease, a disruption of the normal circadian sleep rhythm occurs (Fig. 50-3).

East African trypanosomiasis, caused by *Trypanosome brucei rhodesiense*, causes a more acute infection in contrast to the more chronic West African form. Neurologic symptoms develop rapidly after just a few months or weeks.

DIAGNOSIS

An African sleeping sickness diagnosis is not an easy one to establish in the early phases of the disease when there may not be any CSF changes. Patients are classified as early- or late-stage disease based on CSF findings: those with a CSF WBC >5/mm, often with mild lymphocytic pleocytosis (rarely above 400/mL) and an increased protein content accompanied by a high level of IGM or with trypanosomes demonstrated in CSF seen, are in late-stage disease. Electroencephalography (EEG) can aid in the diagnosis by demonstrating the characteristic impairment in vigilance.

Although visualization of the trypanosome on peripheral smear is the gold standard for diagnosis, immunological tests such as the ELISA and IFA for antibody levels in the CSF are relatively sensitive and specific for the diagnosis of West African trypanosomiasis. However, no reliable serologic tests for East African trypanosomiasis are currently available for practical diagnostic use.

THERAPY

Treatment of African trypanosomiasis is handicapped by the lack of effective nontoxic drugs. Drugs used for early-stage *T. rhodesiense* infection, such as suramin, do not cross the blood–brain barrier. Therefore the risk of disease progression to the neurologic stage exists despite therapy of earlier disease. The most widely used drug is melarsoprol; this is highly toxic because of its own predisposition to cause a toxic encephalopathy. There

are also reports of high relapse rates with standard treatment with melarsoprol.

Intravenous eflornithine is an alternative, less toxic drug recommended in areas where the resistance to melarsoprol is greater than 15%. However, it is more expensive and more difficult to administer because it requires longer intravenous injection as opposed to melarsoprol, which requires five intramuscular injections. However concerns about the development of resistance to monotherapy have prompted clinical trials using combination eflornithine and nifurtimox. Other drugs such as suramin do not cross the blood–brain barrier, and therefore the risk of progression of the disease to the neurologic stage exists despite therapy of earlier disease.

CYSTICERCOSIS

Clinical Vignette

A 29-year-old Asian man, a native Chinese previously living in northern India before he immigrated to the United States 10 years ago, presented to the emergency department after having several witnessed tonic-clonic seizures. He had complained of intermittent mild headaches over the prior week and had no significant past medical history.

On presentation he was postictal; his temperature was 38.5° C (101.3° F). His right pupil was minimally larger than the left, and there was no papilledema. He was intubated during a subsequent seizure for airway protection.

Brain CT revealed a single hypodense area lateral to the right lateral ventricle. Spinal fluid analysis indicated normal results, including a negative Gram stain. Plain radiographs of his extremities showed multiple small calcific densities in the soft tissues, and a serum cysticercosis immunoblot was positive. He was treated with albendazole and dexamethasone, and his seizures resolved.

EPIDEMIOLOGY

Cysticercosis is a relatively common cause of seizure disorders, particularly in individuals from Central and South America, including those who have immigrated to the United States. It may occur in both immunocompromised and nonimmunocompromised individuals. It results from infection with the larval form of the porcine tapeworm *Taenia solium*. Humans acquire the adult tapeworm by eating undercooked pork and become infected with the larval stage (cysticercus) by ingesting tapeworm eggs. Eggs hatch within the small intestine, burrow into venules, and are carried to distant sites, including the CNS and muscle. Because the larvae are relatively large, they may lodge in the subarachnoid space, ventricles, or brain tissue (Fig. 50-4).

CLINICAL PRESENTATION

Symptoms may not occur for 4–5 years, when larvae die and provoke an inflammatory response. Cysts within the cerebrum may mimic brain tumors, leading to a variety of focal symptoms.

Ovum of *Taenia solium* (pork tapeworm); indistinguishable from that of *T. saginata* (beef tapeworm)

Cysticercus (larval stage) of pork tapeworm; fluid-filled sac (bladder) containing scolex (head) of worm

T. solium ova hatch after ingestion by hogs; embryos migrate to hog tissues and form cysticerci. When humans eat infested pork, intestinal tapeworms develop. However, if humans ingest ova instead of larvae, or if ova reach stomach by reverse peristalsis from intestinal worm, human cysticercosis may occur.

Cysticercosis of brain

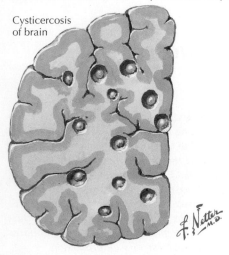

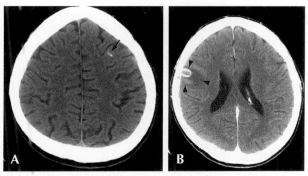

A, Focal calcified cortical mass in left frontal convexity (arrow). **B,** Axial post-enhanced cranial CT image demonstrates rim enhancing lesion with surrounding edema in right frontal convexity (arrowheads).

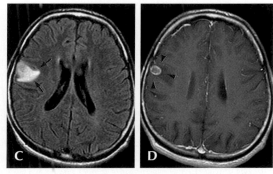

C and **D** Axial FLAIR image demonstrates considerable edema associated with the right frontal convexity mass (arrows), and rim enhancement is noted on the T1-weighted fast spin echo post–gadolinium-enhanced image (arrowheads).

Figure 50-4 Cysticerosis.

Intra-ventricular cysts may lead to CSF obstruction with signs of hydrocephalus. On other occasions, subarachnoid space cysts may lead to symptoms of a chronic meningitis and arachnoiditis.

DIAGNOSIS

Old nonviable cysts eventually calcify, simplifying detection. MRI or contrast-enhanced CT may reveal signs of CNS infection. Serum or CSF serologic study and biopsy of subcutaneous cysts or skeletal muscle calcifications support the diagnosis.

THERAPY

Albendazole or praziquantel are the therapies of choice for cysticercosis. Steroids are used to decrease inflammation. Traditional anticonvulsants are indicated to control seizures.

EOSINOPHILIC MENINGITIS

The two major helminths causing acute eosinophilic meningoencephalitis are *Angiostrongylus cantonensis* and *Gnathostoma spinigerum*. These two pathogens are widespread in the tropics, especially Southeast Asia and Central America, and are contracted from the ingestion of contaminated food substances. Other common parasitic pathogens that may rarely cause

meningoencephalitis are *Trichinella spiralis*, *Toxocara canis*, and filarial species (including loa loa and *Mansonella perstans*).

TRICHINOSIS

Trichinosis occurs secondary to *Trichinella spiralis*, an intestinal nematode. Human disease most typically occurs after ingestion of contaminated meats, particularly homemade pork sausage or, rarely, bear. These meats contain cysts that harbor the *T. spiralis* larvae that were originally liberated within the stomach by action of gastric enzymes. Subsequently the females are fertilized and then burrow into the intestinal mucosa, eventually reaching the blood supply after traversing the lymphatic system. These larvae have a propensity to survive only in skeletal or cardiac muscle tissue, where they become encysted and eventually calcify. These are passed on from animals to humans after the latter's consumption of the infected tissue.

Shortly after ingestion, one may develop significant upper gastrointestinal distress with nausea and vomiting (Fig. 50-5). Periorbital edema may develop but may be relatively transient, disappearing in few days. If heavily infested pork is ingested, this is soon followed by severe generalized myalgia and sometimes an overwhelming encephalomyelitis and fever not unlike acute bacterial meningitis. Cardiac and diaphragmatic muscle is also at risk and may lead to a fatal outcome when severely infested by the trichinella organism. Very rarely there may be cerebral

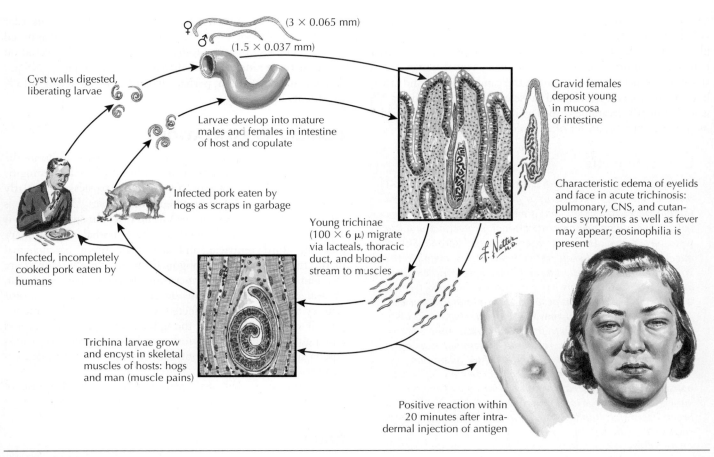

Figure 50-5 Trichinosis.

infestation leading to seizures. Major clinical clues to diagnosis include history of periorbital edema, overwhelming myalgia, and a blood count demonstrating a marked leukocytosis with a very marked degree of eosinophilia (>700 cells/mm³).

A more chronic form of trichinosis typically presents with a modest low-grade myalgia. There is also a predilection to involvement of cranial nerve–innervated muscles. This may lead to diplopia, difficulty chewing and swallowing, and dysarthria. Although any extremity muscle may be affected, usually there is a maximal proximal involvement. Initial biopsy may demonstrate an inflammatory myopathy. Once diagnosis is confirmed, usually by skeletal muscle biopsy—sometimes requiring a half gram of tissue to isolate a cyst—treatment is initiated. Corticosteroids, at 40–60 mg of prednisone daily, combined with thiabendazole is the treatment of choice. This leads to recovery in most patients. However, specific therapy is not necessary per se in less severely affected patients, particularly those presenting with only mild myalgia.

SCHISTOSOMIASIS

Schistosoma japonicum and *S. mansoni* are the most common trematodes to affect the nervous system. Schistosomiasis has a global distribution within tropical areas such as the Nile and Amazon river basins. Unwary bathers, particularly those from Europe or North America, become infected when bathing in

inviting local rivers and lakes. (One might think that the crocodile population would dissuade these individuals from enjoying these otherwise cooling and inviting waters!)

The host snails are in plentiful supply; the parasite enters the body through the skin, leading to "swimmer's itch." Neurologic symptoms may occur a few months later in about 5% of the exposed population. Typically this leads to an acute myelopathy near the conus medullaris. Cerebral infestation results in seizures.

Complement fixation or liver/rectal mucosa biopsy provide the best diagnostic methodology.

Treatment with praziquantel is often very efficacious. However, it must be expeditiously initiated with acute myelopathy patients; if not, a permanent paraplegia may result. In contrast, cerebral schistosomiasis patients may become seizure free.

NEUROSARCOIDOSIS

This is a systemic granulomatous disorder without a specific identified microorganism in contrast to tuberculosis, histoplasmosis, and coccidiomycosis, where Koch's postulates are fulfilled. However, neuro-sarcoidosis (NS) has many similarities to these processes with its propensity for leptomeningeal seeding and its various consequences. These particularly include involvement of the cranial nerves such as the optic, trigeminal, facial, and acoustic. Intraparenchymal brain involvement is particularly likely to occur in the pituitary but may occur at almost any place within the neuraxis, such as the cerebral or cerebellar hemisphere, mimicking a tumor. Similarly spinal nerves are at risk; this is especially prominent at the cauda equina. And lastly, both the peripheral nerves and muscles may be affected. As NS is an eminently treatable disorder, it is imperative to consider its presence in a broad set of neurologic disorders.

Clinical Vignette

A 32-year-old gentleman with a history of insulin-dependent diabetes mellitus, working as a defense contractor, noted fatigue, decreased libido, and diminished potentia. Endocrinologic evaluation demonstrated a high prolactin and a low testosterone level. He was treated with testosterone. Subsequently he developed problems climbing stairs, hiking in the White Mountains, as well as a self-limited rash. He then noted diminished hearing in his left ear; this was initially treated with antibiotics. When this progressed to a total hearing loss, an autoimmune mechanism was proposed. Mood irritability developed, followed by left facial numbness that became bilateral. A gait disorder, recurrent trigeminal neuralgia, and photophobia occurred 2 months before admission.

This pleasant gentleman appeared chronically ill; he was nauseated and occasionally vomiting during our initial evaluation. Neurologic examination showed him to have a broad-based gait, tandem ataxia, a deaf left ear and distal weakness in the left leg.

Laboratory examination demonstrated elevated serum creatine kinase in the range of 1000 IUs (normal < 205). CSF demonstrated a lymphocytic pleocytosis with 46–55 white blood cells, a protein of 263 mg/dL, and glucose of 46 mg/dL. His CSF angiotensin-converting enzyme (ACE) was positive 4.6 units (with the ULN ≤2.5). However, this was normal in his serum.

Brain magnetic resonance imaging (MRI) demonstrated enhancement near his pituitary gland and the trigeminal nerve at the fossa ovale. Lymphadenopathy was identified in both the chest at the hilum, and intraabdominally in the retroperitoneal regions on CT scanning. Gallium scan identified perihilar and lacrimal gland uptake. A mediastinal node biopsy identified non-caseating granulomas with lymphocytes, plasma cells, mast cells, epithelioid cells and macrophages compatible with sarcoidosis.

Therapy with prednisone 60 mg daily was initiated. His symptoms and findings gradually and totally resolved over a 6-month period as his dosage was carefully weaned. His only residual is permanent hearing loss in his left ear. Otherwise, he is now a very active person with no other limitations.

In summary, this gentleman presented with pituitary dysfunction manifested by diminished gonadal function and subsequent multiple cranial nerve as well as cerebellar involvement and a subclinical myopathy.

EPIDEMIOLOGY

The lifetime risk of developing systemic sarcoidosis is 2.4% in the African-American population, almost three times greater than Caucasians, who have a 0.85% lifetime likelihood of developing this disorder. This is a relatively benign disorder overall, and as many as 66.7% of patients eventually diagnosed with sarcoidosis are asymptomatic. Often this is discovered on a routine chest radiograph identifying hilar adenopathy. NS per se is much less common, perhaps having an incidence of 5–15% of patients diagnosed.

CLINICAL PRESENTATION

This depends on the propensity of NS to primarily infiltrate the meninges with inflammatory cells leading to a pachymeningitis and thus producing various cranial nerve palsies, particularly the optic, trigeminal, facial and auditory nerves. When there is extension of this process along Virchow–Robin spaces, there is a predilection for involvement of the hypothalamus pituitary axis, the third ventricle, and eventually brain parenchymal involvement. Early on, hypogonadism or hypothyroidism are frequent presentations. On occasion, lower bulbar, cerebellar, or spinal cord involvement occurs. The peripheral motor sensory unit may also be affected with granulomas, and mononuclear cells developing in the epineurium, perineurium, and endoneurium often in an asymmetric fashion leading to a cauda equina syndrome or a mononeuritis multiplex. Various degrees of a myopathy may occur.

Systemic signs that often provide clues to the diagnosis of NS include erythema nodosum, uveitis, and hepatomegaly.

DIAGNOSIS

A definitive diagnosis requires a tissue specimen, most typically a hilar node biopsy as illustrated by the above vignette. Often one can gain supportive clues from a cranial MRI, particularly with its high sensitivity especially involving the leptomeninges. However, this has a low specificity, as it may mimic MS in its propensity for some white matter involvement. At other times, MRI may demonstrate lesions mimicking a tumor (Fig. 50-6). The CSF is abnormal in 80% of NS patients, not only a cellular response but also an elevated ACE, something that may only be positive here rather than the serum. Chest radiographs are positive in more than half of the patients. Chest CT is sometimes positive when routine chest radiographs are normal. Lastly an otherwise unexplained hypercalcemia as well as abnormal liver function tests may also give further hint that NS is present.

THERAPY

Corticosteroids are the cornerstone of therapy. In general, they are very effective, either commencing orally with 20–60 mg daily or intravenously with methylprednisolone. There are no randomized trials. MRI is helpful in gauging potential therapeutic responses. The best results often occur in patients with cranial or peripheral nerve presentation. The presence of MRI enhancement suggests the presence of active inflammation with good prognosis with corticosteroids, whereas lack of the same may be compatible with fibrosis and chronicity and thus a lesser chance of a good therapeutic response.

A prime problem is the tendency for relapses to occur during tapering. There is no good data for the various steroid-sparing agents such as methotrexate, azathioprine, and mycophenolate.

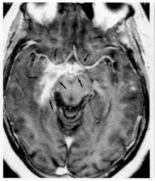
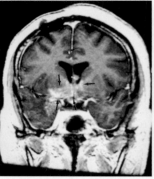
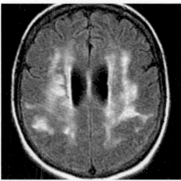
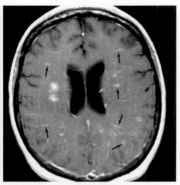

A. and **B.** Axial and coronal T1-weighted fast spin echo imaging following gadolinium demonstrate intense enhancement of hypothalamic region, adjacent basal ganglia, right temporal lobe, and dura (arrows).

C. Axial FLAIR image demonstrates a patchy confluent pattern of involvement of white matter, paraventricular, central with extension into subcortical hemispheric white matter.

D. Axial T1-weighted fast spin echo image following gadolinium shows some globular enhancement but also a linear pattern consistent with infiltration of Virchow-Robin spaces (arrows).

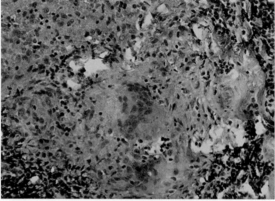

E. Hilar node biopsy. Noncaseating granuloma with lymphocytes, macrophages, epitheloid, mast, and plasma cells compatible with sarcoidosis.

Figure 50-6 Neurosarcoidosis: MRI and Pathology.

OVERVIEW OF FUNGAL INFECTIONS

Cryptococcus neoformans and *Coccidioides immitis* are the most common fungi responsible for central nervous system fungal disease. These two fungi together with *Histoplasma capsulatum* are capable of causing disease in both healthy individuals and immunocompromised hosts. As cryptococcal disease is discussed in Chapter 51, this section primarily discusses CNS disease caused by *H. capsulatum* and *C. immitis*.

HISTOPLASMOSIS

Clinical Vignette

A 30-year-old, right-handed male insurance agent was evaluated for intermittent twitching of his right hand for 3 months. The patient was currently in good health; however, 3 years earlier he experienced an episode of disseminated histoplasmosis when he was working in Ohio trapping rodents in the outdoors. He was treated with itraconazole for 9 months, with apparent cure of his disease. On a recent routine medical examination, a mild neutropenia with a WBC count of 2800/mm and borderline thrombocytopenia

were noted. A bone marrow biopsy revealed rare granulomas but negative culture for H. capsulatum.

Neurologic examination demonstrated a slight intention tremor of his right hand with difficulty writing. His general physical examination was completely normal. Brain MRI revealed two brain abscesses: a large one in the cerebellum causing a mild midline shift and another in the right frontal cerebral cortex. His urine Histoplasma antigen was positive at 4.6 ELISA units. HIV antibody was negative.

He underwent a biopsy and debulking of his cerebellar lesion, and the fungal smear showed many yeast forms of Histoplasma. The patient was treated for twelve months with voriconazole. He responded well with a rapid normalization in his urinary Histoplasma antigen; however he had a persistent neutropenia.

EPIDEMIOLOGY

In the United States, histoplasmosis is primarily acquired in the endemic areas of the Ohio and Mississippi river valleys. This occurs from the inhalation of spores of *H. capsulatum* found in the soil contaminated by fecal material from chickens, starlings, and bats. Travelers to other countries where histoplasmosis is also found have acquired it after exposure in caves inhabited by infected bats or from inhalation from spores found in the soil.

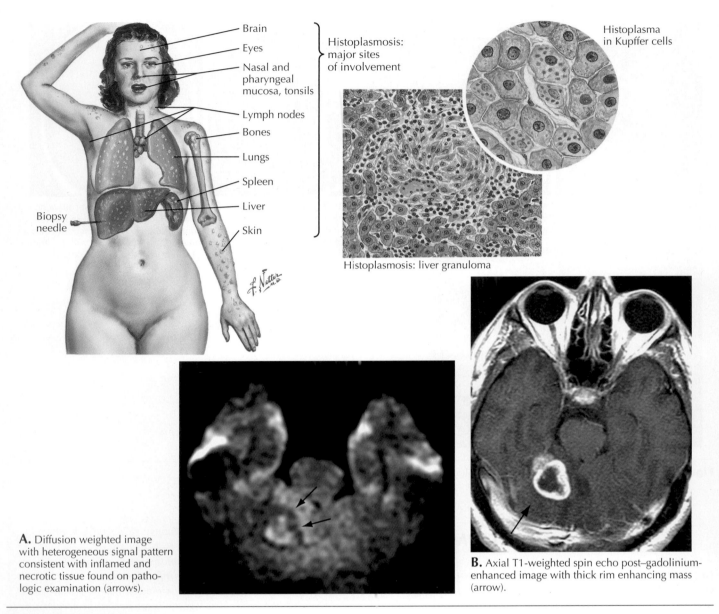

Histoplasmosis: major sites of involvement

- Brain
- Eyes
- Nasal and pharyngeal mucosa, tonsils
- Lymph nodes
- Bones
- Lungs
- Spleen
- Liver
- Skin

Biopsy needle

Histoplasma in Kupffer cells

Histoplasmosis: liver granuloma

A. Diffusion weighted image with heterogeneous signal pattern consistent with inflamed and necrotic tissue found on pathologic examination (arrows).

B. Axial T1-weighted spin echo post–gadolinium-enhanced image with thick rim enhancing mass (arrow).

Figure 50-7 Histoplasmosis.

Most infections are asymptomatic, but symptomatic disease may occur even in the normal host. Disseminated disease tends to occur in infants, the elderly, and patients with hematologic malignancies and HIV infection (where disseminated disease is usually diagnosed in patients with CD4 counts less than 200 cells/mm^3).

CNS histoplasmosis is a manifestation of disseminated disease and is uncommon in North America. It mimics tuberculosis with parenchymal involvement occurring as single or multiple focal granulomas (Fig. 50-7). Granulomatous basilar meningitis may also occur. Abscess formation is rare except in immunocompromised hosts. Patients usually present with signs and symptoms of subacute meningitis with fever, stiff neck, and photophobia. Focal neurologic deficits are more common in CNS histoplasmosis than either cryptococcosis or coccidioidomycosis.

DIAGNOSIS

Isolation of *H. capsulatum* is difficult from the CSF; cultures of bone marrow, blood, and urine are more likely to be positive. The more rapid detection of Histoplasma antigen in blood, urine, or CSF is often diagnostic of disseminated histoplasmosis and can be followed to negativity with antifungal therapy. A false-positive test for serum Histoplasma antigen may be present in disseminated coccidioidomycosis.

THERAPY

There is no clearly defined therapy that is most effective for CNS histoplasmosis. Initial therapy with liposomal amphotericin followed by itraconazole for at least 1 year is suggested. High rates of relapse of up to 40% occur with shorter periods of therapy. The newer azoles, such as voriconazole and posaconazole, are also effective in vitro and may obviate the unreliable blood levels achieved by itraconazole. HIV-positive patients with histoplasmosis need to stay on suppressive itraconazole therapy unless their CD4 count exceeds 150 cells/mm³.

COCCIDIOIDOMYCOSIS

Clinical Vignette

A 68-year-old California woman developed intermittent fever, weight loss, and occasional confusion a few months after a trip around the world that included traveling to West Africa and Brazil. She subsequently had headache and stiff neck and saw her local doctor, who found her with a temperature of 37.7° C (99.8° F), minimally confused but no meningismus, that is, a stiff neck. There were no other significant physical findings.

Chest radiograph revealed mediastinal lymphadenopathy with some fibrosis in the right upper lobe. Her PPD was negative. A lumbar puncture demonstrated a CSF WBC count of 112/mm³, a protein of 80 mg/dL, and glucose of 45 mg/dL. Brain MRI showed basilar meningitis. Her complement fixation titer to C. immitis was 1:8 in the CSF. Her CSF culture did not grow any fungal organisms.

She was started on 800 mg of intravenous fluconazole and intrathecal amphotericin. Mild right-sided hydrocephalus developed but it did not progress with continued therapy. Her symptoms cleared over the next several months with improvement of her MRI. She completed a course of 6 months of intrathecal amphotericin until her CSF parameters normalized and her complement fixation titer became negative. She is being continued on 400 mg of oral fluconazole. It is anticipated that because of her advanced age, she would require this drug lifelong.

EPIDEMIOLOGY

C. immitis is found in soil only in the Western Hemisphere, particularly in the southwestern United States, the northern Pacific coast of Mexico, Guatemala, Honduras, and Venezuela. Aerosolized arthroconidia are inhaled and frequently infect individuals asymptomatically in endemic areas. About 0.5% of exposed patients will develop disseminated disease via lymphatic or vascular spread to the skin, bone, meninges, and genitourinary tract. CNS involvement develops in 33–50% of patients with disseminated disease. Sometimes the neuraxis is the only site of symptomatic disease. Risk factors for dissemination include older age, pregnancy, and immunosuppression (including HIV infection).

CLINICAL FEATURES

When there is central nervous system involvement, this infection causes a subacute to chronic meningitis with a predilection for the basilar meninges. Here a progressive fibrosing granulomatous reaction occurs. This may result in hydrocephalus that eventually requires shunting. Focal space-occupying lesions are rare. C. immitis is recovered in CSF in only 50% of patients with known meningitis.

DIAGNOSIS

Confirmation of the presence of coccidiomycosis is presumptively made in patients with chronic meningitis if the complement fixing antibody to C. immitis is positive in the CSF and any titer or the serum complement fixation titer to C. immitis is positive at 1:16.

THERAPY

Treatment with high-dose fluconazole (400–800 mg/day) in uncomplicated cases is preferred by many physicians. In patients with high antibody titers in the CSF or who are immunosuppressed, this is often best accompanied by intrathecal administration of amphotericin. Patients who respond to oral fluconazole should probably continue on this regimen indefinitely. Those who do not respond initially to the azoles should be started on intrathecal amphotericin. Central nervous system vasculitis is another complication of coccidioidal meningitis. This may respond to the addition of high-dose steroids.

EVIDENCE

Bos MM, Dvereem S, van Engelen BGM, et al. A case of neuromuscular mimicry. Neuromuscular Disorders 2006;16:510-513.

Galgiani JN, Ampel NM, Blair JE, et al. Practice guidelines for the management of coccidioidomycosis. Clin Infect Dis 2005;41:1217-1223.

Kaiboriboon K, Olsen TJ, Hayat GR. Cauda equina and conus medullaris syndrome in sarcoidosis. Neurologist 2005;11:179-183.

Kellinghaus C, Schilling M, Lüdemann P. Neurosarcoidosis: clinical experience and diagnostic pitfalls. European Neurology 2004;51:84-88.

Lejon V, Buscher P. Cerebrospinal fluid in human African trypanosomiasis: a key to diagnosis, therapeutic decision and post-treatment follow-up. Tropical Medicine & International Health 2005;10(5):395-403.

Neurologic involvement in falciparum malaria. J Watch Neurology 2007;2007:3-3.

Stitch A, Abel PM, Krishna S. Clinical review of human African trypanosomiasis. Br Med J 2002;325:203-206.

Terushkin V, Stern BJ, Judson MA, et al. Neurosarcoidosis: presentations and management. Neurologist 2010;16(1):2-15. Review

Wheat LJ, Musial CE, Jenny-Avital E. Diagnosis and management of central nervous system histoplasmosis. Clin Infect Dis 2005:40;844-853.

ADDITIONAL RESOURCES

Centers for Disease Control Division of Parasitic Disease—African trypanosomiasis: http://www.cdc.gov/ncidod/dpd/parasites/trypanosomiasis/default.htm Accessed February 5, 2009.
Coccidioidomycosis: http://www.idsociety.org/content.aspx?id=9200#cocc
Fungal Infections: http://www.idsociety.org/content.aspx?id=9200
Histoplasmosis: http://www.idsociety.org/content.aspx?id=9200#hist
Practice Guidelines of the Infectious Diseases Society of America. Available at: http://www.idsociety.org/Content.aspx?id=9088. Accessed February 5, 2009. Evidence-based statements developed to assist practitioners and patients in making decisions about appropriate health care for specific clinical circumstances. Guidelines for treatment of infections by organ system and organism may be found here.
World Health Organization—African trypanosomiasis: http://www.who.int/topics/trypanosomiasis_african/en/ Accessed February 5, 2009. www.medicalecology.org/diseases/d_african_trypano.htm

Infections in the Immunocompromised Host

Daniel P. McQuillen, Donald E. Craven, and H. Royden Jones, Jr.

51

*I*mmunocompromised hosts are particularly susceptible to infections from a wide spectrum of bacterial pathogens (including those endemic to specific geographic areas), mycobacterial diseases, opportunistic viruses or fungi and, less commonly, parasites. In addition, certain infections are more likely to occur in relation to the onset of immune suppression, the duration of immune compromise, or the type of immune suppression. Some pathogens, such as neurocysticercosis, also occur in nonimmunocompromised hosts.

PROGRESSIVE MULTIFOCAL LEUKOENCEPHALOPATHY (JC VIRUS)

Clinical Vignette

A 65-year-old man with a history of follicular lymphoma initially treated with conventional chemotherapy 4 years previously was given three courses of rituximab for maintenance therapy because of persistence of clonal changes in his bone marrow. He developed confusion, dysarthria, and aphasia after the third course. MRI revealed nonenhancing lesions in the posterior and frontal lobes and left centrum semiovale. Peripheral blood PCR was positive for JC virus, but CSF was negative.

Brain biopsy demonstrated changes characteristic of progressive multifocal leukoencephalopathy (PML). His peripheral blood demonstrated a CD4 count of 100. Treatment with cidofovir was ineffective as the patient's clinical condition worsened with progressive aphasia and confusion, urinary and fecal incontinence, flaccid paralysis of the left arm, accompanied by radiologic progression with mass effect. He died 3 months after presentation.

EPIDEMIOLOGY

JC virus is a human polyomavirus (a small nonenveloped virus with a circular, double-stranded DNA genome). Infection is acquired during childhood and persists in the kidney. JC virus is the cause of PML, a rare demyelinating disease of immunosuppressed patients. PML causes rapidly progressive focal neurologic deficits without signs of increased intracranial pressure. PML is most often an AIDS-defining illness, although it occurs in other immunocompromised settings such as long-term corticosteroid or methotrexate (MTX) therapy. Although one may usually consider such in more chronic settings of the immunocompromised, we have seen one instance of an individual who developed and subsequently died of PML 9 months after commencing MTX therapy. Recently, several cases of PML are reported in patients treated with the monoclonal antibodies natalizumab for multiple sclerosis and Crohn disease as well as

rituximab. This has significantly limited the utilization of natalizumab, a medication that initially was felt to be the most promising therapy ever developed for MS patients. The incidence of PML in HIV-infected patients has decreased after the introduction of highly active antiretroviral therapy (HAART) therapy; however, HAART may "uncover" PML, with it developing within 6 months of commencement of this therapy.

PML occurs most commonly in systemic lupus erythematosus among the various rheumatologic disorders.

CLINICAL PRESENTATION

PML has a variable presentation depending on which part of the brain is initially infected. The temporal profile and clinical symptomatology are no different in HIV patients than in those with other immunodeficiencies, such as acute leukemias. Common neurologic scenarios include a progressive hemiparesis, visual field deficits, aphasia, and cognitive impairment. Occasional patients present with a pure cerebellar truncal and/or appendicular ataxia, or cranial nerve deficits. Late in the course of PML, affected patients develop severe neurologic deficits, including cortical blindness, quadriparesis, profound dementia, and coma.

Lesions may be primarily located in the cerebral white matter or sometimes in the cerebellum and brainstem (Fig. 51-1). Spinal cord involvement is rare but is reported. However, survival remains poor once PML is diagnosed. As there is no specific antiviral medication effective for PML, the main focus should be on prophylactic measures to avoid immunodeficiency.

DIAGNOSIS

MRI scans reveal hypodense, nonenhancing lesions of the cerebral white matter. The severity of clinical findings is often greater than is suggested by the extent of involvement on computed tomographic (CT) scan. The latter may even be normal. MRI typically helps to differentiate brain tumors, especially lymphoma, or abscesses in the immunocompromised. A spongiform encephalopathy caused by a prion, Creutzfeldt–Jakob disease, is a fatal infectious disease that sometimes presents with a progressive cerebellar syndrome or various focal cerebral lesions. However, this does not have a predilection for immunocompromised hosts.

PCR has been used to amplify JC virus DNA in CSF samples (sensitivities range from 60% to 100%). CSF cell count and chemistry results are usually normal. EEG may reveal focal slowing or may be normal early in the course of PML.

A definitive diagnosis of PML requires identification of the characteristic pathologic changes on brain biopsy: multiple asymmetric foci of demyelination at various stages of evolution

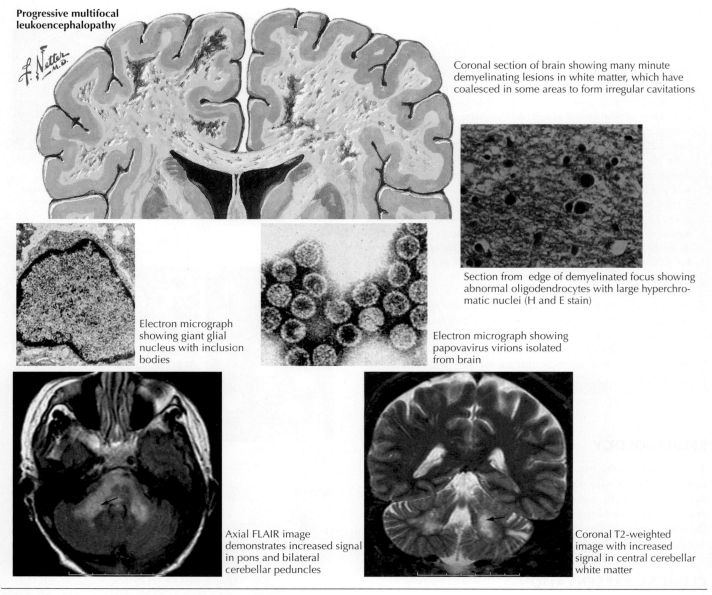

Progressive multifocal leukoencephalopathy

Coronal section of brain showing many minute demyelinating lesions in white matter, which have coalesced in some areas to form irregular cavitations

Section from edge of demyelinated focus showing abnormal oligodendrocytes with large hyperchromatic nuclei (H and E stain)

Electron micrograph showing giant glial nucleus with inclusion bodies

Electron micrograph showing papovavirus virions isolated from brain

Axial FLAIR image demonstrates increased signal in pons and bilateral cerebellar peduncles

Coronal T2-weighted image with increased signal in central cerebellar white matter

Figure 51-1 Progressive Multifocal Leukoencephalitis.

in the cerebral white matter. The oligodendrocytes demonstrate characteristic cytopathic effects, including nuclear enlargement, loss of normal chromatin pattern, and intranuclear accumulation of deeply basophilic homogenous staining material. Electron microscopy reveals polyomavirus particles in enlarged oligodendrocyte nuclei (see Fig. 51-1).

THERAPY

Unfortunately, there is no specific antiviral therapy effective for PML. Although there were some preliminary studies suggesting that cidofovir, a nucleoside analog active against polyomaviruses, might have therapeutic potential, recent results from a large multi-institutional trial are disappointing. We continue to have an overriding need for an effective PML therapy. Marked clinical and radiographic improvement in HIV-infected patients with PML has been seen after treatment with combination HAART regimens that include a protease inhibitor. Aggressive

antiretroviral treatment of underlying HIV infection seems to be the most reasonable therapeutic approach to management in HIV-infected patients, as patients receiving HAART therapy have a lower incidence of PML. The opportunity for treatment may be better with the natalizumab-induced PML patient in that steroid pulse therapy led to clinically significant recovery in one patient. Unless the accompanying underlying immune deficit can be reversed as noted above, PML typically progresses to death fairly rapidly.

CRYPTOCOCCUS

Some pathogens commonly found in healthy hosts may cause meningitis in immunocompromised patients; *Cryptococcus neoformans* and *Listeria monocytogenes* are two organisms particularly prone to such.

Clinical Vignette

A 34-year-old man presented with a month-long history of constant increasingly intense headaches having recently been evaluated for the same complaint at two other hospitals. The headache was accompanied by intermittent photophobia, nausea, and vomiting. Two weeks previously, an ulcerating lesion on his cheek was unsuccessfully treated with doxycycline for possible rickettsial infection. He also had a 20-pound weight loss.

He was lethargic but able to answer simple questions. Temperature was 39.4° C (102.9° F). Mild nuchal rigidity was present. No focal neurologic findings were present.

His CSF was hazy in color with an elevated opening pressure, 29 WBC (22% neutrophils, 54% lymphocytes, and 20% monocytes), a protein of 50 mg/dL, and glucose of 9 mg/dL (concomitant serum glucose 125). India ink staining of his CSF demonstrated multiple encapsulated yeast forms. The cryptococcal antigen was positive 1:1024. HIV testing was negative; however, his CD4 count was low (100 cells/mm³). Previously, he helped his father raise homing pigeons. Despite intravenous amphotericin B and 5-flucytosine, oral fluconazole, and daily spinal taps, he suffered some loss of vision because of effects of increased intracranial pressure. He was subsequently discovered to have a B-cell lymphoma.

EPIDEMIOLOGY

This chronic, subacute, and, rarely, acute CNS infection is caused by *Cryptococcus neoformans*, a yeast-like fungus. Distributed worldwide in soil, fruits, and matter contaminated by pigeon excreta, this organism probably enters the body through the lungs and then disseminates to all organs (Fig. 51-2). Mild, self-limited infections are common.

CLINICAL PRESENTATION

Cryptococcal disease can develop in both healthy and immunocompromised patients. Chronic meningitis is the most common presentation. These patients are often afebrile and have no more than minimal nuchal rigidity. Clinically this disorder usually presents insidiously over a matter of months with symptoms of low-grade headache, nausea, irritability, somnolence, and clumsiness. Cranial nerve involvement occurs in 20% of patients characterized by diminished visual acuity sometimes with papilledema, diplopia, and facial numbness. Dementia may occur in some secondary to direct cerebral involvement.

DIAGNOSIS

Examination of the CSF demonstrates an elevated opening pressure, a lymphocytic leukocytosis with a WBC count of 40–400/mm³, increased CSF protein concentration, and a decreased glucose level in 50% of patients. Although India ink preparations can define the organism, specific cultural isolation of *C. neoformans* is the best diagnostic test. Lacking such definitive

Cryptococcosis

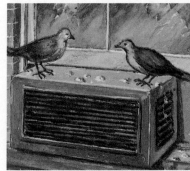

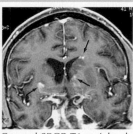

Coronal SPGR T1-weighted image post–gadolinium enhanced demonstrates multiple small enhancing lesions in bilateral basal ganglia (arrows).

Infection is by respiratory route. Pigeon dung and air conditioners may be factors in dissemination.

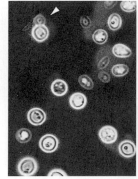

India ink preparation showing budding and capsule

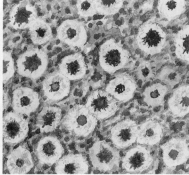

Accumulation of encapsulated cryptococci in subarachnoid space (PAS or methenamine-silver stain)

Listeriosis

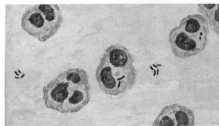

Smear of CSF showing white blood cells and *Listeria* organisms, which appear as gram-positive rods. They may be very short, to resemble cocci, and they often orient in palisades suggestive of Chinese characters. They cause severe purulent meningitis, most commonly in immunocompromised patients or newborns.

Figure 51-2 Cryptococcosis and Listeriosis.

confirmation, diagnosis is made by culturing or identifying the organism with periodic acid-Schiff or methenamine-silver stain in a CNS specimen. PCR is not yet available. Latex agglutination for detection of cryptococcal capsular antigen (in serum and CSF) is also available and is helpful in monitoring therapy response. Urine cultures are positive in approximately 33% of patients.

THERAPY

Treatment is best carried out with at least a 2-week course of intravenous amphotericin B with or without flucytosine.

Thereafter, oral fluconazole is administered for at least 6 weeks. Maintenance therapy is recommended for patients with either HIV or AIDS until immune reconstitution occurs with combination antiretroviral therapy.

LISTERIOSIS

EPIDEMIOLOGY

Listeria monocytogenes is a gram-positive rod that has pathologic connotations in neonates and immunocompromised adults. The bacterium is widespread and is isolated from soil, water, animal feed, and sewage.

CLINICAL PRESENTATION

This organism must always be suspected in patients with either AIDS or those individuals receiving long-term prednisone or azathioprine therapy who develop acute meningitis. Neurologic presentation is similar to that of any acute bacterial meningitis. Headache, fever, meningismus, and, occasionally, seizures and focal symptomatology predominate.

DIAGNOSIS

CSF identification of *gram-positive rods* in association with a polymorphonuclear leucocytosis and a concomitant low CSF glucose level (50% of serum glucose) are the cornerstones to recognition of this uncommon form of bacterial meningitis (see Fig. 51-2).

THERAPY

Ampicillin and gentamicin are the treatments of choice.

NOCARDIOSIS

EPIDEMIOLOGY

Nocardia are present in the soil and decaying vegetable matter. This bacterium is one of two usually benign microorganisms that can lead to a focal cerebritis especially when it occurs within an immunosuppressed clinical setting. The other is a parasite, toxoplasmosis; it is discussed in the last section of this chapter. When *Nocardia asteroides* leads to a brain abscess, it enters through the respiratory tract, even though the pulmonary focus may not be prominent. Because the initial pulmonary focus is suppurative and not well localized, this allows the infection to spread to the brain.

CLINICAL PRESENTATION

Various focal clinical signs occur apropos to the site of organism sequestration in the brain. In the absence of a contiguous abscess, meningitis is infrequent.

DIAGNOSIS

Brain biopsy is the most reliable diagnostic technique if the diagnosis cannot be made by evaluation of pulmonary or skin lesions (Fig. 51-3). Nocardia are weakly acid-fast and can be stained with the modified Ziehl–Neelsen method. They may be isolated on Sabouraud's medium or brain–heart infusion agar, but growth may not be visible for 2–4 weeks.

THERAPY

Sulfonamides are the drugs of choice for nocardiosis. Therapy should continue for at least 3 months or several weeks after clinical resolution of the lesion.

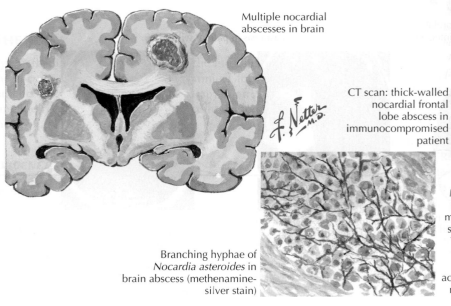

Multiple nocardial abscesses in brain

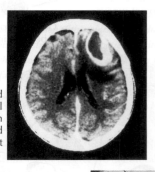

CT scan: thick-walled nocardial frontal lobe abscess in immunocompromised patient

Branching hyphae of *Nocardia asteroides* in brain abscess (methenamine-silver stain)

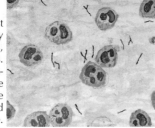

Modified acid-fast organisms as they may appear in pus, sputum, or tissues. They may be mistaken for tubercle bacilli but are actually fragmented nocardial hyphae.

Figure 51-3 Nocardiosis.

Threlkeld SC, Hooper DC. Update on management of patients with Nocardia infection. Curr Clin Top Infect Dis 1997;17:1-23. *Comprehensive review of diagnosis and management of CNS nocardiosis.*

Wenning W, Haghikia A, Laubenberger J, Clifford DB, Behrens PF, Chan A, Gold R. Treatment of progressive multifocal leukoencephalopathy associated with natalizumab. N Engl J Med 2009 Sep 10;361(11):1075-1080.

ADDITIONAL RESOURCE

Practice Guidelines of the Infectious Diseases Society of America. Available at: http://www.idsociety.org/Content.aspx?id=9088. Accessed April 28, 2011. *Evidence-based statements developed to assist practitioners and patients in making decisions about appropriate health care for specific clinical circumstances. Guidelines for treatment of infections by organ system and organism may be found here.*

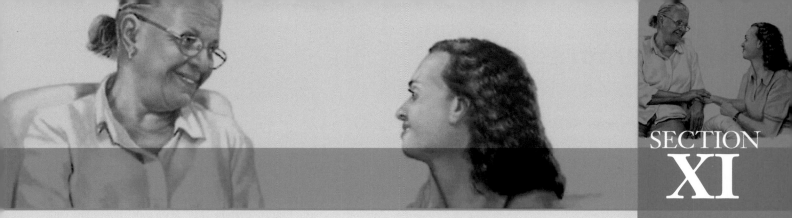

Neuro-oncology

Brain Tumors

52

Lloyd M. Alderson, Peter K. Dempsey, and G. Rees Cosgrove

Clinical Vignette

A 47-year-old self-employed father presented to the emergency department having difficulty discriminating coins in his pocket. He had been skiing that day and was concerned enough to seek medical attention on his way home. His general health was excellent. The only abnormality on his neurologic examination was confined to his right hand. Here he demonstrated loss of two-point discrimination in his fingers, inability to identify numbers traced on right palm, and to identify common objects such as a safety pin, paper clip, or various coins with these fingers. All of these maneuvers were normal for his left hand.

Magnetic resonance imaging (MRI) demonstrated a large 4 × 6-cm high-grade gadolinium-enhancing cystic, vascular tumor with a large amount of peritumor edema in his high left parietal lobe. Stereotactic needle biopsy demonstrated a glioblastoma multiforme (GBM). Radiation and chemotherapy was given. Within a few months, he began to develop seizures; his right hand became weak. He eventually became obtunded and died just 15 months after presentation.

*B*rain tumors are a relatively common neurologic disorder particularly when one combines primary central nervous system (CNS) lesions and those metastatic to the brain and its leptomeninges. Taken together, these tumors are some of the most common cerebral disorders in adults, second only to Alzheimer disease, stroke, and multiple sclerosis. In children with the exception of leukemia, primary brain tumors are the most common malignancy. Glioblastoma multiforme (GBM) arising from within the glial cell matrix occurs in all age groups but typically after age 65 years. A higher age at onset is the most significant predictor of poor outcome. GBM is the most devastating of CNS malignancies; there are very few 2-year survivors. Glial cell tumors comprise more than two thirds of all primary brain tumors. Meningiomas are the next most common tumor and are the prototype of the various primary benign brain tumors.

Although one might think that the temporal profile of a patient's illness may sometimes suggest either a benign or malignant process, one cannot depend on this history to make a differential diagnosis. Brain tumors typically present with four clinical scenarios: (1) focal cerebral or cranial nerve deficits that are gradually progressive over a few weeks to many months, (2) seizures, (3) headache and signs of increased intracranial pressure primarily demonstrating papilledema and sixth-nerve palsies, or (4) stroke mimic, that is, with an apocalyptic onset. Personality changes, evolving language dysfunction, focal loss of sensory discrimination or motor limitation such as a clumsy hand, and ataxic gait are focal signs that usually accurately define the site of the tumor. However, there are certain *false localizing* signs that may lend to initial confusion.

When a slowly enlarging, previously asymptomatic cerebral tumor decompensates, certain *false localizing signs* may cause diagnostic confusion. Transtentorial uncal-parahippocampal herniation occurs, with the offending hemisphere herniating medially through the tentorium cerebri, compressing the contralateral corticospinal tract carrying motor fibers. These fibers originating in the opposite motor cortex control movement on the same side of the body as the site of the tumor. For example, a very large right-sided tumor affects the left corticospinal tract carrying right-sided motor fibers, leading to a paradoxical ipsilateral hemiparesis. Similarly, another false localizing sign occurs when a large herniating tumor compresses the opposite third nerve, thus leading to pupillary dilatation contralateral to the side of the lesion. Today, these clinically confusing signs are less likely to occur with earlier MRI diagnosis of these tumors before they reach a critical mass to cause these herniation syndromes.

The occurrence of a new-onset seizure in an adult must always lead to diagnostic consideration of a brain tumor. It is estimated that 30% of brain tumors present in this fashion. The tumor types and their locations are essential determinants significantly influencing seizure characteristics. Brain tumors with a high risk for epilepsy include slow-growing low-grade gliomas, multiple metastases, and various developmental tumors.

The availability of magnetic resonance imaging (MRI) makes the differentiation relatively simple for those occasional brain tumors that present so acutely that they mimic a stroke. MRI primarily provides morphological and functional information, including tumor localization, vascular permeability, cell density, and tumor perfusion. Today the concurrent employment of positron emission tomography (PET) enables the assessment of molecular processes, such as glucose consumption, expression of nucleoside and amino acid transporters, as well as alterations of DNA and protein synthesis. The value of combining these two modalities is now being studied. Perhaps such will eventually allow one to differentiate a focal "tumefactive" demyelinating lesion from the much more common glioma. At present, it is necessary to perform a stereotactic brain biopsy to make this tissue diagnosis before embarking on a specific therapeutic protocol. Eventually the combined MRI/PET paradigm may also offer important therapeutic implications.

Despite tremendous advances in both the understanding of the biology of malignant gliomas and new neuro-oncologic therapies, the prognosis remains very poor. However, new anti-angiogenic agents are demonstrating some therapeutic promise for recurrent malignant gliomas leading to consideration of them as primary therapeutic agents. Prophylactic cranial irradiation is now being utilized to prevent or delay the occurrence of brain metastases, particularly in patients with high incidence of brain metastases such as small cell lung carcinoma.

MALIGNANT BRAIN TUMORS

When confronted with a patient with a brain tumor, the first priority is to determine whether this lesion arises from within the brain itself, that is, intraparenchymal, or is it a metastasis. Primary brain tumors are commonly solitary and frequently have irregular margins. Intraparenchymal tumors variously arise from glial, ependymal, or lymphoid cells as well as blood vessels. Gliomas are the most common tumors of glial origin; however, both astrocytes and oligodendrocytes can also form tumors. In contradistinction, primary neuronal tumors are very rare, particularly in adults. Metastatic tumors are often multiple, with gadolinium enhancement on MRI and sharply defined borders. The most common primary cancers that metastasize to the brain are lung, breast, skin (particularly melanoma), and kidney.

Traditionally, microscopic features have been the primary means of glial cell tumor classification. However, current study of the molecular events responsible for glioma genesis is beginning to have an impact not only on the diagnostic classification of these tumors but also treatment selection as well as overall prognosis for specific glioma types. Small molecule inhibitors and monoclonal antibodies may eventually provide targeted therapies selectively blocking newly appreciated aberrant growth signaling pathways within gliomas.

GLIOMAS

Epidemiology

The chance of developing a primary malignant brain tumor in the United States is small relative to the chance of developing a tumor of the lung, breast, colon, or prostate. The majority of these are gliomas. Data collected by the Central Brain Tumor Registry of the U.S. (CBTRUS) and Surveillance, Epidemiology, and End Results consortia demonstrates an adult incidence of 5.1 gliomas per 100,000 person-years; almost 50% of these

are glioblastoma. Brain cancer incidence rises with age, peaking at 65–70 years. For glioblastoma alone, the highest incidence is at age 62 years. Men are significantly more likely to develop a glioma (M:F = 1.8). Brain cancer incidence also varies regionally; the incidence in Hawaii is roughly half that of New England, and globally the incidence of brain tumors in Israel is roughly eight times that of Japan. Although some studies suggest that Caucasians are more predisposed to gliomas than African or Asian populations, diminished health care availability in non-Westernized socioeconomic settings may be the primary mechanism explaining this discrepancy rather than genetic susceptibility differences. Gliomas, like most cancers, are usually a random event and rarely have a familial predisposition. However, having a first-degree relative with a glioma doubles a patient's risk but this risk is still small. Rarely, gliomas occur as part of an inherited disorder such as neurofibromatosis types 1 and 2 and tuberous sclerosis. There are no well-defined environmental toxins, with the exception of previous brain irradiation, that predispose patients to glioma.

Pathology

Gliomas typically exhibit features of astrocytes, or oligodendrocytes, or both (mixed glioma) (Fig. 52-1). Microscopically, gliomas appear as diffusely infiltrating cancers of three types: astrocytic, oligodendroglial, and oligoastrocytic (combining the morphologic features of both oligodendroglioma and astrocytoma).

The World Health Organization uses a three-tiered classification system based on histologic criteria that divides these tumors into low-grade glioma, anaplastic glioma, and glioblastoma multiforme (Table 52-1). Low-grade tumors may contain a high density of almost normal-appearing cells. Here the percentage of cells that are dividing (as determined by mib-1 or KI-67 staining) is often 2% or less. Anaplastic gliomas exhibit more atypical cells, with pleomorphic nuclei having growth rates in the 5–10% range but no evidence of necrosis. Gliomas

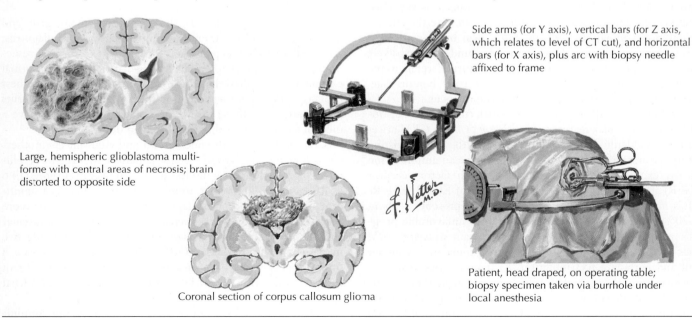

Large, hemispheric glioblastoma multiforme with central areas of necrosis; brain distorted to opposite side

Side arms (for Y axis), vertical bars (for Z axis, which relates to level of CT cut), and horizontal bars (for X axis), plus arc with biopsy needle affixed to frame

Coronal section of corpus callosum glioma

Patient, head draped, on operating table; biopsy specimen taken via burrhole under local anesthesia

Figure 52-1 Gliomas.

Table 52-1 Grades of Gliomas

	Low-Grade Glioma	Anaplastic Glioma	Glioblastoma
Grade	Grade II	Grade III	Grade IV
Symptom duration	Years	Months	Weeks
Age at diagnosis	5–30	30–50	>50
MRI enhancement	—	+/–	+ +
Pathology	Hypercellular	Anaplastic	Necrosis, endothelial cell proliferation
Mitotic index (Ki-67)	<2%	5–10%	>10%
Treatment	Observe	Radiation therapy and chemotherapy	Radiation therapy and chemotherapy
Survival	5–10 years	3–4 years	12 months

with high growth rates (>10% mitotic figures) and necrosis are classified as glioblastoma multiforme (GBM). The less common pilocytic astrocytomas are a separate category of glioma that are histologically characterized by Rosenthal's fibers, usually occur in children, and often have a good prognosis if surgical resection can be achieved. Tumor grade is the most reliable predictor of prognosis. Even if the lesion cannot be safely excised, a needle biopsy is often indicated. Gliomas are not staged as other cancers are because they rarely metastasize outside the CNS. Analysis of tumor samples for genetic abnormalities can help predict response to therapy and will likely lead to a better classification system for gliomas. This classification is valuable prognostically; low-grade gliomas have median survivals of 5–15 years, anaplastic gliomas 2–5 years, and GBM 12–18 months.

GLIOBLASTOMA

These extremely malignant tumors frequently present with seizures, aphasia, or other focal symptomatology, pointing to the specific areas of pathologic origin. Very infrequently, a glioma may manifest itself more globally, *gliomatosis cerebri*, wherein there is widespread dissemination of neoplastic cells globally through a hemisphere or even the entire brain per se. These relatively rare patients may present with cognitive or personality changes. On other occasions, even though the patient presents relatively acutely with focal findings, the clinician is surprised to find a diffusely invasive malignant tumor despite the clinical presentation compatible with an acute focal brain pathology. This is the very common, most aggressive, and the least likely of the gliomas to respond to therapy. "Multiforme" refers to the tumor's gross appearance. Often areas of necrosis, hemorrhage, and fleshy tumor exist within the same tumor focus.

Two types of GBM (Grade IV astrocytomas) are distinguished by molecular features. The classic *primary GBM* arises relatively suddenly in an older person with no preexisting history. Characteristically, primary GBM have an amplification and overexpression of the epidermal growth factor receptor (EGFR) and ligand (EGF). A mutated form of EGFR, EGFR-vIII is another hallmark of primary GBM, present in about 15–20% of cases. EGFRvIII may confer an unfavorable prognosis. p53 mutations are uncommon. Classically *secondary GBM* arises gradually from a low-grade astrocytoma in a younger adult and harbors a p53 mutation. As it undergoes anaplastic transformation, the secondary GBM accumulates other genetic derangements, most notably, mutation of the Rb gene, deletion of the tumor suppressor gene p16/CDKN2A, and amplification of CDK4.

When clinical behavior and genetic abnormalities of GBM tumors are reviewed, a developmental dichotomy emerges. Younger patients with GBM sometimes have a longer history of symptoms or a history of a lower-grade glioma, suggesting that the tumor developed from a lower-grade precursor, whereas older patients with GBM tend to have relatively sudden symptom onset, suggesting that the malignancy did not evolve from a less aggressive tumor. Genetic analysis of GBM samples from older patients frequently reveals overexpression of the epidermal growth factor receptor and loss of 10q. Tumor samples from younger patients are more likely to show mutations in p53, RB, overexpression of the platelet-derived growth factor receptor, and loss of 19q—changes often seen in lower-grade gliomas.

Diagnosis, Treatment, and Prognosis

MRI is the most specific diagnostic modality (Fig. 52-2). On most occasions, one sees focal heterogeneous irregular-margined cystic mass lesions with perilesion edema, gadolinium rim enhancement, and often enough mass effect to produce a transtentorial herniation. In contrast, the occasional patients with gliomatosis cerebri have a characteristic diffusely abnormal MRI picture characterized by multiple areas of subtle white matter enhancement with extension into the cortical mantle, extending far beyond what their clinical presentation usually dictates (Fig. 52-3).

Even with early diagnosis, the prognosis remains grim and most patients will fail therapy within 12 months of diagnosis. The first treatment step is to perform as wide a surgical resection as is functionally tolerable. Younger patients with a normal examination who have had a gross total resection have the best prognosis. Postoperative radiation therapy (RT) clearly benefits many patients as those GBM patients who receive RT have a median survival twice that of those who did not.

Combining RT with concomitant and adjuvant chemotherapy is now the standard of care for patients with GBM. RT plus temozolomide leads to a modest benefit in overall survival (14.6 vs. 12.1 months). However, more importantly, there is a significant increase in the percentage of those surviving 2 or more years (26.5% vs. 10.4%). Bevacizumab, an antagonist of vascular endothelial growth factor, has recently proven safe and effective in patients with recurrent GBM. Recent reports indicate a 6-month progression-free survival of 46%. It is now an urgent priority to determine how best to use this new tool and what agents might work synergistically with it.

When patients have failed these Food and Drug Administration (FDA)–approved treatments, a clinical trial should be

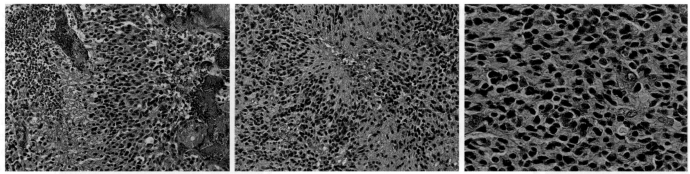

Glioblastoma cerebri. Dense population of astrocytes with malignant nuclear features, palisaded around area of necrosis

Glioblastoma

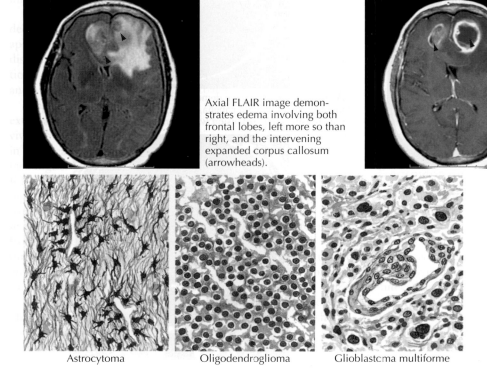

Axial FLAIR image demonstrates edema involving both frontal lobes, left more so than right, and the intervening expanded corpus callosum (arrowheads).

T1-weighted, post–gadolinium-enhanced image shows rim-enhancing lesions with irregular margins and central hypointensity. This central hypointensity represents necrosis, and the enhancing region represents the more active regions within this butterfly glioma.

Astrocytoma   Oligodendroglioma   Glioblastoma multiforme

Figure 52-2 Glioma MRI and Pathology.

considered. Molecular research is defining a number of potential glioma cell targets. These are mostly second messenger molecules involved in pathways that enhance cell proliferation or inhibit programmed cell death. The goal is to treat a selected group of patients whose tumors overexpress the specific target of the treatment drug.

LOW-GRADE GLIOMA

Clinical Vignette

This 34-year-old right-handed woman presented with generalized seizures. Several months earlier, she noted episodes of an unusual smell but these did not cause her immediate concern. Brain MRI demonstrated a right temporal lobe lesion, bright on T2 and FLAIR imaging but

hypointense on T1, with no evidence of enhancement after gadolinium (Fig. 52-4). The patient was treated with oxcarbazepine and admitted to the hospital. Open biopsy was nondiagnostic but subsequent temporal lobectomy revealed an oligodendroglioma with a Ki-67 index of 3.8%. Postoperatively, the patient was treated with monthly temozolomide for 1 year. She is now receiving no treatment and has been clinically and radiographically stable for 2 years.

Clinical Presentation/Pathology

Low-grade gliomas (LGGs) are slow growing with a symptom history that can extend from months to years. Although easily defined by MRI (see Fig. 52-4), LGGs often do not enhance with gadolinium. Their course is usually relatively stable for several years before eventually progressing. At time of diagnosis,

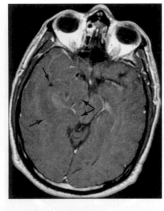

A. Axial FLAIR image demonstrates slight expansion and increased T2 signal involving the medial aspect of the right temporal lobe with the insula and posterior temporal expansion slightly distorting midbrain (arrows).

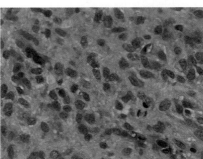

C. A low-power image of anaplastic astrocytoma shows a tumor with high cellularity, but no areas of necrosis or endothelial proliferation are present. (H&E, original magnification 100x)

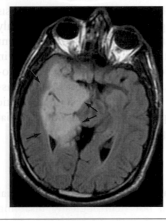

B. T1-weighted fast spin echo image following gadolinium enhancement shows some slight heterogeneity with medial hypointensity which may represent small cystic or degenerative regions with equivocal surrounding enhancement (arrows).

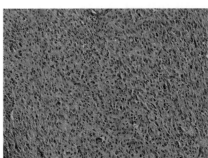

D. A high-power image shows crowded atypical astrocytic cells with irregular nuclei and frequent mitotic figures. (H&E, original magnification 400x)

Figure 52-5 Glioma, Anaplastic Astrocytoma.

evaluation typically demonstrates *monoclonal B cells*. Patients with AIDS or iatrogenically related *immunosuppression* much more commonly develop a PCNSL. Histologically, this is a *polyclonal B cell* tumor that is associated with activation of Epstein–Barr virus.

MRI in PCNSL patients usually demonstrates a homogeneously enhancing lesion(s) often adjacent to a ventricle (Fig. 52-6). A positive cerebrospinal fluid (CSF) cytology is typically found in 25–50% of these individuals. Systemic PCNSL involvement is rare; therefore computed tomography (CT) or MRI scanning of the chest, abdomen, and pelvis is not warranted. Biopsy is essential to make the diagnosis. A large resection is usually not indicated as most of these tumors respond well to chemotherapy and/or RT. In some immunocompetent patients these enhancing brain lesions can disappear either spontaneously or with corticosteroid therapy. For this reason, if PCNSL is suspected, biopsy should be performed prior to treatment with corticosteroids.

PCNSL is markedly sensitive to therapy in *immunocompetent patients*; median survival is often in excess of 3 years. There are two approaches to treatment. The first involves high-dose intravenous (IV) methotrexate as a single agent. The second combines a lower dose of IV methotrexate with ara-C, intrathecal methotrexate, and whole brain RT. This approach is well tolerated in younger patients; however, significant cognitive toxicity occurs in patients older than age 60 years. *Immunosuppressed*

patients are less likely to benefit from chemotherapy and treatment with RT alone. If possible, consideration should be given to reversing the immunosuppression.

OTHER PRIMARY BRAIN TUMORS

Ependymoma

These are unusual tumors of glial origin that can arise anywhere within the neuraxis. The floor of the fourth ventricle is the most common intracranial site for an ependymoma to develop. Histologically, ependymomas often have a cellular appearance characterized by a pseudo-rosette perivascular pattern. There is also a more malignant version with an anaplastic appearance; although unlike gliomas, anaplasia may not confer poor prognosis. Myxopapillary ependymoma is a variant that occurs within the filum terminale at the end of the spinal cord.

MRI is the study of choice (Fig. 52-7). Surgical resection is the primary treatment; however, tumor location determines whether a complete resection is achievable. The extent of tumor resection is the most important indicator of the eventual clinical course. Surgical resection of a myxopapillary ependymoma frequently results in a cure. Indicators of poor prognosis include incomplete resection and CSF spread. Such patients require either local or craniospinal RT. Chemotherapy is seldom used at the time of diagnosis.

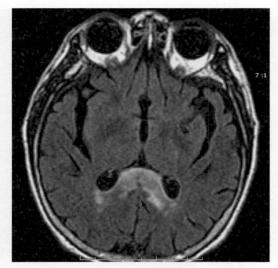

A. Axial FLAIR image demonstrates increased signal within a diffusely expanded splenium of the corpus callosum.

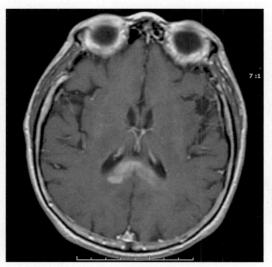

B. Axial T1-weighted, post–gadolinium-enhanced image shows enhancement within the same region.

Figure 52-6 Primary CNS Lymphoma.

Medulloblastoma

These are a class of uncommon primitive neuroectodermal tumors that usually occur in the posterior fossa, often in the midline. Typically, these patients present with double vision, ataxia, hydrocephalus, nausea, and vomiting (Fig. 52-8). These tumors comprise 3% of all primary brain tumors and are significantly more prominent in children. Brain MRI usually reveals a homogeneously enhancing mass situated in the roof of the fourth ventricle, often with some degree of hydrocephalus. Pathologically, medulloblastomas are characterized by sheets of small, poorly differentiated cells with minimal cytoplasm.

Medulloblastomas require both surgical and radiation therapy. When one is able to surgically remove more than 90% of the tumor mass, there is usually an improved survival. Because of this tumor's propensity to spread along the leptomeninges

and throughout the CSF, patients need to undergo evaluation of the entire craniospinal axis to establish the extent of disease. If such has occurred, additional treatment is usually required. External beam RT is directed at the areas identified, often the entire brain and spine. Chemotherapy is then given. This combination therapy is associated with improved survival.

Cerebellar Astrocytoma

Most childhood primary brain tumors are in the glioma family, and many of these occur within the cerebellum (Fig. 52-9). Pilocytic astrocytomas are the most common posterior fossa variant. These tend to arise within the cerebellar hemisphere. A second form of cerebellar astrocytoma, the diffuse or fibrillary form, often arises in the midline and produces obstruction of the fourth ventricle and hydrocephalus. Cerebellar astrocytomas are often cystic in appearance, with an enhancing mural nodule.

Surgical resection can sometimes be curative, particularly with pilocytic astrocytomas. Incompletely resected tumors often require postsurgical irradiation. The survival rate of patients with cerebellar astrocytomas is often very significantly better than those with supratentorial glial tumors.

Pontine Glioma

These serious tumors primarily occur in childhood but are on rare occasions found in adults. They tend to be higher grade tumors that expand the pons and infiltrate into the surrounding tissue (Fig. 52-10). Presenting symptoms are consistent with their location, namely, hydrocephalus from fourth ventricle obstruction, or long tract signs from impairment of corticospinal axonal pathways. Isolated cranial neuropathies, particularly sixth and seventh nerve lesions, may also occur from compression of brainstem nuclei. The infiltrative nature of these tumors often precludes any degree of significant surgical resection. Unfortunately RT is usually ineffective at achieving long-term growth control.

METASTATIC BRAIN TUMORS

Clinical Vignette

A 52-year-old right-handed woman physician had a 2-week history of clumsiness using her right hand, particularly noticeable while performing electromyographies. Neurologic evaluation revealed moderate weakness and clumsiness of her right hand and a hint of a right central facial weakness. She had a 30 pack-year history of tobacco abuse but had discontinued this habit 8 years earlier.

Gadolinium-enhanced brain MRI demonstrated multiple, round ring-enhancing lesions consistent with metastases. As she had no known primary lesion identified during this evaluation, a stereotactic biopsy of a lesion close to the surface demonstrated small cell carcinoma consistent with lung cancer. It took another 4 months before the presumed primary lung lesion was identified with chest CT. She was treated with whole brain RT followed by systemic chemotherapy. Although she had initial symptomatic

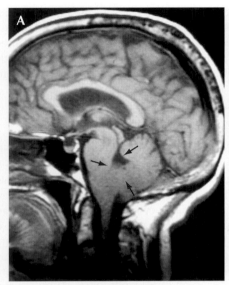

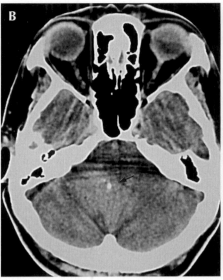

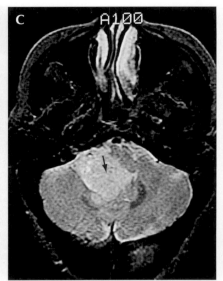

A. Sagittal T1-weighted fast spin echo shows mass within the posterior fourth ventricle and somewhat ill-defined extending into the vallecula and adjacent brainstem (arrows).

B. Axial T1-weighted fast spin echo following intravenous gadolinium shows modest diffuse enhancement. An area of increased signal is associated with a small calcification (arrow).

C. Axial FLAIR shows this central right-sided mass, moderately T2-weighted bright extending into right lateral recess.

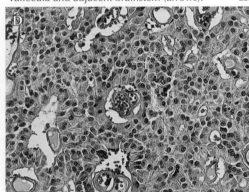

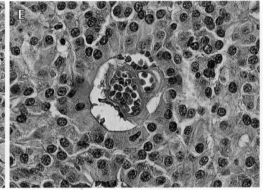

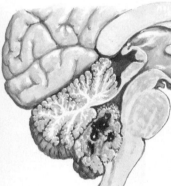

D.-E. Uniform population of epithelioid cells, palisaded around a central blood vessel.

Ependymoma of 4th ventricle protruding into cisterna magna

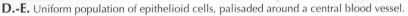

Figure 52-7 Ependymoma.

improvement, her difficulties returned, focal motor seizures developed followed by a dense hemiparesis. She died within 18 months despite three extensive and heroic attempts to achieve remission with focused beam radiosurgery.

For the medical oncologist and internist, metastatic brain tumors are the most common neuro-oncologic challenge. Of all cancer patients, 25% develop CNS metastases, usually after the primary tumor has been diagnosed, but occasionally as the initial sign as noted in this vignette. Typically CNS metastases are either a single or multiple solid tumors compressing the brain and spinal cord, or more diffusely with leptomeningeal infiltration of cancer cells throughout the CSF and neuraxis, especially involving spinal and cranial nerve roots.

Lung cancer is the most common primary tumor that metastasizes to the CNS (50%), followed by breast (33%), colon (9%), and melanoma (7%) (Fig. 52-11). The interval between the primary diagnosis and presentation of a CNS metastasis depends on the tumor type. For lung cancer, the median interval is 4 months; for breast cancer, 3 years. CNS metastasis is an indicator of poor prognosis and portends a survival of <6 months for most patients.

Clinical Presentation and Diagnosis

As with primary CNS malignancies, clinical presentation depends on the tumor site. The onset can be almost precipitous, mimicking a stroke, or can be indolent, with gradual development of focal neurologic deficit: motor, sensory, language, visual, gait, or coordination. In other instances, patients may have focal or generalized seizures or present with nonspecific symptoms, perhaps suggesting increased intracranial pressure, such as positional headaches, cranial neuropathies, and rarely nausea, vomiting, or both.

Gadolinium-enhanced MRI typically demonstrates the presence of focal metastases. When there is a hemorrhagic

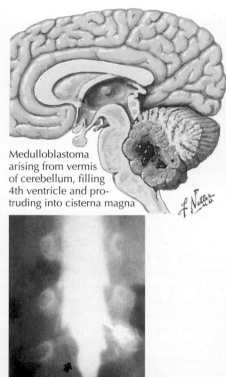

Medulloblastoma arising from vermis of cerebellum, filling 4th ventricle and protruding into cisterna magna

CT scan showing enhancing medulloblastoma in region of 4th ventricle; obstructive hydrocephalus indicated by dilated temporal horn (arrows)

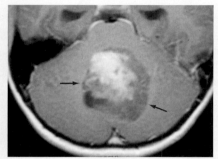

Axial post contrast T1-weighted brain MR: Large, hetero-geneously enhancing intra-fourth ventricular mass lesion (arrows).

Postoperative lumbar metrizamide myelogram showing lumbar seeding of tumor evidenced by nonfilling of S1 root on right side (arrow)

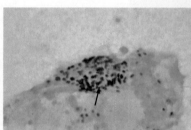

Positive CSF cytologic findings in patient with medulloblastoma; malignant tumor cells clumped on Millipore filter

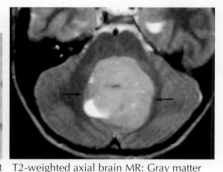

T2-weighted axial brain MR: Gray matter isointense large intraventricular mass lesion (arrows).

Diagnostic images courtesy Tina Young Poussaint, MD, Children's Hospital, Boston.

Figure 52-8 Medulloblastoma.

component, an underlying melanoma is most often responsible. Typically, a number of melanoma patients have forgotten their seemingly innocuous and remote skin lesion or thought it irrelevant as there is often a major delay in the eventual presentation of the metastasis in comparison to the time of its initial removal.

Meningeal gadolinium enhancement portends the presence of carcinomatous leptomeningeal invasion with the important exception of the low pressure syndrome (see below). The malignant enhancement usually has a very irregular character in contrast to the very smooth enhancement seen with the very benign low pressure syndrome (see Fig. 52-23). CSF cytologic analysis, in most instances of leptomeningeal cancer, demonstrates an increased number of malignant cells, thus confirming the diagnosis. Sometimes the initial CSF in this setting is negative. Here, if there is a high clinical suspicion, one must make repeated spinal taps. On one occasion we had a patient who required six different CSF cytologic examinations before a specific diagnosis could be made.

Treatment

Although treatment is clearly palliative, most metastatic brain cancer patients benefit some from CNS-directed therapy. Whole brain RT is indicated for most of these individuals. The patient with an isolated, single brain lesion, who has no evidence of systemic recurrence, is a candidate for surgical resection. On

occasion, the pathology is totally unexpected in that some resected solitary lesions, initially thought to be a metastasis prove to have an entirely different pathology, including benign tumors such as a meningioma. Focal radiation is helpful only in patients with one to two lesions who are otherwise stable. In the occasional patient having a solitary brain metastasis and who has received surgery or focal RT, it is reasonable to withhold whole brain RT until there is evidence of tumor progression in the brain. Rarely there is a symptom-free interlude of a number of years after the initial resection of an isolated metastasis.

Treatment of carcinomatous meningitis involves direct infusion of chemotherapeutic agents, either methotrexate or cytarabine, directly into the CSF via lumbar puncture or preferably a ventricular reservoir. This is a palliative treatment at best; the overall prognosis is usually just a matter of months once malignant leptomeningeal invasion is confirmed.

Therapy and Future Directions

Treatment of malignant brain tumors remains challenging and often unsuccessful. Advances in therapy are being made in the field of imaging, where PET and MR spectroscopy are often able to distinguish recurrent tumors from necrotic, posttreatment change. Image guidance in the operating room allows for smaller, more precisely located incisions and provides real-time information on the extent of tumor resection.

Child with ataxia, wide gait, tendency to fall, headache, and vomiting

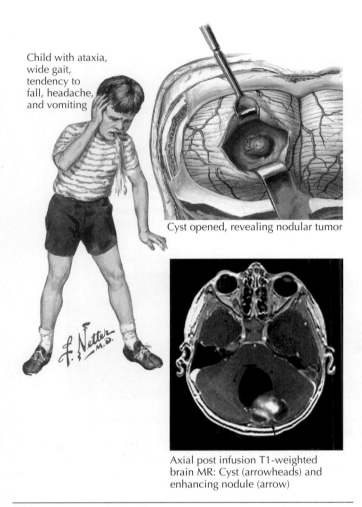

Cyst opened, revealing nodular tumor

Axial post infusion T1-weighted brain MR: Cyst (arrowheads) and enhancing nodule (arrow)

Figure 52-9 Cystic Astrocytoma of Cerebellum.

responding to the modest simple analgesics that she had previously used. She was unaware of any precipitating factors. Her family physician evaluated her; she also reported that recently her marriage had fallen apart when it became widely acknowledged in her small local community that her husband was having multiple affairs. She was very embarrassed and had become socially withdrawn. Her practitioner requested a neurologic consultation. Subsequently this neurologic consultant determined that her examination was normal. A diagnosis of tension stress headache was made. Amitriptyline was prescribed prophylactically. She was referred to a marriage counselor.

The headaches became increasingly bothersome, at times awakening her from her sleep; she had periods of helplessness and spells of crying. She was switched to a selective serotonin reuptake inhibitor for presumed increasing depression. However, she was not convinced of the diagnosis and sought another neurologic opinion. Her history remained unchanged. The only possible abnormal finding on neurologic examination was a subtle suggestion of a left central facial weakness. When this was called to her attention as to whether this finding was new or just a normal asymmetry, neither she nor her accompanying sister had previously noted this, suggesting that this was a significant observation. Contrast-enhanced brain CT demonstrated a homogeneously enhancing mass overlying the right frontal cortex. Brain MRI confirmed its superficial location. There was concomitant dura mater enhancement within the area immediately adjacent to the tumor. A meningioma was identified at surgery; a complete surgical resection was successfully performed. Postoperatively, her headaches ceased.

Radiotherapy remains the mainstay for treating malignant brain neoplasms. Stereotactic radiosurgery is being used more frequently to provide additional doses to previously irradiated tissue, improving the control of tumor growth.

Perhaps the greatest improvements in treating gliomas are the novel chemotherapy treatments, such as temozolomide, that are showing promise in controlling tumor growth. Gene therapy and other targeted, biochemically based treatments are also showing promise.

BENIGN BRAIN TUMORS

MENINGIOMAS

Clinical Vignette

A 48-year-old healthy woman, mother of two young adult children and a respected school teacher, had a history of chronic intermittent low-grade generalized headaches with a family history of migraine. Recently she noted that her headaches were occurring more frequently. These were not

Demographics

Meningiomas typically occur in middle-aged and older individuals, especially women, but do occur at any age. Approximately 15–20% of intracranial tumors are meningiomas. These tumors may present at any level of the neuraxis; they are primarily located intracranially, typically found at the parasagittal falx cerebri separating the two hemispheres, the meninges covering the hemispheres, along the sphenoid ridge medial skull base, and the olfactory groove along the anterior skull base. Meningioma is typically a benign lesion arising from arachnoid meningeal cells.

Classically, these are slow-growing tumors attaining large size before becoming symptomatic; however, occasionally they seem to grow much more rapidly, especially during pregnancy. Meningiomas arising adjacent to the frontal lobe are particularly prone to being clinically silent because of the disproportionately large size of this part of the brain where there is much more tissue to be "forgiving." Such a slowly enlarging lesion can gradually compress brain tissue without producing definitive symptoms in this "clinically silent" part of the brain. A good example occurs when a meningioma affects the prefrontal cortex. Subtle personality changes gradually develop that are only appreciated in retrospect. However, if the tumor lies adjacent to overtly functional brain tissue, such as the motor cortex, symptoms may present relatively early (Fig. 52-12).

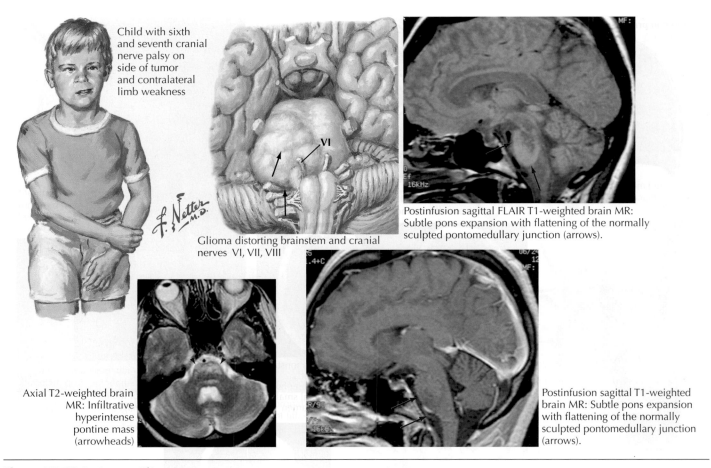

Child with sixth and seventh cranial nerve palsy on side of tumor and contralateral limb weakness

VI

Glioma distorting brainstem and cranial nerves VI, VII, VIII

Postinfusion sagittal FLAIR T1-weighted brain MR: Subtle pons expansion with flattening of the normally sculpted pontomedullary junction (arrows).

Axial T2-weighted brain MR: Infiltrative hyperintense pontine mass (arrowheads)

Postinfusion sagittal T1-weighted brain MR: Subtle pons expansion with flattening of the normally sculpted pontomedullary junction (arrows).

Figure 52-10 Brainstem Glioma.

Clinical Presentation

Meningiomas usually have an ingravescent course, presenting with a variety of symptoms such as long-standing headache, personality change, particularly disinhibition when involving the prefrontal cortex, various types of focal seizures, gait difficulties, or varied cranial nerve palsies as simple as unilateral loss of smell with olfactory groove lesions. On rare occasions, meningiomas may have a precipitous onset mimicking a stroke or even a brief transient ischemic attack. Today many relatively small and clinically silent meningiomas are first identified incidentally on CT and MRI during evaluation of unrelated events, such as for evaluation of posttraumatic injury. Presumed meningiomas located at the base of the skull near blood vessels need to be differentiated from cerebral aneurysms. These lesions are best evaluated with magnetic resonance angiography (MRA) to distinguish these disorders prior to consideration for possible neurosurgery.

Treatment

A decision to treat meningiomas rests on several factors. Because many are initially asymptomatic, it is important to determine that subsequently appearing neurologic symptoms arise from the lesion per se. Given the typical slow growth of these benign tumors when the patient continues to be asymptomatic,

radiographic follow-up is recommended on an annual to biannual basis. No treatment is necessary for those individuals who remain asymptomatic when follow-up CT and MRI demonstrate no change in tumor size or configuration. When the patient develops progressive symptoms or follow-up imaging indicates increasing size of the tumor, surgical resection is in order.

The surgical complexity is directly related to tumor site; those on the brain convexity or along the falx cerebri are often easily resected. Skull base tumors located near blood vessels and cranial nerves often present a surgical challenge when the meningioma becomes entwined with these structures. Radiation therapy, chemotherapy, or both are rarely used to treat typical benign meningiomas. Antiprogesterone agents to slow the growth of the meningiomas are being investigated.

PITUITARY ADENOMA

Clinical Vignette

Bilateral galactorrhea developed in a 32-year-old woman. Her menses had stopped a few months earlier and she thought she was pregnant; however, pregnancy testing was negative. Otherwise, she was in excellent health. Three

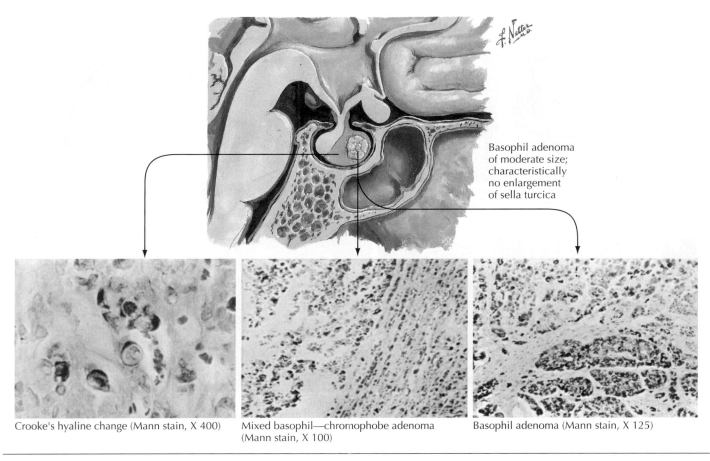

Basophil adenoma of moderate size; characteristically no enlargement of sella turcica

Crooke's hyaline change (Mann stain, X 400)

Mixed basophil—chromophobe adenoma (Mann stain, X 100)

Basophil adenoma (Mann stain, X 125)

Figure 52-14 Basophilic Adenoma Cushing Disease.

skull, and hands. Cushing disease with truncal obesity, cervical buffalo hump, moon-like flushed facies, proximal muscle weakness, hypokalemia, and glucose intolerance occurs when pituitary adenomas primarily secrete adrenocorticotropic hormone, leading to increased circulating serum cortisol (Fig. 52-14).

Chromophobe adenomas are not endocrinologically productive; however when an adenoma develops here initially these tumors may be clinically silent. Although histologically benign, pituitary adenomas may have serious consequences when undiagnosed early on because their proximity to the optic nerves, the optic tracts, the cavernous sinus, and the temporal lobe tip may lead to significant neurologic consequences. The nonendocrinologically active tumors frequently reach a large size before symptoms develop (Fig. 52-15). Typically, their diagnosis depends on the presentation of mass effect symptoms. Bitemporal visual field cuts result when pituitary macroadenomas extend above the sella and compress the overlying optic chiasm.

Pituitary apoplexy is a relatively rare clinical presentation for pituitary adenomas. Classically, this is an acute-onset severe headache associated with significant visual impairment and decreased mental status. Sometimes this may well mimic a ruptured intracranial aneurysm. The cause is often a hemorrhage into a preexisting pituitary adenoma (Fig. 52-16).

Diagnostic Approach

Patients with suspected pituitary adenomas are evaluated with a combination of imaging and endocrinologic studies. Brain MRI is the best radiographic modality to identify pituitary tumors. Sella expansion, diminished enhancement within the sella, and shifting of the pituitary stalk to one side are all clues for a possible pituitary microadenoma In contrast, macroadenomas (measuring >25 mm) extend above the sella or into the cavernous sinus on either side of the sella and are easily identified with MRI (see Fig. 52-16). A thorough endocrine evaluation includes serum levels of prolactin, follicle-stimulating hormone and luteinizing hormone, cortisol, and growth hormone and thyroid function parameters.

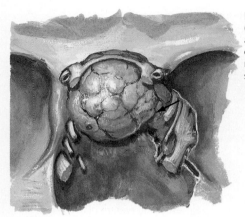

Invasive (malignant) adenoma; extension into right cavernous sinus

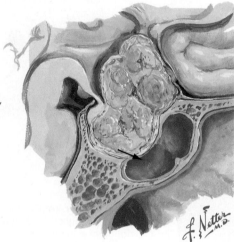

Large acidophil adenoma; extensive destruction of pituitary substance, compression of optic chiasm, invasion of third ventricle and floor of sella

Nonfunctioning

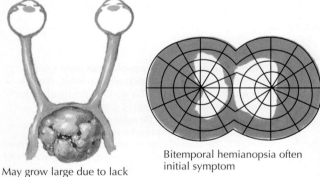

May grow large due to lack of early endocrine symptoms; optic chiasm compressed

Bitemporal hemianopsia often initial symptom

Figure 52-15 Pituitary Macroadenoma.

Treatment

Initially many pituitary adenoma patients primarily require medical therapy. Prolactin secreting tumors are often successfully controlled with bromocriptine, a dopamine agonist that suppresses prolactin production and concomitantly decreases tumor volume. Growth hormone–secreting tumors are often controlled with octreotide, a somatostatin analog. Small, nonsecreting pituitary tumors may often be observed for endocrine dysfunction or signs of growth with combined clinical and MRI modalities.

Endocrinologically active tumors that cannot be controlled with medication are a prime indication for surgical treatment as are patients harboring a macroadenoma producing mass effect. The surgery is primarily performed using a transsphenoidal approach through the nasal cavity and the sphenoid sinus, wherein the contents of the sella can be visualized and the tumor can be removed, often sparing the pituitary gland.

Postoperatively, these patients require follow-up for signs of hypopituitarism. This is particularly important for those individuals presenting with Cushing disease. Subsequent to surgery, their adrenocorticotropic hormone secretion is diminished. These patients usually require postoperative and sometimes lifelong steroid replacement. Pituitary adenoma surgery is associated with concomitant sodium balance and fluid intake problems leading to hyponatremia with polydipsia and polyuria. This necessitates careful follow-up and sometimes treatment with desmopressin acetate (DDAVP) to replace the naturally occurring antidiuretic hormone (ADH). This is a synthetic analogue of the natural pituitary hormone 8-arginine vasopressin, an ADH affecting renal water conservation.

CRANIOPHARYNGIOMA

Craniopharyngiomas are uncommon tumors thought to arise from a remnant of the brain's embryologic development, namely, the Rathke pouch. These histologically benign cystic lesions, often occurring in the region of the sella, hypothalamus, or third ventricle, comprise 2–3% of all intracranial tumors. There is a greater incidence in children. Typically the presenting symptoms include visual impairment, pituitary dysfunction, and hydrocephalus.

The radiographic features of craniopharyngiomas distinguish them from other tumors of the suprasellar region (Fig. 52-17). Cystic changes, variable-contrast enhancement, and calcification seen on CT occur frequently.

Surgery is the treatment of choice for symptomatic craniopharyngiomas. The suprasellar location limits tumor access, making incomplete resections common. Resection is also difficult because of the intense glial reaction of the surrounding brain, causing adherence to critical brain structures and nearby blood vessels. As with pituitary surgery, craniopharyngioma resection may also have a difficult postoperative course, particularly with endocrine dysfunction. Although radiation therapy and possibly radiosurgery can decrease recurrence rates, craniopharyngiomas have a high rate of local recurrence.

A. Grade of sella turcica enlargement and/or erosion

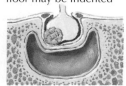 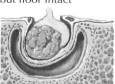 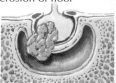 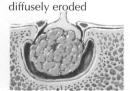

Enclosed adenomas

I. Sella normal, floor may be indented

II. Sella enlarged, but floor intact

Invasive adenomas

III. Localized erosion of floor

IV. Entire floor diffusely eroded

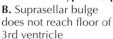

B. Type of suprasellar extension

A. No suprasellar extension of tumor

B. Suprasellar bulge does not reach floor of 3rd ventricle

C. Tumor reaches 3rd ventricle, distorting its chiasmatic recess

D. Tumor fills 3rd ventricle almost to interventricular foramen (of Monro)

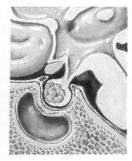 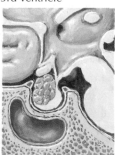 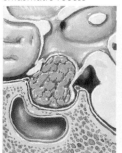 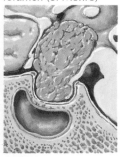

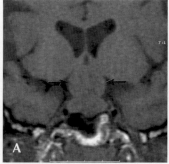 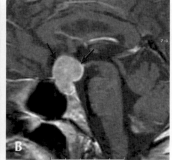

Large pituitary tumor. (**A**) Coronal T1-weighted and (**B**) sagittal T1-weighted post–gadolinium-enhanced images show a dumbbell-shaped tumor within a moderately enlarged sella with a larger component protruding above and posterior to the sella with elevation and distortion of the optic chiasm.

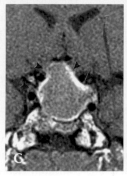 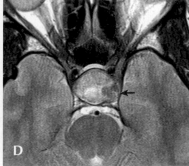

Pituitary apoplexy in a 44-year-old man presenting with severe headache, diplopia, photophobia, nausea and vomiting. (**C**) Coronal T1-weighted post gadolinium-enhanced fast spin echo imaging demonstrates a large intrasellar mass with peripheral enhancement (arrowheads) and upward displacement of the optic chiasm. (**D**) The central nonenhanced component shows a very heterogeneous signal pattern on axial T2-weighted imaging with more compression of the left cavernous sinus (arrow) and represents a hemorrhagic necrotic pituitary adenoma.

Figure 52-16 Pituitary Adenoma Gradation vis-à-vis Sella Enlargement.

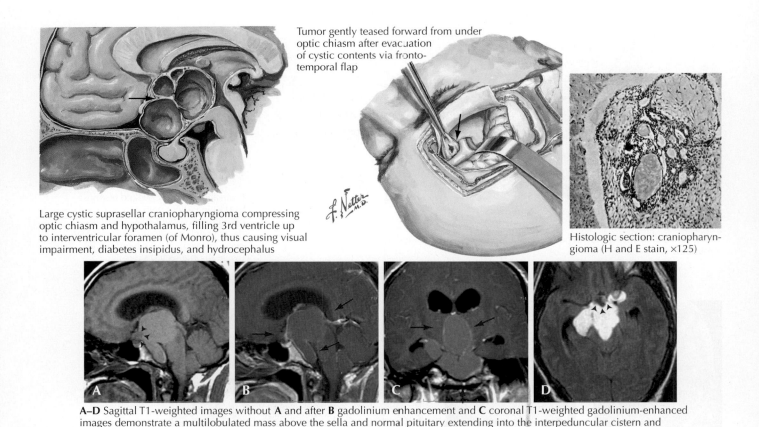

Tumor gently teased forward from under optic chiasm after evacuation of cystic contents via fronto-temporal flap

Large cystic suprasellar craniopharyngioma compressing optic chiasm and hypothalamus, filling 3rd ventricle up to interventricular foramen (of Monro), thus causing visual impairment, diabetes insipidus, and hydrocephalus

Histologic section: craniopharyn-gioma (H and E stain, ×125)

A–D Sagittal T1-weighted images without **A** and after **B** gadolinium enhancement and **C** coronal T1-weighted gadolinium-enhanced images demonstrate a multilobulated mass above the sella and normal pituitary extending into the interpeduncular cistern and into the prepontine cistern. The posterior portion above the sella is solid (arrowheads), whereas the remainder is cystic with faint rim enhancement. The T2-weighted axial image **D** shows the darker solid component (arrowheads) and the T2-bright cystic portions.

Figure 52-17 Craniopharyngioma.

ACOUSTIC NEUROMAS/ VESTIBULAR SCHWANNOMA

Clinical Vignette

A previously healthy 42-year-old Army chaplain noted that he could no longer hear well on the telephone using his left ear or understand a colleague when there was much ambient noise particularly from other conversations. In retrospect, he had experienced mild progressive ringing in this ear. Initially this was attributed to chronic loud noise exposure while assigned to an artillery brigade. Although this gradually worsened over several years, it was not until his telephone difficulties led him to test himself that he found he could no longer appreciate the sound of a watch ticking. He was otherwise totally well. His only abnormal finding on neurologic examination was grossly diminished hearing in his left ear.

Audiometric examination revealed markedly decreased high-frequency appreciation and diminished speech discrimination in his left ear. Gadolinium MRI demonstrated a homogeneously enhancing 2 × 1.5-cm mass within the left cerebellar pontine angle. This emanated from his internal auditory canal and was associated with mild pontine distortion.

Demographics

Acoustic neuromas are the second most common of the benign brain tumors. These comprise approximately 6–8% of all primary intracranial neoplasms. There is a 2% incidence within the general population. Most commonly, acoustic neuromas present between ages 40 and 60 years. With the exception of patients who have genetically determined neurofibromatosis type II, it is unusual to see a patient have an acoustic neuroma become clinically recognized before age 20 years. The non–genetically determined acoustic neuromas predominantly develop unilaterally. In contrast, those occasional patients with type II neurofibromatosis often have bilateral acoustic neuromas. These benign tumors arise from the Schwann cells of the vestibular nerve within the eighth cranial nerve complex (Fig. 52-18).

Clinical Presentation

The classic history is illustrated in the above clinical vignette. Patients typically report a slowly progressive, unilateral hearing loss associated with tinnitus. This is consistent with the innate slow growth of a benign acoustic neuroma (also referred to as a vestibular schwannoma).

Although acoustic neuromas arise from the vestibular portion of cranial nerve (CN) VIII, hearing loss is usually the most prominent symptom. Anatomically, CN-VII (facial) is closely

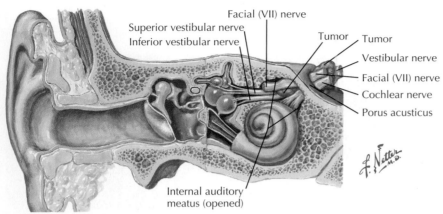

Small neurinoma arising from superior vestibular nerve in internal auditory meatus and protruding into posterior fossa

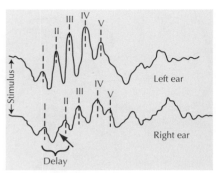

Brainstem auditory evoked response (BAER) in patient with acoustic neurinoma on right side. There is delay in action potentials of cochlear nerve (wave I) and cochlear nuclei (wave II) on affected side.

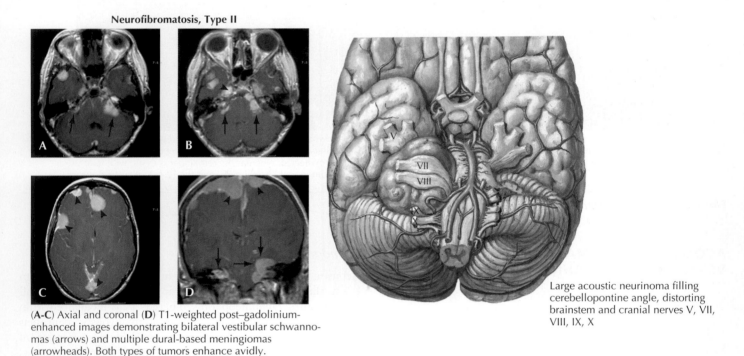

Neurofibromatosis, Type II

(**A-C**) Axial and coronal (**D**) T1-weighted post–gadolinium-enhanced images demonstrating bilateral vestibular schwannomas (arrows) and multiple dural-based meningiomas (arrowheads). Both types of tumors enhance avidly.

Large acoustic neurinoma filling cerebellopontine angle, distorting brainstem and cranial nerves V, VII, VIII, IX, X

Figure 52-18 Acoustic Neuroma.

related to CN-VIII; however, it is almost unheard of for an acute facial nerve palsy to be the initial presenting symptom of an acoustic neuroma. Because of the eighth nerve's relation to the vestibular nerve within the cerebellopontine angle, adjacent to the brainstem and cerebellum, patients with very large acoustic neuromas may also have gait instability and sometimes associated headaches, but these individuals do not present with acute vertigo. Later on an acoustic neuroma may sometimes lead to pressure on either the trigeminal (fifth) cranial nerve or its adjacent brainstem, affecting CN-V function with a resultant ipsilateral facial sensory loss and a diminished corneal reflex. Occasionally very large tumors may impair the CSF circulation near the fourth ventricle, leading to hydrocephalus.

During clinical examination, cranial nerve evaluation is the key to this diagnosis and of utmost importance. Hearing loss

from CN-VIII involvement is the hallmark finding for acoustic neuromas. Lateral gaze nystagmus is occasionally noted when testing extraocular movements. Larger tumors may cause CN-VII and CN-V impairment as previously summarized. It is most unusual to have any lower cranial nerve involvement or clinically significant enough brainstem compression to lead to either a hemiparesis or hemisensory loss.

Diagnostic Studies

MRI is the primary diagnostic modality. Its clarity, resolution, and ability to scan in multiple planes allow for three-dimensional assessment. Because lesion size and its relation to adjacent neurologic structures, such as the pons and various cranial nerves, often determine treatment, MRI is also a therapeutically very

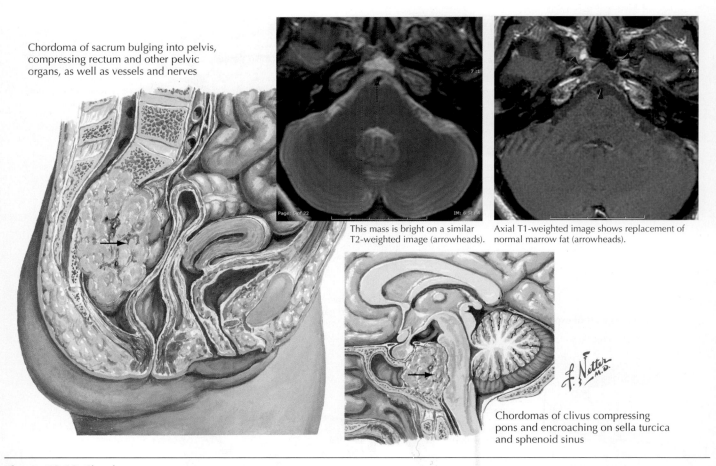

Chordoma of sacrum bulging into pelvis, compressing rectum and other pelvic organs, as well as vessels and nerves

This mass is bright on a similar T2-weighted image (arrowheads).

Axial T1-weighted image shows replacement of normal marrow fat (arrowheads).

Chordomas of clivus compressing pons and encroaching on sella turcica and sphenoid sinus

Figure 52-19 Chordomas.

crucial investigational modality. Typically, these well-demarcated, homogeneously enhancing tumors arise within the cerebellar pontine angle and extend into the internal auditory canal (see Fig. 52-18).

Treatment

Surgery is the traditional and primary therapeutic modality; stereotactic radiosurgery is occasionally used. Acoustic neuromas often grow slowly. It is reasonable to observe some tumors temporally, if clinically warranted, particularly with elderly patients presenting with unilateral hearing loss who also have multiple other medical issues. Often the better part of valor here is to just follow the patient with serial imaging. When MRI evidence demonstrates significant tumor growth or patients have progressively worsening symptoms, especially in addition to hearing loss, surgical intervention is indicated.

Surgical resection of acoustic neuromas is often performed concomitantly using both neurosurgery and otorhinolaryngology specialists. The surgical goal is tumor resection and preservation of CN-VII and CN-VIII function when at all possible. This approach is particularly important with large-volume tumors exhibiting brainstem compression. Hearing preservation in patients with these large acoustic neuromas is often impossible because the cochlear nerve becomes indistinguishable from the tumor. Success rates for hearing preservation vary directly with tumor volume. When CN-VII is densely adherent to the tumor capsule, a subtotal resection is often indicated, because facial nerve preservation is more important than complete surgical removal.

Stereotactic radiosurgery involves a single nonsurgical treatment using high-dose radiation to a precisely localized three-dimensional volume. This modality can control approximately 80–85% of acoustic tumors. It retains many of the same risks as conventional surgery but is an excellent option for patients with small tumors (2–3 cm) who have no useful hearing. Control of tumor growth is achieved and operative risks are avoided. With improved imaging, acoustic neuromas are being detected earlier; therefore, greater potential exists to achieve a complete cure early on in the natural history of the acoustic neuroma.

OTHER BENIGN INTRACRANIAL TUMORS

Chordoma

These are very rare usually benign tumors that have embryologic elements similar to intervertebral disks. Typically, chordomas develop either on the clivus of the skull base or the sacrum (Fig. 52-19). Intracranial chordomas arise from within the skull bone and cause local destruction. Concomitantly these tumors enter the intradural space, where they sometimes affect the brainstem and cranial nerves.

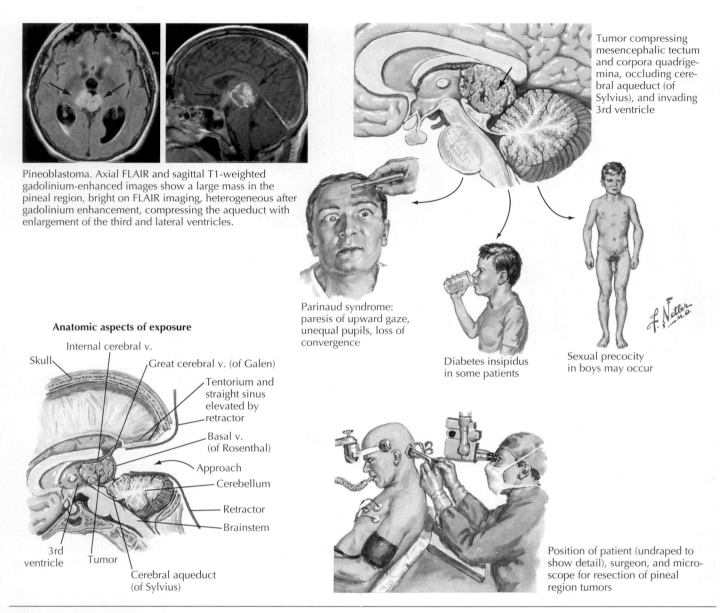

Pineoblastoma. Axial FLAIR and sagittal T1-weighted gadolinium-enhanced images show a large mass in the pineal region, bright on FLAIR imaging, heterogeneous after gadolinium enhancement, compressing the aqueduct with enlargement of the third and lateral ventricles.

Tumor compressing mesencephalic tectum and corpora quadrigemina, occluding cerebral aqueduct (of Sylvius), and invading 3rd ventricle

Parinaud syndrome: paresis of upward gaze, unequal pupils, loss of convergence

Diabetes insipidus in some patients

Sexual precocity in boys may occur

Anatomic aspects of exposure

Internal cerebral v.

Skull

Great cerebral v. (of Galen)

Tentorium and straight sinus elevated by retractor

Basal v. (of Rosenthal)

Approach

Cerebellum

Retractor

Brainstem

3rd ventricle

Tumor

Cerebral aqueduct (of Sylvius)

Position of patient (undraped to show detail), surgeon, and microscope for resection of pineal region tumors

Figure 52-20 Pineal Region Tumors.

The histology of typical chordomas is characterized by, large, mucus-filled cells called physaliferous cells. Very uncommonly, a few chordomas demonstrate features of frank malignancy. Additionally their aggressive local invasion of bone mimics a locally malignant process. The tumors that lead to significant bony destruction often recur locally at a high rate, thus making a surgical cure difficult to achieve. Nevertheless, surgical resection is often used initially, but complete resection is often impossible because of local anatomic constraints. Although radiation therapy is generally used, the role of this modality for treatment of residual tumor is unclear. Radiosurgery and proton beam irradiation have been proposed, but their benefit is also uncertain. Chemotherapy is not of value for treatment of chordomas.

Pineal Region Tumors

Tumors occurring in the region of the pineal gland are uncommon, comprising approximately 1% of intracranial tumors. These neoplasms, having a histologically mixed benignancy, include germ cell tumors, glial neoplasms, and pineal parenchyma tumors (Fig. 52-20). Germ cell origin tumors are the most common, usually occurring in younger patients. Gliomas can arise from within the pineal gland itself or from the glial cells in the surrounding tissue. In this region, glial tumors tend to be of lower grade. Tumors arising from the pineal parenchyma comprise approximately 20% of pineal region tumors.

These neoplasms are further classified into pineoblastomas and pineocytomas. *Pineoblastomas* are poorly differentiated

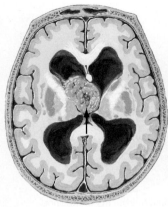

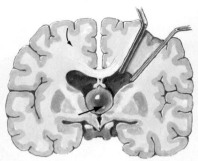

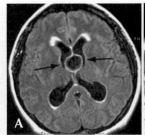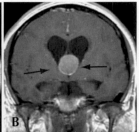

Subependymoma of anterior horn of left lateral ventricle obstructing interventricular foramen (of Monro), thus producing marked hydrocephalus

Colloid cyst of 3rd ventricle and surgical approach via right prefrontal (silent) cerebral cortex. May also be approached through corpus callosum (arrow). Note enlarged lateral ventricles (posterior view).

Colloid cyst. (**A**) Axial, FLAIR and (**B**) coronal, T1-weighted gadolinium-enhanced images demonstrate a round cystic mass in the region of the foramina of Monro, with dilatation of the lateral ventricles. The signal characteristics are variable. This cyst is hypointense on T2-weighted images and bright on T1-weighted imaging, with minimal peripheral enhancement.

Figure 52-21 Intraventricular Tumors.

tumors that can spread throughout the cerebrospinal fluid pathways or directly into adjacent brain parenchyma. *Pineocytomas* are usually well-encapsulated cellular tumors that do not invade surrounding tissue. A mixed form of pineal parenchymal tumor contains features of both pineocytoma and pineoblastoma. Teratomas, embryonal carcinomas, endodermal sinus tumors, and choriocarcinomas are also found in the pineal region.

With the increasing use of MRI, asymptomatic pineal region cysts are identified more commonly. These cysts are usually incidental findings and rarely require any treatment. Serial MRI scans are used to track any growth over time.

Colloid Cysts

These are histologically benign third ventricle tumors that arise from embryologic development remnants. The cells lining the walls of the cyst are ciliated. Third ventricular lesions of this type typically do become symptomatic during adulthood but can be seen in children. Posturally precipitated headaches, with concomitant symptoms and signs of hydrocephalus are the most common clinical presentations for colloid cysts. Because of their inherent intraventricular location, these cysts lead to CSF obstruction at the foramina of Monro (Fig. 52-21).

Colloid cysts occasionally are associated with sudden death presumably from an acute hydrocephalus; however, most patients present with a more gradual temporal profile. Although the diagnosis is typically suggested by recurrent posturally triggered headaches, MRI or CT is ideal for confirming the presence of a cystic-appearing intraventricular mass.

Treatment of symptomatic colloid cysts is usually surgical, and complete resection is often possible. Care must be exercised during surgical resection because the fornix, adjacent to the tumor, can be injured, resulting in severe memory impairment. If surgery for resection is not possible, CSF diversion through shunting can often relieve the symptoms of hydrocephalus.

With the increased use of MRI, many more cystic tumors within the third ventricle are being described. These asymptomatic lesions are followed with serial scans; treatment is reserved for those patients whose cysts increase in size.

DIFFERENTIAL DIAGNOSIS
Pseudotumor Cerebri/Idiopathic Intracranial Hypotension, Intracranial Hypotension, and Other Brain Lesions

> ### Clinical Vignette
>
> *An obese 42-year-old woman presented with a 2-month history of increasingly severe headaches and intermittent double vision. Her headaches were exacerbated by postural changes, particularly bending forward or jarring in the car. Bilateral limitation of adduction of her eyes compatible with sixth cranial nerve paresis and modest papilledema (Fig. 52-22) were noted on neurologic examination. Brain imaging demonstrated diminished size of her lateral ventricles. Cerebrospinal fluid (CSF) pressure was 350 mm CSF (normal < 180 mm CSF); it was otherwise normal.*

This case is representative of a rather uncommon syndrome known as idiopathic intracranial hypertension, i.e., pseudotumor cerebri (PTC). This usually occurs in obese young women who are otherwise healthy. Clinically PTC is primarily characterized by progressively severe, poorly defined headaches, often with diplopia. Transient visual obscurations and pulsatile tinnitus may also occur. On neurologic examination these patients are typically awake, alert, have papilledema, sometimes a lateral rectus muscle weakness, but no focal neurologic deficits. By definition MRI is normal or demonstrates small lateral ventricles. PTC by definition is associated with increased CSF pressure (250–500 mm CSF).

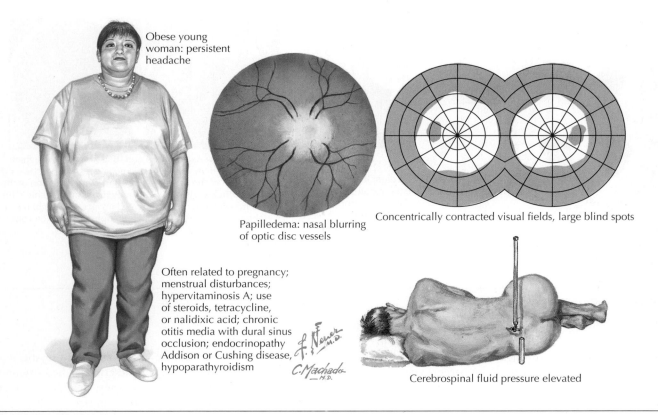

Obese young woman: persistent headache

Papilledema: nasal blurring of optic disc vessels

Concentrically contracted visual fields, large blind spots

Often related to pregnancy; menstrual disturbances; hypervitaminosis A; use of steroids, tetracycline, or nalidixic acid; chronic otitis media with dural sinus occlusion; endocrinopathy Addison or Cushing disease, hypoparathyroidism

Cerebrospinal fluid pressure elevated

Figure 52-22 Pseudotumor Cerebri.

Although idiopathic PTC has no identifiable etiology, certain predisposing factors need to be considered, including oral contraceptives, corticosteroids, estrogens and progestational therapies, NSAIDs, hypervitaminosis A, various antibiotics (tetracycline, minocycline, nitrofurantoin, ampicillin, or nalidixic acid), anesthetic agents (ketamine and nitrous oxide), amiodarone, and perhexiline.

Other neurologic disorders may occasionally present with a PTC clinical picture. These include leptomeningeal diseases such as chronic infectious or granulomatous processes, that is, tuberculosis, metastatic cancer or lymphoma seeding, cerebral venous sinus obstruction, and various endocrinologic disorders, for example, myxedema, hypoparathyroidism, and Addison and Cushing diseases. There are very rare reports of a PTC picture presumed to be related to extremely elevated CSF protein levels, particularly with Guillain–Barré syndrome or primary spinal cord malignancies.

Treatment

Discontinuation of an offending medication will reverse the PTC syndrome on the rare occasion such is identified. Most importantly one needs to be concerned by the fact that chronic increased intracranial pressure leads to loss of visual acuity. This is secondary to swelling of the optic nerve head, that is, papilledema. It is measured by frequent and formal visual field testing to identify increasing size of the blind spots. This is essential to prevent permanent visual loss with PTC. Potential treatments include weight loss, low-salt diet, diuretics, and symptomatic headache control. When PTC continues to evolve with progressive visual compromise, more aggressive therapy is indicated, including optic nerve sheath fenestration or one of the various CSF shunting procedures.

Intracranial Hypotension (Low-CSF-Pressure Syndrome)

Clinical Vignette

A vigorous previously healthy 60-year-old physician, who had recently developed severe depression, requiring both a serotonin reuptake inhibitor as well as unilateral electric shock therapy (EST), developed increasingly severe posturally exacerbated headaches. When these were greatly exacerbated while he was a passenger in a small float plane as it landed bouncing over the water, he went to a neurologist. His examination was normal. Postgadolinium MRI demonstrated leptomeningeal enhancement but no mass lesions. CSF pressure was too low to measure. No known relation with the EST was identified. He then recalled having a relatively severe closed head injury 3 weeks earlier when he forcefully struck his forehead on an unexpectedly low-set barn door frame. A 20-mL extradural blood patch was empirically injected at his mid-lumbar spine. The headaches gradually and totally cleared within 2 weeks.

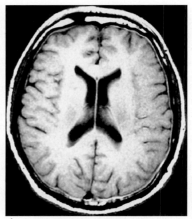

A. Axial FLAIR image with dural thickening.

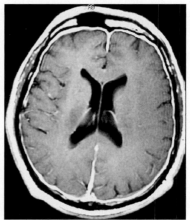

B. Axial T1-weighted, gadolinium-enhanced image with striking enhancement of the thickened dura.

Figure 52-23 Intracranial Hypotension.

Classic low-CSF-pressure headaches are severe, exacerbated by postural factors, and often mimic the ball valve effect seen in some intraventricular brain tumors. Most commonly, these occur subsequent to a diagnostic lumbar puncture, spinal anesthesia, or a seemingly benign closed head injury. MRI with gadolinium is essential to the diagnosis (Fig. 52-23). When there is no history of a spinal tap or significant head trauma, this clinical setting, as well as the MRI, somewhat mimics various leptomeningeal neoplastic or inflammatory lesions. The MRI imaging with low pressure headache syndrome has a smooth enhancement in contrast to serpiginous irregular enhancement seen with neoplastic infiltration. The CSF analysis primarily helps make this differentiation. Occasionally introduction of a radioisotope into the CSF will identify a source of CSF leak that may require surgical repair. In many of these instances, no site of potential spinal fluid leak is identified. As in the above vignette, a spinal blood patch can provide relief and a therapeutic diagnosis; however, it is not universally successful and in rare instances the patient may have permanent incapacitation not being able to raise his/her head, preventing one from pursuing an occupation or even many routine activities of daily living.

Other Intracranial Lesions

Subdural hematomas, herpes encephalitis, brain abscess, and arteriovenous malformations may all have a clinical presentation similar to a brain tumor. There are other rare disorders both of demyelinating nature that require consideration in the differential diagnosis of brain tumors. Occasional patients have MRI findings mimicking a malignant glioma, but stereotactic biopsy demonstrates a primary monofocal acute inflammatory demyelination (see Chapter 46). These lesions usually are self-limited and occur in the setting where there is no prior clinical or MRI evidence of multiple sclerosis. Fortunately these are often responsive to corticosteroids. Subsequently, new lesions may appear in different portions of the cerebral cortex. An acute disseminated encephalomyelitis (ADEM) and acute hemorrhagic leukoencephalopathy (AHL) are two acute postinfectious demyelinating disorders; the former is more likely to respond to corticosteroids and the latter frequently has a fulminate course (see Chapter 47).

Progressive multifocal leukoencephalopathy (PML) may also present in a fashion similar to a brain tumor in immunocompromised hosts receiving long-term immunosuppressive therapy or in patients with HIV (see Chapter 51).

FUTURE DIRECTIONS

Treatment of benign intracranial tumors has improved with better MRI imaging and the development of new surgical techniques that exploit bone removal rather than brain manipulation. These skull base techniques allow for exposure and resection of tumors in previously inaccessible locations within the skull. Intraoperative monitoring of cranial nerve function is being used more frequently to limit the morbidity of these operations.

Improvements in stereotactic radiosurgery continue to allow for tumor growth control while causing fewer radiation adverse effects. Further research into the relation of hormonal receptors in meningiomas may someday allow for a medical means of controlling these tumors.

ADDITIONAL RESOURCES

Ahsan H, Neugut AI, Bruce JN. Trends in incidence of primary malignant brain tumors in USA, 1981-1990. Int J Epidemiol 1995;24(6):1078-1085.

Berger MS, Hadjipanayis CG. Surgery of intrinsic cerebral tumors. Neurosurgery. 2007 Jul;61(Suppl. 1):279-304.

Binder DK, Horton JC, Lawton MT, et al. Idiopathic intracranial hypertension. Neurosurgery 2004;54:538-551.

Black PM. Meningiomas. Neurosurgery 1993;32:643-657.

Castrucci WA, Knisely JP. An update on the treatment of CNS metastases in small cell lung cancer. Cancer J 2008 May-Jun;14(3):138-146.

Ciric I. Long-term management and outcome for pituitary tumors. Neurosurg Clin N Am 2003;14:167-171.

Daumas-Duport C, Scheithauer BW, O'Fallon J, et al. Grading of astrocytomas: a simple and reproducible method. Cancer 1988;62:2152-2165.

Dietrich J, Norden AD, Wen PY. Emerging antiangiogenic treatments for gliomas—efficacy and safety issues. Curr Opin Neurol 2008 Dec;21(6):736-744.

Gutrecht JA, Berger JR, Jones HR, et al. Monofocal acute inflammatory demyelination (MAID): a unique disorder simulating brain neoplasm. South Med J 2002;95:1180-1186.

Karim AB, Afra D, Cornu P, et al. Randomized trial on the efficacy of radiotherapy for cerebral low-grade glioma in the adult: European Organization for Research and Treatment of Cancer Study 22845 with the Medical Research Council study BRO4: an interim analysis. Int J Radiat Oncol Biol Phys 2002;52(2):316-324.

Kennedy PG. Viral encephalitis: causes, differential diagnosis, and management. J Neurol Neurosurg Psychiatry 2004;75(Suppl. 1):i10-i15.

Koss SA, Ulmer JL, Hacein-Bey L. Angiographic features of spontaneous intracranial hypotension. AJNR Am J Neuroradiol 2003;24:704-706.

Larijani B, Bastanhagh MH, Pajouhi M, et al. Presentation and outcome of 93 cases of craniopharyngioma. Eur J Cancer Care (Engl) 2004;13: 11-15.

Maarouf M, Kuchta J, Miletic H, et al. Acute demyelination: diagnostic difficulties and the need for brain biopsy. Acta Neurochir (Wien) 2003; 145:961-969.

MacFarlane R, King TT. Acoustic neurinoma: vestibular schwannoma. In: Kaye AH, Larz Jr ER, editors. Brain Tumors. Philadelphia, Pa: Churchill Livingstone; 1995. p. 577-622.

Mason WP, Cairncross JG. Invited article: the expanding impact of molecular biology on the diagnosis and treatment of gliomas. Neurology 2008 Jul 29;71(5):365-373.

Mathiesen T, Grane P, Lindgren L, et al. Third ventricle colloid cysts: a consecutive 12-year series. J Neurosurg 1997;86:5-12.

Menezes AH, Gantz BJ, Traynelis VC, McCulloch TM. Cranial base chordomas. Clin Neurosurg 1997;44:491-509.

Mokri B. Headaches caused by decreased intracranial pressure: diagnosis and management. Curr Opin Neurol 2003;16:319-326.

Ohgaki H. Epidemiology of brain tumors. Methods Mol Biol 2009;472: 323-342.

Prados MD, Scott C, Curran Jr WJ, et al. Procarbazine, lomustine, and vincristine (PCV) chemotherapy for anaplastic astrocytoma: A retrospective review of radiation therapy oncology group protocols comparing survival with carmustine or PCV adjuvant chemotherapy. J Clin Oncol 1999 Nov;17(11):3389-3395.

Rapport RL, Hillier D, Scearce T, et al. Spontaneous intracranial hypotension from intradural thoracic disc herniation: case report. J Neurosurg 2003;98(Suppl.):282-284.

Raschilas F, Wolff M, Delatour F, et al. Outcome of and prognostic factors for herpes simplex encephalitis in adult patients: results of a multicenter study. Clin Infect Dis 2002;35:254-260.

Tentori L, Graziani G. Recent approaches to improve the antitumor efficacy of temozolomide. Curr Med Chem 2009;16(2):245-257.

Ullrich RT, Kracht LW, Jacobs AH. Neuroimaging in patients with gliomas. Semin Neurol 2008;28(4):484-494.

53

Spinal Cord Tumors

Peter K. Dempsey and Lloyd M. Alderson

*T*he most common spinal cord tumors are metastatic extradural lesions usually but not always occurring in patients with already identified malignancies, either cancers or lymphomas. Their presentation is often relatively acute, usually associated with focal back and/or radicular pain. On occasion, these lesions are the initial clinical manifestation of a heretofore unsuspected systemic malignancy. In contrast, primary intradural spinal cord tumors occur infrequently; typically their presentation is a relatively subtle one, ingravescent in temporal profile. Spinal cord and spinal column tumors are best classified within two categories: *extradural*, occurring outside of the dura, and *intradural*, contained within the dura mater (Table 53-1; Fig. 53-1).

Intradural tumors are further categorized as *extramedullary* or *intramedullary*, depending on their relationship to the spinal cord. *Intradural extramedullary* tumors, usually meningiomas or schwannomas, generally arise outside of the spinal cord parenchyma. These are initially clinically silent; however, with time these tumors surreptitiously enlarge. Once a critical mass is reached, spinal cord compression occurs and symptoms develop. In contrast, *intradural intramedullary* tumors, such as gliomas and ependymomas, originate within parenchyma of the spinal cord. As these intramedullary malignancies primarily expand, important neurologic pathways and cell populations are subsequently compromised and eventually destroyed.

Extradural tumors generally are derived from metastatic lesions to vertebral bodies with extension into the epidural space, causing external compression of the thecal sac and its contents. Primary bony vertebral tumors also occur, both malignant, such as myeloma, and benign, including hemangiomas and osteoid osteomas.

EXTRADURAL SPINAL TUMORS

Clinical Vignette

A 62-year-old postal carrier presented with midthoracic pain and rapidly progressive weakness and numbness in both legs and difficulty initiating his urine stream. During the preceding 6 weeks, he intermittently awakened with midthoracic vertebral pain that increasingly radiated to his epigastrium. This was particularly precipitated by lifting, bending, or straining at stool. An initial gastrointestinal evaluation was normal. Twenty-four hours before admission, he began to experience progressive difficulty standing, walking, and voiding. The morning of this evaluation, he was unable to get out of bed on his own and was totally unable to void. During the past 3 months, he had noted an increasingly irritating cough; he was a 60-pack-year smoker.

Neurologic examination demonstrated a T9 "cord level" to both pinprick and temperature. Muscle stretch reflexes were absent at the knees and ankles, and plantar stimulation was flexor. There was mild tenderness to palpation over the lower thoracic spine. He became incontinent of urine. Rectal sphincter tone was lax.

Spinal radiographs revealed destruction of the T9 vertebral body. Magnetic resonance imaging (MRI) demonstrated a soft tissue mass involving most of the T9 vertebral body, extending into the pedicle, with epidural extension of the tumor into the spinal canal leading to marked compression of the spinal cord. Immediate dexamethasone and subsequent radiation therapy was unsuccessful in reversing his clinical course. Chest radiograph (Fig. 53-2) demonstrated a left main stem bronchus tumor that on biopsy proved to be a primary small cell lung cancer.

Spinal neoplasms are predominantly secondary to metastatic cancer. This occurs in up to one third of cancer patients. Lung, breast, prostate, and lymphoma are the most common metastatic lesions leading to spinal cord compression.

CLINICAL PRESENTATION

Severe focal vertebral pain is frequently the presenting symptom of a metastatic spinal cancer (Fig. 53-2). Unfortunately, back pain is such a ubiquitous complaint that the serious nature of a newly occurring pain is often not appreciated even when there is no history of recent trauma. Sometimes, it is difficult to distinguish pain of a metastatic spinal tumor from the much more common mechanical, degenerative, or osteoarthritic musculoskeletal lower back and/or nerve root disorders. However, pain of metastatic spinal cancer origin is often persistent, frequently unrelated to posture, and tends to increase at night. In contrast to more common mechanical back pain, this pain can be of more recent origin.

Progressive neurologic symptoms often vary and are related to the precise level of spinal column involvement; typically the temporal profile is relatively rapid. Tumors at the cervical and thoracic spinal cord levels present with progressive weakness, numbness, and sphincter dysfunction at levels below the tumor. Sphincter difficulties are nonspecific symptoms per se that may develop with tumors at any spinal level. On occasion, bladder and bowel dysfunction per se may be the initial presenting symptom related to a conus medullaris tumor at the distal tip of the spinal cord. The essential message is that whenever sphincter problems develop in a patient with a known cancer, one needs to be alert to the potential of a spinal metastasis. Examination usually reveals hyperreflexia, Babinski signs, and other long tract signs at spinal levels below the tumor involvement.

When evaluating patients with recent-onset sphincter difficulties and suspicion for a metastatic lesion, it is important to recognize that differentiation of conus medullaris lesions, at the spinal cord tip, versus those within the cauda equina may be difficult. Classically when the clinical findings are symmetric and relatively equally involving both lower extremities, the

Table 53-1 Classification of MRI Abnormalities*

Extradural Extramedullary	Intradural Extramedullary	Intradural Intramedullary
Disc disease	Neurinoma	Syringomyelia
Metastatic carcinoma	Meningioma	Tumor
Lymphoma	Intracranial tumor seeding	Ependymoma
Sarcoma	Ependymoma	Glioma
Plasmacytoma	Medulloblastoma	Hemangioblastoma
Primary bone tumor	Glioma	Myelitis
Scar	Cauda equina lesions	Edema
Abscess	Scarring	Lipoma
Hemangioma	Hypertrophic neuropathy	Rare lesions
Rare lesions	Rare lesions	Abscess
Hemorrhage	Lymphoma	Hematoma
Neurilemmoma	Metastasis	Varix with AVM
Meningioma	Hemangioblastoma	Lymphoma
Chordoma	Lipoma	Neuroblastoma
	Dermoid	Metastasis
	Epidermoid	
	Cyst	
	Clot	

*Dermoid or epidermoid, teratoma, lipoma, and cysts are often associated with spinal dysraphism. In this setting, many tumors are intradural, although they may involve all three areas.

Extradural tumors

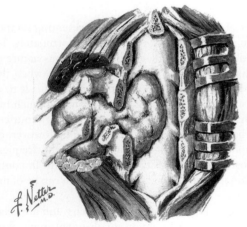

Lymphoma invading spinal canal via intervertebral foramen, compressing dura mater
and spinal cord

Intradural extramedullary tumors

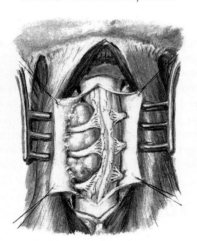

Meningioma compressing spinal cord
and distorting nerve roots

Intramedullary tumors

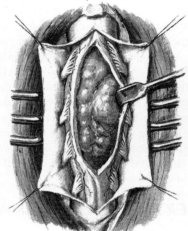

Astrocytoma exposed by longitudinal
incision in bulging spinal cord

Figure 53-1 Classification of Spinal Tumors.

conus medullaris is much more likely the site of the specific pathology. In contrast, cauda equina lesions often lead to an asymmetric distribution of signs and symptoms because not all nerve roots within the cauda equina are equally affected.

Typically, the course of extradural metastatic spinal tumors is more rapid than intradural tumors. It is not unusual for these lesions to have an almost precipitous onset, often producing rapidly evolving motor and sensory deficits within just a few hours to a day or so (Fig. 53-3). A prior diagnosis of either a cancer or a lymphoma will alert the astute clinician to the precise pathophysiologic nature of the spinal lesion. However,

occasionally a spinal metastasis may be the initial presentation of a metastatic malignancy.

DIAGNOSTIC APPROACH

MRI is the standard for evaluating potential metastatic spine lesions, especially those with evolving cord compression. When an MRI is contraindicated, such as with a patient who has a pacemaker, CT myelogram is still a very useful and valid study. An initial preliminary spinal tap is best avoided in these patients as such can change pressure dynamics when there

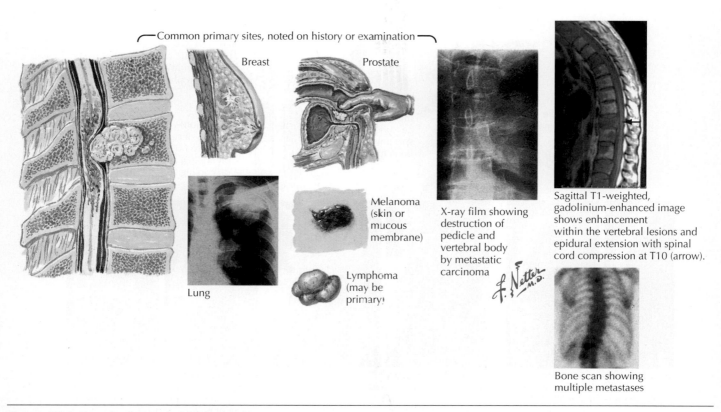

Common primary sites, noted on history or examination

Breast

Prostate

Melanoma (skin or mucous membrane)

Lung

Lymphoma (may be primary)

X-ray film showing destruction of pedicle and vertebral body by metastatic carcinoma

Sagittal T1-weighted, gadolinium-enhanced image shows enhancement within the vertebral lesions and epidural extension with spinal cord compression at T10 (arrow).

Bone scan showing multiple metastases

Figure 53-2 Extradural Metastatic Spinal Tumors.

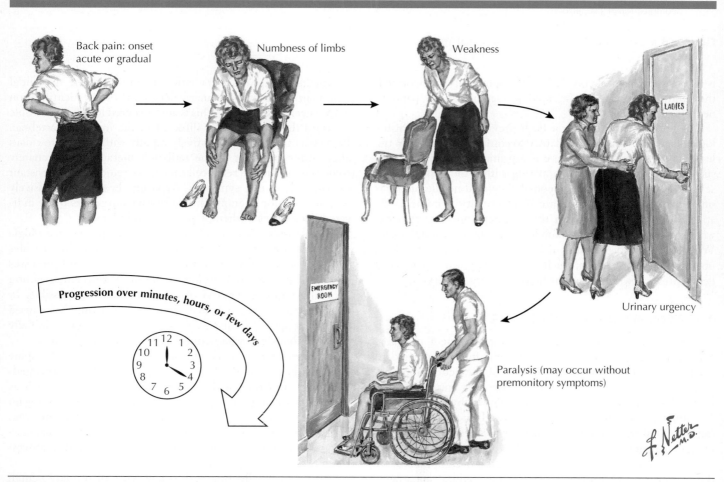

Back pain: onset acute or gradual

Numbness of limbs

Weakness

Urinary urgency

Progression over minutes, hours, or few days

Paralysis (may occur without premonitory symptoms)

Figure 53-3 Clinical Profile: Acute Spinal Cord Decompensation with an Epidural Tumor.

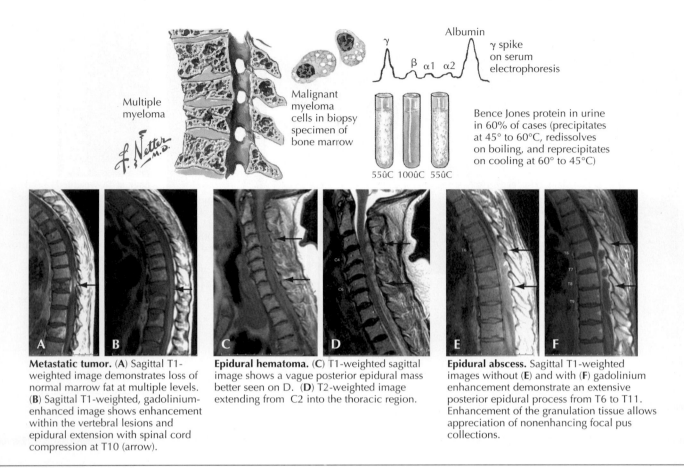

Multiple
myeloma

Malignant
myeloma
cells in biopsy
specimen of
bone marrow

Albumin

γ spike
on serum
electrophoresis

Bence Jones protein in urine
in 60% of cases (precipitates
at 45° to 60°C, redissolves
on boiling, and reprecipitates
on cooling at 60° to 45°C)

55ûC 100ûC 55ûC

Metastatic tumor. (A) Sagittal T1-weighted image demonstrates loss of normal marrow fat at multiple levels. **(B)** Sagittal T1-weighted, gadolinium-enhanced image shows enhancement within the vertebral lesions and epidural extension with spinal cord compression at T10 (arrow).

Epidural hematoma. (C) T1-weighted sagittal image shows a vague posterior epidural mass better seen on D. **(D)** T2-weighted image extending from C2 into the thoracic region.

Epidural abscess. Sagittal T1-weighted images without **(E)** and with **(F)** gadolinium enhancement demonstrate an extensive posterior epidural process from T6 to T11. Enhancement of the granulation tissue allows appreciation of nonenhancing focal pus collections.

Figure 53-4 Extradural Primary Malignant Spinal Tumors.

is an obstructing focal cord lesion. If a spinal tap is performed, this study can precipitate a rapid worsening of the patient's neurologic deficits.

If a primary cancer has not been previously found, a histologic diagnosis becomes mandatory to confirm the nature of the lesion. In some instances, there is a primary bony malignancy such as multiple myeloma originating within the vertebrae per se (Fig. 53-4). Today percutaneous CT-guided needle biopsy is often the most useful procedure if no primary is immediately apparent such as occurred in this chapter's opening vignette, where a routine chest radiograph led to a diagnostic lung biopsy. When there is no evidence of a primary lesion identified, an open surgical procedure, such as neurosurgical spinal cord decompression with a conjoint biopsy, is very important.

TREATMENT AND PROGNOSIS

There are three primary indications for treatment of spinal column metastatic disease: (1) to prevent further spinal cord destruction, (2) to prevent progression of the neurologic deficits, and (3) to control pain. Typically large-dose corticosteroids, that is, 10–20 mg of dexamethasone, followed by 4–6 mg every 4–6 hours, are administered at diagnosis and continued throughout the initial treatment stages for their protective effect on the neural elements.

Focused radiation therapy and/or surgical decompression are the two primary treatment modalities for epidural metastases. When the patient's neurologic examination demonstrates serious neurologic compromise, radiation therapy may be the initial treatment of choice, particularly depending on the identification of the specific pathology. This is administered locally in multiple fractions that are precisely directed to the involved vertebrae. Pain relief often occurs relatively rapidly within just a few days after commencement of the radiation therapy. Unfortunately some tumors such as renal cell cancer are radiotherapy-resistant tumors. Here the symptoms typically evolve progressively despite radiation therapy. In this setting, surgery is often indicated once the radiotherapy per se is completed.

On occasion, patients who present with specific neurologic symptoms and signs are best treated with surgery. This provides for rapid decompression of the neural elements and preserves previously unaffected neurologic function. Surgical intervention generally requires removal of as much tumor as possible. In many instances, when spinal column destruction has caused significant spinal instability, fusion and/or grafting is initially required followed by subsequent radiotherapy to the area.

Prognosis for patients with metastatic disease to the spine depends on their clinical status upon presentation. Individuals who have presented with a severe neurologic deficit such as paraplegia existing at least 24–36 hours often do not regain significant neurologic function. However, many patients who present with acute deterioration, still retaining some distal neurologic function, who undergo rapid evaluation and treatment often experience improvement.

Very occasionally, one finds a few types of primary benign bony vertebral tumors. Although histologically these are not

Osteoid osteoma

Hemangioma

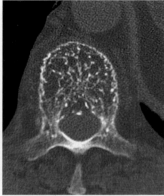

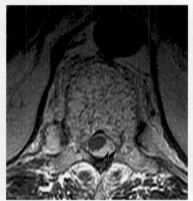

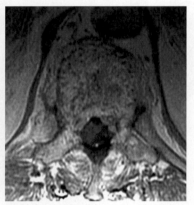

Axial CT demonstrates coarsened trabeculae interspersed with fat lucency. Intraosseous hemangioma involving whole vertebral body with small epidural extension

Axial T2-weighted fast spin echo image demonstrates mixed intensity pattern within vertebral body with left anterolateral epidural extension (arrow). Intraosseous hemangioma with small epidural extension (arrow)

Axial T1-weighted fast spin echo post–gadolinium-enhanced image shows a heterogeneous but generally bright signal pattern within the vertebral body similar to the nonenhanced T1 image; however there is enhancement of the epidural component (arrow). Intraosseous hemangioma with small epidural extension (arrow)

Figure 53-5 Extradural Primary Benign Spinal Tumors.

malignant as are most extradural tumors, these lesions may reach a critical mass, causing vertebral collapse and spinal cord compression (Fig. 53-5). Usually these benign tumors have a less aggressive clinical course; however, once they reach a critical mass, they may portend serious threat to spinal cord function. Uncommonly, surgical decompression is indicated.

INTRADURAL EXTRAMEDULLARY TUMORS

Intradural extra-axial (extramedullary) tumors originate within the dural sleeve of the spinal column but outside of the spinal cord, that is, intradural extramedullary. These lesions primarily arise within the leptomeninges or the nerve roots. Additionally, one may find meningiomas within this age group.

Clinical Vignette

This 41-year-old woman noted the occasional appearance of tingling in her right leg that was particularly prominent when she played tennis. She had no significant back pain. Her initial detailed neurologic examination was perfect. MRI of the lumbosacral spine was normal. A follow-up appointment was scheduled for 2 months. However, within just a few weeks, she noted persistent right leg numbness particularly present when she shaved her leg. On self-testing, she became cognizant of diminished touch sensation in a pre-tibial distribution. Lumbar spine MRI was normal.

Subsequently, her walking began to be limited as her left foot seemed to turn in after walking a few blocks.

Repeat neurologic examination demonstrated a slightly spastic gait, subtle weakness of the left iliopsoas, more brisk muscle stretch reflexes on the left, a left Babinski sign, and a subtle cord level to pin and temperature sensation at T6 on the right.

MRI confirmed the presence of a large intradural extramedullary tumor compressing the spinal cord. An encapsulated benign meningioma was surgically removed. She had an excellent recovery with no clinical residua.

There was a seeming paradox here in that even when the patient developed clinical symptoms, her neurologic examination was initially normal. And then as her symptoms became more specific and subtle abnormalities appeared on neurologic examination, her MRI demonstrated very marked spinal cord compression with a very significant-sized tumor. The clinical temporal profile of meningiomas is to gradually enlarge, subtly compressing the spinal cord. This tissue is amazingly resilient when the pathologic process is a very ingravescent one. Here the initial symptoms were relatively benign, with intermittent leg numbness precipitated by exercise and body heat. Such a setting, in the face of a normal lumbar MRI, suggested the possibility of early multiple sclerosis.

Continued observation was therefore important, as were patient instructions to call with any new symptomatology and return for follow-up within a few months. On this occasion,

Intradural extramedullary tumor (meningioma) compressing spinal cord and deforming nerve roots

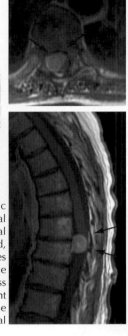

Thoracic meningioma: axial and sagittal T1-weighted, gadolinium images show that the enhancing mass occupies the right anterior 70% of the spinal canal

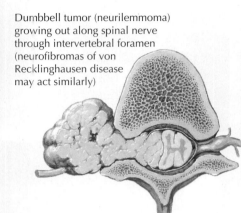

Dumbbell tumor (neurilemmoma) growing out along spinal nerve through intervertebral foramen (neurofibromas of von Recklinghausen disease may act similarly)

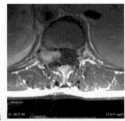

Foraminal neurolemmoma seen on axial T1-weighted, gadolinium-enhanced image (arrowheads)

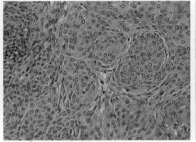

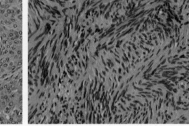

A. Meningioma. Meningioma with a meningothelial pattern showing cells with syncytial features in lobulated groups (H&E, original magnification 200X)

B. Schwannoma (neurilemmoma). Antoni B pattern in a schwannoma showing spindle cells arranged in fascicles (H&E, original magnification 200X)

Figure 53-6 Intradural Extramedullary Primary Spinal Tumors.

subsequent neurologic examination demonstrated a subtle sensory cord level and contralateral corticospinal dysfunction, typical of a classic *Brown–Sequard syndrome* indicating a specific level of spinal cord dysfunction (see Chapter 44). Focused spinal MRI at a higher level led to the diagnosis of this treatable lesion.

Intradural extramedullary tumors are most commonly meningiomas (Fig. 53-6A) arising from within the dura per se, or are nerve sheath tumors. The latter are classified into two main groups, schwannomas, about 65% (Fig. 53-6B), and neurofibromas. Both often have a similar gross appearance and require microscopic analysis for differentiation. Neurofibromas have less dense cellular structure (Antoni B pattern) and often contain nerve elements. Usually benign, these lesions occur as a solitary finding or as multiple nodules throughout the body. Type I neurofibromatosis (von Recklinghausen disease) is a familial condition with two or more neurofibromas, associated neurocutaneous findings such as café-au-lait spots, and axillary freckling. Nerve sheath tumors such as schwannomas typically develop in middle-aged women. These lesions are benign, slow-growing tumors that gradually lead to significant clinical symptomatology especially when these originate near the spinal cord. Type I neurofibromatosis (von Recklinghausen disease) is an autosomal dominant disorder often associated with optic gliomas, and Lisch nodules of the iris, along with certain skeletal abnormalities. Type II neurofibromatosis is most frequently associated with bilateral hearing loss due to neurofibromas of the eighth cranial nerve and are not associated with spinal cord

compression (see Chapter 52). Schwannomas have a dense pattern on microscopic analysis and may be found at the level of the nerve root.

Clinical Vignette

A 36-year-old man reported a several-month history of progressive numbness on the lateral left foot. There was no associated back or leg pain, leg weakness, contralateral leg symptoms, or sphincter dysfunction. Neurologic examination demonstrated sensory loss to light touch and pin prick in the left S1 dermatome. He had full strength in both lower extremities. Muscle stretch reflexes were notable for an absent left Achilles reflex.

An intradural mass was demonstrated at the left S1 level with MRI. There was no bony destruction, but the nerve root foramen was widened compared with the contralateral side. Given the progressive evolution of his clinical difficulties, he underwent surgical resection. Histologic analysis revealed a schwannoma, that is, a nerve sheath tumor.

CLINICAL PRESENTATION

If a single nerve root is involved without invasion of the spinal cord or cauda equina, symptoms mimic a radiculopathy but often without the typical pain such as seen with either sciatica or Herpes zoster, that is, shingles. When these intradural extra-medullary tumors develop, their initial symptoms are not always associated with significant neurologic signs at the first clinical evaluation. The evanescent symptoms may lead the clinician to consider the possibility of multiple sclerosis. Eventually, patients with a spinal lesion develop neurologic signs reflecting posterior column, spinothalamic, and corticospinal tract dysfunction.

TREATMENT

The management of intradural, extramedullary nerve sheath tumors is dictated by the clinical scenario. Patients presenting with neurologic deficits are best managed by surgical resection. Often, intradural extramedullary nerve sheath tumors can be completely resected without a resultant neurologic deficit. The nerve fascicle upon which the tumor arises can usually be separated from other fascicles, avoiding nerve root injury. Although the fascicle is amputated when the tumor is resected, the patient often has no deficit. Radiation and chemotherapy are not required for these benign tumors. If an intradural extramedullary tumor is incidentally discovered, having no associated symptoms or signs; observation is often appropriate as many of these lesions have benign courses.

INTRADURAL INTRA-AXIAL TUMORS

Tumors that originate and grow within the substance of the spinal cord are designated as intra-axial lesions, that is, "intradural, *intramedullary*" neoplasms (Fig. 53-7). These account for ~15% of all primary intradural tumors occurring in both children and adults.

Clinical Vignette

A young woman, known to be an avid athlete, noted a few months' history of right leg clumsiness; difficulty walking, often catching her foot; losing her balance; and experiencing some associated numbness. Her symptoms gradually increased. Subsequently, similar but milder symptoms developed in her left leg. There were no other associated symptoms and particularly no back or neck pain.

Neurologic examination demonstrated mild right leg weakness, increased muscle stretch reflexes, a right Babinski sign, with loss of position and vibratory sensation in the right leg and diminished pinprick and temperature sensation on the left up to a T7 level.

A T6 intra-axial spinal cord mass lesion was demonstrated with thoracic spine MRI. There was extensive T2 signal change within the cord, extending rostrally and caudally to the lesion. Further, similar imaging of the brain and distal spinal cord was normal as were visual evoked potentials. A lumbar puncture, performed to further exclude a primary central nervous system demyelinating process such as multiple sclerosis demonstrated an elevated protein level (96 mg/dL). However, there were no oligoclonal bands present. Cell counts were normal.

At surgical exploration, an anaplastic spinal cord astrocytoma was found. A complete resection was not attempted because of the infiltrative nature of these tumors. Unfortunately, her symptoms continued to progress postoperatively, leaving her paraplegic and incontinent. These tumors do not respond to other treatment modalities such as radiation or chemotherapy.

Although relatively quite rare, primary intradural intramedullary tumors always need to be considered in the differential diagnosis of any patient with possible primary spinal forms of multiple sclerosis. The majority of intramedullary spinal cord malignancies have a primary glial cell source: either an ependymoma or astrocytoma. Spinal cord astrocytomas are more infiltrative and nonencapsulated. Hemangioblastomas, lipomas, and dermoid, epidermoid, and metastatic tumors are among the other extremely rare intramedullary spinal cord tumors.

CLINICAL PRESENTATION

Intramedullary tumors often present with progressive painless neurologic decline over several weeks. The above vignette demonstrated a classic Brown–Sequard syndrome characterized by unilateral hemimotor weakness, diminished position and vibratory sensation ipsilateral to the lesion, and loss of pain and temperature in the contralateral lower extremity. This classic presentation is typically seen in tumors predominantly occupying one side of the spinal cord. A "pure" Brown–Sequard syndrome is rare, as most patients with intradural intramedullary lesions have a mixed clinical presentation affecting both sides of the spinal cord (Fig. 53-7).

TREATMENT

Total resection of ependymomas is occasionally a possibility as the surgeon may find that a tissue plane exists between the tumor and the normal spinal cord, allowing precise removal of the tumor. In contrast, astrocytoma cells have a tendency to more diffusely infiltrate other previously normal tissue, making any thought of a clean surgical extraction totally impossible. Additionally, the highly organized architecture of the spinal cord makes manipulation and resection of the malignant tissue extremely difficult if not impossible. Therefore, the current recommendation is to perform a primary biopsy and possibly a limited resection when dealing with presumed astrocytomas. Recent technological developments in the operating room, including ultrasound, intraoperative MRI, and ultrasonic aspirators, may eventually lead to improved surgical outcomes.

Although both chemotherapy and radiation therapy are advocated for treatment of spinal cord astrocytomas, the results are no more than equivocal. In contrast, ependymomas that are thought to have been completely resected do not require radiation and chemotherapy. Often the best course for such a patient is a period of careful observation with clinical and MRI follow-up.

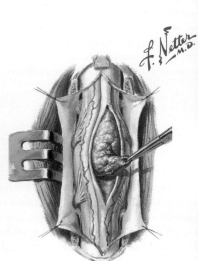
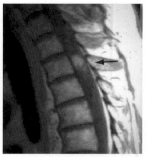
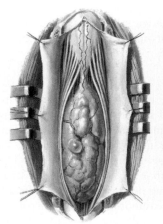
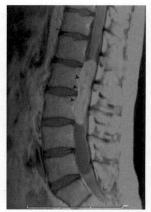
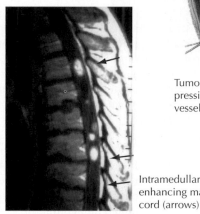

Astrocytoma on gadolinium-enhanced T1-weighted image with diffuse cord enlargement and focal enhancement (arrow)

Intramedullary tumor and myelogram showing widening of spinal cord

Intramedullary metastases: multiple enhancing masses within the spinal cord (arrows)

Tumor of filum terminale compressing cauda equina: enlarged vessels feed tumor

Ependymoma of filum with cyst: sagittal T1-weighted, gadolinium-enhanced image with large, moderately enhancing mass (arrowheads) and cyst distal to it (thin arrows)

Figure 53-7 Intradural Intramedullary Primary Spinal Cord Tumors.

FUTURE DIRECTIONS

The major issue and challenge relates to finding medically successful treatment modalities for the primary glial cell spinal tumor groups, particularly the astrocytomas. Advances in their treatment are occurring in several areas. Imaging, such as MRI, is being employed earlier as a screening tool in many patients with spine-related symptoms. Minimally invasive techniques and advances in instrumentation are improving surgical treatment. Intraoperative monitoring procedures provide improved outcomes for patients undergoing surgical resection of intra- and extramedullary tumors. Stereotactic radiosurgery, usually confined to treating intracranial pathology, is now being developed to administer high-dose radiation with surgical precision to lesions within the spine.

ADDITIONAL RESOURCES

Albanese V, Platania N. Spinal intradural extramedullary tumors. Personal experience. J Neurosurg Sci 2002;46(1):18-24.

Avanzo M, Romanelli P. Spinal radiosurgery: technology and clinical outcomes. Neurosurg Rev 2009 Jan;32(1):1-13.

Bowers DC, Weprin BE. Intramedullary spinal cord tumors. Curr Treat Options Neurol 2003;5(3):207-212.

Cole JS, Patchell RA. Metastatic epidural spinal cord compression. Lancet Neurol 2008 May;7(5):459-466. Review.

Conti P, Pansini G, Mouchaty H, et al. Spinal neurinomas: retrospective analysis and long-term outcome of 179 consecutively operated cases and review of the literature. Surg Neurol 2004;61(1):34-44.

George R, Jeba J, Ramkumar G, et al. Interventions for the treatment of metastatic extradural spinal cord compression in adults. Cochrane Database Syst Rev. 2008 Oct 8;(4):CD006716.

Gibson CJ, Parry NM, Jakowski RM, et al. Anaplastic astrocytoma in the spinal cord of an African pygmy hedgehog (Atelerix albiventris).Vet Pathol 2008 Nov;45(6):934-938.

Minehan KJ, Brown PD, Scheithauer BW, et al. Prognosis and treatment of spinal cord astrocytoma. Int J Radiat Oncol Biol Phys 2008 Aug 5. *This consecutive series of patients with spinal cord astrocytoma were treated at Mayo Clinic Rochester between 1962 and 2005. RESULTS: A total of 136 consecutive patients were identified. Of these 136 patients, 69 had pilocytic and 67 had infiltrative astrocytoma. The median follow-up for living patients was 8.2 years (range, 0.08-37.6), and the median survival for deceased patients was 1.15 years (range, 0.01-39.9). The extent of surgery included incisional biopsy only (59%), subtotal resection (25%), and gross total resection (16%). The results of our study have shown that histologic type is the most important prognostic variable affecting the outcome of spinal cord astrocytomas. Surgical resection was associated with shorter survival and thus remains an unproven treatment. Postoperative radiotherapy significantly improved survival for patients with infiltrative astrocytomas but not for those with pilocytic tumors.*

White BD, Stirling AJ, Paterson E, et al. Diagnosis and management of patients at risk of or with metastatic spinal cord compression: summary of NICE guidance. Guideline Development Group. BMJ 2008 Nov 27;337:a2538.

Cerebrovascular Diseases

Anatomic Aspects of Cerebral Circulation

Claudia J. Chaves

54

The brain and meninges are supplied by arteries derived from the common carotid artery (CCA) and vertebrobasilar system (Fig. 54-1). The right CCA usually originates from the brachiocephalic trunk, whereas the left CCA originates directly from the aortic arch. Both vertebral arteries (VAs) originate from the subclavian arteries. The morphologic variants of the CCA and VAs usually are not clinically significant.

The CCA bifurcates at approximately the level of the sixth cervical vertebrae into the external and internal carotid arteries. The external carotid artery (ECA) supplies the neck, face, and scalp. The internal carotid artery (ICA) and its branches are mostly responsible for the arterial supply of the anterior two thirds of the cerebral hemispheres (anterior circulation).

The vertebrobasilar and posterior cerebral arteries (PCAs) supply blood to the brainstem, cerebellum, occipital lobes, and posterior portions of the temporal and parietal lobes (posterior circulation).

THE CAROTID ARTERY SYSTEM

External Carotid Artery

At its origin, the ECA deviates anteriorly and medially in relation to the ICA in the neck and provides many branches to the neck (superior thyroid, ascending pharyngeal arteries) and face (lingual and facial arteries). As the artery ascends, occipital and posterior auricular branches supply the scalp in their named areas. The occipital artery, however, also has several meningeal branches that supply the posterior fossa and dura. Within the substance of the parotid gland, the ECA divides into its two terminal branches, the superficial temporal and maxillary arteries. The superficial temporal artery is the main supply to the scalp over the frontoparietal convexity and its underlying muscles. The more proximal branches also supply the masseter muscle. The superficial temporal artery is commonly involved in giant cell arteritis, an important consideration in the elderly with headaches, and can be palpated anterior to the tragus and in the temporal area (Chapter 11).

The maxillary artery supplies the face and, through its middle meningeal branch, provides most of the blood supply to the dura mater covering the brain. The middle meningeal artery is often implicated in the formation of epidural hematomas in patients with temporal or parietal bone skull fractures (Chapter 59).

The ECA occasionally has an important role in supplying collateral flow for ICA occlusive disease through anastomoses between its facial, maxillary, and superficial temporal branches and the ophthalmic artery.

Internal Carotid Artery

There are four ICA segments: cervical, petrous, cavernous, and supraclinoid. The cervical segment ascends vertically in the neck, posterior and slightly medial to the ECA. Significant atherosclerotic disease is usually located at the ICA origin, with potential for artery-to-artery embolism, stenosis with eventual occlusion, or both. Unlike the ECA, this segment does not have branches, allowing differentiation between the two vessels on imaging scans.

The ICA enters the skull through the carotid canal within the petrous bone. This petrous segment has two small branches, the caroticotympanic and pterygoid branches, which are usually clinically irrelevant. The cavernous segment, usually called the carotid siphon because of its shape, is the portion of the ICA within the cavernous sinus and provides minor branches supplying the posterior pituitary (meningohypophyseal artery) and the abducens nerve. Of its many branches, the ophthalmic artery is the most significant. The ophthalmic artery arises from the ICA just as it pierces the dura and emerges from the cavernous sinus to pass through the optic canal into the orbit just below and lateral to the optic nerve. It supplies the globe and orbital contents through its 3 major branches: the ocular (central retinal and ciliary arteries), orbital, and extraorbital branches. The ophthalmic artery forms extensive anastomoses with branches of the ECA. The supraclinoid segment is the last portion of the ICA. It begins when this segment penetrates the dura. The *posterior communicating artery* (P-com) and the *anterior choroidal artery* are the two important branches originating at this level. The ICA then bifurcates into *the anterior cerebral artery* (ACA) and *middle cerebral artery* (MCA).

The P-com is often hypoplastic. When present, it travels posteriorly to communicate with the posterior circulation at the level of the posterior cerebral artery (PCA). The P-com also provides thalamoperforate branches that supply the anteromedial thalamus and parts of the cerebral peduncles. Its presence and size is variable but often serves as an important collateral pathway in extensive cerebrovascular disease allowing flow from the anterior to the posterior circulation or vice versa.

The anterior choroidal artery arises from the posterior surface of the ICA just above the P-com origin. This artery supplies an extensive cerebral area, including the visual system (optic tract, anterior portion of the lateral geniculate body and optic radiations), genu and posterior limb of the internal capsule, basal ganglia (medial globus pallidus and tail of the caudate), the diencephalon (portions of the lateral thalamus and the subthalamic nuclei), the midbrain (substantia nigra and portions of the cerebral peduncle), the medial temporal lobe (uncus, pyriform cortex, amygdala), and the choroidal plexus of the temporal horn and atrium.

The ACA travels medially and anteriorly toward the interhemispheric fissure. It supplies the anterior portions of the basal ganglia and internal capsule and most of the mesial portion of the frontal and parietal lobes. The first segment of the ACA, the A1 segment, begins at the carotid bifurcation and terminates

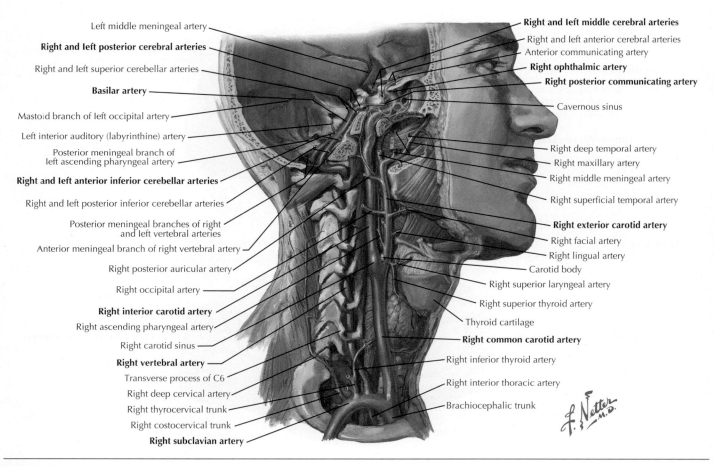

Left middle meningeal artery

Right and left posterior cerebral arteries

Right and left superior cerebellar arteries

Basilar artery

Mastoid branch of left occipital artery

Left interior auditory (labyrinthine) artery

Posterior meningeal branch of
left ascending pharyngeal artery

Right and left anterior inferior cerebellar arteries

Right and left posterior inferior cerebellar arteries

Posterior meningeal branches of right
and left vertebral arteries

Anterior meningeal branch of right vertebral artery

Right posterior auricular artery

Right occipital artery

Right interior carotid artery

Right ascending pharyngeal artery

Right carotid sinus

Right vertebral artery

Transverse process of C6

Right deep cervical artery

Right thyrocervical trunk

Right costocervical trunk

Right subclavian artery

Right and left middle cerebral arteries

Right and left anterior cerebral arteries

Anterior communicating artery

Right ophthalmic artery

Right posterior communicating artery

Cavernous sinus

Right deep temporal artery

Right maxillary artery

Right middle meningeal artery

Right superficial temporal artery

Right exterior carotid artery

Right facial artery

Right lingual artery

Carotid body

Right superior laryngeal artery

Right superior thyroid artery

Thyroid cartilage

Right common carotid artery

Right inferior thyroid artery

Right interior thoracic artery

Brachiocephalic trunk

Figure 54-1 Arteries to Brain and Meninges.

at the level of the anterior communicating artery, which connects opposite A1 segments and constitutes an important collateral pathway in carotid artery occlusive disease. Occasionally, a single A1 exists supplying both medial frontal hemispheres from a single side and is termed an azygous ACA. The recurrent artery of Heubner is the most important branch of the A1 segment and supplies the anteroinferior portion of the head of the caudate, the putamen, and the anterior limb of the internal capsule.

The ACA continues as the A2 segment, where the orbito-frontal branch arises and travels around the genu of the corpus callosum to the orbital and medial surface of the frontal lobe whereas the frontopolar branch supplies the rest of the medial surface of the frontal lobe. The ACA then gives off its two major branches, the pericallosal artery that runs just above the corpus callosum and the callosomarginal artery paralleling the cingulate gyrus. These two arteries supply the mesial portions of the frontal and parietal lobes.

One of the major fail-safe systems within the cerebral circulation is the circle of Willis, formed by the connections between the ACAs, the anterior communicating arteries, the supraclinoid carotid, the P-coms, and PCAs. This vascular network often provides alternative conduits for perfusion avoiding the development of cerebral infarction when a major vessel becomes significantly diseased or occluded, as with cervical ICA atherosclerotic disease. The respective junctions of each

of these vessels in the Circle of Willis is the primary site of berry aneurysm formation—the major cause of subarachnoid hemorrhages.

The MCA originates from the supraclinoid carotid stem and, subsequently, travels laterally to the sylvian fissure as the mainstem M1 segment, giving off lenticulostriate branches to the basal ganglia. As the MCA approaches the sylvian fissure, it usually divides into two large trunks, the superior and inferior divisions. Occasionally, the MCA trifurcates, and a middle trunk is also present. Different branches supply the frontal (orbito-frontal, ascending frontal, precentral, and central branches), parietal (anterior and posterior parietal and angular branches), and temporal (anterior and posterior temporal) lobes. The orbi-tofrontal, ascending frontal, precentral, and central branches usually arise from the superior division of the MCA, whereas the angular, anterior and posterior temporal branches arise from the inferior division. The anterior and posterior parietal branches can arise from either division (Fig. 54-2). The MCA stem or its distal bifurcation point are classic sites where large cerebral artery emboli lodge and are sometimes amenable to emergent intra-arterial thrombolytic therapy.

VERTEBROBASILAR ARTERIES

The *vertebral arteries* (VAs) usually originate from the subclavian arteries on either side (see Fig. 54-1). They have 4 portions: 3

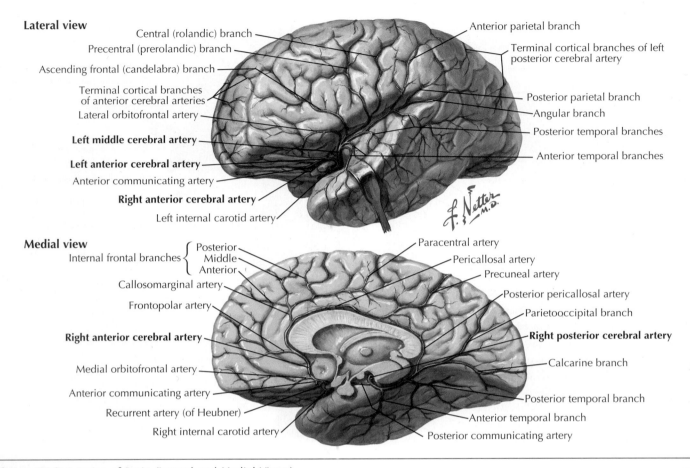

Figure 54-2 Arteries of Brain (Lateral and Medial Views).

extracranial and one intracranial. From their origin, the VAs travel posteriorly (prevertebral segment) and enter the transverse foramen of the sixth cervical vertebrae. They then extend superiorly to exist at C2 (cervical segment), sharply turning posteriorly around the auricular process of the atlas (atlantic segment), then proceeding rostrally, piercing the posterior atlanto-occipital membrane and the dura mater to enter the intracranial cavity through the foramen magnum (intracranial or intradural segment). The vertebral arteries are prone to dissection at their entry and exit sites through the vertebra and are prone to temporal arteritis right at the dural junction.

The intracranial segments course anteriorly lateral to the medulla, then ascend medially to the pontomedullary junction, where they unite at the pontine midline to from the *basilar artery* (Fig. 54-3).

The cervical branches of the VAs give muscular, vertebral body and radicular branches and may serve as collateral conduits in cases of cervical artery compromise or occlusion. The intracranial branches are neurologically more significant and, if diseased, often give definite neurologic syndromes. The first of these are the lateral medullary branches supplying the lateral portions of the medulla. Distally the *posterior–inferior cerebellar arteries* (PICAs) primarily supply the posterior and inferior regions of the cerebellum but also the dorsum of the medulla oblongata. Classic Wallenberg syndrome results from occlusion of medullary arteries of the PICA or penetrator branches of the vertebral arteries.

The anterior spinal artery arises from paired medial VA branches just before the basilar junction unites in the midline to form a single vessel running the full length of the spinal cord caudally in the anteromedial sulcus. It also supplies the medial portions of the medulla; however, adequate collateral circulation in this location makes the medial medullary syndrome rare. In contrast, the anterior spinal artery within the cord is crucial to spinal cord function, and its occlusion leads to an anterior spinal artery syndrome (Chapter 45). The posterior spinal arteries arise from the PICAs or intracranial VAs and run caudally, supplying the posterior and lateral aspect of the spinal cord.

The basilar artery courses rostrally on the anterior surface of the pons, and along the clivus to end at the pontomesencephalic junction providing a number of important branches on its way. The *anterior–inferior cerebellar arteries* (AICAs) usually arise from the midportion of the basilar artery and supply the brachium pontis, lateral pontine tegmentum, flocculus, and anteroinferior portions of the cerebellum. The internal auditory artery may arise from the AICAs or the basilar itself and supplies the vestibular and cochlear structures. The *superior cerebellar arteries* (SCAs) arise from the distal portion of the basilar artery before it bifurcates into the *posterior cerebral arteries* (PCAs). During their course around the midbrain, the SCAs provide branches to the superior lateral pontine tegmentum and the tectum of the mesencephalon. The SCAs then travel toward the cerebellum, supplying the superior vermis, lateral portion of the cerebellar hemispheres and most of the cerebellar nuclei and the cerebellar

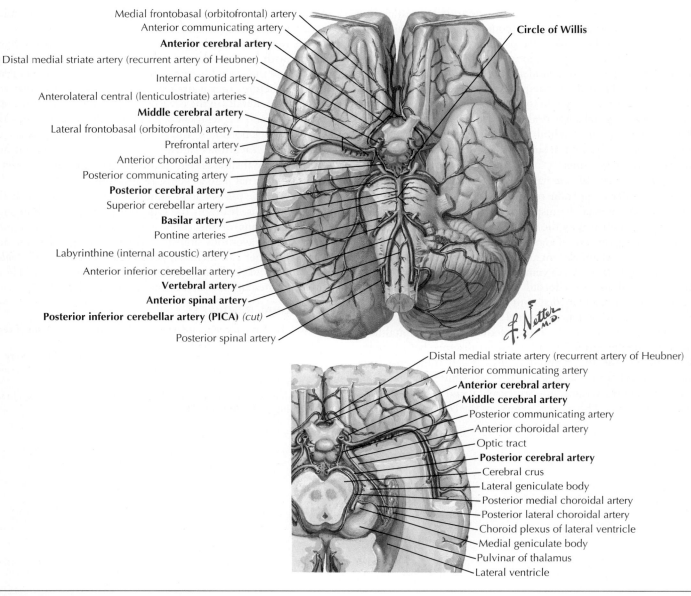

Medial frontobasal (orbitofrontal) artery
Anterior communicating artery
Anterior cerebral artery
Distal medial striate artery (recurrent artery of Heubner)
Internal carotid artery
Anterolateral central (lenticulostriate) arteries
Middle cerebral artery
Lateral frontobasal (orbitofrontal) artery
Prefrontal artery
Anterior choroidal artery
Posterior communicating artery
Posterior cerebral artery
Superior cerebellar artery
Basilar artery
Pontine arteries
Labyrinthine (internal acoustic) artery
Anterior inferior cerebellar artery
Vertebral artery
Anterior spinal artery
Posterior inferior cerebellar artery (PICA) *(cut)*
Posterior spinal artery

Circle of Willis

Distal medial striate artery (recurrent artery of Heubner)
Anterior communicating artery
Anterior cerebral artery
Middle cerebral artery
Posterior communicating artery
Anterior choroidal artery
Optic tract
Posterior cerebral artery
Cerebral crus
Lateral geniculate body
Posterior medial choroidal artery
Posterior lateral choroidal artery
Choroid plexus of lateral ventricle
Medial geniculate body
Pulvinar of thalamus
Lateral ventricle

Figure 54-3 Arteries of Brain: Inferior Views.

white matter. When the basilar artery reaches the level of the cerebral peduncles, it divides into opposite PCAs that loop laterally and posteriorly around the midbrain supplying the medial temporal lobe, portions of the parietal lobe and the occipital lobes. Perforator branches are given off to the thalamus. Distal to the posterior communicating artery, medial and lateral posterior choroidal branches off the PCA supply the posterior portion of the lateral geniculate body, optic tract, pulvinar, hippocampus, and parahippocampal gyrus, as well as the choroid plexus of the lateral and third ventricles.

The basilar artery is particularly prone to atherosclerotic deposition throughout its length, and at its extremes can cause either severe stenosis or occlusion, or formation of a fusiform aneurysm by weakening the vessel wall. The rostral end of the basilar, just before bifurcating into the PCAs, is the site most likely to be occluded by an embolus leading to the classic "top of the basilar" syndrome (Chapter 55). Similarly, this is one of

the most common sites for berry aneurysms within the vertebrobasilar system.

CEREBRAL SINUSES AND VEINS

Surrounded by dura, cerebral sinuses and veins are the venous structures of the brain. They typically contain inpouchings of arachnoid cells, called arachnoid granulations, which allow CSF drainage. These granulations function as one-way valves and are pressure dependent. Malfunction of these valves can occur in subarachnoid hemorrhage or meningitis, leading to normal pressure hydrocephalus. The main venous sinuses include the superior and inferior sagittal sinuses, the straight sinus, the transverse sinuses, the sigmoid sinuses, the occipital sinus, the cavernous sinuses, the superior and inferior petrosal sinuses, and the sphenoparietal sinuses. Acute or subacute cerebral venous thrombosis can be the cause of a wide range of neurologic pathology from isolated chronic headache to venous infarction with seizures to obtundation and coma. Anatomic images and full discussion of this subject are provided in Chapter 56.

The *superior sagittal sinus* is located within the midline of the cerebral hemispheres surrounded by dura and tethered to the inner table of the skull via the pachymeninges. It runs posteriorly from the foramen cecum to the occipitocerebellar junction. The superior sagittal sinus drains the frontal and parietal lobes through the superior cerebral veins, the largest of which is the rolandic vein in the central sulcus. This sinus often drains into the right transverse sinus.

The *inferior sagittal sinus* parallels the corpus callosum, traveling in the inferior portion of the falx cerebri, and drains the region of the medial hemispheres and cingulate gyrus. The *straight sinus* is formed by the intersection of the inferior sagittal sinus and the great vein of Galen. The *vein of Galen* drains many smaller venous channels, including the choroidal, lateral ventricular, and thalamostriate veins and the *basal vein of Rosenthal*. These veins drain the choroid plexus, lateral ventricle, basal ganglia, thalamus, and medial temporal lobes. The straight sinus often drains into the left transverse sinus.

The *transverse sinuses* lie in the grooves of the occipital bone and run laterally and forward for a short distance before diving down to become the sigmoid sinuses. Each transverse sinus receives blood from the superior petrosal sinuses, mastoid and condyloid emissary veins, inferior cerebral and cerebellar veins, and diploic veins. The *sigmoid sinuses* are the continuation of the transverse sinuses and end at the jugular foramina, becoming the internal jugular veins.

The *cavernous sinus* is an intricate venous channel interconnecting with its contralateral partner via intercavernous channels around the infundibulum. The cavernous sinus is important for the structures that it drains and for the structures that run through it. Laterally in the cavernous sinus wall are CN-III, -IV, and -V (V1 and V2 segments), and through its center runs the intracavernous portion of the ICA, the sympathetic plexus, and CN-VI. The cavernous sinuses drain into paired superior and inferior petrosal sinuses that, in turn, drain into the transverse sinus and internal jugular veins, respectively.

The *superior petrosal sinus* connects the cavernous with the transverse sinus. It drains the tympanic cavity, cerebellum, and inferior portions of the cerebrum. The *inferior petrosal sinus* connects the cavernous sinus with the internal jugular vein and drains the inner ear, medulla, pons, and cerebellum. The *sphenopalatine sinuses* lie below the lesser wings of the sphenoid bone and drain the dura mater into the cavernous sinuses.

ADDITIONAL RESOURCES

Damasio, H. A computed tomographic guide to the identification of cerebrovascular territories. Arch Neurol 1983;40(3):138-142.

Netter FM. The Netter Collection of Medical Illustrations. Vol 1: Nervous System. Part 1: Anatomy and Physiology. Teterboro, NJ: Icon Learning Systems; 2001.

Tatu L, Moulin T, Bogousslavsky J. Arterial territories of the human brain. Neurology 1998;50:1699-1708.

Ischemic Stroke

Claudia J. Chaves

55

*I*schemic stroke is the third most frequent cause of mortality in the United States and a common cause of prolonged morbidity. Over time it has become more apparent that ischemic stroke represents a constellation of etiologies and mechanisms that often present with similar symptoms and signs. New technology has improved understanding of stroke pathophysiology that promises to translate into more specific treatments and better outcomes.

The distinction between transient ischemic attacks (TIAs) and strokes based on reversibility or not of ischemic symptoms has become less clinically relevant, because a significant number of patients with transient ischemic symptoms have been found to have strokes on diffusion-weighted imaging. Therefore, the diagnostic approach to patients with transient or persistent ischemic symptoms should be the same, and treatment guided toward the underlying cause of the brain ischemia.

ETIOLOGY AND PATHOPHYSIOLOGY

The most common ischemic stroke etiologies are large artery occlusive disease, cardioembolism, and small vessel disease.

Large Artery Occlusive Disease

Atherosclerosis causes stenosis or occlusion of extracranial and intracranial arteries and is directly responsible for a significant percentage of cerebral ischemic events. Atheroma formation involves the progressive deposition of circulating lipids and ultimately fibrous tissue in the subintimal layer of the large and medium arteries, occurring most frequently at branching points (Fig. 55-1). Plaque formation is enhanced by blood-associated inflammatory factors as well as increased shear injury form uncontrolled blood pressure. Intraplaque hemorrhage, subintimal necrosis with ulcer formation, and calcium deposition can cause enlargement of the atherosclerotic plaque with consequent worsening of the degree of arterial narrowing.

Disruption of the endothelial surface triggers thrombus formation within the arterial lumen through activation of nearby platelets by the subendothelial matrix. When platelets become activated they release thromboxane A_2, causing further platelet aggregation. The development of a fibrin network stabilizes the platelet aggregate, forming a "white thrombus." In areas of slowed or turbulent flow within or around the plaque the thrombus develops further, enmeshing red blood cells (RBCs) in the platelet–fibrin aggregate to form a "red thrombus" (Fig. 55-2). This remains poorly organized and friable for up to 2 weeks and presents a significant risk of propagation or embolization. Either the white or red thrombus, however, can dislodge and embolize to distal arterial branches. Large artery disease can cause ischemic strokes by either intra-arterial embolism as described above and, less commonly, hemodynamic ischemia or hypoperfusion through a significantly narrowed vessel.

Frequent sites for carotid system or anterior circulation atherosclerosis are the origin of the internal carotid artery (ICA), the carotid siphon at the base of the brain (Fig. 55-3), and the main stem of the middle cerebral artery (MCA) and the anterior cerebral artery (ACA). The internal carotid artery at or around the bifurcation is usually affected in Caucasians whereas in Asian, Hispanic, and African-American populations, intracranial atherosclerosis may be more common than carotid disease. In the vertebrobasilar system, the origins of the vertebral arteries in the neck and the distal portion of the intracranial vertebral arteries are the most commonly affected areas. The basilar artery and origins of the posterior cerebral arteries (PCAs) are other sites.

The main risk factors for large artery disease are arterial hypertension, diabetes, hypercholesterolemia, and smoking. Epidemiologic studies have identified hyperhomocysteinemia as a possible risk factor for atherosclerosis, with a twofold greater risk of stroke. However, recent randomized trials have not shown a correlation between moderate reduction of total homocysteine levels and vascular outcomes and theorize it may represent an "innocent bystander" rather than have a direct pathological effect. Further studies are needed to determine if there are subgroups that might benefit from a more aggressive vitamin therapy, particularly over the long term.

Cardiac Embolism

Several types of cardiac disease lead to cerebral embolism: cardiac arrhythmias, ischemic heart disease, valvular disease, dilated cardiomyopathies, atrial septal abnormalities, and intracardiac tumors (Fig. 55-4).

Cardiac arrhythmias including chronic or paroxysmal atrial fibrillation (AF) and sick sinus syndrome (in particular brady-tachycardia syndrome) are the rhythms most associated with cardioembolic event, with stroke often being their first manifestation. Because such arrhythmias are often intermittent, careful and at times repeated monitoring is needed to identify their presence as they pose a significant risk for recurrent stroke.

Within the first 4 weeks of myocardial infarction (MI), particularly with ischemia of the anterior wall, there is a higher risk of embolic stroke. More remote MIs can be a potential embolic source, particularly in patients who develop akinetic segments or left ventricular aneurysms. Mural thrombi are common in patients with dilated cardiomyopathies. Brain embolism is estimated to occur in approximately 15% of these patients.

Rheumatic valvular disease, mechanical prosthetic heart valves, and infective endocarditis are well-known cardiac sources of embolism. Other relatively common abnormalities, mitral valve prolapse, mitral annulus calcification, and bicuspid aortic valve have suspected embolic potential. However, these should be considered as a potential cause of stroke only after other etiologies have been excluded.

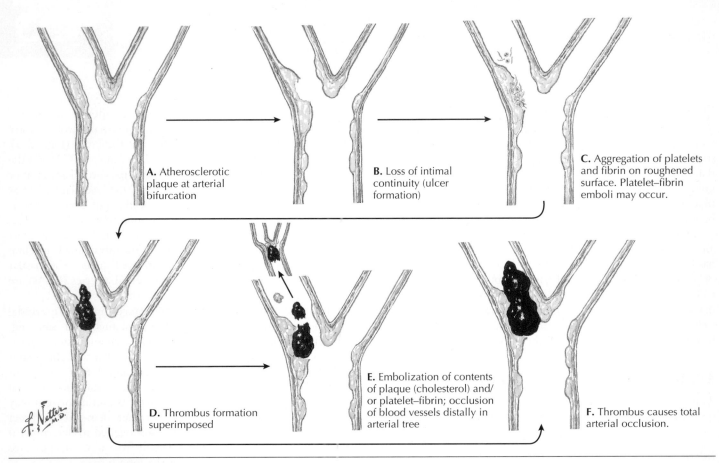

Figure 55-1 Atherosclerosis, Thrombosis, and Embolism.

Patent foramen ovale (PFO) and atrial septal aneurysm are risk factors for stroke. A meta-analysis of case–control studies comparing patients younger than 55 years with ischemic stroke to nonstroke controls showed an odds ratio for stroke of 3.1 for PFO alone and of 6.1 for PFO with an associated atrial septal aneurysm. Potential or presumed mechanisms of stroke included venous "paradoxical embolism," direct embolization from thrombi formed within the PFO or atrial septal aneurysm, and thrombus from atrial arrhythmias thought to be more prevalent in this population.

Atrial myxomas, although rare, are important causes of embolic strokes. These tumor emboli frequently affect the vasa vasorum, leading to the development of multiple and peripheral cerebral aneurysms similar to mycotic aneurysms.

Small Vessel Disease (Lacunes)

The capillary vessel and the end penetrating arteries that supply the basal ganglia, thalamus, internal capsule, and white matter tracts are not prone to atherosclerosis as in the large-caliber cerebral circulation but undergo a characteristic pathologic degeneration in response to endothelial damage. Fibrinoid degeneration with focal enlargement of the vessel wall, foam cell invasion of the lumen, and hemorrhagic rupture through the vessel wall characterize this process known as fibrinoid degeneration or lipohyalinosis. Occlusion of these arteries causes small (1–20 mm), discrete, and often irregular lesions called *lacunes*. As previously alluded to, lacunes do not involve the cortical ribbon and occur most often in the basal ganglia, thalamus, pons, internal capsule, and cerebral white matter and may cause discrete clinical syndromes but often go clinically unnoticed. Arterial hypertension and diabetes are the main risk factors (Fig. 55-5).

Arterial Dissection

Dissection or tear within the extracranial ICA, particularly its pharyngeal and distal segments, or the extracranial vertebral artery, mainly in its first and third segments, are the two commonly affected vessels. Dissection occurring between the intima and media usually causes stenosis or occlusion of the affected artery, whereas dissection between the media and adventitia is associated with aneurysmal dilatation. Congenital abnormalities in the media or elastica of the arteries as seen in Marfan syndrome, fibromuscular dysplasia, and cystic medial necrosis can predispose patients to arterial dissection. Although often associated with acute trauma, arterial dissection may result from seemingly innocuous incidents, such as a fall while hiking or skiing; sports activities, particularly wrestling or diving into a wave; and paroxysms of coughing. The mechanism of stroke involves clot formation in the dissected wall of the vessel with distal propagation or embolization. Also, expansion of the clot in the dissected wall causes progressive narrowing of the lumen, leading to compromised

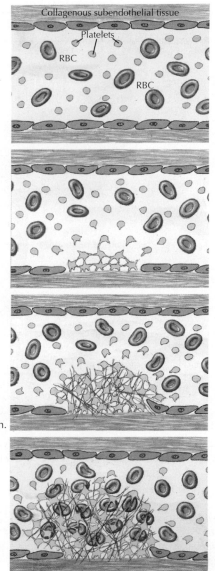

Collagenous subendothelial tissue

Platelets circulating in blood contain thromboxane A$_2$, a substance that promotes their aggregation, while vascular endothelium secretes prostacyclin, an aggregation inhibitor that balances this effect. These products are synthesized after conversion of arachidonic acid into intermediate endoperoxides by cyclooxygenase enzymes.

If endothelial continuity is interrupted by trauma, atherosclerosis, etc., subsurface collagen is exposed to blood and stimulates adhesion of platelets to vessel wall. Platelets then discharge thromboxane A$_2$, causing aggregation of adjacent platelets.

As more platelets aggregate, fibrin network develops and stabilizes mass into "white thrombus," which then retracts into vascular wall. In some cases, endothelium may later heal over with or without narrowing of lumen.

If thrombus develops further, red blood cells become enmeshed in platelet-fibrin aggregate to form "red thrombus," which may grow and block vessel lumen. Either platelet-fibrin aggregates or more fully formed clots may break off, with embolization into distal arterial branches.

Figure 55-2 Role of Platelets in Arterial Thrombosis.

blood flow and hypoperfusion or, ultimately, occlusion (Fig. 55-6).

Less Common Stroke Etiologies

Although frequently considered in the differential diagnosis of ischemic stroke, arteritis is a rare stroke etiology. Usually, CNS vasculitis presents as an encephalopathy with multifocal signs.

Cocaine and amphetamine are the most frequent drugs associated with ischemic strokes. Vasoconstriction and vasculitis are the posited mechanisms.

Hematologic disorders such as polycythemia, sickle cell disease, and thrombocytosis (usually platelets >1,000,000/dL) can cause ischemic strokes by increasing blood viscosity, hypercoagulability, or both. Antithrombin III, protein S, protein C deficiencies, factor V Leiden, and prothrombin gene mutation are usually associated with venous and not arterial thrombosis

but may take on importance in cases of stroke associated with PFO due to passage of venous clots through an intra-atrial defect (paradoxical embolization).

CLINICAL PRESENTATION

Large Artery Occlusive Disease

CAROTID ARTERY DISEASE

Clinical Vignette

A 68-year-old white man with a history of hypercholesterolemia and 50-pack-year smoking presented with transient episodes affecting the right side of his body. During the first episode, he had weakness of his right leg, lasting for about 10 minutes. The second spell happened 1 week later and

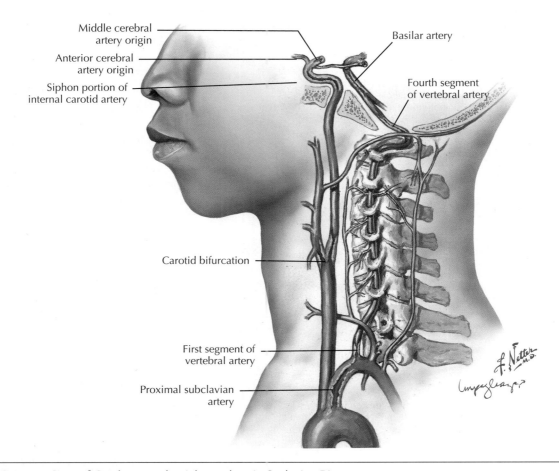

Middle cerebral artery origin

Anterior cerebral artery origin

Siphon portion of internal carotid artery

Basilar artery

Fourth segment of vertebral artery

Carotid bifurcation

First segment of vertebral artery

Proximal subclavian artery

Figure 55-3 Common Sites of Cerebrovascular Atherosclerotic Occlusive Disease.

was characterized by speech difficulties, right facial drop, and right arm weakness that lasted for 2 hours. The patient came to the emergency department (ED) 3 days later. Brain magnetic resonance imaging (MRI) with diffusion-weighted imaging demonstrated two small strokes in the left frontal lobe, one in the ACA territory and the second one in the MCA distribution. Magnetic resonance angiography (MRA) of the head and neck was remarkable for a 70–80% stenosis of the left ICA, confirmed by carotid ultrasound. The patient was started on antiplatelet treatment and a statin. Smoking cessation education was provided. A right carotid artery endarterectomy was successful, with no subsequent TIAs.

Clinical Vignette

A 70-year-old white man with arterial hypertension and high cholesterol presented with 1 month of recurrent 1- to 2-minute episodes of left extremities shaking that occurred only on standing. His blood pressure (BP) was 110/80 mm Hg, and neurologic examination showed a left pronator drift, but was otherwise normal.

Head computed tomography (CT) showed small strokes in the arterial border zone between the right MCA and ACA and right MCA and PCA distributions. Head and neck computed tomography angiography (CTA) demonstrated a right

ICA occlusion. CT perfusion showed hypoperfusion in the right MCA territory, worse in the border zone areas. Collateral flow through the right ophthalmic, anterior communicating, and posterior communicating arteries was detected by transcranial Doppler and conventional angiogram. Patient was started on antiplatelet treatment as well as a statin drug and his antihypertensive medication dose was decreased, with a subsequent increase in the systolic BP to 140–150 mm Hg. No further episodes occurred.

The above vignettes illustrate the two mechanisms of stroke or TIA in large artery atherosclerotic disease, intra-arterial embolism (the first vignette) and hypoperfusion (the second vignette). Identification of the exact mechanism has important therapeutic implications.

TIAs are common in patients with carotid artery disease and usually precede stroke onset by a few days or months. TIAs caused by intra-arterial embolism from a carotid source may not be stereotypical. TIA symptoms vary, depending on which ICA branch is involved. For example, patients can have a first episode of a transient right leg weakness and weeks later have another spell characterized by expressive aphasia, right facial droop and weakness of the right hand. This depends on the destination of the emboli. In the first example, the ACA territory is the

Cardiac Sources of Cerebral Emboli

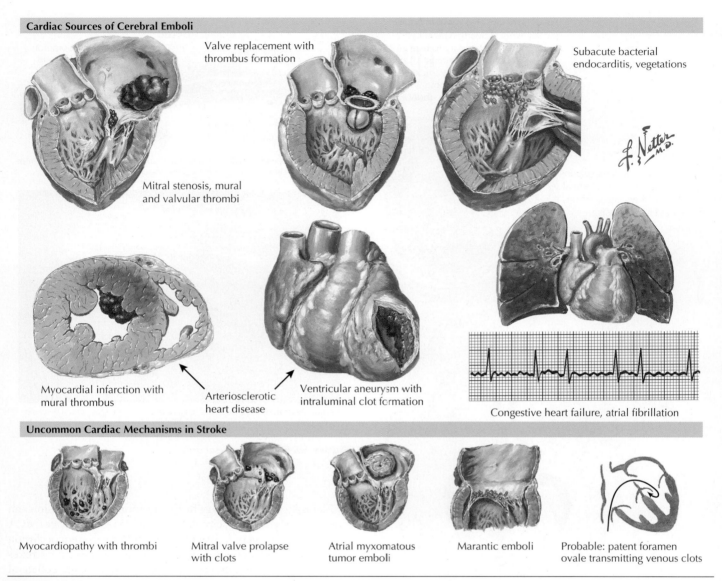

Valve replacement with thrombus formation

Subacute bacterial endocarditis, vegetations

Mitral stenosis, mural and valvular thrombi

Myocardial infarction with mural thrombus

Arteriosclerotic heart disease

Ventricular aneurysm with intraluminal clot formation

Congestive heart failure, atrial fibrillation

Uncommon Cardiac Mechanisms in Stroke

Myocardiopathy with thrombi

Mitral valve prolapse with clots

Atrial myxomatous tumor emboli

Marantic emboli

Probable: patent foramen ovale transmitting venous clots

Figure 55-4 Cardiac Embolism.

destination and in the later example, the MCA territory. In contrast, hemodynamic "limb-shaking" TIAs as in the second vignette presented above are often stereotypical and posturally related and are usually seen in patients with high-grade ICA stenosis or occlusion. In this classic example of a hemodynamic ischemia, patients present with recurrent, irregular, and involuntary movements of the contralateral arm, leg, or both, usually triggered by postural changes and lasting a few minutes. These spells likely represent intermittent loss of cortical control and paralysis and differ from a focal seizure in which the movements are more regular and rhythmic and usually correlate with focal repetitive cortical hyperactivity seen on electroencephalogram.

Another important clue to ICA disease is episodes of transient monocular blindness (TMB). *TMB* refers to the occurrence of temporary unilateral visual loss or obscuration that is classically described by careful observers as a horizontal or vertical "shade being drawn over one eye," but most frequently as a "fog" or "blurring" in the eye, lasting 1–5 minutes. It often occurs spontaneously but at times is triggered by position

changes. Positive phenomena such as sparkles, lights, or colors evolving over minutes are more typical of migrainous phenomena and help to differentiate such benign visual changes from the more serious TMB, a frequent harbinger of cerebral infarct within the carotid artery vasculature. Rarely, with critical ipsilateral internal carotid stenosis, gradual dimming or loss of vision when exposed to bright light, such as glare of snow on a sunlit background, can be reported and is due to limited vascular flow in the face of increased retinal metabolic demand. Besides carotid atherosclerosis, other etiologies of TMB include cardiac embolism and intrinsic ophthalmic artery disease due to processes such as atherosclerosis or arteritis (see Giant cell or Temporal arteritis in Chapter 11), as well as decreased retinal perfusion from glaucoma or increased intraocular pressure. It is not uncommon that homonymous field deficits are reported by patients as monocular visual loss off to the affected side, and careful questioning as to whether each eye was checked independently and whether the visual difficulty involved the perception of a quadrant or one half of the visual world is essential.

Small (100-μm) artery within brain parenchyma showing typical pathologic changes secondary to hypertension. Vessel lumen almost completely obstructed by thickened media and enlarged to about 3 times normal size. Pink-staining fibrinoid material within walls.

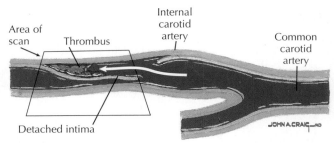

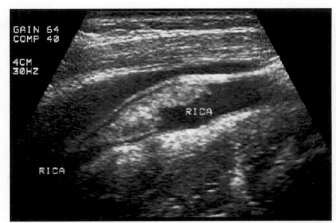

Intimal tear allows blood flow to dissect beneath intimal layer, detaching it from arterial wall. Large dissection may occlude vessel lumen

Carotid dissection: Ultrasound of the carotid artery with clot formed between layers of the artery (near the upper RICA label).

Figure 55-6 Arterial dissection.

Lacunar infarcts in base of pons interrupting some corticospinal (pyramidal) fibers. Such lesions cause mild hemiparesis.

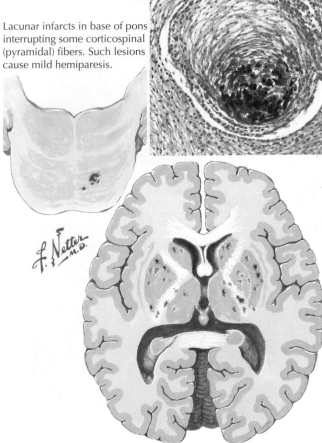

Multiple bilateral lacunes and scars of healed lacunar infarcts in thalamus, putamen, globus pallidus, caudate nucleus, and internal capsule. Such infarcts produce diverse symptoms.

Figure 55-5 Lacunar Infarction.

For example, patients with left occipital infarctions or transient ischemia may report right-sided vision loss, but further questioning reveals that they were unable to read the right side of street signs or a license plate and while covering the "unaffected" left eye the seemingly abnormal right eye had retained vision within the distribution of the unaffected left homonymous field (Fig. 55-7).

As in the first vignette, strokes from intra-arterial embolism from ICA disease are usually cortically based. Symptoms depend on whether branches of the MCA, ACA, or both are involved. The PCA territory may rarely be affected by intra-arterial emboli from ipsilateral ICA stenosis or occlusion in patients with anomalous normal vascular variants as in a persistent fetal PCA.

Neurologic findings vary by the location of the occlusion and presence of collateral circulation (Fig. 55-8). A large MCA stroke is usually seen in patients with MCA main stem occlusion without good collateral flow, whereas deep or parasylvian strokes are the most common presentation when enough collateral flow is present over the convexities.

Contralateral motor weakness involving the foot more than the thigh and shoulder, with relative sparing of the hand and face is the typical presentation of distal ACA branch occlusion. Conversely, prominent cognitive and behavioral changes associated with contralateral hemiparesis predominate in patients with proximal ACA occlusions and the involvement of the recurrent artery of Huebner (caudate and interior limb of internal capsule infarct).

Hemodynamic strokes usually involve the border zone territory between ACA and MCA (anterior border zone), MCA and PCA (posterior border zone), or between deep and superficial perforators (subcortical border zone) and cause typical clinical symptoms outlined in Table 55-1.

INTRACRANIAL MCA AND ACA DISEASE

Clinical Vignette

A 70-year-old woman with history of diabetes mellitus and hypercholesterolemia presented to the ED reporting mild

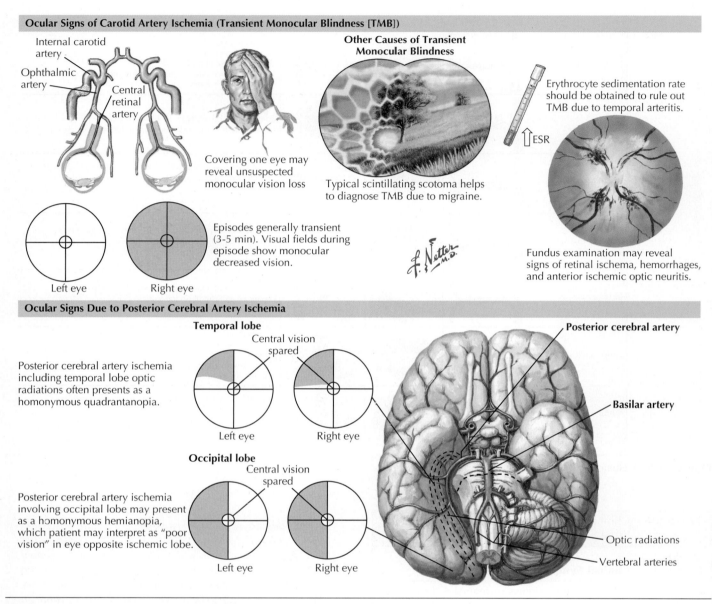

Ocular Signs of Carotid Artery Ischemia (Transient Monocular Blindness [TMB])

Internal carotid artery

Ophthalmic artery

Central retinal artery

Covering one eye may reveal unsuspected monocular vision loss

Episodes generally transient (3-5 min). Visual fields during episode show monocular decreased vision.

Left eye

Right eye

Other Causes of Transient Monocular Blindness

Typical scintillating scotoma helps to diagnose TMB due to migraine.

Erythrocyte sedimentation rate should be obtained to rule out TMB due to temporal arteritis.

↑ESR

Fundus examination may reveal signs of retinal ischema, hemorrhages, and anterior ischemic optic neuritis.

Ocular Signs Due to Posterior Cerebral Artery Ischemia

Temporal lobe

Central vision spared

Posterior cerebral artery ischemia including temporal lobe optic radiations often presents as a homonymous quadrantanopia.

Left eye

Right eye

Occipital lobe

Central vision spared

Posterior cerebral artery ischemia involving occipital lobe may present as a homonymous hemianopia, which patient may interpret as "poor vision" in eye opposite ischemic lobe.

Left eye

Right eye

Posterior cerebral artery

Basilar artery

Optic radiations

Vertebral arteries

Figure 55-7 Ocular Signs of Large Vessel Disease.

right-sided weakness first noticed on awakening 2 days previously. The hemiparesis progressed to a right hemiplegia with dysarthria within 48 hours without change in the patient's level of consciousness. Head CT demonstrated a stroke involving the left centrum semiovale. Head CTA showed a distal M1 segment stenosis. Patient was started on an antiplatelet treatment and a statin. Pharmacologic treatment for her diabetes was maximized. Once stable, patient was transferred to a rehabilitation facility with partial recovery of her motor deficits.

This vignette describes a classic course of subcortical infarct from poor perfusion of the lenticulostriate vessels secondary to a fixed lesion in the ipsilateral MCA. The patient's symptoms evolved from relatively mild hemiparesis to complete paralysis within 2 days. Unlike large MCA infarctions, there was no

impairment of the patient's level of consciousness despite the progressive nature of the neurologic deficit. In contrast, large cortical MCA lesions may also evolve over 2–4 days but due to development of cerebral edema and increased intracranial pressure, altered level of consciousness and even coma are commonly seen.

Intrinsic occlusive disease of the MCA and ACA are more common in Asians, Hispanics, and African Americans than in Caucasians and are more common in women than in men. Arterial hypertension, diabetes, and smoking are the most common risk factors, with a lower incidence of high cholesterol, coronary artery disease, and peripheral vascular disease. Although TIAs can occur, they are not as common as in patients with ICA disease and usually occur over a shorter period of hours or days. When strokes occur, initial symptoms are typically noticed on awakening and often fluctuate during the day, supporting a hemodynamic mechanism.

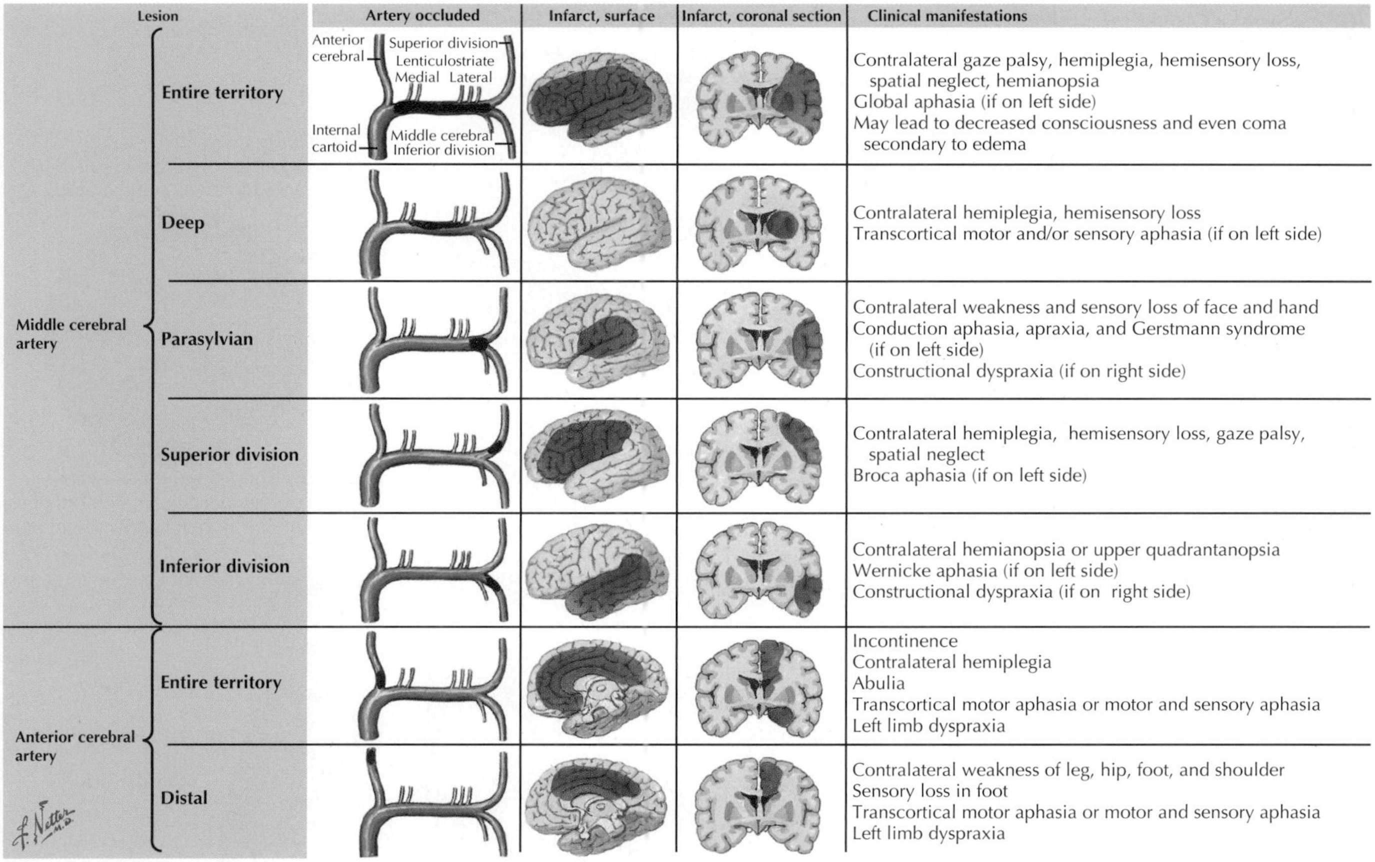

Lesion		Artery occluded	Infarct, surface	Infarct, coronal section	Clinical manifestations
Middle cerebral artery	Entire territory	Anterior cerebral — Superior division, Lenticulostriate, Medial Lateral. Internal cartoid — Middle cerebral Inferior division			Contralateral gaze palsy, hemiplegia, hemisensory loss, spatial neglect, hemianopsia Global aphasia (if on left side) May lead to decreased consciousness and even coma secondary to edema
	Deep				Contralateral hemiplegia, hemisensory loss Transcortical motor and/or sensory aphasia (if on left side)
	Parasylvian				Contralateral weakness and sensory loss of face and hand Conduction aphasia, apraxia, and Gerstmann syndrome (if on left side) Constructional dyspraxia (if on right side)
	Superior division				Contralateral hemiplegia, hemisensory loss, gaze palsy, spatial neglect Broca aphasia (if on left side)
	Inferior division				Contralateral hemianopsia or upper quadrantanopsia Wernicke aphasia (if on left side) Constructional dyspraxia (if on right side)
Anterior cerebral artery	Entire territory				Incontinence Contralateral hemiplegia Abulia Transcortical motor aphasia or motor and sensory aphasia Left limb dyspraxia
	Distal				Contralateral weakness of leg, hip, foot, and shoulder Sensory loss in foot Transcortical motor aphasia or motor and sensory aphasia Left limb dyspraxia

Figure 55-8 Occlusion of Middle and Anterior Cerebral Arteries.

Table 55-1 Clinical Symptoms in Patients with Border Zone Strokes

Stroke Location	Clinical Symptoms
Anterior border zone	Contralateral weakness (proximal > distal limbs and sparing face), transcortical motor aphasia (left-sided infarcts), mood disturbances (right-sided infarcts)
Posterior border zone	Homonymous hemianopsia, lower-quadrant-anopsia, transcortical sensory aphasia (left-sided infarcts), hemineglect, and anosognosia (right-sided infarcts)
Subcortical border zone	Brachiofacial hemiparesis with or without sensory loss, subcortical aphasia (left-sided infarcts)

VERTEBROBASILAR DISEASE

Clinical Vignette

A 76-year-old white man with a history of hypercholesterolemia and a previous myocardial infarction had acute onset of vertigo associated with vomiting and gait difficulties 2 days before presentation. On admission, he had sudden onset of slurred speech and lack of right arm coordination. Head CT demonstrated an old right posterior–inferior cerebellar artery (PICA) stroke and a subacute left PICA stroke. Head MRI with diffusion-weighted imaging showed a new right superior cerebellar artery stroke. Head and neck CTA showed occlusion of the left vertebral artery (VA) origin, a hypoplastic right vertebral artery, and an embolus in the middistal portion of the basilar artery. He was started on a statin and on anticoagulation. Clinically, the patient improved significantly.

The vertebral arteries originate from the subclavian arteries in the neck. Stenosis or occlusion of the proximal subclavian arteries and the vertebral arteries at their origin rarely causes symptoms because of the concomitant development of adequate collateral circulation within the neck through the thyrocervical and costocervical trunks and other subclavian artery branches eventually flowing into the distal vertebral artery (see Fig. 55-3). More often, patients with subclavian and concomitant vertebral-origin stenosis have symptoms related only to upper extremity ischemia. They report pain, coolness, and weakness of the ipsilateral arm. Rarely does chronic atherosclerotic disease at the vertebral origins, even when bilateral, cause significant vertebrobasilar system flow reduction to cause symptoms. When stenosis or occlusion of the VA origin leads to TIAs or stroke,

Table 55-2 Clinical Manifestations of Ischemia in the Vertebrobasilar System According to the Artery Involved*

Involved Artery	Ischemic Manifestations
Vertebral or PICA penetrator arteries (Lateral medullary or Wallenberg syndrome)	Ipsilateral limb ataxia and Horner syndrome, crossed sensory loss, vertigo, dysphagia, hoarseness
PICA	Vertigo, nausea, vomiting, gait ataxia
AICA	Gait and limb ataxia, dysfunction of ipsilateral CN-V, -VII, -VIII
SCA	Dysarthria and limb ataxia
PCA right	Contralateral visual field cut and sensory loss, visual neglect, prosopagnosia (inability to recognize faces)
Left	Contralateral visual field cut and sensory loss, alexia without agraphia, anomic or transcortical sensory aphasia, impaired memory and visual agnosia
Top of the basilar syndrome	Rostral brainstem—somnolence, vivid hallucinations, dreamlike behavior, and oculomotor dysfunction. Temporal + occipital regions—hemianopsia, fragments of Balint syndrome, agitated behavior, and amnestic dysfunction

*AICA, anterior inferior cerebellar artery; PCA, posterior cerebral artery; PICA, posterior–inferior cerebellar artery; SCA, superior cerebellar artery

intra-arterial embolism is the commonly recognized mechanism. The embolus usually lodges in the distal vertebral artery, causing a PICA stroke, or passes through, leading to a "top of the basilar syndrome" (Table 55-2).

Distal intracranial VA atherosclerotic disease most often occurs at the level of the penetrators to the lateral medulla and at the take-off to the PICA. Occlusion at this site presents as a Wallenberg syndrome (lateral medullary syndrome) or cerebellar PICA stroke or both. Lateral medullary syndrome progressing into coma and herniation due to an associated large PICA cerebellar infarction is not uncommon and emphasizes the need to investigate and closely observe those with Wallenberg syndromes for unfolding signs of wider neurologic involvement.

Atherosclerosis of the basilar artery most often affects its proximal and mid portions. Patients experience TIAs characterized by transient diplopia, dizziness, incoordination, and weakness affecting both sides at once or alternating between sides over minutes and even hours or days (Fig. 55-9). As in other occlusive large artery disease, some patients with severe basilar stenosis develop prominent headaches in the weeks before focal symptoms commence. The headache is thought to be from developing posterior circulation collateral flow. When stroke occurs, the most commonly affected area is the basis pons, with bilateral, often asymmetric, hemiparesis, pseudobulbar syndrome, abnormalities of eye movements (sixth nerve palsy, unilateral or bilateral internuclear ophthalmoplegia, ipsilateral conjugate gaze palsy, "one and one-half syndrome"), nystagmus, and if the reticular activating system is involved, coma (Fig. 55-10). Presence of coma or altered level of consciousness is dependent on collateral flow to the tegmentum from other vessels. If the pontine and midbrain tegmentum is spared, bilateral motor and sensory signs as well as varying degrees of ophthalmoplegia may be present without altered consciousness, such as in the "locked in" syndrome.

Embolus to the distal basilar artery leads to the classic top of the basilar syndrome (Fig. 55-11). Affected areas are the rostral brainstem (penetrator branches from distal basilar artery), the thalamus (penetrators of the proximal PCAs), and the medial temporal and occipital lobes. Clinical presentation includes bilateral homonymous hemianopsias or cortical blindness,

confusion, vivid-formed visual hallucinations (peduncular hallucinations), and inability to form new memories. In contrast, emboli moving past the basilar tip cause only unilateral PCA occlusions, with isolated homonymous hemianopsias.

Most PCA infarcts are either cardioembolic or from intra-arterial embolism. Intrinsic PCA stenosis can occur but is rare. Clinical symptoms consist of transient episodes of hemivisual loss with, at times, associated contralateral sensory symptoms that precede the stroke onset by weeks or days. When headaches occur, they are often retro-orbital or around the brow. In addition to visual and sensory abnormalities, patients with left PCA strokes often have concurrent anomic or transcortical sensory aphasia, impaired memory, associative visual agnosia (recognition) and, when involving the posterior commissure, alexia without agraphia (inability to read with preserved writing). Patients with right PCA stroke often have associated visual neglect and prosopagnosia (difficulty in recognizing familiar faces or specific items of a recognizable group). Bilateral parieto-occipital damage (Balint syndrome) leads to inability to view a grouped visual stimulus as a whole (asimultanagnosia), loss of accurate visual fixation and ocular tracking (optic apraxia), and impaired precision pointing to a visual target ("optic ataxia"). Bilateral occipital cortex injuries produce an inability to recognize all visual stimuli, often with absent insight into the deficit (cortical blindness or Anton syndrome).

Cardioembolic Disease

Clinical Vignette

A 59-year-old physician suddenly had difficulty driving; his wife noted that their car almost hit objects off to the right side. When questioned, he agreed that he was having difficulty seeing to the right. When this did not improve overnight, he was evaluated in the ED, revealing a dense right homonymous hemianopsia. Otherwise, neurologic and general physical examination were normal. Brain CT demonstrated a left occipital lobe hypodensity compatible with PCA infarction. MRI confirmed these findings, and MRA

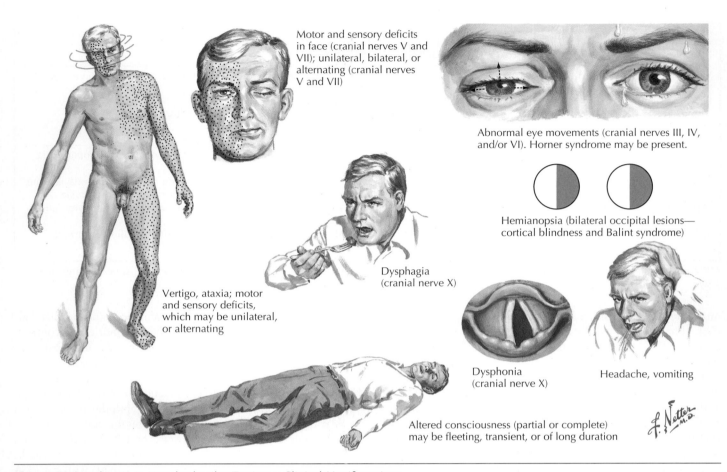

Motor and sensory deficits in face (cranial nerves V and VII); unilateral, bilateral, or alternating (cranial nerves V and VII)

Abnormal eye movements (cranial nerves III, IV, and/or VI). Horner syndrome may be present.

Hemianopsia (bilateral occipital lesions—cortical blindness and Balint syndrome)

Dysphagia (cranial nerve X)

Vertigo, ataxia; motor and sensory deficits, which may be unilateral, or alternating

Dysphonia (cranial nerve X)

Headache, vomiting

Altered consciousness (partial or complete) may be fleeting, transient, or of long duration

Figure 55-9 Ischemia in Vertebrobasilar Territory: Clinical Manifestations.

revealed a left PCA origin occlusion. A 48-hour Holter monitor demonstrated paroxysmal AF. Warfarin sodium was administered with careful monitoring. His right homonymous hemianopsia did not improve and he was told not to drive. Otherwise, he successfully compensated for this loss of vision.

Atrial fibrillation, paroxysmal or chronic, is one of the most common sources of cardiac brain embolism and accounts for up to 15–20% of all ischemic stroke. The incidence of atrial fibrillation in the population older than age 65 years is estimated at around 6%, but most patients do not experience embolic events. Risk factors that predispose to stroke or embolization from nonvalvular atrial fibrillation include age older than 75 years, hypertension, ejection fraction below 35%, and congestive heart failure. Conditions such as coronary artery disease, thyrotoxicosis, and female gender may represent other factors that play a lesser role. Multiple risk factor increase the likelihood of major stroke up to sevenfold and should be strongly considered for antithrombotic treatment. Those who present with TIA or stroke hold the highest risk or recurrence around 12% a year for the first year, then 5–6% yearly thereafter. Atrial flutter, although a more organized cardiac arrhythmia, still predisposes to emboli formation and should be approached in the same fashion as atrial fibrillation.

Strokes secondary to cardiac sources typically present with acute onset of focal neurologic deficits, such as sudden loss of hand control or drooping of the mouth, often associated with language dysfunction, if involving the dominant hemisphere, or neglect if involving the nondominant hemisphere. Cerebral emboli are most clinically apparent during the day, and patients often provide a precise time of stroke or TIA onset. Cardioembolic stroke typically occurs during the waking hours with patient activity, in contrast to intra-arterial thrombosis or artery-to-artery embolism that often occur in sleep when rheological factors may favor increased coagulation. The anterior carotid circulation receives 80% of cerebral blood flow and is four times more likely than the posterior vertebrobasilar circulation to be affected with emboli. Furthermore, a history of TIAs, strokes, or both, affecting both carotid and vertebrobasilar territories increases the suspicion of cardiac embolism. The vessels more often affected by cardiac emboli are the MCA and its branches, followed by the distal portion of the intracranial vertebral artery, distal basilar (top of the basilar syndrome), and the PCA territory.

Emboli from recent MI typically are more likely to occur within the first 2 weeks of the acute event. Patients with anterior wall myocardial infarctions may develop segmental hypokinetic myocardial wall defects or even aneurysms. Such lesions provide a potential nidus for platelet aggregation with subsequent embolus formation.

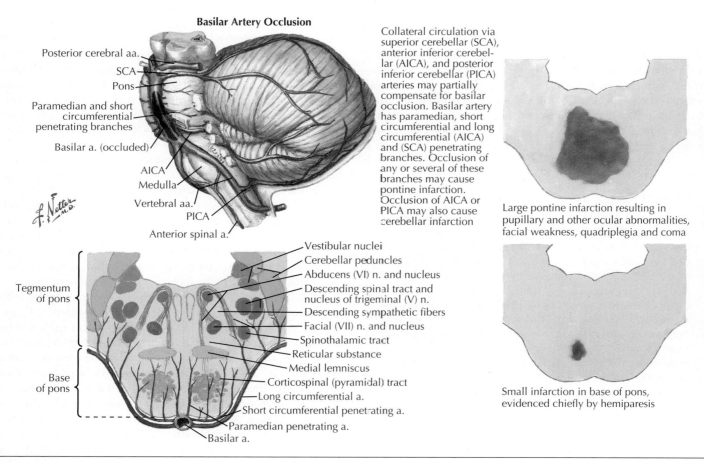

Figure 55-10 Basilar Artery Occlusion.

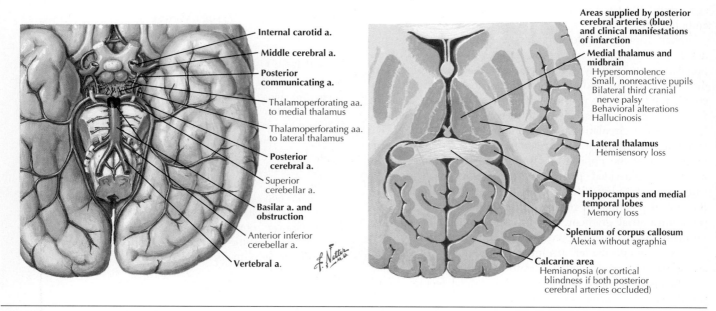

Figure 55-11 Occlusion of "Top Basilar" and Posterior Cerebral Arteries.

Infective endocarditis presents with TIA or stroke in approximately 15% of cases, but eventually 30% of patients are likely to experience a major neurologic complication throughout the course of the illness. Individuals with valvular heart disease are particularly at risk for developing endocarditis after any procedure that leads to transient bacteremia, even those as innocuous as dental cleaning, and should be treated beforehand with prophylactic antibiotics. Intravenously illicit drug use is also a major risk for infective endocarditis because of the reuse of nonsterilized needles. Endocarditis commonly presents with systemic symptoms, such as fever, weight loss, and malaise as well as signs of a new-onset or changing cardiac murmur, petechial rash, microemboli to the nail beds (splinter hemorrhages) and conjunctiva, tender nodules or erythematous lesions in the palms and finger pads (Osler nodes and Janeway lesions), and retinal emboli with exudate (Roth spots). Microemboli affecting the brain diffusely often present as an encephalopathy rather than with focal neurologic findings and may be hard to diagnose in the setting of chronic medical illness.

Clinical Vignette

A previously healthy 41-year-old woman had a right facial droop and difficulty speaking 1 day after she had made a continuous 10-hour car trip. At the ED, neurologic examination confirmed right central facial weakness and a mild mixed expressive and receptive aphasia. Cardiac examination and an electrocardiograph were normal. Brain MRI with diffusion-weighted imaging showed a small left insular stroke. Head and neck MRA results were normal. Transesophageal echocardiography (TEE) showed a patent foramen ovale (PFO), and her hypercoagulable screen was remarkable for protein S deficiency. Symptoms gradually improved, clearing completely within 72 hours.

Despite a clinically normal initial cardiac examination, the TEE confirmed a congenital intra-atrial heart defect. The symptom complex acuity was consistent with a cardioembolic source, justifying a careful heart evaluation. In patients of this age group, PFO is the most likely associated condition with embolic stroke.

Patent foramen ovale and, less encountered atrial septal defects, are common and occur in up to one fourth of the population and usually do not cause cardiac symptoms. This intra-arterial connection is a remnant of the intrauterine fetal circulation that allows placental oxygenated blood to bypass the fetal unaerated lung vasculature directly to the left atrium and fetal systemic circulation. This conduit, which usually closes within a few months of birth, remains partially patent in a large proportion of the population. Any venue that predisposes to increased right-sided pulmonary and right atrial pressures (squatting, straining, lifting, coughing, etc.) would have the theoretical potential of transiently reversing the usual left-to-right intra-atrial gradient, and prompt venous clots that are normally dissolved or filtered in the pulmonary circulation, to cross directly into the left atrium and subsequently the cerebral and systemic arterial circulation. Another presumed mechanism is turbulent or stagnant flow in and around the defect itself, with subsequent clot formation and propagation. PFOs are usually detected by Doppler echocardiography. After a brief delay, intravenous agitated saline or colloid injections are seen as echodense air bubbles crossing the intra-atrial septum from right to left. This is often aided by a Valsalva maneuver that transiently increases right-sided atrial pressure with respect to the left. Transesophageal echocardiography holds a higher sensitivity as compared to a transthoracic approach and is considered the test of choice. PFO has been shown to be more common in young

adults with cryptogenic stroke as compared to the general population and as compared to those with identifiable sources of stroke. Being a common finding, the presence of a PFO as a cause of paradoxical embolism in cryptogenic stroke remains however presumptive, and other situational, hematologic, and anatomic factors likely come into play that make the PFO clinically relevant. For example, a paradoxical embolism becomes more suspicious in a young patient with a prior history of deep venous thrombosis who presents with a stroke after a bout of coughing from an upper respiratory tract infection during a period of relative immobility. As illustrated in the vignette, patients at risk include those who are nonambulatory from prolonged illness or even seemingly inconsequential settings, such as during prolonged transoceanic flights or car trips where venous flow in the legs is diminished or stagnant. Those with coagulation disorders, either hereditary or acquired such as with hormone replacement therapy or pregnancy, are also at a higher risk. Studies show that the incidence of an associated hypercoagulable hematologic abnormality is higher in patients with cryptogenic stroke and PFO than the general population. Coagulation studies and a search for deep vein thrombosis should be included in the workup for all young patients with cryptogenic stroke and an associated PFO. Anatomic considerations also come into play. A PFO with an associated atrial septal aneurysm (>10 mm protrusion into either atrium) holds a much higher risk of recurrence of up to 19.2% over 4 years even when treated with antiplatelets. A large-size PFO (>1 cm) with many microbubbles crossing the intra-arterial septum, especially without the aid of a Valsalva maneuver, likely represents a high risk of recurrence.

Lacunar Small Vessel Disease

Clinical Vignette

A 71-year-old woman with poorly controlled arterial hypertension developed subacute-onset, initially stuttering, left hemiparesis over 48 hours. She presented 2 weeks later when she had not fully recovered. There was no history of headache, sensory loss, visual changes, or language dysfunction. Neurologic examination demonstrated a pure motor hemiparesis, brisk right-sided muscle stretch reflexes, and a right Babinski sign.

Brain MRI showed a lacuna within the right pons. MRA of the head and neck were normal. The patient was started on antiplatelet treatment and gradually improved during a 2-week stay at the rehabilitation unit, but remained with a slight tendency to circumduct the leg while walking, even 6 months later.

Lacunar strokes affecting the internal capsule, thalamus, striatum, or brainstem (see Fig. 55-5) can often be clinically distinguished from embolic disease by the tendency toward a more insidious onset, with deficits progressing or stuttering on over 2–4 days. Additionally, lacunar deficits have a relatively typical distribution; they affect the entire side of the body with motor and/or sensory symptoms without cortically based

Table 55-3 Most Frequent Lacunar Syndromes and Their Locations

Clinical Syndrome	Location
Pure motor stroke: weakness equally involving face, arm, and leg	Internal capsule (posterior limb) or basis pontis
Pure sensory stroke: numbness or paresthesia equally involving face, arm, leg and usually trunk	Lateral thalamus (posteroventral nucleus)
Ataxic hemiparesis: weakness and incoordination in the arm and/or leg	Basis pontis or internal capsule
Dysarthria—clumsy hand: facial weakness, severe dysarthria and dysphagia, slight weakness, and clumsiness of the hand	Basis pontis
Rare sensorimotor stroke: combination of pure motor/pure sensory symptoms and findings	Thalamus internal capsule

findings or visual changes. This is in contrast to middle cerebral artery cortical branch occlusions that tend to have a brachiofacial distribution often associated with other cognitive and/or visual signs.

Patients experiencing lacunar strokes can present with TIA in up to 15–20% of instances. TIAs are stereotypical, and tend to cluster over 2–5 days, at times occurring frequently over a 24-hour period and in a crescendo fashion. Signs and symptoms vary according to the location of the ischemia (Table 55-3).

Hypertension and diabetes are the most important risk factors, and proper treatment of these conditions is essential to prevent further strokes.

Arterial Dissection

Clinical Vignette

A 42-year-old man with no vascular risk factors presented with acute-onset left-sided weakness and numbness. Symptoms were preceded by severe nonspecific right-sided neck and retro-orbital pain for 1 week after he had had a relatively inconsequential fall. Examination revealed evidence of a spastic left hemiparesis and hemineglect of the left arm more than the leg. Head CT showed a complete right MCA stroke, and CTA showed tapering of the right ICA 2 cm above the bifurcation, suggestive of arterial dissection. Patient was treated with heparin and subsequently with warfarin. Repeated CTA 6 months later showed complete recanalization of the right ICA. Warfarin was discontinued and the patient was placed on antiplatelet treatment.

Extracranial carotid artery dissection occurs predominantly in patients aged 20–50 years. The characteristic clinical presentation is unilateral neck or face pain followed a few days later by acute onset of neurologic signs. In patients with carotid dissection, pain is usually referred to the eye, temple, or forehead.

Ipsilateral Horner syndrome occurs in 40–50% of patients and is due to distension or pressure against the oculosympathetic fibers running along the internal carotid artery to the eye. Pulsatile tinnitus is common. Often, a history of minor trauma exists (violent coughing, cervical manipulation, whiplash injury, etc.) in the days preceding symptom onset. As in the preceding vignette, benign traumatic events can cause a slight intima tear in the carotid or vertebral arteries, leading to platelet fibrin aggregation with potential for developing artery-to-artery emboli.

Similar to the carotid artery within the neck, the extracranial VA has a significant potential for sustaining traumatic dissection. Dissection usually occurs in the distal extracranial portion at C1–C2, also called the *third segment*, just before it penetrates the dura at the skull base. In those patients, pain is referred to the neck or back of the head and usually precedes the onset of neurologic signs by days and rarely weeks.

TIAs are more common in ICA than on VA dissections. In ICA dissection, TIAs usually involve the ipsilateral eye and cerebral hemisphere. Symptoms of VA dissection are of dizziness, diplopia, gait unsteadiness, and dysarthria. In extracranial ICA and VA dissections, strokes usually affect the MCA and distal VA territories (PICA and lateral medullary). The mechanism of stroke relates to artery-to-artery embolization from clot accumulation and eventual rupture through the media into the vessel lumen. Also progressive true lumen narrowing with hypoperfusion occurs as does eventual occlusion, often following a flurry of successive TIA before the final stroke.

DIAGNOSTIC APPROACH

For every patient evaluated with ischemic stroke or TIA, the location of the lesion and mechanism should be investigated thoroughly to better predict potential complications and to most effectively direct treatment. CT and MRI brain scanning have greatly enhanced our ability to diagnose and follow neurologic disease as well as guide treatment. Noninvasive arterial imaging with CTA and MRA have largely replaced catheter angiography in the initial evaluation of cerebrovascular disease and show great promise in advancing acute stroke care (Fig. 55-12).

Anatomic Site

Although the precise anatomic location of an acute TIA or stroke can frequently be deduced by the history and neurologic examination, confirmation with an imaging study is needed and often provides more specific etiologic information that can direct potential treatment. In addition, intracerebral hemorrhages, subdural hematomas, or other structural lesions including benign and malignant tumors are occasionally found on brain CT and MRI in patients presenting with seemingly typical cerebrovascular events.

Brain CT examination, with its immediate availability in most hospitals and short scanning time, is usually the initial study performed in individuals presenting with an acute focal neurologic deficit. Its sensitivity to detect the presence of a primary cerebral hemorrhage or a hemorrhagic infarct is a crucial starting point in determining the future course of action

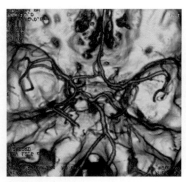

A. 3-D reconstructed image of the Circle of Willis on computed tomography angiography (CTA).

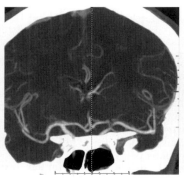

B. Reconstructed CTA images of coronal intercerebral vessels.

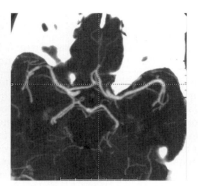

C. Reconstructed CTA images of axial intercerebral vessels.

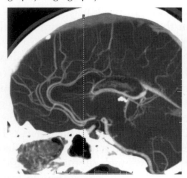

D. Reconstructed CTA images of sagittal intercerebral vessels.

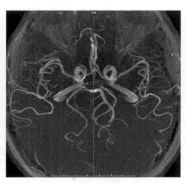

E. Reconstructed magnetic resonance angiography (MRA) composite of all proximal vessels.

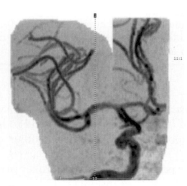

F. Reconstructed magnetic resonance angiography (MRA) of the right internal carotid circulation.

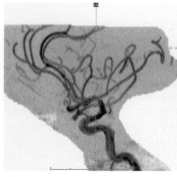

G. Reconstructed magnetic resonance angiography (MRA) of the right internal carotid circulation.

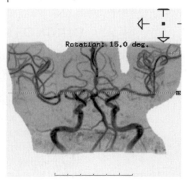

H. Reconstructed magnetic resonance angiography (MRA) composite of all proximal vessels.

Figure 55-12 Intracranial Arterial Imaging with CT and MRI.

such as the use of thrombolytics, the need for surgical intervention, and the degree of blood pressure control. The head CT is often normal in the first few hours of an ischemic stroke. However, in some cases, the presence of an acute arterial occlusion can be detected by the presence of a localized intraluminal hyperdense signal, often seen in patients with MCA occlusion (Fig. 55-13A), even when the brain parenchyma shows no evolving processes. Head CT may also show early infarct changes characterized by sulcal effacement or loss of gray–white matter differentiation (Fig. 55-13B). Such findings have important therapeutic implications. A CT angiogram can confirm the presence of a thrombus (Fig. 55-13C) and help guide further intervention concerning intravenous or intra-arterial tissue plasminogen activator (t-PA), anticoagulation, and management of blood pressure.

Diffusion-weighted MRI is the most sensitive and specific test for acute ischemia, and abnormalities have been demonstrated as early as 1 hour after symptom onset. Combined with concomitant perfusion scanning information, the ischemic penumbra (area of brain with compromised cerebral perfusion but without established infarction) can be defined, and decision concerning the risk and feasibility of reperfusion intervention can now be made more effectively and safely. Other MRI sequences, such as FLAIR and T2-weighted imaging, can show the area of stroke, often 6–12 hours after onset of symptoms (Fig. 55-13D and E).

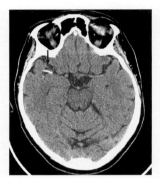

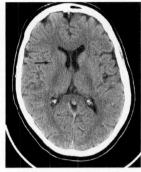

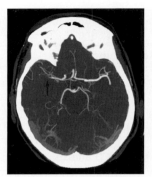

A. Axial CT scan demonstrates increased density in distal right M1 segment (arrow); a hyperdense MCA sign.

B. Axial CT scan 2 cm higher demonstrates normal insular ribbon and imperceptible change in right basal ganglia (arrow)

C. Computed tomography angiography (CTA) shows opacification of a few branches proximal to the previously demonstrated clot and expected obstruction of distal right M1 segment (arrow)

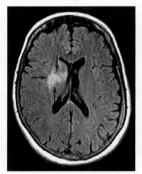

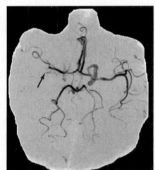

D. Axial FLAIR image 11 hours later demonstrates edema in the ischemic basal ganglia (arrows) where restricted diffusion was also noted.

E. MR angiography shows obstruction of distal right M1 segment similar to CTA (arrow)

Figure 55-13 Acute Ischemic Infarct with a Right Middle Cerebral Artery Clot.

Table 55-4 Comparison of Neurologic Imaging Techniques*

Imaging Method	Advantages	Disadvantages
MRI/MRA	DWI and PWI demonstrate the area of stroke and the area at risk (penumbra), respectively.	Prolonged test (30–60 min); patient must cooperate or sedation is required. Cannot be performed in patients with PCM. MRA can overestimate tight stenosis as an occluded vessel.
CTA/CTP	Images can be obtained rapidly (<5 min).	Patient must have normal renal function because CTA and CTP require high doses of contrast, 100 and 50 mL, respectively.
Ultrasonography of the neck	Easy to perform, can be done at the bedside	No detailed information about the vertebral arteries or the intracranial vessels.
TCD	Easy to perform, even at the bedside	Poor transtemporal windows limit the information about the intracranial vessels.

*CTA, computed tomography angiography; CTP, computed tomography perfusion; DWI, diffusion-weighted imaging; PCM, pacemaker; PWI, perfusion-weighted imaging; TCD, transcranial Doppler

Etiologic Mechanism

To define the specific pathophysiologic mechanism for a TIA or stroke, patency of the extracranial and intracranial arteries, the character of their endothelial surface, and the adequacy of cerebral perfusion are required.

Complete assessment of cardiac function is essential and includes the electrical stability of the cardiac rhythm, myocardial contractility, valvular status, and whether a PFO is present. TEE provides more sensitivity and anatomic details and is preferred over the transthoracic approach for valvular lesions, intra-atrial abnormalities (PFO and ASD), and aortic arch disease. Ultrasound of the carotid arteries at their bifurcation in the neck and transcranial Doppler of the intracranial vessels can functionally assess cerebral flow and determine the presence of critically stenotic extracranial or circle of Willis arteries, respectively. Carotid ultrasound helps characterize the carotid plaque as "soft" consisting of cholesterol deposits and clot, which is more prone to ulceration and artery-to-artery embolization, or "hard" where the vessel wall has fibrosed and calcified over time, making it a less likely source of distal embolization. MRA or CTA of the head and neck is appropriate to assess patency of intracranial and extracranial arteries. The more recent addition of perfusion scanning helps define the effect of any stenotic lesion upon regional blood flow (Table 55-4).

Table 55-5 Guidelines for Imaging in Ischemic Stroke/TIA Apropos Patient Renal Function and Pacemaker Presence*

Normal Renal Function	Presence of PCM	Abnormal Renal Function
CT of the head, CT perfusion, and CTA of head and neck	CT of the head, CT perfusion, and CTA of head and neck	CT of the head, TCD and US
or	or	or
MRI of the head + DWI/PWI, MRA of the head and neck	CT of the head, TCD and US	MRI of the head MRA of head and neck without use of contrast
or		
CT of the head, TCD and US		

*CTA, computed tomography angiography; DWI, diffusion-weighted imaging; PCM, pacemaker; PWI, perfusion-weighted imaging; TCD, transcranial Doppler; US, ultrasonography

Information gathered from imaging studies allows differentiation of three primary carotid or vertebrobasilar stroke mechanisms: large artery disease with intra-arterial embolism, small vessel disease, and large artery disease with hemodynamic ischemia.

Renal failure or pacemaker devices limit the imaging studies that can be performed in patients with TIAs and strokes (Table 55-5). Gadolinium-based contrast agents have recently been linked to the development of nephrogenic systemic fibrosis and nephrogenic fibrosing dermopathy, often with serious and irreversible skin or organ pathology in patients with moderate to end-stage renal disease. The mechanism is unclear but thought to be due to stimulation of tissue fibrosis similar to that seen in scleroderma or eosinophilia-myalgia syndrome.

A hypercoagulable screen, including protein C, protein S, antiphospholipid antibodies (anticardiolipin antibodies and lupus anticoagulant), factor II DNA, factor V Leiden or protein C resistance, antithrombin III, and homocysteinemia are part of the evaluation of patients younger than 50 years and in patients of any age without identifiable risk factors. It should be kept in mind that most inherited coagulopathies are more associated with systemic and cerebral venous thrombosis rather than arterial stroke and a direct relation cannot be made. Other factors such as smoking, hormonal therapy, and the presence of a PFO may make them more relevant in cases of ischemic stroke without any other clear source.

TREATMENT

The treatment of ischemic TIAs and strokes can be divided into identification and treatment of vascular risk factors, primary and secondary stroke prevention, treatment of the acute phase of stroke, surgical treatment and rehabilitation.

Identification and Treatment of Vascular Risk Factors

Well-documented and modifiable risk factors for strokes, such as hypertension and diabetes, should be regularly screened in all patients with or without history of prior TIAs and strokes and appropriately treated according to the 2006 American Heart Association/American Stroke Association (AHA/ASA) guidelines, which include dietary changes, increased physical activity, and pharmacologic treatment.

Statins have been approved for prevention of ischemic strokes or TIAs in patients with elevated cholesterol, comorbid coronary artery disease, or evidence of an atherosclerotic origin. Treatment should aim for a target low-density lipoprotein cholesterol (LDL-C) level of <100 mg/dL and for high-risk patients with multiple risk factors an LDL-C <70 mg/dL is usually recommended.

Since the publication of the Stroke Prevention by Aggressive Reduction in Cholesterol Levels (SPARCL) trial, statins have been recommended for patients with atherosclerotic ischemic stroke or TIA even without known coronary heart disease to reduce the risk of both subsequent stroke and cardiovascular events. This trial showed a 5-year absolute risk reduction of 2.2% for the combination fatal and nonfatal stroke and of 3.5% absolute risk reduction for major cardiovascular events in patients receiving 80 mg of atorvastatin as compared with placebo. The two treatment groups have no significant differences in the incidence of serious adverse events; however, there were slightly more hemorrhagic strokes in the atorvastatin group as compared with placebo (55 vs. 33). Hemorrhagic strokes were more frequent in men, older patients, with hemorrhagic stroke as an entry event, and in patients with stage 2 hypertension (systolic BP ≥ 160 mm Hg, diastolic BP ≥ 100 mm Hg) at the last visit just prior to the hemorrhagic stroke. There was no relationship between the hemorrhagic risk and the LDL cholesterol levels.

Smoking cessation is recommended, and avoidance of environmental tobacco smoke for stroke prevention should be considered in all patients.

Primary and Secondary Stroke Prevention

PRIMARY PREVENTION

Aspirin is the only antiplatelet agent that has been studied for primary stroke prevention. Five trials have examined the effects of daily or every-other-day aspirin for the primary prevention of cardiovascular events over periods of 4–7 years. Most participants were men older than 50 years. Meta-analysis from these studies showed that aspirin therapy reduced the risk of CHD by 28% but without any significant effect on total mortality and stroke. Most of the data for primary prevention in women comes from The Women's Health Study. This study showed a nonsignificant reduction for a first major vascular event (nonfatal MI, nonfatal stroke, or cardiovascular death) in women older than age 45 years treated with low-dose aspirin as compared with placebo but a 17% reduction in the stroke risk. The most consistent benefit was for women aged 65 years or older at study entry, among whom the risk of major cardiovascular event or stroke was reduced by 26%, including a 30% reduction of risk of ischemic stroke. Analysis of the subgroups showed a reduction in stroke for those women with history of hypertension, diabetes, hyperlipidemia, or a 10-year cardiovascular risk equal to or greater than 10. Based on the above data, the 2006 guideline update from the AHA/ASA for primary prevention of ischemic stroke recommends the use of low-dose aspirin for cardiovascular prophylaxis among patients whose risk is sufficiently high.

Anticoagulation with warfarin is indicated for primary stroke prevention in patients with atrial fibrillation who have valvular heart disease, particularly mechanical valve. For patients with nonvalvular AFIB, stratification according to stroke risk following CHADS2 (congestive heart failure, hypertension, age >75 years, diabetes mellitus, and prior strokes and TIAs) is recommended. The score gives 1 point for each risk factor and 2 points for strokes and TIAs. Nonvalvular atrial fibrillation patients with CHADS2 score of 0–1 have an annual stroke risk of approximately 1%, and aspirin treatment only is recommended. For patients with a CHADS2 score of 2 (2.5% annual stroke risk) and CHADS2 equal to or greater than 3 (annual stroke risk >4%), anticoagulation is recommended in the absence of contraindications. It is generally recommended that the target international normalized ratio be in the range of 2.0–3.0. Monitored closely within this range, warfarin is generally found to be safe and effective although there continues to be a higher rate of major bleeding complications compared to aspirin. Aspirin treatment alone holds modest benefit for stroke prevention in atrial fibrillation and should be considered in patients who cannot take warfarin.

SECONDARY PREVENTION

The benefit of antiplatelets for secondary prevention in patients with a prior history of noncardioembolic stroke or TIA, more specifically, atherosclerotic, lacunar, or cryptogenic stroke, is well established. The most common antiplatelet agents used are aspirin, clopidogrel, and a combination of dipyridamole and low-dose aspirin.

Aspirin is the oldest antiplatelet drug and probably the most often prescribed drug worldwide. It inhibits the cyclooxygenase enzyme preventing production of thromboxane A_2, a stimulator of platelet aggregation. A meta-analysis published in 2002 by the Antithrombotic Trialist's Collaboration supports the benefits of aspirin for prevention of ischemic stroke and cardiovascular events. This meta-analysis showed that patients at high risk for cardiovascular disease treated with antiplatelets (primarily aspirin) have a 25% relative risk reduction in nonfatal stroke as compared with placebo. The dose of aspirin for secondary stroke prevention varies from 20 to 1300 mg in the different trials. However, most studies have found that 50–325 mg of aspirin a day is as effective as higher doses, with less bleeding complications.

Clopidogrel is a thienopyridine that inhibits ADP-dependent platelet aggregation. In the CAPRIE trial (Clopidogrel versus Aspirin in Patients at Risk of Ischemic Events), patients with recent stroke, MI, or peripheral vascular disease were randomly assigned to 75 mg/day of clopidogrel or 325 mg/day of aspirin. The primary end point (composite outcome of stroke, MI, or vascular death) was significantly reduced with clopidogrel as compared with aspirin, with a relative risk reduction of 8.7%. Of note, most of the benefit in this trial was observed in the subgroup of patients with peripheral vascular disease. Clopidogrel had a favorable side effect profile as compared with aspirin, with a slightly lower frequency if GI bleeding and slightly higher frequency of rash and diarrhea.

Despite its proven benefits on stroke prevention, ticlopidine, another thienopyridine, is rarely used because of its potentially serious side effects of severe neutropenia and thrombotic thrombocytopenic purpura (TTP).

Dipyridamole inhibits platelet aggregation induced by the phosphodiesterase. The combination of low-dose aspirin (50 mg) and sustained-release dipyridamole (400 mg/day) for secondary stroke prevention has been shown to be more effective than either drug alone. The relative risk reduction of stroke compared to placebo in the European Stroke Prevention Study (ESPS-2) was 37% for the combination between aspirin and dipyridamole, 18.1% for aspirin, and 16.3% for dipyridamole. Similar benefits were later reported in the European/Australasian Stroke Prevention in Reversible Ischemia Trial (ESPRIT).

Interestingly, the combination of aspirin and clopidogrel for stroke prevention does not show any benefit over treatment with clopidogrel alone (MATCH [Management of Atherothrombosis with Clopidogrel in High-risk patients] trial) or aspirin alone (CHARISMA [Clopidogrel for High Atherothrombotic Risk and Ischemic Stabilization, Management, and Avoidance] trial), and has a significantly increased risk of life-threatening bleeding complications. Therefore, the combination of clopidogrel and aspirin is not recommended for stroke prevention at this time.

The recent results of the Prevention Regimen for Effectively Avoiding Second Strokes trial (PROGRESS trial) comparing clopidogrel with the combination of aspirin and dipyridamole in more than 20,000 patients with recent atherothrombotic ischemic stroke showed no statistical difference between the groups in the primary outcome of recurrent stroke. Also, the main secondary composite endpoint of stroke, myocardial infarction or vascular death, was similar between the two treatment groups.

Warfarin inhibits vitamin K–dependent coagulation factor synthesis (II, VII, IX, X, proteins C and S). Warfarin has a significant benefit compared with placebo for secondary stroke prevention in patients with AF with an annual stroke rate of 4% in patients receiving warfarin compared with 12% in patients receiving placebo.

According to the WARSS trial, warfarin was not superior to aspirin for prevention of recurrent ischemic strokes or death in patients with a prior noncardioembolic ischemic strokes. Most patients in this trial had small vessel disease (56%) or stroke of unclear etiology (26.1%). Warfarin also showed no advantage over aspirin for prevention of ischemic stroke or vascular death in patients with symptomatic intracranial artery stenosis (WASID trial) and was associated with significantly higher rates of adverse events.

The best treatment for stroke prevention in patients with extracranial dissections remains unclear. The 2006 AHA/ASA guidelines recommend the use of either warfarin or antiplatelets for 3–6 months in patients with extracranial vessel dissections. Beyond 3–6 months, long-term antiplatelet is reasonable for most patients, but anticoagulation may be considered for those with recurrent ischemic events.

For patients with ischemic strokes or TIAs and a PFO, antiplatelet therapy is reasonable to prevent recurrent events. However, warfarin may be preferable for patients with an underlying hypercoagulable state and for those with anatomic features associated with higher recurrence rates such as large PFOs with a vigorous and spontaneous right-to-left atrial shunting and those associated with atrial septal aneurysms. Currently, there is insufficient evidence to support PFO closure in patients with a first-time cryptogenic stroke, and randomized trials comparing the effectiveness of PFO closure versus conventional medical treatment in preventing stroke recurrence are ongoing.

Treatment of the Acute Phase

Acute treatment of patients with ischemic stroke includes general measures, thrombolysis in selected patients, and antiplatelet treatment in patients not treated with thrombolytics.

Deep venous thrombosis prophylaxis, monitoring and control of BP and blood sugars, aggressive treatment of hyperthermia and any associated infection, strict fluid management, and aspiration precautions are basic, but important measures in the first few days of acute stroke.

Despite the high prevalence of arterial hypertension following a stroke, its optimal management has not been well established. High levels of blood pressure in the acute setting of a stroke can increase the risk of hemorrhagic transformation, cerebral edema, and further vascular damage. However, aggressive treatment of the blood pressure can reduce cerebral blood flow in the area of ischemia, increasing the infarct size. The Stroke Council of the AHA recommends for patients not eligible for thrombolytic treatment to withhold treatment with antihypertensive agents unless the diastolic blood pressure is >120 mm Hg or systolic blood pressure is >220 mm Hg. For thrombolytic-eligible patients, systolic blood pressure should be maintained below 180 mm Hg and diastolic below 105 mm Hg during and up to 24 hours after the treatment in order to prevent parenchymal hemorrhage. Intravenous beta blockers and calcium channel blockers such as labetalol and nicardipine, respectively, are first-line agents to control blood pressure levels in those patients. For patients with diastolic blood pressure higher than 140 mm Hg, sodium nitroprusside is the drug of choice.

A randomized double-blind trial of IV recombinant tissue plasminogen activator (rt-PA) in patients with ischemic stroke treated within the first 3 hours of symptom onset showed a 12% absolute (32% relative) increase in the number of patients with minimal or no disability at 3 months in the rt-PA group. The benefit was present for all the different stroke subtypes analyzed. Similar benefits of early treatment with rt-PA within a 3-hour window were also shown in a subpopulation analysis of patients in the ATLANTIS (Alteplase Thrombolysis for Acute Noninterventional Therapy in Ischemic Stroke) trial.

Box 55-1 Contraindications for IV rt-PA*

Strong Contraindications for IV rt-PA

1. Symptoms minor or rapidly improving
2. Other stroke or serious head trauma within the past 3 months
3. Major surgery within the past 14 days
4. Known history of intracranial hemorrhage
5. Sustained systolic BP >185 mm Hg
6. Sustained diastolic pressure >110 mm Hg
7. Symptoms suggestive of subarachnoid hemorrhage
8. Gastrointestinal or urinary tract hemorrhage within 21 days
9. Arterial puncture at noncompressible site within 7 days
10. Received heparin within 48 h and had increased PTT
11. Platelet count <100,000 μL
12. CT: evidence of brain hemorrhage or mass effect: suspected large infarct (more than $\frac{1}{3}$ territory of MCA)

Relative Contraindications

1. Seizure at onset of stroke
2. Serum glucose <50 mg/dL or >400 mg/dL
3. Hemorrhagic eye disorder
4. Myocardial infarction in the previous 6 weeks
5. Suspected septic embolism
6. Infective endocarditis
7. INR >1.7

*INR, international normalized ratio; PTT, partial thromboplastin time; rt-PA, recombinant tissue plasminogen activator

---

This treatment, since approved by the Food and Drug Administration (FDA), has become the standard of care for acute ischemic stroke, and all patients arriving to the hospital within the first 3 hours of symptom onset should be considered for IV rt-PA administration after appropriately screening for thrombolytic contraindications (Box 55-1).

In contrast to studies of patients treated within the 3-hour window, most clinical trials of intravenous t-PA in unselected patients presenting after 3 hours of symptoms onset have not shown any clear benefit. However, recent studies using MRI screening criteria have shown a favorable outcome in patients with a baseline diffusion and perfusion mismatch. In theory, the region of hypoperfused but potentially viable brain around an irreversibly damaged area of tissue, may respond favorably to thrombolytic therapy beyond the typical 3-hour window provided the infarcted core is small. The EPITHET trial (Echoplanar Imaging Thrombolytic Evaluation Trial) that evaluated IV t-PA versus placebo in the 3–6-hour window in patients evaluated with advanced neuroimaging showed increased perfusion and a trend toward reduced infarct size in threatened tissue but did not translate into an across-the-board clinical benefit. The ECASS III (European Cooperative in Acute Stroke Study) IV t-PA trial, however, excluded patients at high risk of bleeding and large deficits and supports extending the thrombolytic window to 4.5 hours in patients younger than 80 years with moderate stroke severity who are not taking warfarin or other anticoagulants.

Ultrasound-enhanced intravenous thrombolysis is a promising treatment, but so far remains to have a proven advantage and further study is needed regarding its safety and effectiveness.

Patients with large artery occlusions and severe strokes show only a limited response to intravenous thrombolytics and considerably higher rates of intracerebral hemorrhage. Intra-arterial thrombolysis holds promise in improving the outcomes of these patients, and studies show a recanalization rate of major cerebral vessel occlusions of 50% as compared to around only 25% with intravenous therapy alone. A review of the available data on intra-arterial thrombolysis shows a possible reduction of mortality and more favorable outcomes with this type of therapy, though with an increased risk of hemorrhagic complications as compared to standard intravenous therapy, especially when higher doses of heparin are used during the angiographic procedure. Overall, although promising, there is currently no evidence that intra-arterial thrombolysis is better than intravenous treatment, and IV therapy should not be withheld from eligible patients except in the setting of a comparative trial. Intra-arterial t-PA can, however, be considered in patients who do not qualify for IV t-PA and for those with major intracranial vessel occlusion (basilar artery or mainstem MCA syndromes) outside the 3-hour window but within 6 hours.

The combination of IV and IA thrombolysis has been studied and is based on the idea of uniting the advantages of both treatments: early intervention with IV thrombolysis and higher rates of recanalization with the use of intra-arterial therapy. Earlier trials show a better recanalization rate but with no improvement in clinical outcome when compared with intra-arterial treatment alone. Recent studies (Interventional Management of Stroke Study [IMS]) showed a 56% rate of recanalization in patients treated with the combination; however, similar outcomes and rate of symptomatic hemorrhage are seen as in the NINDS (National Institute for Neurological Disorders and Stroke) IV t-PA treatment group. Further studies are necessary to assess safety and efficacy of combined IA and IV thrombolysis.

Mechanical clot disruption and endovascular embolectomy have been used in the acute treatment of ischemic stroke, with or without intra-arterial thrombolysis. The MERCI (Mechanical Embolus Removal in Cerebral Ischemia) device, a corkscrew-like coil that retrieves the thrombus, is approved by the FDA for clot removal in selected patients. Even though the MERCI trial showed a higher rate of recanalization, there was no evidence of better outcome at 90 days as compared with historical controls from the Prourokinase for Acute Ischemic Stroke II study (PROACT II) Study. The risk of symptomatic intracranial hemorrhage (8%) was similar to that with IV t-PA in the NINDS trial (6.4%).

In patients that are ineligible for thrombolysis, treatment with heparin, low-molecular-weight heparin and aspirin may be considered. Aspirin (160 mg or 325 mg daily) is the only antiplatelet agent that has shown a small but statistically significant reduction in risk of early recurrent ischemic stroke, death and disability when given within 48 hours after ischemic stroke, regardless of the stroke subtype.

Abciximab, unfractionated heparin, LMW heparins, and heparinoids have not been shown to reduce rate of stroke recurrence, mortality, or stroke-related mortality when used within the first 48 hours of stroke onset. Regarding stroke subtype, the TOAST (Trial of ORG 10172 in Acute Stroke) trial showed a possible benefit of IV danaparoid in patients with large artery disease; however, this observation requires prospective validation before it can be given any weight.

Surgical Treatment

Carotid endarterectomy (CEA) for prevention of ischemic stroke has been performed since the early1950s, but it was only in the 1990s that several large-scale trials were performed comparing this type of surgery against best medical treatment in patients with internal carotid artery stenosis.

For the symptomatic patients, evidence from the North American Symptomatic Carotid Endarterectomy Trial (NASCET) and the European Carotid Surgery Trial (ECST) support CEA for severe (70–99%) symptomatic stenosis over best medical treatment, with a 17% absolute risk reduction and a 65% relative risk reduction of ipsilateral stroke at 2 years. CEA was not indicated for patients with stenosis less than 50%. For the symptomatic patients with stenosis between 50 and 69%, CEA is moderately useful and can be considered in selected patients. There is increasing evidence that specific plaque morphological features, such as "soft" noncalcific plaque with intraplaque hemorrhage and ulceration, increase the risk of stroke, and CEA may be a treatment option in symptomatic patients with only moderate degrees of ICA stenosis. NASCET showed that in symptomatic patients with stenosis of 50–69%, the 5-year rate of ipsilateral stroke in the surgical group was 15.7% compared to 22.2% among those treated medically.

For patients with asymptomatic ICA stenosis from 60 to 99%, evidence from the Asymptomatic Carotid Atherosclerosis Study (ACAS) and Asymptomatic Carotid Surgery Trial (ACST) showed a modest benefit favoring CEA, with an absolute risk reduction at 5 years of 5.9% and 5.4%, respectively. The stroke risk reduction was more prominent in men and independent of the degree of stenosis or contralateral disease. Therefore, it is reasonable to consider CEA for asymptomatic stenosis of 60–99% if the patient has a life expectancy of at least 5 years and if the rate of perioperative stroke or death for the institution or particular surgeon can be reliably kept to less than 3%.

Carotid endarterectomy is one of the more common vascular procedures, with rates of perioperative mortality or stroke below 1% now achieved in many centers or practices (Fig. 55-14). A complication rate of less than 3–5% is thought to ensure overall patient benefit and most go home 1 or 2 days following surgery. Postoperative cranial neuropathies, cardiac complications, hyperperfusion syndrome with intracranial hemorrhages and rarely seizures can also occur but are rare.

Rehabilitation

Advances in basic and clinical research have shown that the human brain is capable of significant recovery after stroke, provided appropriate rehabilitation treatment is applied at the right amount and time. Several new techniques have become available in the past decade, such as task-specific therapy, robotic-assisted rehabilitation, and constraint-induced movement therapy with ongoing studies about their short- and long-term efficacy.

Task-specific therapy is specifically designed to deal with loss of particular abilities and seems to be more efficacious than traditional approaches for patients with motor deficits. Robotic-assisted rehabilitation, especially for the upper extremities, has been shown to reduce even severe motor impairment in stroke patients. Constraint-induced movement therapy, where the

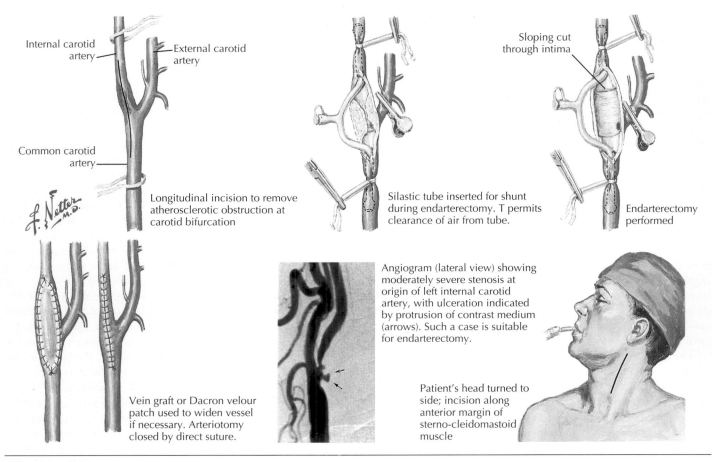

Figure 55-14 Endarterectomy for Extracranial Carotid Artery Atherosclerosis.

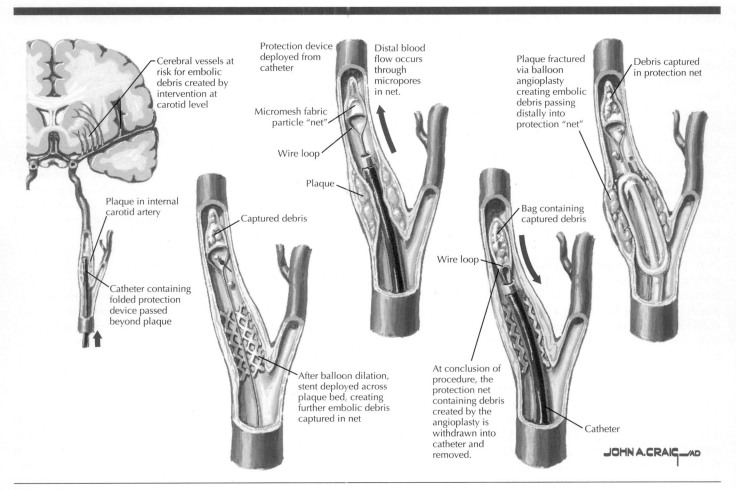

Figure 55-15 Endovascular Balloon Angioplasty and Stenting.

unaffected arm is restrained while the paralyzed limb is left to perform intense exercises over 2 consecutive weeks, has shown a statistically and clinically significant improvement in motor arm function as compared with traditional therapy. Persistent benefits up to 2 years have been reported.

FUTURE DIRECTIONS

Modern technology has improved the understanding of stroke and TIA pathophysiology, which will translate into a more rational therapeutic approach.

Emerging therapies being evaluated for secondary prevention of atherothromboembolism include P2Y12 ADP receptor antagonists, thromboxane receptor antagonists, and thrombin receptor antagonists. The oral direct thrombin antagonist Dabigatran has recently emerged as an alternative to warfarin for atrial fibrillation with similar efficacy in stroke prevention and a decreased incidence of major bleeding complications in general. Unlike with warfarin, frequent dose adjustments and blood monitoring are not needed. Although Dabigatran promises to replace warfarin in the future, its current disadvantages include higher cost and slightly increased MI rates; also, it remains unclear how to best reverse its effects in cases of emergency.

Endovascular techniques, such as angioplasty and stents (Fig. 55-15), will likely change the management approach for some patients with extracranial and intracranial disease. The recent Carotid Revascularization Endarterectomy versus Stenting Trial (CREST) shows similar outcomes with carotid artery stenting (CAS) and CEA for the treatment of symptomatic and asymptomatic carotid stenosis (vascular event or death: 7.2% vs 6.8% at 2.5 years). However, 30-day stroke rates were significantly higher for stenting (4.1% vs 2.3%), whereas MI rates were higher for CEA (2.3% vs 1.1%). The choice of procedure therefore depends on a careful consideration of co-morbidities, individual risks, institutional experience, and patient preference.

Angioplasty and stents have also been used for intracranial artery stenosis in patients who failed medical treatment, but results are mixed. Although effective in reducing recurrence of symptoms when successful, the complication rate of intracranial procedures remains high and its durability is in question. Future randomized studies are needed to determine its benefit.

EVIDENCE

Adams H, Adams R, Del Zoppo G, et al. Guidelines for the early management of patients with ischemic stroke. 2005 Guidelines Update. A scientific statement from the Stroke Council of the American Heart Association/American Stroke Association. Stroke 2005;36:916-921. *This article presents an update on the guidelines for the acute treatment of patients with ischemic stroke.*

Adams R, Albers G, Alberts MJ, et al. Update to the AHA/ASA recommendations for the prevention of stroke in patients with stroke and transient ischemic attack. Stroke 2008;39:1647-1652. *Recent update of prior guidelines for stroke and TIA prevention with emphasis on antithrombotic use and statin therapy*

Chaturvedi S, Bruno A, Feasby T, et al. Carotid endarterectomy—An evidence-based review. Report of the Therapeutics and Technology Assessment Subcommittee of the American Academy of Neurology. Neurology 2005;65:794-801. *The authors provide an excellent evidence-based review of the efficacy of carotid endarterectomy for stroke prevention in asymptomatic and symptomatic patients with internal carotid artery stenosis.*

Goldstein LB, Adams R, Alberts MJ, et al. Primary prevention of ischemic stroke. A Guideline from the American Heart Association/American Stroke Association Stroke Council. Stroke 2006;37:1583-1633. *Extensive review of the evidence on various stroke risk factors with recommendations for reduction of stroke risk*

Sacco RL, Adams R, Albers G, et al. Guidelines for prevention of stroke in patients with ischemic stroke or transient ischemic attacks. A statement for healthcare professionals from the American Heart Association/American Stroke Association council on stroke. Stroke 2006;37:577-617. *This article presents guidelines for secondary prevention of strokes and TIAs.*

ADDITIONAL RESOURCE

Caplan LR. Stroke: A Clinical Approach. 3rd ed. Boston, Mass: Butterworth-Heinemann; 2000. *This single-authored book written by a leader in the field focuses on all aspects of diagnosis and treatment of patients with stroke.*

56

Cerebral Venous Thrombosis

Gregory J. Allam

Clinical Vignette

A 45-year-old man with a history of bipolar disorder and binges of alcohol abuse gradually developed global headaches that suddenly worsened over a 6-day period. He presented to the emergency room reporting excruciating headaches, especially while lying flat or after coughing. He described visual blurring and transient visual dimming while straining or getting up abruptly. He was slightly inattentive but had no focal weakness or numbness on examination. Ophthalmoscopy showed bilateral severe papilledema with peripapillary flame-shaped hemorrhages but no visual field loss. Computed tomographic (CT) scan of the brain showed hyperdensity in the sagittal sinus and the left transverse sinus. Cerebrospinal fluid (CSF) fluid analysis was normal but the opening pressure was elevated. Magnetic resonance imaging (MRI) of the brain showed no acute stroke or hemorrhage, but magnetic resonance venography (MRV) showed partial occlusion of the sagittal sinus, left transverse sinus, and the left jugular vein. He later admitted to drinking heavily and smoking just before his headaches worsened. There was no evidence of malignancy, and initial coagulation studies were normal. He was treated with warfarin and acetazolamide with no evidence of progressive visual loss and ultimately resolution of the headaches. Serial MRVs showed partial recanalization of the occluded cerebral sinuses and he was eventually taken off warfarin. He was admitted about 6 months later with recurrent episodes of shortness of breath and palpitations and was found to have multiple small pulmonary emboli and deep vein thrombosis. A repeat hypercoagulability screen revealed a lupus anticoagulant, and a newly available test showed the presence of a prothrombin gene mutation. He was advised to stay on warfarin life-long.

Clinical Vignette

A 34-year-old man presented to the hospital after 1 week of increasing occipital headache, stiff neck, and chills. Brain CT and CSF analysis were normal; however, the patient was admitted to the hospital for worsening confusion and behavioral changes. Soon after admission, he had a generalized tonic-clonic seizure and underwent intubation.

A brain MRI demonstrated bilateral frontal hemorrhagic infarctions with edema and a sagittal sinus thrombosis. Because of obtundation and signs of increased intracranial pressure (ICP), mannitol and an IV heparin infusion were started. A continuous intrasinus infusion of urokinase was given over 2 days. The thrombosis resolved, and he recovered consciousness.

Eventually, the patient was discharged from the hospital on warfarin and anticonvulsants, with only minor left-sided

sensory changes and mild left leg weakness. Unfortunately, he did not continue the prescribed anticoagulants and was readmitted 20 days later with pleuritic chest pain and shortness of breath. Bilateral deep vein thrombosis and a pulmonary embolism were diagnosed. An infrarenal inferior vena cava filter was inserted, and anticoagulation was resumed. The patient had a positive test result for anticardiolipin antibodies. This led to the diagnosis of an anticardiolipin antibody syndrome, confirming the need for long-term systemic anticoagulation.

When venous drainage of the brain is compromised, arterial flow creates back-pressure into tissue capillaries causing capillary congestion, interstitial edema, decreased tissue perfusion, and ultimately ischemia. Eventually capillary rupture causes hematoma formation. This process of cerebral venous congestion followed by infarction (not conforming to strict arterial territories) and hemorrhage is the hallmark of cerebral sinus thrombosis. The causes of cerebral venous thrombosis vary (Box 56-1), but many relate to transient or permanent hypercoagulable states, with dehydration acting as a common precipitating event. A thorough investigation for such etiologies is crucial to directing long-term treatment and anticipating potential comorbidities.

Attention should be given to signs of meningitis, such as fever, stiff neck, and rash. Examining the ears, sinuses, and face for infection or discharge may provide clues to possible septic venous thrombosis. Physical evidence or a history of head or neck trauma is important. Ocular pain, proptosis, and chemosis, often with combinations of cranial neuropathies, are significant signs that may indicate a basal skull or cavernous sinus thrombosis.

ANATOMY

Although complex, cerebral venous system anatomy is best considered in three levels: the dural-based posterosuperior group, the dural anteroinferior or basal group, and the deep veins of the brain.

The dura is formed of two layers, one abutting the inner calvarium and the other forming the outer meningeal covering. These layers separate in the midsagittal and transverse planes, forming dural venous sinuses ultimately draining into the jugular veins. A single superior sagittal sinus joins the often asymmetric but paired transverse sinus at the confluence of sinuses or torcular herophili (Fig. 56-1). The transverse sinuses run laterally from the occipital bone to the middle cerebral fossa along the tentorium cerebelli. The right is often larger and is continuous with the superior sagittal sinus whereas the left curves out laterally as an extension of the single midline straight sinus. The straight sinus runs downward from near the splenium of the corpus callosum to the occipital protuberance. The sigmoid sinus curves down toward the skull base from the transverse sinus and joins the inferior petrosal sinus at the jugular foramen to form the jugular vein.

The straight sinus (Figs. 56-1 through 56-4) is formed by the splayed falx layered over the cerebellar tentorium. The inferior sagittal sinus runs in the fold of the lower arch of the falx cerebri and joins the cerebral vein of Galen in the proximity of the posterior horns of the lateral ventricles to form the straight sinus. The superior and inferior sagittal sinuses provide drainage for the cerebral hemispheres.

The great cerebral vein of Galen drains, through paired internal cerebral veins, the brainstem, cerebellum, posterior frontal and anterior parietal lobes, and thalamus; through the

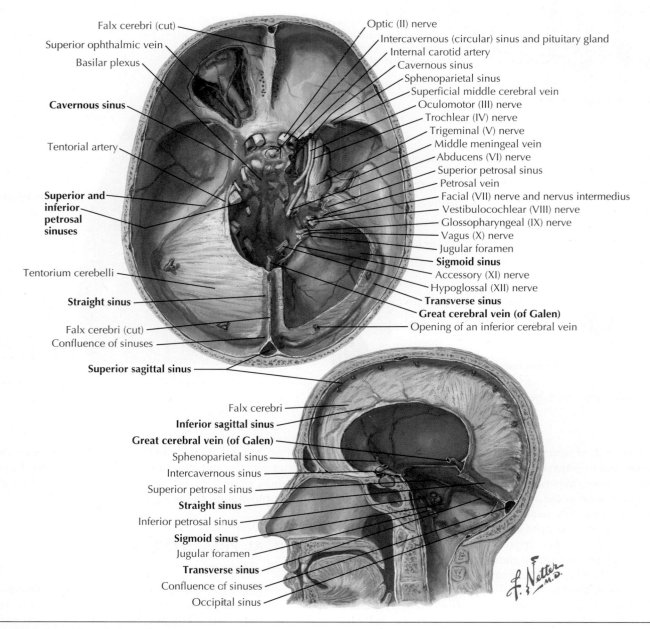

Figure 56-1 Dura Mater Venous Sinuses.

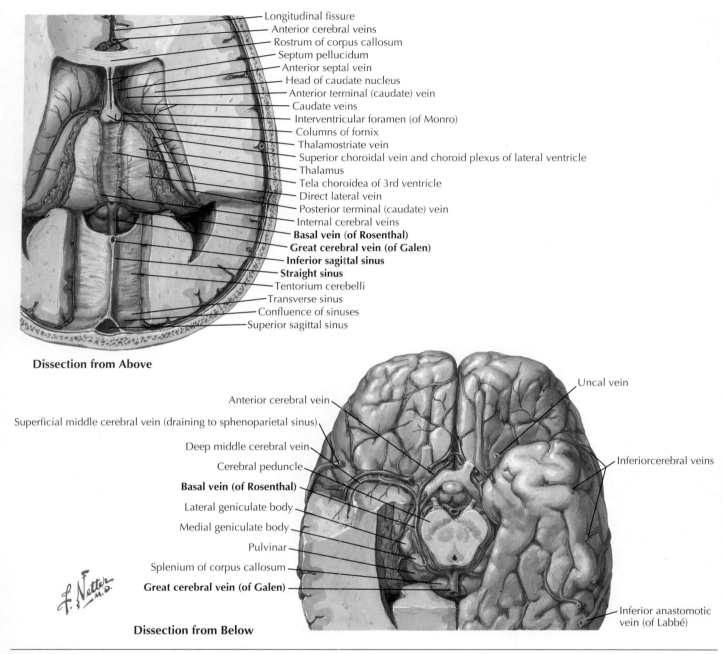

Longitudinal fissure
Anterior cerebral veins
Rostrum of corpus callosum
Septum pellucidum
Anterior septal vein
Head of caudate nucleus
Anterior terminal (caudate) vein
Caudate veins
Interventricular foramen (of Monro)
Columns of fornix
Thalamostriate vein
Superior choroidal vein and choroid plexus of lateral ventricle
Thalamus
Tela choroidea of 3rd ventricle
Direct lateral vein
Posterior terminal (caudate) vein
Internal cerebral veins
Basal vein (of Rosenthal)
Great cerebral vein (of Galen)
Inferior sagittal sinus
Straight sinus
Tentorium cerebelli
Transverse sinus
Confluence of sinuses
Superior sagittal sinus

Dissection from Above

Anterior cerebral vein
Superficial middle cerebral vein (draining to sphenoparietal sinus)
Deep middle cerebral vein
Cerebral peduncle
Basal vein (of Rosenthal)
Lateral geniculate body
Medial geniculate body
Pulvinar
Splenium of corpus callosum
Great cerebral vein (of Galen)

Uncal vein
Inferiorcerebral veins
Inferior anastomotic vein (of Labbé)

Dissection from Below

Figure 56-2 Deep and Subependymal Veins of Brain.

paired basal vein of Rosenthal, it drains the limbic system, hippocampus, and mesencephalon.

The cavernous sinus runs posteriorly at the brain base from the sphenoid bone in the area of the superior orbital fissure to the petrous temporal bone. Cavernous sinus tributaries include cerebral veins and the ophthalmic vein. The cavernous sinus drains along the medial upper layer of the tentorium and through the superior petrosal sinus, coursing posteriorly to the transverse sinus. The cavernous sinus houses the carotid artery; the oculomotor, trochlear, and abducens nerves; and the ophthalmic division of the trigeminal nerve (Fig. 56-5). A mesh of venous sinuses around the pituitary and the anterior skull base connects the two cavernous sinuses across the midline. The

superior petrosal sinus drains the anterior brainstem and the anterior superior and inferior cerebellar hemispheres. Below the tentorium, along the skull base, the inferior petrosal sinus links the cavernous sinus to the sigmoid sinus (Fig. 56-1).

CLINICAL PRESENTATION

General Aspects

The neurologic presentation of cerebral venous thrombosis is protean. General features depend on the location of venous thrombosis and the abruptness of occlusion. In most patients, the earliest sign is an evolving, constant, diffuse headache that

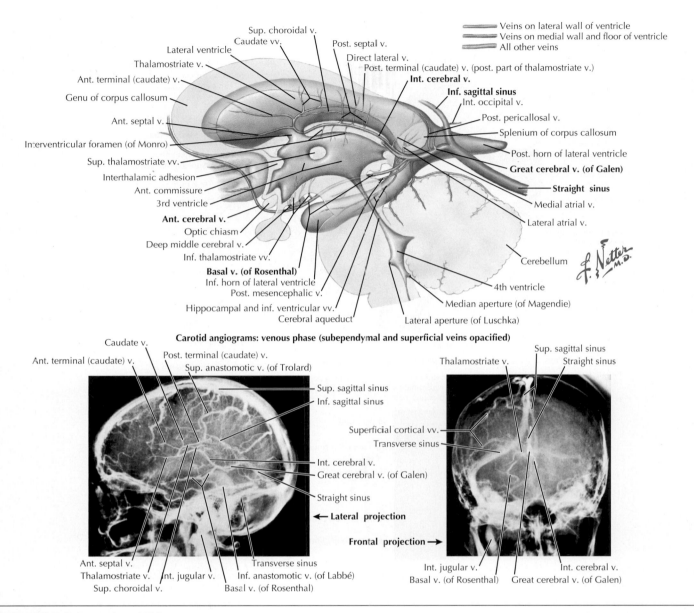

Figure 56-3 Subependymal Veins.

worsens with recumbency. Blurred vision from papilledema is often present but, unless persisting for weeks, rarely leads to significant or permanent visual loss. Sudden brief spells of visual obscuration can occur with abrupt positional changes and are thought to represent transiently decreased perfusion of swollen optic nerves. Slowed cognition or encephalopathy without localized brain lesions or focal neurologic signs may occur with long-standing cerebral thrombosis of gradual evolution, as seen in the first vignette presented above.

In patients who have a more abrupt onset of cortical vein or superficial venous sinus thrombosis, cortically based often hemorrhagic lesions with focal neurologic signs and focal or generalized seizures develop. With involvement of the deep cerebral veins or more than two thirds of the superior sagittal sinus, obtundation followed by coma with decorticate or decerebrate posturing are presenting signs reflecting bihemispheric, bithalamic basal ganglionic, or brainstem dysfunction. Combinations

of painful cranial neuropathies with little involvement of consciousness occur with basal skull (jugular vein, cavernous, or petrosal sinus) sinus thrombosis.

Specific Clinical Presentations

In **superior sagittal sinus thrombosis** (SSST), increased venous pressure from decreased drainage initially causes generalized headaches with paroxysms of pain occurring with any Valsalva-like maneuver, that is, coughing, sneezing, straining, lifting, or bending. Blurred vision may occur secondary to optic nerve head edema or associated exudates involving the macula. Permanent visual compromise is unusual and only happens when papilledema persists for weeks. Light-headedness, transient blindness, and tinnitus can occur with sudden head elevation from a lying or bending position, similar to pseudotumor cerebri.

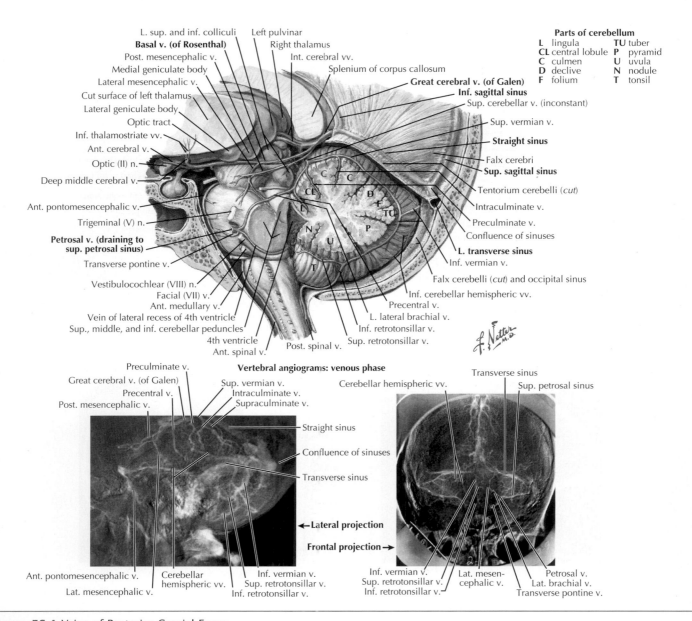

Figure 56-4 Veins of Posterior Cranial Fossa.

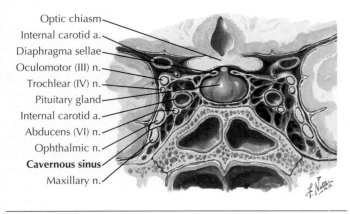

Figure 56-5 Cavernous Sinus and Its Cranial Nerves.

Intracerebral cortically based hemorrhages, common with SSST, are often associated with focal neurologic signs and seizures. Confusion, behavioral changes, somnolence, and coma may occur as thrombosis propagates within the sinus and ICP increases. These signs usually develop after the clot extends into the posterior third of the sinus. In most cases of SSSTs, one of the lateral sinuses is concomitantly involved (Fig. 56-6).

Occasionally, **isolated cortical vein thrombosis** is seen without sagittal sinus involvement. The clinical picture is again one of headaches, focal neurologic dysfunction, and seizure, however without increased ICP or papilledema. Underlying causes are similar to sagittal sinus thrombosis, and treatment follows the same principles. Neuroimaging shows isolated, often hemorrhagic, ischemic lesions that are not confined to a cerebral artery territory.

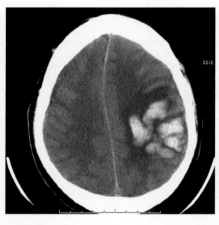

A. CT 2 days after admission showing left posterior frontal parietal patchy hemorrhage within the ischemic region.

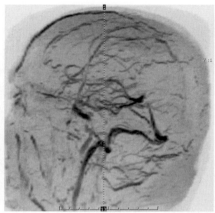

B. Magnetic resonance venography (MRV) demonstrates absence of flow in posterior sagittal sinus and some cortical veins.

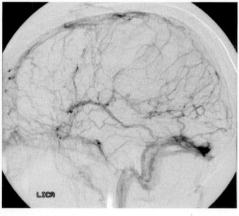

C. Digital angiogram, venous phase confirms the MRV findings.

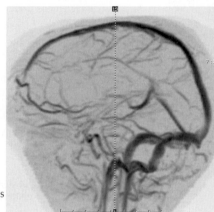

D. Normal MRV for comparison.

Figure 56-6 Sagittal Sinus Thrombosis.

Deep cerebral vein thrombosis is present in 40% of superior sagittal sinus cases and is more likely to produce coma, pupillary abnormalities, ophthalmoplegia, and increased ICP than SSST alone. Sole or predominant deep venous system involvement mostly occurs in children but is reported in adults with presentations ranging from isolated drowsiness or obtundation to coma with bilateral posturing and ocular abnormalities. Survivors experience bilateral weakness, rigidity, dystonia or athetosis, memory loss, personality changes, and various neuropsychologic disturbances.

Base of the skull sinus thrombosis has a clinical presentation of painful cranial neuropathies. *Cavernous sinus thrombosis* is often septic from facial, orbital, or middle ear infections with eye pain, proptosis, and chemosis as frequent features (Fig. 56-7). Varying degrees of ophthalmoplegia are present secondary to involvement of CN-III, -IV, and -VI running through the lateral portion of the cavernous sinus. The ophthalmic division of the trigeminal nerve (V1) also courses through this sinus, and forehead sensory changes are occasionally seen. Inferior petrosal sinus thrombosis, often septic, causes retro-orbital pain, trigeminal V1 sensory changes, and abducens nerve palsy (Gradenigo syndrome; CN-V, -VI). Localized thrombosis involving the internal jugular vein may be an extension of transverse or sigmoid sinus thrombosis or may result from catheterization or trauma. This often presents with CN-IX, -X, and -XI dysfunction (jugular foramen or Vernet syndrome).

DIAGNOSTIC APPROACH

All patients with cerebral venous thrombosis should be examined for a hypercoagulable state. In addition to prothrombin time, partial thromboplastin time and platelet count, blood studies now commonly include protein C and S quantification, lupus anticoagulant, anticardiolipin antibodies, homocysteine levels, and DNA testing for factor V (Leiden factor) and prothrombin gene mutation.

Lumbar puncture often shows an opening pressure greater than 200 mm H_2O. The CSF protein is increased but the glucose content, unless there is associated meningitis, is usually normal. CSF RBCs, xanthochromia, and pleocytosis are commonly seen, especially in cases of septic sinus thrombosis and in cases associated with meningitis. Normal CSF analysis, although rare, does not exclude the diagnosis.

Acutely, brain CT without contrast is obtained to assess for intracranial hemorrhage. It may reveal irregularly shaped paramedian cortical venous infarctions that do not conform to defined arterial distributions. The "empty delta sign," where contrast partially fills the sinus, leaving an unenhanced island of clot within the occipital confluence, occurs in 50% of cases. Over the hemispheric convexities, thrombosed cortical vessels sometimes appear as hyperintense coiled or serpiginous signals. Diffuse edema and narrowed lateral ventricles may be apparent with or without hemorrhagic lesions.

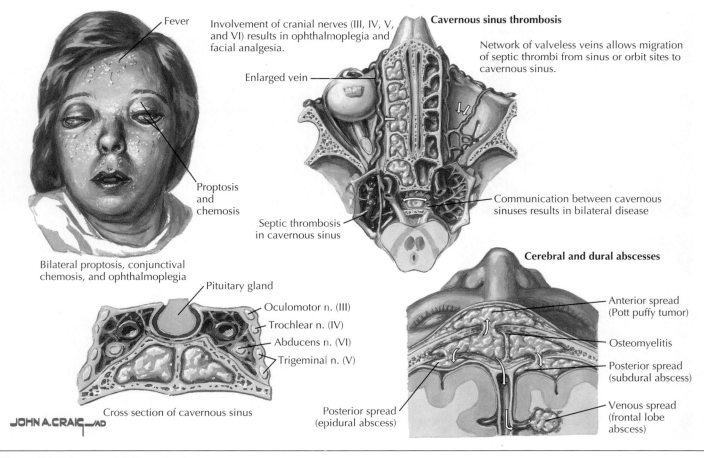

Fever

Involvement of cranial nerves (III, IV, V, and VI) results in ophthalmoplegia and facial analgesia.

Cavernous sinus thrombosis

Enlarged vein

Network of valveless veins allows migration of septic thrombi from sinus or orbit sites to cavernous sinus.

Proptosis and chemosis

Septic thrombosis in cavernous sinus

Communication between cavernous sinuses results in bilateral disease

Bilateral proptosis, conjunctival chemosis, and ophthalmoplegia

Pituitary gland

Oculomotor n. (III)

Trochlear n. (IV)

Abducens n. (VI)

Trigeminal n. (V)

Cross section of cavernous sinus

JOHN A. CRAIG—AD

Cerebral and dural abscesses

Anterior spread (Pott puffy tumor)

Osteomyelitis

Posterior spread (subdural abscess)

Venous spread (frontal lobe abscess)

Posterior spread (epidural abscess)

Figure 56-7 Intracranial Complications.

MRI and MRV have largely replaced angiography as standard imaging techniques to confirm cerebral sinus thrombosis (see Fig. 56-6). Cerebral angiography with a prolonged venous phase is now reserved for cases not clearly diagnosed by MRI or CT and for patients requiring intrasinus thrombolysis.

Cerebral sinus thrombosis is often a clinical diagnosis based on a detailed history and corroborating physical findings. Imaging studies, however, have become crucial in the management of these patients from confirming the diagnosis to guiding treatment and to help in predicting the clinical course and outcome.

TREATMENT

The management of sagittal sinus thrombosis consists of hydration, anticoagulation, and the treatment of any underlying cause. Because dehydration enhances clot propagation, early volume repletion is of utmost importance. Heparin is given to make the partial thromboplastin time double the control value. Anticoagulation is indicated despite hemorrhagic infarctions because the overall outcome is improved and intracranial hemorrhage is rarely worsened. Low-molecular-weight heparin has also been used with safety and efficacy. Close clinical follow-up and repeated brain CT scanning, however, are advised to monitor the size and location of cerebral hemorrhages throughout the course of treatment. Warfarin is given for long-term anticoagulation and is started after 24 hours of intravenous

heparin treatment or after the patient is stable. When indefinite anticoagulation is not needed, the duration of warfarin treatment remains unclear; accepted practice is 3–6 months.

After the precipitating cause is resolved, it is best to confirm that headache and papilledema are controlled and that MRV shows, at least, partial recanalization of the sagittal sinus before discontinuing oral anticoagulants. Seizures occur in the acute phase in up to 30% of patients and are usually focal but can be generalized. Recurrent seizures should be treated promptly because they can cause increased intracranial pressure, clinical deterioration, and increased mortality. Up to 10% of patients may experience pulmonary embolism. This is suspected when respiratory deterioration and increased oxygen needs suddenly occur.

If deterioration continues despite IV anticoagulation, many advocate a more invasive approach with in situ clot thrombolysis. A femoral venous catheter thread through the jugular vein to the transverse or sagittal sinus is used. An initial attempt at partial thrombolysis is usually followed by a continuous 12-hour intra-sinus infusion. Numerous case series have shown significant neurologic recovery with only a minor increase in bleeding complications. Monitoring hematomas remains necessary because expanding hemorrhagic infarcts may cause shift and herniation, necessitating acute treatment of increased ICP with osmotic agents or hyperventilation. Surgical evacuation of intracranial hemorrhage is rarely required. To decrease potential bleeding complications, rheolytic mechanical thrombectomy catheters alone or in combination with low doses of thrombolytic agents have been pursued with some success. Numerous cases of thrombolytic treatment have been described where significant clinical improvement occurred even in patients with several hemorrhagic infarcts and days of obtundation or coma.

PROGNOSIS AND LONG-TERM COMPLICATIONS

With anticoagulation, about 80% of patients have good recovery with little or no residual disability. Poor outcomes correlate with rapid deterioration after admission, coma or obtundation on presentation, involvement of the deep venous system, and multiple cerebral hemorrhages, especially if present for days. Before the advent of anticoagulation, the mortality rate was 30–50%. A mortality rate of 6–10% remains in the acute phase. Aggressive treatment with intrasinus thrombolysis, especially in those with evidence of evolving venous infarctions and progressive obtundation, may improve outcomes and decrease the rate of early mortality but, to date, there are no randomized controlled studies to support its routine use.

Long-term complications include focal or generalized seizures, headaches, and papilledema with visual loss, with approximately 10% rate of occurrence for each. Seizures may necessitate continued anticonvulsant therapy despite resolution of all other symptoms and sinus recanalization. Headache usually resolves with increasing recanalization and better venous drainage and often does not necessitate long-term therapy. The recurrence rate of cerebral thrombosis and other thrombotic events, such as deep vein thrombosis or pulmonary embolism, is estimated around 2–5%, with the majority of these patients likely requiring lifelong anticoagulation with warfarin.

Papilledema, when present, should be followed with serial visual fields by an ophthalmologist. If not controlled, progressive visual loss (arcuate mid–peripheral field constriction and central visual loss with widening blind spot) is a danger, secondary to gradual optic nerve atrophy. Treatment of papilledema involves lumboperitoneal shunting, serial spinal taps, carbonic anhydrase inhibitors, or optic nerve fenestration into the orbit to relieve locally increased CSF pressure that otherwise would be transmitted to the optic nerve. Optic nerve fenestration is safe, has few complications, and rarely reoccludes. It is done unilaterally, with positive effects on both eyes. The exact mechanism is unknown but is not thought to relate to general reduction of overall CSF pressure, although many cases still demonstrate high lumbar puncture pressures after fenestration.

ADDITIONAL RESOURCES

Baker MD, Opatowsky MJ, Wilson JA, et al. Rheolytic catheter and thrombolysis of dural venous sinus thrombosis: a case series. Neurosurgery 2001;48:487-494.

De Bruijn SF, De Haan RJ, Stam J. Clinical features and prognostic factors of cerebral venous sinus thrombosis in a prospective series of 59 patients. For The Cerebral Venous Sinus Thrombosis Study Group. J Neurol Neurosurg Psychiatry 2001;70:105-108.

DeBruijn SF, Stam J. Randomized placebo-controlled trial of anticoagulation treatment with low molecular weight heparin for cerebral sinus thrombosis. Stroke 1999;30:481-482. *Of those treated with nadroparin 13% had a bad outcome compared to 21% in the placebo group. There were no new symptomatic intracranial hemorrhagic complications even though many patients in the treatment group initially presented with ICH.*

Einhaupl KM, Villringer A, Meister W, et al. Heparin treatment in sinus venous thrombosis. Lancet 1991;338:597-600. *Randomized controlled study terminated after 20 patients because of a significant advantage in favor of heparin over placebo in angiographically proven cases of cerebral venous thrombosis.*

Ferro JM, Canhão P, Stam J, et al. ISCVT Investigators. Prognosis of cerebral vein and dural sinus thrombosis: results of the International Study on Cerebral Vein and Dural Sinus Thrombosis (ISCVT) Stroke 2004 Mar;35(3):664-670. *Large multinational prospective observational study that shows good recovery in 79% of patients. A subgroup of men with venous hematomas, low Glasgow coma scores, deep venous involvement and malignancy tended to do worse.*

Ferro JM, Lopes MB, Rosas MJ, et al. Long-term prognosis of cerebral vein and dural sinus thrombosis: results of the VENOPORT study. Cerebrovasc Dis 2002;13:272-278.

Haley EC, Brasmear HR, Barth JT, et al. Deep cerebral venous thrombosis: clinical, neuroradiological and neuropsychological correlates. Arch Neurol 1989;46:337-340.

Horton JC, Seiff SR, Pitts LH, et al. Decompression of the optic nerve sheath for vision-threatening papilledema caused by dural sinus occlusion. Neurosurgery 1992;31:203-212.

Mehraein S, Schmidtke K, Villringer A, et al. Heparin treatment in cerebral sinus and venous thrombosis: patients at risk of fatal outcome. Cerebrovasc Dis 2003;15:17-21.

Preter M, Tzourio C, Ameri A, et al. Long-term prognosis in cerebral venous thrombosis: follow-up of 77 patients. Stroke 1996;27:243-246.

Wasay M, Bakshi R, Kojan S, et al. Nonrandomized comparison of local urokinase thrombolysis versus systemic heparin anticoagulation for superior sagittal sinus thrombosis. Stroke 2001;32:2310-2317.

Subarachnoid Hemorrhage

57

Clemens M. Schirmer and Carlos A. David

Clinical Vignette

A 66-year-old woman suddenly experienced a terrible temporal pain radiating into her forehead. The headache was so severe that she almost lost consciousness. She became nauseated, vomited, and felt disoriented. Her family called emergency medical services and had her brought to the emergency room. There, she was noted to be arousable but sleepy and confused. She had nuchal rigidity, photophobia, but no focal motor deficit. An unenhanced head computed tomography (CT) showed subarachnoid hemorrhage centered in the right sylvian fissure but no brain parenchymal abnormalities. Angiography demonstrated a ruptured middle cerebral artery aneurysm that was successfully clipped the next morning. The patient's postoperative course was uneventful (Figs. 57-1 and 57-2).

Clinical Vignette

A 44-year-old postal worker presented with severe headache and nuchal rigidity to an emergency room. Unenhanced head CT revealed a subarachnoid hemorrhage centered in the basal cisterns, and further evaluation with catheter angiography revealed a large aneurysm arising from the basilar artery tip. After consultation between the neurosurgeon and the interventional neuroradiologist, the decision to perform endovascular coil embolization was made and the procedure was carried out successfully. The patient recovered fully after a 3-week hospital stay but required a second procedure after 6 months when follow-up angiography demonstrated a reexpansion of the neck of the aneurysm (Figs. 57-3 and 57-4).

Subarachnoid hemorrhage (SAH) refers to bleeding beneath the arachnoid coverings of the brain surface and within the contained cisterns. The incidence is about 6–8 per 100,000 in most countries in the northern hemisphere and is highest between the fifth and seventh decades of life. The multiple etiologies for SAH are classified into primary aneurysmal and spontaneous nonaneurysmal mechanisms. Ruptured intracranial aneurysm is the most preponderant cause of spontaneous SAH, accounting for up to two thirds of all cases. One study of acute SAH in more than 6300 patients demonstrated that 51% of the patients had ruptured intracranial aneurysm. Nonaneurysmal SAHs include arteriovenous malformations (AVMs), angiographically occult vascular malformations (cavernous malformation or angioma), idiopathic and iatrogenic coagulopathies, bacterial endocarditis, venous thrombosis, inflammatory processes such as granulomatous angiitis, arterial dissections, occasional tumors, hypertension, and drug abuse. In addition, pathologic processes within the spinal canal, such as spinal

AVMs and spinal neoplasms, especially myxopapillary ependymomas, can rarely lead to SAH. Despite the normal neurologic examination results and head CT in the vignette, the patient's history was so compelling for a ruptured aneurysm or **warning leak** that her neurologist proceeded with the evaluation to find a large treatable berry aneurysm.

Subarachnoid hemorrhage is a catastrophic neurologic event having a precipitous onset, frequently without any premonitory warning. In North America, 28,000 patients per year experience a ruptured aneurysm. Slightly more than half die shortly after rupture. Among those who survive to reach a hospital, there is an additional 20–25% chance of further ruptures within the first 2 weeks, and the overall mortality during the first month is approximately 50%. Of those patients who survive, only about 30% will have a favorable outcome.

Aneurysmal SAH, although catastrophic, can often be treated successfully. When an aneurysm is identified before rupture, treatment can be curative, preventing the devastating effects of a SAH. Recognition of SAH, accurate diagnosis, and timely treatment are essential.

Crucial points in the history of patients with a recent headache are the abruptness of pain onset and the severity of discomfort. Lack of abnormality on the neurologic examination does not exclude a symptomatic aneurysm, and therefore, a detailed history and careful evaluation of such patients is essential. Furthermore, a mild hemorrhage as in the first vignette, may not be observed on CT after just 24 hours. Therefore, in spite of a negative head CT, cases in which there is still a high suspicion of a ruptured aneurysm would require angiography to identify the aneurysm and avoid rebleeding with its associated 50% mortality rate.

CLINICAL PRESENTATION

The classic symptom of SAH is the "worst headache of one's life." Headaches associated with aneurysm rupture are frequently sudden in onset and often described as a severe thunderclap, excruciating and unbearable. The headache peaks rapidly and is frequently associated with pain extending across the head and toward the neck. The headache is usually global, with a constant viselike ache but occasionally throbbing. Unilateral aches or a retro-orbital stab-like pain, even fleetingly, raise the suspicion of a possible posterior communicating artery aneurysm.

Nausea and vomiting, neck pain, and altered consciousness are often associated with the headache. Approximately 30% of patients are found to be confused and lethargic after the ictus. During the moment of rupture, one fourth of patients become comatose and up to 40% have transient loss of consciousness.

Seizure-like activity may be observed. The incidence of true seizure activity in patients with SAH is estimated at 20%. Seizures in SAH are most commonly associated with middle cerebral artery (MCA) and anterior communicating artery

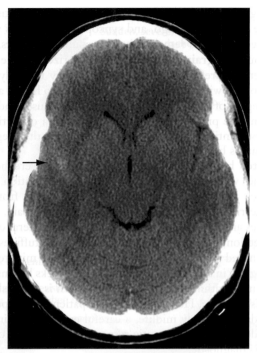

A. Axial CT exam shows subarachnoid hemorrhage lateralized to the right extending into the right sylvian fissure (arrow).

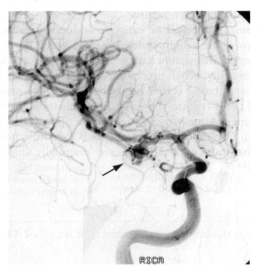

B. Frontal digital subtraction angiogram showing large right middle cerebral artery aneurysm (arrow).

Figure 57-1 Right Middle Cerebral Artery Aneurysm.

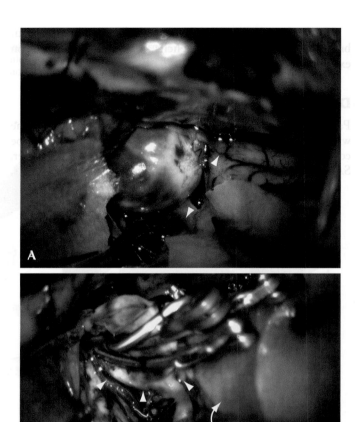

Right-sided pterional approach depicting large bulging MCA aneurysm (arrowheads) before **(A)** and after **(B)** surgical clipping. Aneurysm has been decompressed with surgical clips at its base with preservation of the parent artery (arrowheads).

Figure 57-2 Middle Cerebral Artery Aneurysm Clipping.

(ACA) aneurysmal rupture causing intracerebral hematomas. Unfortunately, many patients recall having a sentinel hemorrhage or warning leak with a fleeting but severe headache within the 2–3 weeks before the major ictus. This headache is somewhat milder and usually not associated with meningismus; it is often ignored until the catastrophic return of a major rupture. When evaluating patients with SAH or sudden severe headache, special attention should be focused on the level of consciousness, focal neurologic signs such as hemiparesis or cranial nerve palsies, and signs of meningismus (Fig. 57-5). Meningismus frequently occurs, associated with nuchal rigidity. Brudzinski's maneuver is an excellent means of evaluating meningismus; the examiner flexes the patient's neck, precipitating hip flexion, knee flexion, and hamstring pain. Diplopia (due to abducens or oculomotor nerve palsies) and visual loss (chiasmal or optic nerve involvement) are caused by either cranial nerve compression from the aneurysmal dome or aneurysmal rupture and increased intracranial pressure (Fig. 57-6).

Examination of the optic fundi frequently discloses retinal or preretinal hemorrhage, subhyaloid hemorrhages, and occasional papilledema. Hemorrhage into the vitreous results in Terson syndrome, with scarring and epiretinal membrane formation (macular pucker) and eventually visual loss or distortion. Terson syndrome is a frequent cause of visual loss in SAH, which often goes unnoticed until the patient regains consciousness 1–2 weeks later. It is often related with more severe subarachnoid bleeds that cause loss of consciousness and papilledema. Its association with ACA aneurysms is less clear. The long-term prognosis for vision in this situation is fairly good; however, a vitrectomy is occasionally required.

A. Cranial neuropathies

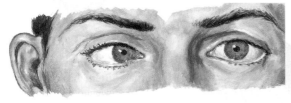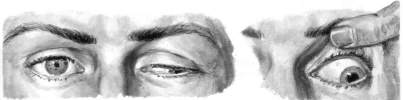

Abducens nerve palsy: affected eye turns medially. May be first manifestation of intracavernous carotid aneurysm. Pain above eye or on side of face may be secondary to trigeminal (V) nerve involvement.

Oculomotor nerve palsy: ptosis, eye turns laterally and inferiorly, pupil dilated. Common finding with cerebral aneurysms, especially carotid-posterior communicating aneurysms.

B. Visual field disturbances

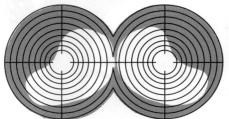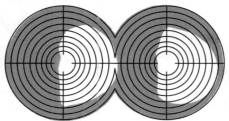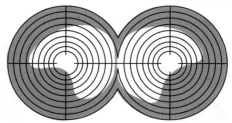

Superior bitemporal quadrantanopia caused by supraclinoid carotid aneurysm compressing optic chiasm from below

Right (or left) homonymous hemianopsia caused by compression of optic tract. Unilateral amaurosis may occur if optic (II) nerve is compressed.

Inferior bitemporal quadrantanopia caused by compression of optic chiasm from above

C. Retinal changes

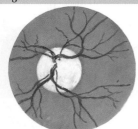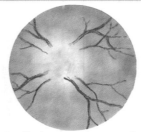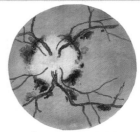

Optic atrophy may develop as result of pressure on optic (II) nerve from a supraclinoid carotid, ophthalmic, or anterior cerebral aneurysm.

Papilledema may be caused by increased intracranial pressure secondary to rupture of cerebral aneurysm.

Hemorrhage into optic (II) nerve sheath after rupture of aneurysm may result in subhyaloid hemorrhage, with blood around disc.

Figure 57-6 Ophthalmologic Manifestations of Cerebral Aneurysms.

PATHOPHYSIOLOGY

Intracranial Aneurysms

Subtypes of intracranial aneurysms include saccular or berry, fusiform, dissecting, traumatic, and infectious (mycotic) aneurysms. Frequently associated with an SAH, saccular aneurysms are by far the most common type. They are spherical in shape but frequently have asymmetric outpouching and multilobulated characteristics that are felt to be potential rupture sites for the aneurysm. The aneurysmal fundus or body is connected to the parent vessel via a small neck region, and as the aneurysm grows, this neck region may broaden and incorporate normal branching vessels.

Intracranial aneurysms characteristically occur at branch points of major cerebral arteries. Almost 85% of aneurysms are found in the anterior circulation and 15% within the posterior circulation (Fig. 57-8). Overall, the most common sites are the anterior communicating artery followed by the posterior communicating artery and the middle cerebral artery bifurcation. Within the posterior circulation, the most preponderant site is at the top of the basilar artery bifurcation into the posterior cerebral arteries.

Aneurysms are frequently classified according to size, with small being less than 10 mm, large 10–25 mm, and giant aneurysms larger than 25 mm. At presentation, most aneurysms are small, with only 2% found to be giant. Giant aneurysms are more likely to cause compressive symptoms on the optic chiasm, cranial nerves, and brainstem depending on location. Rarely involvement of tributary vessels, either due to aneurysmal expansion or cavitary clot, may lead to ischemic symptoms as well (Fig. 57-9). Although controversy remains regarding the association of size and the incidence of rupture, 7 mm seems to be the minimal size at the time of rupture. Overall, ruptured aneurysms tend to be larger than unruptured aneurysms.

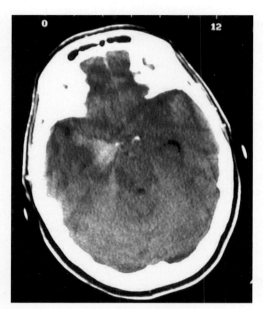

Unenhanced axial CT of the brain with SAH centered in the right sylvian fissure

Figure 57-7   Subarachnoid Hemorrhage.

Table 57-1	Hunt–Hess Grading Scale for Berry Aneurysms
Grade	**Description**
1	Asymptomatic, or mild headache and slight nuchal rigidity
2	Moderate to severe headache, nuchal rigidity, no neurologic deficits other than cranial nerve palsies.
3	Mild focal deficit, lethargy, confusion
4	Stupor, hemiparesis, central neurologic signs
5	Deep coma, decerebrate rigidity, moribund appearance

Aneurysms occur in approximately 5% of the adult population, somewhat more commonly in women. The causes of intracranial aneurysm formation and rupture are not well understood; however, it is thought that intracranial aneurysms form over a relatively short period and either rupture or undergo changes resulting in a stable unruptured aneurysm. Pathologic examination of ruptured aneurysms obtained at autopsy demonstrates disorganization of normal vascular architecture with loss of the internal elastic lamina, and reduced collagen content. In contrast, unruptured aneurysms have nearly twice the collagen content of the normal arterial wall, resulting in increased thickness of the aneurysmal dome, which may be responsible for the observed relative stability and low rupture rate.

RUPTURED ANEURYSMS

The peak incidence of aneurysmal SAH is in the sixth decade of life. Only 20% of aneurysm ruptures occur in patients aged between 15 and 45 years. No predisposing activity has been identified, and aneurysmal SAH is equally distributed in sleep, routine daily activities, and strenuous activity.

Nearly 50% of patients who have an SAH, when properly questioned, relate a history of a **warning leak with headache** or symptoms around 2–3 weeks before the major hemorrhage. Nearly half of these individuals die before arriving to the hospital. Many of the initial survivors succumb to a recurrent hemorrhage after presenting to the hospital. The peak incidence of subsequent hemorrhage occurs in the first 24 hours, but the subsequent daily risk continues such that approximately 20–25% have rebled within the first 2 weeks of presentation. Mortality associated with the second hemorrhage is nearly 70%.

RISK FACTORS

Risk factors associated with aneurysmal rupture include cigarette smoking, oral contraceptive use, alcohol consumption, pregnancy, and childbirth. Possible diurnal blood pressure variations are associated with a circadian rhythm for aneurysm rupture. Most ruptures occur early in the morning or evening, but few occur in the middle of the night. There also may be a predisposition to occur during the winter months or when there are drastic changes in barometric pressure. The most likely cause of rupture is hemodynamic stress associated with biomechanical and structural weakness within the blood vessel and aneurysmal wall.

Perimesencephalic Subarachnoid Hemorrhage

Of patients presenting with spontaneous SAH, approximately 15–20% have negative arteriograms. Repeated arteriography may discern another 7% of patients. However, a specific subset of individuals displays SAH with a specific CT distribution of blood over the anterior aspect of the brainstem or perimesencephalic regions. *Benign perimesencephalic SAH* typically occurs in nonhypertensive younger males who generally do well. Although the clinical presentation is similar to that of an aneurysmal SAH, symptom onset is more gradual and patients appear less ill. When these patients have a typical presentation and characteristic CT findings and a good-quality angiogram that is negative, a follow-up arteriogram is not always needed. The cause of benign perimesencephalic SAH is unknown but is postulated to be caused by rupture of bridging vessels across the perimesencephalic cistern.

MANAGEMENT

Complications of the Ruptured Aneurysm

Specific therapeutic issues pertain to ruptured aneurysms and SAH; primarily the prevention of rebleeding, management of increased intracranial pressure (ICP) and hydrocephalus, and the treatment of potential cerebral vasospasm. Associated medical sequelae lead to other management issues noted below.

REBLEEDING

Rebleeding is the major cause of poor outcome after SAH. A second hemorrhage is associated with 70% mortality rate. If

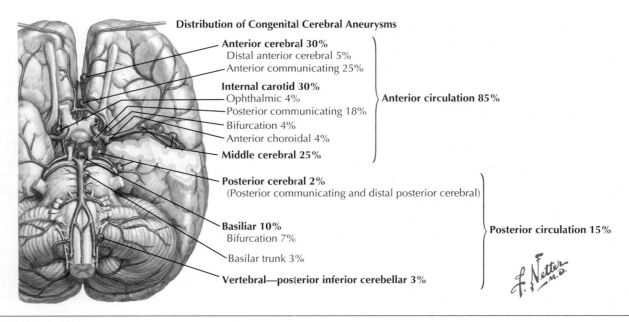

Distribution of Congenital Cerebral Aneurysms

Anterior cerebral 30%
Distal anterior cerebral 5%
Anterior communicating 25%

Internal carotid 30%
Ophthalmic 4%
Posterior communicating 18%
Bifurcation 4%
Anterior choroidal 4%

Middle cerebral 25%

} **Anterior circulation 85%**

Posterior cerebral 2%
(Posterior communicating and distal posterior cerebral)

Basiliar 10%
Bifurcation 7%
Basilar trunk 3%

Vertebral—posterior inferior cerebellar 3%

} **Posterior circulation 15%**

Figure 57-8 Typical Sites of Cerebral Aneurysms.

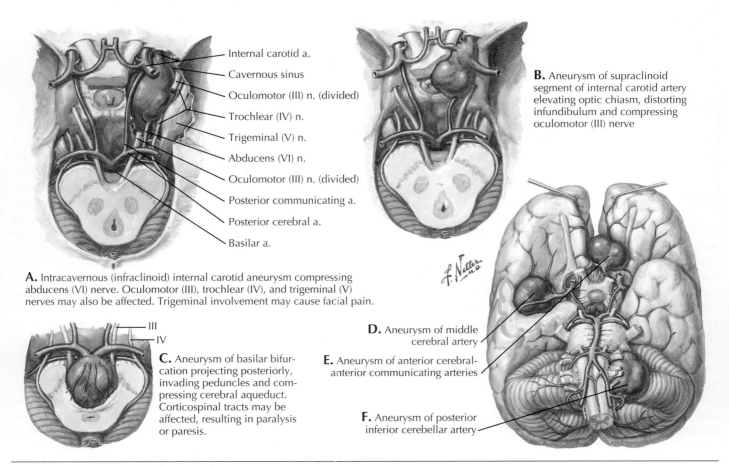

Internal carotid a.

Cavernous sinus

Oculomotor (III) n. (divided)

Trochlear (IV) n.

Trigeminal (V) n.

Abducens (VI) n.

Oculomotor (III) n. (divided)

Posterior communicating a.

Posterior cerebral a.

Basilar a.

B. Aneurysm of supraclinoid segment of internal carotid artery elevating optic chiasm, distorting infundibulum and compressing oculomotor (III) nerve

A. Intracavernous (infraclinoid) internal carotid aneurysm compressing abducens (VI) nerve. Oculomotor (III), trochlear (IV), and trigeminal (V) nerves may also be affected. Trigeminal involvement may cause facial pain.

III
IV

C. Aneurysm of basilar bifurcation projecting posteriorly, invading peduncles and compressing cerebral aqueduct. Corticospinal tracts may be affected, resulting in paralysis or paresis.

D. Aneurysm of middle cerebral artery

E. Aneurysm of anterior cerebral-anterior communicating arteries

F. Aneurysm of posterior inferior cerebellar artery

Figure 57-9 Giant Cerebral Aneurysms.

untreated, the risk of subsequent aneurysm rupture is approximately 4% in the first 24 hours and 1.5% per subsequent day, leading to approximately 27% incidence of subsequent aneurysmal rupture within the first 2 weeks of hemorrhage. The rebleeding rate decreases to 3–5% per year. The major goal in SAH treatment is to prevent rebleeding, ideally by methods designed to obliterate the aneurysm. Although the rebleeding risk can be somewhat decreased pharmacologically in the short term, the only definitive prevention is direct obliteration using surgical or endovascular techniques. Previous beliefs regarding the timing of aneurysm occlusion have been replaced by a general attitude that early and expeditious aneurysm occlusion, when feasible, must be performed.

HYDROCEPHALUS

Up to 25% of patients with SAH develop secondary acute hydrocephalus, independent of grade that worsens if left untreated. There is no consensus on the management of hydrocephalus and intraventricular hemorrhage. However, external ventricular drainage is recommended in conjunction with early aneurysm occlusion. Many patients can be weaned off the ventricular drainage later in their hospital course. Chronic hydrocephalus develops in 25% of patients who survive aneurysmal rupture. Of patients with acute hydrocephalus who require ventricular drainage, approximately one half will ultimately require a ventricular–peritoneal shunt.

CEREBRAL VASOSPASM

Cerebral vasospasm, a poorly understood phenomenon, is the most feared and difficult issue associated with SAH. This represents a pathologic change within the cerebral vessels leading to vascular narrowing with decreased cerebral blood flow and subsequent stroke. Vasospasm is correlated with poor clinical grade and larger degrees of hemorrhage. It is thought that vessel spasm and narrowing is the result of RBC degradation and lysis within the subarachnoid space with resultant imbalance between vascular relaxing and constricting factors in CSF. Typically, vasospasm develops about the fourth day after SAH and usually peaks between 7 and 10 days but may occur up to 3 weeks following bleeding.

Management includes the use of calcium channel blockers such as nimodipine, decreasing ICP with ventricular drainage, and augmenting cerebral circulation and perfusion through narrowed vessels. The latter is best achieved with **triple-H therapy**, consisting of hypervolemia, hemodilution, and hypertensive therapy. Hypervolemia is easily achieved using volume expanders, such as albumen and crystalloid fluids. Hemodilution frequently occurs passively or with phlebotomy with an optimum hematocrit goal between 30% and 33%. Hypertensive therapy, when needed, may be instituted using α-adrenergic agonists such as phenylephrine hydrochloride. The goal is to prevent the development of permanent neurologic deficits by reversing deficits as they occur. Transcranial Doppler ultrasonography is of value for detecting the presence and degree of vasospasm and for monitoring its response to therapy. Transcranial Doppler ultrasonography provides real-time information regarding blood flow velocities, which correlates with the degree of vessel spasm.

Occasionally, ischemic deficits continue to develop despite aggressive triple-H therapy. In this setting, endovascular maneuvers, such as intracranial angioplasty, intraarterial papaverine (a direct smooth muscle relaxant) or, more recently, intraarterial calcium channel blakers such as verapamil, can be used with excellent, albeit transient, results. The voltage-gated calcium channel blocker nimodipine has been shown to decrease rates of infarctions related to vasospasm by about a third in patients with no neurologic deficits on presentation. There is no evidence that it reduces the frequency of medium or large vessel vasospasm directly, and its effect may be through enhancing cerebral blood flow through increasing microvascular and collateral flow. Its use in critically ill patients must be weighed against its potential effects of excessively lowering the blood pressure and the difficulty of administration (60 mg PO qid for 3 weeks).

SYSTEMIC COMPLICATIONS

Subarachnoid hemorrhage concomitantly results in a catastrophic assault on the entire physiologic system, and patients are frequently critically ill, requiring a multisystem therapeutic approach.

At the moment of SAH, experimental evidence suggests that a **massive surge in ICP** overcomes MAP, resulting in a momentary **global arrest in cerebral circulation**. As the increased ICP begins to wane, the circulation is reinstated, at which point a small fibrin plug is created, sealing the aneurysm and preventing further bleeding.

The sudden ICP increase affects the hypothalamus and when combined with the associated global ischemia, there is a **massive neuroendocrine response** to a **catecholamine surge** consequently leading to possible cardiac and pulmonary injury. **Cardiac abnormalities** may be identified on ECG in up to 50% of patients at admission, including T-wave abnormalities, ST-segment depressions, prominent U waves, or prolongation of the QT interval. Cardiac arrhythmias and myocardial injury may develop.

Other patients may present with **acute respiratory distress syndrome** from massive pulmonary edema, termed *neurogenic pulmonary edema*. It may result in associated hypoxia and may contribute to the overall system failure.

There is usually associated acute **hypertension**, likely as part of the Cushing response, secondary to increased ICP. This reflexive mechanism is protective as it maintains mean arterial pressure and cerebral circulation in the face of a dramatic increase in ICP. Management of hypertension in this setting requires treatment of the increased ICP, such as ventricular drainage of the CSF, rather than the use of antihypertensive medications and an abrupt drop in blood pressure.

Frequently, abnormalities of **electrolytes** are also noted, particularly hyponatremia. Usually associated with a salt wasting state rather than a syndrome of inappropriate antidiuretic hormone, hyponatremia should be managed accordingly. The mechanism is not totally clear but likely involves increased renal natriuresis as a result of heightened sympathetic tone and the release of cerebral natriuretic peptide. Unlike SIADH, the urine volume remains high and treatment entails both intravascular fluid and sodium replacement, at times with hypertonic fluids. Mineralocorticoids have also been reported to be useful.

are occluded or injured is completed just before clipping. Once secured, the aneurysm can be punctured to allow it to collapse and relieve mass effect if present. Adjuncts to the surgical treatment of aneurysms are beyond the scope of this text but include temporary clipping, cerebral bypasses, aneurysmorrhaphy, and, in some cases, full hypothermic cardiac arrest. With microsurgical technology and various temporary and permanent aneurysm clips available and the establishment of skull base and revascularization techniques, management of once inoperable lesions has become routine.

Endovascular Therapy

The treatment for ruptured intracranial aneurysms requires multidisciplinary efforts; the core team consists of an interventional neuroradiologist, vascular neurosurgeon, neurointensivists, and rehabilitation specialists. Recently the endovascular approach has emerged as an alternative treatment modality for selected aneurysms. In the treatment of complex large and giant aneurysms, endovascular therapy may serve as an adjunct to surgical interventions.

Although there are singular reports of aneurysm treatments from Ciniselli, Moore, and Werner in the last 150 years that resemble modern endovascular therapy, the current treatment modality was originally devised by Guglielmi in 1990 using platinum coils that were detached within the aneurysm dome using an electrolytic mechanism. Approved by the Food and Drug Administration in 1991, the device became known as Guglielmi detachable coil (GDC). Presently coils that incorporate other materials and utilize alternative detachment mechanisms are available in the United States.

The international subarachnoid aneurysm trial (ISAT) is currently the only large-scale international prospective randomized controlled trial (RCT) comparing surgical clipping with endovascular treatment of ruptured aneurysms. The authors demonstrated a 24% relative and 7.4% absolute reduction of death or dependency at 1 year in favor of coiling. A number of criticisms of this publication have been made, specifically the applicability of the findings to the practice pattern found in the United States and a perceived imbalance between the experience of the endovascular practitioners and the surgeons in the study.

Endovascular treatment for ruptured intracranial aneurysms is usually conducted under general anesthesia. Systemic heparinization during the procedure is preferred by some but is not universally accepted. A 6 or 7 French guide catheter is introduced via the femoral artery into the internal carotid artery (ICA) or vertebral artery to provide a stable platform. A microcatheter is advanced over a microguidewire coaxially through the guide catheter into the aneurysm, and a series of soft platinum coils are deployed sequentially until radiographic occlusion of the aneurysm dome is achieved. Coils used for aneurysm embolization are usually MR compatible, and MR imaging may be used for noninvasive follow-up imaging.

The shape, size, and neck diameter of the aneurysm in relation to the parent vessel determine whether or not its dome can be successfully occluded. Larger or odd-shaped aneurysms with wide necks are more difficult to occlude completely. In ISAT the proportions of completely, subtotally (with remnants at the neck), and incompletely occluded aneurysms at follow-up were

66%, 26%, and 8%, respectively. It is not clear what the risk of rebleeding is from a small neck remnant following either endovascular coil embolization or rarely surgical clipping. Post-clip angiography shows that only 4–10% of aneurysms have any major remnant while coiling achieves complete aneurysm occlusion in only 50% of cases. When near-complete occlusions are included, this level increases to 85–90%. Another limitation to endovascular procedures is an approximately 16–32% aneurysm recurrence depending on the location, degree of compaction, and morphology of the aneurysm when primarily treated (Fig. 57-12). Patients may require repeated treatment or even surgical intervention with removal of the coils.

More recent modifications in device technology aim to achieve safer and more durable treatment of a larger proportion

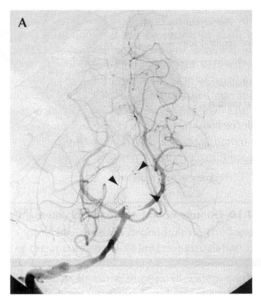

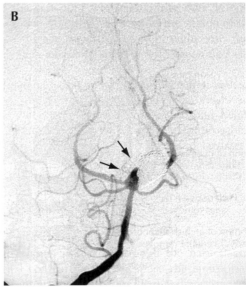

AP vertebral artery angiogram showing compaction of coils in a basilar tip aneurysm over time and regrowth of the aneurysm base (patient in the second vignette).

Figure 57-12 Basilar Tip Aneurysm Re-expansion.

of aneurysms, including those with a wide neck or complex shape that were not readily amenable to occlusion with GDC platinum coils alone. These include complex coil shapes that conform better to irregular aneurysm geometries, balloon remodeling techniques (a nondetachable balloon catheter deployed across the aneurysm neck and inflated to prevent herniation of the coils into the parent vessel), stent-assisted coil embolization, bioactive coils coated with polyglycolic polylactic acid to enhance thrombus formation and organization, platinum coils coated with a polymeric hydrogel that swells when in contact with blood to achieve greater packing density, and radioactive coils. Liquid embolization systems with high-density Onyx (Ethyl-vinyl alcohol copolymer mixed with micronized tantalum powder) deliver a mass of highly viscous and cohesive material into the aneurysm, ideally leading to complete occlusion of the aneurysm and covered stents aimed to restore the parent vessel wall in its entirety. Many of these technologies have been studied in selected patients and are currently under review for approval in the United States.

Interval posttreatment angiographic follow-up, either with noninvasive CT or MR angiography or catheter angiography, is mandatory and should be performed lifelong. There are no clear guidelines regarding the most appropriate follow-up intervals, and an individualized approach may be taken.

Overall procedure-related morbidity is 6–19%, and mortality 1–2%. Procedural complications include aneurysm rupture (2–5%) potentially leading to worse outcome or death, thromboembolic events (5–9%), parent vessel occlusion (2.5%), coil migration 0.5%, and significant groin hematomas (0.6%).

Long-term complications of coil embolization include recanalization and coil compaction. Even after complete radiographic occlusion of the aneurysm, only about 25–35% of its volume consists of coils, with the rest being thrombus. About 10% of coiled aneurysms will require a second treatment after recanalization to ensure stability. The risk of rebleeding has been documented at 0.2% per patient year with a mean follow-up of 4 years, similar to the rebleeding rates after neurosurgical clipping.

The risk of postoperative epilepsy, though low in absolute terms, is lower after endovascular treatment compared to craniotomies. The relative risk reduction of coiling compared to surgery at 1 year is 47.9%, and the absolute risk reduction is 3.9%.

Embolization materials are more expensive than aneurysm clips, but health economic data emerging from the ISAT suggests that these excess costs are offset by shorter hospital stays, fewer dependent survivors, less requirement for rehabilitation, and possibly reduced neuropsychological impact. The development and clinical experience with the Guglielmi detachable coil technology is extensive, and follow-up is available beyond 10 years. In many patients, aneurysm endovascular coil occlusion is a valuable alternative to surgery. Overall, 82% of patients experience favorable outcomes.

ADDITIONAL RESOURCES

Allen GS, Ahn HS, Preziosi TJ, et al. Cerebral arterial vasospasm—a controlled trial of nimodipine in patients with subarachnoid hemorrhage. N Engl J Med 1983;308:619-624. *This study was conducted in intact neurologically stable patients. Extrapolating these findings to those presenting with deficits and critically ill patients requires caution.*

Bederson JB, Ward I, Wiebers DO, et al. Recommendations for the management of patients with unruptured intracranial aneurysms: a statement for healthcare professionals from the Stroke Council of the American Heart Association. Stroke 2000;31:2742-2750.

Eskridge J, Song J, and participants. Endovascular embolization of 150 basilar tip aneurysms with Guglielmi-detachable coils: results of the food and drug administration multi-center clinical trial. J Neurosurg 1998;89:81-86.

International Study of Unruptured Intracranial Aneurysms Investigators. Unruptured intracranial aneurysms: risk of rupture and risk of surgical intervention. N Engl J Med 1998;339:1725-1733.

International Subarachnoid Hemorrhage Aneurysm Collaborative Group. International Subarachnoid Aneurysm Trial (ISAT) of neurosurgical clipping versus endovascular coiling in 2,143 patients with ruptured intracranial aneurysms: a randomized trial. Lancet 2002;360:1267-1274. *Pivotal randomized study that has established the use of endovascular coiling as a less invasive, safe and efficacious alternative to surgical clipping.*

MacDonald RL, Wallace MC, Kestle JR. The role of angiography following aneurysm surgery. J Neurosurg 1993;79:826-832.

Intracerebral Hemorrhage

58

Kinan K. Hreib

Clinical Vignette

A 72-year-old woman with history of hypertension noticed tingling in the right arm. Within 30 minutes, her right leg buckled and she fell. Her husband helped her up and she was able to walk without support. She rested, but within an hour, she developed speech difficulties and more definite right-sided weakness.

She was brought to the emergency department (ED) and was noted to have mild right arm weakness and some word-finding difficulties. Her blood pressure was 140/80 mm Hg. She got up to go to the bathroom, walked approximately 10 ft, and collapsed on the floor. She was then globally aphasic, with left gaze deviation (i.e., paralysis of gaze to the right) and right hemiplegia. Within 10 minutes, she became gradually unresponsive.

She was intubated for airway protection and taken for brain CT scanning, which demonstrated a large left putaminal hemorrhage. Soon thereafter, she had bilaterally dilated fixed pupils. The vestibular-ocular reflexes were lost. Within another 10 minutes, she was determined brain dead.

The preceding vignette demonstrates the classic presentation of a primary intracerebral hemorrhage (ICH with a rapidly evolving focal neurologic deficit). Its progressively increasing size led to increased intracranial pressure with coma from downward herniation of the uncus onto the brainstem and ultimately irreversible neurologic damage. The only means to prevent ICH is appropriate therapy of its major risk factor, hypertension.

There are two forms of intrinsic cerebral hemorrhage, primary ICH, which has a predilection to affect the striatum, thalamus, midbrain, pons, and cerebellum, and subarachnoid hemorrhage (Chapter 57). ICH comprises approximately 10% of all strokes in the Caucasian population and up to 20% in the Asian population. Over the past several years, improved treatment of hypertension has decreased the number of patients experiencing ICH.

Hypertension is a major risk factor for intracerebral hemorrhages in patients between the ages of 40 and 70. A small proportion of intracerebral hemorrhages in patients older than age 60 years is not directly related to hypertension and is primarily caused by amyloid angiopathy. Furthermore, the increased use of oral anticoagulant therapy in the elderly population has led to higher rates of warfarin-associated ICH. Warfarin anticoagulation increases the risk of intracerebral hemorrhage fivefold, and some studies have estimated that 18% of intracerebral hemorrhages admitted to the hospital are related to its use. Of interest is that most bleeds in patients on warfarin occur when the INR is within the recommended therapeutic limits. Secondary, less common causes of intracerebral hemorrhages include primary and metastatic tumors of the brain and in younger individuals cerebral hemorrhage associated with underlying arterial venous malformation or cavernous angioma.

PATHOPHYSIOLOGY OF HYPERTENSISVE PRIMARY ICH

Intracranial hemorrhage is a rapidly evolving process that may progress over hours or days. The pressure effects of the initial hemorrhage lead to mechanical disruption and tearing of surrounding vessels with subsequent gradual expansion of the hematoma out from the original center. Rebleeding is the most feared early complication of ICH and occurs in approximately 40% of patients. Rebleeding usually occurs within the first 24 hours but, on occasion, has been reported up to a week later. The underlying pathological mechanism of primary hypertensive ICH is attributable to either the formation of miliary microaneurysms or primary arteriolar degeneration (lipohyalinosis and weakening of the blood vessel intima and media wall layers) (Fig. 58-1). The presence of miliary aneurysms is directly related to hypertension but is not necessarily the initial site of bleeding, and cases of hypertensive ICH outside the areas of microaneurysms have been noted. This suggests that degeneration of the arteriolar smooth muscle wall is likely an important factor in the evolution of ICH. Hypertensive intracerebral hemorrhages have a predilection to occur in the basal ganglia and the thalamus. The arterioles in these structures are likely more vulnerable to degenerative changes brought on by diffuse, large pressure pulses over time.

Although hypertension is considered an important risk factor for ICH, studies are inconsistent in estimating the exact risk of ICH in hypertensive patients. It has been noted in some studies that up to 90% of patients with ICH have evidence of hypertension at the time of presentation. Other important risk factors include smoking, alcohol consumption, black race, and low total serum cholesterol levels. The latter is likely to be an anomaly of population studies. Patients with ICH and concomitantly low serum cholesterol levels tend to be older than age 80 years and, on average, have higher diastolic pressures. The effect of lower cholesterol levels, particularly LDL, on increasing the incidence of ICH is likely small and the mechanism remains unclear; whether it is causative or an epiphenomenon of another process warrants further investigation.

CLINICAL PRESENTATION

Intraparenchymal hemorrhages vary in presentation depending on the site of the bleeding (Fig. 58-2). In approximately 60% of patients, neurologic symptoms develop gradually or stepwise over a period of hours. To some extent, the location and size of the hematoma predict clinical outcome.

Headache occurs at presentation in approximately 40% of patients with ICH. Less commonly, headache develops within a

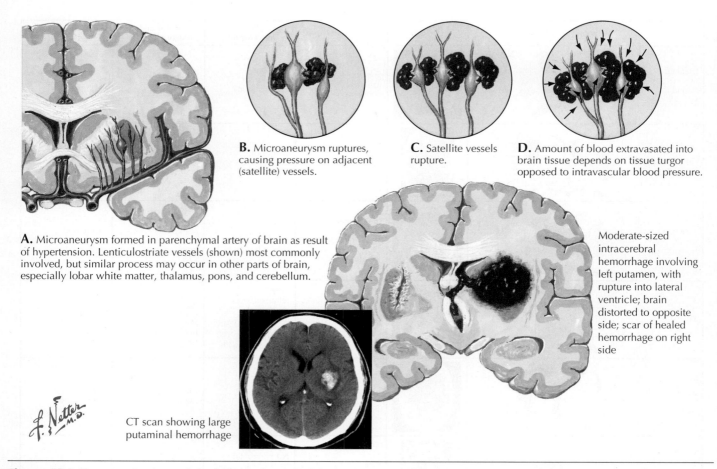

B. Microaneurysm ruptures, causing pressure on adjacent (satellite) vessels.

C. Satellite vessels rupture.

D. Amount of blood extravasated into brain tissue depends on tissue turgor opposed to intravascular blood pressure.

A. Microaneurysm formed in parenchymal artery of brain as result of hypertension. Lenticulostriate vessels (shown) most commonly involved, but similar process may occur in other parts of brain, especially lobar white matter, thalamus, pons, and cerebellum.

Moderate-sized intracerebral hemorrhage involving left putamen, with rupture into lateral ventricle; brain distorted to opposite side; scar of healed hemorrhage on right side

CT scan showing large putaminal hemorrhage

Figure 58-1 Hypertensive Intracerebral Hemorrhage: Pathogenesis.

few days after the ictus. Intracerebral hemorrhages presenting with headache are often located at the brain surface or within the cerebellum. Depression in the level of consciousness and vomiting occur in 50% of patients, particularly those with large cerebellar bleeds. Seizures occur at onset in up to 10% and are seen most commonly with lobar bleeds in the anterior circulation. There are rare incidences of patients with deep hemorrhages having seizures. The subsequent risk for seizures in ICH patients is up to 29% for those with lobar hemorrhages but only 4% for those with deep hemorrhages. Other symptoms seen in association with ICH include low-grade fever without obvious infection, cardiac arrhythmias, and dysautonomia, especially with pontine bleeds. A description of some of the most common symptoms at different sites of ICH follows.

Deep Supratentorial Hemorrhage

PUTAMINAL HEMORRHAGES

The most common site of ICH is the putamen, and these are classified into anterior, middle, and posterior lesions. Anterior putaminal hemorrhage often causes motor weakness due to compression of the anterior limb of the internal capsule. If the ICH is on the left, abulia and aphasia are common accompaniments. When the lesion occurs on the right, significant behavioral changes can occur, including disinhibition, poor insight

and judgment, and occasionally violent behavior. Caudate hemorrhages are associated with similar behavioral and cognitive changes. Studies suggest that these behaviors result from frontal lobe disconnection. Often, deficits from small anterior putaminal hemorrhages are reversible.

A hemorrhage within the midputamen, however, results in severe deficits, often with poor recovery. In this case, ICH compresses and undercuts nearby cortical structures, causing global aphasia if involving the left hemisphere and severe neglect if involving the right. With posterior putaminal hemorrhages, a combination of sensory-motor deficits, visual field difficulties, limb ataxia, and behavioral changes often results. Some putaminal hemorrhages not extending into the globus pallidus present with short-lived hemichorea or hemiballismus, although a variety of other abnormal involuntary movements have been described. Large or medially located putaminal hemorrhages and head of the caudate hemorrhages can dissect toward the ventricle, with resultant intraventricular hemorrhage and the development of acute obstructive hydrocephalus with rapid deterioration due to increased intracranial pressure. Primary intraventricular hemorrhage, in contrast, does not affect surrounding brain tissue, and most cases present as a nonlocalizing rapidly progressive syndrome of nausea, vomiting, stupor, and seizure. In less acute cases, the patient presents with headaches, confusion, and somnolence.

Pathology	CT scan	Pupils	Eye movements	Motor and sensory deficits	Other
Caudate nucleus (blood in ventricle)		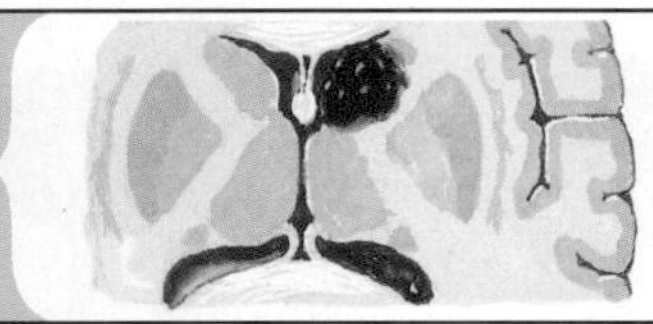 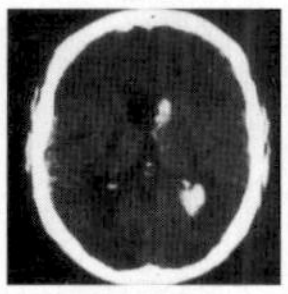 Sometimes ipsilaterally constricted	Conjugate deviation to side of lesion; slight ptosis	Contralateral hemiparesis, often transient	Headache, confusion
Putamen (small hemorrhage)		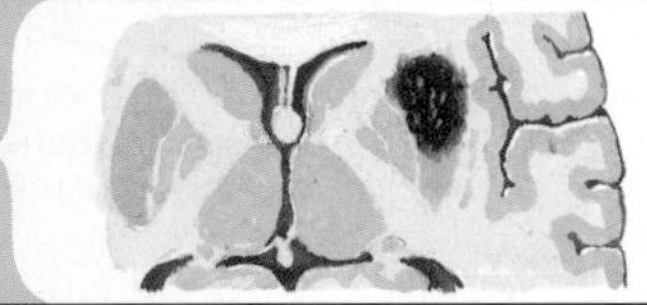 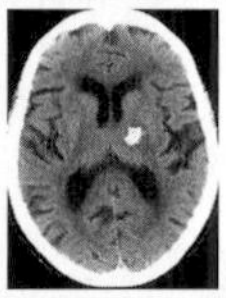 Normal	Conjugate deviation to side of lesion	Contralateral hemiparesis and hemisensory loss	Aphasia (if lesion on left side)
Putamen (large hemorrhage)		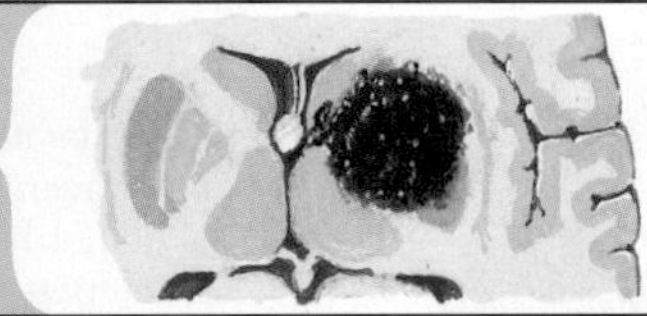 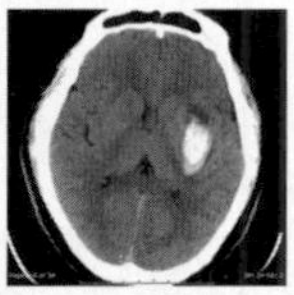 In presence of herniation, pupil dialated on side of lesion	Conjugate deviation to side of lesion	Contralateral hemiparesis and hemisensory loss	Decreased consciousness
Thalamus		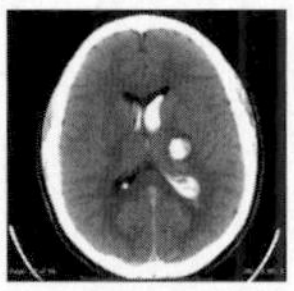 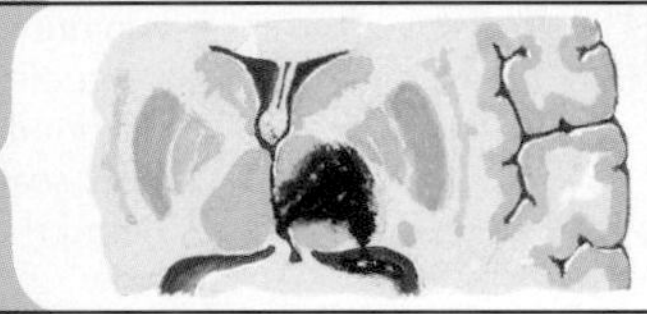 Constricted, poorly reactive to light bilaterally	Both lids retracted; eyes positioned downward and medially; cannot look upward	Slight contralateral hemiparesis, but greater hemisensory loss	Aphasia (if lesion on left side)
Occipital lobar white matter		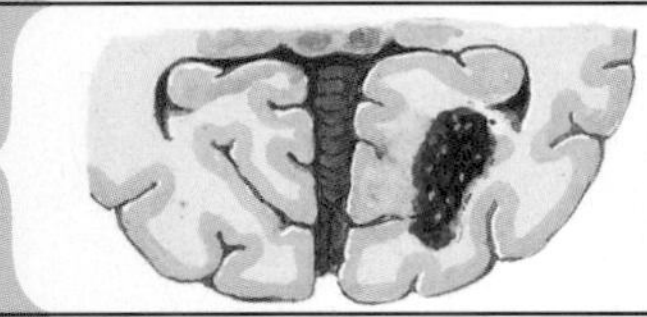 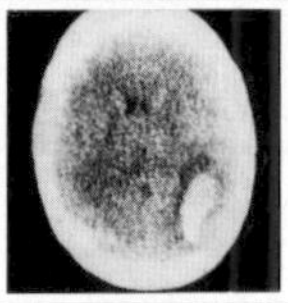 Normal	Normal	Mild, transient hemiparesis	Contralateral hemianopsia
Pons		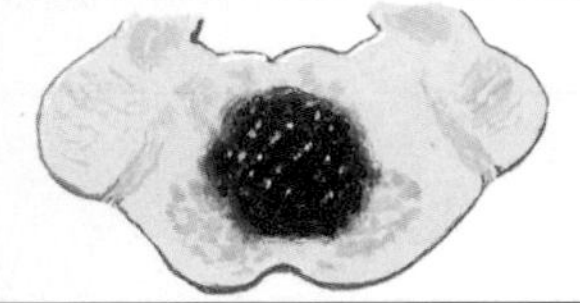 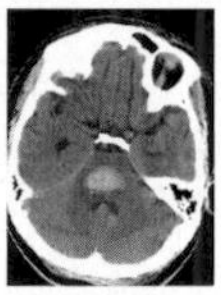 Constricted, reactive to light	No horizontal movements; vertical movements preserved	Quadriplegia	Coma
Cerebellum		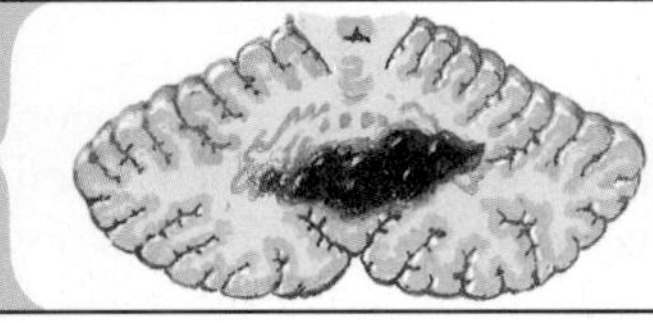 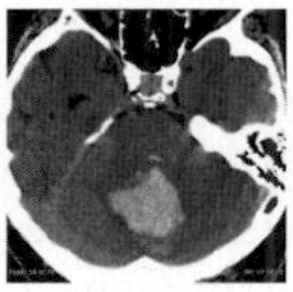 Slight constriction on side of lesion	Slight deviation to opposite side; movements toward side of lesion impaired, or sixth cranial nerve palsy	Ipsilateral limb ataxia; no hemiparesis	Gait ataxia, vomiting

Figure 58-2 Intracerebral Hemorrhage: Clinical Manifestations Related to Site.

THALAMIC HEMORRHAGES

Clinically, thalamic ICHs are classified into posterior–inferior, posterior–lateral, and dorsal–medial. Somnolence is one of the most common presentations of medial–posterior and inferior thalamic bleeds and can be profound as a result of bilateral disruption of the rostral reticular activating system. If the hemorrhage dissects anteriorly, often persistent hypokinetic behavior results from disconnection of the frontal lobe. With inferior–lateral thalamic hemorrhage, there is weakness and clumsiness and, occasionally, tremors and choreoathetoid movements. Tremors are likely related to disruption of projections from the cerebellum and dentate nucleus. Disruption of the fibers of the ansa lenticularis are likely responsible for the choreoathetoid movements.

More lateral thalamic hemorrhages involving the ventral posteromedial and ventral posterolateral thalamic nuclei primarily cause unilateral sensory symptoms but occasionally motor involvement when the hemorrhage extends laterally to involve the internal capsule. Eye movement abnormalities, small pupils, ptosis, chorea, and dystonia also occur. Hematomas involving the dorsal-medial thalamic area present with prominent memory problems and behavioral changes thought to relate to dissociated frontal cortex, cingulate gyrus, and amygdalar connections. Speech and language deficits are the least consistent symptoms of thalamic hemorrhages. Paraphasia, naming difficulties, or a perceived inability to comprehend, with preservation of repetition, is typical of thalamic aphasia. In patients with right thalamic hemorrhage, deficits mimic cortical lesions with neglect or hemi-inattention, vivid visual, and, less often, auditory hallucinations can occur in the days following thalamic ICH.

SUPERFICIAL LOBAR HEMORRHAGES

After the putamen, the most common site of primary ICH is one of four locations in the cerebral cortex. The parietal and occipital areas are most frequently involved. In general, hypertension is an important risk factor for all ICH regardless of location, but whether blood pressure plays a lesser role in the contribution of lobar versus subcortical hemorrhages remains inconclusive. Primary amyloid angiopathy frequently underlies nonhypertensive intracerebral lobar hemorrhage. Other less common causes include vascular malformations, primary and metastatic malignancies, sympathomimetic drugs, anticoagulants, irreversible antiplatelet and fibrinolytic agents, and sinus thrombosis with venous infarctions and bleeds.

Lobar hemorrhages often present with headaches and vomiting. Seizures at the onset of lobar hemorrhage are common, particularly those within the posterior parietal or frontal lobe. Functionally, patients with lobar hemorrhage may have better outcomes than those with deep hemorrhages. However, prognosis depends on hematoma size, level of consciousness at presentation, and presence of intraventricular blood. Mortality rates range from 12 to 30% in superficial lobar hemorrhages compared to 25–42% in deep basal ganglionic and thalamic hemorrhages and up to 97% in pontine hemorrhages.

- **Frontal hematomas.** Intracranial hemorrhages in the superior aspect of the frontal lobe are usually small and cause weakness in the contralateral leg. Inferior frontal hemorrhages are larger, causing a depressed level of consciousness, hemiplegia, hemisensory deficits, and horizontal gaze paresis. Language output can also be affected. Apathy and abulia occur with superior mesial lesions and may be prominent.
- **Parietal hematomas.** With right hemispheric hemorrhages, often the most striking clinical presentation is a cortical neglect syndrome, while left hemispheric hemorrhages produce various degrees of aphasia. Extension into subcortical areas often occurs with weakness, and hemianopsia is frequently seen. More medial hemorrhages result in downward pressure on the upper brainstem and can cause obtundation or coma.
- **Occipital hematomas.** Although headaches are prominent in many lobar hemorrhages, those occurring with occipital hemorrhage are particularly severe. The most obvious neurologic deficit is a homonymous hemianopsia but some patients present with other visual changes, including flashes of bright lights and palinopsia (afterimages). Other deficits indicative of more anteriorly located hemorrhage include visual extinction, dysgraphia, and dyslexia. Occipital hematomas are the least likely to be related to hypertension.
- **Temporal hematomas.** Neurologic deficits in temporal hematomas differ depending on the side involved. Fluent aphasia, often associated with paraphasia and poor comprehension, is the most prominent deficit from isolated left temporal lobe hemorrhage. In contrast, right temporal hemorrhages are often associated with relatively minor problems, most commonly confusion. Other neurologic symptoms depend on whether there is extension into the surrounding subcortical areas or adjacent frontal lobe.

Infratentorial Hemorrhages

CEREBELLAR HEMORRHAGE

Clinical Vignette

A 58-year-old woman with substantial history of arterial hypertension presented to the ED with a 1-hour duration of acute-onset headache, gait unsteadiness, and left arm incoordination. On examination, the patient was alert and oriented but had left-sided dysmetria, gait ataxia, and left CN-VI and CN-VII palsies. Her BP was 200/110 mm Hg. Urgent head CT showed a 3-cm cerebellar hemorrhage with slight compression of the fourth ventricle. Antihypertensive treatment aiming for a MAP of 100–120 mm Hg was initiated.

Within 30 minutes after the CT scan, the patient's level of consciousness deteriorated, necessitating intubation. She was brought immediately to the operating room for evacuation of the hematoma and responded well. One month later, her examination was remarkable for only mild clumsiness of the left arm and a slightly wide-based gait.

As in the preceding vignette, patients with cerebellar hemorrhages can deteriorate rapidly, even "in front of one's eyes," but can still respond exceptionally well with expeditious surgical intervention. Most cerebellar hemorrhages are associated with hypertension. However, approximately 10% of primary cerebellar hemorrhages are caused by AVM, tumors, blood dyscrasias and the use of warfarin anticoagulation. Headache, spinning vertigo, nausea, vomiting, and, most commonly, unsteady gait characterize the typical presentation. Some headaches are occipital, but many involve the orbital and supraorbital areas. The most reliable symptoms of a hemispheric cerebellar hemorrhage include headache, vomiting, nystagmus, ipsilateral limb ataxia with, at times, ipsilateral peripheral CN-VI and CN-VII palsies and horizontal nystagmus.

The less common vermian hemorrhages often resemble a pontine hemorrhage and can progress rapidly to coma, making it difficult to identify specific early clinical signs that can differentiate one from the other. Cranial nerve palsies are related to involvement of adjacent pontine structures or stretching secondary to increased cerebellar pressure. In hypertensive bleeds involving the vermis or the cerebellar hemispheres, the superior cerebellar artery is most often involved.

Unlike supratentorial bleeds, in which a small hemorrhage is often well tolerated, infratentorial ICH within the posterior fossa often leads to rapid neurologic deterioration and death. Close monitoring in an ICU for 36–48 hours, when the risk of deterioration is at its highest, is therefore recommended for most patients. Rebleeding, rupture into the fourth ventricle, and accelerated hemorrhagic edema, alone or in combination, often lead to a devastating outcome. Hemorrhages larger than 3 cm may extend into the fourth ventricle and lead to the development of acute hydrocephalus and require ventriculostomy placement. The threshold for surgical evacuation of the hematoma should be low and considered at the earliest sign of deterioration. The major goal is decompression of the posterior fossa to prevent blockage of the fourth ventricle and compression of the adjacent brainstem. Fortunately, if impending brainstem compression is recognized early, there are often only minimal residual deficits after surgery, even with extensive cerebellar evacuation and decompression. The potentially positive recovery from cerebellar hemorrhages and decompressive surgery reflects that the deep cerebellar nuclei, crucial for gait coordination and balance, are often spared from direct damage.

PONTINE/MIDBRAIN HEMORRHAGE

Pontine and midbrain hemorrhages are relatively uncommon but have the most devastating outcome compared with other sites of primary intracranial hemorrhages. Three distinct vascular territories dictate the clinical presentation. The paramedian penetrators, arising directly from the basilar trunk, are the primary arteries supplying the midline pons or midbrain. ICH in this location causes bilateral damage and is often fatal. Sudden onset of deep coma, quadriparesis, ophthalmoplegia, and bilateral papillary abnormalities are the presenting signs.

Another group of small arteries, the short circumferential penetrators, courses laterally, supplying the lateral basis pontis, where a hemorrhage may predominantly cause unilateral bulbar symptoms with profound dysphagia. The third important group of vessels, the long circumferential arteries, arises from the anterior–inferior cerebellar artery and primarily supplies the lateral tegmentum. ICH within this segment leads to relatively minor symptoms, including facial numbness and ataxia secondary to involvement of the spinal trigeminal and vestibular nuclei. However, involvement of the intrinsic pontine nuclei, such as the cochlear and facial nuclei, are also affected, which leads to a more serious outcome.

Pontine hemorrhages often have a relatively gradual clinical presentation evolving over hours. Neurologic deficits, including horizontal gaze palsies, miotic sluggishly reactive pupils, quadriparesis, and coma, are the expected clinical signs. Certain unique eye findings, including ocular bobbing and the one-and-a-half syndrome, provide excellent diagnostic clues to pontine hemorrhages. Some patients also exhibit twitching of the limbs and face and rippling of torso muscles. Dysautonomia with irregular pulse, erratic breathing patterns, and an increase in body temperature have also been observed. Vivid, sometimes frightening, formed hallucinations, called peduncular hallucinosis, occur relatively often in patients with involvement of the midbrain tegmentum.

SECONDARY INTRACEREBRAL HEMORRHAGE

ICH not directly caused by hypertension is encountered with vascular malformations, hemorrhagic transformation of ischemic stroke, anticoagulants, as well as fibrinolytic agents or irreversible antiplatelet therapy (Box 58-1). Primary amyloid angiopathy is often the underlying cause of nonhypertensive lobar hemorrhage. Less common causes include primary and metastatic malignancies, sinus thrombosis with venous infarctions and bleeds, acquired or inherited coagulopathies, induced or autoimmune vasculitides and systemic granulomatous disorders, central infectious processes, and trauma (Box 58-2).

Box 58-1 Common Causes of Intracerebral Hemorrhage

1. Primary intracerebral hemorrhage
   Hypertension
   Idiopathic
2. Vascular malformations
   Aneurysm
   Arteriovenous malformation
   Cavernous angioma
3. Embolic infarct
4. Anticoagulant therapy

Box 58-2 Uncommon Causes of Intracerebral Hemorrhage*

1. Endocarditis
2. Venous sinus thrombosis
3. Malignancy: primary, metastatic
4. Blood diathesis
   DIC, ITP, TTP
   Leukemia
   Multiple myeloma
   Sickle cell disease
5. Other hematologic disorders, particularly coagulopathies
   Hemophilia
   von Willebrand factor deficiency
   Afibrinogenemia
6. Vasculitis
   Polyarteritis nodosa
   Systemic lupus erythematosus
   Wegener granulomatosis
   Takayasu arteritis
   Temporal arteritis
   Chemical vasculitis
   Primary CNS vasculitis
   Sympathomimetics (amphetamine, cocaine, phenylpropanolamine)
7. Systemic disorders
   Sarcoidosis
   Behçet syndrome
   CNS infections, particularly herpes zoster
8. Trauma

*DIC, disseminated intravascular coagulation; ITP, idiopathic thrombocytopenic purpura; TTP, thrombotic thrombocytopenic purpura.

In most cases of ICH, especially when hypertension is absent, follow-up imaging studies are essential to investigate the possibilities of underlying predisposing pathology. Contrast-enhanced brain MRI scanning performed about 3 months later, after extravasated blood has been allowed to reabsorb, may uncover an underlying lesion initially obscured by the acute hematoma.

Occult vascular malformations were possibly the most underdiagnosed causes of lobar hemorrhages prior to CT and MRI scanning and were frequently missed by early angiography due to the presence of clot and mass effect on the brain. They were diagnosed only during surgical or pathologic specimen inspection after hematoma removal. The most common occult vascular lesions include small AVMs and cavernous angiomas (Fig. 58-3A–D).

Thalamic Hemorrhage Secondary to AVM

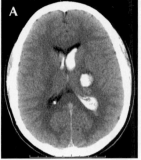

CT with left thalamic hemorrhage and blood in ventricles.

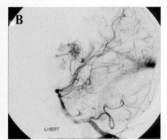

Lateral view; vertebral angiogram with thalamic AVM

Cavernous Hemangioma

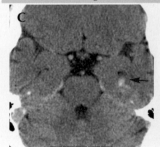

CT with small acute hemorrhage in the left medial temporal lobe close to the lateral ventricular horn (arrow).

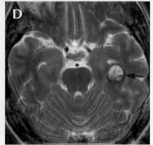

T2-weighted MR with variable intensity pattern and black halo (paramagnetic effect of iron, Fe^{3+}) (arrow).

Hemorrhagic Transformation With Intravenous tPA Therapy.

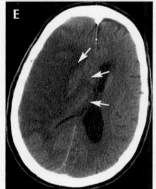

Axial CT showing large right MCA territory infarction (hypodensity) with moderate mass effect.

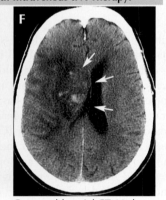

Comparable axial CT 11 days post stroke and intravenous tPA therapy showing multiple small petechial hemorrhages (arrows).

Figure 58-3 Common Causes of Intracerebral Hemorrhage.

Hemorrhagic brain infarct (HBI), in contrast to primary intracranial hemorrhage, is a secondary phenomenon that occurs as a result of ischemic damage to both the brain parenchyma and the vessel wall distal to the site of occlusion. The vascular wall endothelium and the blood–brain barrier are subsequently damaged and leak with reperfusion as they no longer tolerate normal arterial pressure. Petechial bleeding and, at times, gross hemorrhage through the damaged vessel into the infarcted area may be seen (Fig. 58-3E&F). It is estimated that

---

Box 58-3 Tumors Causing Intracerebral Hemorrhage*

Primary CNS
Mixed glioma
Epidermoid cyst
Pituitary adenoma
Oligodendroglioma
Ependymoma
Choroid plexus papilloma
Meningioma
Craniopharyngioma
Glioblastoma
Astrocytoma

Metastatic
Melanoma
Kidney
Lung
Breast
Osteogenic sarcoma
Ovary
Colon

*In order of frequency.

petechial bleeding develops in more than 50% of patients with embolic infarcts. Although it is often implied that cardioembolic strokes are more likely to be associated with development of HBI, some investigators suggest that any large infarct, regardless of mechanism, is predisposed to such bleeding. The use of IV heparin or heparinoid for secondary stroke prevention also promotes the development of HBI. However, the presence of petechial hemorrhage without frank hematoma formation does not seem to worsen neurologic outcome.

Along with typical subarachnoid hemorrhage, *aneurysmal rupture* can, at times, cause intraparenchymal hematoma with focal neurologic signs (Fig. 58-4A&B). The location of the blood often hints to the site of the aneurysm. Lateral temporal lobe hematomas suggest MCA aneurysmal rupture while medially located bleeds are associated with carotid artery aneurysms. Frontal hematomas indicate anterior communicating artery aneurysm. Posterior communicating artery aneurysms cause thalamic hemorrhages, often with intraventricular extension.

Primary or metastatic *brain tumors* can lead to ICH (Box 58-3; Fig. 58-4C&D). A single small hemorrhage from a metastatic lesion, as can be seen with melanomas or hypernephromas, may be difficult to distinguish from primary ICH unless evidence of other lesions is identified. Other clues, such as an atypical cortical or subcortical location of the bleed, irregular margins, and unexpected contrast enhancement of the lesion must prompt further investigations to exclude systemic disorders. A detailed dermatologic examination may reveal irregularly pigmented lesions, suggesting melanoma, and ultrasound or body CT scan may uncover a renal tumor.

Antithrombotic- and Anticoagulant-Induced ICH

The question of whether aspirin promotes ICH remains unclear, but the Physicians' Health Study, a randomized, double-blinded,

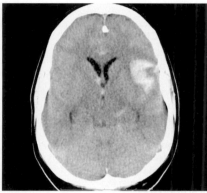

A. CT with blood in left sylvian fissure.

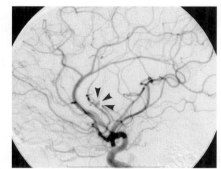

B. Lateral left internal carotid angiogram with small distal MCA aneurysm (arrowheads).

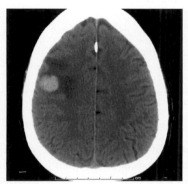

C. CT showing dense right frontal subcortical mass with edema representing a hemorrhagic colon cancer metastasis.

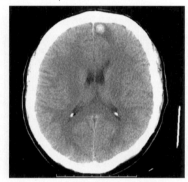

D. CT showing small left frontal hemorrhage in a patient with leukemia and bleeding diathesis.

Figure 58-4 Uncommon Causes of Intracerebral Hemorrhage.

placebo-controlled trial looking at aspirin in cardiovascular disease, suggested a trend toward increased risk. There were 2.1% hemorrhagic strokes in the treatment group and 1.1% in the placebo group. This increase was not seen in many other clinical trials testing the benefits of aspirin for the prevention of stroke. Several trials using warfarin for stroke prevention in patients with atrial fibrillation have demonstrated intracerebral bleeding rates of 0.5–1.8 per year. The highest risk for bleeding was seen in patients older than age 75 years. The combination of warfarin and aspirin suggested similar rates of systemic bleeding, approximately 2.4 per year, and no difference in rates of ICH. The use of intravenous heparin in the setting of acute stroke has not been systematically studied as to benefit or complications. A few studies have suggested no risk of ICH whereas others indicated a risk of approximately 2%, especially when heparin is used in the setting of an acute stroke. The International Stroke Trial used subcutaneous heparin at 12,500 U twice daily versus 5000 U twice daily or a combination of subcutaneous heparin and aspirin. At 14 days, the risk of ICH was 1.8% for the high heparin dose and 0.7% for the low heparin dose. Rates were similar when heparin was combined with aspirin. Heparinoid formulations as well have shown a risk of ICH of 2.4% versus 0.8% for controls.

Amyloid Angiopathy

Amyloid angiopathy is an uncommon arteriolar and venular vasculopathy with hyaline eosinophilic depositions and subsequent weakness of the vessel wall and microaneurysm formation. It is the cause of ICH in 10% of patients age 60 years or older and 20% in patients older than age 70 years. The usual areas of ICH are lobar, both in the subcortical area and the cortex, routinely sparing the basal ganglia, the thalamus, and the brainstem. In the Dutch and Icelandic familial forms of amyloid angiopathy, the mean age for ICH occurrence is as young as 30 years of age. In contrast to the nonfamilial form, ICH in the familial forms of amyloid angiopathy may also affect the brainstem and the cerebellum along with the more typical cortical and subcortical loci.

MRI evidence of previous asymptomatic small hemorrhages is encountered in many patients (Fig. 58-5). However, cases of rapidly successive, small intracranial hemorrhages within a short time period with progressive disability and death have been described. The presence of subcortical white matter disease seen on CT or MRI scans may be a reflection of chronic ischemia from amyloid-laden arterioles. These changes may suggest a higher risk for future hemorrhages and therefore a more cautionary approach to anticoagulation or the potential use of thrombolytic agents is advised.

Endocarditis

The true incidence of endocarditis is unknown. Rheumatic heart disease was formerly the primary cause of bacterial endocarditis, with the most common agent being *Streptococcus viridans*. More virulent forms of endocarditis have emerged as the use of intravenous drugs has increased. Furthermore, the use of

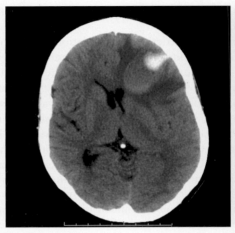

A. CT with moderate-sized left frontal hematoma with edema.

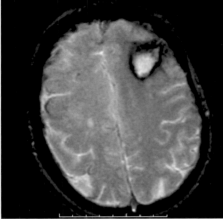

B. GRE MRI shows high-intensity lesion with a hypointense rim representing blood products.

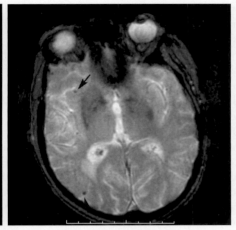

C. GRE MRI showing multiple small paramagnetic lesions consistent with multiple small previous hemorrhages (arrows).

Figure 58-5 Amyloid Angiopathy.

implanted long-term catheters or other similar devices, particularly in hemodialysis or immunocompromised patients, has increased the risk of infection. Native valve acute endocarditis usually has an aggressive course, with *Staphylococcus aureus* and group B streptococci the typical organisms. Underlying structural valve disease need not be present.

Subacute endocarditis due to alpha-hemolytic streptococci or enterococci usually occurs in the setting of structural valve disease and has a more indolent course. *Staph. aureus* and fungal infections are surpassing streptococcal bacteria as causes for valvular infection. Mitral and aortic valves are especially vulnerable. The mitral valve is more consistently associated with neurologic complications than is the aortic valve. In one study, more than 28% of those with bacterial endocarditis had neurologic complications. Mortality was 77% with staphylococcal infections and 36% with streptococcal infections. Cerebral infarctions occurred in up to 50% of patients, ICH occurred in 2.1%, and subarachnoid hemorrhage in 0.8%.

Bacterial mycotic aneurysms are often small and located peripherally, unlike berry and fungal mycotic aneurysms found at the bifurcations in the circle of Willis. Corresponding ICH is therefore typically located superficially in the more distal part of the vessels. However, the more peripheral locations are not necessarily less devastating than the more typical deeper hemorrhages. The presumed hemorrhage mechanism is pyogenic arteritis resulting in blood vessel wall erosion and rupture or rupture of mycotic aneurysm (present in only 12% of patients). Patients receiving anticoagulation as treatment of a presumed ischemic stroke were more likely to suffer hemorrhages. ICH occurred in 24% of patients receiving anticoagulation in the setting of ischemic infarcts or TIAs caused by endocarditis. Repeated blood culture and transesophageal echocardiography are the cornerstones of diagnosis in endocarditis and, if both are positive, have a sensitivity higher than 90%.

Varied clinical profiles of TIA, stroke, and subarachnoid hemorrhage typify the presentation of an atrial myxoma. Therefore, a cardiac embolic evaluation, including transesophageal echocardiography and electrocardiography, are needed.

Vasculitis

Although systemic necrotizing vasculitides, usually associated with peripheral complication such as mononeuritis multiplex, are rarely the cause of cerebral infarction or hemorrhage, primary CNS angiitis is commonly associated with both. The disease course is subacute and presents with mental status changes, headaches, focal deficits, and seizures. Systemic lupus erythematosus is another disorder with a variable degree of CNS involvement. Autopsy series, however, suggest a high frequency of subarachnoid hemorrhage and, to a lesser extent, intracerebral and subdural hemorrhages.

Moyamoya

Moyamoya is a rare primary angiopathy of unknown etiology associated with cerebral vascular occlusive disease due to fibrocellular thickening of the intima and thinning of the media. The carotid siphons and the proximal middle cerebral arteries are typically involved with numerous small vessels developing around the site of occlusion, usually at the base of the circle of Willis. Two forms of Moyamoya exist, the familial and atherosclerotic form. The familial form is most commonly seen in Japan and affects children aged around 10 years. These children often experience recurring bouts of hemiplegia or aphasia. Some symptoms may stutter or progress over a few weeks. The atherosclerotic form occurs in older patients, who may present with recurring TIAs or ICHs. Early in the disease, symptoms may be difficult to interpret, and MRI findings are often unspecific. Careful observation for flow voids within the major vessels may demonstrate abnormalities that can prompt further investigation with angiography. ICH occurs mostly in the older-patient form because of small friable vessels sprouting within the basal ganglia.

Arteriovenous Malformation

Prevalence of arteriovenous malformation (AVM) is unknown, but estimates range from 1 to 2 per 100,000 individuals. Luckily only 10% become symptomatic from bleeding. Patients often present with headaches, TIA-like spells and seizures. The risk of bleeding from an AVM is estimated at 3% per year. However, the risk of rebleeding in the first year is as high as 30%. AVM with associated aneurysmal lesions, poorly developed venous drainage, and location near the ventricles hold a higher risk for bleeding. Management of symptomatic AVMs includes surgical decompression and removal of the AVM, if it is accessible. Other interventions include a combination of catheter-based intervention plus surgery. Small vascular malformations may be treated with focused radiation, although the latter approach may take years to obliterate the malformation. Brain swelling and hemorrhage may complicate treatment because of altered flow dynamics. Some experts advocated treatment of the malformation in stages to allow the brain and the malformation to adjust gradually to changes in blood flow.

Cerebral Cavernous Angioma

This vascular malformation is either inherited or sporadic. Single lesions are seen in the sporadic form whereas the inherited form often presents with multiple lesions. In the familial form of the disease, three genes have been identified, *CCM1/KRIT1*, *CCM2/MGC4607*, and *CCM3/PDCD10*. Large clusters of family members with cavernous angioma have been identified in Hispanic-American families. Often this condition presents with TIA-like spells, seizures, or headaches. Lesions that are diagnosed on MRI are frequently shown to have bled in the past. When bleeding from cavernous angioma is significant, the morphologic features of the lesion may be obscured, making diagnosis acutely difficult. Repeat imaging studies, once there is some resolution of the hematoma, may ultimately help reveal the lesion.

MANAGEMENT AND PROGNOSIS

Many ICH patients initially presenting with a modest neurologic deficit may rapidly worsen during the first 24 hours. Serial CT scans demonstrate that ICH can recur or worsen even up to 7 days after the ictus. As in the first vignette of this chapter, recurrent or progressive ICH is often rapid and fatal, particularly if the hemorrhage extends to the ventricular system and produces acute hydrocephalus. Sudden volume increase, and mass effect from enlarging ICH compromises the surrounding microvasculature and leads to both mechanical and ischemic tissue damage to the surrounding brain structures. Tissue shifts compounded by evolving vasogenic cerebral edema over 24 hours may lead to transtentorial herniation. Excessive increases in blood pressure, concomitant infection, fever, hyperglycemia or hypoglycemia, and other medical conditions all worsen outcome. The initial management of ICH, after ensuring adequate ventilation and hemodynamic stability, involves correcting coagulopathies, treating hypertension, and addressing the possibility of increased intracranial pressure. In patients with intraventricular blood and early hydrocephalus, placement of a temporary external drain should be considered. Beyond these basics principles, the best treatment of ICH remains unclear and quite variable from center to center and in different countries. Although some advocate invasive techniques for

hematoma evacuation, others rely mostly on medical treatment and supportive care.

At present, there are no strict recommendations for blood pressure control in the setting of primary hypertensive ICH. There is evidence to indicate that elevated BP greater than 210 mm Hg is associated with recurrent or expanding ICH but lower BP measurement may not be. Indeed, far too aggressive lowering of BP may lead to a potential drop in cerebral perfusion pressure (CPP), especially in the presence of elevated ICP, and cause secondary ischemia with worsening outcomes. The present guidelines set by the American Heart Association/American Stroke Association council suggest definite treatment of SBP above 210 mm Hg or of MAP of 150 mm Hg with a continuous infusion of a titratable IV medication such as nicardipine, a beta-blocker, or nitroprusside if needed. For measurements below this level but above 180 mm Hg systolic or MAP of 130 mm Hg and in the presence of suspected ICP, a decrease of BP to keep the CPP above 60 mm Hg is recommended. If ICP is not present, careful monitoring with an attempt to avoid hypertensive episodes is suggested. It is often useful to obtain patients' prior BP measurements from outpatient records or from primary care providers if available. This may help guide blood pressure control by providing a sense of where each individual patient's BP range of cerebral autoregulation was before the ICH.

Surgical Trial in Intracerebral Hemorrhage (STICH, 2005) was a multicenter international prospective randomized trial to compare early surgery with initial conservative treatment for patients with spontaneous supratentorial intracerebral hemorrhage. In this study, no overall benefit from early surgery when compared to conservative treatment could be demonstrated. Surgery demonstrated slightly better outcome (26.1% vs. 23.8%), but survival rates appeared to be similar in surgically and medically treated patients. Subgroup analysis suggested that large hemorrhages, older age, and blood in the ventricles predicted poor outcome. Also the subgroup with superficial bleeds and no intraventricular hemorrhage tended to fare better with surgery than with medical treatment alone (49% vs. 37%). The outcome from surgery likely depends on several factors, including the fact that deep-seated basal ganglia or thalamic hemorrhages are difficult to evacuate without disrupting surrounding normal structures and exacerbating brain damage, especially with open craniotomy. A trial to evaluate the role of early surgery in superficial supratentorial lobar hematomas without intraventricular hemorrhage is ongoing. However, when a nondominant hemispheric or cerebellar ICH threatens impending herniation and before the patient's level of consciousness significantly deteriorates, emergent surgery may be lifesaving and may provide a reasonably good recovery, especially in younger patients.

Patients who have small hematomas (smaller than 30 cm³) seem to do generally well without surgical evacuation. However, larger hematomas (larger than 60 cm³) do poorly, even when evacuated surgically. Hematomas between 30 and 40 cm³ may do best after surgical evacuation. There is no evidence that minimally invasive surgery (microsurgery or endoscopy) hold any advantage over open craniotomy, and the advantage of these technique is yet to be determined. A few neurosurgical studies have investigated the benefits of evacuating deep hematomas using a continuous infusion of thrombolytic agents and suction method. Thrombolytic agents such as tissue plasminogen activator have been infused into the hematoma. Although they produce more rapid hematoma resolution, the long-term clinical outcome seems unchanged. Generally, the therapeutic approach must be individualized.

Rebleeding and hematoma expansion is a common cause of acute deterioration and holds up to a 70% risk of death or unfavorable outcome. Prevention of hemorrhage progression, therefore, has become a central theme in the acute treatment of primary ICH. To that end, pro-coagulants, such as activated Factor VII, have been tested in patients with intracerebral hemorrhage (Factor Seven for Acute Hemorrhagic Stroke [FAST]). Activated Factor VII initiates the clotting cascade by binding to the surface of platelets and generating aX, which, in turn, induces surface thrombin formation. This reaction is specific to the site of bleeding as Factor VII works in the presence of tissue factor released at the site of injured tissue. A safety study in 2005 demonstrated that patients treated within 3 hours of presentation with activated Factor VII had the hematoma increase only by 11–16% compared to a 29% increase in the placebo group. Mortality in this Phase II trial decreased from 29 to 18%. Clotting events such as myocardial infarctions, deep venous thrombosis, pulmonary emboli, and ischemic strokes increased from 2% to 7%. A Phase III trial demonstrated that Factor VIIa did indeed decrease ICH volume, but failed to show a clinical effect with mortality and severe disability rates found comparable in the treatment groups and the placebo group. It was postulated that age might have played a role in diluting out the result and that relatively healthy individuals below the age of 70 years may be the ideal patients to respond to such treatments. At this time, however, no pharmacological treatment is available to limit the expansion of the spontaneous intracerebral hemorrhage in the absence of a coagulopathy.

Expansion of the hematoma or rebleeding in patients taking warfarin is another difficult management issue. Obviously, reversing the effects of warfarin is the first step in trying to limit bleeding. The administration of vitamin K and fresh-frozen plasma is often given acutely, but the benefits are not realized for another 24 hours. Some have advocated the use of prothrombin complex concentrate a (conglomerate of high levels of vitamin K–dependent factors) or activated Factor VII to help reverse the effects of warfarin. However, as mentioned previously, there is a significantly increased risk of thromboembolic events, and there are no studies at this time to help guide such treatment.

SUMMARY

The overall mortality of patients with ICH is approximately 50% with lobar and basal ganglionic bleeds and up to 75% when involving the brainstem. Of those who survive, only half will achieve independent living. Initial presentation is predictive of outcome. Individuals who present with coma and signs of herniation have poor prognoses. Rapid increase in intracranial pressure with concurrent brainstem Duret hemorrhages leads to irreversible reticular activating system damage and coma. Patients in whom intraventricular blood leads to hydrocephalus do not fare well either, with 90% suffering poor outcomes or death.

The size of the initial hematoma, as defined by CT, is also predictive. There is a mortality rate of approximately 50–75% in patients with more than 40 mL of blood on CT at presentation. If the patient survives the bleed, the ultimate neurologic recovery depends on the hemorrhage location and residual deficits.

ADDITIONAL RESOURCES

Caplan LR. Caplan's Stroke: A Clinical Approach. 3rd ed. Woburn, Mass: Butterworth-Heinemann; 2000.

Broderick J, Connolly S, Feldmann E, et al. Guidelines for the management of spontaneous intracerebral hemorrhage in adults: 2007 update: a guideline from the American Heart Association/American Stroke. Stroke 2007 Jun;38(6):2001-2023. *Evidence-based guidelines to help manage intracerebral hemorrhage and its complications.*

Dennis MS. Outcome after brain haemorrhage. Cerebrovasc Dis 2003; 16(Suppl 1):9-13.

Fisher CM. Pathological observations in hypertensive cerebral hemorrhage. J Neuropathol Exp Neurol 1971;30:536-550.

Garcia JH, Ho KL. Pathology of hypertensive arteriopathy. Neurosurg Clin North Am 1992;3:497-507.

Garibi J, Bilbao G, Pomposo I, et al. Prognostic factors in a series of 185 consecutive spontaneous supratentorial intracerebral haematomas. Br J Neurosurg 2002;16:355-361.

Kaneko M, Tanaka K, Shimada T, et al. Long term evaluation of ultra-early operation for hypertensive intracerebral hemorrhage in 100 cases. J Neurosurg 1983;58:838-842.

Kase CS. Intracerebral hemorrhage: non-hypertensive causes. Stroke 1986;17:590-595.

Mayer SA. Intracerebral hemorrhage: natural history and rationale of ultra early hemostatic therapy. Intensive Care Med 2002;28(Suppl 2): S235-S240.

Mayer SA, Brun NC, Begtrup K et al. Recombinant activated factor VII for acute intracerebral hemorrhage. N Engl J Med 2005:352(8):777-785.

Mayer SA, Brun NC, Begtrup K, et al. Efficacy and safety of recombinant activated factor VII for acute intracerebral hemorrhage. N Engl J Med 2008 May 15;358(20):2127-2137. *Treatment with rFVIIa within 4 hours of ICH reduced hematoma volume growth but did not improve survival or functional outcome. Also, there were higher rates of arterial thrombotic events in the higher-dose group.*

Morgenstern LB, Frankowski RF, Shedden P, et al. Surgical treatment for intracerebral hemorrhage (STICH): a single-center, randomized clinical trial. Neurology 1998:51(5):1359-1363. *This clinical study has influenced our approach to surgical evacuation of ICH with most neurosurgeons and neurologists considering it as generally showing lack of benefit for hematoma evacuation. However, a subset of patients with superficial ICH and no intraventricular blood emerged as potentially benefiting from surgical evacuation and are currently being randomized to STICH II.*

Skidmore CT, Andrefsky J. Spontaneous intracerebral hemorrhage: epidemiology, pathophysiology, and medical management. Neurosurg Clin North Am 2002;13:281-288.

Woo D, Broderick JP. Spontaneous intracerebral hemorrhage: epidemiology and clinical presentation. Neurosurg Clin North Am 2002;13: 265-279.

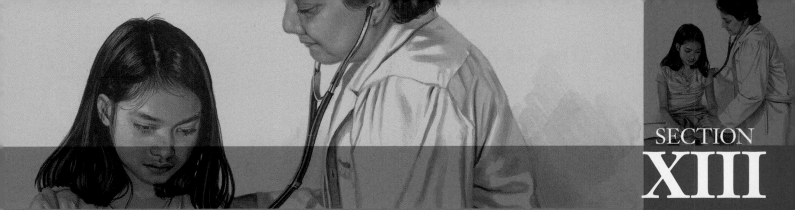

Trauma

Trauma to the Brain

Carlos A. David and Jeffrey E. Arle

59

Traumatic brain injury (TBI), occurring worldwide in relation to various types of civilian and armed forces accidents, is one of the most common mechanisms for serious lifelong morbidity or mortality. Within the United States, one person sustains a head injury every 15 seconds. The societal loss is devastating as the majority of these injuries involve individuals entering adulthood with great promise only to be cut down, often with irretrievable injuries that leave them dependent for their remaining lives. For example, within the United States there are 2 million cases of traumatic head injury annually; 100,000 die within hours, 500,000 require hospital stays, and up to 100,000 have permanent disability. Whether it is a cycling, skiing, or relatively uncommon contact sports injury, or result of an impulsive acceleration while negotiating a challenging roadway to impress peers with one's driving prowess, or on a battlefield such as currently occurs in Iraq or Afghanistan, the consequences are the same: a very promising or accomplished life has lost all its future potential. Various head injury classification systems exist. These include (1) *severity* (mild, moderate, severe), mechanism (closed vs. penetrating), (2) *skull fractures* (depressed vs. nondepressed), (3) presence of *intracranial lesions* (focal vs. diffuse), and (4) *hemorrhages*, that is, extra-axillary epidural or subdural, subarachnoid, or focal parenchymatous lobar, or brainstem Duret hemorrhage.

Clinical Vignette

An otolaryngologist requested an expeditious neurologic evaluation of a very vigorous octogenarian who was so fit that he downhill skied 3 weeks earlier; this patient reported recent-onset sense of "spinning vertigo" and cloudiness of vision, precipitated by sudden standing or neck extension. Additionally, he was experiencing new-onset headaches that were becoming increasingly severe and were awakening him from his sleep. Concomitantly he was having difficulty with mental concentration and hand coordination, as well as a feeling of "weak legs." On further questioning, he recalled that 7 weeks earlier he had slipped on the ice, striking his occiput, while helping to push an auto out of a snow bank.

On examination, he had moderately severe difficulty performing tandem gait (something most healthy 70-year-olds often cannot perform, but this was probably abnormal in this athletic man). The remainder of his neurologic examination was normal. Head computed tomography (CT) demonstrated large biparietal subdural hematomas. Bilateral craniotomies were performed, draining both hematomas. Except for a few focal motor sensory seizures, occurring only in the immediate postoperative period and responding well to phenytoin, his recovery was otherwise excellent.

Comment: This gentleman presented a classic history for subdural hematoma. Initially he had disregarded a

moderately significant closed head injury as there were no immediate sequelae other than for a modest scalp contusion. He was symptom-free for 5 weeks. This patient's initial symptoms were not very impressive because his brain compensated well. Despite a careful neurologic examination, the tandem ataxia was his only neurologic abnormality. This could easily be dismissed as appropriate for age; however, the entire clinical picture was classic for a subdural hematoma until proven otherwise as defined by the CT scans.

GENERAL PRINCIPLES OF HEAD INJURY CARE

The initial management of severe head injuries, as for any serious trauma victim, includes the "ABC" evaluation for *Airway, Breathing, and Circulation* and a careful general and neurologic examination.

- A—airway: Suction to free pharynx from blood and other material; intubate after cervical spine evaluation.
- B—breathing: Evaluate rate, rhythm, and breath sounds; ventilate to raise PaO_2 and reduce $PaCO_2$ (to lower intracranial pressure [ICP]); monitor arterial blood gas levels.
- C—circulatory status: Start intravenous infusion of normal saline solution, followed by blood if indicated; obtain immediate laboratory work and x-rays; administer steroids and phenytoin, plus pressor agent if required (shock rarely due to head injury alone; search for cause).

Concomitantly, the patient's general level of responsiveness must be assessed using the Glasgow Coma Scale (Fig. 59-1). The lowest possible score of 3 means that individuals have no ability to open the eyes, no motor response to verbal command or direct stimuli, and no verbal response to the physician's questions, giving a score of 1 or nil for each of the three components. The highest possible score is 15. Soft tissue injuries are commonly associated with more severe head injuries. A complete examination of the exterior surface of the face and head is vital. Blood loss can be extensive given the location of blood vessels within the dense connective tissue of the scalp, which decreases retraction of cut vessels and promotes bleeding.

SKULL FRACTURES

These can be located in the calvaria (vault) and/or the basal skull. Fractures of the cranial vault carry a 20 times greater incidence of intracranial hematoma in comatose patients and a 400 times greater incidence in conscious patients. Basal skull fractures, often difficult to identify on head CT, can present with pathognomonic signs, including raccoon or Panda bear eyes, battle signs (ecchymosis over the mastoid), and cerebrospinal fluid (CSF) leakage from the nose, throat, or ears (Fig. 59-2).

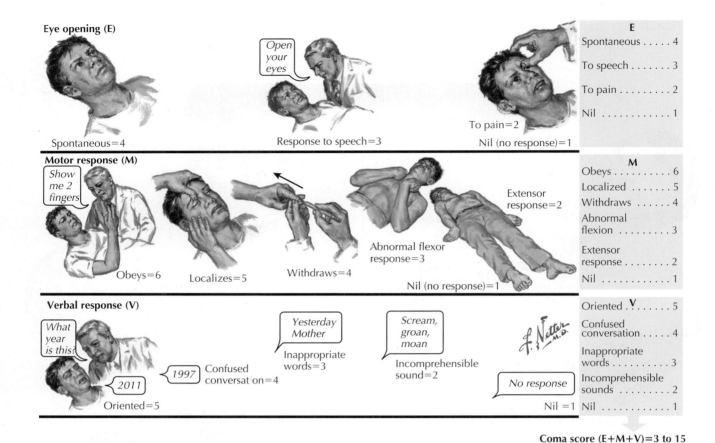

Figure 59-1 Glasgow Coma Scale.

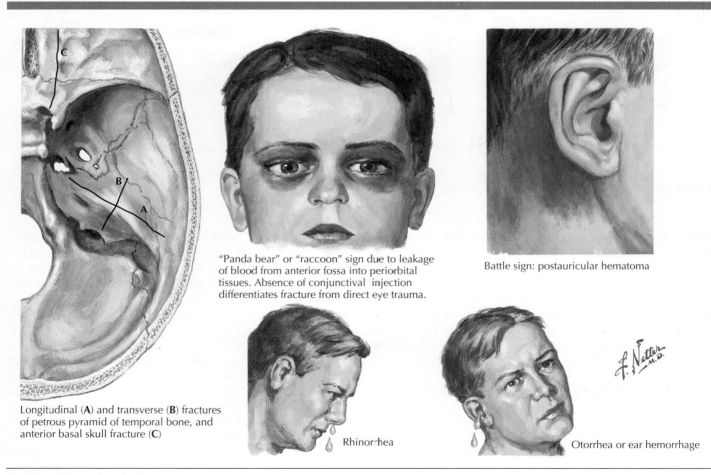

"Panda bear" or "raccoon" sign due to leakage of blood from anterior fossa into periorbital tissues. Absence of conjunctival injection differentiates fracture from direct eye trauma.

Battle sign: postauricular hematoma

Longitudinal (**A**) and transverse (**B**) fractures of petrous pyramid of temporal bone, and anterior basal skull fracture (**C**)

Rhinorrhea

Otorrhea or ear hemorrhage

Figure 59-2 Basilar Skull Fractures.

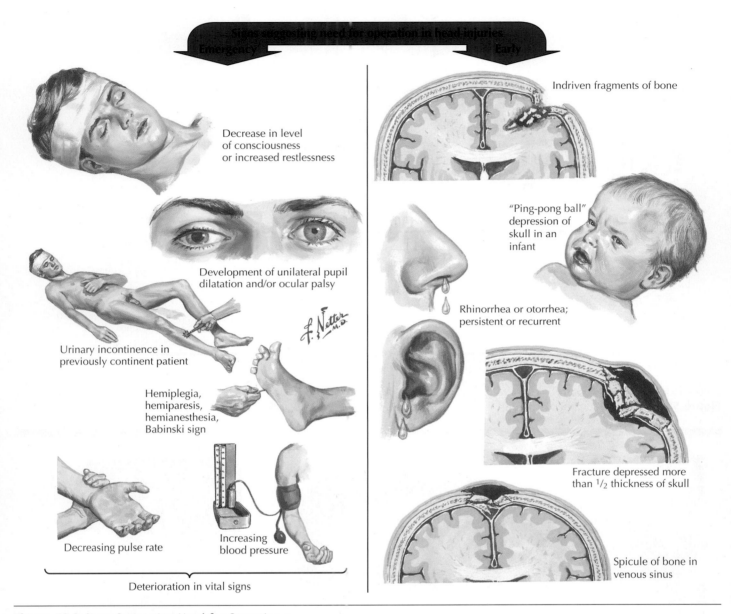

Figure 59-3 Signs Suggesting Need for Operation.

Most leaks resolve spontaneously. Persistent leaks necessitate operative treatment (Fig. 59-3).

Depressed fractures, and those along the temporal bone, are more commonly associated with injury to the brain or blood vessels. A fracture line across the middle meningeal artery may predispose to an epidural hematoma. Open fractures with their communication between the intracranial vault and the external environment are associated with higher risks of spinal fluid leaks and infection (Fig. 59-4).

EXTRA-AXIAL TRAUMATIC BRAIN INJURIES

Traumatic Subarachnoid Hemorrhage

This is the most common sequela of TBI and is typically associated with other types of intracranial lesions. Subarachnoid hemorrhage (SAH) can range from clinically insignificant to fatal.

These SAH blood products can obstruct CSF reabsorption, leading to increased intracranial pressure (ICP) with hydrocephalus. Treatment of SAH often involves placement of ventricular drains and shunting systems for secondary hydrocephalus.

Epidural Hematomas

These represent an acute blood collection contained between the dura and inner table of the skull. These occur in approximately 2% of TBIs (Fig. 59-5). Epidural hematomas (EHs) most commonly develop in the temporal and parietal regions; 90% of EH are associated with a skull fracture. Arterial lacerations, particularly of the middle meningeal artery (Fig. 59-6) or, less commonly, venous injuries, initiate the formation of hematomas. Contiguous lacerations of the dura mater allow this blood into the epidural space.

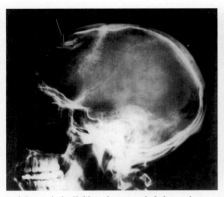

Left lateral skull film showing left frontal depressed skull fracture

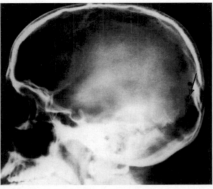

Left lateral skull film revealing occipital depressed skull fracture

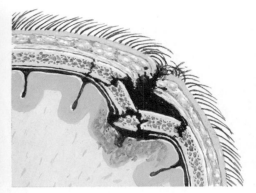

Compound depressed skull fracture. Note hair impacted into wound

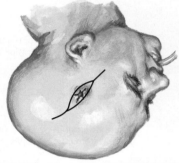

Elliptical incision with extensions to remove devitalized skin and pericranium

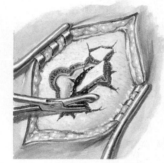

Burr hole placed at margin of fracture to facilitate elevation of depressed bone fragments. Bone edges, dura, and brain then debrided

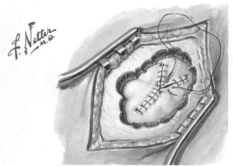

Watertight dural closure. Optionally, bone fragments may be cleaned and wired in place Skin is closed in one layer

Figure 59-4 Compound Depressed Skull Fractures.

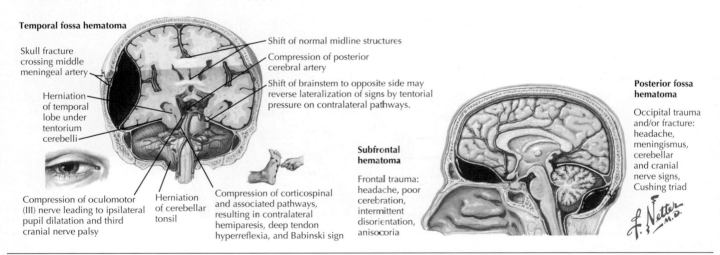

Temporal fossa hematoma

Skull fracture crossing middle meningeal artery

Herniation of temporal lobe under tentorium cerebelli

Compression of oculomotor (III) nerve leading to ipsilateral pupil dilatation and third cranial nerve palsy

Herniation of cerebellar tonsil

Shift of normal midline structures

Compression of posterior cerebral artery

Shift of brainstem to opposite side may reverse lateralization of signs by tentorial pressure on contralateral pathways.

Compression of corticospinal and associated pathways, resulting in contralateral hemiparesis, deep tendon hyperreflexia, and Babinski sign

Subfrontal hematoma

Frontal trauma: headache, poor cerebration, intermittent disorientation, anisocoria

Posterior fossa hematoma

Occipital trauma and/or fracture: headache, meningismus, cerebellar and cranial nerve signs, Cushing triad

Figure 59-5 Epidural Hematoma.

Immediately after the closed head injury, the patient "typically" experiences an initial but relatively brief loss of consciousness secondary to the primary concussive injury. This is then followed by a lucid interval with return of wakefulness. Subsequently, as the torn vessels leak, an epidural hematoma develops and enlarges, leading to a rapid lapse into coma. Sometimes this entire process may transpire from injury, to transient loss of consciousness, and to a brief period of a "paradoxically reassuring alertness," only to have a devastating, often irreversible, coma develop within just 1 hour after the blunt head injury (see Fig. 59-3). However, this classic presentation occurs in less than one third of affected individuals. The actual rate of symptom progression depends on the type of associated brain injuries, their etiology, and the subsequent precise rate of blood accumulation within the epidural space.

Cranial CT imaging usually demonstrates a hyperdense, biconvex collection between the skull and brain (Fig. 59-7). On occasion, the initial CT is normal as the hematoma has yet to

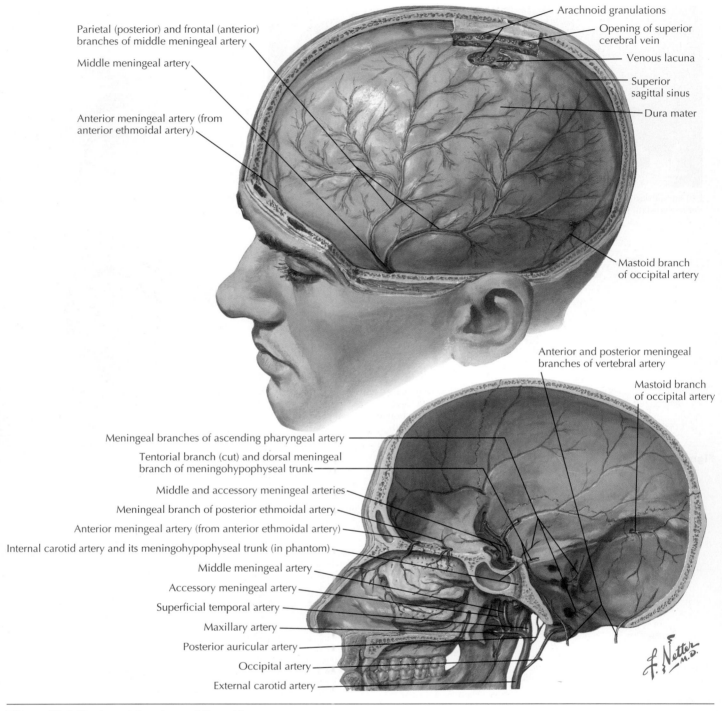

Arachnoid granulations

Opening of superior cerebral vein

Venous lacuna

Superior sagittal sinus

Dura mater

Mastoid branch of occipital artery

Parietal (posterior) and frontal (anterior) branches of middle meningeal artery

Middle meningeal artery

Anterior meningeal artery (from anterior ethmoidal artery)

Anterior and posterior meningeal branches of vertebral artery

Mastoid branch of occipital artery

Meningeal branches of ascending pharyngeal artery

Tentorial branch (cut) and dorsal meningeal branch of meningohypophyseal trunk

Middle and accessory meningeal arteries

Meningeal branch of posterior ethmoidal artery

Anterior meningeal artery (from anterior ethmoidal artery)

Internal carotid artery and its meningohypophyseal trunk (in phantom)

Middle meningeal artery

Accessory meningeal artery

Superficial temporal artery

Maxillary artery

Posterior auricular artery

Occipital artery

External carotid artery

Figure 59-6 Meningeal Arteries and Dura Mater.

develop to a size that is definable. Thus when the patient is "at risk," it is essential to be prepared to repeat the CT scan at the slightest change in clinical status. Once the EH is identified, emergency surgical evacuation is indicated. Any failure to recognize an epidural hematoma has a most significant mortality depending on patient age, time of treatment, hematoma size, and associated injuries.

Acute Subdural Hematoma

These blood collections are located between the brain parenchyma and the dural membranes and are classified by their temporal profile. *Acute subdural hematomas* (SDHs) occur in 15% of TBI patients; these are seven to eight times more common than epidural hematomas. Older individuals are at greater risk because as the brain ages, there is an innate atrophy of the

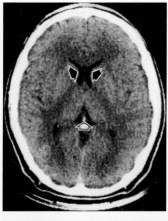

A. Normal brain. CT scan demonstrating normal anatomy at level of frontal horns of lateral ventricles (black arrows). Pineal gland (white arrow) is in normal midline location.

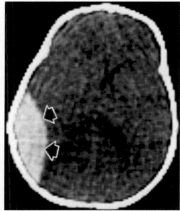

B. Epidural hematoma. CT scan demonstrating hyperdense right parietal epidural hematoma (black arrows), which has assumed classic biconvex lens configuration secondary to adherence of dura to inner table of skull. Other structures are compressed and shifted.

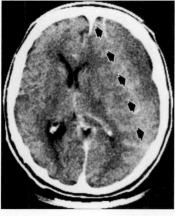

C. Subacute subdural hematoma. CT scan demonstrating large isodense mass over left cerebral convexity. Compressed cerebral cortex (black arrows) shows enhanced density delineating inner border of subacute subdural hematoma. Normal structures are shifted across midline.

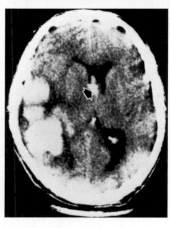

D. Acute intracerebral hematoma. CT scan demonstrating hyperdense mass in right parietotemporal area. Large acute intracerebral hematoma has shifted lateral ventricle toward midline. Blood is visualized within ventricular system (black arrow).

Figure 59-7 CT and Angiogram of ICH.

cerebral cortex. Thus in seniors, as the brain "normally" lessens in volume, an increasing space develops within their subdural compartment. In turn this leads to increased stretch on the bridging veins between the skull and the cerebral surface (Fig. 59-8). When any individual sustains direct head trauma, the brain parenchyma accelerates and decelerates in relation to fixed dural structures. This leads to a tearing of the now anatomically stretched veins that form a "bridge" between the cerebral cortex and the skull. Similarly concomitant injury to cortical arteries can also lead to bleeding into the subdural space (Fig. 59-9).

CLINICAL PRESENTATION AND DIAGNOSIS

The initial severity of the injury determines the patient's clinical presentation; this varies from neurologically intact, to altered mental states, subsequently associated with pupillary inequality and motor weakness, and eventually becoming comatose with signs of decorticate or decerebrate posturing. The lucid interval, a classical finding with epidural hematoma, is also commonly seen with acute SDH. Brain CT is the initial test of choice for detecting SDH and concomitant brain injuries. An acute SDH is recognized by its hyperdense crescent-shaped image between the brain and skull (see Fig. 59-7). Unlike epidural hematomas, SDHs typically cross skull suture lines, and sometimes extend along the falx cerebri. Head CT sometimes underestimates the size of the SDH given the similar imaging density of the nearby bone.

TREATMENT AND PROGNOSIS

If the patient has mental status changes or signs of focal cerebral compromise, beginning treatment of acute SDH as rapidly as possible with medical management for increased ICP and the associated cerebral edema using mannitol is very useful. Surgical intervention with a craniotomy is appropriate for individuals whose SDHs have mass effect, leading to focal neurologic deficits. Once a significant SDH is defined, surgical evacuation of the clot must be expeditiously performed. A burr-hole trephine evacuation is inadequate because the clot is often already more viscous than normal blood. Increased postoperative ICP occurs in almost 50% of SDH patients, and thus the initial medical management must be continued (Fig. 59-10). Residual and recurrent hematomas are also postoperative concerns.

An acute SDH is often associated with a poor outcome. The combination of the hematoma with other injuries, particularly those affecting the brain parenchyma, is associated with a 50% mortality rate. Of those patients who do survive a significant number have permanent mental and physical disabilities. Outcomes are strongly predicted by patient age and initial presentation. Mortalities of 20% are recorded for individuals younger than 40 years, but this number increases to 65% for those older than this. This is a devastating lesion in senior citizens as there is an 88% mortality for octogenarians. The initial consciousness level also provides a prognostic guide. Conscious patients have a mortality rate of less than 10%, whereas unconscious patients have 45–60% mortality.

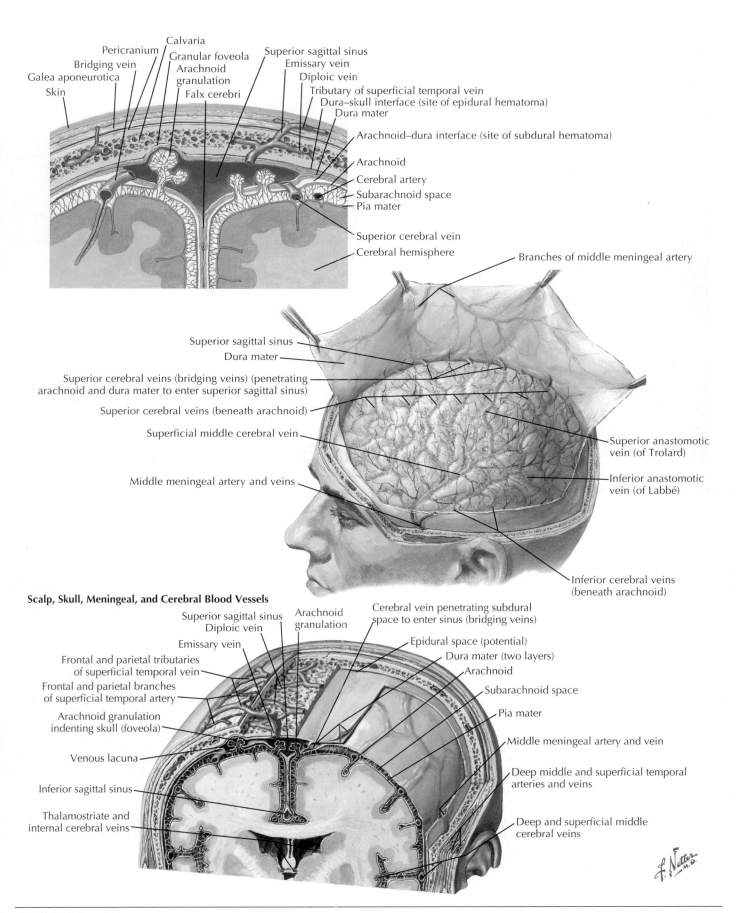

Calvaria
Pericranium
Granular foveola
Bridging vein
Arachnoid granulation
Galea aponeurotica
Falx cerebri
Skin

Superior sagittal sinus
Emissary vein
Diploic vein
Tributary of superficial temporal vein
Dura–skull interface (site of epidural hematoma)
Dura mater

Arachnoid–dura interface (site of subdural hematoma)

Arachnoid
Cerebral artery
Subarachnoid space
Pia mater

Superior cerebral vein
Cerebral hemisphere

Branches of middle meningeal artery

Superior sagittal sinus
Dura mater
Superior cerebral veins (bridging veins) (penetrating arachnoid and dura mater to enter superior sagittal sinus)
Superior cerebral veins (beneath arachnoid)
Superficial middle cerebral vein

Middle meningeal artery and veins

Superior anastomotic vein (of Trolard)
Inferior anastomotic vein (of Labbé)

Inferior cerebral veins (beneath arachnoid)

Scalp, Skull, Meningeal, and Cerebral Blood Vessels

Superior sagittal sinus
Diploic vein
Arachnoid granulation
Cerebral vein penetrating subdural space to enter sinus (bridging veins)
Emissary vein
Epidural space (potential)
Frontal and parietal tributaries of superficial temporal vein
Dura mater (two layers)
Frontal and parietal branches of superficial temporal artery
Arachnoid
Subarachnoid space
Arachnoid granulation indenting skull (foveola)
Pia mater
Venous lacuna
Middle meningeal artery and vein
Inferior sagittal sinus
Deep middle and superficial temporal arteries and veins
Thalamostriate and internal cerebral veins
Deep and superficial middle cerebral veins

Figure 59-8 Superficial Cerebral Veins and Diploic Veins.

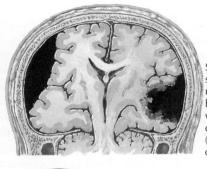

Section showing acute subdural hematoma on right side and subdural hematoma associated with temporal lobe intra-cerebral hematoma ("burst" temporal lobe) on left

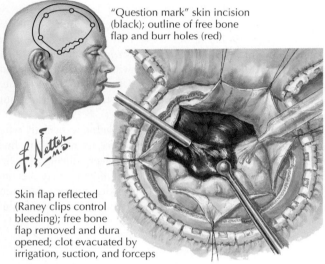

"Question mark" skin incision (black); outline of free bone flap and burr holes (red)

Skin flap reflected (Raney clips control bleeding); free bone flap removed and dura opened; clot evacuated by irrigation, suction, and forceps

Figure 59-9 Acute Subdural Hematoma.

CHRONIC SUBDURAL HEMATOMA

These subdural blood collections commonly appear 2–3 weeks after an often seemingly innocuous injury, as illustrated in the initial vignette. Their incidence is 1–2 per 100,000 persons each year. Most chronic SDH patients are older than 50 years. Chronic alcoholics or patients with coagulopathies, particularly from iatrogenic sources such as anticoagulants, are more prone to bleeding with relatively minor trauma such as striking one's head on the door frame on entering an automobile.

Initially, relatively minor amounts of blood enter the subdural space after trauma or spontaneous hemorrhages. Subsequently, over a few weeks' interval these blood products lead to a membrane formation at both the inner and outer aspects of the hematoma. Eventually, these membranes are prone to low-grade bleeding and thus lead to slow enlargement of the SDH. Concomitantly a higher osmotic pressure develops within the subdural hematoma leading to an osmotic gradient that promotes passage of CSF into the initial SDH and consequently this mass lesion gradually enlarges. The clinical course is variable and not predictable. If the SDH reaches a critical size to compromise brain function, symptoms will develop. In contrast, a number of SDHs will slowly reabsorb without ever becoming symptomatic.

CLINICAL PRESENTATION AND DIAGNOSIS

The presentation may range from subtle focal signs of cerebral compromise as determined by the site of injury such as aphasia, focal weakness or sensory loss, confusion, or seeming early dementia with bifrontal lesions, to those symptoms of the various herniation syndromes. A high clinical suspicion of SDH must always occur especially with the at-risk individual whenever there is remote history of head trauma. CT is the study of choice (see Fig. 59-7). Occasionally, a brain MRI serendipitously leads to a diagnosis of SDH in patients presenting with stroke-like or seizure-type symptoms.

TREATMENT AND PROGNOSIS

Medical management and observation is recommended for individuals with subtle clinical symptoms and signs: discontinuation of anticoagulant medications, close observation in a hospital or by a reliable adult, and serial CT. Surgical therapy is advisable for any chronic SDH that is causing significant mass effect or is associated with significant clinical morbidity. Up to 45% of chronic SDHs reaccumulate. Postsurgical mortality is approximately 10%. Unlike acute SDH, most chronic subdural patients are able to return to their previous levels of functioning although about 10% may develop seizures.

INTRA-AXIAL TRAUMATIC INJURIES

Cerebral Contusions

These are the second most common of the TBI lesions. Usually the frontal and temporal lobes are affected. Basically a contusion is a bruise to the brain tissue per se. These lesions are composed of hemorrhage, infarcted tissue, and necrosis. *Coup* lesions are those found under the sites of direct injury; *contrecoup* lesions are located at sides opposite to impact secondary to brain tissue necrosis and edema sites, where the brain decelerates against the skull (often the frontal and temporal poles). Cortical contusions are most common, but they also will occur within the deep white matter.

Clinical presentation varies widely and is predicated on the location and size of the lesion. Many brain contusions enlarge during the first few days after injury. This can become very significant in patients who sustain high-impact trauma. Surgical intervention is usually not required for intracerebral contusions, especially for small, deep subcortical contusions; these are generally managed medically. However, larger lobar contusions with significant signs of mass effect sometimes require craniotomy and evacuation. Temporal lobe contusions are potentially the most dangerous given their location near the brainstem. Repeat CT scanning is essential to follow these lesions. Mortality rates for cerebral contusions range from 25% to 60%.

Intraparenchymal Hematomas

About a quarter of head injury patients develop intraparenchymal hematomas: these are well demarcated areas of acute hemorrhage. The basic pathophysiology is similar to contusions. Most (90%) occur within the frontal and temporal lobes. Shear injury leads to deep cerebral white matter hematomas. Two thirds of intraparenchymal hematomas are also associated with concomitant subdural or epidural hematomas (see Fig. 59-9). An intraventricular hemorrhage, often complicated by hydrocephalus, may also commonly develop.

Depending on the severity of the injury, almost half of these patients present with a loss of consciousness. Other signs and symptoms relate to the size and location of the hemorrhage.

Medical management is the treatment of choice for deep or small hemorrhages and for unstable patients. Surgical resection is indicated for large superficial lobar hematomas associated with clinical signs of mass effect. Ventricular CSF drains also serve to monitor their ICP. These provide a means to follow neurologically severely compromised patients.

Mortality rates vary from 25% to 75% in patients with an intraparenchymal hemorrhage. The eventual outcome of those who survive depends on their level of consciousness at presentation, size and location of hematoma, and severity of concomitant injuries. Lastly, age is a very important determiner of morbidity. The teenager may eventually have his or her posttraumatic parenchymal hemorrhage reabsorbed without significant residual neuronal damage. In contrast, the senior citizen may already have sustained age-related neuronal compromise and thus have a much diminished prognosis for reasonable return to a productive life.

Diffuse Axonal Shear Injury

The combination of rotational acceleration and deceleration of the brain during traumatic impact results in shearing of both diffuse axonal pathways and small capillaries. High-speed motor vehicle accidents are the most common etiology in the civilian population. Very microscopic, penetrating blood vessels are damaged at multiple levels including the corticomedullary junction, corpus callosum, internal capsule, deep gray matter, and upper brainstem, leading to numerous small hemorrhagic foci. Early on, conventional CT scanning will not demonstrate any abnormality related to this type of lesion. The microhemorrhages may be best seen on gradient echoT2-weighted sequences (Fig. 59-11). Later there may be nonspecific white matter hyperintense lesions with atrophic changes. Shear injury is very commonly associated with other intraaxial and extraaxial traumatic insults, including focal hematomas. Shear injury is a major prognostic contributor to overall head injury morbidity.

Often the initial brain CT is unremarkable, especially when there is no concomitant hematoma, as there are no specific findings associated with shear injury. However, during the first 48–72 hours after the injury, cerebral edema may become obvious. Small areas of punctate contusions can also be found in areas of diffuse axonal injury. The most common MRI finding

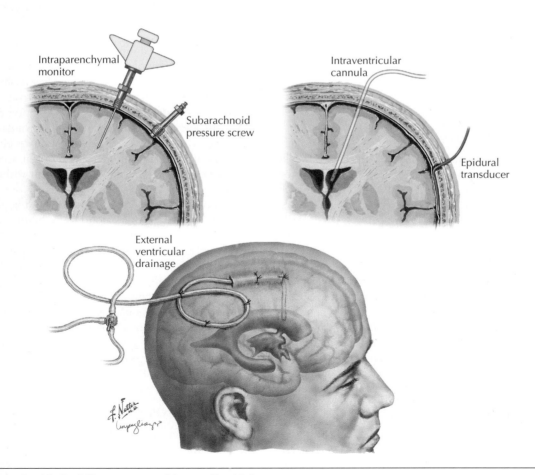

Figure 59-10 Intensive Medical Management of Severe Head Injury.

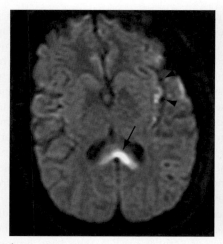
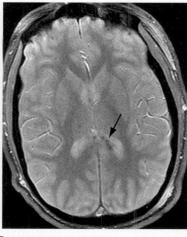
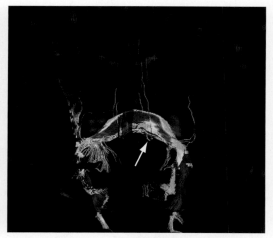

A. Restricted diffusion is quite prominent in left splenium of corpus callosum (arrow) and less so involving left insular white matter (arrowheads).

B. Paramagnetic signal within corpus callosum on gradient echo image confirms associated petechial hemorrhage (arrow).

C. Axial diffusion tensor image shows disruption of fibers (arrow).

Figure 59-11 Shear Injury.

is the presence of multifocal areas of abnormal signal (bright on T2-weighted images) at the white matter in the temporal or parietal corticomedullary junction or in the splenium of the corpus callosum.

Patients with diffuse axonal injury often develop cerebral edema, with resulting increased ICP. Pressure monitors are required in patients whose clinical examination results are not reliable. Intraparenchymal monitors are usually used because the ventricles are often so compressed that ventricular catheter placement is difficult (see Fig. 59-11).

It is this group of patients who may remain comatose for extended periods. This clinical picture is classified as a persistent vegetative state (Chapter 16). This entity carries an extremely poor prognosis (Fig. 59-12).

POSTERIOR FOSSA LESIONS

Cerebellar and posterior fossa traumatic brain lesions account for only 5% of post-TBI sequelae. Epidural hematomas, SDH, and intracerebellar hematomas are the most common traumatic lesions at this level. Because of the limited space within the posterior fossa, strategically placed lesions at this level can rapidly lead to early neurologic decline secondary to both brain-stem compression and acute hydrocephalus. Careful assessment of patients for these injuries is critical, especially in high-risk individuals with basal skull fractures. MRI is the study of choice for detecting posterior fossa damage. Normal bony architecture, as imaged with brain CT, frequently prevents identification of posterior fossa lesions artifacts in patients with TBI. Therefore, evacuation of the hematoma with posterior fossa craniectomy is the primary treatment modality when there is a critical mass lesion (Fig. 59-13). In contrast, a ventricular drain is adequate for intraventricular bleeds.

Condition is called *persistent* when it lasts without change for more than 1 month.

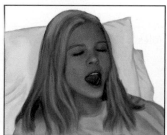
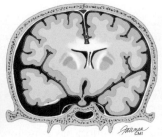

Patients may startle, look about, or yawn, but none of these actions are in conscious response to a specific stimulus.

Subarachnoid hemorrhage

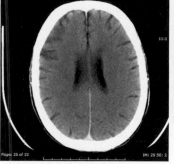
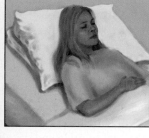

Noncontrast brain CT demonstrating ominous sign of diffuse brain injury and possible prelude to a persistent vegetative state: sulcal effacement (diffuse edema) and subtle disappearance of normal differentiation between gray and white matter.

Figure 59-12 Persistent Vegetative State.

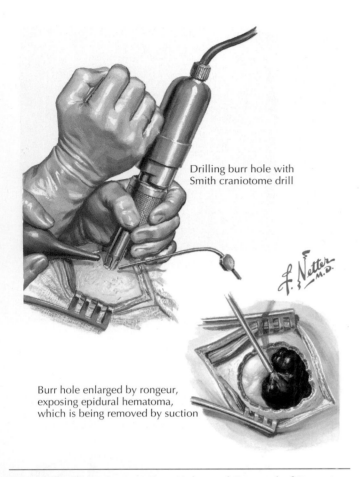

Drilling burr hole with
Smith craniotome drill

Burr hole enlarged by rongeur,
exposing epidural hematoma,
which is being removed by suction

Figure 59-13 Exploratory Burr Holes and Removal of Posterior Fossa Hematoma.

TRAUMATIC BRAIN INJURY IN MILITARY COMBAT SETTINGS

Significant effort has gone into defining appropriate guidelines of care for traumatic brain injury (TBI) since 1990. In 2005, Guidelines for Field Management of Combat-Related Head Trauma was offered by the Brain Trauma Foundation and also provides levels of evidence found in published literature supporting its conclusions. Nearly all of the supporting scientific literature is Class III evidence. Combat brain trauma tends to occur from high-velocity rifle rounds (as opposed to handguns) and penetrating shrapnel and debris, with or without blast injury. Yet, although there are differences in the circumstances and nature of brain traumas that occur within combat, the same general principles for managing both initial and ongoing care for TBI should be adhered to. This includes the maintenance of PO_2 >90 mm Hg and systolic blood pressure >90 mm Hg, the use of mannitol or hypertonic saline if there is evidence of severe neurological dysfunction (Glasgow Coma Scale [GCS] score <8) to help reduce ICP, and the avoidance of hypocapnia (PCO_2 <30–35 mm Hg) in all but the acute setting of impending herniation. Differences between combat and civilian care may include limited ability to obtain an adequate exam or history, delay in transportation of patient, or no access to the patient. Inability to secure an area may require assessment of the casualty while under heavy fire. Chemical or radioactive contamination

may require medical personnel to don protective clothing that can severely limit assessment, and finally the tactical plans may hamper mobilization of appropriate resources. Supply of bandages, fluids, and medications alone for field medics who are under siege for days or even weeks at a time may be extremely difficult. Not all aspects of the care and assessment of neurologic injuries in a combat setting are negative relative to the civilian world. The dedication of medics for saving casualties and "leaving no one behind" is extraordinarily high and is an important foundation to support the confidence of combat soldiers. Soldiers are among the most physiologically robust and compliant of patients, and medics' acts of fearlessness to provide care in the battlefield setting are legendary.

One main difference between the civilian and combat setting is the need for multicasualty triage in the field; this is one of the primary responsibilities of combat medics, who have limited ability, if any, to provide mechanical ventilation or ICP management. Measurement of GCS serves to assess severity of TBI and outcome and may be a useful baseline measure for triage decisions. However, its use is only helpful once casualties reach a military hospital level of assessment. Moreover, reliability of combat medics, and even military physicians, in measuring GCS has been shown to be poor compared to civilian personnel, as Emergency Medical Services/paramedics have more medical training.

Recent experience in Afghanistan and Iraq by U.S. neurosurgeons has led to a more aggressive surgical approach in handling brain trauma: aggressive cranial decompression to help manage brain edema, including bilateral hemicraniectomies to allow the brain to swell without pressure from the fixed cranial volume. This minimizes the need for intensive ICP medical management in these initial combat hospital facilities. If patients survived this acute care, better and longer-term management and ultimately cranioplasty repair could be performed at better-equipped facilities in higher-level settings.

OVERALL TREATMENT PROTOCOLS

TBI is one of the primary medical challenges of the current Iraq and Afghanistan wars. Significant effort has gone into further definition of guidelines for their care. In 2005, Guidelines for Field Management of Combat-Related Head Trauma were published. Nearly all supporting scientific literature is Class III evidence. None is Class I. Combat brain trauma tends to occur from high-velocity rifle rounds (as opposed to handguns) and penetrating shrapnel and debris, with or without blast injury. It is debatable whether civilian outcome studies, where injury etiology is typically different, can be used to draw conclusions for combat-related brain trauma.

However, although there are clearly differences in the setting, circumstances, and nature of the typical combat TBI, it was found that the same general principles for managing both initial and ongoing care are applicable. These include the maintenance of PO_2 >90, systolic blood pressure >90, the use of mannitol or hypertonic saline with evidence of severe neurologic dysfunction (generally GCS score <8) to help reduce ICP, and the avoidance of hypocapnia (PCO_2 <30–35) are vital. Surgery is indicated where there is a focal decompressible lesion in the acute setting of impending herniation.

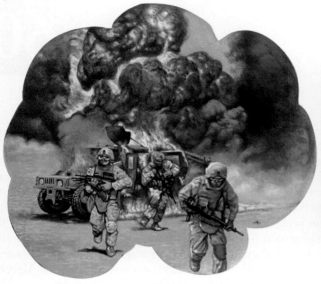

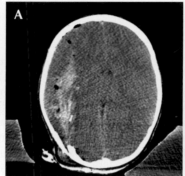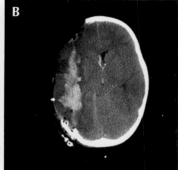

Infant hit by IED (improvised explosive device) with brain injury in the right hemisphere **(A). B** shows the hemicraniectomy performed to mitigate brain injury from swelling

Figure 59-14 Brain Injury in Military Combat.

Recent military experience has led to a more aggressive surgical approach in handling brain trauma. Because two surgeons were often working together in a highly efficient and staffed operating theater environment, in many cases receiving severe head trauma within minutes of the injury, even the soldier with a low GCS score underwent aggressive cranial decompression to help manage brain edema (Fig. 59-14). This minimizes the need for intensive ICP medical management in these initial combat hospital facilities. It will take time and long-term follow-up to eventually evaluate the prognosis for useful brain recovery with such aggressive and bolder therapeutic approaches.

A recent civilian study with TBI demonstrated that decompressive craniectomy is associated with a better-than-expected functional outcome in patients having medically uncontrollable ICP and/or brain herniation. This therapeutic approach was compared with outcomes in other previously reported control cohorts. Thus, there is a very pressing need to standardize treatment of TBI. It is estimated that the *annual fiscal savings* in the United States would include $262 million in medical costs and $3.84 billion in lifetime societal costs. This is absolutely staggering as it puts into perspective what the annual economic loss must be for management of acute traumatic brain injury.

LONG-TERM PROGNOSIS OF TRAUMATIC BRAIN INJURY

Typically it is often difficult to accurately determine a patient's eventual functional outcome despite the physician's desire to answer this very critical issue for the patient's family. Although it is relatively easy to identify individuals at both ends of the trauma severity spectrum, it is more difficult in the gray middle-zone area. Useful factors include injury severity, the initial Glasgow Coma Scale score, response to therapy, global that is shear versus focal injuries, associated injuries, age, medical comorbidities, and the ability to rapidly commence medical and surgical interventions. The final degree of neurologic recovery often stabilizes 6 months to 1 year after TBI.

ADDITIONAL RESOURCES

Aarabi B. Surgical Outcome in 435 Patients who sustained missile head wounds during the Iran-Iraq War. Neurosurgery 1990;27:692-695.

Aarabi B, Taghipour M, Alibaii E, et al. Central Nervous System Infections after Military Missile Head Wounds. Neurosurgery 1998;42:500-509.

Brain Trauma Foundation, American Association of Neurological Surgeons, Joint Section on Neurotrauma and Critical Care.

Chesnut RM. Management of brain and spine injuries. Crit Care Clin 2004;20:25-55.

Fakhry SM, Trask AL, Waller MA, et al. Management of brain-injured patients by an evidence-based medicine protocol improves outcomes and decreases hospital charges. J Trauma 2004;56:492-500.

Faul M, Wald MM, Rutland-Brown W, et al. Using a cost-benefit analysis to estimate outcomes of a clinical treatment guideline: testing the Brain Trauma Foundation guidelines for the treatment of severe traumatic brain injury. J Trauma 2007 Dec;63(6):1271-1278.

Guidelines for Field Management of combat-related head trauma, Brain Trauma Foundation, New York, NY, 2005.

Guidelines for the management of severe traumatic brain injury. Brain Trauma Foundation; American Association of Neurological Surgeons; Congress of Neurological Surgeons. J Neurotrauma 2007;24(Suppl. 1):S1-106. *A detailed overview.*

Personal communication, Brett Schlifka, MD, Maj, USA, 2006.

Riechers GR, Ramage A, Brown W, et al. Physician knowledge of the Glasgow Coma Scale. J Neurotrauma 2005;22(11):1327-1334.

Trauma to the Spine and Spinal Cord

Stephen R. Freidberg and Subu N. Magge

60

Clinical Vignette

On a winter's morning, this vigorous hypertensive, 68-year-old musician, went to pick his newspaper off his icy driveway. He was next found lying on the ground barely able to move any extremity with the exception of some spontaneous, brief dystonic posturing of his right arm. He had no recall of what occurred. Admission to a local hospital led to a diagnosis of a brainstem stroke.

When there was no sign of improvement after 48 hours, his son-in-law, a Lahey colleague, had him transferred to our hospital. Neurologic examination demonstrated an alert, articulate gentleman with absolutely normal brainstem function, full visual fields, and normal optic fundi. He had a severe spastic quadriparesis, and bilateral Babinski signs. There was a dense spinal cord level; he had absolutely no appreciation of touch, temperature, or pin sensation below the C6 dermatomes.

Magnetic resonance imaging (MRI) of the cervical spinal cord demonstrated a large herniated midline disc compressing the spinal cord at the C5–C6. An emergency anterior cervical diskectomy and fusion adequately decompressed the spinal cord. During the subsequent 6 months, he had a slow but marvelous recovery, fully regaining almost all his neurologic function.

Comment:

This patient was most fortunate having a physician in his family who did not accept the initial diagnosis. Senior citizens are very prone to cervical spine fracture dislocation injuries particularly from such simple things as a fall in the home or on the ice as occurred here. Furthermore subsequent history led to yet another diagnosis of a cardiac arrhythmia. In retrospect it was thought that this arrhythmia led to a brief loss of consciousness, precipitating the fall that provoked his catastrophic cervical spine injury. Although acute spinal cord lesions are not often considered in the differential of a "brainstem stroke," the demonstration of the "spinal cord level" at the time of the neurologic examination was the keystone to the diagnosis. This observation differentiated our patient's clinical diagnosis from the initial impression of a brainstem stroke. This patient's eventual excellent recovery was totally dependent on his consulting neurologic physician's most careful clinical evaluation.

Traumatic spinal cord injury (TSCI) secondary to spinal column trauma is one of the most devastating human injuries in terms of morbidity, changes in the normal activities of daily living, and severe economic costs to the patient, family, and society. The recognition of the seriousness of spinal cord injury dates back to antiquity. It was noted in the Edwin Smith Surgical Papyrus dating to the 17th century BC. The recent major interest in stem cell research has brought hope to many TSCI individuals; however, no matter how promising one might think these techniques may prove to be, it is likely that successful clinical application of these technologies are many years removed. These patients and their physicians need to be realistic and take heart in the plethora of current research into rehabilitation problems and the opportunity to adequately confront the long-term medical, social, psychological, urological, and skin issues that they are faced with going forward. Unfortunately, war settings such as have recently occurred in Iraq and Afghanistan always lead to a major influx of TSCI patients.

When one reflects on the greatly shortened life spans that TSCI individuals faced 50 years ago, today's survivors are a marvel to both their own courage as well as many medical advances. In spite of the neurologic injury, most TSCI patients are able to live active, productive lives. The Americans with Disabilities Act of 1990 has removed many physical barriers to wheelchair accessibility and has prevented discrimination in the workplace. To watch the wheelchair paraplegics come to the finish line of the Boston marathon speaks to these triumphs.

Major trauma centers evaluate two to three TSCI individuals out of every 100 patients brought to their emergency departments. The very high mortality (50%) associated with TSCI occurs mainly at the initial accident scene. Most often, these patients are accidentally injured while in an automobile (Fig. 60-1) or on a motorbike, particularly motorcycles. This type of injury also predisposes the patient to multiple-organ damage, for example, brain shear injury and/or intracerebral or subdural/epidural hematoma, cardiac tamponade, or a ruptured aorta, often leading to their very substantial fatality rate. In contrast, nonvehicular spinal cord injuries often occur with falls in (Fig. 60-2) or near the home (Fig. 60-3).

These patients have a 16% mortality rate if they survive to get to the hospital. Young men sustain 85% of TSCI, and thus there is a high correlation with alcohol, motor vehicle accidents, or athletic injuries usually from contact sports or on occasion skiing, diving, or trampolines. In the older population, individuals having significant predisposing cervical spinal spondylosis and/or stenosis are much more likely to develop TSCIs, a central cord injury (Fig. 60-2), from relatively simple falls on stairs or precipitously while navigating icy walkways.

The dollar cost per year is estimated at $4 billion to care for the acute and long-term needs of the patient with TSCI. The costs to the patient and family are incalculable as their problems will last a lifetime. The patient with a spinal cord injury must adjust to limited mobility, psychiatric issues, urological problems, pulmonary difficulty, skin breakdown, sexual dysfunction, and frequently the inability to perform his or her job. The higher within the spinal cord the level of neurologic injury, the more difficult will be the patient's adjustment to the injury. Clearly, TSCI is a condition where the opportunity for

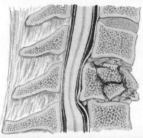
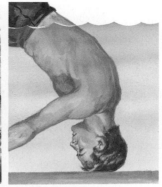

Use of seat belt could have prevented this injury.

Mechanism. Vertical blow on head as in diving or surfing accident, being thrown from car, or football injury

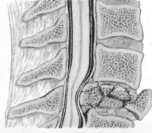

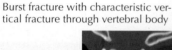
Burst fracture with characteristic vertical fracture through vertebral body

More severe trauma explodes vertebral body. Posteriorly displaced bone fragments frequently produce spinal cord injury.

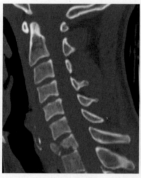
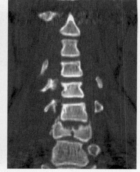
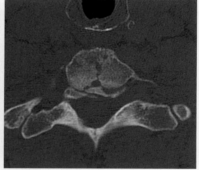

Sagittal CT reconstruction shows compressed comminuted fracture of C7 vertebral body with minimal posterior displacement into the spinal canal.

Coronal CT reconstruction showing disrupted C7 vertebral body.

Axial CT demonstrates comminuted fracture of the vertebral body with sparing of the posterior arch.

Figure 60-1 Cervical Spine Injury: Compression.

prevention far exceeds the potential for treatment. The patient in the opening vignette of this chapter was extremely fortunate and is not an example of the typical course of TSCI. The American Association of Neurological Surgeons sponsors an effective and aggressive program, *Think First*. This program has brought the very meaningful message of prevention to more than 8 million high school and elementary school pupils in almost all of the United States and seven foreign countries.

PATHOPHYSIOLOGY

Different types of trauma can lend themselves to severe spinal cord injury. One of the most well-known, particularly among adolescents, is that related to diving or vehicular trauma leading to compression damage to the spine and concomitantly the spinal cord (see Fig. 60-1). The more senior population is primarily subject to TSCI in relation to seemingly simple falls in

the home (see Fig. 60-2); similarly, alcoholics or abusers of other drugs are also at significantly increased risk of spinal cord trauma (see Fig. 60-3).

In addition to the various types of trauma to the vertebrae per se (Fig. 60-4), there may be gross external cord trauma varying from a simple contusion to a total severing of the proximal from the distal cord, and there is often very significant intramedullary microvascular thrombosis. This is associated with hemorrhage and necrosis secondary to infarction. The hemorrhage is probably venous in origin. Toxic excitatory amines produced by the trauma worsen the secondary injury.

INITIAL MANAGEMENT

Many spinal cord injuries, particularly of vehicular or wartime origin, have a number of other important associated clinical accompaniments equally demanding immediate focus and

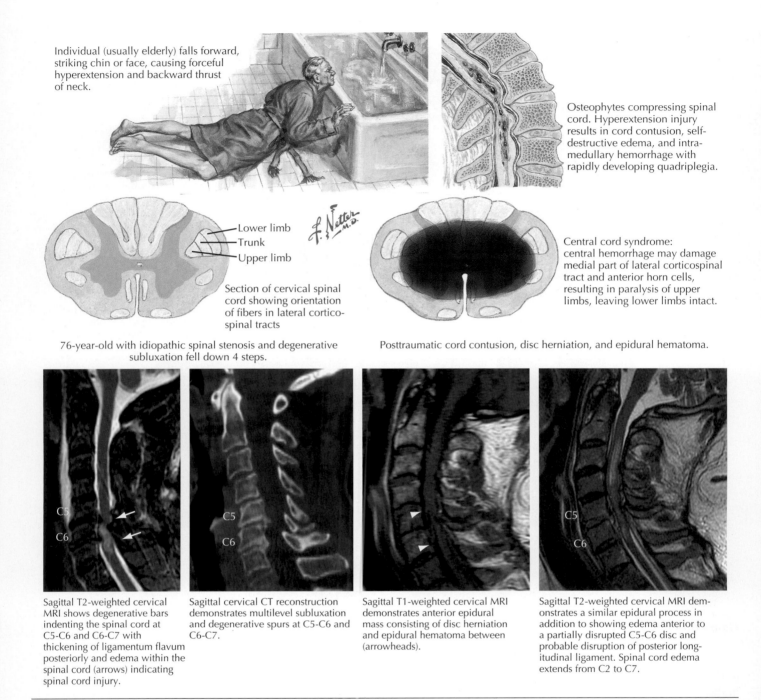

Individual (usually elderly) falls forward, striking chin or face, causing forceful hyperextension and backward thrust of neck.

Osteophytes compressing spinal cord. Hyperextension injury results in cord contusion, self-destructive edema, and intra-medullary hemorrhage with rapidly developing quadriplegia.

Lower limb
Trunk
Upper limb

Section of cervical spinal cord showing orientation of fibers in lateral cortico-spinal tracts

Central cord syndrome: central hemorrhage may damage medial part of lateral corticospinal tract and anterior horn cells, resulting in paralysis of upper limbs, leaving lower limbs intact.

76-year-old with idiopathic spinal stenosis and degenerative subluxation fell down 4 steps.

Posttraumatic cord contusion, disc herniation, and epidural hematoma.

C5
C6

C5
C6

C5
C6

Sagittal T2-weighted cervical MRI shows degenerative bars indenting the spinal cord at C5-C6 and C6-C7 with thickening of ligamentum flavum posteriorly and edema within the spinal cord (arrows) indicating spinal cord injury.

Sagittal cervical CT reconstruction demonstrates multilevel subluxation and degenerative spurs at C5-C6 and C6-C7.

Sagittal T1-weighted cervical MRI demonstrates anterior epidural mass consisting of disc herniation and epidural hematoma between (arrowheads).

Sagittal T2-weighted cervical MRI demonstrates a similar epidural process in addition to showing edema anterior to a partially disrupted C5-C6 disc and probable disruption of posterior long-itudinal ligament. Spinal cord edema extends from C2 to C7.

Figure 60-2 Cervical Spine Injury: Hyperextension.

intervention. Thus, usually it is not possible to focus on the problems of spine and spinal cord trauma per se as isolated clinical phenomena in such settings. Frequently multisystem injuries are concomitantly present, leading to issues such as hypotension, hypoxia, infection, and the need for surgery on other organ systems. Each and every one of these factors complicates the treatment of the spine injury. The ABCs of Advanced Trauma Life Support, that is, *Airway, Breathing, and Circulation*, demand immediate medical attention. Because any degree of hypotension and hypoxia will further the intrinsic spinal cord injury, it is absolutely essential that everything be done to

minimize any subsequent injury to the contused spinal cord secondary to inadequate blood supply and/or oxygen (Fig. 60-5).

DIAGNOSTIC APPROACH

Cervical Spine

Most trauma patients require spinal computed tomographic (CT) examination especially with the alert patient who complains of neck pain, and/or tenderness even when he or she has no obvious neurologic deficits. While the neck is still from the occiput through T1. Whenever this traditional imaging is questionable or just inadequate, thin-cut CT scanning with reconstruction through the questionable areas must be performed. In addition, when caring for any head trauma patient requiring CT, the scanning must always be carried through the cervical spine.

Whenever there is any neurologic injury, an MRI (see Fig. 60-2) is performed before removing the collar or instituting therapy. An MRI will elegantly provide evidence of any spinal cord injury, nerve root pressure, disc herniation, and ligamentous soft tissue injury. A normal examination makes it safe to remove the collar support and allow for early mobilization. This mitigates the possibility of skin breakdown if the patient unnecessarily remains in a hard cervical collar for prolonged periods of time. Formal MRI imaging may not be necessary if the trauma victim is alert, has no neck pain or tenderness, full painless range of motion of the neck, a normal neurologic examination, and no evidence of alcohol or illicit drug use,.

In the circumstance of the neurologically intact patient with definite posttraumatic neck pain, but whose cervical radiographs and/or CT are normal, it is still essential to evaluate for the possibility of a subtle but unstable fracture dislocation with potential for severe cord injury. Here one must obtain dynamic, lateral flexion/extension radiographs or fluoroscopy. These required neck excursions can be performed by the cooperative patient. However, in the setting when the patients are not cooperative or are obtunded, these individuals must be kept in rigid collar until flexion–extension films can be performed passively by a neurosurgeon, orthopaedic spine surgeon, neuroradiologist, or other experienced trauma physician.

Thoracic, Thoracolumbar, and Lumbar Spine

For injuries to the thoracic, thoracolumbar, and lumbar spines, plain radiograph, CT, and MRI scanning are all used. MRI is a mandatory examination whenever there is any question of injury to the spinal cord or disc rupture. Plain bony radiographs may point to and demonstrate any specific vertebral injuries. However, to see the extent of the fracture and/or any spinal canal compromise by bone, CT scanning reconstruction is the study of choice.

TREATMENT

Immediate

Treatment begins at the accident scene. EMT personnel are trained to safely extract injured patients from the accident location. This may include individuals within or those thrown from a motor vehicle, the presence of a football helmet, or an elderly person who has just taken a fall and is found in an awkward position in the bathroom. Immediate spine immobilization is mandatory; the patient is placed on a back board with his or her neck in a collar, taped to the board with the spine stabilized to prevent secondary injury (see Fig. 60-5). This position must be maintained until the entire spine is clinically, and usually radiologically, cleared by appropriate physicians. Because of spinal instability, 4% of patients with TSCI deteriorate after initial

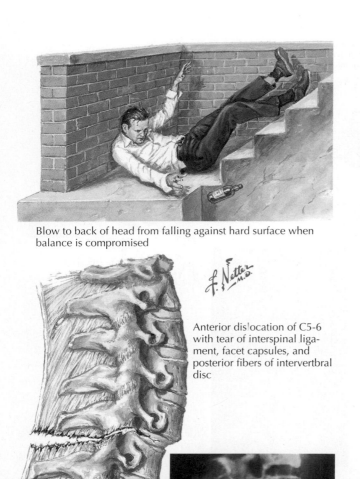

Blow to back of head from falling against hard surface when balance is compromised

Anterior dislocation of C5-6 with tear of interspinal ligament, facet capsules, and posterior fibers of intervertbral disc

X-ray film (lateral view) showing bilateral interfacet dislocation at C5-6 (arrow)

Figure 60-3 Cervical Spine Injury: Hyperextension Flexion-Rotation.

immobilized, if modern CT scanning is available, spinal CT is indicated. This examination is very rapid and is so elegant that it is our procedure of choice (see Fig. 60-1 and 60-2). It is definitely more useful than plain radiographs as it offers the opportunity to provide reconstruction of the CT data in sagittal, coronal, or any angled plane desirable to the physician. The elegance of modern CT scanning far surpasses the utilization of plane spine radiographs performed with portable technique in the emergency department. However, in settings lacking the rapid CT scan capabilities, standard radiographic imaging still provides very important initial screening for fracture dislocations. This three-view cervical spine study must include lateral, anteroposterior, and open-mouth views of the odontoid. It is essential to visualize the entire cervical spine

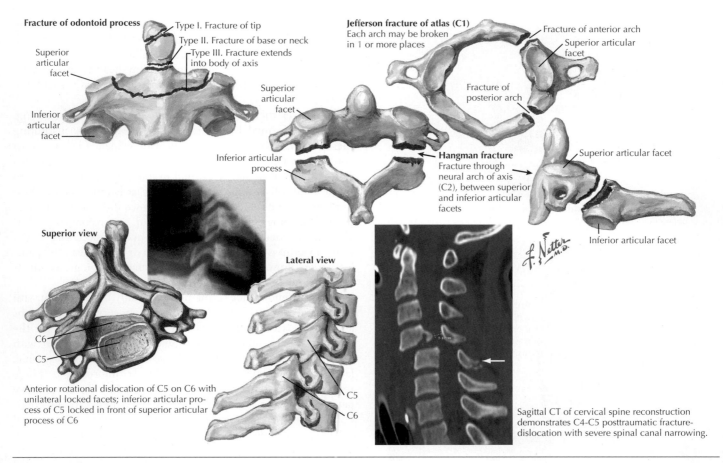

Figure 60-4 Fracture and Dislocation of Cervical Vertebrae.

attempts at treatment. Nonoperative spinal stabilizing techniques include a collar, craniocervical traction, a halo, a rotating frame, or rocking bed (Fig. 60-6).

Corticosteroids

Therapeutic guidelines published in 2002, vis-à-vis immediate medical treatment of spinal cord injury, established a consensus that there is insufficient evidence to support initiating corticosteroid treatment as a standard despite the then traditional and widespread use of this medication. This controverts a 1990 document sponsored by the National Acute Spinal Cord Injury Study. Corticosteroids are sometimes mentioned currently as a TSCI *treatment option* **"that should be undertaken only with the knowledge that the evidence suggesting harmful side effects is more consistent than any suggestion of clinical benefit."** In fact, the Canadian Neurosurgical Society states that steroids are *contraindicated for spinal cord trauma*.

Surgery

When spinal cord neural compression is documented or bony spine misalignment is evident, neurosurgical and/or orthopedic surgery intervention must be immediately considered. The degree of neural compression is assessed by CT and MRI. Significant spinal cord or nerve root compression requires surgical decompression and stabilization. The issue of stability can be difficult to evaluate. There is disagreement among neurosurgeons regarding the timing of surgery. Earlier surgical decompression and stabilization are championed by some when there is a partial lesion, especially with residual autonomic function, as this greatly improves the potential for neurologic improvement.

In contrast, the outlook for improvement with a complete spinal cord lesion is very poor. However, some neurosurgeons feel that early surgery and stabilization, even with complete lesions, allows for early mobilization and rehabilitation, possibly reducing the significant morbidity of prolonged bedrest. Early surgery may also be indicated for facet fractures to improve nerve root function. Other neurosurgeons are more conservative and wait until the patient's neurologic recovery has plateaued before any surgery. It is generally thought that regardless of the timing, surgical decompression and fusion provides better neurologic results than nonoperative treatment even after a long delay. This applies to both spinal cord and/or nerve root injury.

Controversy continues to exist as to whether early surgery with complete cord injury improves neurologic function compared to late surgery. In summary, the goals of surgery are twofold: to decompress the neural elements and to stabilize the spine. This allows the best chance for early mobilization. There are also specific evaluation and therapeutic approaches necessary depending on the anatomical site of injury.

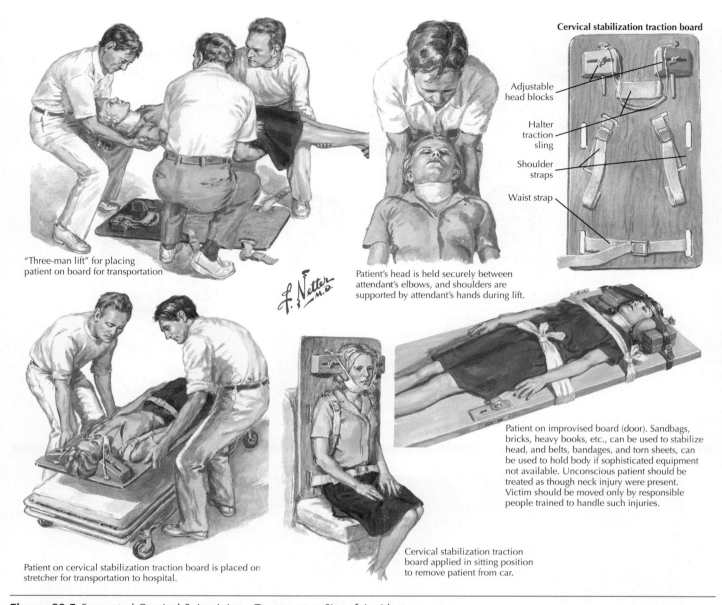

"Three-man lift" for placing
patient on board for transportation

Patient's head is held securely between
attendant's elbows, and shoulders are
supported by attendant's hands during lift.

Cervical stabilization traction board

Adjustable
head blocks

Halter
traction
sling

Shoulder
straps

Waist strap

Patient on improvised board (door). Sandbags,
bricks, heavy books, etc., can be used to stabilize
head, and belts, bandages, and torn sheets, can
be used to hold body if sophisticated equipment
not available. Unconscious patient should be
treated as though neck injury were present.
Victim should be moved only by responsible
people trained to handle such injuries.

Patient on cervical stabilization traction board is placed on
stretcher for transportation to hospital.

Cervical stabilization traction
board applied in sitting position
to remove patient from car.

Figure 60-5 Suspected Cervical Spine Injury: Treatment at Site of Accident.

ATLANTO-AXIAL (C1–2)

In the cervical spine, open-mouth odontoid films are used to demonstrate the relationship of the lateral masses of C1 with the articular pillars of C2. The "rule of Spence" states that if the sum of the overhang of both C1 lateral masses on C2 is greater than 7 mm, then the transverse ligament is likely disrupted, resulting in C1–2 instability. Treatment typically involves halo vest immobilization or occipitocervical fusion (see Fig. 60-4).

Dens fractures are subclassified (see Fig. 60-4). Type 1 fractures occur through the tip of the dens above the transverse ligament. They are quite rare and may be associated with atlantoaxial instability, necessitating arthrodesis. Type 2 fractures, the most common, occur through the base of the dens and are usually unstable (Figs. 60-4 and 60-6).

There is considerable controversy regarding treatment. The primary indications for surgery include a displacement of the dens greater than 6 mm, instability in a halo, and painful

non-union. Otherwise, this treatment consists of immobilization in a halo or hard cervical collar. Type 3 fractures occur through the body of C2 and are usually stable, healing with immobilization in a hard collar or halo vest (see Fig. 60-6).

Traumatic spondylolisthesis of the axis caused by bilateral fractures of the C2 pars interarticularis is known as "hangman's fracture." Judicial hangings (executions) caused injury by hyperextension and distraction (Fig. 60-8). Today these injuries are caused by hyperextension and axial loading.

Type 1 hangman's fractures have minimal angulation and less than 3-mm subluxation. These are considered stable. Treatment involves fracture reduction and stabilization in a hard collar or halo. *Type 2 hangman's fractures* have 4 mm or more subluxation. These are usually unstable and require reduction and stabilization in halo. *Type 3 hangman's fractures* involve marked disruption of C2–3 posterior elements and wide subluxation. These injuries are often fatal. They require open reduction and

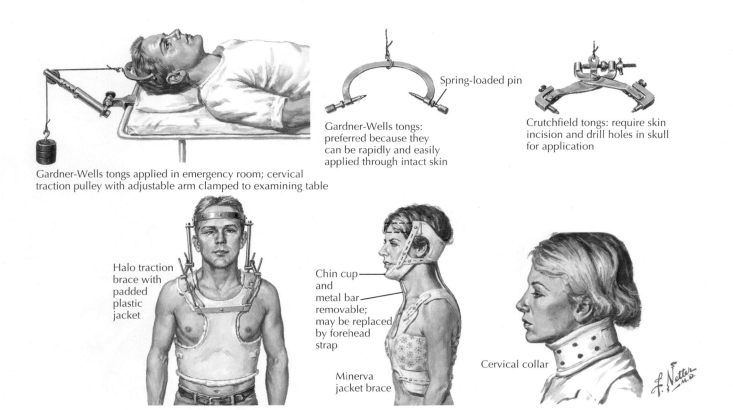

Figure 60-6 Cervical Spine Injury: Traction and Bracing.

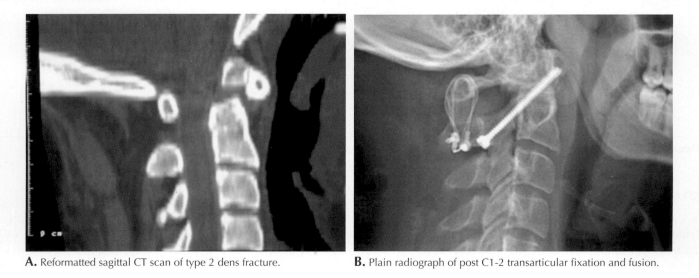

A. Reformatted sagittal CT scan of type 2 dens fracture.   **B.** Plain radiograph of post C1-2 transarticular fixation and fusion.

Figure 60-7 Dens Fracture of Cervical Spine.

stabilization via C2–3 anterior discectomy and fusion or posterior C1–3 fusion.

SUBAXIAL CERVICAL SPINE

Subluxation is defined by neutral spinal radiographs demonstrating instability with greater than 3.5 mm or angulation greater than 11 degrees. Injuries resulting in stable fractures usually heal well with immobilization in hard collar or halo.

Grossly unstable injuries require surgical stabilization (see Fig. 60-8, Fig. 60-9).

THORACOLUMBAR SPINE

Approximately 64% of spine fractures occur at the thoracolumbar junction (Fig. 60-10). These can be successfully repaired; however, the degree of initial, spinal cord or cauda equina injury usually determines the long-term prognosis.

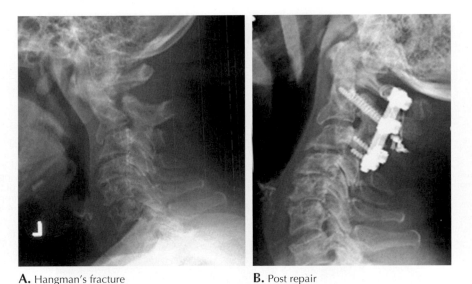

A. Hangman's fracture

B. Post repair

Figure 60-8 Plain Radiograph of Hangman's Fracture: Cervical Spine.

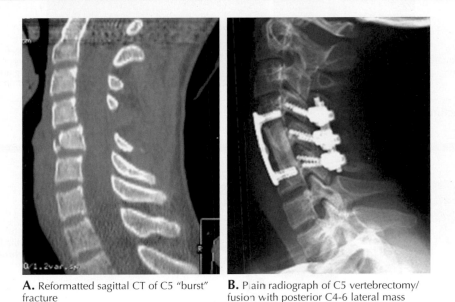

A. Reformatted sagittal CT of C5 "burst" fracture

B. Plain radiograph of C5 vertebrectomy/ fusion with posterior C4-6 lateral mass fixation/fusion

Figure 60-9 Non-Axial Burst Fracture: Cervical Spine.

PROGNOSIS

Spinal cord injury remains an absolutely devastating life-altering injury. When there is complete loss of neurologic function, clinical improvements allowing return to some activities of daily living are totally dependent on the availability of superior physiatric rehabilitation medical principles rather than anatomic spinal cord regeneration. Obviously whenever there is a complete spinal cord transection, there is no possibility for any specific return of clinical neurologic function. However, the presence of a partial lesion, with even residual autonomic function, provides some potential for a degree of certain neurologic functions.

Early patient mobilization is mandatory; it is a primary treatment goal. Deconditioning and morbidity are associated with any significant bedrest. This also makes the patient more susceptible to major complications, particularly deep venous thrombosis (DVT) and/or phlebitis, pneumonia, and skin breakdown. Interestingly the incidence of DVT appears to be relatively low (2–3%) and not influenced by use of heparin.

Fortunately, patients with TSCI now have many entrees back into a normal life. Many hold full-time jobs, including being teachers, physicians, or attorneys (Fig. 60-11). They can marry and have children as better understanding of sexual function in the spinal injury patient has led to excellent counseling and means to perform adequately in this setting. Lastly many athletic endeavors are now available as best exemplified by the many wheelchair participants in the marathon (see Fig. 60-11).

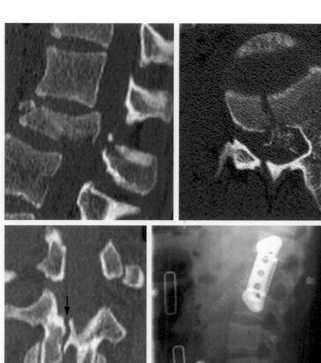

A. Midsagittal CT reconstruction showing markedly compressed and disrupted L1.

B. Axial CT demonstrates fracture in vertebral body, retropulsed fragment occupying the anterior aspect of the spinal canal, and disruption of the posterior arch.

C. Coronal CT reconstruction demonstrates fracture in posterior arch (arrow).

D. Reformatted sagittal CT scan of vertebrectomy and fusion using anterior titanium mesh cage and anterior plate.

Figure 60-10 Burst Fracture: Lumbar Spine.

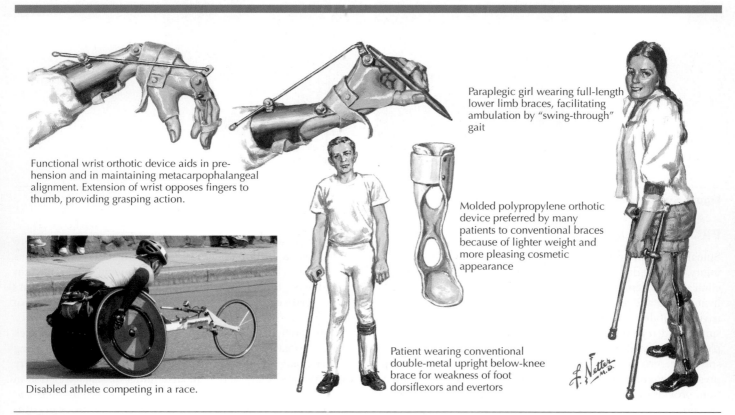

Functional wrist orthotic device aids in prehension and in maintaining metacarpophalangeal alignment. Extension of wrist opposes fingers to thumb, providing grasping action.

Paraplegic girl wearing full-length lower limb braces, facilitating ambulation by "swing-through" gait

Molded polypropylene orthotic device preferred by many patients to conventional braces because of lighter weight and more pleasing cosmetic appearance

Disabled athlete competing in a race.

Patient wearing conventional double-metal upright below-knee brace for weakness of foot dorsiflexors and evertors

Figure 60-11 Cervical Spine Injury: Rehabilitation of Patient.

ADDITIONAL RESOURCES

Agarwal NK, Mathur N. Deep vein thrombosis in acute spinal cord injury. Spinal Cord 2009;47:769-772.

Eyster EF, Watts C. An Update of the National Head and Spinal Cord Injury Prevention Program of the American Association of Neurological Surgeons and the Congress of Neurological Surgeons. Clinical Neurosurgery 1992;38:252-260.

Groopman J. The Reeve Effect. The New Yorker Nov 10, 2003;82-93.

Hadley MN, Argires PJ. The acute/emergent management of vertebral column fracture-dislocation injuries. Neurosurgical Emergencies, Volume II, American Association of Neurological Surgeons 1994;Chapt 15:249-262.

Hugenholtz H. Methylprednisolone for acute spinal cord injury: not a standard of care. Canadian Medical Association journal 2003;168:1145.

Hurlbert RJ. Methylprednisolone for acute spinal cord injury: an inappropriate standard of Care. J Neurosurgery 2000;93(Suppl. 1):1-7.

Kim SU, de Vellis J. Stem cell-based cell therapy in neurological diseases: A review. J Neurosci Res 2009;87:2183-2200.

Lo B, Parham L. Ethical issues in stem cell research. Endocr Rev 2009;30:204-213.

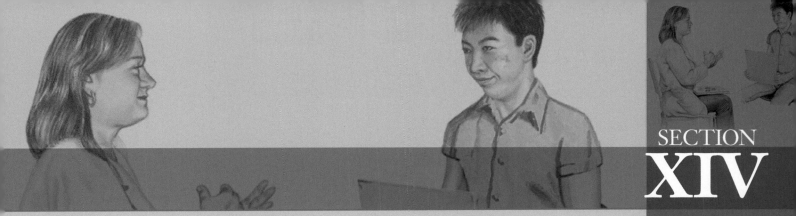

Radiculopathies and Plexopathies

Cervical Radiculopathy

Stephen R. Freidberg and Subu N. Magge

61

Clinical Vignette

A 42-year-old woman presented with a 2-week history of increasingly severe neck pain with radiation to the back of her right upper arm. In retrospect, she had developed very acute right medial scapula pain 4 weeks earlier after carrying a heavy briefcase to a meeting; this discomfort improved within 10 days. However, she then developed the cervical and right arm discomfort; this was associated with numbness and tingling in her second and third fingers. She was an active tennis player and tried to play despite her discomfort but noted difficulty serving as she could not fully extend her arm. Her family physician initially treated her for "bursitis" and suggested she might also have an emerging carpal tunnel syndrome because of the hand paresthesiae. However, when the pain suddenly worsened she consulted a neurologist. The neurologist elicited a 2-year history of similar but milder intermittent pain and numbness, especially after driving long distances. Neurologic examination demonstrated modest right triceps weakness with an absent right triceps muscle stretch reflex. A trial of physical therapy was ineffective, and her symptoms significantly worsened after an afternoon of raking leaves. Further neurologic evaluation demonstrated more severe triceps weakness. A magnetic resonance imaging (MRI) of the cervical spine demonstrated a herniated disc at C6–7. A neurosurgeon performed a posterior laminoforaminotomy and microdiscectomy. This provided immediate relief of her radicular pain. Her triceps strength improved to normal in the ensuing 3 months.

This vignette illustrates the classic history of a C7 nerve root irritation. More than 80% of these radiculopathies resolve spontaneously with conservative therapy. However, on occasion the patient experiences increasingly severe pain and progressive weakness. Unresolved pain and significant weakness are the two primary indications for cervical spine surgery.

Cervical radiculopathy, due to compression of a cervical nerve root, is a common clinical problem. It affects most adult age groups and is uncommon in adolescents and children. The symptoms may be relatively minor and chronic, or acute pain, which may be associated with weakness and sensory disturbance. Although on most occasions the cervical root symptoms have a spontaneous onset, not infrequently, the symptoms begin with a specific precipitating incident, such as trauma.

CLINICAL PRESENTATION

The clinical presentations of cervical radiculopathy depend on the specific root involved. It is unusual to have multiple nerve roots compressed at one time. The usual symptoms are pain, motor weakness, and sensory disturbance. Neck and/or medial scapular pain commonly occur with cervical root compression; shoulder or arm pains are often present. Typical clinical findings include both arm weakness and sensory disturbance appropriate to the affected nerve root (Fig. 61-1). Neck movement often exacerbates the radicular pain and may result in an electric shock–like sensation (Fig. 61-2). Very rarely, pressure on the spinal cord as well as the nerve root may result in concomitant evidence of myelopathy. In any patient with cervical radiculopathy, clinical examination requires careful evaluation for evidence of a myelopathy by making certain the neurologic examination does not demonstrate a spastic gait with enhanced muscle stretch reflexes, a Babinski sign, and evidence of a spinal cord sensory level.

Of the various cervical radiculopathies, C7 nerve root is the most commonly affected. It exits the spinal canal between C6 and C7. Typically, compression leads to pain in the posterior arm. Unlike C5 and C6 lesions, C7 has little functional overlap with other roots. C7 innervates the triceps muscle, which extends the elbow (see Fig. 61-2). Unless patients perform activities that demand extension of the elbow, such as hammering for a carpenter, serving in tennis, rowing, or performing pushups, many individuals with a C7 radiculopathy are unaware of significant triceps weakness. In order to best ascertain the presence of triceps weakness, the examiner must ask the patient to flex the arm at the elbow to 90 degrees and then have the patient try to extend against resistance. In contrast, if one first asks the patient to extend his arm fully, relatively subtle degrees of weakness will be missed. In repose, gravity extends the elbow in most cases. Sensory loss in C7 radiculopathy usually extends to the index and middle fingers (Table 61-1).

The C6 nerve root exits the spine between C5 and C6 vertebrae. Compression here leads to pain in the medial scapula and into the arm frequently to the lateral side of the forearm, as well as the hand and into the thumb. Motor loss overlaps with C5 root and there is weakness in the proximal arm muscles, particularly the biceps, with difficulty flexing the arm and abducting the arm at the shoulder. Sensory changes affect the thumb and index finger.

C8 is the lowest of the cervical roots, exiting the spinal column between the C7 and T1 vertebrae. When this nerve root is compressed, the pain radiates from the neck into the medial forearm and into the medial hand. If there is significant C8 compromise, patients develop weakness of their intrinsic hand muscle function. They also often complain of numbness and demonstrate sensory change in the medial hand as well as the fourth and fifth digits.

C5 is the least frequent level for radiculopathy. The C5 nerve root exits the spine between the C4 and C5 vertebral bodies. Compression of the C5 root produces pain within the medial scapula and into the upper arm; the pain rarely radiates below the elbow. There may be weakness of the deltoid resulting in difficulty carrying out tasks with the arm elevated (see Fig.

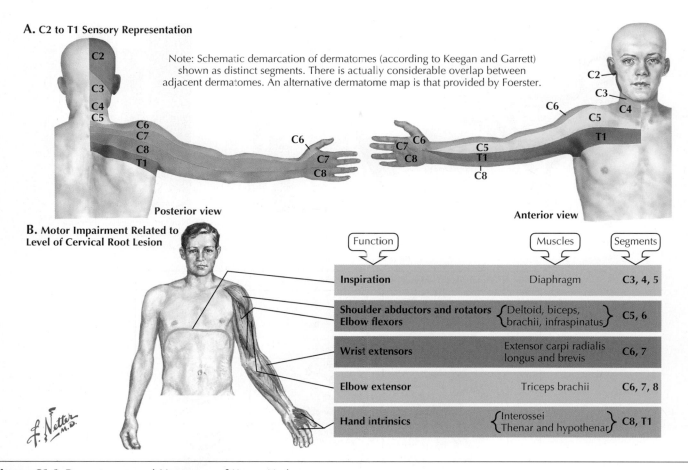

A. C2 to T1 Sensory Representation

C2
C3
C4
C5
C6
C7
C8
T1

Note: Schematic demarcation of dermatomes (according to Keegan and Garrett) shown as distinct segments. There is actually considerable overlap between adjacent dermatomes. An alternative dermatome map is that provided by Foerster.

C6
C7
C8

Posterior view

C2
C3
C4
C5
C6
T1
C5
T1
C8

C6
C7
C8

Anterior view

B. Motor Impairment Related to Level of Cervical Root Lesion

Function	Muscles	Segments
Inspiration	Diaphragm	C3, 4, 5
Shoulder abductors and rotators / Elbow flexors	Deltoid, biceps, brachii, infraspinatus	C5, 6
Wrist extensors	Extensor carpi radialis longus and brevis	C6, 7
Elbow extensor	Triceps brachii	C6, 7, 8
Hand intrinsics	Interossei / Thenar and hypothenar	C8, T1

Figure 61-1 Dermatomes and Myotomes of Upper Limb.

61-2). Sensory loss will be over the shoulder and upper arm and is often minimal (see Table 61-1).

When evaluating a patient with a suspected radiculopathy, it is important to define the temporal profile as well as the degree of progression of the symptoms. Has there been slow progression or rapid worsening? Has there been a plateau or improvement in the condition? How long have the symptoms persisted? The severity and quality of the pain and its provocative factors provide other useful information. In particular, does the arm pain worsen with movement of the neck? Is the pain of an electric quality? It is important to palpate the axilla or supraclavicular fossa, as a mass there could suggest the presence of an extraspinal tumor (Fig. 61-3) or a tumor of the brachial plexus (Fig. 61-4).

DIFFERENTIAL DIAGNOSIS

A modest number of pathologic conditions affect the cervical spine and require consideration in the evaluation of the individual with neck pain associated with limb muscle weakness and sensory loss. Radiculopathy secondary to ruptured cervical disc is the most common cause (Fig. 61-5). Degenerative encroachment of the neural foramen from cervical spondylitic disease is another common cause. Primary or secondary neoplastic tumors of the cervical spine or vertebral infection can mimic disc

herniation. Metastatic extradural tumor is the most common neoplasm within the cervical spine; the common sites of origin are breast, lung, prostate, and myeloma. The intradural extramedullary tumors, that is, schwannoma and meningioma, are also considerations. In contrast, intramedullary lesions, including a tumor or syrinx, usually present with symptoms of myelopathy. Spinal infection, especially epidural abscess, has increased in frequency; this may be due to sepsis associated with infection in the skin, wounds, urinary tract, and dental manipulation; there is a higher incidence in drug abusers and immune-suppressed patients. Patients with spinal infection usually have a great deal of spine and root pain and may have significant myelopathy. The presence of myelopathic signs, in this clinical setting, demands urgent surgical decompression. Furthermore, these patients frequently have significant spinal instability, which must be a consideration when planning surgery.

On occasion, a lesion in the brachial plexus may be confused with a cervical radiculopathy. Neoplasms, either cancers or lymphoma invading the medial brachial plexus, may mimic a C8 radiculopathy; this also occurs with occult superior sulcus apical lung tumors (Pancoast syndrome). Schwannomas are the most common primary nerve tumors arising from the brachial plexus. Brachial plexitis (Parsonage–Turner syndrome) may mimic a C5 radiculopathy. Other diagnostic considerations include ulnar neuropathy and the rare neurogenic thoracic outlet syndrome.

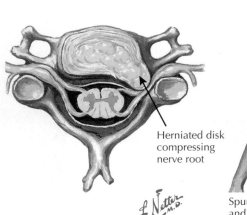
Herniated disk compressing nerve root

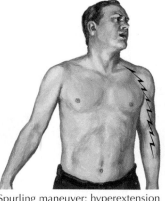
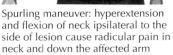
Spurling maneuver: hyperextension and flexion of neck ipsilateral to the side of lesion cause radicular pain in neck and down the affected arm

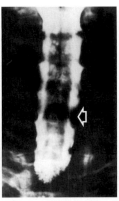
Myelogram (AP view) showing prominent extradural defect (*open arrow*) at C6-7

Level	Motor signs (weakness)	Reflex signs	Sensory loss
C5	Deltoid	0	
C6	Biceps brachii	Biceps brachii — Weak or absent reflex	
C7	Triceps brachii	Triceps brachii — Weak or absent reflex	
C8	Interossei	0	

Figure 61-2 Cervical Disc Herniation: Clinical Manifestations.

Table 61-1 Cervical Nerve Roots and Primary Clinical Findings

Root	Motor Weakness	Sensory Loss	Reflex Loss
C5	Deltoid	Around shoulder	None
C6	Biceps	Thumb and index finger	Biceps and brachioradialis
C7	Triceps	Index and middle finger	Triceps
C8	Intrinsic muscles of hand	Fourth and fifth fingers	None

DIAGNOSTIC APPROACH

Approximately 80% of patients with cervical radiculopathy improve spontaneously, and therefore imaging is often unnecessary. MR imaging studies of the spine are important in patients with unusual presentations or those who do not improve. To ensure there is no mismatch between symptoms and imaging findings, evaluate the studies carefully. It is not uncommon for asymptomatic patients to have significant abnormalities on imaging that are of no consequence. The clinical findings must correlate with imaging abnormalities in order to consider surgical treatment.

It is common practice to omit standard cervical radiographs but these may have some clinical value. Such images provide excellent visualization of the degree of spondylosis and disc degeneration and are of great importance to detect the presence of kyphosis. Flexion and extension lateral views of the spine are important in defining the presence of abnormal movement between the vertebrae.

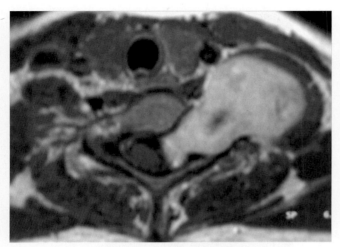

Axial T1-weighted post-gadolinium MR image demonstrating a dumbbell-shaped tumor, a schwannoma, exiting the spine through the left enlarged C6-7 foramen. This mass was palpable in the supraclavicular fossa.

Figure 61-3 Extraspinal Tumor.

MRI is the imaging modality of choice for evaluating the spine and spinal cord. Occasionally open MRI or CT myelography are good options for claustrophobic patients. Imaging studies will demonstrate the nerve root compression caused by disc herniation or spondylosis. A bright signal in the spinal cord on the T2-weighted image is indicative of an injury to the cord (Fig. 61-6). Additionally, it is possible to visualize tumors within the vertebrae or epidural space. Intradural tumors have a well-defined relationship to both the nerve root and spinal cord; MRI clearly demonstrates these lesions. Extramedullary tumors usually readily enhance with gadolinium; in contrast, intramedullary tumors are often difficult to differentiate from intrinsic spinal cord demyelinating lesions such as multiple sclerosis.

Spinal computed tomography (CT) has limited value when used as a stand-alone diagnostic modality. However, CT used in conjunction with myelography is particularly useful in patients unable to have an MRI (e.g., because of cardiac pacemakers). Standard myelography followed by postmyelogram CT will show nonfilling of nerve root sleeves or direct compression of the nerve roots (see Fig. 61-2). It may also demonstrate pressure on the spinal cord (extramedullary lesions) as well as pathology within the cord (intramedullary lesions). CT is particularly effective for demonstration of ossification of the posterior longitudinal ligament (OPLL). Additionally reconstructed spinal CT is an excellent study when attempting to understand complex spinal deformities. We recommend electrodiagnostic studies if there is conflict between the clinical story and imaging findings or if a diagnosis other than radiculopathy is suspected, for example, brachial plexopathy.

TREATMENT AND PROGNOSIS

The choice of therapy for a cervical radiculopathy depends on the clinical presentation of the patient. Because most individuals improve spontaneously, early imaging and active treatment are rarely necessary unless there is significant weakness or signs of a concomitant myelopathy. Approximately 80% of patients with

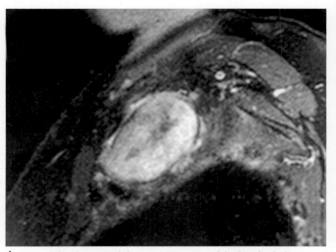

A. T1-weighted post-gadolinium MR image of the brachial plexus demonstrating a large enhancing mass.

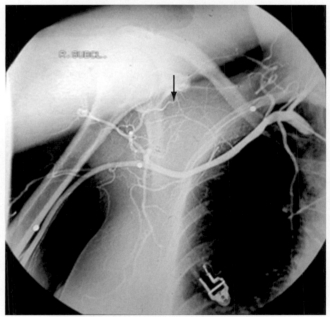

B. Angiogram demonstrating downward displacement of the subclavian artery.

Figure 61-4 Desmoid Tumor.

cervical radiculopathy secondary to either disc herniation or foraminal narrowing will improve spontaneously within 3 months. Heavy activity is restricted in individuals with acute nerve root compression. This particularly applies to activity that exerts tension on the cervical nerve roots leading to protective muscle spasm, with consequent worsening of the pain. Examples include carrying a heavy briefcase, heavy lifting, or making a bed, etc. These patients are reexamined within few weeks. Occasionally, muscle relaxants, simple analgesics, or anti-inflammatory agents are helpful adjuncts. Narcotics are used for severe pain, usually only for a limited period. Usually these modalities are successful. The good results of these conservative treatments and similarly of treatments such as traction, acupuncture, chiropractic manipulation and massage, probably owe their therapeutic success to the natural history of the condition.

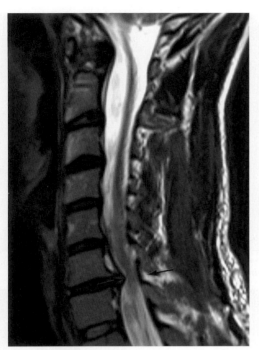

A. Far right lateral sagittal T2-weighted MR image demonstrates large disc herniation at C6-C7 (arrows).

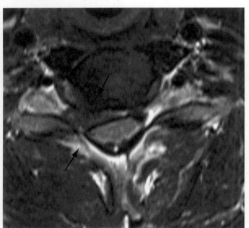

B. Axial T2-weighted MR image at C6-C7 shows the disc herniation extending from the left side across into the right lateral recess with slight deformity of the anterior aspect of the cervical spinal cord (arrows).

Figure 61-5 Large Right Lateral C6-C7 Disc Herniation.

For those patients with unremitting severe pain, or with significant neurologic deficit, or with evidence of myelopathy MRI is mandatory. If there is evidence of cervical disc herniation and the finding is appropriate to the clinical examination, surgery is an option.

Spine surgeons differ on the best surgical means to repair a ruptured lateral cervical disc, either an anterior or posterior approach. One approach involves anterior neck dissection, complete removal of the disc, and reconstruction commonly with spinal fusion. For a lateral disc herniation, a posterior medial

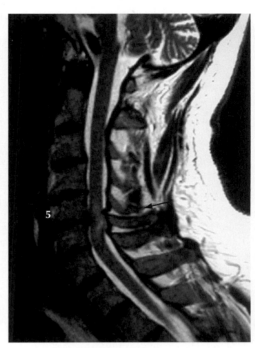

Sagittal T2-weighted MR image demonstrating marked stenosis at C5-6. There is an altered bright signal at that level within the spinal cord (arrow).

Figure 61-6 Cervical Spinal Stenosis.

facetectomy, with elevation of the nerve root and removal of the ruptured disc fragment is an option. The posterior approach is more uncomfortable than the anterior approach for the patient, but the exposure of the nerve root is superior and the patient does not have the potential long-term problems of fusion. An anterior approach is used for midline disc herniations causing cord and/or root symptoms.

If imaging demonstrates a diagnosis such as tumor or infection, then treatment is appropriately tailored. In the near future, replacement of the degenerative disc by an artificial disc may become a therapeutic option. Arthroplasty may prevent the late development of stress-related degenerative changes that can occur at levels adjacent to a fusion.

ADDITIONAL RESOURCES

Albert TJ, Murrell SE. Surgical management of cervical radiculopathy. J Am Acad Orthop Surg 1999 Nov-Dec;7(6):368-376.

Freidberg SR, Pfeifer BA, Dempsey PK, et al. Intraoperative computerized tomography scanning to assess the adequacy of decompression in anterior cervical spine surgery. J Neurosurg (Spine 1) 2001;94:8-11.

Guzman J, Haldeman S, Carroll LJ, et al. Clinical practice implications of the bone and joint Decade 2000-2010. Task Force on Neck Pain and Its Associated Disorders: from concepts and findings to recommendations. Spine 2008 Feb 15;33(Suppl. 4):S199-213. Review.

Levine MJ, Albert TJ, Smith MD. Cervical radiculopathy: diagnosis and nonoperative management. J Am Acad Orthop Surg 1996 Nov;4(6): 305-316.

Wirth FP, Dowd GC, Sanders HF, et al. Cervical discectomy. A prospective analysis of three operative techniques. Surg Neurol 2000 Apr;53(4): 340-346.

Lumbar Radiculopathy

Stephen R. Freidberg and Subu N. Magge

62

Clinical Vignette

A 53-year-old man had a history of occasional, severe episodes of low back pain radiating down his buttock and posterior left thigh that began with an athletic injury at age 17. Typically, he experienced exacerbations every few years that lasted a few days. Precipitating factors included sitting for prolonged periods, activities such as jogging, or playing hockey. In general he "toughed out" these exacerbations by forcing himself out of bed in the morning despite the pain, and continuing with his usual activities and being careful not to suddenly bend over. If his symptoms persisted, it was necessary to use simple analgesics, low-dose muscle relaxants, and to "take it easy." After a weekend of skiing, he developed severe left sciatica that progressively worsened over a 3-day period. The pain was excruciating, kept him up at night and did not respond to the usual medications. Getting out of bed in the morning was very painful and he had to force himself up despite the "paralyzing" pain. He noticed left foot drop with paresthesiae over his great toe. Straining or coughing further exacerbated the discomfort. He went to see a neurosurgeon; en route, routine jolting of the car significantly exacerbated the pain. Neurologic exam demonstrated a left foot drop, marked lumbosacral paravertebral muscle spasm, diminished lumbar lordosis, and an inability to tolerate straight leg raising on the left. Magnetic resonance imaging (MRI) demonstrated an extruded disc fragment at L4–5 interspace with compression of the left L5 root. A micro-hemi-laminectomy was performed, the disc fragment removed, and the nerve root decompressed. The sciatic pain was relieved the next morning.

Comment: This patient's course was typical for an intermittent, recurrent, subacute lumbosacral radiculopathy; his intermittent symptoms had always improved with conservative therapy. The sudden onset of an acute severe radiculopathy secondary to disc extrusion with excruciating pain and the rapid development of a foot drop over a few days led to successful surgical intervention.

Lumbosacral radiculopathy, frequently called "sciatica," is one of the most common neurologic afflictions, typically affecting 1% of the population/year. Most individuals with sciatica experience some degree of chronic low back pain. These symptoms are a major cause of disability and are the primary cause of workers' compensation disability in the United States.

CLINICAL PRESENTATION

Sciatic pain may occur acutely or evolve more gradually; when the onset is sudden, it may be spontaneous or related to a specific incident, sometimes a seemingly trivial event, such as bending over to make a bed. The symptoms may be minor and clinically inconsequential or significant requiring urgent evaluation and treatment (Fig. 62-1). Depending on the specific nerve root involved, the pain may be classic sciatica with radiation down the posterior aspect of the leg into the foot, as is seen with compression of the L5 or S1 roots (Figs. 62-2 and 62-3). At higher levels, with L3 or L4 root compression, the pain may radiate to the anterior thigh. The clinical signs of lumbar radiculopathy are due to the specific level of involvement (Table 62-1), and the most common levels of nerve root irritation are L5 and S1 roots, followed less commonly by L4 and L3 roots. It is rare to have involvement of the higher roots (L1 and L2).

In the adult, the spinal cord ends between L1 and L2; therefore the nerve root compressed by disc herniation depends upon whether the lesion is medial in the spinal canal or lateral in the neural foramen. The exiting root passes around the pedicle cephalad to the disc space. Therefore a lesion occurring at the disc space in the spinal canal compresses the passing root, the root with the next lower number. For example, a medial disc rupture in the spinal canal at L4–5 will compress the L5 root, whereas less commonly the disc rupturing laterally in the neural foramen will compress the L4 root.

ETIOLOGY

The most frequent cause of lumbar radiculopathy is a herniated lumbar disc, due to herniation of the nucleus pulposus, usually occurring with an equal frequency at the lowest two levels, L4–5 and L5–S1 (Figs. 62-4 and 62-5; see Fig. 62-1). Only ~5% of lumbar disc herniations occur at higher levels. Herniation is the last manifestation of disc degeneration that is an ongoing process in all humans. Hence, disc herniation is uncommon in youth, although occasionally teenagers and rarely toddlers have symptomatic herniations. Disc herniation occasionally occurs with spinal stenosis and may be the cause of rapid deterioration. Most lumbar radiculopathies are unilateral; bilateral sciatica has an ominous significance, suggesting compression of the cauda equina; these patients are at risk for loss of sphincter functions as well as sexual function in males. Early recognition is essential, as even after expeditious decompression, sphincter control and potency may not always return. Rarely spondylosis with foraminal encroachment resulting from disc degeneration may cause radiculopathy.

DIFFERENTIAL DIAGNOSIS

Spinal stenosis is becoming more prevalent with the increasingly aging population. It rarely occurs before age 60 years, although individuals with achondroplasia or other congenital processes, with narrow spinal canals caused by shortened pedicles, are predisposed to premature spinal stenosis. Spondylosis is the primary pathologic process, characterized by hypertrophy of the ligaments and facet joints (Fig. 62-6). Patients may develop single or multilevel spinal canal compression of the lumbosacral nerve roots; L3–4 and L4–5 interspaces are the most commonly affected levels; it is rare at L5–S1, unless there is subluxation of

Peripheral annulus fibrosus and posterior longitudinal ligament supplied with nociceptors (small unmyelinated nerve fibers with free or small capsular-type nerve endings). Nociceptors connect to sinuvertebral nerve and/or to somatic afferent nerves carried within the sympathetic chain to the upper lumbar levels, which lead to dorsal root ganglion in spinal nerve root.

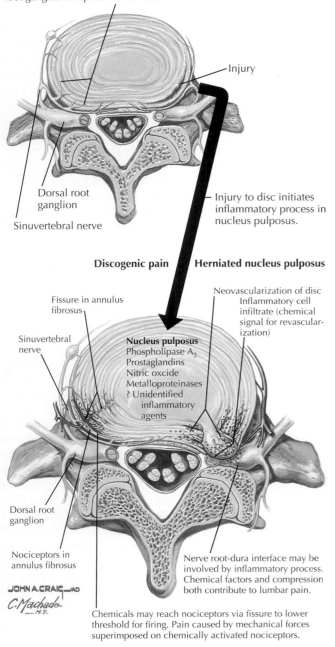

Injury

Dorsal root ganglion

Sinuvertebral nerve

Injury to disc initiates inflammatory process in nucleus pulposus.

Discogenic pain   **Herniated nucleus pulposus**

Fissure in annulus fibrosus

Neovascularization of disc Inflammatory cell infiltrate (chemical signal for revascularization)

Sinuvertebral nerve

Nucleus pulposus
Phospholipase A₂
Prostaglandins
Nitric oxcide
Metalloproteinases
? Unidentified inflammatory agents

Dorsal root ganglion

Nociceptors in annulus fibrosus

Nerve root-dura interface may be involved by inflammatory process. Chemical factors and compression both contribute to lumbar pain.

JOHN A. CRAIG—AD
C. Machado—M.D.

Chemicals may reach nociceptors via fissure to lower threshold for firing. Pain caused by mechanical forces superimposed on chemically activated nociceptors.

Figure 62-1 L4-5 Role of Inflammation in Lumbar Pain.

the vertebral bodies. Characteristically, the patient has a neurogenic claudication pain pattern mimicking arteriosclerotic occlusive (ASO) disease of the legs. Most individuals become symptomatic with standing or ambulating (Fig. 62-6). They are able to walk a set distance and then feel the need to sit; relief is usually rapid with sitting. Characteristically patients are more comfortable flexed at the waist; thus walking uphill may be easier than walking downhill, as spinal hyperextension

associated with walking downhill may precipitate symptomatology. Patients may also be more comfortable leaning forward on a walker or grocery cart. Often the patient has a normal neurologic exam; occasionally, with long-standing symptomatic spinal stenosis, there may be neurologic deficits.

The primary issue is often the differentiation of spinal stenosis from vascular claudication. The demographic population for both conditions is similar. Individuals with spinal stenosis tend to have pain of a more dysesthetic burning character in contrast to the squeezing tight discomfort typical for ASO. Another useful differentiating point on history is that those with spinal stenosis can ride a bicycle long distances, whereas arteriosclerotic patients are limited as if they are walking. Unlike patients with disc herniations, patients with spinal stenosis are typically comfortable at rest, showing no signs of paraspinal spasm, difficulty with straight leg raising testing, or problems bending forward. Plain radiographs provide a good inexpensive means to recognize severe spondylotic changes. MRI is the diagnostic modality of choice. Computed tomographic (CT) myelography is helpful if the patient cannot tolerate MRI. For individuals who have relatively modest symptomatology, there is no urgency to proceed with surgery. However, once the patient is limited in walking, or is uncomfortable even when seated, a wide decompressive laminectomy and foraminotomy at appropriate spinal levels brings significant relief for a high percentage of patients. For patients whose stenosis may be associated with spondylolisthesis, spinal fusion is indicated.

Spondylolisthesis, the anterior slippage of the superior vertebral body with respect to the inferior is another common cause of lumbar root compression, resulting in low back pain (Figs. 62-6A and B), radiculopathy symptoms, and sometimes cauda equina syndrome. The two common causes of spondylolisthesis involve spinal degenerative (spondylotic) changes and congenital defects of the vertebral pars interarticularis. Patients with degenerative spondylolisthesis tend to be older, whereas those with a pars defect usually present in their third or fourth decade with significant lumbar and root pain, usually related to postural change.

Although relatively uncommon, synovial cysts may produce symptoms identical to disc herniation. The cysts develop from hypertrophy of synovial tissue in the facet joint. Neurosurgeons may encounter these cysts pushing into the paraspinal muscles when reflecting them for exposure of the spine. In this location, they indicate degenerative joint disease, but by themselves are not symptomatic. When cysts become intraspinal they may compress the nerve root; synovial cysts create a surrounding inflammatory reaction and therefore must be carefully dissected from the dura of the nerve roots. Resection of lumbar epidural synovial cysts usually relieves patients' pain.

Epidural infections occur secondary to disc surgery or via hematogenous spread. Unlike metastatic tumors that primarily involve the vertebral bodies, abscess involves the disc space, with secondary spread to the adjacent vertebral bodies. Back pain from disc space and vertebral body involvement and secondary nerve root pain are usually very severe. Common causative organisms in the United States are coagulase-positive and -negative Staphylococcus from surgical or hematogenous spread. Gram-negative organisms from urinary sepsis may also be causative agents. Intravenous drug users and

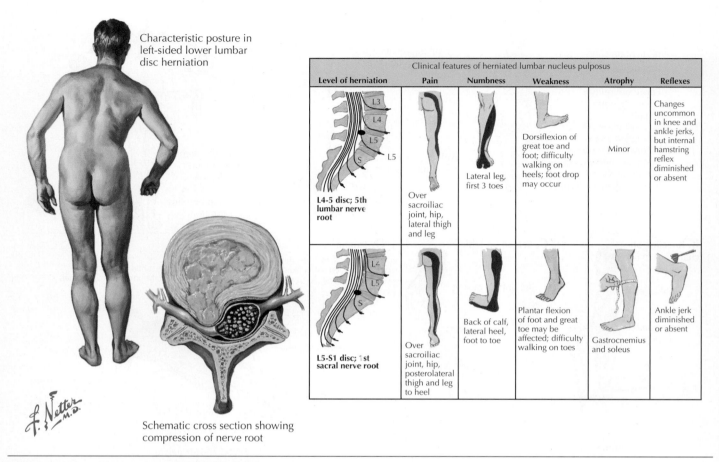

Characteristic posture in left-sided lower lumbar disc herniation

Schematic cross section showing compression of nerve root

Clinical features of herniated lumbar nucleus pulposus					
Level of herniation	Pain	Numbness	Weakness	Atrophy	Reflexes
L4-5 disc; 5th lumbar nerve root	Over sacroiliac joint, hip, lateral thigh and leg	Lateral leg, first 3 toes	Dorsiflexion of great toe and foot; difficulty walking on heels; foot drop may occur	Minor	Changes uncommon in knee and ankle jerks, but internal hamstring reflex diminished or absent
L5-S1 disc; 1st sacral nerve root	Over sacroiliac joint, hip, posterolateral thigh and leg to heel	Back of calf, lateral heel, foot to toe	Plantar flexion of foot and great toe may be affected; difficulty walking on toes	Gastrocnemius and soleus	Ankle jerk diminished or absent

Figure 62-2 Lumbar Disc Herniation: Clinical Manifestations.

immunocompromised patients have higher incidences of epidural abscess. Worldwide, the most common cause of spinal infection is tuberculosis. The incidence of spinal TB appears to be increasing with the increasing incidence of HIV positivity in susceptible populations.

Neoplasms may be a cause of lumbosacral pain. Metastatic extradural cancers to the spine are the most common tumors. Primary bone tumors and intradural primary and metastatic tumors may also mimic discogenic disorders. The common cancers that metastasize include prostate, breast, lung, melanoma, and myeloma. Usually symptoms begin with spine pain that worsens gradually; root pain starts once neural elements become involved and may worsen rapidly. Evaluation and treatment in this situation is urgent, as recovery after treatment may not be complete. Schwannoma, meningioma, myxopapillary ependymoma, and lipoma are the common lumbar spinal intradural tumors (Fig. 62-7). The symptoms of schwannoma, meningioma, and ependymoma are gradually progressive. Patients with a lipoma, a congenital tumor, may have a history of baseline neurologic deficits with a slow, later progression.

DIAGNOSTIC APPROACH

The evaluation of patients having their initial bout of acute sciatica or low back pain does not routinely require any diagnostic testing. Most individuals recover spontaneously. However, for those who do not fit the classic pattern of nerve root compression or acute low back strain, and for patients who do not improve, neurodiagnostic testing is necessary.

Lumbar spine plain radiographs, including lateral flexion and extension views, serve two purposes: the anatomy of the spine with its degenerative changes is demonstrated, as are subluxations and instability and destructive lesions in the vertebral bodies, and disc space can be seen. MRI is the primary spinal imaging modality (Figs. 62-5 and 62-6). Good-quality MRI demonstrates disc herniation or spinal stenosis and identifies the rare tumor or infection. However, on occasion, for technical reasons, MR imaging may not be successful; for example, the patient may have moved during imaging; obesity or claustrophobia may be other impediments. Myelogram with CT continues to be a valuable adjunct to the diagnostic repertoire, especially when MRI is contraindicated (e.g., pacemaker) or not tolerated. Myelography with water-soluble contrast, followed by axial CT scanning, can demonstrate nerve root filling or lack thereof with more clarity than MRI. Sagittal and coronal reconstructions of CT data give excellent additional information. Electrodiagnostic studies are invaluable in those situations where data from imaging are difficult to interpret or where other superimposed conditions, for example polyneuropathy, coexist.

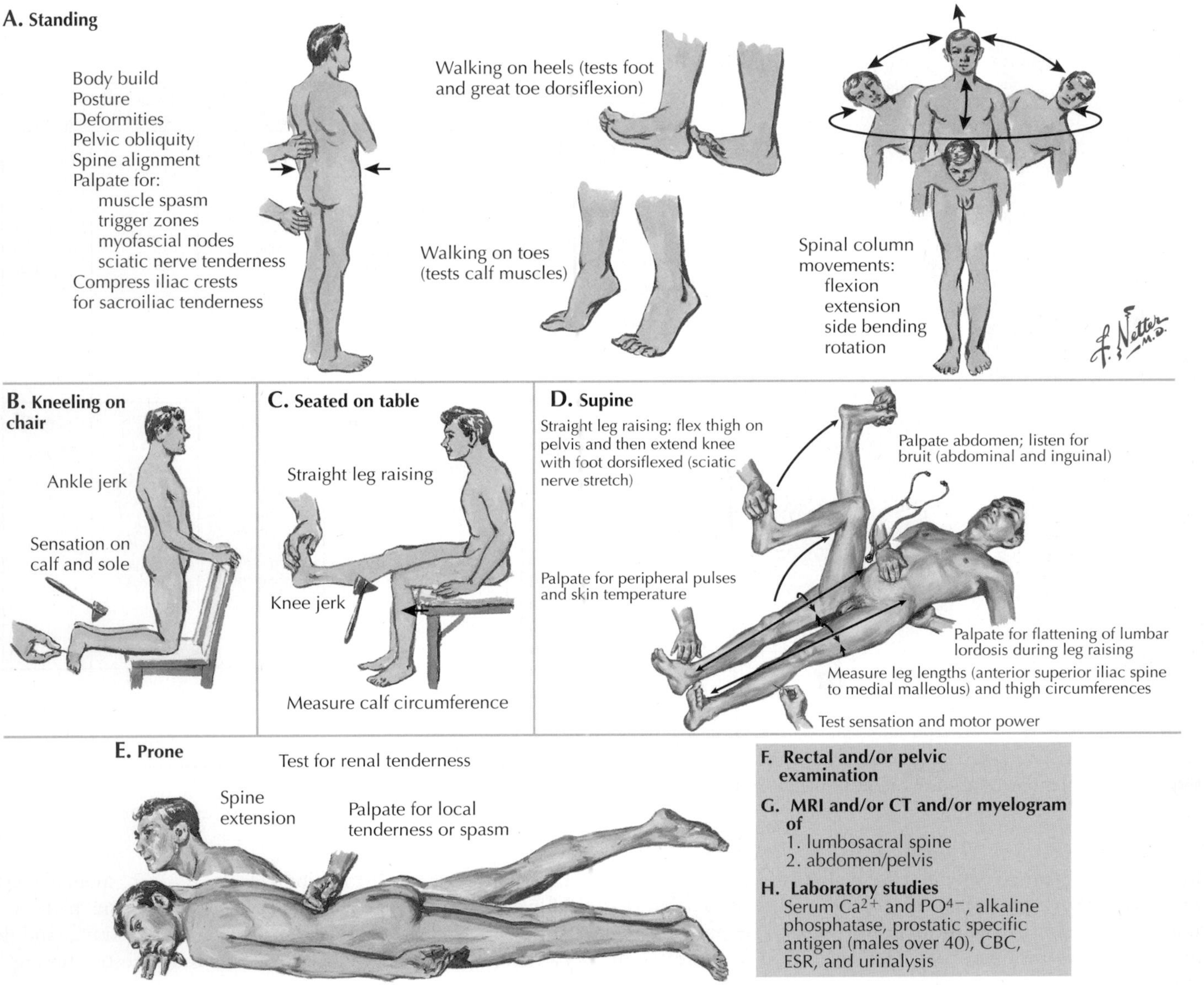

A. Standing

Body build
Posture
Deformities
Pelvic obliquity
Spine alignment
Palpate for:
    muscle spasm
    trigger zones
    myofascial nodes
    sciatic nerve tenderness
Compress iliac crests
for sacroiliac tenderness

Walking on heels (tests foot
and great toe dorsiflexion)

Walking on toes
(tests calf muscles)

Spinal column
movements:
    flexion
    extension
    side bending
    rotation

B. Kneeling on chair

Ankle jerk

Sensation on
calf and sole

C. Seated on table

Straight leg raising

Knee jerk

Measure calf circumference

D. Supine

Straight leg raising: flex thigh on
pelvis and then extend knee
with foot dorsiflexed (sciatic
nerve stretch)

Palpate for peripheral pulses
and skin temperature

Palpate abdomen; listen for
bruit (abdominal and inguinal)

Palpate for flattening of lumbar
lordosis during leg raising

Measure leg lengths (anterior superior iliac spine
to medial malleolus) and thigh circumferences

Test sensation and motor power

E. Prone

Test for renal tenderness

Spine
extension

Palpate for local
tenderness or spasm

**F. Rectal and/or pelvic
examination**

**G. MRI and/or CT and/or myelogram
of**
    1. lumbosacral spine
    2. abdomen/pelvis

H. Laboratory studies
Serum Ca^{2+} and PO^{4-}, alkaline
phosphatase, prostatic specific
antigen (males over 40), CBC,
ESR, and urinalysis

Figure 62-3 Examination of Patient with Low Back Pain.

Table 62-1 Nerve Root Signs of Lumbar Radiculopathy

Root	Motor Weakness	Sensory Loss	Muscle Stretch Reflexes
L3	Iliopsoas/quadriceps	Anterior thigh	KJ diminished but still present
L4	Quadriceps	Anterior thigh to below knee	KJ absent
L5	Tibialis anterior	Dorsum and medial foot	Internal hamstring
S1	Gastrocnemius	Lateral aspect of foot, sole, and heel	AJ absent

KJ, knee jerk; AJ, ankle jerk.

TREATMENT

Treatment of lumbar radiculopathy is usually successful if the history, physical exam, and imaging correlate. Most acute episodes of back pain or nerve root pain, without significant neurologic deficit, only require judicious rest and simple analgesics. Strict bed rest is not necessary because it may lead to rapid deconditioning; it may also predispose to more serious complications, such as deep venous thrombosis, pulmonary embolism, and rarely fatal paradoxical cerebral emboli. Patients need to be encouraged to get up as much as possible, but to avoid activities that exacerbate their symptoms. When patients have recovered from their acute symptoms, they can begin a judicious exercise

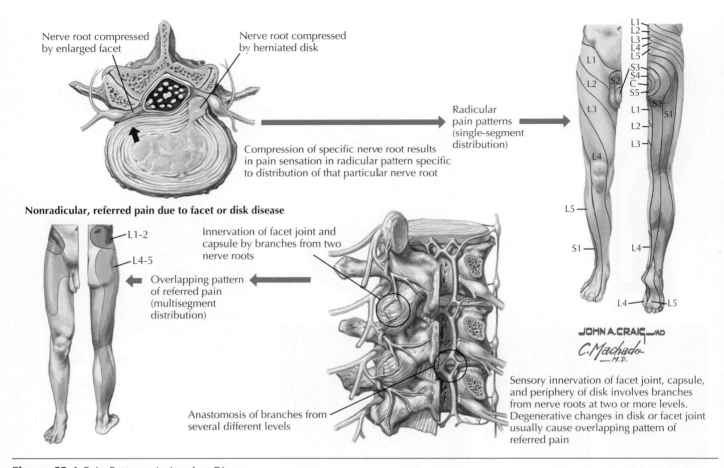

Nonradicular, referred pain due to facet or disk disease

Compression of specific nerve root results in pain sensation in radicular pattern specific to distribution of that particular nerve root

Radicular pain patterns (single-segment distribution)

Innervation of facet joint and capsule by branches from two nerve roots

Overlapping pattern of referred pain (multisegment distribution)

Anastomosis of branches from several different levels

Sensory innervation of facet joint, capsule, and periphery of disk involves branches from nerve roots at two or more levels. Degenerative changes in disk or facet joint usually cause overlapping pattern of referred pain

Figure 62-4 Pain Patterns in Lumbar Disease.

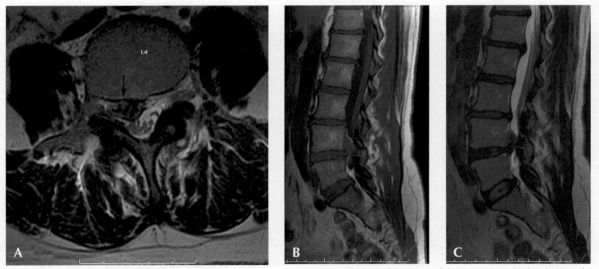

(A) Axial T2-weighted image at L4 shows large hypointense mass in the right lateral recess and foramen. T1-weighted (B) and T2-weighted (C) sagittal MR images show mass extending cephalad from the L4-5 disc (arrowheads).

Figure 62-5 Disc Extrusion.

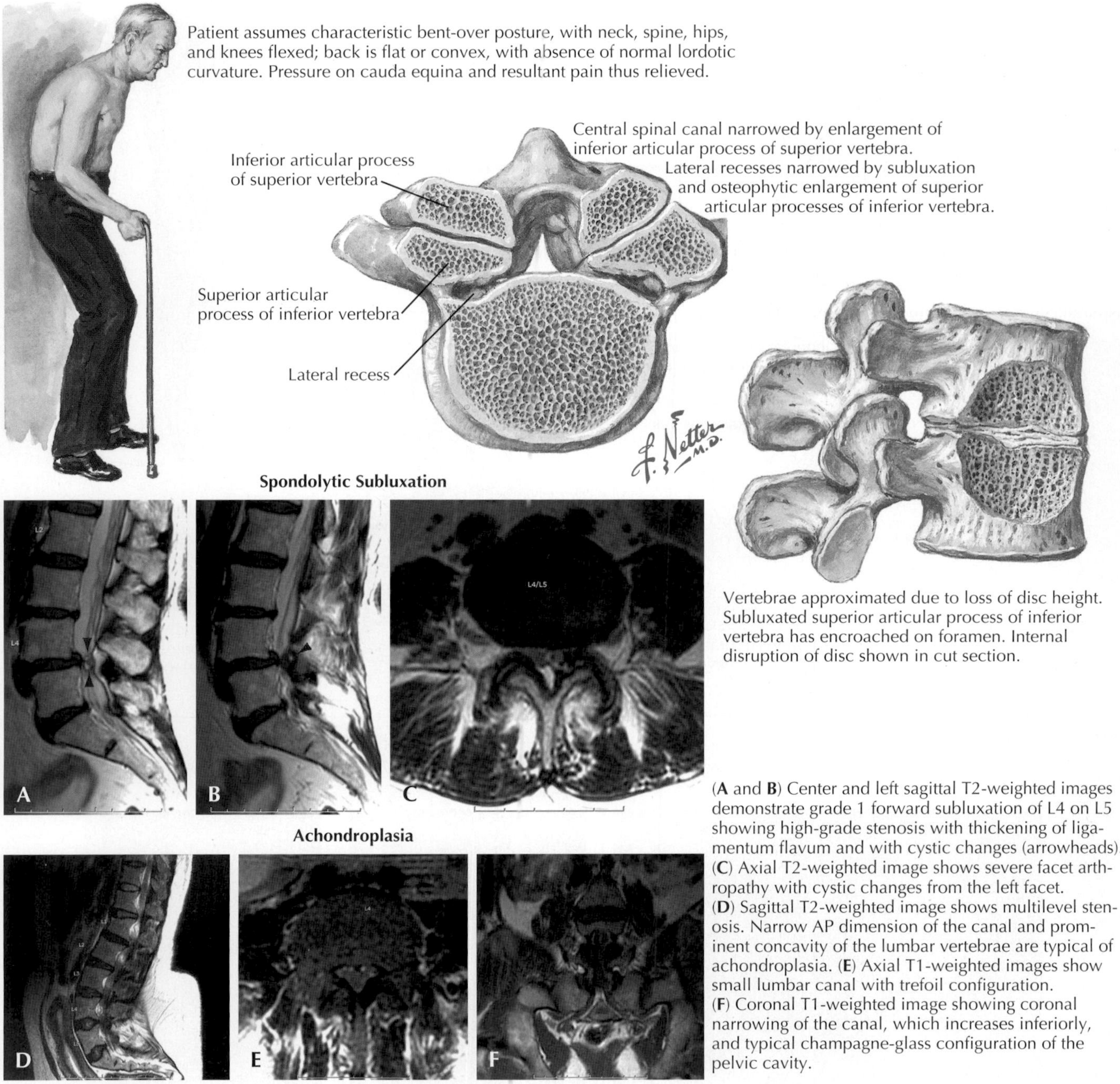

Patient assumes characteristic bent-over posture, with neck, spine, hips, and knees flexed; back is flat or convex, with absence of normal lordotic curvature. Pressure on cauda equina and resultant pain thus relieved.

Inferior articular process of superior vertebra

Central spinal canal narrowed by enlargement of inferior articular process of superior vertebra.
Lateral recesses narrowed by subluxation and osteophytic enlargement of superior articular processes of inferior vertebra.

Superior articular process of inferior vertebra

Lateral recess

Spondolytic Subluxation

Vertebrae approximated due to loss of disc height. Subluxated superior articular process of inferior vertebra has encroached on foramen. Internal disruption of disc shown in cut section.

Achondroplasia

(**A** and **B**) Center and left sagittal T2-weighted images demonstrate grade 1 forward subluxation of L4 on L5 showing high-grade stenosis with thickening of ligamentum flavum and with cystic changes (arrowheads).
(**C**) Axial T2-weighted image shows severe facet arthropathy with cystic changes from the left facet.
(**D**) Sagittal T2-weighted image shows multilevel stenosis. Narrow AP dimension of the canal and prominent concavity of the lumbar vertebrae are typical of achondroplasia. (**E**) Axial T1-weighted images show small lumbar canal with trefoil configuration.
(**F**) Coronal T1-weighted image showing coronal narrowing of the canal, which increases inferiorly, and typical champagne-glass configuration of the pelvic cavity.

Figure 62-6 Lumbar Spinal Stenosis.

program, graduating to a full fitness exercise program. Analgesics and anti-inflammatory medication including occasional use of steroids may help patients. With this approach, 80% of patients improve within 3 months. This is the natural history of discogenic nerve root compression, and care is advised when evaluating therapeutic claims for other treatment modalities such as chiropractic manipulations or acupuncture. For patients with more chronic, nondisabling pain, lifestyle changes with weight loss and health club membership are the best approach, although unfortunately, few patients successfully change their behavior patterns.

When acute symptoms do not improve, or the chronic degenerative disc-related pain persists, surgery is an option (Fig. 62-8). An important indication for surgery is the presence of a significant persistent neurologic deficit such as foot drop. However, severe or chronic unrelenting nerve root pain that disrupts a patient's life is a common reason to proceed with nerve root decompression. When advising patients who are making decisions about surgery, they should be clear that postponing surgery would not place them in neurologic jeopardy, but that the discomfort will likely persist. Surgical goals for patients with degenerative disease or disc rupture

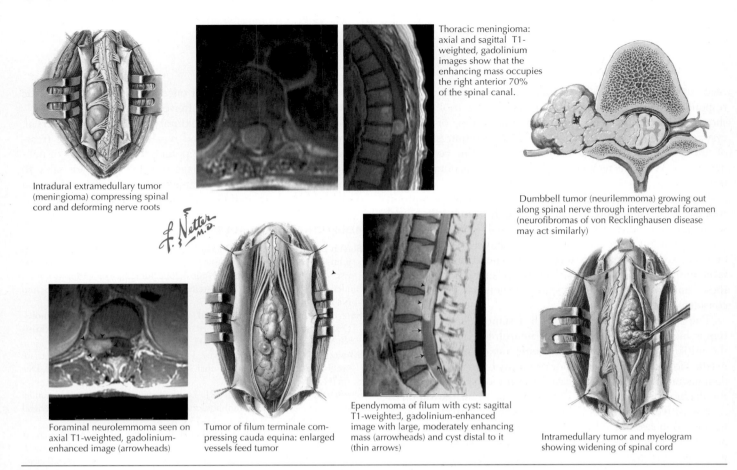

Thoracic meningioma: axial and sagittal T1-weighted, gadolinium images show that the enhancing mass occupies the right anterior 70% of the spinal canal.

Intradural extramedullary tumor (meningioma) compressing spinal cord and deforming nerve roots

Dumbbell tumor (neurilemmoma) growing out along spinal nerve through intervertebral foramen (neurofibromas of von Recklinghausen disease may act similarly)

Foraminal neurolemmoma seen on axial T1-weighted, gadolinium-enhanced image (arrowheads)

Tumor of filum terminale compressing cauda equina: enlarged vessels feed tumor

Ependymoma of filum with cyst: sagittal T1-weighted, gadolinium-enhanced image with large, moderately enhancing mass (arrowheads) and cyst distal to it (thin arrows)

Intramedullary tumor and myelogram showing widening of spinal cord

Figure 62-7 Intradural Spinal Tumors.

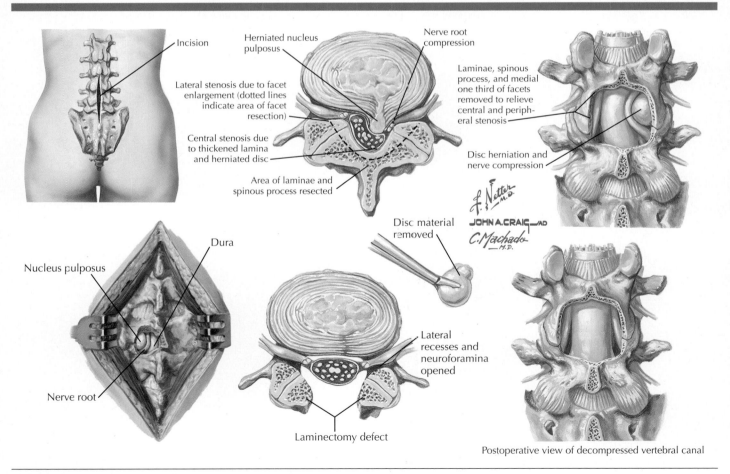

Incision

Herniated nucleus pulposus

Nerve root compression

Lateral stenosis due to facet enlargement (dotted lines indicate area of facet resection)

Laminae, spinous process, and medial one third of facets removed to relieve central and peripheral stenosis

Central stenosis due to thickened lamina and herniated disc

Disc herniation and nerve compression

Area of laminae and spinous process resected

Disc material removed

Dura

Nucleus pulposus

Nerve root

Lateral recesses and neuroforamina opened

Laminectomy defect

Postoperative view of decompressed vertebral canal

Figure 62-8 Laminectomy and Discectomy.

relate to the pain's origin. If the patient has root pain with corresponding root compression on imaging, the root or roots should be decompressed, and the herniated disc or synovial cyst removed. Surgery for an extruded disc requires removal of the extruded fragment with freeing of the compressed nerve root. With this technique, >90% of patients obtain symptomatic relief.

If posture-related lumbar pain is the primary symptom, root decompression alone will not resolve the symptoms. Spinal segmental instability, with abnormal spinal motion, can also cause significant pain secondary to intermittent compression of nerve roots. It can also increase degeneration around the facet joints and disc annulus, causing primary back pain. In these uncommon instances, spinal fusion is a reasonable consideration.

The treatment of a patient with a tumor depends on the tumor histology and the extent of neurologic involvement. If the initial presentation of a metastatic tumor is in the spine, needle biopsy of the spinal tumor or biopsy of an obvious tumor demonstrated in the lung, breast, prostate, or skin can provide the diagnosis. Radiotherapy is appropriate when the tumor is radiosensitive, the spine is stable, and there is relatively minimal neural compression. However, if these considerations are not met, surgery is indicated. A major destructive lesion involving most of the vertebral body and both pedicles usually requires a 360-degree decompression and fusion. Neurologic

deterioration can be rapid, and once paresis has occurred, the patient may not recover, even after emergency surgery.

Appropriate therapy of an epidural infection is controversial. Some reports demonstrate good results with antibiotic treatment. However, because of the potential for rapid loss of neurologic function, surgical drainage of frank pus is advisable to reduce pain and to prevent paraplegia. Rapid deterioration can occur in patients treated nonoperatively with antibiotics.

ADDITIONAL RESOURCES

Berven S, Tay BB, Colman W, Hu SS. The lumbar zygapophyseal (facet) joints: a role in the pathogenesis of spinal pain syndromes and degenerative spondylolisthesis. Semin Neurol 2002 Jun;22(2):187–196.

Binder DK, Schmidt MH, Weinstein PR. Lumbar spinal stenosis. Semin Neurol 2002 Jun;22(2):157–166.

Katz JN, Dalgas M, Stucki G, et al. Degenerative lumbar spinal stenosis. Diagnostic value of the history and physical examination. Arthritis Rheum 1995 Sep;38(9):1236–1241.

Schultz IZ, Crook JM, Berkowitz J, et al. Biopsychosocial multivariate predictive model of occupational low back disability. Spine 2002 Dec 1;27(23):2720–2725.

Storm PB, Chou D, Tamargo RJ. Lumbar spinal stenosis, cauda equina syndrome, and multiple lumbosacral radiculopathies. Phys Med Rehabil Clin N Am 2002 Aug;13(3):713–733, ix.

Winstein JN, Lurie JD, Tosteson TD et al. Surgical vs nonoperative treatment for lumbar disk herniation: the Spine Patient Outcomes Research Trial (SPORT) a randomized trial. JAMA 2006 Nov 22;296(20):2441-2450.

Vascular, Rheumatologic, Functional, and Psychosomatic Back Pain

H. Royden Jones, Jr.

63

Clinical Vignette

A 55-year-old lumber yard foreman with history of hyper-cholesterolemia, prior 30 pack-year smoking, and depression, began to experience bilateral left > right leg pain primarily precipitated with walking. The pain ceased whenever he stopped and rested for a few minutes ... he did not even need to sit. With time, his pain was precipitated with significantly shorter distances, getting to the point where he could not go more than 100–150 yards without having to stop to relieve his discomfort. At rest he felt fine. He could not obtain an effective erection. This initially appeared to be a classic picture of intermittent claudication secondary to primary vascular disease.

However, all of his peripheral pulses were normal. Doppler arterial evaluation was normal. His symptoms progressed; he could not mow his lawn or take walks and he felt weak climbing stairs. Lumbar spinal MRI and EMG were normal.

He was than referred to us for a possible myopathy or spinal stenosis. His neurologic examination was perfect. All peripheral pulses were normal, and Doppler arterial studies, lumbar spinal MRI and EMG were normal.

Vascular consultants did not feel that he had peripheral vascular disease. Psychiatric consultation found no psychosomatic component. Exercise Doppler suggested mild decreased flow on the right.

A repeat examination now demonstrated his peripheral pulses were no longer present. He now had a bruit over his left femoral artery CT angiogram demonstrated severe stenosis of the proximal left femoral and iliac artery (Fig. 63-1). Angioplasty and stenting led to immediate pain relief.

Comment: This patient had classic intermittent claudication precipitated by exercise and totally relieved by rest. This almost always implies peripheral atheromatous disease. With his initially normal peripheral arterial evaluation he was thought to have a neurologic mechanism; however, this was not confirmed.

Reevaluation demonstrated that he now had a femoral artery bruit. CT angiography identified proximal intrapelvic arterial compromise despite normal traditional techniques.

This case particularly emphasizes the importance of revisiting the history and the examination with any patient whose clinical picture is not initially confirmed by traditional studies. The neurologist must always look at potential nonneurologic mechanisms whenever forming a differential diagnosis.

Clinical Vignette

A 28-year-old milkman, who lifted many heavy milk cases daily, presented with low back pain. This had begun 1 year earlier after lifting an extra-large load, "wrenching" his back. Subsequently he noted gradually increasingly severe and eventually almost incapacitating low back pain that occasionally radiated into his buttocks and posteriorly down his right leg. He also noted increasingly more limiting early morning back and hip stiffness that gradually "loosened up" after he worked an hour.

During the previous few months, his difficulties had progressed significantly. He now felt unable to finish his daily job responsibilities. Therefore he applied for workers' compensation.

Neurologic examination demonstrated complete loss of lumbar lordosis, significantly diminished chest excursion of only 1.5 cm (normal 3–6 cm), and mildly positive right straight leg testing. His neurologic examination was otherwise normal. An aortic diastolic murmur was presnt on cardiac examination.

Spinal and hip radiographs demonstrated typical findings of ankylosing spondylitis. These included significant sacroiliac joint sclerosis (Fig. 63-2). A serum HLA-B27 test was positive. A rheumatologist concurred with the diagnosis and began appropriate therapy.

Comment: This patient sought care for a presumed job-related injury. Instead, a diagnosis of a serious rheumatologic disorder, namely ankylosing spondylitis, was made. If that diagnosis had not been appreciated at his age, eventually this would have led to serious spinal ankylosis with significant spinal immobility and possibly serious pulmonary compromise. Despite this early diagnosis of such a treatable condition, paradoxically this patient was disappointed with his care bacause he was no longer entitled to workman's compensation!

The frequency of work- and accident-related back pain sometimes seems to be reaching pandemic proportions among workers performing heavy labor. Very often patients present with many potential causes for their back pain. These not only represent the classic well-defined organic mechanisms, such as lumbosacral nerve root compression, or ischemic compromise, but aditionally there may be many occupation-related

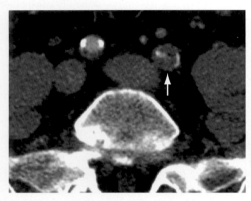

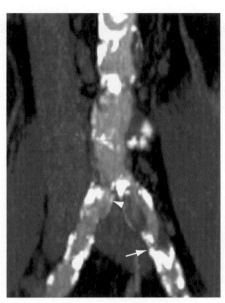

A. Axial CTA demonstrates total occlusion of left common iliac artery (arrow).

B. Coronal CTA reconstruction demonstrates beginning of high-grade stenosis from mixed plaque (arrowhead) to total occlusion (arrow).

Figure 63-1 Total Obstruction of Left Common Iliac Artery.

symptoms wherein overt or covert psychologic factors combine to provide a confusing milieu. Secondary gain issues are commonly confounding factors. It is vital not to impugn patients' veracity by applying pejorative labels such as "hysteric," "a crock," "functional," "litiginous," or even "having psychological overlay." Too often, these labels have led to inadequate evaluations, and serious illness is occasionally overlooked, as initially occurred in both of the above vignettes.

Sincere physicians often encounter difficulties dealing with disingenuous patients seeking a "free ride" or a "green poultice" (Fig. 63-3). Most often secondary gain is the primary motivating factor, particularly with the perspective of a generous workers' compensation settlement. However, the examining neurologist must carefully evaluate each patient to search for a specific neurologic or other illness, as many patients understandably look for a simple explanation for their troubles—and it is easy to blame the workplace. Often the symptoms become embellished, not uncommonly subconsciously, to prove that a "work-related injury" truly exists. Very often these patients tend to focus on their backs, seeking to prove the presence of a post-traumatic mechanically related disorder. They most definitely want to have their neurologist diagnose a specific work-related neurologic disorder as in the second vignette.

Back pain patients may have psychosomatic features, but as with many organic disorders other primary psychologic disorders require consideration. These include depression,

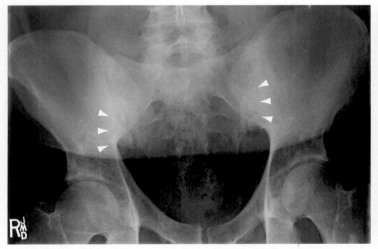

A. A. Digital frontal radiograph of pelvis showing fusion (arrowheads).

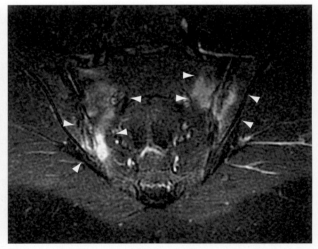

B. T2-weighted fat-saturated coronal oblique view of sacrum demonstrates augmented T2 signal related to both SI joints (arrowheads).

Figure 63-2 Fusion of Sacroiliac Joints in 28-Year-Old Man with Ankylosing Spondylitis.

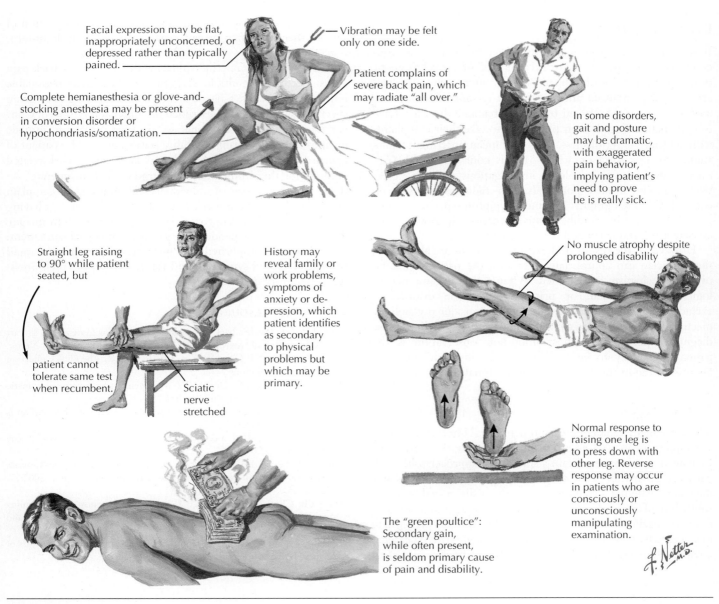

Facial expression may be flat, inappropriately unconcerned, or depressed rather than typically pained.

Vibration may be felt only on one side.

Patient complains of severe back pain, which may radiate "all over."

Complete hemianesthesia or glove-and-stocking anesthesia may be present in conversion disorder or hypochondriasis/somatization.

In some disorders, gait and posture may be dramatic, with exaggerated pain behavior, implying patient's need to prove he is really sick.

Straight leg raising to 90° while patient seated, but

History may reveal family or work problems, symptoms of anxiety or depression, which patient identifies as secondary to physical problems but which may be primary.

No muscle atrophy despite prolonged disability

patient cannot tolerate same test when recumbent.

Sciatic nerve stretched

Normal response to raising one leg is to press down with other leg. Reverse response may occur in patients who are consciously or unconsciously manipulating examination.

The "green poultice": Secondary gain, while often present, is seldom primary cause of pain and disability.

Figure 63-3 Somatoform Back Disorders.

conversion disorder, psychophysiologic disorder, chronic pain syndrome, hypochondriasis, factitious disorder, and even schizophrenia. As the physician gains the patient's confidence during the interview and examination, certain life stressors may become apparent, including family, job, personal issues, and inappropriate use of medications or even street drugs.

NEUROLOGIC EXAMINATION

Each patient requires a comprehensive general neurologic examination, not only to evaluate the affected extremity and back but also to confirm that other neurologic systems and anatomic structures such as joints or vessels are healthy. There are specific clinical testing means that help distinguish an organic lesion from one that is embellished or inconsistent. The straight leg raise is an excellent example. A patient with organic

nerve root compression becomes uncomfortable when lying supine while the physician attempts to bring the patient's leg to the perpendicular and is similarly affected when seated for a similar maneuver. Stretch on the sciatic nerve and its already compromised origins within the L5–S1 nerve roots initiates the discomfort. In contrast, an inconsistent response is often noted wherein individuals seeking secondary gain report pain with movement in the supine but not the seated posture.

Another example is the well-known observation that when denervation occurs with significant peripheral nerve injury, it is followed by significant muscular atrophy. Such is generally lacking in the nonorganic setting. However, the quadriceps femoris is an exception; it may undergo significant disuse atrophy without a true peripheral nerve injury. Other useful clues and testing modalities can help to verify psychosomatic back pain (see Fig. 63-3).

EVALUATION

It is absolutely essential to carefully investigate patients' concerns even when the clinician "is confident" of a psychosomatic or compensation disorder diagnosis. Too often such individuals are compartmentalized and put in the *compensation diagnostic mode* only to later be found to have a treatable disorder. Each of these patients needs their physicians to take their complaints with appropriate seriousness. This may mean ordering imaging studies such as MRI or, when MRI is contraindicated, CT/myelography, neurophysiologic investigations including electromyography, evoked potentials, hip radiographs, and on occasion CT angiography. Finding a symptom-specific organic lesion that can be readily treated occasionally rewards the conscientious physician and patient alike.

However, if the results of these investigations are all normal, the physician can appropriately reassure the patients that no organic mechanism is identified. When a true organic neurologic, musculoskeletal, or primary psychiatric disorder is excluded, only then should the physician consider psychologic mechanisms or secondary gain. A number of clues help in these diagnoses; perhaps the most important observation is the patient's tendency to be "consistently inconsistent" in some features of the history or neurologic examination.

TREATMENT

There are many rehabilitative and behavioral interventions that are supportive as well as often therapeutic for these patients. One needs to always maintain a supportive approach with such patients, no matter what the final diagnosis. This does not depend on whether a conversion disorder is diagnosed or a very subtle hint of a lumbosacral disc protrusion is suggested. Neither requires specific therapy especially a surgical one. Appropriate management combines reassurance, rehabilitative medicine techniques, group therapy, and, in the more refractive instances,

individual psychiatric intervention. An eclectic combination of various therapies often provides an improvement in long-term outcomes.

Unfortunately, some individuals with chronic low back pain are subjected to multiple surgeries for less than reasonable indications. Thus they have no chance of improving because no specific lesion such as an extruded disc has been removed. Concomitantly these surgeries, per se, are then utilized to provide justification for granting disability status per se. The patient of course feels "there must have been" an organic work-related etiology for their difficulties if a surgeon "had to operate" on them. Another subset of individuals will continue to complain until a legal settlement is reached. They are identified as having the "green poultice syndrome" (see Fig. 63-3, bottom image). This is of course dependent on gaining a financial settlement; once that is accomplished it is not uncommon to see a rapid resolution of their symptoms and ability to return to their previous activities of daily living!

ADDITIONAL RESOURCES

Hayes J. Psychosomatic back complaints. In: Nervous System. Vol 1. Part II: Neurologic and Neuromuscular Disorders. Prepared by Frank Netter. West Caldwell, NJ: Ciba; 1986. p. 198. Jones HR. The Ciba Collection of Medical Illustrations.

Henningsen P, Zipfel S, Herzog W. Management of functional somatic syndromes. Lancet 2007;369:946-955.

Lindstrom-Hazel D. The backpack problem is evident but the solution is less obvious. Work 2009;32:329-338.

Murphy PL, Volinn E. Is occupational low back pain on the rise? Spine 1999;24:691-697.

Schultz IZ, Crook JM, Berkowitz J, et al. Biopsychosocial multivariate predictive model of occupational low back disability. Spine 2002;27: 2720-2725.

Storm PB, Chou D, Tamargo RJ. Lumbar spinal stenosis, cauda equina syndrome, and multiple lumbosacral radiculopathies. Phys Med Rehabil Clin North Am 2002;13:713-733, ix.

Tubach F, Beauté J, Leclerc A. Natural history and prognostic indicators of sciatica. J Clin Epidemiol 2004;57:174-179.

Brachial and Lumbosacral Plexopathies

Ted M. Burns, Monique Ryan, and H. Royden Jones, Jr.

64

Clinical Vignette

A 54-year-old man developed acute-onset right thigh, hip, and buttock pain. He also noted right knee "buckling" when he stepped off a curb, resulting in a fall. He also noted right foot drop. Paresthesias developed over the right thigh, shin, and foot. He required oral narcotics for pain relief.

His past medical history was remarkable for type II diabetes mellitus, for which he took an oral hypoglycemic. His blood sugars had been under fair control. His review of systems was remarkable for a 30-pound weight loss over the past 3 months, which he attributed to renewed efforts at dieting. He doesn't smoke or drink heavily. He is an attorney. Family history is negative.

His general examination was unremarkable. His neurologic examination was notable for moderate weakness of right hip flexion, hip extension, knee extension, and ankle dorsiflexion. He has an absent right knee and ankle reflex, but reflexes are normal on the left lower extremity and upper extremities. Sensory testing demonstrates reduced vibration sensation at the right great toe and ankle. His gait is hesitant and reveals a right foot drop.

Electromyography (EMG) demonstrated borderline right peroneal and tibial compound motor action potentials with normal velocities and distal latencies. The sural and superficial peroneal sensory nerve action potentials were absent on the right and normal on the left. Active denervation was present in right femoral and sciatic innervated muscles, and to a lesser extent in lumbosacral paraspinals and gluteal muscles.

Magnetic resonance imaging (MRI) of the lumbosacral spine and pelvis was unremarkable, except for signal changes in denervating muscles. Lumbar puncture demonstrated an elevated cerebrospinal fluid (CSF) protein with normal cell count. Glycosylated hemoglobin was slightly elevated but otherwise his laboratory studies were normal.

He was diagnosed with diabetic lumbosacral radiculoplexus neuropathy (also known as diabetic amyotrophy). After discussion of the pros and cons he was prescribed an empiric treatment trial of intravenous methylprednisolone.

The most important diagnostic tool for the evaluation of a possible plexopathy is a thorough and accurate history. The history-taking must be aided by a solid understanding of the risk factors for development of brachial or lumbosacral plexopathy. The most common etiologies of plexopathy are trauma, surgery (e.g., related to arm or leg positioning, injury with regional anesthetic block), birth injury, inherited genetic mutations (e.g., hereditary neuralgic amyotrophy), a primary autoimmune process (e.g., Parsonage–Turner, also known as neuralgic amyotrophy), previous radiotherapy, and neoplastic invasion (Fig. 64-1; Table 64-1). Systemic vasculitis and peripheral nerve sarcoidosis are other uncommon etiologies. Diabetes mellitus is a risk factor for an immune-mediated lumbosacral (and less often, brachial) plexopathy, that is, diabetic lumbosacral radiculoplexus neuropathy (diabetic LRPN) secondary to microvasculitis. Thus, if a prior or concomitant history of any of these risk factors (e.g., previous surgery, trauma, or family history, diabetes) is present, the clinician should strongly consider that etiology yet not necessarily forget to consider other plausible etiologies. It is also helpful to remember that recent infection, vaccination, and parturition are triggers for the immune-mediated plexopathies, especially brachial plexopathies (e.g., hereditary neuralgic amyotrophy and neuralgic amyotrophy). There are often other clues about etiology found in the symptomatology of the plexopathy. For example, the abrupt, spontaneous onset of shoulder and upper extremity symptoms favors an immune-mediated (e.g., microvasculitic) mechanism, such as that seen with hereditary neuralgic amyotrophy, neuralgic amyotrophy and diabetic cervical radiculoplexus neuropathy (diabetic CRPN), whereas a more gradual or insidious onset of symptoms would point toward neoplastic invasion or postradiotherapy plexopathy. Immune-mediated plexopathies (e.g., diabetic LRPN or neuralgic amyotrophy) usually begin with severe pain, lasting days to weeks, followed by the development of weakness a few days to a few weeks later. Radiation-associated plexopathy (e.g., for breast cancer) usually presents with much less pain than plexopathy due to malignancy or due to immune-mediated mechanism. Radiation-induced brachial or lumbosacral plexopathy usually presents more gradually and can occur months to decades after radiotherapy. Recurrent, painful brachial plexopathy is most typical of hereditary neuralgic amyotrophy. The recognition of accompanying symptoms is also important. For example, weight loss is a common accompaniment of diabetic LRPN or diabetic CRPN, as well as plexopathies secondary to neoplasm or a more systemic process such as vasculitis.

In the case presented above, the temporal evolution was of an abrupt-onset neuropathic process that caused motor and sensory dysfunction. The neuropathic process involved one lower extremity. The pain was so severe that the patient required narcotics. The patient had not experienced antecedent trauma, surgery, or radiotherapy. There was no family history of plexopathy. These factors suggested that an immune-mediated plexopathy was likely. Furthermore, the clinical setting was remarkable for diabetes mellitus and significant weight loss, and as diabetes mellitus is believed to be a risk factor for immune-mediated plexopathy and many of these patients experience contemporaneous weight loss, this diagnosis was most likely. Thus, the most likely etiology in this patient was DLRPN. Additional evaluation, including examination, electrodiagnostic testing and imaging, further supported the diagnosis (Fig. 64-2).

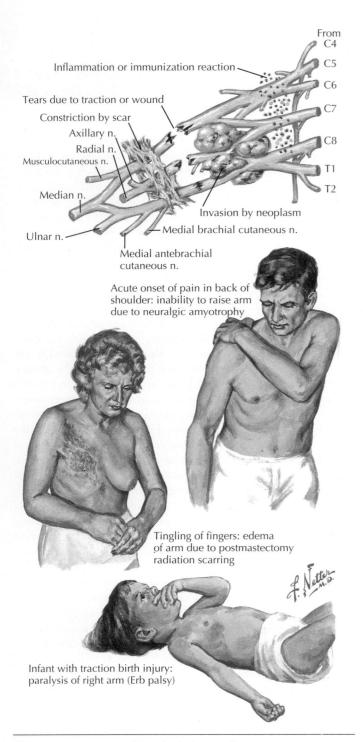

Figure 64-1 labels:

From
C4
C5
C6
C7
C8
T1
T2

Inflammation or immunization reaction

Tears due to traction or wound

Constriction by scar

Axillary n.

Radial n.

Musculocutaneous n.

Median n.

Ulnar n.

Invasion by neoplasm

Medial brachial cutaneous n.

Medial antebrachial cutaneous n.

Acute onset of pain in back of shoulder: inability to raise arm due to neuralgic amyotrophy

Tingling of fingers: edema of arm due to postmastectomy radiation scarring

Infant with traction birth injury: paralysis of right arm (Erb palsy)

Figure 64-1 Causes of Brachial Plexopathy.

Table 64-1 Brachial Plexus Etiologies

Mechanism	Examples	Comments
Trauma, traction	Motorcycle injury, cardiothoracic surgery	Often severe degree, poor prognosis
Stinger	Football etc.	Good prognosis
Perinatal	Mixed mechanisms	Generally good prognosis
Idiopathic	Autoimmune?	Self-limited
Hereditary	Genetically determined	Recurrent, benign
Malignancy	Infiltration of tumor cells	Poor prognosis
Radiation	RoRx-induced ischemia	Prognosis guarded but not suggestive of recurrent tumor
Knapsack, rucksack, etc	Compression	Usually self-limited
Thoracic outlet	Entrapment	Rare, confused with CTS
Heroin induced	Indeterminate	

CTS, carpal tunnel syndrome; RoRx, radiation therapy.

disturbances, caused by disruption of the sympathetic fibers traversing the lower trunk to the superior cervical ganglia of the brachial plexus, may be present and include trophic skin changes, edema, reflex sympathetic dystrophy (complex regional pain syndrome), and Horner syndrome (miosis, ptosis, ipsilateral facial anhidrosis).

Upper plexus lesions of the lumbar plexus cause weakness of thigh flexion, adduction, and leg extension. Lower sacral plexus lesions result in weakness of thigh extension, knee flexion, and foot dorsiflexion and plantar flexion, and sensory changes. Complete lumbosacral plexopathy produces weakness and muscle atrophy throughout the lower extremity, with total areflexia and anesthesia. Concurrent autonomic loss results in warm, dry skin and peripheral edema.

In addition to considering etiologies for plexopathy, the clinician needs to consider whether processes that may be mimicking plexopathy are likely considerations. The presence of neuropathic pain can reasonably exclude pure motor processes, such as motor neuronopathies (e.g., amyotrophic lateral sclerosis), disorders of neuromuscular junction transmission (e.g., myasthenia gravis), and myopathies. Orthopedic injuries can sometimes mimic plexopathy, usually only when symptoms are relatively mild; the examination and electrodiagnostic testing usually identifies the plexopathy. The most important mimic of plexopathy is polyradiculopathy; nerve root lesions also present with both weakness and pain. The mechanism of nerve root injury may be structural (e.g., neural foraminal stenosis or disk herniation), infectious (e.g., Lyme neuroborreliosis), or neoplastic (e.g., carcinomatous meningitis).

ANATOMY

Brachial Plexus

The brachial plexus is formed from the ventral rami of cervical roots 5–8 and thoracic root 1 (Fig. 64-3). The ventral rami of

CLINICAL PRESENTATION

Plexus lesions commonly result in unilateral or asymmetric extremity muscle weakness and sensory complaints that do not conform to the distributions of single roots or nerves. Brachial plexopathies cause shoulder girdle weakness if the upper plexus is involved and hand weakness if the lower, or medial plexus is principally involved. Sensory loss is usually variable but follows a similar pattern; for example, a medial plexus lesion causes numbness of the fourth and fifth fingers. Autonomic

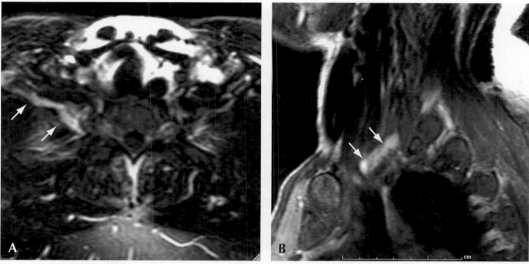

Axial (**A**) and sagittal (**B**) T1-weighted post gadolinium-enhanced images of the brachial plexus showing enhancement around the right brachial plexus (arrows).

Figure 64-2 Parsonage-Turner brachial plexitis.

the fifth and sixth cervical roots together form the upper trunk, the seventh cervical root ventral ramus becomes the middle trunk, and the eighth cervical and first thoracic root ventral rami join to become the lower trunk. The trunks of the brachial plexus are located above the clavicle between the scalenus anterior and scalenus medius muscles, in the posterior triangle of the neck, posterior and lateral to the sternocleidomastoid muscle. The dorsal scapular, long thoracic, and suprascapular nerves originate from the brachial plexus above the clavicle. Behind the clavicle and in front of the first rib, each trunk separates into anterior and posterior divisions. The anterior divisions of the upper and middle trunks unite to become the lateral cord, whereas the anterior division of the lower trunk forms the medial cord. The posterior divisions of all three trunks unite to become the posterior cord. The three cords are named for their positions relative to the axillary artery. Below the clavicle, the upper extremity nerves arise from the cords. From the lateral cord arises the musculocutaneous, the lateral head of the median, and the lateral pectoral nerves. From the medial cord comes the ulnar, the medial head of the median, the medial pectoral, and the medial brachial and medial antebrachial nerves. From the posterior cord arise the radial, axillary, subscapular, and thoracodorsal nerves.

Lumbosacral Plexus

The femoral nerve, innervating the iliopsoas and the quadriceps femoris muscles, is the predominant derivative of the lumbar portion of the lumbosacral plexus (Fig. 64-4). Its sensory supply includes the anterior and lateral thigh, and the medial foreleg as the saphenous nerve. The obturator nerve innervating the adductor magnus also originates from the lumbar plexus. The sacral portion of the lumbosacral plexus innervates the remainder of the lower extremity muscles, including posterior thigh and buttocks muscles and all leg musculature below the knee.

The superior and inferior gluteal nerves, the most proximal nerves originating from the sacral derivative of the lumbosacral plexus, innervate the gluteal muscles (medius, minimus, and maximus). The sciatic nerve innervates the hamstring group and bifurcates into the peroneal and tibial nerves, providing all motor innervation below the knee. The sciatic nerve provides sensory innervation to the posterior thigh and the entire leg below the knee, with the exception of the medial foreleg, which is supplied only by the saphenous nerve. The peroneal nerve is derived from the lateral portion of the sciatic nerve within the thigh; it supplies only one muscle above the knee, the short head of the biceps femoris. This site provides a means to differentiate electrodiagnostically atypical proximal peroneal or sciatic nerve lesions from common peroneal nerve compression or entrapment syndromes at the fibular head. The peroneal nerve bifurcates into the superficial and deep peroneal nerves, the latter innervating all anterior compartment muscles. The superficial peroneal motor nerve supplies the lateral compartment. The tibial nerve, the other primary sciatic nerve derivative, supplies the calf. The superficial peroneal sensory, the sural, and the medial and lateral plantar nerves are the primary superficial sensory nerves below the knee, in addition to the saphenous.

DIAGNOSTIC APPROACH

The neurologic examination should focus on identifying any motor, sensory, and reflex impairment referable to the different components of the plexus. A diminished or absent biceps reflex would be expected for a brachial plexopathy involving the upper trunk, for example. Weakness involving the hand and wrist would point toward lower trunk/medial cord brachial plexus involvement. In addition to localizing a lesion to particular trunks and cords, the examination can sometimes help determine whether lesions are preganglionic (e.g., root avulsion) or postganglionic (e.g., upper trunk plexopathy). Weakness of the

Comparison of Embryonic Limb Organization to the Plan of the Brachial Plexus

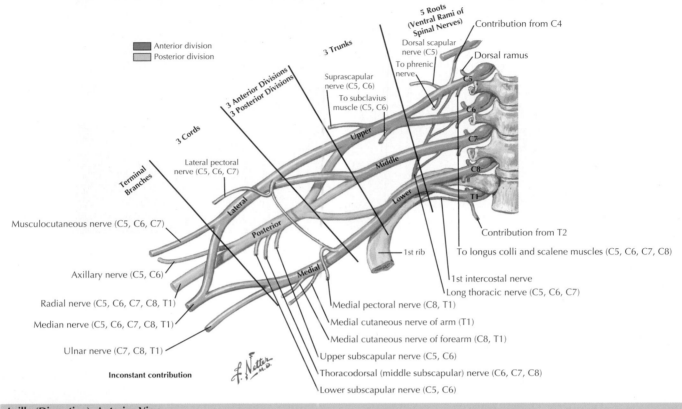

Axilla (Dissection): Anterior View

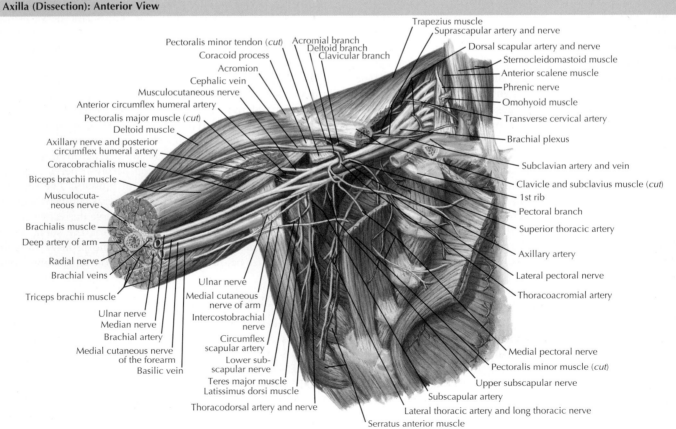

Figure 64-3 Anatomy of Brachial Plexus.

Lumbar Plexus

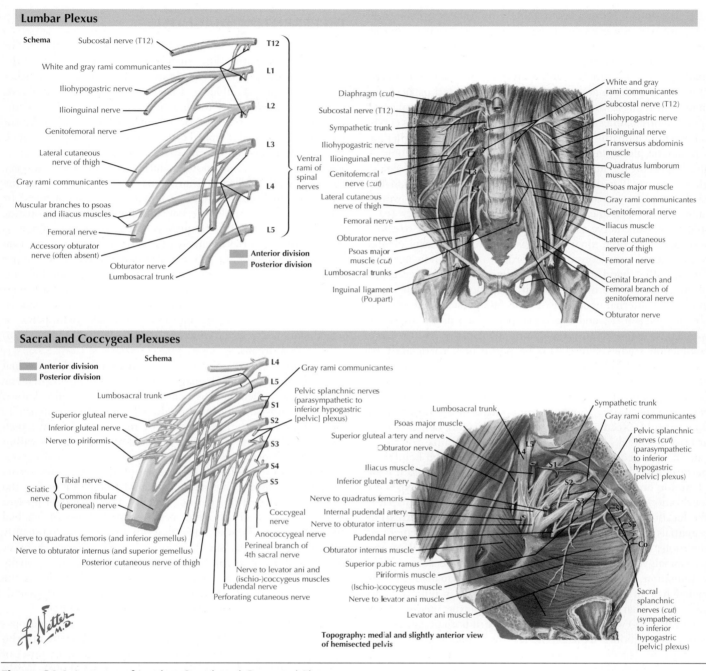

Figure 64-4 Anatomy of Lumbar, Sacral, and Coccygeal Plexuses.

rhomboid muscles (from C4 and C5 roots) and the serratus anterior muscle (from C5, C6, and C7 roots) would suggest involvement as proximal as the cervical root. Needle examination of these muscles and cervical paraspinal muscles, discussed below, will be helpful also in determining where the lesions are along the length of the nerve.

Electrodiagnostic (EDX) testing helps confirm the diagnosis and localization of a suspected plexopathy. Rarely, nonneuropathic processes (e.g., rotator cuff tendinitis, hip fracture) can mimic plexopathy, in which case EDX testing and the neurologic examination will be normal. More commonly, EDX testing serves to confirm localization of a neuropathic process to the

plexus. A watershed for the localization of plexopathies is the dorsal root ganglia (DRG), with lesions involving segments proximal to the DRG (e.g., root) classified as preganglionic lesions, whereas those distal to the DRG (e.g., trunk) are labeled as postganglionic lesions. Assessment of sensory nerve action potentials (SNAPs) is very helpful with this localization because the preservation of SNAPs favors a preganglionic lesion (e.g., radiculopathy) whereas the diminution or loss of SNAPs favors a postganglionic lesion (e.g., plexopathy). For a unilateral plexopathy, the SNAP abnormality should be on the side of the lesion, and for asymmetric plexopathies, the SNAP abnormalities should theoretically be more severe on the more affected side. Side-to-side differences in SNAP amplitude of greater than 50% are typically considered significant, but repeat testing at the same sitting to confirm that this finding is not simply technical is advisable, particularly given the significance of such a finding for localization. Differentiating preganglionic (e.g., radiculopathy) from postganglionic plexopathy is a particularly important request when trying to differentiate a structural (e.g., spinal stenosis), infectious (e.g., Lyme), or carcinomatous cervical polyradiculopathy from a plexopathy. Determining whether a traumatic plexus injury is preganglionic or postganglionic is also important for surgical management. For instance, preganglionic lesions (e.g., root avulsions) are generally not amenable to direct plexus repair with nerve grafting and hence would more likely be surgically treated with a nerve transfer (e.g., spinal accessory nerve to suprascapular nerve in order to allow shoulder abduction, ulnar nerve fascicle to flexor carpi ulnaris to the musculocutaneous nerve in order to allow elbow flexion). On the other hand, postganglionic lesions (e.g., upper trunk plexopathy) may be directly repaired at the plexus with nerve grafting or internal neurolysis. In the case presented above, the absent sural sensory and superficial peroneal sensory responses were consistent with a postganglionic plexopathy. Motor nerve conduction studies should also be performed, particularly to look for low CMAP amplitudes over muscles innervated by affected nerves. Needle examination helps localize the lesion, both longitudinally (i.e., where along the length of the nerve or root) and specifically to which components of the plexus (e.g., upper trunk). Needle examination should *ideally* be performed at least 2–3 weeks after onset in order to maximize what data can be collected from the study, but it still can be helpful to perform a study earlier than that because reduced recruitment of motor unit potentials of weak muscles can still help with localization. Abnormalities on needle examination can map out the location of the plexus lesions. The presence of fibrillation potentials in paraspinal muscles would point to involvement of the roots; however, the absence of fibrillation potentials in the paraspinals does not exclude radiculopathy because needle examination of paraspinal muscles will be normal in an estimated half of patients with radiculopathy. It is important to also note that patients with radiculoplexus neuropathies (e.g., DLRPN) will demonstrate evidence of both preganglionic and postganglionic damage, hence the name radiculoplexus neuropathy. Needle examination can also sometimes assist in determining etiology. For example, plexopathies secondary to radiotherapy are sometimes associated with myokymic discharges on needle study, whereas plexopathies due to another cause (e.g., neoplasm) are much less likely to reveal myokymic discharges.

Routine radiographs, CT, and MRI of the lumbosacral spine and pelvis are often required to exclude inflammatory or mass lesions within the spine or pelvis. CSF examination may be indicated to exclude infection. CSF protein is increased in approximately 50% of patients with idiopathic lumbosacral plexopathy. In vasculitic lumbosacral plexopathy, nerve biopsy may reveal ischemic nerve injury caused by microvasculitis or vasculitis. Histopathologic evidence of vasculitis is frequently seen on biopsy of patients with DLRPN, although often the clinical context and other ancillary studies provide enough evidence of the diagnosis so that a nerve biopsy can be avoided.

DIFFERENTIAL DIAGNOSIS

Trauma is the most common pathophysiologic mechanism for a brachial plexopathy. The superficial anatomic location of the brachial plexus with close proximity to bony and vascular structures within the shoulder and neck predisposes it to this risk. Traumatic mechanisms for brachial plexopathy include compression, traction, ischemia, laceration, or a combination. Motor vehicle accidents, high-speed cycling accidents, gunshot or knife wounds, and falls can be causative. Some events may be iatrogenic; for example, positioning during cardiothoracic surgery that maximally abducts the arm, may cause stretching of the lateral brachial plexus. Sporting activities causing "burners" or "stingers" are common mechanisms for brachial plexopathy. Despite their relative frequency, their pathophysiology is unclear; these injuries are likely caused by compression, traction or both, usually of the C5–6 cervical nerve roots and upper trunk of the brachial plexus. Trauma to the lumbosacral plexus, on the other hand, is uncommon because the nerves are relatively immobile and protected by the vertebrae, psoas muscle, and pelvis. Most traumatic injuries are associated with pelvic or acetabular fractures, frequently with soft-tissue injuries to other pelvic organs.

Neuralgic amyotrophy (also known as idiopathic brachial plexus neuropathy or Parsonage–Turner syndrome) and diabetic lumbosacral radiculoplexus neuropathy (DLRPN; also known as diabetic amyotrophy) are thought to be autoimmune in origin. Both conditions are likely caused by microvasculitis, in which case the autoimmune attack is directed at small vessels within and near the nerves of the roots, plexus and proximal nerves. Neuralgic amyotrophy of the brachial plexus sometimes occurs after a viral illness, vaccination, or mild trauma or during the immediate postpartum period. Usually, these patients present with relatively acute shoulder pain and partial loss of brachial plexus function. Typically, neuralgic amyotrophy predominantly affects nerves of the shoulder girdle muscles, although other portions of the plexus and its terminal branches are occasionally involved, especially the anterior interosseous segment of the median nerve. Approximately one third of patients with neuralgic amyotrophy have bilateral, asymmetric involvement.

DLRPN is the most common cause of lumbosacral plexopathy (Fig. 64-5). DLRPN typically presents in older patients who have type 2 diabetes mellitus, with abrupt or subacute onset of hip and thigh severe pain (see case presentation above). Weakness and muscle atrophy occur within a week or two, often at the time the pain begins to improve. Muscle stretch reflexes may be lost, especially at the knee. DLRPN often begins unilaterally but frequently progresses to bilateral involvement. This monophasic disorder is usually significantly disabling and is commonly associated with unexplained weight loss. Like neuralgic amyotrophy, DLRPN is thought to originate from peripheral nerve microvasculitis. Idiopathic lumbosacral radiculoplexus neuropathy (LRPN) is a rare primary plexopathy that occurs in nondiabetics. It is also manifested by rapid onset of pain, leg weakness, and atrophy. Patients often experience a viral illness 1–2 weeks before symptoms begin. Lumbar plexus involvement often affects the most proximal musculature, causing weakness of the iliopsoas, quadriceps, and adductor muscles. Often, significant recovery occurs within 3 months.

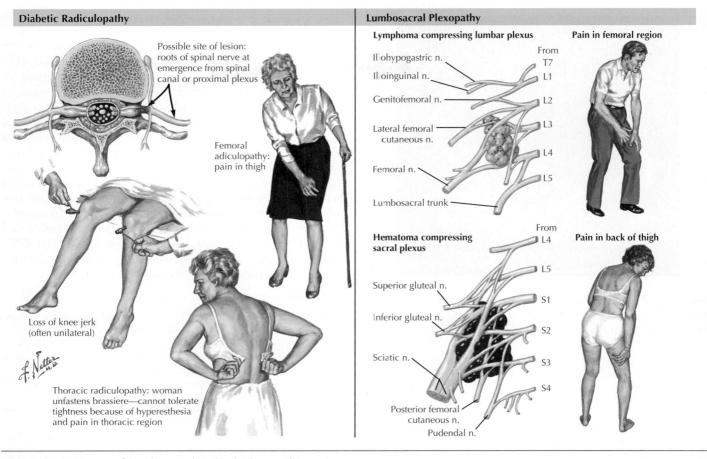

Diabetic Radiculopathy

Possible site of lesion: roots of spinal nerve at emergence from spinal canal or proximal plexus

Femoral radiculopathy: pain in thigh

Loss of knee jerk (often unilateral)

Thoracic radiculopathy: woman unfastens brassiere—cannot tolerate tightness because of hyperesthesia and pain in thoracic region

Lumbosacral Plexopathy

Lymphoma compressing lumbar plexus

Iliohypogastric n.
Ilioinguinal n.
Genitofemoral n.
Lateral femoral cutaneous n.
Femoral n.
Lumbosacral trunk

From T7
L1
L2
L3
L4
L5

Pain in femoral region

Hematoma compressing sacral plexus

Superior gluteal n.
Inferior gluteal n.
Sciatic n.
Posterior femoral cutaneous n.
Pudendal n.

From L4
L5
S1
S2
S3
S4

Pain in back of thigh

Figure 64-5 Causes of Lumbosacral Radiculoplexopathies.

Hereditary neuralgic amyotrophy (also known as hereditary brachial plexus neuropathy) is an autosomal dominant disorder characterized by periodic, often recurrent, episodes of unilateral or asymmetric pain, weakness, atrophy, and sensory alterations in the shoulder girdle and upper extremity. Genetically, many cases of HBPN are caused by mutations in the SEPT9 gene. Hereditary neuralgic amyotrophy is also believed to be an immune-mediated disorder and likely a microvasculitis with a strong genetic predisposition caused by an inherited SEPT9 mutation.

Malignant tumors, particularly apical lung or postradiation breast cancer, are common causes of brachial plexus lesions (Fig. 64-6). With apical lung tumors, the lesion may insidiously advance, causing numbness in the fourth and fifth fingers, weakness in the ulnar and median hand intrinsic muscles, and Horner syndrome (Pancoast tumor). Often, pain is significant, secondary to neoplastic infiltration of the brachial plexus. This clinical constellation sometimes precedes recognition of the lung tumor. Every patient who smokes and presents in this fashion requires a chest CT or MRI. Tumors occasionally invade the lumbosacral plexus by primary extension from pelvic, abdominal, or retroperitoneal malignancies (see Fig. 64-5). Pain in the distribution of the affected nerves is the cardinal symptom. Late symptoms and signs may include numbness and paresthesias, weakness and gait abnormalities, and lower extremity edema. Retroperitoneal

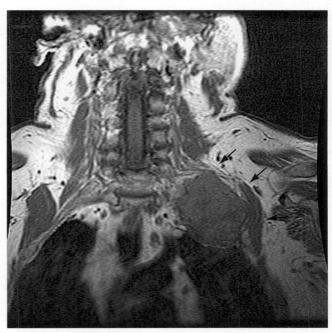

Coronal T1-weighted image demonstrates large left apical lung mass extending into brachial plexus (arrows).

Figure 64-6 Apical lung tumor invading left brachial plexus.

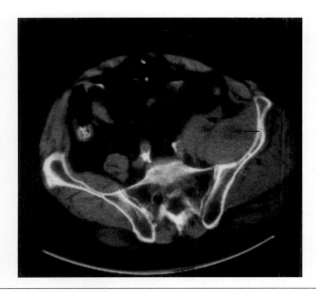

Figure 64-7 Large hematoma involves the left iliacus and psoas muscles (arrow) and adjacent region, likely involving the lumbar plexus and femoral nerve.

hematomas can compress the lumbar or sacral plexuses or both. Patients present with unilateral pelvic or groin pain; the patient preferentially has the hip flexed to minimize pressure on the plexus (Fig. 64-7). This condition is typically a complication of anticoagulation therapy, or less commonly bleeding diatheses, and immediate surgical decompression can be beneficial.

Compressive lumbosacral plexopathies may also occur from a number of other mechanisms, including late pregnancy or childbirth and abdominal aortic aneurysms. A retroperitoneal infection such as a psoas abscess rarely affects the lumbosacral plexus. Radiation-induced lumbosacral plexopathies develop months to years after radiotherapy to pelvic malignancies. The lumbar plexus is more commonly affected in radiation-induced lesions, whereas the sacral plexus is more frequently affected by neoplastic plexopathies. Painless weakness develops at a variable rate, ultimately causing asymmetric but significant weakness of both lower extremities. Paresthesias and pain are common but usually mild. Sphincter involvement is rare.

TREATMENT AND PROGNOSIS

Treatment of plexus lesions comprises management of the primary condition. Careful glucose control may hasten DLRPN recovery and improve outcome. The efficacy of steroids or intravenous immunoglobulin in the acute or subacute phase of DLRPN is not proven, although anecdotal reports suggest clinical benefit and some evidence is emerging that the pain and other neuropathic symptoms may respond to these treatment options. Most traumatic lesions are treated conservatively, although pelvic fractures and gunshot wounds may necessitate surgery. No effective treatment exists for radiation-induced brachial or lumbosacral plexopathy. Oncologic intervention is necessary for neoplastic brachial or lumbosacral plexopathy. Symptomatic pain management is usually necessary. Pain control with narcotics is often necessary in the acute phase of DLRPN, LRPN, neuralgic amyotrophy, hereditary neuralgic amyotrophy, traumatic plexopathy, and neoplastic plexopathies.

ADDITIONAL RESOURCES

Dyck PJ, Norell JE, Dyck PJ. Microvasculitis and ischemia in diabetic lumbosacral radiculoplexus neuropathy. Neurology 1999;53:2113-2121.

Dyck PJ, Norell JE, Dyck PJ. Non-diabetic lumbosacral radiculoplexus neuropathy: natural history, outcome and comparison with the diabetic variety. Brain 2001;124:1197-1207.

Ferrante MA. Brachial plexopathies: classification, causes, and consequences. Muscle Nerve 2004;30:547-568.

Lederman RJ, Wilbourn AJ. Postpartum neuralgic amyotrophy. Neurology 1996;47:1213-1219.

Moghekar AR, Moghekar AB, Karli N, et al. Brachial plexopathies. Etiology, frequency and electrodiagnostic localization. J Clin Neuromusc Dis 2007;9:243-247.

Parsonage MJ, Turner JWA. Neuralgic amyotrophy. The shoulder-girdle syndrome. Lancet 1948;973-978.

Rubin DI. Diseases of the plexus. Continuum 2008;14:156-181.

Suarez GA, Giannini C, Bosch EP, et al. Immune brachial plexus neuropathy: suggestive evidence for an inflammatory immune pathogenesis. Neurology 1996;46:559-561.

Triggs W, Young MS, Eskin T, et al. Treatment of idiopathic lumbosacral plexopathy with intravenous immunoglobulin. Muscle Nerve 1997;20:244-246.

Tsairis P, Dyck PJ, Mulder DW. Natural history of brachial plexus neuropathy. Report on 99 patients. Arch Neurol 1972;27:109-117.

Van Alfen N. The neuralgic amyotrophy consultation. J Neurol 2007;254:695-704.

Van Alfen N, van Engelen BGM. The clinical spectrum of neuralgic amyotrophy in 246 cases. Brain 2006;129:438-450.

Verma A, Bradley WB. High dose intravenous immunoglobulin therapy in chronic progressive lumbosacral plexopathy. Neurology 1994;44:248-250.

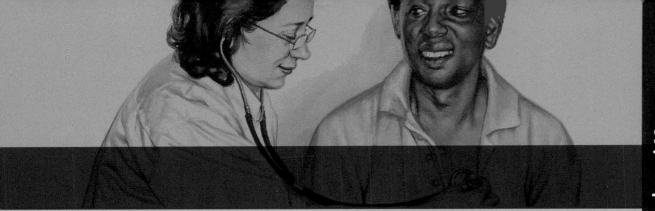

Mononeuropathies

Mononeuropathies of the Upper Extremities

Gisela Held and Miruna Segarceanu

65

MONONEUROPATHIES OF THE SHOULDER GIRDLE

Mononeuropathies of the shoulder girdle are relatively uncommon and can be challenging to diagnose. Unlike other mononeuropathies, pain is often the cardinal symptom, and shoulder pain and weakness, real or perceived, can originate from mononeuropathies, but also from cervical disc disease, disorders of the musculoskeletal system, or vascular causes. True weakness can be difficult to separate from impaired effort due to pain. Shoulder muscles might appear weak in rotator cuff or other tendon tears in the absence of nerve injury.

Shoulder girdle mononeuropathies are caused by the following mechanisms: stretch, transecting injury, brachial plexus neuritis with patchy involvement of isolated nerves, direct compression, or entrapment. The history should help define the precise location of the pain, positions and activities that provoke pain, the time of day of maximal discomfort, and any precipitating injury. Paresthesias or sensory loss, particularly if well defined within a recognized single nerve distribution, usually indicates peripheral nerve pathology. Atrophy can be related to axon loss or occasionally prolonged disuse; sometimes the clinical distinction is difficult. Shoulder motion is evaluated for abnormal dynamics of the glenohumeral, acromioclavicular, and scapulothoracic joints.

DORSAL SCAPULAR NEUROPATHIES

Clinical Vignette

A 27-year-old professional weight lifter complained about difficulty exercising. He had trouble getting his wallet out of the right back pocket of his pants. Examination revealed weakness of the right rhomboid muscles without noticeable muscle atrophy. There was scapular winging with lateral displacement of the scapula, most pronounced during elevation of the arm. Electrophysiologic testing disclosed active and chronic denervation–reinnervation changes in the right rhomboids. Testing of other arm and shoulder muscles was normal.

The dorsal scapular nerve receives fibers from the C5 nerve root. It innervates the levator scapulae and the rhomboideus major and minor muscles, which assist in stabilization of the scapula, rotation of the scapula in a medial–inferior direction, and elevation of the arm (Fig. 65-1). Rhomboid weakness can lead to scapular winging, which is most prominent when the patient raises the arm overhead. Possible etiologies of injury to this nerve include shoulder dislocation, weightlifting, and entrapment by the scalenus medius muscle.

LONG THORACIC NEUROPATHIES

Clinical Vignette

A 57-year-old left-handed woman underwent a left mastectomy for breast cancer. Immediately following the surgery, she noted an aching pain in the left posterior shoulder area. After discharge from the hospital, she had difficulty using the left arm. In particular, she complained of being unable to get dishes from the kitchen cabinets. She was not aware of sensory loss. Electrodiagnostic testing 3 weeks later showed evidence of acute denervation changes in the left serratus anterior muscle, consistent with a mononeuropathy of the long thoracic nerve.

The long thoracic nerve originates directly from C5–C7 roots, before the formation of the brachial plexus. It innervates the serratus anterior muscle and has no cutaneous sensory representation (Fig. 65-2). Weakness of the serratus anterior is debilitating, because it stabilizes the scapula for pushing movements and elevates the arm above 90 degrees. This is the most common cause of scapular winging; it is best recognized by having the patient push against a wall. The inferior medial border is the most prominently projected away from the body wall. A dull shoulder ache may accompany this neuropathy. When severe acute pain occurs with the onset of scapular winging, brachial plexus neuritis should be considered.

The long thoracic nerve may be damaged by mechanical factors, including repetitive or particularly forceful injuries to the shoulder or lateral thoracic wall and by surgical procedures including first rib resection, mastectomy, or thoracotomy. It is one of the most common nerves to be affected by acute brachial neuritis, solely or in combination with others.

Scapular winging can also be related to scapular fracture and avulsion. Because they are surgically correctable, it is important to distinguish them from a primary long thoracic nerve injury. Furthermore, scapular winging can be caused by weakness of the trapezius (resulting from injury of the spinal accessory nerve) or the rhomboid muscles (resulting from a dorsal scapular nerve lesion). Inspection of the posterior shoulder region can provide diagnostic clues. Although the scapula is typically displaced medially in long thoracic nerve lesions, lateral deviation points to weakness of the trapezius or rhomboids. Scapular winging is a predominant feature in patients with facioscapulohumeral muscular dystrophy, where its bilateral representation and the other associated clinical features distinguish it from long thoracic nerve palsy.

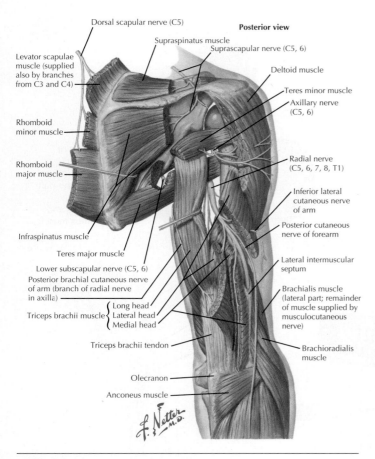

Dorsal scapular nerve (C5)

Posterior view

Suprascapular muscle

Suprascapular nerve (C5, 6)

Levator scapulae muscle (supplied also by branches from C3 and C4)

Deltoid muscle

Teres minor muscle

Axillary nerve (C5, 6)

Rhomboid minor muscle

Radial nerve (C5, 6, 7, 8, T1)

Rhomboid major muscle

Inferior lateral cutaneous nerve of arm

Posterior cutaneous nerve of forearm

Infraspinatus muscle

Teres major muscle

Lateral intermuscular septum

Lower subscapular nerve (C5, 6)
Posterior brachial cutaneous nerve of arm (branch of radial nerve in axilla)

Brachialis muscle (lateral part; remainder of muscle supplied by musculocutaneous nerve)

Triceps brachii muscle { Long head / Lateral head / Medial head }

Triceps brachii tendon

Brachioradialis muscle

Olecranon

Anconeus muscle

Figure 65-1 Radial Nerve in Arm and Nerves of Posterior Shoulder.

SUPRASCAPULAR NEUROPATHIES

Clinical Vignette

A 25-year-old right-handed woman was evaluated for dull right shoulder pain and weakness. The symptoms were most noticeable during overhead activities. She had no sensory loss, and no injury had preceded the onset of her symptoms. Examination disclosed tenderness to palpation at the spinoglenoid notch. Shoulder position was normal; range of motion was full. Motor examination was significant for weakness of external shoulder rotation and mild atrophy of the infraspinatus muscle overlying the scapula. Reflexes and sensory examination were normal. These findings of infraspinatus atrophy, weak external rotation of the shoulder, and point tenderness over the spinoglenoid notch were consistent with a focal suprascapular neuropathy. Electromyography (EMG) demonstrated active denervation changes confined to the infraspinatus muscle consistent with the clinical diagnosis. A magnetic resonance image (MRI) of the right shoulder revealed a cystic lesion at the spinoglenoid notch, which was confirmed by surgical exploration.

The suprascapular nerve emerges from the upper trunk of the brachial plexus, receiving fibers from C5 and C6 roots. It does not have any cutaneous innervation. The suprascapular nerve first provides innervation to the supraspinatus muscle, a

shoulder abductor, and then to the infraspinatus, a shoulder external rotator (see Fig. 65-1). The suprascapular nerve may be injured at the suprascapular notch, before the innervation of the supraspinatus muscle, or distally at the spinoglenoid notch, affecting the infraspinatus alone (see Fig. 65-2). The most common site of entrapment is at the suprascapular notch, under the transverse scapular ligament. Acute-onset cases result from blunt shoulder trauma, with or without scapular fracture, or from forceful anterior rotation of the scapula. The suprascapular nerve may also be affected by brachial plexus neuritis in isolation or with other nerves. Suprascapular neuropathies of insidious onset often occur subsequent to callous formation after fractures, from entrapment at the suprascapular or spinoglenoid notch, by compression from a ganglion or other soft tissue mass, or by traction caused by repetitive overhead activities such as volleyball or tennis.

AXILLARY NEUROPATHIES

Clinical Vignette

A 72-year-old man had pain and weakness of the right arm following a fall. Evaluation in the emergency room disclosed an anterior dislocation of the right shoulder, which was reduced. Despite treatment, the patient continued to have difficulty raising the arm above the head. Electrodiagnostic testing several weeks later showed reduced recruitment pattern of motor unit action potentials in the right deltoid and teres minor muscles. The EMG was suggestive of stretch injury with demyelinating nerve injury without evidence of axon loss. The patient recovered spontaneously over the course of the following month.

The axillary nerve, along with the radial nerve, is a terminal branch of the posterior cord of the brachial plexus. It innervates the deltoid and the teres minor and provides sensory innervation to the lateral upper part of the shoulder via the superior lateral brachial cutaneous nerve of the arm (Figs. 65-1 and 65-3). In lesions of the axillary nerve, shoulder abduction is weakened and cutaneous sensibility of the lateral shoulder diminishes, overlapping the C5 dermatome. Because the teres minor is not the predominant external rotator of the shoulder, clinical isolation and testing are difficult. EMG may be necessary to define neurogenic injury to this muscle. Most axillary neuropathies are traumatic, related to anterior shoulder dislocations, humerus fractures, or both. Recognition of nerve injury may be delayed because of the shoulder injury. Acute axillary neuropathies can result from blunt trauma or as a component or sole manifestation of brachial plexus neuritis.

MUSCULOCUTANEOUS NEUROPATHIES

Clinical Vignette

A 43-year-old woman presented to the laboratory for routine blood work after her annual physical examination. During phlebotomy in the right antecubital fossa, she experienced

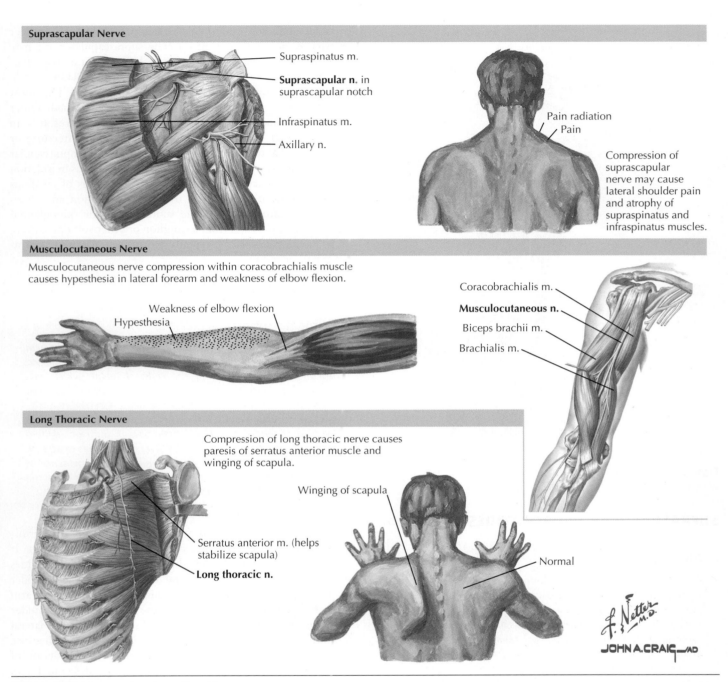

Figure 65-2 Neuropathy about Shoulder.

a sharp pain, radiating from the elbow to the wrist, which persisted for several days. She then developed numbness of the right lateral forearm. She had no weakness. Nerve conduction studies showed an absent sensory nerve action potential of the lateral antebrachial cutaneous nerve. The needle examination was normal.

The musculocutaneous nerve originates directly from the lateral cord of the brachial plexus. It innervates the coracobrachialis, biceps brachii, and brachialis muscles and terminates in its cutaneous branch, the lateral antebrachial cutaneous nerve. Isolated musculocutaneous neuropathies are rare. They have

been reported in weight lifters, after surgery, and after prolonged pressure during sleep. Damage to the musculocutaneous nerve results in weakness of forearm flexion and supination and sensory loss of the lateral volar forearm (see Fig. 65-2). The biceps reflex is diminished, but the brachioradialis reflex (same myotome, different nerve) is preserved. More commonly, injury to this nerve occurs as part of a more widespread traumatic injury, usually involving the proximal humerus. The musculocutaneous nerve can also be preferentially involved in acute brachial plexus neuritis. Distal lesions of the lateral antebrachial cutaneous nerve may result from attempted cannulation of the basilic vein in the antecubital fossa. Rupture of the biceps tendon is a significant differential diagnostic consideration of musculocutaneous neuropathy.

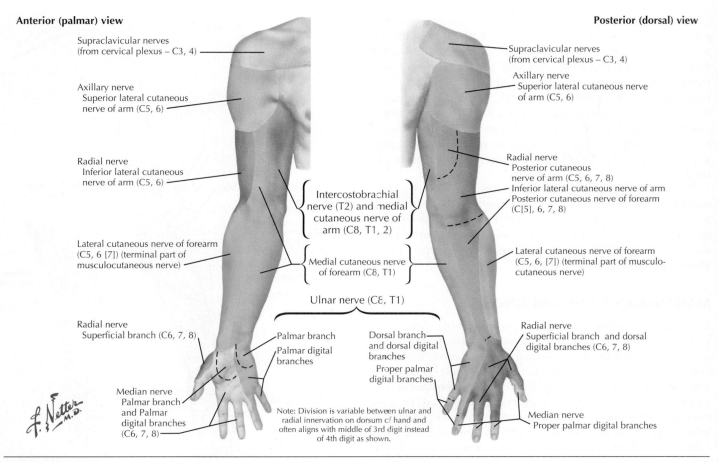

Anterior (palmar) view

Supraclavicular nerves
(from cervical plexus – C3, 4)

Axillary nerve
Superior lateral cutaneous
nerve of arm (C5, 6)

Radial nerve
Inferior lateral cutaneous
nerve of arm (C5, 6)

Lateral cutaneous nerve of forearm
(C5, 6 [7]) (terminal part of
musculocutaneous nerve)

Radial nerve
Superficial branch (C6, 7, 8)

Median nerve
Palmar branch
and Palmar
digital branches
(C6, 7, 8)

Palmar branch
Palmar digital
branches

Intercostobrachial
nerve (T2) and medial
cutaneous nerve of
arm (C8, T1, 2)

Medial cutaneous nerve
of forearm (C8, T1)

Ulnar nerve (C8, T1)

Dorsal branch
and dorsal digital
branches

Proper palmar
digital branches

Note: Division is variable between ulnar and
radial innervation on dorsum of hand and
often aligns with middle of 3rd digit instead
of 4th digit as shown.

Posterior (dorsal) view

Supraclavicular nerves
(from cervical plexus – C3, 4)

Axillary nerve
Superior lateral cutaneous nerve
of arm (C5, 6)

Radial nerve
Posterior cutaneous
nerve of arm (C5, 6, 7, 8)
Inferior lateral cutaneous nerve of arm
Posterior cutaneous nerve of forearm
(C[5], 6, 7, 8)

Lateral cutaneous nerve of forearm
(C5, 6, [7]) (terminal part of musculocutaneous nerve)

Radial nerve
Superficial branch and dorsal
digital branches (C6, 7, 8)

Median nerve
Proper palmar digital branches

Figure 65-3 Cutaneous Innervation of the Upper Limb.

DIFFERENTIAL DIAGNOSIS

The most common etiologies of shoulder pain are injuries to glenohumeral, subacromial, and acromioclavicular regions. Pain often may be reproduced by local pressure or provocative movements and positions. Rotator cuff tears can mimic nerve injury because of apparent weakness of shoulder abduction (supraspinatus) and external rotation (teres minor and infraspinatus). Motor neuron disease may begin in the shoulder region. It must be considered in the differential diagnosis of weakness without associated pain or sensory signs and symptoms. C5 radiculopathy also enters the differential diagnosis in patients reporting shoulder pain sometimes extending into the upper arm with weakness and numbness. This pain might originate within the scapular region and not the neck. Having patients flex their neck laterally in the direction of the symptomatic limb may reproduce the pain. Patients with C5 weakness have problems with shoulder abduction (deltoid and supraspinatus muscles), external rotation (infraspinatus), and arm flexion (biceps brachii). The biceps stretch reflex is often diminished. Paresthesias or sensory loss occurs in a discrete patch on the lateral proximal arm overlying the deltoid muscle.

DIAGNOSTIC APPROACH

EMG is the primary diagnostic tool in the evaluation of suspected shoulder mononeuropathies. It is particularly helpful to identify mononeuropathies affecting the shoulder girdle for several reasons. Neurogenic injury may go unsuspected because pain is the predominant symptom. Weakness may be hidden by the observation of normal strength within unaffected muscles performing similar functions, for example, supraspinatus weakness obscured by normal deltoid function. Conversely, nerve injury may be suspected because of apparent weakness caused by tendon rupture, only to be refuted by the absence of denervation on needle EMG. Although theoretically nerve conduction studies can be performed on the musculocutaneous and axillary nerves, their value is limited by technical factors. These nerves are typically accessible at only one stimulation site, precluding the determination of conduction velocities and accurate identification of conduction block. However, demyelination with conduction block may be suspected when a normal compound muscle action potential is obtained from a weak muscle; often, this finding portends an excellent prognosis. This conclusion should be reached cautiously because the same pattern may result from axon loss when the study is performed within the first week after injury, before wallerian degeneration has taken place.

Needle EMG can identify even subtle axon loss by the detection of fibrillation potentials. The evaluating physician and the electromyographer should always examine the patient and consider every potential neuropathic cause of shoulder pain. Otherwise, uncommon neuropathies can easily be overlooked.

A common clinical dilemma occurs with patients who have nontraumatic shoulder girdle mononeuropathies. It is difficult to differentiate a primary idiopathic lesion from a limited form of brachial plexus neuritis and to determine whether entrapment or a related process necessitating surgical exploration is involved. A thorough clinical and electrodiagnostic examination is thus required. Subtle clinical or electrodiagnostic evidence of involvement of muscles innervated by a different nerve usually suggests that a conservative approach is indicated, as this constellation of findings speaks against compression of a single nerve.

Routine radiographs are useful to detect scapular fractures secondary to acute injuries, which sometimes predispose patients to suprascapular neuropathies or serratus anterior dehiscence from the scapula. MRI can define insidious-onset neuropathies that may be caused by expanding masses, for example, a ganglion cyst in the spinoglenoid notch.

MANAGEMENT AND PROGNOSIS

Unfortunately, shoulder bracing provides little benefit to patients with shoulder girdle weakness. Exercises to strengthen other shoulder girdle muscles may provide partial functional compensation. If nerve transection from acute penetrating injury is suspected, surgical exploration and primary anastomosis should be considered, although results are mixed. In acute nonpenetrating injury, exploration can be considered after 3–6 months, provided no clinical or electrodiagnostic evidence of reinnervation exists. Nerve grafting is an option if unanticipated nerve transection is found. For insidious-onset neuropathies without defined cause, imaging should be considered to exclude ganglion cysts or other masses. If no mass is demonstrable and the patient shows no evidence of improvement, exploration may be considered, particularly at potential sites of entrapment such as the suprascapular or spinoglenoid notches.

Despite apparent axonal injury in brachial plexus neuritis, there is a good prognosis for functional recovery. Unfortunately, this recovery typically takes 6 months to 2 years. The prognosis for direct compressive injury is less predictable and probably depends on reinnervating distance, patient age, and attendant comorbidities. Stretch injuries and entrapment have the highest likelihood of a significant demyelinating component, with excellent outcome being the rule, particularly if entrapment is recognized and removed before significant axon loss occurs.

MEDIAN MONONEUROPATHIES

The anatomy of the median nerve is important in understanding the signs and symptoms of entrapment lesions at the level of the wrist, versus the more proximal lesions. The median nerve provides essential motor and sensory function to the lateral aspect of the hand (Fig. 65-4). It supplies the intrinsic hand muscles of most of the thenar eminence and innervates several forearm muscles. Its major sensory role is to provide innervation for the thumb, index, and middle fingers and the lateral half of the ring finger.

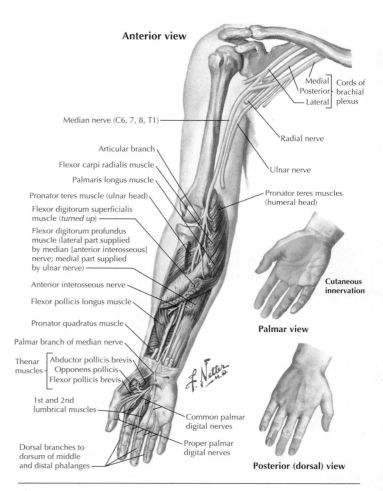

Figure 65-4 Median Nerve.

The median nerve is formed by lateral and medial cord fibers of the brachial plexus. The lateral cord carries mainly sensory fibers from C6–C7 roots and provides the sensory innervation to the thumb and the first two and a half fingers. It also contains motor fibers from the C6-C7 roots, which contribute to the innervation of the forearm muscles. The medial cord carries motor fibers from the C8-T1 roots that innervate the thenar eminence. The distal median nerve at the wrist is the primary site of clinical involvement in carpal tunnel syndrome. More proximal lesions at the elbow are far less common.

DISTAL MEDIAN ENTRAPMENT

Clinical Vignette

A 45-year-old factory worker presented with a 3-year history of intermittent right hand tingling. Initially, this had occurred only in the morning on awakening. In recent months, his symptoms had awoken him at night, interfering with his sleep. He reported that "all" digits were affected and that the paresthesias were sometimes accompanied by aching of the wrist and forearm. Shaking of the hand relieved the discomfort. There was no decline of hand strength. Neurologic examination disclosed minimal weakness of right thumb abduction without loss of thenar eminence bulk. Results of reflex and sensory examinations were normal, including 2-point discrimination and graded monofilament touch. The symptoms were reproduced by nerve percussion over the median nerve at the wrist (Tinel sign).

Etiology and Epidemiology

Carpal tunnel syndrome (CTS) is common and associated with high economic costs. The lifetime risk of acquiring CTS might be as high as 10%, with an approximate annual incidence of 0.3% and a peak in the 6th decade. CTS is more than three times more prevalent in women than in men and often affects both hands. The incidence is substantially increased in the working population, particularly blue-collar workers. Carpal tunnel syndrome has been associated with numerous other conditions, such as pregnancy, endocrine disorders (hypothyroidism, acromegaly, diabetes), rheumatoid arthritis, sarcoid, hemodialysis, and amyloidosis. However, most of the cases are idiopathic, related to repeated stress to the nerve, followed by edema, ischemia, and demyelination of the median nerve at the wrist. If the trauma is severe or prolonged enough, axonal loss ensues.

Clinical Presentation and Testing

Median nerve entrapment at the wrist commonly presents with intermittent symptoms, including pain and paresthesias in the hand and forearm. The symptoms tend to occur on awakening or at night, and they are often provoked by certain postures or activities such as reading or driving (Fig. 65-5). The perception that paresthesias may affect all digits (rather than just the lateral three and a half innervated by the median nerve) is likely related to the greater cortical representation of the thumb and first two fingers. As CTS progresses, persistent numbness ensues, alerting the patient that the precise sensory distribution involves the volar surface of the first three and a half digits. The neurologic examination, particularly in mild CTS cases, may offer few clues. It is helpful in severe cases, in which atrophy of the thenar eminence is common. Median hand functions, primarily thumb abduction and opposition, are weak. Having the patient supinate the forearm so the palm is flat, and then raise the thumb vertically against resistance, tests the abductor pollicis brevis muscle. Forearm muscles supplied by the median nerve proximal to the flexor retinaculum are spared in CTS.

Provocative tests offer supportive but not diagnostic evidence in suspected CTS (Fig. 65-6). A positive Tinel sign consists of an electric, shooting sensation (not just local discomfort) radiating into the appropriate digits with wrist percussion. Tinel and Phalen maneuvers (reproduction of paresthesias on forceful flexion of the wrist) should be performed with nonleading questions to improve response credibility. It is recommended that the Phalen maneuver be maintained for at least 1 minute before determining that the result is negative. The pressure test may be the most reliable of the three maneuvers; pressure is placed over the carpal tunnel (proximal palm, not wrist) for 20–30 seconds, attempting to reproduce paresthesias in a median nerve distribution.

Differential Diagnosis

Diagnosis of CTS is usually straightforward, although other conditions may mimic CTS. The assessment of the patient needs to incorporate clinical and electrophysiologic data, as more than 10% of the asymptomatic general population might have abnormal nerve conduction parameters suggestive of CTS. The most common differential diagnosis is a C6–C7 radiculopathy, in which numbness occurs in a similar distribution, that is, digits 1 through 3. Patients with a radiculopathy usually have neck or radicular pain. Nerve conduction studies and needle EMG can differentiate these entities. Although the muscles of both thenar and hypothenar eminence originate from the C8 root, its sensory territory is confined to the medial aspect of the hand and arm. The C8 root also innervates the flexor digitorum profundus of digits 4 and 5 and the extensor indicis proprius muscles via the ulnar and radial nerves, respectively. Ulnar neuropathies have an entirely different pattern of motor and sensory loss.

Carpal tunnel syndrome virtually never presents with predominant motor symptoms. If thumb abduction is weak, evidence of other motor involvement should be sought to confirm a different lesion. Weakness and atrophy confined to the median forearm muscles suggest a proximal median nerve lesion, particularly at the elbow (pronator syndrome). If more widespread weakness is demonstrated, with the absence of sensory signs or symptoms, motor neuron diseases or multifocal motor neuropathy require diagnostic consideration.

A more widespread polyneuropathy should be excluded. This can occur particularly in patients with diabetes, who may not be as aware of sensory loss in their feet compared with their hands. Clinical examination and EMG usually clarify this issue. Plexopathies typically produce motor and sensory dysfunction within multiple nerve distributions in a single extremity and pain in the shoulder region. They rarely enter the CTS differential diagnosis. Although it is uncommon for CNS disorders to produce sensory signs and symptoms within the distribution of a single peripheral nerve, occasionally cervical spinal cord lesions, such as cervical spinal stenosis or intrinsic cord tumors, and very rarely focal frontoparietal brain lesions, may mimic CTS. Vitamin B_{12} deficiency and syringomyelia are considerations in patients with bilateral hand numbness.

Management

Data regarding the natural history of CTS is scarce. Twenty to 30% of hands appear to improve spontaneously over 1–2 years, but this might in part be due to lifestyle changes, and long-term follow-up is not available. There are few randomized controlled trials comparing different treatment modalities. Treatment recommendations are further complicated by conflicting data as to whether clinical features or electrophysiological parameters can predict treatment outcome.

Conservative therapies should be considered first, as carpal tunnel release surgery carries a risk of potentially serious complications, such as reflex sympathetic dystrophy (complex regional pain syndrome), injury to the median palmar cutaneous

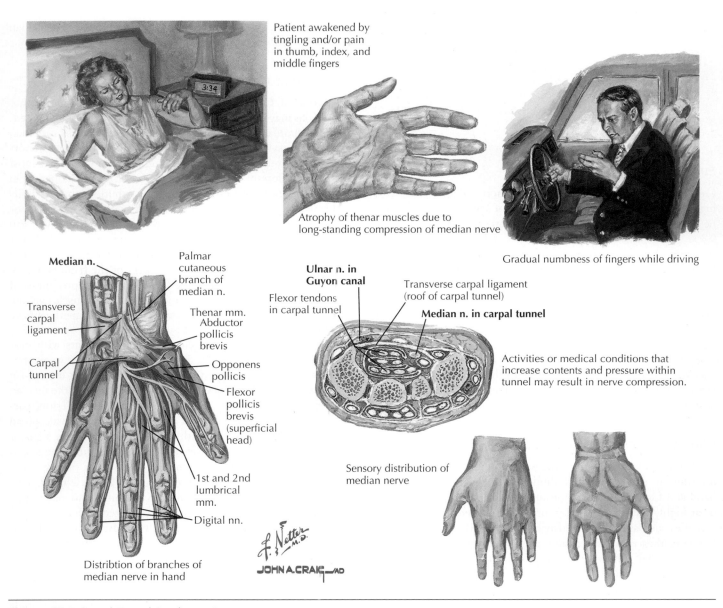

Patient awakened by tingling and/or pain in thumb, index, and middle fingers

Atrophy of thenar muscles due to long-standing compression of median nerve

Gradual numbness of fingers while driving

Median n.

Palmar cutaneous branch of median n.

Transverse carpal ligament

Thenar mm. Abductor pollicis brevis

Carpal tunnel

Opponens pollicis

Flexor pollicis brevis (superficial head)

1st and 2nd lumbrical mm.

Digital nn.

Distribtion of branches of median nerve in hand

Ulnar n. in Guyon canal

Flexor tendons in carpal tunnel

Transverse carpal ligament (roof of carpal tunnel)

Median n. in carpal tunnel

Activities or medical conditions that increase contents and pressure within tunnel may result in nerve compression.

Sensory distribution of median nerve

Figure 65-5 Carpal Tunnel Syndrome–I.

branch, and hypertrophic scar. Ergonomic workplace alterations and avoidance of offending activities or positions are generally recommended. Neutral wrist splints, typically worn at night, initially help more than 50% of patients by maximizing the carpal tunnel diameter and minimizing nerve pressure, which is better than the natural remission rate. Local steroid injections may provide temporary pain relief with an initial success rate almost as good as surgical therapy. However, this is rarely a permanent solution, as there are frequent relapses requiring repeated injections, and there is the possible risk of flexor tendon rupture. Nonsteroidal anti-inflammatory drugs, vitamin B$_6$, and diuretics are of no proven benefit.

Surgical decompression is offered to patients with increasingly annoying sensory symptoms and progressive abnormalities on neurologic examination and electrophysiological testing (see Fig. 65-6). Although published success rates vary significantly, the average surgical success rate is 75%; 8% of patients may worsen after surgery. Long duration of symptoms, increasing age, and the presence of workers compensation claims appear to be associated with poorer outcome. Patients with moderate electrophysiological abnormalities appear to do best, and the success rate of surgery in the absence of nerve conduction abnormalities is only 51%. Occasionally, patients present with end-stage CTS and absent motor responses on nerve conduction studies. Resolution of pain is the only realistic goal of surgical intervention for these patients. Meaningful return of thenar strength is less likely this late in the course of the neuropathy. Endoscopic techniques are being used in carpal tunnel decompression but the relative benefit of this technique compared with traditional decompressive surgery is not known.

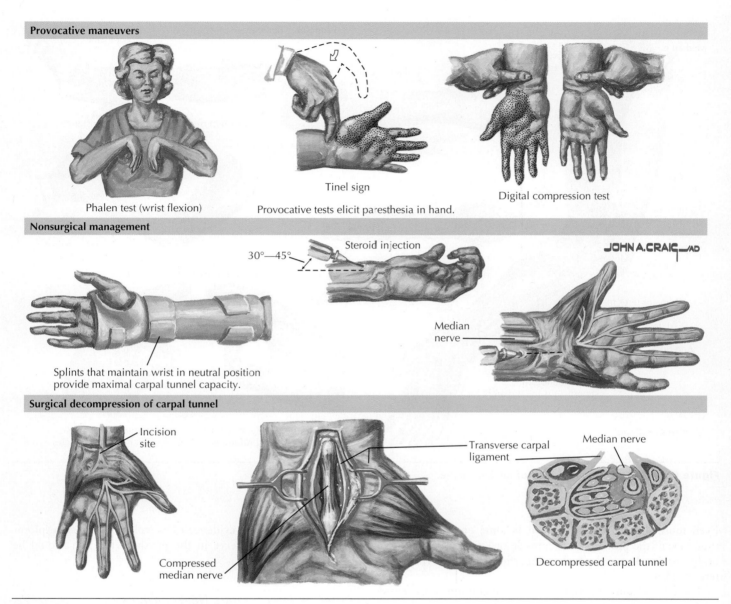

Provocative maneuvers

Phalen test (wrist flexion)

Tinel sign

Provocative tests elicit paresthesia in hand.

Digital compression test

Nonsurgical management

Steroid injection

30°—45°

JOHN A.CRAIG—AD

Splints that maintain wrist in neutral position provide maximal carpal tunnel capacity.

Median nerve

Surgical decompression of carpal tunnel

Incision site

Compressed median nerve

Transverse carpal ligament

Median nerve

Decompressed carpal tunnel

Figure 65-6 Carpal Tunnel Syndrome–II.

PROXIMAL MEDIAN NEUROPATHIES

Clinical Vignette

A 36-year-old secretary complained of difficulty holding a pen and snapping her fingers to music for 6 months. The onset of weakness had been preceded by an aching pain in the volar forearm. There was no sensory loss. The patient had delivered healthy twins 3 months prior to presentation. Neurologic evaluation demonstrated weakness of the flexor pollicis longus muscle and the median-innervated portion of the flexor digitorum profundus, manifested by the inability to flex the distal phalanx of the thumb and the index and long fingers.

EMG confirmed active and chronic denervation in the flexor pollicis longus, flexor digitorum profundus 2 and 3, and pronator quadratus muscles. MRI of the forearm showed evidence of atrophy in the muscles supplied by the anterior interosseous nerve, but no other abnormalities were detected. Surgical exploration revealed entrapment of the anterior interosseous nerve by the deep head of the pronator teres muscle.

Median neuropathies arising rostral to the most proximal muscle innervated by the median nerve (the pronator teres) occur at a frequency of less than 1% of that of CTS. In a very small proportion of the population, there is a bony spur that originates from the shaft of the medial humerus, proximal to the medial epicondyle. A tendinous band called the ligament of Struthers stretches between these two structures and may represent a site of compression for the median nerve. More distally, in the antecubital fossa, the median nerve may become entrapped beneath the lacertus fibrosus, a fibrous band that runs between the tendon of the biceps and the proximal flexors of the forearm.

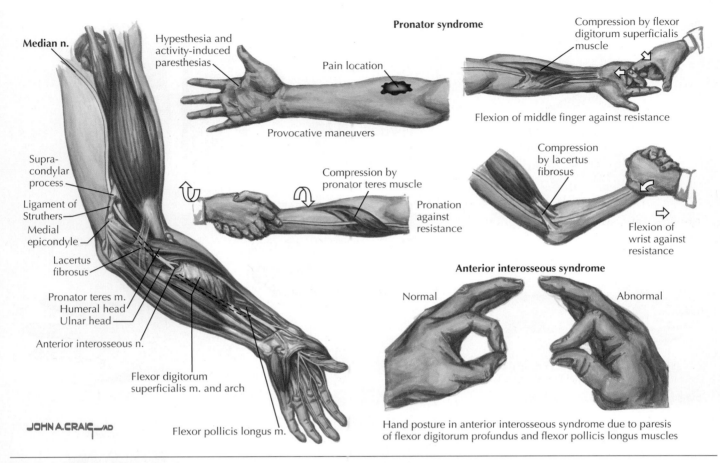

Figure 65-7 Proximal Compression of Median Nerve.

Even more distally, the nerve can become entrapped in the substance of the pronator teres muscle or beneath the sublimis bridge of the flexor digitorum superficialis muscle (pronator teres syndrome).

The clinical and electrophysiologic recognition of weakness in the distribution of the forearm muscles innervated by the median nerve is the diagnostic key (Fig. 65-7). When the median nerve lesion is most proximal, the pronator teres muscle is involved and may be atrophied. Clinical features also include pain in the volar forearm exacerbated by physical activity. There is weakness of thenar muscles and sensory loss in the thumb, index finger, long finger, and lateral aspect of the ring finger.

Mechanical lesions within the axilla, secondary to shoulder dislocation or penetrating injury, may also affect the proximal median nerve, although concomitant injury of other nerves often exists. More distal lesions of the proximal median nerve include humeral fractures, elbow dislocations, tourniquet compression, and forms of penetrating trauma, such as catheterization of the antecubital veins.

EMG is the crucial initial study. Imaging studies, particularly MRI of the elbow region, are indicated when EMG results are positive. Focal lesions, such as the bony origin of a ligament of Struthers or a venous infarction secondary to tourniquet compression, may be defined on neuroimaging.

Conservative treatment consists of rest and anti-inflammatory medications. In patients with severe symptoms

and electrodiagnostic evidence of axonal loss, surgical exploration of the median nerve in the proximal forearm should be considered.

Anterior Interosseous Neuropathies

The anterior interosseous nerve is the largest motor branch of the median nerve. It does not supply any sensory innervation to the skin, but does carry sensory fibers to the muscles of the forearm and interosseous membrane. It arises about 5–6 cm below the elbow. The muscles supplied by the anterior interosseous nerve are flexor pollicis longus, flexor digitorum profundus to the second and third digits and pronator quadratus. Possible etiologies for anterior interosseous neuropathy are aberrant fibrous bands, fractures, compression by the deep head of the pronator teres muscle, pregnancy, brachial plexus neuritis, which might present as a multifocal neuropathy, or idiopathic.

Anterior interosseous neuropathy usually presents with nonspecific pain in the proximal forearm. The motor symptoms include weakness of forearm pronation with the elbow flexed and weakness of distal phalanx flexion of the thumb, the index finger, and the long finger. Affected persons cannot form a circle by pinching their thumb and index finger. This presentation is similar to more proximal median neuropathies but without involvement of the pronator teres. Furthermore, there is no sensory involvement.

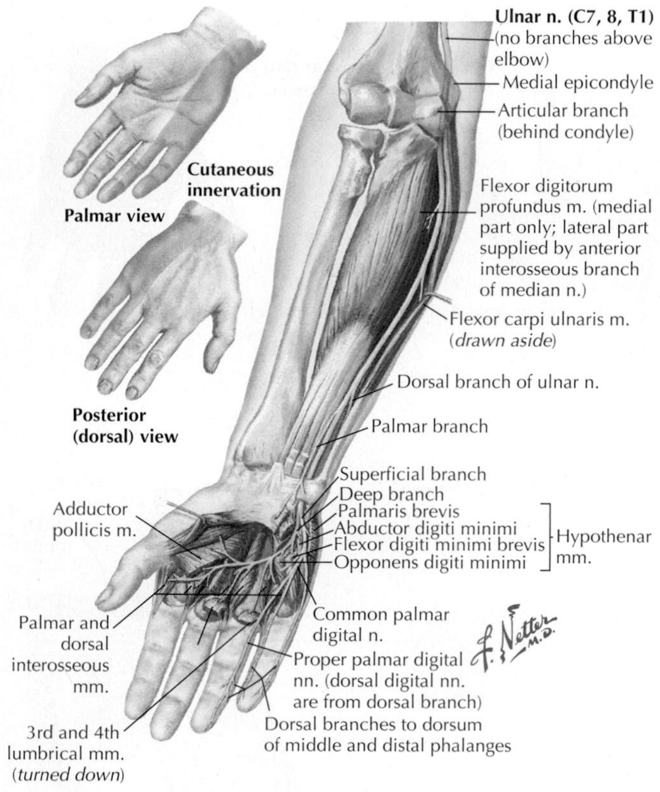

Figure 65-8 Ulnar Nerve.

The treatment, depending on etiology, may be nonsurgical or surgical. Rest, anti-inflammatory medications, and splints can help. Surgical treatment includes exploration of the nerve.

ULNAR MONONEUROPATHIES

The ulnar nerve primarily innervates intrinsic hand muscles, including all hypothenar muscles (Fig. 65-8). The muscles of the thenar eminence supplied by the ulnar nerve are the adductor pollicis and part of the flexor pollicis brevis. Only two forearm muscles have ulnar innervation, the flexor carpi ulnaris and the medial part of the flexor digitorum profundus. The ulnar nerve also supplies sensation to the medial one and a half fingers (the medial aspect of digits 4 and 5), on the dorsal surface sometimes the medial two and a half fingers (see Figs. 65-3 and 65-8). Manifestations of ulnar neuropathies vary with location and severity. Progressive motor deficits lead to the classic "claw hand," with hyperextension of the fourth and fifth metacarpophalangeal joints and flexion of the proximal and distal interphalangeal joints (Fig. 65-9). This is most pronounced when the patient is asked to open the hand because of the unopposed action of radial nerve–innervated muscles. Similar to its median counterpart, the ulnar nerve is typically affected at two anatomic loci, the elbow and wrist, however, in reverse frequency. The majority of ulnar nerve lesions occur at the elbow (Fig. 65-10).

PROXIMAL LESIONS

Clinical Vignette

A 55-year-old man presented to the emergency room afraid he was having a heart attack. He had suddenly experienced sharp, shooting pain radiating from the left elbow distally, associated with tingling of the hand. Upon further questioning, the patient mentioned occasional tingling of digits 4 and 5 of the left hand for several years. He was an avid reader and frequently read with his elbows resting on his desk.

The neurologic examination revealed decreased light touch in the left ring finger and little finger, splitting the ring finger. There was minimal weakness of finger abduction, and a Tinel sign at the left elbow was present.

Electrodiagnostic testing showed a demyelinating left ulnar neuropathy at the elbow.

Proximal ulnar neuropathies are second only to CTS in frequency. Etiologies include external compression or entrapment at the elbow after remote elbow trauma (tardy ulnar palsy), and entrapment just distal to the elbow joint (cubital tunnel syndrome, Fig. 65-11).

Numbness and paresthesias of the fifth and sometimes half of the fourth digit are the rule and may be provoked by having the patient maintain a fully flexed elbow posture for 30 to 60 seconds. Sensory signs or symptoms should not extend proximal to the wrist, in which case a C8 radiculopathy has to be considered in the differential diagnosis. Weakness of the intrinsic muscles of the hand is more common in ulnar neuropathies than in CTS. Clinically apparent involvement of ulnar forearm muscles is rarely detected. Sometimes, there is associated aching of the elbow or forearm pain. The diagnosis is confirmed by EMG. High-resolution sonography can be helpful, when precise localization of the lesion by EMG is difficult, but is not routinely performed.

DISTAL LESIONS

Clinical Vignette

A 40-year-old jackhammer operator noted progressive wasting of muscle bulk in the right hand. He had no pain or sensory loss. He had read about his symptoms on the Internet, and he became concerned he might have Lou-Gehrig's disease.

On neurologic examination, the patient had difficulty holding a piece of paper between the right thumb and index finger. While attempting to do so, he flexed the distal phalanx of the thumb (Froment sign). There was atrophy of the first dorsal interosseous muscle, and fasciculations were observed within this muscle. Abduction of the little finger was of normal strength, and no sensory deficits were demonstrated.

Electrodiagnostic testing was consistent with a distal left ulnar neuropathy involving only the deep motor branch. The patient regained some strength after switching jobs.

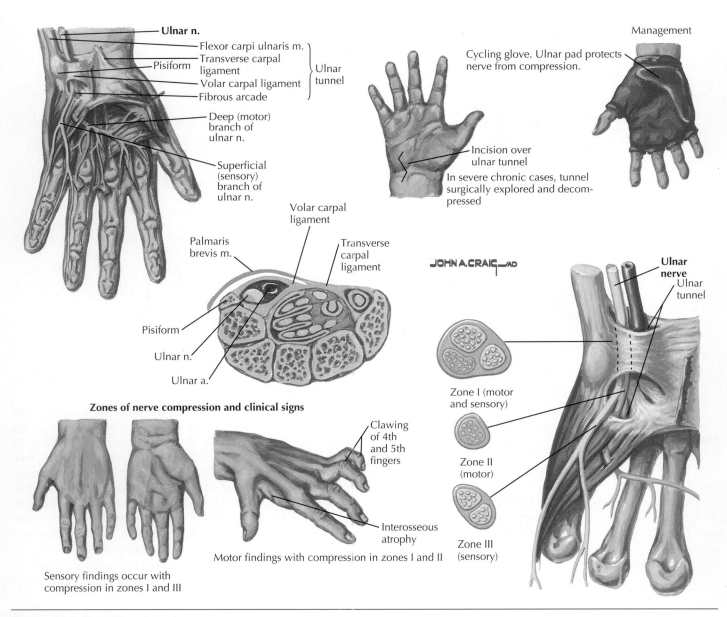

Figure 65-9 Ulnar Tunnel Syndrome.

Ulnar neuropathies at the level of the wrist or palm are less common than proximal lesions. The nerve might become entrapped at the level of the ulnar tunnel or the Guyon canal. Common causes are trauma, ganglion cysts, rheumatoid arthritis, and wrist fractures. Depending on the exact site of injury, there may or may not be associated sensory symptoms (see Fig. 65-9). Sensory loss on the dorsal aspect of the medial hand points to a more proximal ulnar neuropathy with involvement of the dorsal ulnar cutaneous nerve.

Ulnar neuropathies in the palm distal to the Guyon canal present with weakness confined to the ulnar muscles on the lateral aspect of the hand, particularly thumb adduction. This is secondary to weakness of the adductor pollicis, the only thenar muscle not primarily innervated by the median nerve. The first dorsal interosseous muscle is also affected, whereas abduction of the little finger may be preserved. The accompanying intrinsic muscle atrophy and the lack of sensory deficits sometimes prompt consideration of motor neuron disease. Lesions in the palm usually result from local trauma and repetitive injury, for example, from bicycling or from occupations that use tools requiring significant intermittent pressure over the distal ulnar motor fibers (i.e., electricians, clam or oyster shuckers, and pizza cutters). EMG is essential for diagnosis. When the pressure is discontinued, significant recovery of function can occur.

DIFFERENTIAL DIAGNOSIS

Motor neuron disease is a primary consideration in patients presenting with asymmetric painless atrophy of the hand intrinsics. One key differentiating feature between motor neuron disease and an ulnar nerve lesion is the frequent involvement of the abductor pollicis brevis muscle in motor neuron disease; this is innervated by the median nerve.

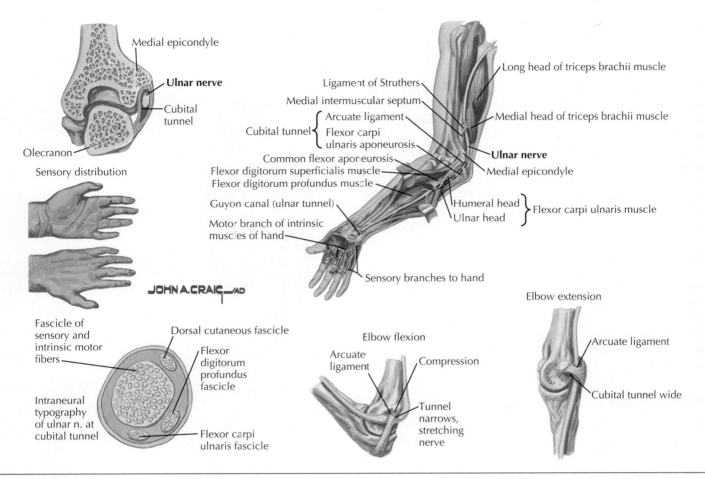

Figure 65-10 Compression of Ulnar Nerve.

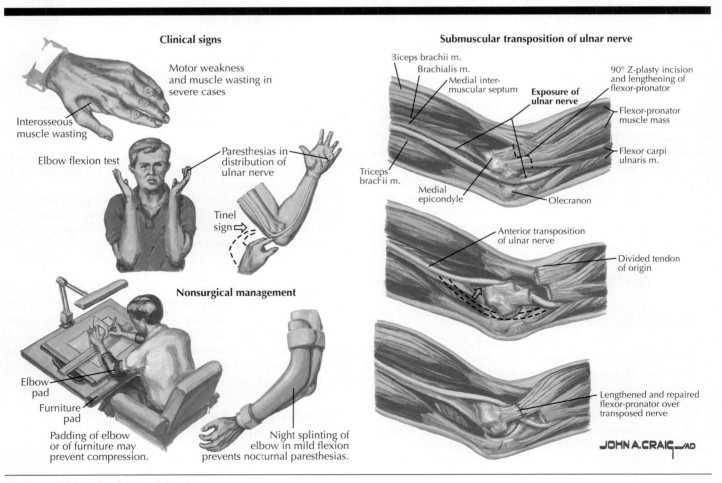

Figure 65-11 Cubital Tunnel Syndrome.

Lower brachial plexus injuries are accompanied by motor and sensory dysfunction in the distribution of multiple peripheral nerve territories within a single extremity. Historically, thoracic outlet syndrome, a distal T1 radiculopathy or proximal lower trunk brachial plexopathy, was considered a common cause of upper extremity neurologic symptoms. Thoracic outlet syndrome is now recognized as a rare condition that is more likely to mimic an ulnar neuropathy than CTS. Perhaps many cases of CTS were erroneously diagnosed and treated as thoracic outlet syndrome before the recognition of the frequency of CTS in the late 1950s and early 1960s. EMG defined the relative frequency of these lesions.

C8 radiculopathies are less common than C7 or C6 radiculopathies but can easily be confused with an ulnar neuropathy because of their overlapping sensory territory. Medial forearm numbness and weakness of non–ulnar innervated C8 muscles (i.e., the thenar eminence, the flexor pollicis longus, and the extensor indicis proprius) provide the major diagnostic distinctions.

MANAGEMENT

Conservative treatment consists of avoiding the stretch produced by a fully flexed elbow via a padded splint that prevents further direct nerve pressure. More than 50% of patients with mild nerve compression might recover with conservative therapy, although data on long-term outcome is limited. Surgical management of ulnar lesions is not as well defined as with CTS. It is even less clear who is likely to benefit from surgery, and there is no consensus on which surgical procedure is appropriate. Persistent pain, progressive motor deficits, and to a lesser extent failure to improve after 3–6 months of conservative management are reasons to consider surgery. Once sensory ulnar nerve conductions can no longer be obtained, recovery of sensory function after surgery becomes less likely. With tardy ulnar palsy, surgeons typically transpose the nerve away from the offending epicondylar groove, often with concomitant epicondylectomy (see Fig. 65-11). This procedure is associated with some risk, particularly in patients with diabetes, because the microvasculature of the nerve can be easily compromised. For cubital tunnel lesions in the absence of trauma or prior surgical procedure involving the elbow, anterior transposition seems to offer no advantage over simple decompression of the nerve.

RADIAL NEUROPATHIES

Clinical Vignette

An 82-year-old man was seen in urgent consultation for a possible stroke. He had awoken in his chair during the late morning with weakness of the right arm. The night prior, he had taken a sleeping pill for the first time in his life.

The neurologic examination revealed weakness of elbow flexion in the semi-pronated position (brachioradialis muscle), wrist extension, and finger extension. The brachioradialis reflex was absent, whereas the triceps reflex and triceps strength were preserved. There was sensory loss to

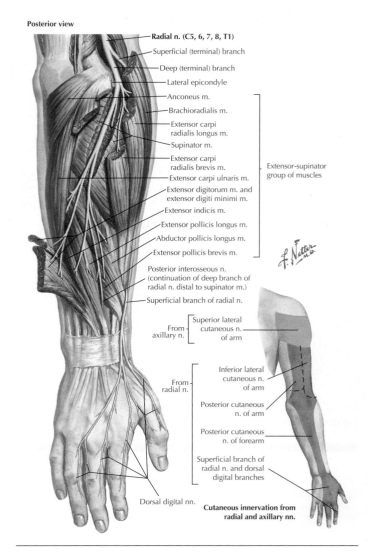

Posterior view

Radial n. (C5, 6, 7, 8, T1)
Superficial (terminal) branch
Deep (terminal) branch
Lateral epicondyle
Anconeus m.
Brachioradialis m.
Extensor carpi radialis longus m.
Supinator m.
Extensor carpi radialis brevis m.
Extensor carpi ulnaris m.
Extensor digitorum m. and extensor digiti minimi m.
Extensor indicis m.
Extensor pollicis longus m.
Abductor pollicis longus m.
Extensor pollicis brevis m.

Extensor-supinator group of muscles

Posterior interosseous n. (continuation of deep branch of radial n. distal to supinator m.)
Superficial branch of radial n.

From axillary n.
Superior lateral cutaneous n. of arm

From radial n.
Inferior lateral cutaneous n. of arm
Posterior cutaneous n. of arm
Posterior cutaneous n. of forearm
Superficial branch of radial n. and dorsal digital branches

Dorsal digital nn.

Cutaneous innervation from radial and axillary nn.

Figure 65-12 Radial Nerve in Forearm.

light touch and pinprick on the dorsal aspect of the forearm and dorsolateral hand.

Electrodiagnostic testing performed on the day of presentation was suggestive of an acute right radial neuropathy at the spiral groove. At the time of his follow-up visit 4 weeks later, the patient had completely recovered.

The radial nerve is formed by fibers from all three trunks of the brachial plexus, hence from roots C5 to T1. It primarily supplies the extensor muscles of the arm, forearm, and fingers and one flexor of the arm, the brachioradialis (see Fig. 65-1). It also provides the sensory innervation to the dorsal arm, the dorsolateral aspect of the hand, and the dorsum of the first three and a half, sometimes two and a half fingers (Fig. 65-12).

PREDOMINANT MOTOR RADIAL NEUROPATHIES

Radial neuropathies most commonly occur at the midhumeral level near the spiral groove, secondary to external compression

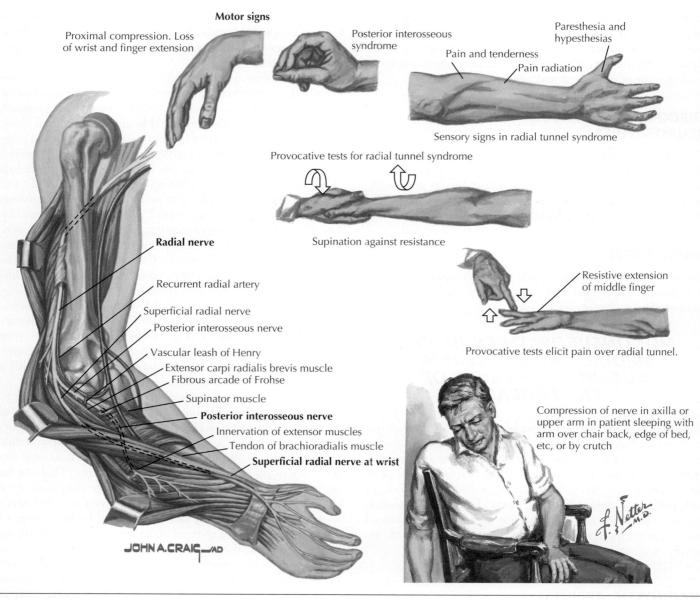

Motor signs

Proximal compression. Loss of wrist and finger extension

Posterior interosseous syndrome

Pain and tenderness

Pain radiation

Paresthesia and hypesthesias

Sensory signs in radial tunnel syndrome

Provocative tests for radial tunnel syndrome

Supination against resistance

Radial nerve

Recurrent radial artery

Superficial radial nerve

Posterior interosseous nerve

Vascular leash of Henry

Extensor carpi radialis brevis muscle

Fibrous arcade of Frohse

Supinator muscle

Posterior interosseous nerve

Innervation of extensor muscles

Tendon of brachioradialis muscle

Superficial radial nerve at wrist

Resistive extension of middle finger

Provocative tests elicit pain over radial tunnel.

Compression of nerve in axilla or upper arm in patient sleeping with arm over chair back, edge of bed, etc, or by crutch

JOHN A. CRAIG—AD

Figure 65-13 Radial Nerve Compression.

(Fig. 65-13). This can occur as a result of impaired consciousness during anesthesia or due to drug or alcohol intoxication ("Saturday night palsy"). These lesions primarily present with wrist and finger drop but little or no pain. Sensory signs and symptoms are often elusive. Elbow extension is spared because the branches of the triceps originate proximal to the spiral groove. The brachioradialis reflex is typically diminished or lost, whereas the triceps and biceps reflexes are unaffected. A potentially confounding examination feature is apparent weakness of ulnar innervated finger abduction that appears concomitant with wrist drop. The full strength of these ulnar muscles requires at least partial wrist extension. Testing the strength of finger abduction while placing the hand and forearm flat on a hard and flat surface circumvents this problem and prevents false localization.

The posterior interosseous nerve is analogous to the anterior interosseous nerve because it is a distal, predominantly motor branch of a major peripheral nerve trunk. Posterior interosseous neuropathies commonly occur with fractures of the proximal radius and sometimes have a delayed onset. The posterior interosseous nerve can also be compromised by soft tissue masses. A syndrome of pain and weakness in the muscles innervated by the posterior interosseous nerve may occur in patients who perform repetitious and strenuous pronation/supination movements, which in some instances leads to intermittent posterior interosseous nerve compression by the fibrous edge of the arcade of Frohse (the proximal aspect of the supinator muscle). Entrapment may also develop secondary to a hypertrophied or anomalous supinator muscle. The extensor carpi radialis longus and brevis and the brachioradialis muscles are innervated by branches exiting the radial nerve before the origin of the posterior interosseous nerve; therefore, finger drop, rather than wrist drop as with a more proximal radial nerve lesion, is the dominant manifestation. The extensor carpi ulnaris, however, is weak, which leads to radial deviation of the hand during wrist extension. There is no sensory loss. Pain near the lateral epicondyle of the humerus, extending distally, may occur, as the posterior interosseous nerve gives off sensory fibers supplying the interosseous membrane and joints of the forearm.

PREDOMINANT SENSORY RADIAL NEUROPATHIES

The superficial radial nerve, a primary distal sensory branch, may be injured in isolation with external pressure at the wrist, for example, with handcuff injuries. These lesions are readily recognized by the distribution of sensory symptoms on the dorsolateral portion of the hand. Weakness does not occur.

MANAGEMENT

Radial neuropathies usually result from monophasic external compression. They are almost always treated conservatively and successfully.

MONONEUROPATHIES OF THE MEDIAL AND POSTERIOR CUTANEOUS NERVES OF THE FOREARM

Isolated injuries of the medial cutaneous nerve of the forearm are rare (see Fig. 65-3). Sensory symptoms in the medial volar forearm are more commonly a result of more proximal injuries to the lower trunk or medial cord of the brachial plexus or to the C8 nerve root. Nerve injuries at these levels are associated with additional clinical findings, particularly hand weakness. Sensory symptoms on the posterior forearm from isolated injuries to the posterior cutaneous nerve of the forearm are equally rare.

DIAGNOSTIC APPROACH TO MONONEUROPATHIES

EMG and Nerve Conduction Studies

Myelin loss manifests electrodiagnostically in three ways: focal slowing, differential slowing (also known as temporal dispersion), and conduction block. Focal slowing occurs when all nerve fibers are affected, approximately to the same extent, in one precise anatomic area. Impulse transmission is slowed uniformly in all fibers at that location. When patients have evidence of differential slowing, that is, temporal dispersion, demyelination is typically multifocal, varying in severity in different fibers within the same nerve. Temporal dispersion is the EMG hallmark of acquired demyelinating polyneuropathies, such as Guillain–Barré syndrome, and is not typically seen in focal mononeuropathies. Primary conduction block is consistent with a demyelinating process in one or more locations that is sufficient to prohibit impulse transmission across involved sections of affected nerve fibers, and this causes clinical weakness. Because axonal integrity is not compromised, muscle wasting does not occur. Since unmyelinated fibers are also not affected,

pain and thermal sensation are relatively spared. Conduction block commonly occurs with ulnar neuropathies at the elbow, radial neuropathies at the spiral groove, and peroneal neuropathies at the fibular head.

With motor axonal disruption, the axon is separated from the anterior horn cell and degenerates. Myofibers are deprived of the trophic influence provided by that axon, with resultant atrophy greater than that produced by disuse. Abnormal spontaneous activity characterized by fibrillation potentials and positive sharp waves appears on needle examination, and the number of activated motor unit potentials decreases. Similarly, the loss of unmyelinated axons mediating nociceptive, thermal, and autonomic functions usually produces clinical features different from primary demyelinating insults. These are characterized by loss of pain and thermal perception, hypersensitivity to touch, changes in sweat production, and sometimes vasomotor changes secondary to focal dysautonomia. Clinical features of axon loss can be superimposed upon those associated with the demyelinating component of the nerve injury.

The various mononeuropathies do not have identical pathophysiologic signatures. Some, such as CTS, are initially characterized by focal slowing (Fig. 65-14), whereas others may preferentially produce a demyelinating conduction block, such as an ulnar neuropathy at the elbow, or axon loss as with a primary laceration, or a combination of the above.

EMG and nerve conduction studies provide the means to confirm the existence, location, pathophysiology, and severity of most mononeuropathies. However, electrodiagnosis has important limitations. Ideally, the injured nerve needs to be accessible to stimulation at multiple levels, including at least one site proximal to the site of a demyelinating lesion. This can be technically difficult, even impossible, with proximal nerve segments that are deep and in close proximity to other nerve elements. Localization can also be predicted by the pattern of muscles demonstrating changes of denervation on needle examination. However, the major limitation of this methodology is anatomic as nerve branching is erratic. For example, the ulnar nerve has no branches in the upper arm, two near the elbow, and then none until the hand. The other limitation is selective fascicular involvement, whereby a nerve injury at a given location may not result in denervation of all muscles innervated distal to that injury. Understandably, a false estimate of nerve injury location may result.

False-positive results can result from cold limb temperature, failure to recognize normal anatomic variants, or poor technique. Caution is required not to overcall on the basis of borderline data. Ideally, the presence of abnormalities in two concordant parameters enables conclusive diagnosis. False-negative results also occur. Approximately 10% of patients with clinical histories strongly suggestive of CTS might have normal electrodiagnostic evaluations.

Other Testing Modalities

Although most mononeuropathies occur secondary to recognizable compression, stretch, or entrapment mechanisms, some seem to be idiopathic. Additional testing, particularly MRI, may be diagnostic when mononeuropathies develop in atypical locations or under unusual circumstances.

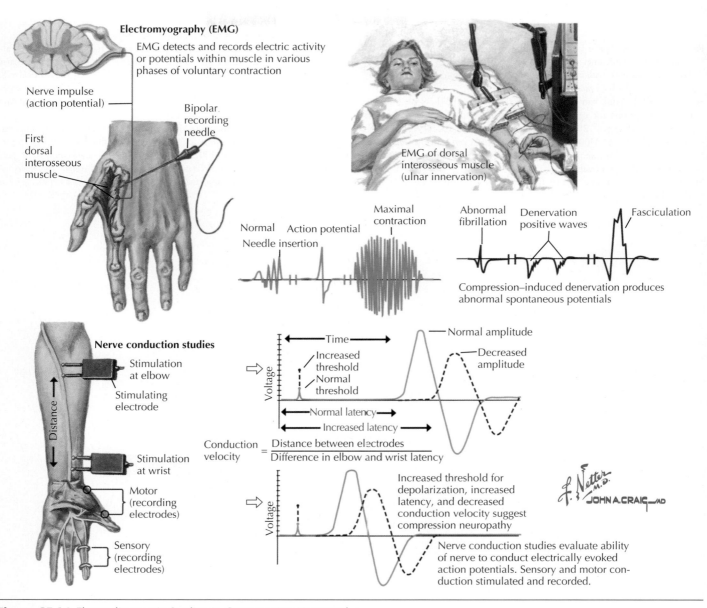

Electromyography (EMG)

EMG detects and records electric activity or potentials within muscle in various phases of voluntary contraction

Nerve impulse (action potential)

First dorsal interosseous muscle

Bipolar recording needle

EMG of dorsal interosseous muscle (ulnar innervation)

Normal Action potential

Needle insertion

Maximal contraction

Abnormal fibrillation Denervation positive waves Fasciculation

Compression–induced denervation produces abnormal spontaneous potentials

Nerve conduction studies

Stimulation at elbow

Stimulating electrode

Distance

Stimulation at wrist

Motor (recording electrodes)

Sensory (recording electrodes)

Time

Increased threshold
Normal threshold

Normal amplitude

Decreased amplitude

Voltage

Normal latency

Increased latency

$$\text{Conduction velocity} = \frac{\text{Distance between electrodes}}{\text{Difference in elbow and wrist latency}}$$

Voltage

Increased threshold for depolarization, increased latency, and decreased conduction velocity suggest compression neuropathy

Nerve conduction studies evaluate ability of nerve to conduct electrically evoked action potentials. Sensory and motor conduction stimulated and recorded.

Figure 65-14 Electrodiagnostic Studies in Compression Neuropathy.

PROGNOSIS OF MONONEUROPATHIES

Prognosis primarily depends on whether the injury has a demyelinating or axonal pathophysiologic mechanism or both. If axonal, recovery depends on the number of axons damaged, the persistence or resolution of the causative insult, the distance between the site of injury and the innervated muscle or cutaneous region, and the patient's age and comorbidities. Demyelinating lesions usually resolve spontaneously after removal of focal compression or entrapment.

ADDITIONAL RESOURCES

American Association of Neuromuscular and Electrodiagnostic Medicine. Available at: http://www.aanem.org. Accessed June 13, 2011. *The information on this website includes a list of suggested reading for physicians as well as educational material for patients with various neuromuscular disorders.*

Bland JDP. Do nerve conduction studies predict the outcome of carpal tunnel syndrome? Muscle Nerve 2001;24:935-940. *This study examines factors influencing the outcome of surgical carpal tunnel decompression.*

Bland JDP. Treatment of carpal tunnel syndrome. Muscle Nerve 2007;36:167-171. *This review article summarizes the current knowledge about different treatment modalities for carpal tunnel syndrome.*

Dumitru D, Amato A, Zwarts M. Electrodiagnostic Medicine. 2nd ed. Philadelphia, PA: Hanley&Belfus; 2002. *This textbook is an excellent reference for physicians interested in disorders of the peripheral nervous system and electrophysiological techniques.*

Marshall S, Tardif G, Ashworth N. Local corticosteroid injection for carpal tunnel syndrome. Cochrane Database of Systematic Reviews 2007;Issue 2. Art. No.: CD001554. DOI: 10.1002/14651858.CD001554.pub2. *This article reviews data from 12 randomized or quasi-randomized studies regarding the effectiveness of local corticosteroid injection for carpal tunnel syndrome.*

O'Connor D, Marshall S, Massy-Westropp N. Non-surgical treatment (other than steroid injection) for carpal tunnel syndrome. Cochrane Database of Systematic Reviews 2003; Issue 1. Art. No.: CD003219. DOI: 10.1002/14651858.CD003219. *This review article evaluates the effectiveness of conservative treatment options (other than corticosteroid injection) for* carpal tunnel syndrome based on data from 21 randomized or quasi-randomized studies.

Padua L, Padua R, Aprile I, et al. Multiperspective follow-up of untreated carpal tunnel syndrome. A multicenter study. Neurology 2001;56:1459-1466. *The authors evaluate the natural history of untreated carpal tunnel syndrome over a 10-15 month follow-up period.*

Scholten RJPM, Mink van der Molen A, Uitdehaag BMJ, et al. Surgical treatment options for carpal tunnel syndrome. Cochrane Database of Systematic Reviews 2007;Issue 4. Art. No.: CD003905. DOI: 10.1002/14651858.CD003905.pub3. *The authors compare the outcome of various surgical techniques for carpal tunnel syndrome, including data from 33 randomized controlled trials.*

Sunderland S. Nerves and Nerve Injuries. 2nd ed. Edinburgh, Scotland: Churchill Livingstone; 1978. *This outstanding textbook provides a detailed description of the anatomy and physiology of peripheral nerves and outlines the various mechanisms of nerve injury in great depth.*

Verdugo RJ, Salinal RS, Castillo J, et al. Surgical versus non-surgical treatment for carpal tunnel syndrome. Cochrane Database of Systematic Reviews 2003;Issue 3. Art. No.: CD001552. DOI: 10.1002/14651858. CD001552. *The authors summarize two randomized controlled trials comparing surgical treatment of carpal tunnel syndrome with splinting and pool data from both trials for secondary outcomes.*

Zlowodzki M, Chan S, Bhandari M, et al. Anterior transposition compared with simple decompression for treatment of cubital tunnel syndrome. J Bone Joint Surg A 2007;89:2591-2598. *This meta-analysis of four randomized controlled trials compares the efficacy of simple decompression with anterior transposition of the ulnar nerve in compression neuropathies at the elbow.*

Mononeuropathies of the Lower Extremities

66

Gisela Held and Miruna Segarceanu

SCIATIC NEUROPATHIES

Clinical Vignette

An 82-year-old frail woman fell in her home. She sustained a hip fracture, which necessitated surgical repair. Postoperatively, she received anticoagulation. Two days later, she had discomfort in her right buttock and hip and foot weakness. Within 24 hours, marked buttock pain and paralysis of all muscles below the right knee and numbness developed. Computed tomographic (CT) scan revealed pelvic hematoma. Despite surgical drainage of 2 L of blood, there was little improvement in sciatic nerve function. Electromyography (EMG) confirmed a primary sciatic neuropathy.

The sciatic nerve is the body's largest nerve, receiving contributions primarily from the L5, S1, and S2 nerve roots, but also carrying L4 and S3 fibers (Fig. 66-1). It has two primary divisions: the laterally situated more superficial peroneal nerve and the more medially placed tibial nerve (see Fig. 66-1). These separate into two distinct nerves in the mid- to distal thigh. The sciatic nerve and its branches innervate the hamstrings (biceps femoris, semimembranosus, and semitendinosus muscles), distal adductor magnus, anterior and posterior lower leg compartments, and intrinsic foot musculature. Through sensory branches of the tibial nerve (sural, medial and lateral plantar, and calcaneal) and the superficial peroneal nerve, the sciatic nerve also supplies sensation to the skin of the entire foot and the lateral and posterior lower leg.

ETIOLOGY

Sciatic neuropathies can be due to hip arthroplasty, pelvic or femoral fractures, or posterior dislocation of the hip. Like femoral neuropathies, they are sometimes caused by a prolonged lithotomy position, presumably from stretching of the nerve in individuals who are anatomically predisposed. Occasionally, sciatic neuropathies develop from external pressure in patients who are comatose or immobilized for protracted periods such as with drug overdose. They may result from traumatic mechanisms including misplaced injections into the inferior medial quadrant of the buttock. Mass lesions including nerve sheath tumors and external compression from hematoma, aneurysm, endometriosis, and other mechanisms have been described. Sciatic neuropathies may occur in patients with systemic vasculitis.

CLINICAL PRESENTATION

Acute sciatic neuropathies typically present with distal leg weakness, pain, and sensory loss. Foot pain is a frequent complaint. Because of predominant affliction of the peroneal division, the weakness often manifests itself as foot drop and needs to be differentiated from a common peroneal neuropathy at the fibular head. Weakness of the more proximal muscles (hamstrings) and of foot plantar flexion and inversion (gastrocnemius, tibialis posterior) helps differentiate between the two entities. The ankle jerk and internal hamstring reflex are usually depressed or absent. Sensory loss and dysesthesia of the sole and dorsum of the foot and posterolateral lower leg are common.

DIFFERENTIAL DIAGNOSIS

A lumbosacral plexus lesion is the primary consideration in most patients with sciatic neuropathies, when findings clearly encompass a territory outside the peroneal nerve. Diminished sensation on the posterior thigh points to a concomitant neuropathy of the posterior femoral cutaneous nerve, which exits the greater sciatic foramen in proximity to the sciatic nerve. Injury to the perineal branches of this nerve leads to sensory loss on the scrotum or labia majora. Hip extension and abduction should be preserved in sciatic neuropathies. When clinical or EMG evidence suggests gluteal muscle involvement, primary lesions within the pelvis, such as benign tumors, for example, schwannoma, or malignant processes, particularly, lymphoma are considerations.

Piriformis syndrome is a poorly understood disorder that is phenomenologically similar to the thoracic outlet and tarsal tunnel syndromes. The piriformis muscle lies deep to the gluteal muscles; it originates from the sacral spine and attaches to the greater trochanter of the femur. The sciatic nerve passes posterior to the piriformis muscle. It is postulated that acute or chronic injury of the muscle may cause irritation of the sciatic nerve, resulting in posterior thigh and gluteal pain. Patients with an aberrant course of the nerve through the muscle are particularly predisposed to this condition. Objective clinical or electrodiagnostic evidence of sciatic neuropathy is not seen in most patients in whom piriformis syndrome is suspected.

PERONEAL NEUROPATHIES

Clinical Vignette

A 44-year-old woman presented with right foot drop and numbness of the dorsum of the right foot. She had first

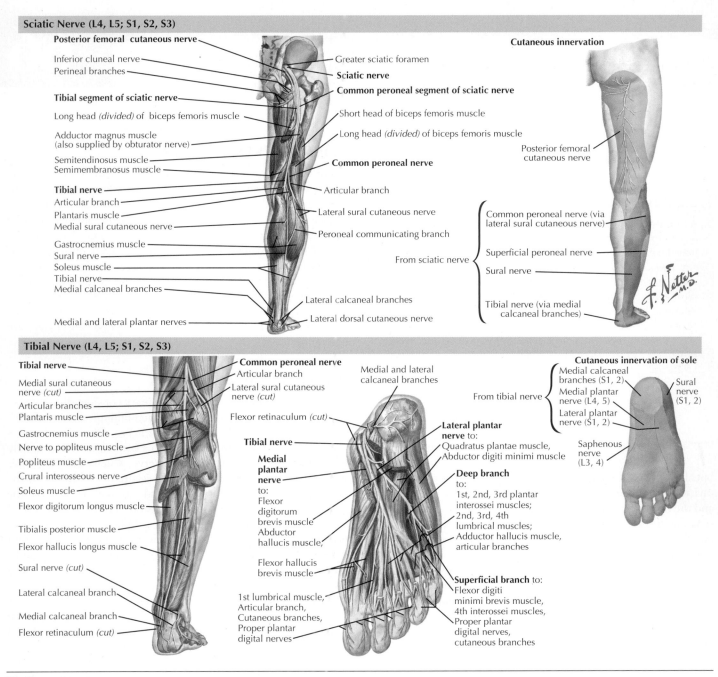

Figure 66-1 Sciatic, Peroneal, and Tibial Nerves.

noted difficulty walking 7 weeks earlier when she tripped over a curb and fell. She had intentionally lost 70 pounds over the last year. To accomplish this, she had done frequent exercises in a squatting position on the floor. There was no history of recent trauma to the back or buttock, or of radicular leg pain.

On examination of the patient, there was tenderness to palpation at the proximal lateral knee, but there was no discrete mass. On motor examination, she had weakness in right toe extension, foot dorsiflexion, and foot eversion. Plantar flexion and inversion of the foot, knee flexion, and

hip abduction were preserved. Sensory examination was notable for reduced pinprick and light touch on the dorsum and first web space of the right foot. Muscle stretch reflexes were normal. Nerve conduction studies revealed conduction block on peroneal motor studies across the fibular head; needle electromyography showed a reduced recruitment in peroneal muscles with sparing of the short head of the biceps femoris; this is consistent with a demyelinating peroneal neuropathy. Her weakness improved significantly over the following weeks, and 3 months later, she had recovered completely.

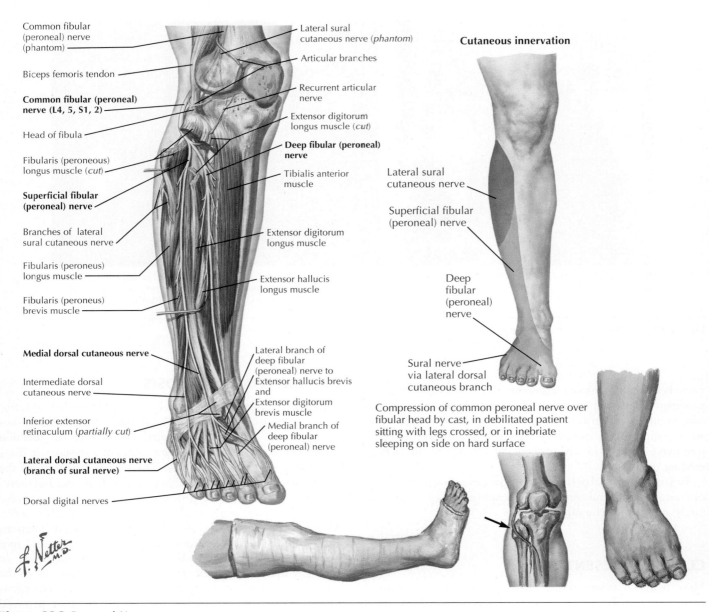

Figure 66-2 Peroneal Nerve.

ETIOLOGY

Axons originating from the L4, L5, S1 and S2 roots, primarily L5 nerve root fibers, come together to form the common peroneal nerve. It is one of the two major divisions of the sciatic nerve and separates from it as a distinct nerve in the mid- to distal thigh. It travels through the popliteal fossa and gives off the lateral sural cutaneous nerve, which unites with the medial sural cutaneous nerve (a branch of the tibial nerve) to form the sural nerve. The lateral cutaneous nerve of the calf also branches off in the popliteal fossa. It provides sensation to the skin of the lateral leg just below the knee. On its course around the fibular head, the common peroneal nerve is very superficial and covered only by skin and subcutaneous tissue. It then pierces through a fibrous, sometimes tight opening in the peroneus longus muscle (fibular tunnel) and divides into superficial and deep branches.

Common peroneal neuropathy is the most frequent lower extremity mononeuropathy. The common peroneal nerve is most susceptible to external compression at the fibular head, where it is very superficial (Fig. 66-2). Predisposing causes include recent substantial weight loss, habitual leg crossing, or prolonged squatting. External devices such as casts, braces, and tight bandages can also cause peroneal neuropathy. Diabetes mellitus, vasculitis, and rarely hereditary tendency to pressure palsy (HNPP) are other etiologic conditions. An acute anterior or lateral compartment syndrome below the knee can also lead to acute common, deep, or superficial peroneal neuropathies. Patients with insidious onset and progressive course require evaluation for mass lesions, including a Baker cyst or ganglion, osteoma, or schwannoma (Fig. 66-3). The common peroneal

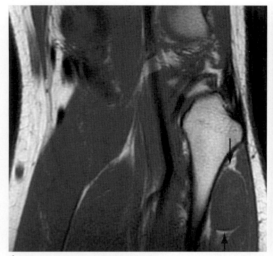 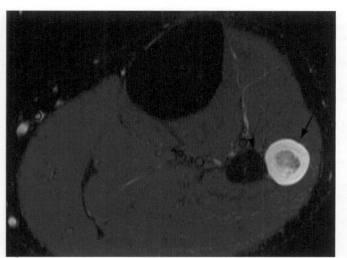

A. Coronal T1-weighted MRI demonstrates an oval mass of left peroneal nerve (arrows)

B. Axial T1-weighted post gadolinium-enhanced fat-saturated MRI demonstrating enhancing peroneal nerve schwannoma with central myxoid degeneration (arrow) near fibula (arrowhead).

Figure 66-3 Peroneal Nerve Schwannoma.

nerve is sometimes injured iatrogenically. Knee positioning and padding to decrease pressure on the peroneal nerve in the operating room and intensive care unit are important to prevent an acute compression neuropathy. Rarely, laceration of the peroneal nerve occurs with arthroscopic knee repair or direct penetrating trauma.

Isolated superficial peroneal neuropathies are uncommon but can result from lateral compartment syndrome, local trauma, or rarely an isolated schwannoma.

CLINICAL PRESENTATION

Most peroneal neuropathies involve the common peroneal nerve at the fibular head causing weakness of foot dorsiflexion and eversion (see Fig. 66-1). Ambulation reveals a "steppage gait" with compensatory hip and knee flexion in order to lift the foot off the floor. The foot might hit the floor with a slap, as the patient has poor control over its movements. With the less frequently occurring deep peroneal neuropathies, there is weakness of the tibialis anterior, extensor hallucis, extensor digitorum longus, and extensor digitorum brevis. Primary superficial peroneal neuropathies cause weakness of the peroneus longus and brevis muscles, which are mainly responsible for foot eversion.

Sensory symptoms are limited to the web space between the first and second toes with deep peroneal neuropathies. Superficial peroneal neuropathies can diminish sensation on the dorsum of the foot and lateral distal half of the leg. Common peroneal sensory symptoms occur on the dorsal foot surface extending up the lateral half of the leg.

EMG involvement of the short head of the biceps femoris is the major distinguishing feature with proximal peroneal division sciatic neuropathies. Biceps femoris function cannot be isolated clinically; therefore, EMG is crucial to diagnosis.

DIFFERENTIAL DIAGNOSIS

Differential diagnoses of peroneal neuropathies include anterior horn cell disease, L5 radiculopathy, lumbosacral trunk or plexus lesions, sciatic neuropathy, or rarely neuromuscular junction disorders. Sciatic neuropathies are sometimes mistakenly diagnosed as peroneal neuropathies. The peroneal division of the sciatic nerve is more superficial than its tibial division and therefore external compressive proximal lesions of the sciatic nerve involve the common peroneal nerve more than the tibial nerve. Most sciatic neuropathies also affect some tibial nerve functions with weakness of knee flexion, foot plantar flexion, and foot inversion. The ankle jerk is characteristically depressed or absent if there is involvement of the tibial component of the sciatic nerve, whereas it is typically unaffected in primary peroneal neuropathies. Sensory loss involves the common peroneal territory described above and the plantar and lateral foot surface. L5 radiculopathy remains a consideration in any patient with a foot drop. Back pain is common with nerve root lesions and is uncommon in peroneal neuropathies; the pain is typically radicular, with buttock, thigh, and leg components sometimes aggravated by positional change. The distribution of weakness is very important; involvement of muscles outside the peroneal nerve territory, such as the tibialis posterior or gluteus medius innervated by the L5 root is critical. Isolated weakness of great toe extension occurs with mild L5 radiculopathy but is uncommon in peroneal neuropathy. In moderate–severe L5 radiculopathies, foot inversion will be weak because of involvement of the tibial nerve innervated posterior tibial muscle. Uncommonly, hip abduction weakness due to involvement of gluteus medius, an L5 muscle supplied by the superior gluteal nerve, is noticeable. Careful evaluation of patients with an L5 root lesion should demonstrate these deficits in addition to weakness of the peroneal innervated muscles. The distribution of sensory symptoms in L5 radiculopathies overlaps significantly with peroneal neuropathies, although L5 nerve root sensory loss may extend more proximally onto the lateral leg. Lumbosacral plexus lesions rarely enter the differential diagnosis of peroneal neuropathies but are a consideration in patients who have a foot drop, proximal lower extremity pain, and motor and sensory findings extending beyond a single peripheral nerve or root distribution. Involvement of hip abduction and extension, clinically and/or by EMG, suggests plexus localization. Polyneuropathy is easily distinguished from peroneal neuropathy, the clinical examination and EMG usually reveal bilateral widespread motor and sensory abnormalities, not confined to a particular nerve or root distribution, muscle tendon reflexes are depressed or absent. The possibility of motor neuron disease exists with insidious onset of a foot drop without pain or sensory findings. Motor neuron disease or amyotrophic lateral sclerosis is a slowly progressive disorder and may be associated with evidence of upper motor neuron dysfunction. In patients with myasthenia, a disorder of neuromuscular transmission, unilateral foot drop is not seen. Distal myopathies may produce foot drop but usually do so bilaterally, and there is often evidence of weakness elsewhere. Unilateral foot drop with or without sensory symptoms can occur with disorders of the spinal cord or parasagittal frontal lobe; these conditions are usually associated with hyperreflexia; magnetic resonance imaging (MRI) is useful to diagnose these conditions.

TIBIAL NEUROPATHIES

Clinical Vignette

A 39-year-old man presented to the emergency room for severe pain and swelling of the right leg associated with difficulty walking. On neurologic examination, there was weakness of right foot plantar flexion and inversion, and flexion of the toes. The ankle jerk was absent. Doppler ultrasound and an MRI of the right knee revealed a ruptured Baker's cyst in the popliteal fossa. Surgical removal of the synovial cyst resulted in resolution of the pain and foot weakness.

Tibial nerve fibers arise primarily from L5, S1 and S2 nerve roots with some contributions from L4 and S3. The tibial nerve leaves the sciatic nerve in the mid- to distal thigh (see Fig. 66-1). The medial sural cutaneous nerve comes off in the popliteal fossa and joins the lateral sural cutaneous nerve (a branch of the common peroneal nerve) in the distal calf to form the sural nerve, which supplies the skin of the lateral aspect of the foot and the posterior lower leg to a variable degree. After innervating the gastrocnemius and soleus muscles, the nerve travels distally between the tibialis posterior and gastrocnemius muscles. It sends branches to the tibialis posterior, flexor digitorum longus, and flexor hallucis longus before entering the tarsal tunnel under the flexor retinaculum. Here, the tibial nerve typically divides into the medial plantar, lateral plantar, and medial calcaneal nerves. Although the medial calcaneal nerve is a purely sensory branch to the medial heel, the medial and lateral plantar nerves are mixed nerves innervating the intrinsic foot muscles as well as the skin of the sole.

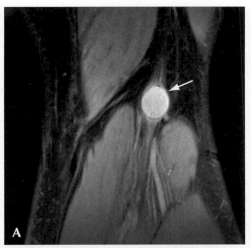

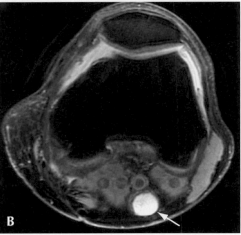

Coronal (**A**) and axial (**B**) proton density fat-saturated MR images demonstrate discrete T2 bright tumor that enlarges the nerve sheath (arrow).

Figure 66-4 Posterior Tibial Neurofibroma.

PROXIMAL LESIONS

Proximal tibial neuropathies may result from Baker's cysts, ganglia, tumors (Fig. 66-4), or rarely indirectly from severe ankle strains, the latter presumably resulting from traction injury. They rarely occur in isolation. They are characterized by weakness of foot plantar flexion and inversion; although flexion, abduction, and adduction of the toes may be affected, these latter functions are difficult to evaluate clinically. The ankle jerk is absent if the neuropathy occurs proximal to the branch points of the gastrocnemius-soleus complex. Sensory loss occurs on the heel and plantar foot surface.

TARSAL TUNNEL SYNDROME

Tarsal tunnel syndrome (TTS), a distal tibial neuropathy, presents primarily with sensory symptoms. It is classified as an entrapment neuropathy of the posterior tibial nerve and of its primary branches, the medial and lateral plantar nerves, at the ankle (See Fig. 66-3). Although well described, there is controversy regarding its prevalence as electrophysiological documentation is infrequent. Whether this reflects its uncommon occurrence or the inadequate sensitivity of diagnostic procedures is unclear. Fractures, ankle sprain, foot deformities due to rheumatoid arthritis or other conditions, varicose veins, tenosynovitis and fluid retention have been implicated as possible etiologies. Patients typically present with burning pain and numbness on the sole of one or both feet. Symptoms may occur while weight bearing and are often exacerbated at night. In well-established instances, examination may disclose intrinsic plantar surface muscle atrophy. However, weakness of these muscles is difficult to appreciate because the more proximal long toe flexors in the leg mask weakness from the involved short toe flexors within the foot. Toe abduction weakness occurs early but is difficult to assess even in healthy individuals. Sensory loss is confined to the sole of the foot; there is sparing of the lateral foot (sural distribution), the dorsum of the foot (peroneal territory), and the instep (saphenous nerve). Muscle stretch reflexes are unaffected. A Tinel sign elicited from the tibial nerve at the ankle is supportive, although not confirmatory.

If TTS results from nerve entrapment, simulating carpal tunnel syndrome, EMG should demonstrate demyelination via prolongation of the distal latencies. However, prolonged tibial motor and mixed nerve distal latencies from the medial and lateral plantar nerves are rarely seen in patients with suspected TTS. Absent mixed nerve responses from the plantar nerves may be seen, but have limited localizing value because they also occur in some seemingly healthy elderly individuals and in those with an underlying polyneuropathy. Fibrillation potentials in tibial innervated foot muscles must be interpreted with similar caution. Imaging in suspected TTS includes radiographs to detect osseous abnormalities involving the tarsal tunnel region and CT, if severe ankle osteoarthritic changes and exostosis are considered.

Initial treatment of TTS is nonoperative, consisting of footwear modification, particularly avoidance of high-heeled and poorly fitting footwear. Anti-inflammatory medications may help. Steroid injections, augmented with lidocaine, can be helpful if flexor tenosynovitis is suspected. Care is taken to avoid an intraneural injection with the unlikely possibility of causing local nerve sclerosis. Hind foot valgus deformities may benefit from orthoses. When nonoperative measures fail in TTS, surgical intervention may be considered. The results of surgical decompression are not always rewarding. Release of the flexor retinaculum and fibrous origin of the abductor hallucis muscle is required. Local flexor tenosynovitis is resected with radical tenosynovectomy. Enlarged and varicose veins are ligated and resected. Postoperatively, an open shoe is used with partial weight bearing for 2 weeks.

FEMORAL NEUROPATHIES

Clinical Vignette

A 63-year-old man with hemophilia presented with right knee buckling a week after a motor vehicle accident. He also complained of dull pain in the right flank radiating into the thigh and knee. He could not raise his right leg off the bed. There was no back pain or sphincter dysfunction. The neurologic examination revealed weakness of the right iliopsoas

and quadriceps muscles, an absent right quadriceps muscle stretch reflex, and diminished sensation to touch and pinprick over the anterior thigh and medial leg below the knee. Pelvic CT demonstrated a hemorrhage of the right iliacus and psoas muscles in the pelvis. Surgery revealed a large hematoma compressing the femoral nerve. This was successfully drained. Postoperatively, the patient gradually improved, regaining significant function within a week.

The femoral nerve comes off the lumbar plexus and is formed by the posterior divisions of the L2–L4 roots (Fig. 66-5). It travels between two important hip flexors, the iliopsoas and iliacus muscles, which it innervates. Approximately 4 cm proximal to the inguinal ligament, the femoral nerve is covered by a tight fascia at the iliopsoas groove. It exits the pelvis by passing beneath the medial inguinal ligament to enter the femoral triangle just lateral to the femoral artery and vein. Here, the nerve separates into the anterior and posterior divisions. The anterior division innervates the sartorius muscle and the anteromedial skin of the thigh via the medial cutaneous nerve of the thigh. The posterior division gives off muscular branches to the pectineus and quadriceps femoris muscles as well as the saphenous nerve, a cutaneous branch to the skin of the inner calf. The nerve can be compressed anywhere along its course, but it is particularly susceptible within the body of the psoas muscle, at the iliopsoas groove, and at the inguinal ligament.

ETIOLOGY

Femoral mononeuropathies are infrequent. Historically, diabetic femoral neuropathies were considered common, although most of these were actually diabetic radiculoplexopathies in which the femoral component dominated. They may represent an autoimmune process, perhaps with a vasculitic component. Vasculitis, such as polyarteritis nodosa, may manifest as mononeuritis multiplex, with acute involvement of the femoral nerve.

Femoral neuropathies occasionally follow prolonged surgeries or childbirth in the lithotomy position, presumably from anatomic predisposition to kinking beneath the inguinal ligament. Iliacus hematoma or abscess, misplaced attempts at femoral artery or vein puncture, or iatrogenic injury after nephrectomy or hip arthroplasty are other recognized causes. Tumors, benign and malignant, may rarely cause femoral neuropathy (Fig. 66-6). Isolated saphenous nerve injuries may result from knee arthroscopy, femoral–popliteal artery bypass surgery, and in the course of coronary artery bypass graft surgery.

CLINICAL PRESENTATION

When the more proximal femoral nerve is involved, weakness of the iliopsoas manifests as limited hip flexion. Mild hip flexion weakness may also occur with more distal femoral nerve involvement from poor function of the rectus femoris, the only head of the quadriceps muscle originating within the pelvis and contributing to hip flexion. Patients with severe quadriceps weakness are unable to extend the leg or lock the knee; when severe, this often interferes with or precludes walking. Initially, mild

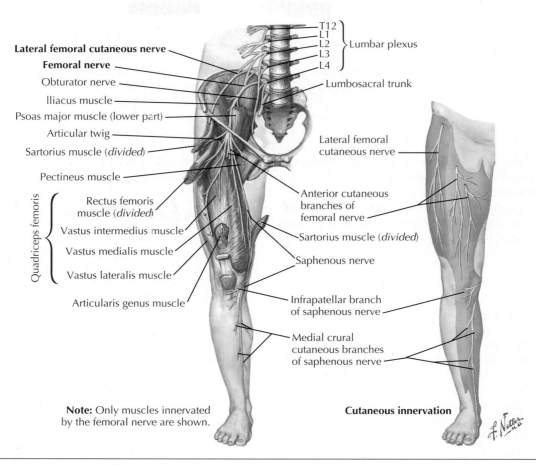

Lateral femoral cutaneous nerve
Femoral nerve
Obturator nerve
Iliacus muscle
Psoas major muscle (lower part)
Articular twig
Sartorius muscle (*divided*)
Pectineus muscle
Quadriceps femoris {
    Rectus femoris muscle (*divided*)
    Vastus intermedius muscle
    Vastus medialis muscle
    Vastus lateralis muscle
}
Articularis genus muscle

T12
L1
L2   } Lumbar plexus
L3
L4
Lumbosacral trunk

Lateral femoral cutaneous nerve

Anterior cutaneous branches of femoral nerve
Sartorius muscle (*divided*)
Saphenous nerve
Infrapatellar branch of saphenous nerve
Medial crural cutaneous branches of saphenous nerve

Lateral femoral cutaneous nerve

Note: Only muscles innervated by the femoral nerve are shown.

Cutaneous innervation

Figure 66-5 Femoral Nerve and Lateral Cutaneous Nerve of Thigh.

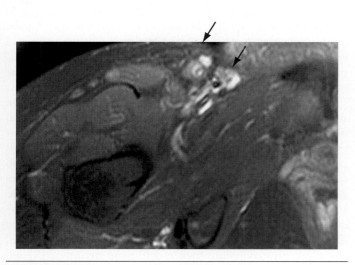

Figure 66-6 Femoral Nerve Neurofibromas in Neurofibromatosis (arrows).

femoral neuropathies may present with difficulty going down stairs because the knee buckles from mild quadriceps weakness. Eversion of the thigh might be impaired because of sartorius weakness. The patellar muscle stretch reflex is almost always diminished or absent in femoral neuropathies. Groin and thigh pain are frequent presenting symptoms. When patients experience sensory symptoms, these typically involve the anteromedial

thigh, and medial lower leg. A pure motor syndrome with quadriceps weakness and atrophy can result from lesions distal to the branching of the saphenous nerve in the thigh.

DIFFERENTIAL DIAGNOSIS

A nerve root lesion at L3–L4 is the most common consideration. Unlike L5–S1 radiculopathies, a herniated nucleus pulposus infrequently involves the level L3–L4. Lumbosacral plexus lesions primarily affecting the lumbar nerves may also mimic femoral neuropathies.

LATERAL FEMORAL CUTANEOUS NEUROPATHY

Clinical Vignette

A 38-year-old woman presented with pain and numbness of the left thigh in her seventh month of pregnancy. She described a burning discomfort extending from the hip to the lateral aspect of the thigh, intensified by standing or walking. There was associated cutaneous hypersensitivity with an aversion to having clothes or bed sheets rub against her. She was unaware of any other precipitating events. Examination demonstrated an elliptically shaped area of sensory loss on the distal half of the left anterolateral thigh. She had no atrophy, weakness, or reflex loss. The symptoms gradually improved in the months following the delivery of a healthy baby.

The lateral femoral cutaneous nerve (LFCN) arises from the second and third lumbar roots and travels through the retroperitoneum. After traversing the psoas muscle, the nerve reaches the iliacus muscle (see Fig. 66-4). Medial to the anterior superior iliac spine, it exits the pelvis under or through the inguinal ligament, the presumed usual site of entrapment. Subsequently, it supplies sensation to the anterolateral thigh.

ETIOLOGY

Meralgia paresthetica is an entrapment mononeuropathy of the lateral femoral cutaneous nerve (Fig. 66-7). Cadaver studies suggest that meralgia paresthetica is primarily an entrapment neuropathy due to "kinking" of the nerve as it passes through the inguinal ligament. Like many mononeuropathies, it is more common in people with diabetes. Meralgia paresthetica often occurs in overweight individuals, especially after sudden gain in weight, or in individuals wearing tight belts and garments. It is usually unilateral. Occasionally, the nerve is injured within the thigh secondary to blunt or penetrating trauma (e.g., a misplaced injection), or rarely, by a soft tissue sarcoma within the thigh.

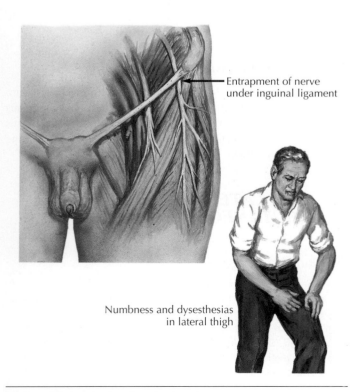

Entrapment of nerve under inguinal ligament

Numbness and dysesthesias in lateral thigh

Figure 66-7 Lateral Femoral Cutaneous Nerve.

CLINICAL PRESENTATION

Often aggravated by standing or walking, symptoms include an uncomfortable positive component (burning, hypersensitivity) and negative features (numbness). Typically, the area of demonstrable sensory loss on examination is smaller than the lateral femoral cutaneous nerve territory in most anatomic diagrams, likely due to significant overlap with adjacent nerves. Because the LCFN is a purely sensory nerve, there are no associated reflex or motor abnormalities, helping to distinguish meralgia from other disorders that deserve diagnostic consideration.

DIFFERENTIAL DIAGNOSIS

Although uncommon, L2 radiculopathy of any etiology, evidenced as weakness and denervation of L2-innervated hip flexors and adductors, is a differential consideration. Sensory symptoms and signs extend over the anterior and medial aspects of the thigh. Lumbar spinal stenosis also tends to be exacerbated by prolonged standing or walking, although it does not cause numbness in this specific distribution.

Disorders of the lumbosacral plexus may mimic meralgia, particularly in patients having insidious onset of invasive or compressive disorders in which pain and other sensory symptoms have no obvious motor component. Retroperitoneal neoplasms or hematomas and abdominal surgery might affect the LCFN; however, they are unlikely to cause isolated meralgia. Instead, concomitant involvement of adjacent nerves usually leads to widespread motor, reflex, and sensory loss, indicating that there may be a plexus lesion rather than a single nerve problem.

Isolated femoral neuropathies are uncommon and unlikely to be confused with meralgia because of the type and distribution of abnormalities. Sensory symptoms involve the anterior and medial thigh and extend to the medial surface of the leg. Weakness of the quadriceps muscle and loss of its stretch reflex are other objective and distinguishing features.

Although the LFCN can be tested by nerve conduction studies in the thigh distal to the inguinal ligament, technical difficulties interfere with detection of mild demyelinating injuries. A response cannot be obtained from all individuals and is particularly difficult to record in overweight individuals who are most susceptible to this syndrome. Nerve conduction studies of the LFCN are of greatest value when a normal response is readily obtained from the asymptomatic side and a low-amplitude or absent response is obtained from the symptomatic side. In patients with atypical symptoms, thigh MRI is indicated to exclude primary lesions such as soft tissue sarcoma. MRI and CT of the retroperitoneum and pelvis should be considered in patients with unexplained LFCN neuropathy. Fasting blood glucose measurement is appropriate in acute-onset, painful LFCN neuropathies without alternative explanation.

MANAGEMENT

The natural history of meralgia varies, but most patients become asymptomatic within 2 years. Others have a more protracted and chronic course. Conservative management includes weight loss and avoidance of tight garments. Medications such as amitriptyline, carbamazepine, gabapentin, and venlafaxine may diminish pain intensity. Injections of local anesthetics and steroids near the anterior superior iliac spine may serve diagnostic and therapeutic roles and are sometimes "curative." Exploration at the presumed entrapment site is used in particularly intractable and lifestyle-altering cases.

OBTURATOR NEUROPATHIES

Clinical Vignette

A 35-year-old woman presented with pain in the right medial thigh and difficulty walking. This had begun 6 months prior, immediately after the delivery of her son. After 8 hours of labor complicated by fetal failure to progress, she had eventually undergone an emergent cesarean section. On neurologic examination she had weakness of the right thigh adductors and a patch of numbness and dysesthesia on the medial surface of the thigh.

The obturator nerve originates from the anterior rami of the L2, L3, and L4 nerve roots (Fig. 66-8). After its course through the pelvis, the nerve exits through the obturator canal and separates into the anterior and posterior divisions. The anterior division supplies the adductor longus, adductor brevis and gracilis muscles, whereas its terminal branch provides sensation to the distal medial thigh. The posterior division innervates the obturator externus, the superior portion of the adductor magnus, and sometimes the adductor brevis.

ETIOLOGY

Obturator neuropathies may be caused by pelvic masses, difficult parturition, or obturator hernias or may be complications of hip arthroplasty or pelvic surgery.

CLINICAL PRESENTATION

Obturator neuropathies are exceedingly uncommon focal nerve lesions that typically present with hip instability. Weakness and denervation are confined to the large hip adductors. Occasionally, they present with pain and sensory symptoms in the medial thigh without obvious weakness.

ILIOHYPOGASTRIC, ILIOINGUINAL, AND GENITOFEMORAL NEUROPATHIES

These mononeuropathies should be considered in the differential diagnosis of dysesthesias of the pelvis and groin without apparent motor deficits.

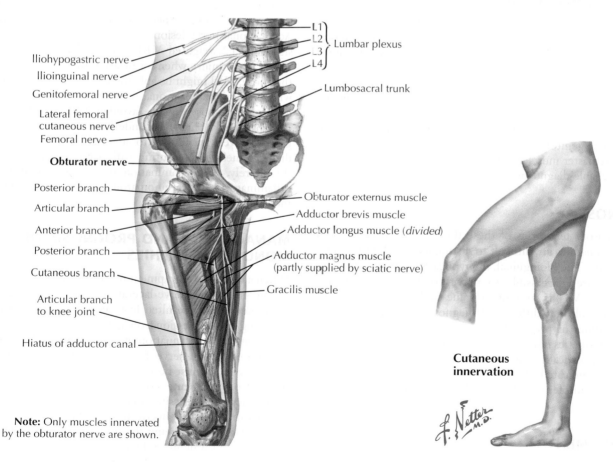

Note: Only muscles innervated by the obturator nerve are shown.

Figure 66-8 Obturator Nerve.

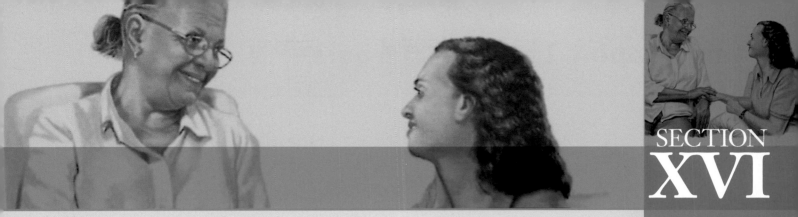

Motor Neuron Disorders

Amyotrophic Lateral Sclerosis

James A. Russell

67

Clinical Vignette

A 62-year-old female first noted difficulty walking over uneven ground. Progressive painless weakness developed over the course of the next 6 months; initially this affected the left leg more than the right, resulting in a number of falls. By the time she was evaluated by a neurologist, she could no longer cut her own food or clip her own finger nails. She denied any pain, sensory disturbance or change in her ability to think, speak, swallow, or breathe.

Her examination revealed normal cognitive function. Cranial nerve examination revealed mild dysarthria, tongue fasciculations, the presence of a jaw jerk, and weakness of neck flexion. All limb muscles were weak, left more than right, more pronounced distally. Intrinsic hand muscles were atrophic. Fasciculations were noted throughout her limbs. Muscle stretch reflexes were brisk despite her weakness and atrophy. Plantar responses were extensor. Sensory examination revealed no abnormalities.

In 1874, Jean-Martin Charcot described a disorder that he named amyotrophic lateral sclerosis (ALS). In France, it is referred to as Charcot disease, whereas motor neuron disease (MND) is the preferred name for the disorder in the United Kingdom. In the United States, ALS is better known as Lou Gehrig's disease.

Charcot's description was of a disorder characterized by loss of voluntary motor function, resulting from degeneration of anterior horn cells, corticospinal tracts, and motor cranial nerve nuclei and cortical motor neurons (Figs. 67-1 and 67-2). ALS is a sporadic disorder (sALS) in the majority of cases. ALS is inherited in 5–10% of cases, i.e., familial ALS (fALS), usually in an autosomal dominant fashion. In general, fALS patients have phenotypes that closely resemble sALS, although fALS may have an earlier onset. In absence of family history, the disorders are clinically indistinguishable.

The incidence of ALS approximates 1.8 in 100,000. The incidence of ALS in men is twice that in women, although this ratio becomes closer to 1:1 in a postmenopausal population. The median age at onset is 55 years of age; this disease may afflict patients in their late teens or in their 90s. The average life expectancy is between 2 and 3 years; in less than 10% of patients, ventilator-independent survival of less than 1 year or greater than 10 years is seen. Half of affected individuals die within 3 years and only a quarter survive 5 years without dependency on invasive mechanical ventilation. Young males and patients with restricted upper motor neuron (UMN) or lower motor neuron (LMN) presentations tend to have a slower course. Primary bulbar (disordered speech and swallowing) presentations tend to disproportionately affect older women and appear to have a more rapid course.

In the United States, it is estimated that at any given time 25,000 patients are diagnosed with ALS. The prevalence of ALS appears to be increasing, perhaps because of an aging population. Other than historical observations identifying an increased incidence on Guam and the Kii peninsula of Japan, there does not appear to be any particular geographic location or ethnic group that has a significantly higher risk of contracting ALS.

ETIOLOGY, GENETICS, AND PATHOGENESIS

The cause of sporadic ALS is unknown. As with other neurodegenerative diseases, it is hypothesized that ALS may result from the dual insult of genetic susceptibility and environmental injury. Attempts to identify predisposing mutations and potential toxic or infectious agents have been unsuccessful to date.

It has been long recognized that a small percentage of patients (fALS) have an autosomal dominant pattern of Mendelian inheritance. A major breakthrough in our understanding of familial ALS took place in 1991 with the identification of cytosolic copper-zinc superoxide dismutase (SOD1) gene mutations on chromosome 21q22.11 in affected individuals in some families. This represents the most frequently identified form of fALS. SOD1 is a free radical scavenger. Recognition of the SOD1 mutation led to the hypothesis that SOD1-fALS was mediated by free radical toxicity. However, SOD1 knock-out mouse with no SOD1 protein do not develop motor neuron disease. In contrast, heterozygote mice become symptomatic and die from a paralyzing disorder. It is thought that SOD1 mutations may injure neurons through conformational changes in the SOD1 protein.

Particularly intriguing has been the recognition of the phenotypic heterogeneity in SOD1 fALS (Table 67-1). About 114 pathologic mutations have been identified within the five exons of the SOD1 gene; each of these mutations may produce a distinct phenotype. The most common mutation found in North America is an alanine for valine (A4V) substitution at codon 4; this typically produces a lower motor neuron dominant phenotype (LMN-D) with a life expectancy approximating 1 year. Table 67-1 summarizes the phenotypic heterogeneity that results from different SOD1 mutations. SOD1 mutations are not fully penetrant. It is estimated that individuals carrying the mutation have an 80% chance of developing disease by age 85 years. SOD1 mutations constitute 20–25% of all individuals with fALS. Other fALS genotypes are listed in Table 67-2. Some of these mutations produce a predominantly lower motor neuron (LMN) or upper motor neuron (UMN) disorder and more closely resemble the phenotypes of spinal muscular atrophy or hereditary spastic paraparesis, respectively.

Mutations that may produce both a frontotemporal lobar degeneration and motor neuron disease occur on chromosomes 9p13.2-21.3, 9q21-q22, and 17q21. A recently identified fALS mutation occurs in the TAR DNA-binding protein, 43

Cerebral Cortex: Efferent Pathways

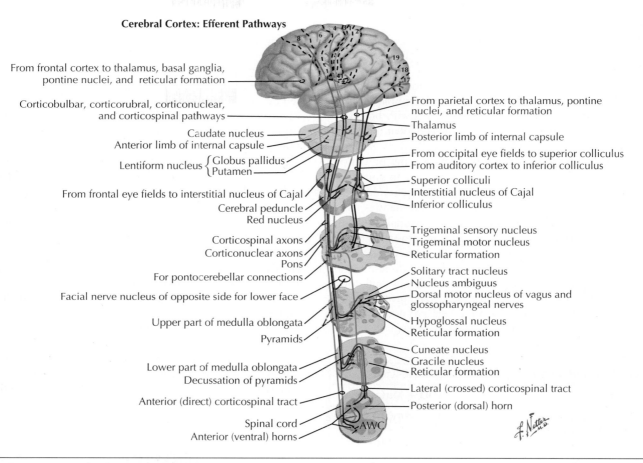

From frontal cortex to thalamus, basal ganglia, pontine nuclei, and reticular formation

Corticobulbar, corticorubral, corticonuclear, and corticospinal pathways

Caudate nucleus
Anterior limb of internal capsule

Lentiform nucleus { Globus pallidus / Putamen

From frontal eye fields to interstitial nucleus of Cajal
Cerebral peduncle
Red nucleus

Corticospinal axons
Corticonuclear axons
Pons

For pontocerebellar connections

Facial nerve nucleus of opposite side for lower face

Upper part of medulla oblongata
Pyramids

Lower part of medulla oblongata
Decussation of pyramids

Anterior (direct) corticospinal tract

Spinal cord
Anterior (ventral) horns

From parietal cortex to thalamus, pontine nuclei, and reticular formation
Thalamus
Posterior limb of internal capsule

From occipital eye fields to superior colliculus
From auditory cortex to inferior colliculus
Superior colliculi
Interstitial nucleus of Cajal
Inferior colliculus

Trigeminal sensory nucleus
Trigeminal motor nucleus
Reticular formation

Solitary tract nucleus
Nucleus ambiguus
Dorsal motor nucleus of vagus and glossopharyngeal nerves
Hypoglossal nucleus
Reticular formation

Cuneate nucleus
Gracile nucleus
Reticular formation

Lateral (crossed) corticospinal tract
Posterior (dorsal) horn

AWC

Figure 67-1 Cerebral Cortex: Efferent Pathways.

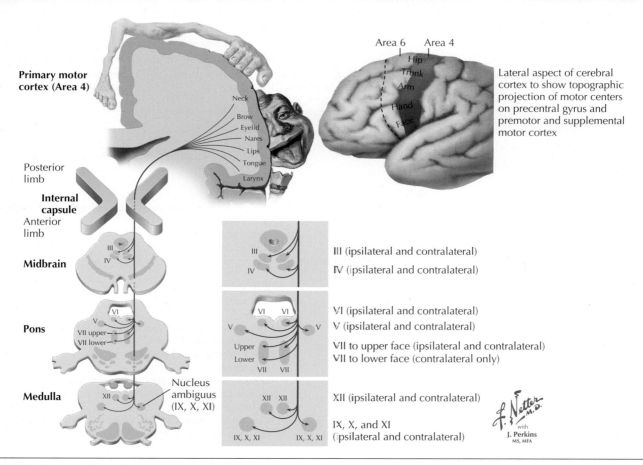

Primary motor cortex (Area 4)

Neck
Brow
Eyelid
Nares
Lips
Tongue
Larynx

Posterior limb

Internal capsule
Anterior limb

Midbrain
III
IV

Pons
VI
V
VII upper
VII lower

Medulla
XII
Nucleus ambiguus (IX, X, XI)

Area 6   Area 4
Hip
Trunk
Arm
Hand
Face

Lateral aspect of cerebral cortex to show topographic projection of motor centers on precentral gyrus and premotor and supplemental motor cortex

III
IV
III (ipsilateral and contralateral)
IV (ipsilateral and contralateral)

VI   VI
V   V
Upper
Lower
VII   VII
VI (ipsilateral and contralateral)
V (ipsilateral and contralateral)
VII to upper face (ipsilateral and contralateral)
VII to lower face (contralateral only)

XII   XII
IX, X, XI   IX, X, XI
XII (ipsilateral and contralateral)
IX, X, and XI (ipsilateral and contralateral)

Figure 67-2 Corticobulbar Fibers.

(TDP-43) gene. Non-amyloid, structurally modified TDP-43 has been recognized as a major constituent of the ubiquitinated inclusions found in cortical neurons of patients with both sporadic (s) and familial (f) forms of frontotemporal lobar degeneration (FTD).

There are many proposed mechanisms for motor neuron death in sALS, including excitotoxicity secondary to glutamate, free radical–mediated oxidative cytotoxicity, mitochondrial dysfunction, protein aggregation, cytoskeletal abnormalities, aberrant activation of cyclo-oxygenase, impaired axonal transport, activation of inflammatory cascades, and apoptosis. Why the motor neurons and corticospinal/bulbar tracts are vulnerable in a selective manner remains unknown. Why the disease begins focally and progresses in a regional fashion is also unknown. One putative hypothesis is that misfolded, toxic protein aggregates may proselytize normal protein in adjacent neurons, analogous to mechanisms proposed for prion diseases.

Whatever the mechanism, ALS is pathologically characterized by loss of myelinated fibers in the corticospinal and corticobulbar pathways (see Fig. 67-2) and loss of motor neurons within the anterior horns of the spinal cord and many motor cranial nerve nuclei. Even in individuals with predominantly UMN or LMN involvement clinically, pathologic involvement of both systems is seen. Patients with associated FTD have preferential lobar atrophy and neuronal loss from these portions of the brain (Fig. 67-3). As a result of anterior horn cell loss, ventral roots become atrophic in comparison to sparing of their dorsal root counterparts (Fig. 67-4). Anterior horn cell loss occurs within virtually all levels of the spinal cord with selective sparing of the third, fourth, and sixth cranial nerves, and Onuf's nucleus within the anterior horn of sacral segments 2–4. There is also cell preservation within the intermediolateral cell columns.

The majority of sALS patients will be found to have ubiquitinated inclusions and Bunina bodies within the central nervous system. The latter are dense granular intracytoplasmic inclusions within motor neurons considered specific for ALS. Additionally in ALS with FTD, spongiform changes of the first and second layers of the frontal cortex have been described.

CLINICAL PRESENTATIONS

The diagnosis of ALS remains a clinical endeavor. EMG and nerve conduction studies and measurements of ventilatory capacity are routinely obtained in ALS suspects. These tests are done to provide diagnostic support for diffuse LMN and ventilatory muscle involvement respectively. Other testing is done with the primary intent of identifying or excluding differential diagnostic considerations. SOD1 mutational analysis provides

Table 67-1 Phenotypic Variation in SOD1 fALS

Phenotype	SOD 1 Mutation
Lower motor neuron predominant	A4V, L84V, D101N
Upper motor neuron predominant	D90A
Slow progression (>10-year survival)	G37R, G41D, G93C, L144S, L144F
Fast progression (<2-year survival)	A4T, N86S, L106V, V148G
Late onset	G85R, H46R
Early onset	G37R, L38V
Female predominant	G41D
Bulbar onset	V148I
Low penetrance	D90A, I113T
Posterior column involvement	E100G

Table 67-2 Current Classification of fALS

Inheritance	Name	Genetics	Phenotype
Dominant inheritance	ALS1	21q22.1 SOD1	Adult onset—multiple phenotypes (see Table 67-3)
	ALS3	18q21	Adult onset
	ALS4	9q34 senataxin	Juvenile onset Slow progression with distal amyotrophy and UMN signs
	ALS6	16q12	Adult onset
	ALS7	20ptel-p13	Adult onset
	ALS8	20q13.33, vesicular associated membrane protein	Adult onset
	ALS-FTD	9q21-22	Adult onset
	ALS with PD & dementia	17q21, microtubule associated tau	Adult onset
	ALS	2p13, dynactin	Adult onset—progressive LMN disease with variable vocal cord and facial weakness
	ALS	TDP-43	Slowly progressive LMN disorder
X-linked	ALSX	XLD—Xp11	Adult onset
Recessive	ALS2	2q ALSIN	Juvenile onset—pseudobulbar and UMN
	ALS5	15q	Juvenile onset—distal amyotrophy, minor spasticity, long term survival
	GM2, gangliosidosis	15q23-24 Hexosaminidase A deficiency	Adult onset—primarily LMN disorder with variable UMN and spinocerebellar features (primarily Ashkenazi)
Mitochondrial	Single case reports	COX1	Predominantly UMN

diagnostic proof in patients with suggestive family histories. Although a small percentage (2%) of seemingly sALS patients will be found to have SOD1 mutations, mutational analysis is not routinely recommended in this population.

The presenting features of ALS are quite variable. Typically, the patient seeks medical care when his or her weakness begins to affect activities of daily living (Fig. 67-5). It is not uncommon for ALS to be misdiagnosed initially and the time between symptom onset and diagnosis is usually months. Unfortunately, there is a tendency to misdiagnose ALS as a potentially treatable

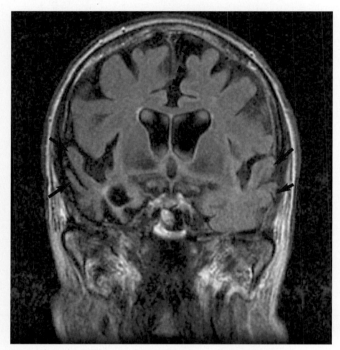

Coronal FLAIR MR image demonstrates ventricular enlargement, especially of the right temporal horn, atrophy of superior and middle temporal gyri (arrow), and prominence of frontal sulci. Notice prominent widening of the interhemispheric fissure (arrowheads). Courtesy of Richard Caselli, MD.

Figure 67-3 Frontotemporal Atrophy.

nerve, nerve root, or spinal cord compressive syndrome or orthopedic condition. A significant percentage of ALS patients may undergo unnecessary surgeries. It should be emphasized that progressive weakness and atrophy in the absence of pain and sensory symptoms rarely represents a surgically treatable condition.

The exclusive motor involvement and the chronologic course serve to distinguish ALS from other neurologic disease. Simultaneous involvement of both UMNs and LMNs and progression both within and outside of the originally involved regions is necessary for a definite clinical diagnosis. LMN involvement may be documented by clinical, electrodiagnostic, or pathologic (muscle biopsy) means. UMN involvement is currently defined by clinical criteria alone. Classic ALS is usually an easy diagnosis for an experienced neurologist. Diagnosis may be delayed in patients with limited clinical evidence of the LMN or UMN involvement, slow disease progression, and confounding neurologic signs from unrelated problems such as sensory loss from mononeuropathies, radiculopathies, and polyneuropathies.

The signature of anterior horn cell loss is painless weakness and atrophy, hypoactive or absent deep tendon reflexes, and fasciculations. Atrophy is best appreciated when it is focal, in contrast to normal muscle bulk elsewhere. It may be difficult to distinguish atrophy from LMN disease resulting from the atrophy of disuse, particularly in the elderly. Suppressed deep tendon reflexes may also be difficult interpret as they may represent a normal variant. In ALS, muscle weakness due to LMN dysfunction occurs in a segmental (myotomal) distribution and spreads in a regional fashion. As an example, a patient with ALS and hand weakness may have all hand muscles innervated by C8–T1 roots affected. Weakness occurring in a nerve distribution should lead to consideration of a different disorder, for example, multifocal motor neuropathy.

Fasciculations seen in many muscles in multiple limbs are ominous and are strongly suggestive of a motor neuron disease. Fasciculations that occur infrequently, or repetitively in one area, are more likely to have a benign origin, particularly in the absence of weakness or atrophy. The absence of fasciculations does not eliminate ALS. They may not be readily visible because of prominent subcutaneous tissue. Physicians often initially

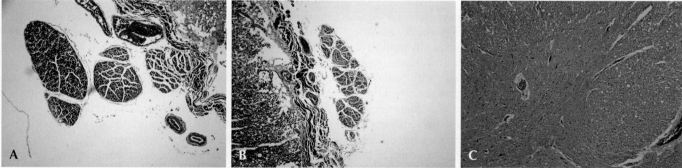

A, Dorsal root (normal), and B, ventral root (atrophic due to loss of lower motor neurons) in amyotrophic lateral sclerosis. C, Ventral gray matter of lumbar spinal cord showing loss of lower motor neurons. (From Amato AA, Russell JA. Neuromuscular Disorders, McGraw-Hill, New York, 2008, pp. 104-105.)

Figure 67-4 Dorsal and Ventral Roots and Ventral Horn.

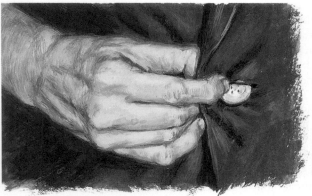

Fine movements of hand impaired; prominent metacarpal bones indicate atrophy of interossei muscles

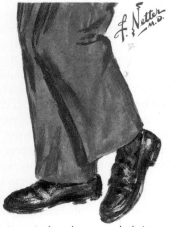

Weak, dragging gait; foot drop or early fatigue on walking

Figure 67-5 Motor Neuron Disease: Early Clinical Manifestations.

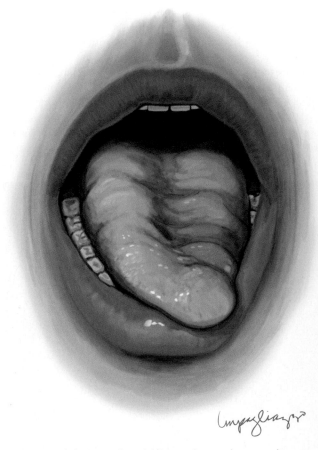

Asymmetric (left greater than right); atrophy, weakness, and fasciculations of the tongue, with deviation to the left on protrusion.

Figure 67-6 Tongue Atrophy in Amyotrophic Lateral Sclerosis.

recognize fasciculations, although the patient in retrospect may recall that they were present for some time. Muscle cramping is a common, albeit nonspecific, manifestation of motor neuron disease. The initiation of cramps during manual muscle testing is common in ALS.

What constitutes clinical signs of corticospinal or corticobulbar tract pathology may be more ambiguous. Spasticity represents a definite UMN sign; Babinski signs if unequivocal are confirmatory of UMN disease. Unfortunately, Babinski signs may not be elucidated in many ALS patients as a result of LMN toe extensor weakness. The Hoffman sign is generally indicative of UMN involvement of the arms, particularly if asymmetric. Hyperactive deep tendon reflexes, particularly with sustained clonus, indicate UMN involvement. The term relative UMN sign has been used to describe the presence of a deep tendon reflex in a weak and atrophic muscle. Reflex spread also implicates UMN disease; finger flexion (C8) occurring in response to brachioradialis tendon percussion (C6), and activation of the contralateral thigh adductors when the insertions of the ipsilateral thigh adductors are percussed (crossed adduction) are two notable examples of this phenomenon. Motor impairment in UMN disease typically results in slowness and incoordination. UMN weakness occurs in a specific pattern: the elbow, wrist,

and finger extensors are weaker than their flexor counterparts in the upper extremity whereas conversely, hip and knee flexors and foot dorsiflexors and evertors are weaker in the lower limb.

Tongue atrophy, fasciculation, and weakness are perhaps the most frequently occurring and recognized manifestations of LMN involvement of cranial nerves. It is important to observe for fasciculations when the tongue is relaxed on floor of the mouth (Fig. 67-6). Tremulousness of the tongue with attempted protrusion may be readily misinterpreted as representing fasciculations. Weakness of both facial and jaw muscles may occur in ALS but they are usually subtle. Weakness of neck extension and neck flexion is common in ALS, and head drop may be a rare presenting feature (Fig. 67-7). Neck drop is commonly associated with posterior neck discomfort and is typically relieved when the neck is supported. Notable for their absence are ptosis and ophthalmoparesis, and symptoms related to sight, hearing, taste, smell, and facial sensation.

Upper motor neuron signs and symptoms in the bulbar region may be more difficult to characterize. The presence of a jaw jerk or snout reflex is considered an indicator of corticobulbar tract dysfunction. An exaggerated gag reflex has a similar implication. One common manifestation of central nervous system involvement in ALS is a pseudobulbar affect, that is, the

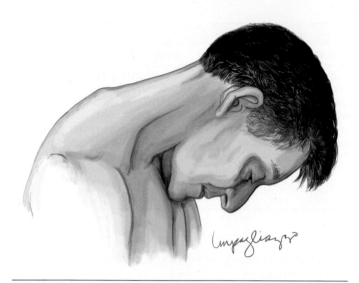

Figure 67-7 Head Drop in Amyotrophic Sclerosis.

tendency to laugh in the absence of happiness and cry in the absence of sadness. The pathologic substrate of this phenomenon is incompletely understood.

Symptoms related to disordered ventilation occur most commonly in the latter stages of ALS but may be the presenting manifestation in approximately 1% of patients. The inability to generate a robust cough, sniff, or sneeze is due to the inability to generate sufficient intrathoracic pressures due to LMN weakness of the internal intercostal or abdominal muscles. Orthopnea implicates diaphragmatic insufficiency due to anterior horn cell disease in the upper segments (C3–C5) of the cervical cord. Paradoxical abdominal movement, that is, outward (rather than the normal inward) movement of the abdominal wall during inspiration, is a helpful clinical sign. Disordered sleep is probably a common manifestation of impaired nocturnal ventilation, and early morning headache represents a fairly ominous indicator of nocturnal carbon dioxide retention.

As previously mentioned, clinical involvement of extraocular muscles and external urethral and rectal sphincters never occurs in ALS. ALS patients with UMN dominant disease may complain of urinary urgency. Traditionally, ALS is considered to be a painless disease. However, discomfort due to impaired mobility, spasticity, and cramping may be prominent. Immobilized upper extremities commonly result in painful adhesive capsulitis of the shoulders. Alteration in gait mechanics from leg weakness may put inordinate stress on the back, hips and knees, potentially exacerbating preexisting degenerative joint disease.

Behavioral and cognitive abnormalities in ALS have been recognized since the 19th century but may be obscured by dysarthria, or blamed on coexisting depression. The frontotemporal dementia (FTD) associated with ALS may precede, coincide, or follow signs and symptoms of motor neuron disease. It may occur in both sporadic and familial disease, and it is now estimated that 20% of ALS patients will fulfill criteria for FTD. The cognitive changes are most prominent in the domain of executive dysfunction and language. Disorganization, impaired planning, mental inflexibility, nonfluent progressive aphasia (word finding), and fluent semantic dementia (word meaning) may dominate the clinical picture. Tests of verbal fluency provide

a sensitive screening method. Normal patients should be able to generate at least 11 words in 1 minute in a defined category, for example, fruits. Behavioral difficulties are typically displayed in social and interpersonal realms. Patients lose the ability to appreciate nonverbal cues as well as the insight to interpret them. Patients may also become withdrawn, disinhibited, and depressed.

The classification of ALS and related motor neuron disease remains confusing. Many would suggest that the standard is based on histopathologic examination, demonstrating degeneration restricted to anterior horn cells, motor cranial nerve nuclei in the pons and medulla, and corticospinal and corticobulbar tracts, with or without the addition of ubiquitinated inclusions and Bunina bodies. The major problem with this approach of course is the impracticality of using autopsy as a diagnostic tool. An additional hurdle is the potential histopathologic involvement of other nonmotor neurologic systems, most notably the association with frontotemporal dementia. Diagnostic dilemmas occur when the course is slow, or when either UMN or LMN signs do not develop until late in the course. Less typical phenotypes of ALS have often been referred to by other names. Progressive bulbar palsy refers to motor neuron disease that initially exclusively affects bulbar function, typically speech and swallowing. Approximately a quarter of ALS patients, often older women, present in this manner. They may have both UMN and/or LMN features confined to lower cranial nerves. Eventually, the vast majority develops limb involvement and incontrovertible ALS.

Of the approximately two-thirds of patients who present with limb-onset disease, about a third will have predominantly or exclusively LMN features. Sporadic cases of pure lower motor neuron disease have been historically referred to as progressive muscular atrophy (PMA). Most PMA patients will develop UMN features, leaving little doubt that they have ALS. There are patients with PMA who progress more slowly than ALS and never develop UMN signs. Some of these patients, usually men, develop profound weakness that is restricted to either the upper or lower extremities for years before progressing to other regions. These syndromes have been referred to as bibrachial amyotrophic diplegia (BAD) and lower extremity amyotrophic diplegia (LAD), respectively. These designations have little practical value other than to alert clinicians that such atypical presentations exist.

The opposite end of the phenotypic spectrum is the patient with UMN predominant disease. Five percent or less of MND patients will present in this manner. Signs and symptoms typically begin in the legs but may start in the arms or bulbar regions. Exclusive UMN disease has historically been referred to as primary lateral sclerosis (PLS). PLS often has a much more protracted course than full-blown ALS. Most series report an average life expectancy of 7–14 years. A certain percentage of patients with PLS eventually develop clinical and electrodiagnostic evidence of LMN disease, and therefore it would be logical to consider PLS as a subtype of ALS until evidence suggests otherwise. PLS patients who devolve into ALS typically do so within 4 years of onset.

The El Escorial criteria were developed in 1990 in El Escorial, Spain, and were modified in 1998 in Airlie House, Virginia, in an attempt to develop consensus criteria for the research

Table 67-3 Differential Diagnosis of ALS

UMN and LMN Features	UMN Dominant Limb Onset	LMN Dominant Limb Onset	Bulbar Onset
Spinocerebellar degeneration	Hereditary spastic paraparesis	Multifocal motor neuropathy	Myasthenia gravis
Hexosaminidase deficiency	Compressive myelopathy	Inclusion body myositis	Kennedy disease
Hereditary spastic paraparesis	HTLV 1 infection	Hirayama disease	Inclusion body myositis
Copper deficiency	Paraneoplastic	Kennedy disease	Oculopharyngeal MD
Dural vascular malformations		Spinal muscular atrophy	Head and neck neoplasms
Polyglucosan disease		Benign fasciculations	Brainstem pathology
Prion disease		Myasthenia gravis	Multi-infarct state
			Chronic meningitis with multiple cranial nerve palsies

diagnosis of ALS. Definite diagnosis according to these criteria requires both UMN and LMN clinical findings in three of the four body regions (cranial, cervical, thoracic, and lumbosacral). In addition to a definite ALS category, there are probable, possible, and laboratory-supported probable ALS categories. The former two are based solely on clinical criteria, whereas the latter allows for consideration of electrodiagnostic evidence of denervation as a surrogate for clinical evidence of LMN disease. In most cases, an experienced neurologist will recognize the inevitability of the ALS diagnosis long before these criteria are fulfilled. Even more dissuasive is the recognition that approximately a quarter of ALS patients will succumb to their disease without fulfilling these criteria.

DIFFERENTIAL DIAGNOSIS

The differential diagnosis of ALS is largely that of other disorders of anterior horn cells, myopathies, disorders of neuromuscular transmission, motor predominant polyneuropathies and myelopathies (Table 67-3). With bulbar onset and predominantly LMN features, myasthenia gravis, inflammatory myopathy particularly inclusion body myositis, X-linked bulbospinal muscular atrophy (Kennedy disease), oculopharyngeal muscular dystrophy, multiple cranial neuropathies, or infiltrative head and neck cancers are the primary considerations. Of these, myasthenia gravis (MG) deserves the most attention. Clues favoring a diagnosis of MG include a weak tongue without atrophy or fasciculations, absence of UMN signs, and presence of ptosis or ophthalmoparesis. Dysphagia, usually without dysarthria, may rarely be the initial or most prominent symptom of the inflammatory myopathies. The pattern of limb weakness, the absence of fasciculations, and UMN signs in these disorders provides distinction from ALS. X-linked bulbospinal muscular atrophy or Kennedy disease may have early or prominent weakness of the throat, tongue, or jaw muscles often associated with fasciculation and may therefore easily be confused with bulbar ALS. A slower evolution of symptoms, the pattern of limb weakness, and the presence of gynecomastia and sensory abnormalities are distinctive features from ALS. Oculopharyngeal muscular dystrophy (OPMD) may be confused with bulbar ALS, although the course of OPMD is typically much longer, with a positive family history and prominent ptosis and ophthalmoplegia on examination. Multiple cranial neuropathies from chronic

meningitis (e.g., cancer, sarcoidosis) are usually associated with sensory dysfunction.

The differential diagnosis of head drop includes chronic inflammatory demyelinating neuropathy, radiation neuropathy, MG, and a wide variety of myopathies, for example, acid maltase deficiency, inflammatory myopathies, primary paraspinal myopathy, mitochondrial myopathy, and adult-onset nemaline myopathy. In addition, the dropped head syndrome may be mimicked by anterocollis resulting from multiple system atrophy and other extrapyramidal disorders. Neuromuscular causes of ventilatory failure in adults include a number of neuropathic disorders, for example, infectious disorders such as poliomyelitis and West Nile virus, Guillain–Barré syndrome, critical illness myoneuropathy, toxic neuropathies, and bilateral phrenic neuropathies. Severe hypophosphatemia and hypokalemia may result in ventilatory muscle weakness. In addition, disorders of neuromuscular transmission and some myopathies may progress to ventilatory insufficiency. MG, botulism and rare envenomations may be associated with diaphragmatic weakness. Acid maltase deficiency can affect ventilation early in the course. The dystrophinopathies, limb girdle dystrophy, myotonic muscular dystrophy, and adult-onset nemaline myopathy may progress to ventilatory failure.

In most series, multifocal motor neuropathy (MMN) is the entity most likely to be confused with LMN presentations of ALS. The distinction is important as MMN represents a potentially treatable disorder. The weakness of MMN occurs in an individual nerve distribution rather than in the myotomal pattern of ALS. Unfortunately, as the disease progresses, the confluence of deficits may preclude the identification of this distinctive multifocal neuropathy pattern. In addition, in keeping with its initial demyelinating pathophysiology, MMN often produces weakness in the absence of atrophy. The clinician may have to rely on electrodiagnostic or serologic testing, and a therapeutic trial of intravenous immunoglobulin to make a confident diagnosis.

Another disorder that may be mistaken as LMN predominant ALS is IBM. IBM presents with asymmetric painless weakness in older males that may affect distal as well as proximal muscles. Wrist and finger flexors, foot dorsiflexors, and quadriceps are often weak. The slow progression and the typical pattern of weakness help distinguish IBM from ALS. The juvenile segmental form of spinal muscular atrophy (Hirayama disease) may be difficult to initially distinguish from ALS. This is a slowly progressive and self-limited LMN disorder affecting young adult men with initial involvement of C8–T1 hand and forearm muscles unilaterally.

Benign fasciculations tend to occur repetitively in a single region of a single muscle over the course of a few seconds to minutes and then disappear. The calves and the orbicularis oculi tend to be particularly affected. Patients may seek medical attention for fasciculations that they describe as being widespread and pervasive. Their examination demonstrates no pathologic alterations in muscle strength, bulk, or tone and no reflex abnormalities. In this context, particularly with a normal EMG examination, the patient can be reassured.

UMN presentations of ALS affecting the limbs have a more extensive differential diagnosis. Cervical spondylotic myelopathy is a major differential diagnostic consideration, particularly in individuals presenting with LMN signs in the arms and UMN features in the legs. The presence of sensory and bladder symptoms and imaging should help distinguish this disorder from ALS. Other causes of myelopathy including ischemic (e.g., dural vascular malformations of the spinal cord), infectious, and inflammatory causes of myelopathy also remain considerations.

The differential diagnosis of ALS also uncommonly includes a number of hereditary and degenerative disorders. Of these, hereditary spastic paraparesis is potentially the most confounding, particularly in those individuals in whom there is no family history. Slow progression, the high arched feet, loss of large fiber sensory perception in the feet, and sparing of upper extremity and bulbar function are distinguishing features. An ALS-like syndrome may occur in certain individuals with hexosaminidase deficiency, typically in compound heterozygotes. A motor neuron syndrome may also accompany the spinocerebellar atrophies, particularly type III (Machado–Joseph disease) or occasionally in prion disorders such as Creutzfeldt–Jakob and Gerstmann–Straussler–Scheinker disease. Polyglucosan disease is a rare heritable disorder of glycogen metabolism that may produce cognitive and genitourinary issues in addition to a motor neuropathy.

Finally, certain toxic, metabolic, infectious, immune-mediated, and paraneoplastic conditions have been reported to mimic ALS. Lead toxicity, hyperthyroidism and parathyroidism, HIV, Lyme disease, and lymphoma are the most notable of these. Recently, serum copper deficiency has been reported as a potential ALS mimic and should receive consideration in anyone with an ALS-like syndrome with unexplained sensory complaints.

DIAGNOSTIC APPROACH

There is no perfect algorithm in the evaluation of an ALS suspect. In a patient with LMN and UMN features that have progressed in a typical pattern and time course, the diagnosis is indisputable. In most cases where ALS is suspected, tests are ordered guided by the clinician's index of suspicion (Table 67-4). In large part, these tests are done to exclude considerations other than ALS.

Virtually every ALS patient undergoes electromyography and nerve conduction studies, collectively referred to as electrodiagnosis (EDX) (Table 67-5). The goal of EDX in ALS is to confirm a pattern of active denervation, chronic denervation, and fasciculation potentials in multiple muscles innervated by multiple segments in multiple regions. According to the modified El Escorial EDX criteria, a definite diagnosis of ALS requires evidence of active denervation (fibrillation potentials and positive sharp waves) in at least three of the following four body regions: cranial, cervical, thoracic, and lumbosacral. In the limbs, at least two different muscles belonging to different nerve and root innervations need to be affected. Involvement in a single cranial muscle is sufficient to satisfy that region's requirements. Thoracic paraspinal muscles are particularly helpful as they are uncommonly denervated in non-ALS disorders. Fasciculation potentials are a supportive but not mandatory

Table 67-4 Testing Considerations for a Suspected ALS Patient

All Patients	LMN Presentations	UMN Presentations	Bulbar Presentations	Selected Patients
EMG/NCS	Anti-GM1 antibodies	MRI brain, cervical, and thoracic spinal cord	MRI brain	HTLV-1
Pulmonary function	Acetylcholine receptor-binding antibodies	CSF examination	Acetylcholine receptor-binding antibodies	Lyme serology
	Muscle-specific kinase antibodies	HSP genotyping	Muscle-specific kinase antibodies	HIV serology
	MRI lumbosacral spine	Serum copper	CSF examination	Hexosaminidase levels
	Serum CK	Serum B_{12}	Serum CK	Androgen receptor gene mutational analysis
		Mammography		Muscle biopsy
		Amphiphysin antibodies		Nerve biopsy
				C26–C22 long-chain fatty acid ratio
				Survival motor neuron gene mutation
				Paraneoplastic antibodies
				Serum copper and ceruloplasmin
				TSH, calcium, PTH

HSP, hereditary spastic paraparesis; CSF, cerebrospinal fluid; TSH, thyroid-stimulating hormone; PTH, parathormone.

Table 67-5 Electrodiagnostic Features of EMG

Pattern of abnormalities	Multisegmental in multiple regions (cranial–cervical–thoracoabdominal–lumbosacral)
Motor conductions	↓ or normal CMAP amplitudes depending on severity, relative preservation of conduction velocities, and distal latencies
Sensory conductions	Normal
F waves and H reflexes	F waves normal or absent, M response of H reflex reduced in amplitude, absent or normal depending on severity. Latencies preserved
Slow repetitive stimulation	May demonstrate decremental response
Spontaneous activity (EMG)	Fibrillation potentials and positive waves necessary for diagnosis, complex repetitive, myotonic, myokymic, and neuromyotonic discharges uncommon and should lead to alternative considerations
MUP morphology	Typically long duration, high amplitude with instability if sought for
MUP recruitment	MUP recruitment reduced, MUP activation may be reduced as well with prominent UMN component.

CMAP, compound muscle action potential; MUP, motor unit potential.

electrodiagnostic feature. Features that would suggest an alternative diagnosis that might mimic ALS need to be excluded; examples include abnormal sensory conductions in Kennedy syndrome, decremental response to repetitive stimulation consistent with myasthenia, conduction block suggestive of multifocal motor neuropathy, or small motor unit potentials suggestive of a myopathy such as IBM. Finally EX may offer insight into the rate of progression, that is, active denervation without chronic denervation and reinnervation, motor unit variability, and a rapid decline in motor unit estimation being electrodiagnostic indicators of a rapidly progressive course.

MR imaging of the brain should be strongly considered in any patient with a bulbar presentation without limb involvement to identify brainstem parenchymal, meningeal, or cranial nerve disorders. Imaging of the cervical and/or thoracic cord would be indicated in patients with predominantly UMN limb involvement without bulbar signs. Lumbosacral MRI with gadolinium enhancement is indicated in purely LMN syndromes affecting the lower extremities to evaluate for conus medullaris or cauda equina pathology. MRI, positron emission tomography (PET) or single-photon emission computed tomographic (SPECT) imaging may support preferential atrophy or hypometabolism of the anterior brain in individuals suspected of having FTLD.

It is important to recognize that elevated serum creatine kinase levels are not specific for myopathy. Approximately two thirds of ALS patients will have creatine kinase elevations, typically in the 300–500 U/L range but occasionally as high as 1000 or more. Antibodies directed at the GM1 ganglioside are found in high titer in 30–80% of patients with MMN. They are typically ordered in patients with LMN syndromes without cranial nerve or UMN findings. Serologic tests for myasthenia, typically acetylcholine receptor binding, may be obtained in patients with bulbar presentations. Other tests, listed in Table 67-4, are used more judiciously in the appropriate clinical context. Many patients with ALS inquire about the possibility of Lyme disease, and Lyme serologies are frequently ordered to lessen these concerns. HIV testing is not done in suspected ALS unless the clinical context would suggest an increased probability of infection. Historically, screening for heavy metals, thyroid and parathyroid disorders, and occult neoplasia was emphasized. Serum copper, ceruloplasmin, and zinc levels should be considered in any patient with weakness and unexplained sensory symptoms.

Testing for the five commercially available fALS genetic tests is performed in patients with suspected ALS in whom there have been other affected family members. Genetic testing is not recommended in apparent sporadic ALS patients unless there are mitigating circumstances. With a known SOD1 mutation in the proband, testing in an asymptomatic family member should only be done after detailed counseling.

Muscle biopsy is rarely done in ALS suspects except to exclude IBM or other myopathies that might mimic ALS. Pulmonary function tests are used to monitor disease progression; forced vital capacity and inspiratory pressure measurements are obtained both in the sitting and supine positions. Forced vital capacity of less than 50% of predicted suggests a 6-month life expectancy and along with a negative inspiratory force of <60 cm H_2O or PCO_2 of >40 mm Hg are indications for the use of positive airway pressure equipment.

MANAGEMENT AND THERAPY

Management of ALS includes disease-specific treatments, symptomatic and supportive treatments, as well as adequate education and counseling. These are summarized in Table 67-6 and are elaborated on in two of the reviews listed in the bibliography. Rilutek is the only FDA-approved and effective pharmacologic agent identified to date. Unfortunately, it prolongs life expectancy on average by 10% without noticeable improvement in function or sense of well-being. Its cost is substantial, and it should be prescribed only after the patient has been informed of its benefits and drawbacks. Patients should be encouraged to participate in clinical trials when available. Many ALS patients utilize alternative health measures. Patients should be informed that any treatment biologically active enough to help is also biologically capable of harm. It is not uncommon for patients to ask for medications that have been touted, but unproven to be effective. If these agents are to be studied in clinical trials, clinicians should discourage their use outside of the trial so as to not subvert enrollment in and/or the integrity of the trial.

An important aspect of the management of ALS patients and their families is the provision of reliable education. It is important to discuss end-of-life issues with a patient at some point before a ventilatory crisis occurs or the ability to communicate is lost. Until an effective treatment is found, the primary goals in ALS management are to provide symptom relief and to maintain independent and safe function. In the later stages of disease, the primary goal shifts to maintenance of comfort. Table 67-6 provides a list of many of these potential interventions (Fig. 67-8). In our clinic, we focus on symptoms referable to the

Table 67-6 Therapeutic Considerations in ALS

Problem	Potential Prescription	Problem	Potential Prescription
ALS	Riluzole 50 mg bid	Contractures	Night splints
ALS	Clinical trials		Botulinum toxin
Sialorrhea (excessive thin secretions)	Glycopyrrolate		Range-of-motion exercises
	Tricyclic antidepressants	Tripping from foot drop	Ankle–foot orthoses
	Robinul		
	Botulinum toxin	Falling secondary to quadriceps weakness	Canes
	Atropine		Crutches
	Salivary gland radiation		Walker
	Scopolamine		Knee–ankle–foot orthoses with mercury switch
	Chorda tympani section		Wheelchair, manual or power
Secretion clearance (thick secretions)	Home suction	Reduced bed mobility	Hospital bed with side-rails and/or trapeze
	Cough assist devices	Bathroom safety and functionality	Stall shower
	Expectorants (e.g., guaifenesin)		Shower chair
	Beta blockers		Transfer bench
	Nebulized n-acetylcysteine and albuterol		Toilet seat extension
	Tracheostomy		Shower and toilet bars
Pseudobulbar affect	Dextromethorphan hydrobromide and quinidine sulfate	House accessibility	Stair lift
	Tricyclic antidepressants		Lift chair or chair lift
	Selective serotonin reuptake inhibitors		Hoyer lift
	Selective serotonin and norepinephrine reuptake inhibitors		Elevators
			Ramps
			Transfer belt
Depression	Tricyclic antidepressants	Improved ADLs	Velcro for buttons and shoelaces
	Selective serotonin reuptake inhibitors		Elastic shoelaces
			Long-handled grippers
	Selective serotonin and norepinephrine reuptake inhibitors		Foam collars for pens and utensils
		Dysphagia— malnutrition	Neck positioning
	Stimulants		Change in food consistency
Laryngospasm	Antihistamines		Liquid thickeners
	H_2 receptor blockers		Percutaneous gastrostomy
	Antacids	Constipation	Bulk and fiber (applesauce–prunes–bran mix)
	Proton pump inhibitors		Stool softeners/cathartics
	Sublingual lorazepam drops		Hydration
Neck drop	Cervical collar (headmaster)	Urinary urgency	Tolterodine
Communication	Assistive augmentative communication (AAC) devices	Cramps	Gabapentin
	Pad and pencil or erasable slates		Tizanidine or baclofen
Hypoventilation	Positive pressure ventilators, e.g. BiPAP		Benzodiazepines
			Phenytoin
	Negative pressure ventilators, e.g. Cuirass		Carbamazepine
			Mexiletine
	Tracheostomy and mechanical ventilation		Primrose oil
			Brewer's yeast
	Morphine sulfate	Safety	Lifeline
	Benzodiazepines		Phone auto dialer
			Home safety evaluation

following domains: pain, sleep, psychosocial issues, speech and swallowing, ventilation, motor function, and miscellaneous issues. As mentioned above, pain occurs commonly in this disease. Prophylactic range of motion should be applied to immobilized body parts. Analgesics including opioids may be required. Impaired sleep has many potential causes in an ALS patient, including discomfort secondary to immobility or cramping, depression, impaired ventilation and bathroom requirements, each of which may be have to be identified and addressed separately.

FUTURE DIRECTIONS

Current ALS research is focusing on the identification of biomarkers in ALS that might allow for improved classification of the motor neuron diseases, earlier and more precise identification of ALS patients, and potential insights into critical pathophysiological mechanisms. In addition, scientists are currently attempting to identify susceptibility genes that would potentially provide additional clues for disease origins and mechanisms. Although stem cell biology offers the hope of replacing

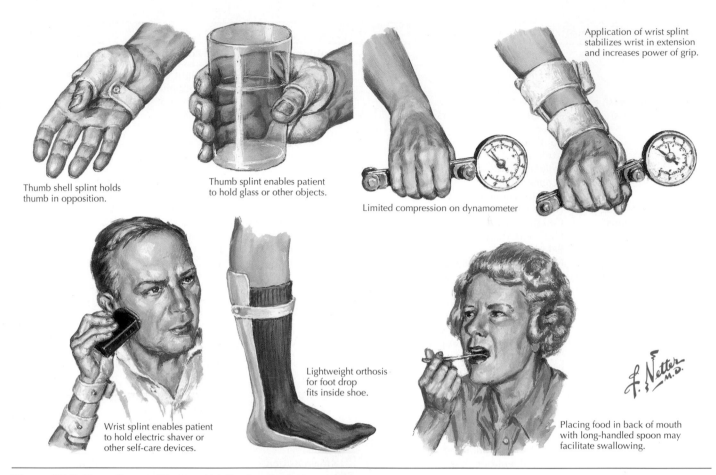

Thumb shell splint holds thumb in opposition.

Thumb splint enables patient to hold glass or other objects.

Application of wrist splint stabilizes wrist in extension and increases power of grip.

Limited compression on dynamometer

Wrist splint enables patient to hold electric shaver or other self-care devices.

Lightweight orthosis for foot drop fits inside shoe.

Placing food in back of mouth with long-handled spoon may facilitate swallowing.

Figure 67-8 Motor Neuron Disease: Habilitation Devices.

degenerating motor neurons, ultimately, identifying the root causes of ALS and eliminating them will provide a realistic means by which to cure this devastating disease.

ADDITIONAL RESOURCES

Amato AA, Russell JA. Neuromuscular Disorders. New York: McGraw Hill; 2008.

Bensimon G, Lacomblez L, Meininger V, et al. A controlled trial of riluzole in amyotrophic lateral sclerosis. N Engl J Med 1994;330:585-591.

Chaudhuri KR, Crump SJ, Al-Sarraj S, et al. The validation of El Escorial criteria for the diagnosis of amyotrophic lateral sclerosis: a clinical-pathological study. J Neurol Sci 1995;129(Suppl.):11-12.

Hand C, Rouleau GA. Familial amyotrophic lateral sclerosis. Muscle Nerve 2002;25:135-159.

Miller RG, Jackson CE, Kasarskis EJ, et al. Practice Parameter update: the care of the patient with amyotrophic lateral sclerosis: drug, nutritional, and respiratory therapies (an evidence-based review): report of the Quality Standards Subcommittee of the American Academy of Neurology. Neurology 2009;73:1218-1226.

Miller RG, Jackson CE, Kasarskis EJ, et al. Practice Parameter update: multidisciplinary care, symptom management, and cognitive/behavioral impairment (an evidence-based review): report of the Quality Standards Subcommittee of the American Academy of Neurology. Neurology 2009;73:1227-1233.

Pasinelli P, Brown RH. Molecular biology of amyotrophic lateral sclerosis: insights from genetics. Nature Reviews 2006;7:710-723.

Rowland L. Diagnosis of amyotrophic lateral sclerosis. J Neurol Sci 1998;160(Suppl.):6-24.

Shaw CE, Al-Chalabi A. Susceptibility genes in sporadic ALS: separating the wheat from the chaff by international collaboration. Neurology 2006;67:738-739.

Strong MJ, Lomen-Hoerth C, Caselli RJ, et al. Cognitive impairment, frontotemporal dementia and the motor neuron diseases. Ann Neurol 2003;54(5):S20-S23.

Other Motor Neuron Diseases and Motor Neuropathies

James A. Russell

68

Clinical Vignette

A 63-year-old man was evaluated for 3 years of slowly progressive symptoms of proximal lower extremity weakness. He first noted difficulty negotiating the high step up from the dock to the deck of his boat. Eleven years prior to his neurologic evaluation for weakness, he had been evaluated for painful enlarged breasts, attributed to alcoholic liver disease. More recently, he had noticed difficulty swallowing and had received the Heimlich maneuver on one occasion. Increasingly, muscle cramping had become an annoyance. His mother was troubled by dysphagia and questionable weakness in later life; a brother, two sons, and a daughter had no symptoms. Examination was remarkable for mild facial, tongue, neck flexor and proximal weakness of upper and lower extremities. Tongue and chin fasciculations were seen. There was a mild postural tremor of the hands. Muscle stretch reflexes were traced at the patellar and biceps tendons but otherwise absent. Sensory examination was normal. There were no upper motor neuron signs. Serum creatine kinase level was modestly elevated to 500 IU/L. On nerve conduction studies (NCS), the amplitudes of sensory nerve action potentials were reduced. Needle electromyography (EMG) demonstrated reduced recruitment of high-amplitude and long-duration motor unit potentials consistent with chronic partial denervation and reinnervation in a generalized distribution. Fasciculation potentials were abundant. No evidence of active denervation was demonstrable. Genetic testing revealed expansion of the CAG trinucleotide repeat (>35 CAGs) in the androgen receptor (AR) gene.

M otor neuron diseases (MNDs) are disorders that produce painless weakness, atrophy, cramps, and fasciculations and are consequent to degeneration of anterior horn cells and selective cranial nerve nuclei. This chapter will address notable MNDs other than ALS.

Many of the disorders discussed in this chapter have known or suspected genetic mechanisms. The spinal muscular atrophies (SMAs) are conceptualized as largely inherited disorders in which there is predominant degeneration of anterior horn cells and selective cranial nerve nuclei. In the childhood SMAs, mutations of a single gene and derangement of a single gene product are responsible for the majority of cases, and the resultant phenotype is fairly homogeneous. In other disorders, for example, hereditary spastic paraplegia (HSP), there are a plethora of recognized genotypes correlating with an almost equally heterogeneous array of phenotypic variations.

Because of the relative rarity of these disorders, societal impact is usually limited. However, as with most hereditary disorders, the impact on individuals and families is substantial. This is particularly true for spinal muscular atrophy type I where parents have to cope with the consequences of a newborn with a lethal illness as well as with the specter that subsequent children are at risk. SMA I, also known as Werdnig–Hoffman disease, is the most common of the SMAs. Its incidence is estimated to be between 4 and 10 in 100,000 live births depending on the geographic cohort studied. After cystic fibrosis, it is the second most common, lethal, recessively inherited disorder of Caucasians.

CLINICAL PRESENTATION

Spinal Muscular Atrophy Types I–IV

Spinal muscular atrophy types I–IV are allelic disorders of the survival motor neuron (SMN) gene 1 located on chromosome 5q12.2-q13.3. When there is more than one affected individual in a given family, the phenotype is typically homogeneous but may be disparate in some cases. In normal individuals, there are two copies each of the SMN1 and SMN2 genes. Both genes produce similar but not identical proteins; the SMN2 gene appears to produce an unstable and rapidly degrading protein that can partially compensate for the lack of the SMN1 protein. There are no known clinical consequences from mutations of the SMN2 gene alone.

It is estimated that 95% of SMA I–III patients are homozygous for deletion of exons 7 and 8 of the SMN1 gene. The remainder are thought to be compound heterozygotes with absence of exons 7 and 8 on one allele and a point mutation of the other SMN1 allele. The severity of the SMA phenotype appears to be related to the number of SMN2 copies available to compensate for deleted SMN1 gene. Homozygotes devoid of SMN1 who harbor two copies of SMN2 tend to manifest as an SMA I phenotype. An increasing number of SMN2 copies correlates with proportionately milder (SMA II-IV) forms of the disease. Individuals homozygous for the SMN1 mutation with five copies of the SMN2 gene have been reported to be asymptomatic. Why motor neurons remain selectively vulnerable to SMN deficiency remains unknown.

Of the multiple SMA phenotypes, the infantile and childhood forms are the most prevalent. SMA type I or Werdnig–Hoffman disease is the most severe form (Fig. 68-1). Clinical manifestations become evident within the first 6 months of life. In contrast to the latter three categories, afflicted children with SMA I never develop the capability of sitting independently. In some cases, recognition of reduced movement occurs in utero or within the first few days of life. Affected infants are hypotonic with a symmetric, generalized, or proximally predominant

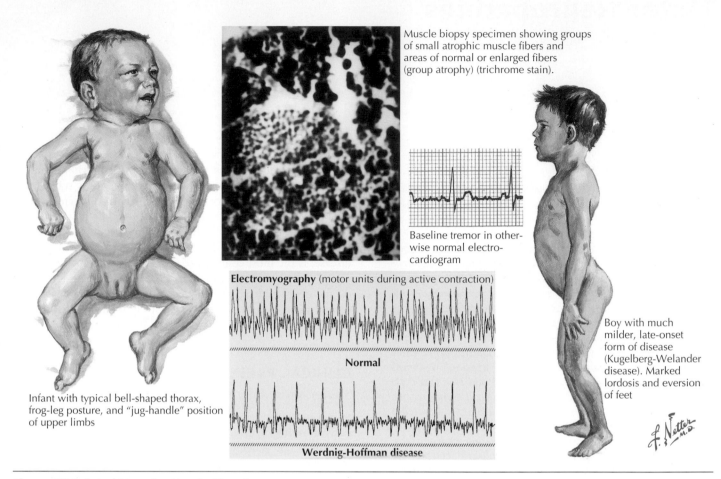

Muscle biopsy specimen showing groups of small atrophic muscle fibers and areas of normal or enlarged fibers (group atrophy) (trichrome stain).

Baseline tremor in otherwise normal electrocardiogram

Electromyography (motor units during active contraction)

Normal

Werdnig-Hoffman disease

Infant with typical bell-shaped thorax, frog-leg posture, and "jug-handle" position of upper limbs

Boy with much milder, late-onset form of disease (Kugelberg-Welander disease). Marked lordosis and eversion of feet

Figure 68-1 Spinal Muscular Atrophy Type 1.

pattern of weakness. Like ALS, facial weakness is typically mild and extraocular muscles are spared. Fasciculations are seen in the tongue but rarely in limb muscles, presumably because of the ample subcutaneous tissue of neonates. Manual tremor, so characteristic of SMA types II and III, is rarely present. Deep tendon reflexes are typically absent. Abdominal breathing, a weak cry, and a poor suck are commonplace. Ventilation difficulties stem primarily from intercostal rather than diaphragmatic weakness. Pectus excavatum and a diminished anteroposterior diameter of the chest are seen. Mild contractures may occur but arthrogryposis is not part of the classic phenotype. Intellectual development is normal. Without mechanical ventilation, death is inevitable, almost always within a year or two. An earlier age of onset correlates with a shorter life expectancy.

SMA type Ia refers to a severe form of neonatal SMA associated with arthrogryposis multiplex congenita and a paucity of movement. Prognosis is poor with ventilatory support required at birth.

The intermediate form or SMA II typically begins between 6 and 18 months of age. The disorder is clinically defined by a child who sits independently but never walks. Postural hand tremor is the only significant phenotypic variance from Werdnig–Hoffman disease. Tongue fasciculations, areflexia, and a generalized to proximally predominant and symmetric pattern of weakness mimic the SMA I phenotype. Approximately 98% of these individuals survive to age 5 and two thirds to age 25. In view of the more protracted course and of wheelchair

dependency SMA II and SMA III patients commonly acquire kyphoscoliosis and joint contractures (Fig. 68-2).

The SMA III or the Kugelberg–Welander syndrome differs from the intermediate form only in the age of onset, milestones achieved, and life expectancy. Affected individuals develop the ability to stand and walk. Onset age is typically 18 months or more. Certain authors have attempted to divide SMA III into type a and type b, based on age at onset of symptoms, with the intention of better defining the natural history in individual patients. In SMA type IIIa, defined as symptom onset before 3 years, it is estimated that 70% will remain ambulatory 10 years after symptom onset. Twenty percent will still ambulate in 30 years after symptom onset. In SMA type IIIb, defined as symptom onset after 3 years, virtually all patients will remain ambulatory in 10 years and 60% at 40 years after symptom onset. Life expectancy extends into the sixth decade and may be normal in many individuals. Initial symptoms are typically related to proximal weakness. Hand tremor, areflexia, and tongue fasciculations are commonplace. Fasciculations in limb muscles are more evident than in SMA types I and II.

Adult-onset SMA IV is a rare, genetically heterogeneous disorder. SMA IV children achieve motor milestones at normal ages. Onset of weakness is typically in the third or fourth decade in the recessively inherited cases. Initial symptoms are typically proximal weakness of the lower extremities, particularly the hip flexors, hip extensors, and knee extensors. Shoulder abductors

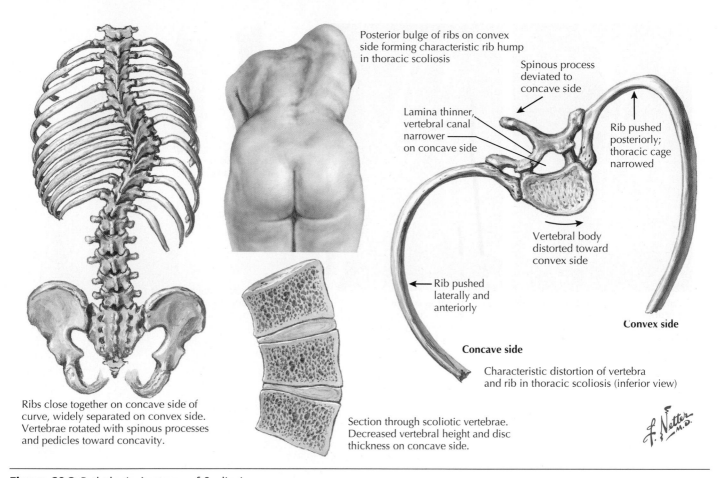

Posterior bulge of ribs on convex side forming characteristic rib hump in thoracic scoliosis

Spinous process deviated to concave side

Lamina thinner, vertebral canal narrower on concave side

Rib pushed posteriorly; thoracic cage narrowed

Vertebral body distorted toward convex side

Rib pushed laterally and anteriorly

Convex side

Concave side

Characteristic distortion of vertebra and rib in thoracic scoliosis (inferior view)

Ribs close together on concave side of curve, widely separated on convex side. Vertebrae rotated with spinous processes and pedicles toward concavity.

Section through scoliotic vertebrae. Decreased vertebral height and disc thickness on concave side.

Figure 68-2 Pathologic Anatomy of Scoliosis.

and elbow extensors are the most frequently affected muscles of the arms. Tongue fasciculations, hand tremor, and in some cases, calf hypertrophy may occur. Life expectancy in SMA IV is normal. Parents with SMA IV have given birth to children with more severe SMA phenotypes.

Spinal Muscular Atrophy with Respiratory Distress (SMARD1)

This is a rare disorder in which infants develop diaphragmatic weakness and ventilatory weakness in addition to hypotonia.

X-Linked Bulbospinal Muscular Atrophy (SBMA)—Kennedy Disease

SBMA is an X-linked disorder associated with an androgen receptor gene mutation. Consequently, it has frequent endocrine as well as neuromuscular consequences, the latter providing the primary source of morbidity.

SBMA is an X-linked, adult-onset disorder that is depicted in the vignette at the beginning of this chapter. It is a disorder almost exclusively of males with a median age of onset of 44 years. Initial symptoms are usually attributable to weakness of bulbar or proximal limb muscles. Younger men, and rarely female carriers, may be symptomatic but may go undiagnosed unless there are other previously diagnosed family members.

As the name implies, the clinical manifestations are largely referable to degeneration of the lower cranial nerve motor nuclei and anterior horn cells of the spinal cord. The weakness progresses insidiously and is proximally predominant and symmetric in pattern. Typically, symptoms referable to the lower extremities have the greatest initial impact. Approximately 10% of the time, the initial symptoms pertain to difficulty with swallowing, chewing, or speaking. Facial weakness is common. Jaw drop due to muscles of mastication may occur as well. Perioral and tongue fasciculations are common and represent helpful clinical clues. Like ALS, ptosis and ophthalmoparesis should suggest an alternative diagnosis. Like other SMAs, postural tremor is common. There is an associated, but frequently asymptomatic, sensory neuropathy that may only be recognized by nerve conduction studies. Clinical heterogeneity exists. Asymmetry of muscle weakness at onset has been emphasized by some authors. Occasionally, rapidly progressive weakness occurs. The median age of wheelchair dependency is 61 years or approximately 15 years after onset of weakness. Women who are heterozygous for Kennedy disease mutation may rarely be symptomatic.

The effects of SBMA are not restricted to the neuromuscular system. Affected males suffer the consequences of androgen insensitivity, including gynecomastia, impotence, testicular atrophy, and potential infertility. There is also an increased incidence of diabetes mellitus.

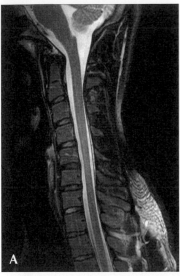 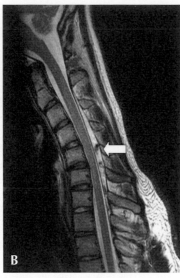 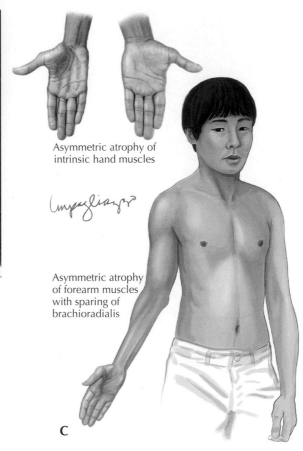

A. and B. Sagittal T2 fast spin echo imaging of cervical spinal cord in (A) neutral and (B) flexion. Note marked expansion of posterior epidural space on flexion with signal voids indicating enlarged veins. **C,** Atrophy of the forearm and intrinsic hand muscles (C7, C8, and T1 myotomes) in Hirayama disease with sparing of brachioradialis.
Courtesy Dr. Devon Rubin, Mayo Clinic.

Asymmetric atrophy of intrinsic hand muscles

Asymmetric atrophy of forearm muscles with sparing of brachioradialis

Figure 68-3 Hirayama Disease.

Juvenile Segmental Spinal Muscular Atrophy—Benign Focal Amyotrophy—Hirayama Disease

Unlike other SMAs, Hirayama disease appears to be a sporadic disorder in the majority of cases. In 1963, Hirayama described a slowly progressive, focal motor neuron disease affecting one, and at times, both upper extremities. In this and subsequent descriptions, males are affected in 60% of cases. Hirayama disease is perhaps best considered as a segmental or regional form of spinal muscular atrophy. Onset is typically between ages 15 and 25 with a range of 2 to 30 years. Although most commonly reported in those of Asian origin, it may occur in any ethnic background.

The characteristic phenotype is the insidious development of atrophy and weakness in C8–T1 muscles of the hand and forearm. It begins unilaterally, typically in the dominant extremity. Over the course of months to years, the weakness may gradually spread to involve more proximal muscles. In a third of cases, there is clinical weakness of the opposite limb. An even higher percentage will have bilateral upper extremity involvement on electrodiagnostic studies. Tendon reflexes in the involved limb may be spared, although neither overt pyramidal or bulbar involvement occurs. Reflex preservation may reflect the restricted nature of the disease and the lack of a reliable C8–T1 muscle stretch reflex. Like many other SMAs, tremor may occur. In most cases, there is an arrest of further progression after 6 years or less. Although a significant decline in affected limb function in the cold is common with all motor neuron diseases, "cold paresis" is particularly emphasized in this population. Hyperhidrosis of the involved limb has been described.

Hirayama disease is less frequently seen in Western populations. Ischemic changes in the cervical spinal cord of a single autopsied case of Hirayama disease led to the hypothesis of a compressive mechanism. In 2000, Hirayama reported the results of dynamic imaging in 73 patients and 20 controls. Ninety-four percent of patients had significant forward displacement and flattening of the posterior surface of the cervical cord during neck flexion (Fig. 68-3). The presumption is that the blood supply to the spinal cord is compromised, with the anterior horn representing the watershed and the most susceptible to ischemia. Other observations that supported this potential mechanism are the frequent asymmetric nature of spinal cord flattening in keeping with the asymmetric disease onset, and the lesser degree to which distortion occurred in older patients in whom progression had arrested. Nonetheless, this pathogenetic hypothesis is not universally accepted.

Scapuloperoneal Form of SMA (Davidenkow Disease)

A scapuloperoneal pattern of weakness may result from either neurogenic or myopathic disorders. The neurogenic form of the scapuloperoneal syndrome has been referred to by the eponym

Table 68-1 Genetics of Spinal Muscular Atrophies

Classification	Chromosome	Gene
SMA I-IV	5q12.2-q13.3	SMN1
SMARD I	11q13.2-q13.4	IGHMBP2
SBMA (Kennedy)	X	Androgen receptor gene
Juvenile segmental SMA (Hirayama)	None identified	None identified
Scapuloperoneal (Davidenkow)	17p11.2	PMP 22

Davidenkow disease. It has been considered to represent a SMA variant even though distal sensory loss was common in Davidenkow's original series. Symptomatic onset typically occurs in late childhood related to asymmetric weakness of scapular fixators or foot dorsiflexors. Weakness typically progresses into a more generalized pattern. Some patients with a neurogenic scapuloperoneal syndrome have been found to have mutations within the *PMP-22* gene. This suggests that the disorder might be more correctly characterized as a hereditary neuropathy.

Distal SMA (Hereditary Motor Neuronopathy, Spinal Forms of Charcot–Marie–Tooth Disease)

Distal SMA (dSMA) is usually inherited in a dominant fashion in one third of cases but may have recessive or X-linked pattern as well. There are numerous genetic loci (Table 68-1). Like hereditary spastic paraparesis, distal SMA can be either "pure" or "complicated" based upon other neurologic system involvement. Complicated phenotypes may include diaphragmatic paralysis, vocal cord paralysis, and arthrogryposis.

Harding and Thomas introduced the concept of dSMA in 1980. The dSMAs have been perceived as progressive, hereditary disorders producing distal symmetric weakness in the absence of either clinical or electrodiagnostic sensory loss. The dSMAs have also been referred to as hereditary motor neuropathies but are considered to be anterior horn cell disorders in view of their pure motor manifestations. Distal SMA strongly resembles Charcot–Marie–Tooth (CMT) disease without sensory involvement. In fact, at least three forms of dSMA are allelic to recessively inherited forms of CMT. Weakness in distal SMA typically predominates in ankle dorsiflexors and evertors and toe extensors. Foot deformities characteristic of CMT are also common. Hand muscles may eventually become involved. There are a number of recognized dSMA genotypes (see Table 68-1).

Poliomyelitis

Poliomyelitis is a viral infection with tropism for gray matter of the spinal cord and motor cranial nuclei. Poliomyelitis translates literally into inflammation of spinal cord gray matter. It is often used synonymously with paralytic polio caused by the polio virus. In this chapter, it will refer to any viral infection with a predilection for anterior horn cells or motor cranial nerve

nuclei. Polio may be either a monophasic or biphasic disease. The initial symptoms are nonspecific, last 1–2 days, and are predominantly constitutional and/or gastrointestinal in nature. They consist of fever, malaise, pharyngitis, headache, nausea, vomiting, and abdominal cramping (Fig. 68-4). In the majority of infected individuals, the illness is self-limited and ends at this point. In individuals who fall victim to the "major" illness, symptoms of brain or spinal cord involvement develop 3 to 10 days subsequent to the initial symptoms. The major illness is defined by CNS involvement with meningoencephalitis, with or without an associated paralytic component. Stiff neck, back pain, and fever are prominent; encephalitis with altered mental status can also be seen.

In individuals destined to develop paralytic disease, myalgias and cramping rapidly evolve into muscle weakness. The progression reaches its nadir within 48 hours of onset. The paralysis is typically asymmetric. It is confined to the limbs and trunk in half of the cases. There is a predilection for lumbosacral segments and proximal more than distal muscles (Fig. 68-5). Ten percent of cases have bulbar weakness only. Children are particularly susceptible to bulbar polio. Motor functions of the 7th, 9th and 10th cranial nerves are most likely to be affected. Ten percent of patients will manifest both spinal and bulbar weakness; ventilatory failure is more common in this group. Affected limbs are flaccid and areflexic. Like virtually all motor neuron disorders, the 3rd, 4th, and 6th cranial nerves are spared. Sensory signs and symptoms are atypical. In keeping with the known pathological involvement of the brainstem tegmentum and hypothalamus in cases with encephalitic components, clinical dysautonomia including fluctuating blood pressure, cardiac arrhythmia, and hyperhydrosis may occur.

The natural history of paralytic polio is variable, dependent in large part on the severity and extent of the initial illness. As in GBS, less than 10% of individuals will die from the acute illness. Acute mortality typically results from ventilatory failure or the complications of immobility. Those who survive typically regain strength inversely proportionate to the severity of the initial illness. The majority of this recovery takes place over the course of weeks to months, presumably due to reinnervation from neighboring motor units not affected by the disease.

The postpolio syndrome (PPS) has been recognized since 1875 but received no more than cursory attention until 1981 when interest escalated in response to the large numbers of people affected by the epidemics of the early 1940s who were now experiencing new symptoms. Current evidence suggests that patients who develop postpolio muscular atrophy do so because of the loss of anterior horn cells that occur as a consequence of normal aging superimposed upon a depleted reserve. There is convincing evidence that some individuals with prior polio may develop slowly progressive weakness (average decline 1%/year) after a protracted period of stability. How frequently this postpolio muscular atrophy (PPMA) occurs as a manifestation of PPS is a matter of some controversy. In one study, 50 prior polio patients were selected from a cohort of 300 patients and followed for 5 years. Sixty percent of this group developed symptoms. Of this symptomatic group, only a third had symptoms attributed to musculoskeletal complaints and none of these had measurable evidence of progressive atrophy and weakness. When PPMA occurs, it typically manifests in the regions most

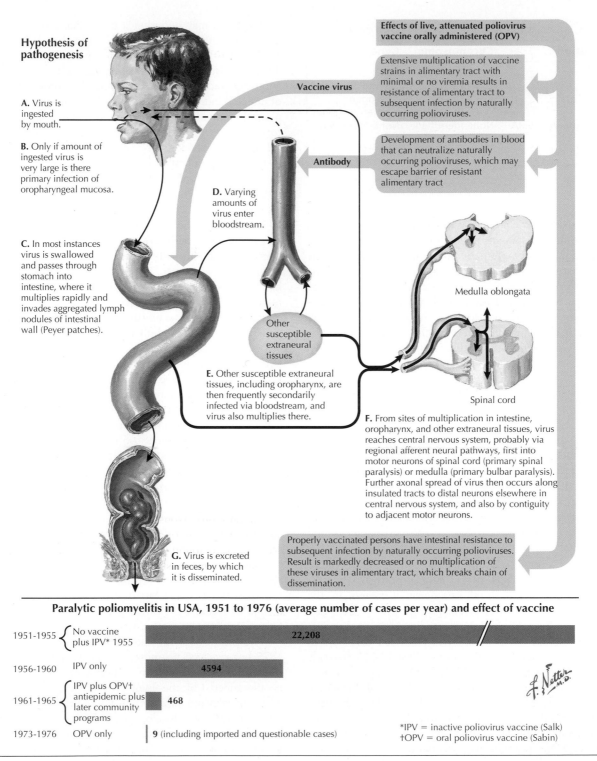

Hypothesis of pathogenesis

A. Virus is ingested by mouth.

B. Only if amount of ingested virus is very large is there primary infection of oropharyngeal mucosa.

C. In most instances virus is swallowed and passes through stomach into intestine, where it multiplies rapidly and invades aggregated lymph nodules of intestinal wall (Peyer patches).

D. Varying amounts of virus enter bloodstream.

Vaccine virus

Antibody

Other susceptible extraneural tissues

E. Other susceptible extraneural tissues, including oropharynx, are then frequently secondarily infected via bloodstream, and virus also multiplies there.

G. Virus is excreted in feces, by which it is disseminated.

Effects of live, attenuated poliovirus vaccine orally administered (OPV)

Extensive multiplication of vaccine strains in alimentary tract with minimal or no viremia results in resistance of alimentary tract to subsequent infection by naturally occurring polioviruses.

Development of antibodies in blood that can neutralize naturally occurring polioviruses, which may escape barrier of resistant alimentary tract

Medulla oblongata

Spinal cord

F. From sites of multiplication in intestine, oropharynx, and other extraneural tissues, virus reaches central nervous system, probably via regional afferent neural pathways, first into motor neurons of spinal cord (primary spinal paralysis) or medulla (primary bulbar paralysis). Further axonal spread of virus then occurs along insulated tracts to distal neurons elsewhere in central nervous system, and also by contiguity to adjacent motor neurons.

Properly vaccinated persons have intestinal resistance to subsequent infection by naturally occurring polioviruses. Result is markedly decreased or no multiplication of these viruses in alimentary tract, which breaks chain of dissemination.

Paralytic poliomyelitis in USA, 1951 to 1976 (average number of cases per year) and effect of vaccine

1951-1955 {	No vaccine plus IPV* 1955	22,208
1956-1960	IPV only	4594
1961-1965 {	IPV plus OPV† antiepidemic plus later community programs	468
1973-1976	OPV only	9 (including imported and questionable cases)

*IPV = inactive poliovirus vaccine (Salk)
†OPV = oral poliovirus vaccine (Sabin)

Figure 68-4 Pathogenesis of Poliomyelitis.

severely afflicted by the initial illness. Ventilatory function may decline, with one study suggesting an approximate 2% loss of vital capacity a year in keeping with the slowly progressive nature of the illness. Criteria have been established to solidify a PPMA diagnosis. These include objective measures of declining strength, muscle atrophy, and fatigue following a documented polio-like illness. This must occur subsequent to a protracted period of stability in absence of an alternative explanation.

There is no "gold standard" to determine which polio victims have developed PPMA. Consequently, estimates of the prevalence of PPS have ranged from 22 to 85%. Signs and symptoms of PPS have been reported to begin as early as 8 years after the initial illness or as late as 71 years with an average of 35 years. The likelihood of developing PPS seems to correlate with both the age of the patient at the time of the initial illness, as well as its severity.

Stages in destruction of a motor neuron by poliovirus

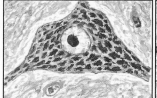

A. Normal motor neuron

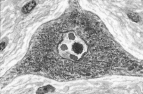

B. Diffuse chromatolysis; three acidophilic nuclear inclusions around nucleolus

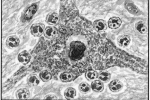

C. Polymorphonuclear cells invading necrotic neuron

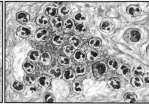

D. Complete neuronophagia

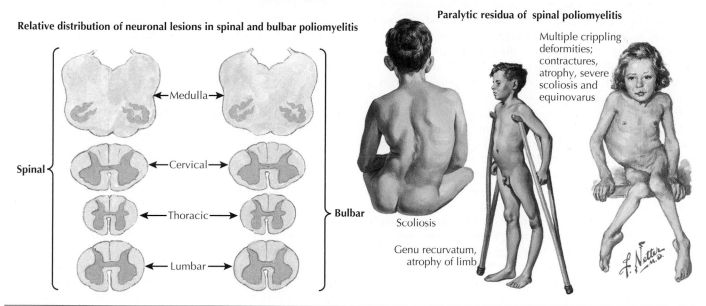

Relative distribution of neuronal lesions in spinal and bulbar poliomyelitis

Medulla

Spinal

Cervical

Thoracic

Bulbar

Lumbar

Paralytic residua of spinal poliomyelitis

Multiple crippling deformities; contractures, atrophy, severe scoliosis and equinovarus

Scoliosis

Genu recurvatum, atrophy of limb

Figure 68-5 Poliomyelitis.

West Nile Virus

West Nile virus (WNV) is a mosquito-borne viral pathogen of the Flavivirus family. Like polio, most infected individuals develop a minor, nonspecific illness that often includes fever, gastrointestinal complaints, back pain, and rash in addition to potential neurologic manifestations. A number of reports have linked WNV to a poliomyelitis-like phenotype that may affect facial as well as limb muscles with or without an associated meningo-encephalitic component. Approximately half of patients will develop flaccid weakness over a 3- to 8-day period that tends to be proximal and asymmetric in distribution. Electrophysiological and pathologic observations have suggested that this weakness originates from anterior horn cell injury. Confounding these observations are reports that the West Nile virus may produce Guillain–Barré and transverse myelitis phenotypes. Like the poliovirus, varying degrees of irreversible paralysis may result. Other agents that have been reported to cause poliomyelitis include enterovirus 71, acute hemorrhagic conjunctivitis, Coxsackie virus group A type 7, echovirus type 6, and the Japanese encephalitis virus. Rabies may also present as a paralytic illness in 20% of cases, with paralysis typically beginning in the bitten extremity.

Multifocal Motor Neuropathy

The majority if not all of the evidence available to date suggests that multifocal motor neuropathy (MMN) is an immune-mediated neuropathy resulting from multifocal myelin loss in peripheral motor axons. This selective vulnerability hypothetically exists because of a glycolipid epitope that is unique to or predominantly found in the myelin of peripheral motor nerves. Although antiganglioside antibodies are found in the serum of 30–80% of individuals with the MMN phenotype, a pathogenetic role for these antibodies remains unproven. Reduction in antiganglioside antibody levels does not correlate with disease responsiveness in all patients. Conversely, patients with the MMN phenotype who are seronegative appear to respond equally well to immunomodulating treatments.

MMN is characterized as a multifocal, pure motor, acquired immune mediated motor neuropathy. Despite this anatomic localization, it is more likely to be considered in the differential diagnosis of a motor neuron disease than a peripheral neuropathy. Like ALS it presents with painless weakness in a single limb, often in distal muscles in the upper extremity. Cramps and fasciculations may occur providing an additional phenotypic overlap with ALS. Like ALS, muscle stretch reflexes may be lost in an affected extremity. The clinical features that are most useful in distinguishing MMN from ALS include slower progression, the absence of unequivocal upper motor neuron signs, weakness without atrophy, nerve rather than segmental pattern of muscle weakness, and absence of signs attributable to cranial nerve dysfunction. The latter have been only reported as a rare consequence of MMN. Unfortunately with disease progression, these diagnostic clues may become obscured. On average, untreated MMN progresses much more slowly than ALS.

Hereditary Spastic Paraplegia

There are in excess of 30 different gene mutations associated with the hereditary spastic paraplegia (HSP) phenotype. Autosomal dominant, recessive, and X-linked modes of transmission are recognized. The multiple genotypes underlying HSP suggest that there is a common mechanism by which mutations of different proteins translate into an identical or near-identical phenotype. A uniform final common pathway, however, is yet to be defined. Proposed mechanisms include disturbances in axon transport, impaired Golgi function, mitochondrial dysfunction, disordered myelin synthesis, and maturational disturbances of the corticospinal tracts. Some of these hypotheses are based upon the intracellular positioning of affected proteins. The pathology of HSP would support its conceptualization as a "dying back myelopathy."

HSP is a slowly progressive upper motor neuron (UMN) disorder of the lower extremities. Like other heritable disorders, other affected family members may not be readily identifiable. The presenting symptoms of HSP occur as a consequence of lower extremity spasticity that is symmetric in its distribution. Patients lose the ability to run or hop early in the course because of increased lower extremity extensor tone and the inability to flex the hip or knee in a facile manner. As a result, stride length is reduced. The legs tend to "scissor," that is, cross over each other because of increased tone of thigh adductor muscles. Circumduction, that is, advancing the leg in a circular rather than a linear motion, is done for compensatory reasons to avoid tripping on a foot that maintains an inverted and plantar flexed posture. Leg strength may be diminished; weakness occurs in an "upper motor neuron" pattern, with hip flexors, knee flexors, and foot dorsiflexors being affected to the greatest extent. Hyperreflexia of the lower extremities is a universal feature, almost always accompanied by extensor plantar responses. Hyperreflexia of the upper extremities with Hoffman's signs and reflex spread are common as well. Weakness, increased tone, impaired coordination or loss of function of the upper extremities, and cranial nerve dysfunction occur infrequently in pure HSP and should lead to consideration of an alternative diagnosis. Posterior column involvement with loss of vibratory sense in a length-dependent pattern in the lower extremities may be seen. Urinary frequency, urgency, and urgency incontinence are common symptoms even within the "pure" forms of the disease. Rectal urgency and incontinence and sexual dysfunction are less common but do occur. High arched feet and hammer toe deformities, a feature of a number of chronic neurologic diseases, are a common feature of the illness. Onset and severity of HSP varies considerably both within and between families. Initial symptoms may be recognized in any decade of life. The reasons for variations of disease onset and severity of affliction, both within and between families of the same genotype, are not currently understood although other "disease-modifying" genes are hypothesized to have a role.

Miscellaneous Causes of Motor Neuron Disease

Motor neuron disease phenotypes have occurred in association with other disorders. Understandably, little is known of the pathogenesis of these disparate and relatively uncommon disorders. Postirradiation neuropathy is frequently a pure motor syndrome; current evidence, including reports of root enhancement on MR imaging in some patients, favors a polyradiculopathy as the proposed pathomechanism. Radiation injury of the peripheral nervous system is typically delayed in onset with an average latency between exposure and symptoms of 6 years. The range, however, is exceedingly broad, with onset latency varying between 4 months and 25 years. Radiation doses typically exceed 4000 cGY in these patients.

Motor neuron disease may rarely occur as a paraneoplastic disorder or as a potential complication in irradiated Hodgkin patients. The latter is referred to as subacute motor neuronopathy to emphasize the presumed anterior horn cell localization. Motor deficits predominate in most cases. In the lower extremity, where bilateral exposure to nerve elements is the norm, the deficits are typically bilateral and asymmetric. Monomelic presentations do occur.

DIFFERENTIAL DIAGNOSIS

The differential diagnosis of the motor neuron diseases includes disorders in which weakness occurs in the absence of significant pain and/or sensory symptoms. This includes other motor neuron diseases including ALS, myopathies, disorders of neuromuscular transmission and occasional peripheral neuropathies in which motor signs dominate. Differential diagnostic considerations vary with each of the disorders described above and depend in large part on age of onset, speed of progression, and pattern of weakness.

The differential diagnosis of infantile SMA I is that of the floppy infant. The majority of these hypotonic neonates will be afflicted with a central nervous system disorder. An alert and appropriately interactive child with diminished or absent deep tendon reflexes would increase the probability of a neuromuscular cause of hypotonia. Within this category, neonatal or congenital myasthenia, neonatal myotonic dystrophy, Pompe disease, nemaline, myotubular or other congenital myopathies, infantile botulism, and rare hypomyelinating neuropathies are the major considerations. SMA II, III, and IV need to be differentiated from a wide variety of myopathic disorders, including the dystrophinopathies, limb-girdle, myotonic and Emery-Dreifuss muscular dystrophies, dermatomyositis, the congenital myopathies, mitochondrial disorders, and lipid and glycogen storage disorders. Chronic inflammatory demyelinating polyradiculoneuropathy would be the primary neuropathic consideration.

Kennedy disease may be misdiagnosed as ALS. The Lambert–Eaton myasthenic syndrome, myasthenia gravis, and myopathy with a similar potential pattern of weakness are other diagnostic possibilities. In view of its propensity to affect older individuals and cause symptomatic dysphagia as well as limb weakness, inclusion body myositis and oculopharyngeal muscular dystrophy are the principal myopathic considerations.

Focal limb onset presentations of motor neuron disease are commonly mistaken as mononeuropathies, radiculopathies, or plexopathies. The absence of pain and sensory symptoms should deflect consideration away from these disorders. The age of onset, the speed of disease progression, and the presence or absence of "bulbar" dysfunction and UMN signs would all aid in the determination of whether ALS, MMN, Hirayama disease, Davidenkow disease, or inclusion body myositis represent the leading consideration.

The distal SMAs are frequently misdiagnosed as the more common CMT disease.

Polio and other "anterior horn cell tropic" viruses enter into the differential diagnosis of other causes of acute generalized weakness in which weakness predominates over sensory symptoms. The Guillain–Barré syndrome, botulism, hypokalemia, and hypophosphatemia and a number of toxic neuropathies are chief considerations in this regard.

The differential diagnosis of HSP includes other causes of spastic paraparesis. Compressive myelopathies, inflammatory, immune-mediated myelopathies such as multiple sclerosis, and neuromyelitis optica deserve consideration. Primary lateral sclerosis (PLS) may provide a source of confusion as it is usually a slowly progressive upper motor neuron disorder. PLS commonly produces functional impairments of the upper extremities and of bulbar function unlike HSP. PLS would not typically include cavus foot deformities or large fiber sensory loss in the feet. Vitamin B_{12} and copper deficiency should be considered as potentially treatable causes of spastic paraparesis. In both cases, these disorders are typically more rapid in their onset as well as dominated by signs of posterior column involvement. The corticospinal tracts may be affected by retroviral infection, and both the HIV and HTLV1 viruses need to be considered in the appropriate clinical context. Other hereditary neurodegenerative disorders that affect the corticospinal tracts, the leukodystrophies, particularly adrenoleukodystrophy in young adult women, and the spinocerebellar atrophies are considerations.

DIAGNOSTIC APPROACH

The diagnostic approach is dependent on the index of clinical suspicion for a given disorder, and the availability and affordability of genetic testing. Of the disorders discussed in this chapter, mutational analysis is currently commercially available for SMA types I–IV, Kennedy disease, and a few of the dominantly inherited forms of HSP. As the cost of this testing is currently substantial, it would be reasonable to utilize these tests only when a high degree of clinical suspicion exists and not as a screening tool.

The majority of tests are performed with a goal of excluding other diagnostic considerations. Electrodiagnostic testing (EDX), that is, EMG and nerve conduction testing, has the greatest utility in this regard and often serves to support if not define an MND diagnosis.

The characteristic pattern in the majority of MNDs is normal sensory nerve conductions, low amplitude or absent compound muscle action potentials in affected limbs, and normal or mildly reduced conduction velocities. The needle exam demonstrates reduced recruitment of motor unit action potential (MUAPs) that are long duration and high amplitude in their morphology, indicative of chronic partial denervation and reinnervation; ongoing denervation in the form of fibrillation potentials and positive waves is also seen. Rarely, one can see fasciculation potentials.

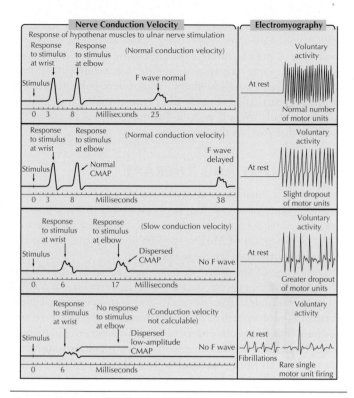

Figure 68-6 Multifocal Motor Neuropathy: Conduction Block on Nerve Conduction Study.

For the most part, the only EDX features that distinguish between the different motor neuron diseases are the distribution of abnormalities and the degree of active versus chronic denervation changes. More chronic disorders such as Kennedy disease or old polio are dominated by features of chronic denervation and reinnervation whereas ALS typically has prominent features of both active and chronic denervation. Kennedy disease is rather unique within the MND spectrum in that sensory nerve action potential amplitudes are often reduced or absent. A key diagnostic feature in MMN is the presence of demyelinating features on motor nerve conductions, particularly the presence of conduction block (Fig. 68-6). Unfortunately, there are a number of reasons why this feature is not always demonstrable.

Creatine kinase is often modestly elevated in many of the MNDs, to levels of 200–500 U/L and occasionally to levels greater than 1000 U/L. Antibodies directed against the GM1 ganglioside are found in high titer in the serum of 30–80% of patients with MMN but are neither sensitive nor specific. MR imaging of proximal nerve may identify focal areas of increased signal that are supportive of an MMN diagnosis. Lumbar puncture is of value if an infectious cause of motor neuron disease is suspected but otherwise has limited value.

Testing in HSP is done primarily to identify or exclude other disorders that may produce a spastic paraparesis. Somatosensory evoked potentials may serve to confirm involvement of the posterior columns and exclude consideration of primary lateral sclerosis.

Prior to the availability of genetic testing, muscle biopsies were routinely performed in Werdnig–Hoffman suspects. A characteristic but nondiagnostic pattern consists of sheets of small rounded atrophic fibers with small islands of hypertrophied type 1 muscle fibers. Muscle biopsy in any MND will demonstrate some pattern of neurogenic atrophy that may include angulated atrophic fibers, target fibers, pyknotic nuclear clumps, and particularly muscle fiber type grouping and grouped atrophy. Usually there is no role for nerve biopsy in any of the disorders discussed in this chapter.

MANAGEMENT AND THERAPY

Unfortunately, management in the majority of these disorders remains symptomatic and supportive, with the primary goals of education, maintenance of safety, and independent function. With the exception of MMN, specific and effective treatments do not currently exist for these disorders.

Knowledge of the defective gene product in SMA I–IV has led to rational therapeutic trials. Ventilatory failure in SMA I and II is inevitable; tracheostomy and long-term mechanical ventilation, and insertion of a percutaneous feeding tube are decisions with enormous emotional consequences to the parents of an affected child. Noninvasive positive pressure ventilation may provide an improved quality and duration of life until a decision regarding tracheostomy is required.

Results of clinical trials utilizing gabapentin, riluzole, acetyl-carnitine and phenylbutyrate on patients affected with SMA I–III are negative, inconclusive, or incomplete to date. Valproic acid can increase the rate of SMN2 transcription. Recently, an observational study demonstrated that valproate appeared to increase strength by a mean of 16% in SMA type III and IV patients. Valproate therapy is not without risk, including liver toxicity and carnitine deficiency. Its use in SMA patients outside of a clinical trial is not recommended.

The development of kyphoscoliosis is a common problem in children with SMA who are wheelchair bound. Spine stabilization is commonly recommended in individuals whose curves exceed 50 degrees and whose vital capacities exceed 40% of predicted. The goals of this intervention are patient comfort and potential stabilization of restrictive pulmonary deficits. A high index of suspicion is maintained for symptoms of impaired nocturnal ventilation and if necessary treated with application of positive airway pressure.

With Hirayama disease, decompression of the cervical spinal cord has been attempted. It is unclear whether this meaningfully affects the natural history of the disease.

Treatment for HSP is supportive. There are a number of different options to reduce spasticity, including oral tizanidine, baclofen, dantrolene, benzodiazepines, intrathecal baclofen, or botulinum toxin injections directly into spastic muscles. The goal of treatment is to improve mobility, augment range of motion, and relieve the discomfort associated with spastic muscles. In an individual who also has considerable underlying weakness, the increased tone of extensor muscles may represent the major source of antigravity resistance. Suppression of this tone may deprive an individual of his or her ability to stand.

Home modification and durable medical equipment are important components of the management of patients with chronic neuromuscular diseases. The goals are to maintain independent mobility and patient safety simultaneously. Ankle–foot orthoses are of great benefit to individual patients. Their primary purpose is to prevent tripping by maintaining the foot in a partially dorsiflexed position. A skilled physical therapist is invaluable to decide whether a cane, Lofstran crutches, a walker or a wheelchair is the best solution for an individual patient. Motorized scooters or power wheelchairs are options for patients who lack the ability to propel a manual chair but who have enough upper extremity function to operate either of these. Although scooters are more attractive to patients, they are often disadvantageous as they require a greater degree of upper extremity function to operate, provide less trunk support, and allow for less additional equipment to be mounted on them. In patients who live in multiple-story dwellings, stair lifts provide a safe option. A skilled occupational therapist is also a valuable aid in maintaining independence in activities of daily living.

FUTURE DIRECTIONS

As most of these disorders are heritable, effective treatment may depend on future technological advances that might allow for the identification and restitution of the affected genes in utero. Truncating the effects of mutated genes pharmacologically and arresting disease progression appears to be another interventional strategy that may be feasible in the near future at least in certain diseases. Reversing the established consequences of these mutations will be a more daunting challenge.

ADDITIONAL RESOURCES

SMA

http://www.mda.org/disease/
www.nlm.nih.gov/medlineplus/spinalmuscularatrophy.html
http://www.ncbi.nlm.nih.gov/sites/entrez?db=omim

HSP

Spastic Paraplegia Foundation, Inc.
209 Park Rd.
Chelmsford MA 01824
Phone: 703-495-9261
community@sp-foundation.org
sp-foundation.org
National Ataxia Foundation
2600 Fernbrook Lane Suite 119
Minneapolis MN 55447
Phone: 763-553-0020
Fax: 763-553-0167
naf@ataxia.org

Bertini E, Burghes A, Bushby K, et al. 134th ENMC International Workshop: Outcome measures and treatment of spinal muscular atrophy 11-13 February 2005. Naarden, The Netherlands. Neuromuscular Disorders 2005;15:802-816.
Chahin N, Klein C, Mandrekar J, et al. Natural history of spinal-bulbar muscular atrophy. Neurology 2008;70;1967-1971.
Harding, AE. Inherited neuronal atrophy and degeneration predominantly of lower motor neurons. In: Dyck PJ, Thomas PK, Griffin JW, Low PA, Poduslo JF, editors. 3rd ed. Peripheral Neuropathy. Philadelphia: W. B. Saunders; 1993. p. 1051-1064.
Irobi J, Dierick I, Jordanova A, et al. Unraveling the genetics of distal hereditary motor neuropathies. Neuromolec Med 2006;8:131-146.

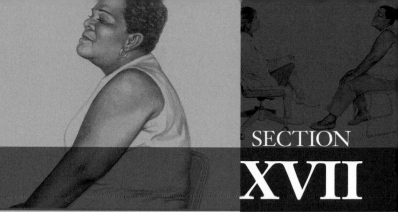

Neuromuscular Hyperactivity Disorders

Stiff Person Syndrome

Ted M. Burns, Juliana Lockman, and H. Royden Jones, Jr.

69

This chapter concentrates on the most common of the very uncommon motor neuron hyperactivity disorders, namely the stiff person syndrome. Two other potentially related syndromes characterized by incomplete relaxation or inhibition of motor neurons—Isaac (Merten) syndrome and neuromyotonia—are discussed in Chapter 70.

Clinical Vignette

A 53-year-old woman with myeloid metaplasia reported a 6-month history of severe back pain, difficulty walking, and occasional falls. No lumbosacral disc disorder could be identified. During the past month, these spasmodic muscle pains of her legs, back, and abdomen were induced by attempting to sit up, stand, or walk. Occasionally, these spasms led to stiffening of her entire body; at their extreme these induced urinary incontinence. At times, the severity of the pain led her to cry out to such a degree that it caused one observer to liken her distress to that of a "bellowing cow"! These outbursts led to her being referred to a psychiatrist.

Neurologic examination demonstrated an anxious and alert middle-aged woman. The primary finding was her spontaneous reaction to the slightest sensory stimuli wherein she totally stiffened, reminding this neurologist (HRJ) of a tetanus patient. Other than hyperlordosis, marked hyperreflexia at her knees and a right Babinski sign, her basic neurologic examination was normal. However, on a neurosurgeon's brusque attempt to get her out of bed to stand, she developed severe painful body spasm and fell into the hospital room wall as if a chain saw had cut her legs off.

Head and cervicothoracic spine magnetic resonance imaging (MRI) and cerebrospinal fluid (CSF) study were normal, as was serum B$_{12}$ level. Nerve conduction studies were normal. Her needle electromyography (EMG) study demonstrated prolonged motor unit activity in contracting muscles during episodes of stiffness and spasm but was otherwise normal. Double-antibody radioimmunoassay demonstrated a high level of serum glutamic acid decarboxylase 65 (GAD-65) antibodies (138 nmol/L; reference range: ≤0.02 nmol/L). The patient was diagnosed with stiff person syndrome (SPS).

Increasing doses of diazepam alleviated symptoms at a dose of 60 mg daily. A course of plasmapheresis treatments followed by prednisone (80 mg daily) led to gradual symptomatic improvement. She was successfully tapered off corticosteroids during a 2-year period and diazepam over 5 years.

The stiff person syndrome (SPS, originally known as the stiff man syndrome) was first described by Moersch and Woltman in 1956. Classic stiff person syndrome is a chronic autoimmune disease characterized by spine and leg rigidity with lumbar hyperlordosis and painful spasms. Women are more often affected than men at a ratio of 2:1. This disorder generally presents in the fourth through sixth decades. Its onset is typically insidious and the course is usually progressive.

Laboratory studies that are classically abnormal in SPS include an elevated serum GAD-65 antibody titers (>20 nmol/L), needle EMG findings of continuous motor unit activity in at least one axial muscle, and normal brain MRI and CSF studies. Variants of SPS include those with focal limb dysfunction (stiff limb syndrome), encephalomyelitis ("SPS Plus"), and those associated with paraneoplastic antibodies, namely, amphiphysin as seen with breast cancer. Although most instances of SPS do not have a family history, at least one instance of such is reported. Interestingly the parent and propositus had a stiff limb variant and the daughter a purely intermittent axial presentation initially diagnosed as hysteria or anxiety disorder because of her presentation with recurrent opisthotonus.

ETIOLOGY

The findings that support an autoimmune basis for SPS are the following: (1) SPS is associated with autoantibodies, both the classic GAD-65 antibodies and a paraneoplastic variant, amphiphysin antibodies; (2) SPS is frequently accompanied by other autoimmune disorders such as type 1 diabetes, thyroiditis, vitiligo, and pernicious anemia; and (3) intravenous immunoglobulin (IVIg) and plasma exchange provide effective treatments for some patients.

The precise pathophysiologic role for the specific antibodies is unclear, although it is speculated that the autoimmune lesions are directed at a site on the inhibitory spinal interneurons (Fig. 69-1). Although a direct relation is inferred, this is not fully substantiated. Factors supporting a direct role for antibodies are (1) the finding of elevated intrathecal GAD antibodies; (2) the antibody concentration correlates with the degree of motor excitability; (3) GAD antibodies, obtained from serum of stiff person patients, inhibit both GAD and GABA synthesis in vitro.

CLINICAL PRESENTATION

Classic SPS

Typically this is characterized by spine and leg rigidity with lumbar hyperlordosis as a key feature (Figs. 69-2 and 69-3). Lower extremity rigidity can cause full extension of the legs, making walking difficult. Patients often also experience superimposed painful spasms that may be precipitated by sudden noise, anxiety, or touch. The spasms can be of such abrupt onset and power that these individuals may unexpectedly and precipitously fall. Patients soon recognize that emotional stress often provokes their spasms. They may develop agoraphobia secondary to the fear of falling in public. Neurologic examination

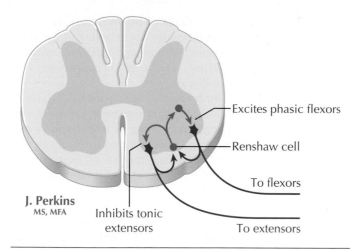

Figure 69-1 Renshaw Cell Bias.

sometimes reveals paraspinal and abdominal musculature contraction with lumbar hyperlordosis and lower limb rigidity. However, these findings are often not present until late in the clinical course. The muscle stretch reflexes may be normal to brisk, with occasionally extensor plantar responses.

Stiff Person Syndrome—Primary Limb Involvement

This variant of stiff person syndrome presents focally with rigidity and spasms involving one or more limbs. In "stiff limb syndrome," motor symptoms predominantly affect the limb distally. In contrast to the more traditional SPS, axial involvement is less prominent. However, significant proximal muscle involvement does eventually occur if the SPS is not diagnosed and treated early. This was illustrated by one of our patients who had spontaneous quadriceps spasms leading to automobile accidents. These were spontaneous and precipitous contractions leading him to suddenly apply excess pressure to the accelerator on one occasion and the brake on another. GAD autoantibody titers are elevated less frequently in these patients. The EMG pattern is even less predictable in these more limited forms.

Stiff Person Syndrome with Encephalomyelitis (SPSE)

Patients with stiff person syndrome with encephalomyelitis typically present with a subacute onset of axial or limb rigidity accompanied by pyramidal tract signs (e.g., abnormally brisk muscle stretch reflexes, Babinski sign), brainstem dysfunction, cognitive decline, and myoclonus. The variant syndrome is often paraneoplastic, and amphiphysin antibodies are frequently present. Paraneoplastic stiff person syndrome is associated with several malignancies, including breast adenocarcinoma, small cell lung cancer, colon cancer, and Hodgkin lymphoma. It is not unusual for the SPS to be the first sign of the underlying malignancy. Thus, when amphiphysin antibodies are positive, it is important to ensure careful follow-up. One patient had two negative mammograms over a 1-year period only to self-discover a breast mass a short time later.

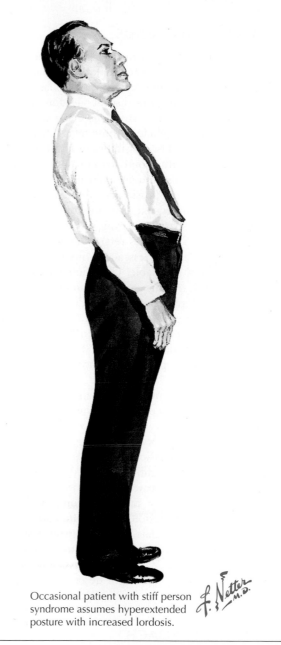

Occasional patient with stiff person syndrome assumes hyperextended posture with increased lordosis.

Figure 69-2 Stiff Person Syndrome.

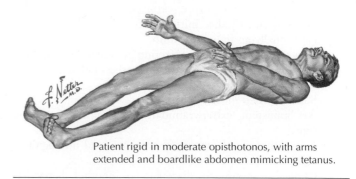

Patient rigid in moderate opisthotonos, with arms extended and boardlike abdomen mimicking tetanus.

Figure 69-3 End-Stage Stiff Person Syndrome.

DIFFERENTIAL DIAGNOSIS

Frequently SPS patients have a history of a number of nondiagnostic visits to a variety of physicians, including a few neurologists. They are often inappropriately labeled as hysteric or having a functional somatoform disorder leading to recurrent psychiatric evaluations. Other erroneous diagnoses sometimes applied to these patients include chronic tetany, tetanus, dystonia, stroke, and arthritis. The possibility of a spinal cord disorder (i.e., a myelopathy with spondylosis or disc herniation), or a basal ganglia disorder also requires consideration.

In any acute setting, the possibility of tetanus must be considered because of the board-like stiffening of the abdomen and the severity of muscle spasms. Sparing of the jaw muscles and absence of trismus in SPS makes tetanus unlikely. Spasms are generally less violent and of less acute onset in SPS than in tetanus, but this is not invariable. Chronic tetanus is rare and typically presents with trismus and risus sardonicus.

Hereditary hyperekplexia or startle disease with startle-induced spasms is a rare disorder caused by mutations in the glycine receptor, a receptor for a major inhibitory central nervous system (CNS) neurotransmitter. Startle-induced spasms may also be seen in focal spinal cord lesions such as tumors or syringomyelia.

Patients with psychogenic muscle contraction or spasm usually have a consistently inconsistent as well as more variable presentation; this diagnosis must only be entertained after long periods of careful observation and recurrent laboratory testing. Such cases occur occasionally but warrant consideration. Other causes of muscular rigidity include disorders of muscle or neuronal membrane hyperexcitability. Two channelopathies with muscle rigidity, namely myotonia congenita and Isaac syndrome, deserve consideration in the differential diagnosis, but neither of these is associated with the pain typically seen with SPS. Multiple sclerosis, poliomyelitis, Lyme disease, spinal myoclonus, tumors, and even strychnine poisoning are also in the differential and might deserve consideration in some cases.

DIAGNOSTIC APPROACH

Stiff person syndrome is primarily a clinical diagnosis, and diagnostic criteria include:

1) Stiffness and rigidity initially affecting axial muscles or occasionally an individual limb.
2) Progressive involvement affecting proximal limb muscles.
3) Abnormal axial posture with increased lumbar hyperlordosis.
4) Superimposed muscle spasms.
5) No brainstem, extrapyramidal, or lower motor neuron signs.
6) No sphincter and sensory disturbance, and no cognitive involvement.
7) Clinical response to diazepam or another benzodiazepine.
8) Markedly elevated GAD-65 autoantibody titers in serum support the diagnosis; 60–90% of classic SPS patients have very high titers of GAD-65 in serum, usually greater than 20 nmol/L. Significantly lower levels of GAD-65 antibodies are frequently seen in type 1 diabetes mellitus, drug-resistant epilepsy, cerebellar degeneration syndromes, and Batten disease.
9) Early on in this disorder EMG is often normal. However, EMG eventually reveals a characteristic abnormality with concomitant and continuous firing of motor unit potentials in both agonist and antagonist muscles in severely affected individuals. The lack thereof of characteristic EMG findings should not be a reason to dismiss the diagnosis.

Other studies will prove to be very important to exclude competing differential diagnostic considerations. Magnetic resonance imaging of the brain and spinal cord is normal but can be useful in identifying mimics of the variant with encephalomyelitis (see below). The cerebrospinal fluid is usually normal but can occasionally demonstrate increased CSF protein, oligoclonal bands, or IgG. It must be emphasized that if one waits until all of the above classic "requisites" for diagnosis of SPS are fulfilled, the opportunity for significant therapeutic control of the potentially future downhill course of this eventually lethal disorder will be missed. This is illustrated by some of the early variants as noted below.

TREATMENT AND PROGNOSIS

Symptomatic Treatment

These medications may be very helpful but do not address the basic autoimmune process in this chronic disorder.

BENZODIAZEPINES

Diazepam is the first-line symptomatic therapy. It was the first pharmacologic agent shown to dramatically alter the clinical course of SPS. Its use is associated with significant clinical improvement in stiffness, frequency of spasms, and ability to ambulate. Benzodiazepines are $GABA_A$ receptor agonists and thus can act to inhibit the excessive MUP firing leading to the painful muscle contraction of SPS. Common side effects include sedation, somnolence, fatigue, and ataxia. Serious side effects include hypotension, respiratory depression, and long-term physical dependence. Much caution is advised if one considers discontinuation of a benzodiazepine. This should involve a carefully monitored and very slow taper with the avoidance of an abrupt withdrawal as it can be lethal, possibly secondary to arrhythmias.

BACLOFEN

Baclofen is also considered a first-line therapy. Baclofen is a $GABA_B$ receptor agonist that also can inhibit the excessive muscle contraction of SPS. Common side effects include constipation, nausea, decreased muscle tone, headache, dizziness, and somnolence. Seizures and even death secondary may occur with abrupt withdrawal of baclofen.

Immunosuppressants/Immunomodulators

CORTICOSTEROIDS

Corticosteroids are the first-line immunosuppressive therapy requiring a high dose (e.g., prednisone 1 mg/kg/d). Once patients become asymptomatic, they usually require long-term maintenance therapy, followed by a gradual taper as tolerated. The usual side affects need to be monitored.

INTRAVENOUS IMMUNOGLOBULIN

Intravenous immunoglobulin (IVIg) is another consideration for SPS patients refractory to symptomatic management with first-line agents. IVIg is generally well tolerated; its biggest downside is cost and availability. Corticosteroids, in contrast, are very inexpensive but generally cause more side effects. It is not clear whether long-term treatment with one modality per se is better than the other.

PLASMA EXCHANGE

Plasma exchange has demonstrated mixed clinical efficacy. It is sometimes considered in combination with first-line agents as a short-term management option.

AZATHIOPRINE

Azathioprine is a reasonable long-term option for patients who fail conventional regimens, but clinical improvement is often delayed 4–6 months after initiation of therapy.

RITUXIMAB

Rituximab, an anti-CD-20 monoclonal antibody that attacks B lymphocytes, has been reported to lead to clinical improvement of SPS. GAD-65 antibodies become undetectable and the EMG normalizes within weeks. However, more studies of Rituximab in SPS need to be performed before it becomes a first-line immunosuppressive choice.

Other Issues

Psychiatric problems commonly accompanying SPS include anxiety, depression, and substance abuse. These may exacerbate both the chronic stiffness and the frequency of spasms. Psychiatric consultation can play an important role in the identification and treatment of such problems.

ADDITIONAL RESOURCES

Amato AA, Cornman EW, Kissel JT. Treatment of stiff-man syndrome with intravenous immunoglobulin. Neurology 2004;44:1652-1654.

Barker RA, Revesz T, Thom M, et al. Review of 23 patients affected by the stiff person syndrome: clinical subdivision into stiff trunk (man) syndrome, stiff limb syndrome, and progressive encephalomyelitis with rigidity. J Neurol Neurosurg Psychiatry 1998;65:633-640.

Burns TM, Jones Jr HR, Phillips II LH, et al. Two generations of clinically disparate stiff man syndrome, confirmed by significant elevations of GAD65 autoantibodies. Neurology 2003;61:1291-1294.

Dalakas MC, Li M, Fujii M, et al. Stiff person syndrome: quantification, specificity, and intrathecal synthesis of GAD 65 antibodies. Neurology 2001;57:780-784.

Lockman J, Burns TM. Stiff-person syndrome. Current Treatment Options Neurol 2007;9:234-240.

Moersch FP, Woltman HW. Progressive fluctuating muscular rigidity and spasm ("stiff-man" syndrome): report of a case and some observations in 13 other cases. Mayo Clin Proc 1956;31:421-427. *The initial and very classic paper with exquisitely detailed patient history*

Other Peripheral Motor Hyperactivity Syndromes

H. Royden Jones, Jr.

70

ISAAC (MERTEN) SYNDROME/QUANTAL SQUANDER, NEUROMYOTONIA

This is another hyperkinetic presumed peripheral nerve hyperexcitability syndrome that occurs even more rarely than the stiff person syndrome. As noted above, there are a number of synonyms. It is a very unusual neurologic disorder also characterized by the continuous firing of peripheral nerves, and thus muscle fibers. It is much more subtle in its presentation. Typically the age of onset is in the teenage years, but it may be seen in adulthood. This appears to be autoimmune in origin (anti–potassium channel antibodies are positive in some patients.) This is a nonspecific finding per se as these antibodies may be found in a variety of neurologic syndromes.

Here the patient first notes what appears to be an almost continuous firing of groups of muscle fibers usually appearing to mimic fasciculations. These occur concomitantly in both agonists and antagonists. The patient often notes a sense of fatigue. Usually there are no significant associated muscle spasms, cramping, or pain; however, in some instances such may occur. The patient may note a degree of weakness because of the inconsistent firing of opposing muscle groups, leading to ineffective mechanical function. Some patients have excessive sweating.

Other than the apparent pseudo-fasciculations and a hint of muscle weakness, the neurologic examination is normal. Diagnosis is suggested when electromyography (EMG) demonstrates continuous firing of normal motor unit potentials without any abnormalities on insertion. These persist even during sleep. A therapeutic trial of phenytoin or carbamazepine most always leads to a complete cessation of all aspects of this syndrome. This therapeutic result serves to confirm the suspected diagnosis. This is a particularly gratifying diagnosis to make as some of these extremely unusual patients may have received an earlier clinical diagnosis of amyotrophic lateral sclerosis (ALS).

CRAMP FASCICULATION SYNDROME

This is a rare peripheral nerve hyperexcitability syndrome that has similarities to Isaac syndrome, but with the added feature of pain and cramps. When EMG is performed, motor nerve stimulation results in a sustained contraction of the activated muscle. Some but not all of these patients may have potassium channel antibodies. Treatment is similar to that for Isaac syndrome.

BENIGN FASCICULATION SYNDROME

These patients seemingly develop the relatively rapid onset of scattered fasciculations that occur much less frequently than those seen in Isaac syndrome. This is obvious by both clinical examination and EMG. The major issue here is the patient who is medically knowledgeable and makes an association between fasciculations and ALS. However, if there is no concomitant clinical weakness and/or muscle atrophy, this almost always is a benign idiopathic entity. Its importance lies in the need for the neurologist to respond immediately to the concern of their medical colleague by performing a very careful clinical evaluation followed an EMG. If both areas are normal, the patients can be told that they have no greater risk to have ALS than any other healthy individual. Often such physicians and nurses have waited to seek expert attention for a matter of months while trying to ignore their symptoms. Finally they become so overwhelmed that they seek help often calling to say that they do have ALS. We look upon this request as a neurologic social emergency in order to immediately allay the angst of our colleagues. The emotional relief that is expressed by these colleagues when they hear the good news is heart warming.

MYOKYMIA

This very uncommon finding is a subcutaneous vermification, or worm-like activity, of just a few muscles. These patients often rarely note these muscle twitches. They are very rhythmic and are basically a quivering under the skin. Typically these are seen in two neurologic conditions.

The most common setting is the patient with prior breast cancer who had a mastectomy many years earlier that was followed soon after surgery by radiation. After a many-year postradiation delay, sometimes as much as 20+ years, the patient begins to note weakness and atrophy in the adjacent arm and hand muscles. With careful inspection one may rarely note the myokymia. However, EMG will demonstrate the spontaneous rhythmic firing of grouped motor unit potentials. These are so unique that they provide strong evidence that the patient's plexopathy is a consequence of radiation.

Subtle peripheral facial nerve lesions associated with a contiguous pontine glioma may also be characterized by myokymia. Here the subcutaneous tissue is so thin that the myokymia is clinically evident to the patient. They may note these adventitious movements when shaving or applying lipstick. In this instance, a magnetic resonance imaging is indicated to search for a pontine mass. On rare occasions, myokymia occurs subsequent to Bell palsy or spontaneously without a specific pathologic lesion.

ADDITIONAL RESOURCES

Benerud MD, Windebank A, Daube J. Long term follow-up of 121 patients with benign fasciculations. Neurology 1993;34:622.

Newsom-Davis J. Neuromyotonia. Rev Neurol 2004;160:85.

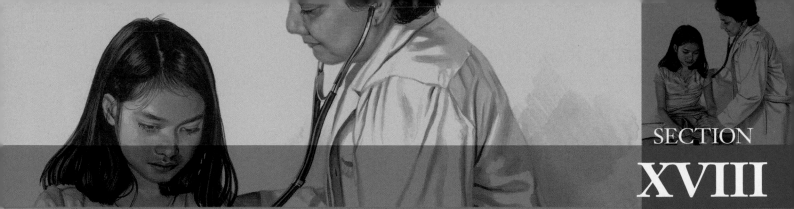

Polyneuropathies

71

Hereditary Polyneuropathies

Monique M. Ryan

Clinical Vignette

A 15-year-old boy presents with frequent tripping and exercise intolerance. He falls frequently and tires easily. He was born at term after an uncomplicated pregnancy. His early developmental milestones were normal until he walked late, at 20 months of age. On examination, he has mild wasting of the distal lower extremities without contractures. He walks well on his toes but cannot walk on his heels. There is mild weakness of ankle dorsiflexion and eversion. The ankle jerks are absent even with reinforcement, but other reflexes are preserved. Sensation is intact. There is no family history of neuromuscular disorders, but on examination his father has high-arched feet with distal weakness and generalized areflexia. Neurophysiologic testing of the patient and his father reveals marked slowing of motor nerve conduction, of the order of 18 m/s, with absent sensory responses. Genetic testing is positive for a duplication of the PMP22 gene on chromosome 17, confirming the clinical diagnosis of Charcot–Marie–Tooth disease type 1A.

The hereditary motor and sensory neuropathies (HMSNs) account for approximately 40% of chronic neuropathies. There are now more than 40 known genes or loci for the various forms of HMSN, which are collectively known as Charcot–Marie–Tooth disease (CMT). About 1 in 2500 persons is affected by CMT. New genes or loci for CMT subtypes are identified very frequently. Less common inherited polyneuropathies are those associated with systemic genetic disorders and inborn errors of metabolism (Table 71-1). Advances in genetic characterization of the inherited neuropathies have afforded greater insight into their biologic basis, and there is increasing interest in therapeutic strategies for these disorders, which can cause lifelong morbidity related to weakness, sensory loss, and orthopedic complications.

ETIOLOGY AND PATHOGENESIS

Charcot–Marie–Tooth disease is commonly divided—on the basis of inheritance, neurophysiologic findings, and histopathology—into demyelinating forms (including dominantly inherited subtypes, CMT1 and CMT3, and autosomal recessive forms, CMT4) and axonal neuropathies (CMT2, which can have either dominant or recessive inheritance). Other forms of CMT include hereditary sensory and autonomic neuropathy (HSAN), which has prominent sensory and autonomic features, and distal hereditary motor neuropathy (dHMN), which has pure motor findings with no clinical or neurophysiologic evidence of sensory deficits.

Regardless of their genetic basis, the final common pathway of all neurologic deficits in the inherited neuropathies is length-dependent axonal degeneration, which accounts for the clinical

findings common to many forms of CMT. Neurophysiologic studies variably demonstrate changes of demyelination, axon loss, or a combination of these findings.

CLINICAL PRESENTATION

CMT generally first manifests in the first decade but progresses slowly, presenting in childhood or early adulthood with an abnormal gait or pes cavus. Less commonly, CMT presents in infancy with hypotonia and delayed motor milestones, or in late adulthood. The cardinal features of the genetic polyneuropathies are distal muscle wasting and weakness, loss of the deep tendon reflexes, and impaired distal sensation. The gait is high-stepping because of foot drop. Nerve hypertrophy may be palpable in the neck or at the elbow (Fig. 71-1) or nerve enlargement may be seen on magnetic resonance imaging (MRI) (Fig. 71-2).

Orthopedic deformities develop in at least two thirds of CMT patients. The most common finding is pes cavus, caused by imbalance between the muscles of the posterior and anterior compartments of the leg. With time, foot deformities become fixed and can cause pain, pressure areas, and stress fractures. Scoliosis and developmental hip dysplasia are less common complications of CMT.

The clinical evaluation should include inquiry as to the family history. Consanguinity suggests a possible recessive inheritance, whereas male-to-male transmission excludes an X-linked condition.

DIFFERENTIAL DIAGNOSIS

A hereditary neuropathy is suggested by a long, slowly progressive course, clinical findings such as pes cavus (which suggests long-standing weakness), and relatively prominent motor deficits without positive sensory phenomena. Acquired neuropathies have a shorter time course, are more likely to be associated with painful sensory phenomena, and may be associated with systemic symptoms or signs.

DIAGNOSTIC APPROACH

Careful clinical evaluation is very important. Often no family history can be obtained, either because a case is sporadic, or because less severely affected relatives have not been diagnosed. Clinical examination and targeted neurophysiologic and genetic testing may reveal relatives to be also affected by hereditary neuropathies.

In patients with suspected neuropathies, the initial investigation will generally be nerve conduction studies and electromyography (Fig. 71-3). CMT is classified as demyelinating if the median nerve motor conduction velocity (MCV) is less than 38 m/s, or axonal (CMT2) if the median MCV is more than 38 m/s. Axonal (neuronal) neuropathies are also associated with low-amplitude sensory and motor responses. Intermediate

Table 71-1 Classification of Inherited Polyneuropathies

	Inheritance	Neurophysiology
Hereditary motor and sensory neuropathy type 1	Autosomal dominant	Demyelinating
Hereditary motor and sensory neuropathy type 2	Autosomal dominant	Axonal
	Autosomal recessive	
Hereditary motor and sensory neuropathy type 3	Autosomal/*de novo* dominant	Demyelinating
Hereditary motor and sensory neuropathy type 4	Autosomal recessive	Demyelinating
Intermediate CMT	Autosomal dominant	Mixed
X-linked CMT	X-linked dominant,	Mixed
	X-linked recessive	
Hereditary sensory and autonomic neuropathies	Autosomal recessive	Axonal
Hereditary motor neuropathies	Autosomal dominant	Axonal
Hereditary neuropathy with liability to pressure palsies	Autosomal dominant	Demyelinating
Other Inherited Neuropathies		
Hereditary neuralgic amyotrophy	Autosomal dominant	Axonal
Familial amyloid polyneuropathy	Autosomal dominant	Axonal
Giant axonal neuropathy	Autosomal recessive	Axonal
Infantile neuroaxonal dystrophy	Autosomal recessive	Axonal
Andermann syndrome	Autosomal recessive	Axonal
Neuropathies Associated with Inborn Errors of Metabolism		
Lipid Disorders		
Cerebrotendinous xanthomatosis	Autosomal recessive	Mixed
Abetalipoproteinemia, hypolipoproteinemia	Autosomal recessive	Demyelinating
Ataxia with vitamin E deficiency	Autosomal recessive	Demyelinating
Peroxisomal Disorders		
Refsum disease	Autosomal recessive	Demyelinating
Adrenomyeloneuropathy	X-linked	Axonal
Mitochondrial Cytopathies		
NARP	Autosomal recessive	Mixed
MNGIE	Autosomal recessive	Mixed
Leigh disease	Autosomal recessive	Mixed
Lysosomal Enzyme Diseases		
Globoid cell leukodystrophy	Autosomal recessive	Demyelinating
Metachromatic leukodystrophy	Autosomal recessive	Demyelinating
Fabry disease	X-linked	Axonal
Tyrosinemia type 1	Autosomal recessive	Axonal
Sphingomyelin Lipidoses		
Niemann–Pick disease type C	Autosomal recessive	Demyelinating
Farber disease	Autosomal recessive	Demyelinating
Porphyrias		
Acute intermittent porphyria	Autosomal dominant	Axonal
Hereditary coproporphyria	Autosomal dominant	Axonal
Variegate porphyria	Autosomal dominant	Axonal
Disorders with Defective DNA Synthesis or Repair		
Ataxia telangiectasia	Autosomal recessive	Axonal
Cockayne syndrome	Autosomal recessive	Demyelinating
Neuropathies Associated with Spinocerebellar Ataxias		
Friedreich ataxia, other SCAs	Autosomal recessive	Axonal
Neuroacanthocytosis	Autosomal recessive	Axonal

MNGIE, mitochondrial neurogastrointestinal encephalopathy; NARP, neuropathy, ataxia, and retinitis pigmentosa; SCA, spinocerebellar ataxia.

forms of CMT have median MCVs in the 25–45 m/s range. In the hereditary demyelinating neuropathies, neurophysiologic abnormalities are generally homogeneous, with uniform slowing of motor and sensory nerve conduction. In contrast, the acquired demyelinating neuropathies (such as Guillain–Barré syndrome and chronic inflammatory demyelinating polyradiculoneuropathy) are characterized by patchy involvement of peripheral nerves with focal slowing, conduction block, and dispersion of motor responses (Fig. 71-4).

CMT can be inherited in an autosomal dominant, autosomal recessive, or X-linked fashion. Many "sporadic" patients have (new) heterozygous mutations in a gene for an autosomal dominant form of CMT. Others have autosomal recessive CMT. In Western populations, about 90% of cases of CMT are either autosomal dominant or X-linked. Recessive CMT is more frequent in populations in which consanguinity is common.

Genetic testing is available for the more common forms of CMT, but for less common phenotypes is often performed only

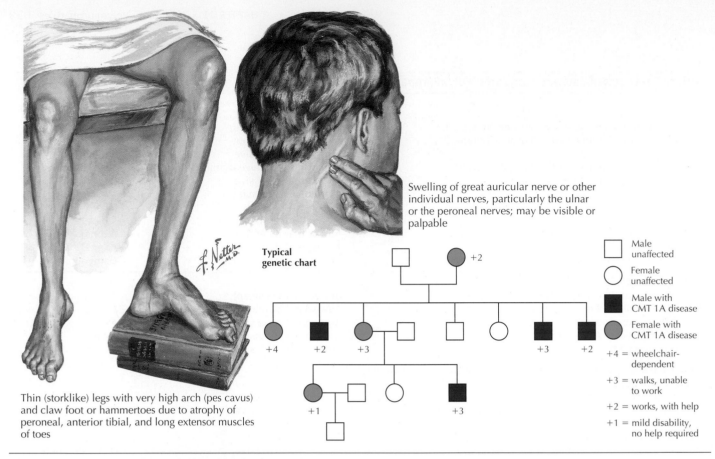

Swelling of great auricular nerve or other individual nerves, particularly the ulnar or the peroneal nerves; may be visible or palpable

Typical genetic chart

Thin (storklike) legs with very high arch (pes cavus) and claw foot or hammertoes due to atrophy of peroneal, anterior tibial, and long extensor muscles of toes

☐ Male unaffected

○ Female unaffected

■ Male with CMT 1A disease

● Female with CMT 1A disease

+4 = wheelchair-dependent

+3 = walks, unable to work

+2 = works, with help

+1 = mild disability, no help required

Figure 71-1 Findings in Charcot–Marie–Tooth Disease.

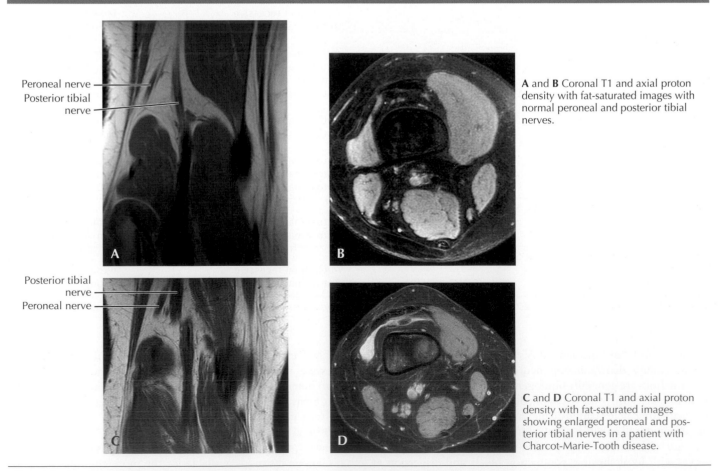

Peroneal nerve
Posterior tibial nerve

Posterior tibial nerve
Peroneal nerve

A and **B** Coronal T1 and axial proton density with fat-saturated images with normal peroneal and posterior tibial nerves.

C and **D** Coronal T1 and axial proton density with fat-saturated images showing enlarged peroneal and posterior tibial nerves in a patient with Charcot-Marie-Tooth disease.

Figure 71-2 MRI Findings in Charcot–Marie–Tooth Disease, with Normal Comparison.

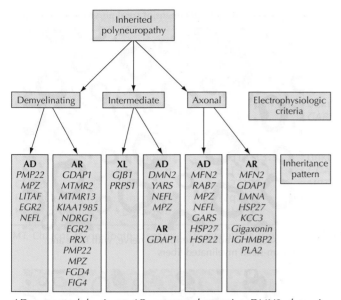

Figure 71-3 Classification of Charcot–Marie–Tooth Disease.

AD, autosomal dominant; AR, autosomal recessive; DMN2, dynamin 2; EGR2, early growth response 2; FGD4, frabin; FIG4, sac domain-containing inositol phophatase 3; GARS, glycyl-tRNA synthetase; GDAP1, ganglioside-induced differentiation-associated protein 1; GJB1, gap junction protein beta 1; HSP22, heat shock 22 kDa protein 8; HSP27, heat shock 27 kDa protein 1; IGHMBP2, immunoglobulin mu binding protein 2; KIAA1985, K1AA1985 protein; KCC3, potassium-chloride cotransporter 3; LITAF, lipopolysaccharide-induced tumor necrosis factor; LMNA, lamin A/C; MFN2, mitofusin 2; MPZ, myelin protein zero; MTMR2, myotubularin-related protein 2; MTMR13, myotubularin-related protein 13; NDRG1, N-myc downstream-regulated gene 1; NEFL, neurofilament light polypeptide 68 kDa; PLA2, phospholipase A2; PMP22, peripheral myelin protein 22; PRPS1, phosphoribosylpyrophosphate synthetase I (PRPS1); PRX, periaxin; RAB7, RAS-associated protein RAB7.

on a research basis. Specific genetic diagnoses enable evaluation of relatives, prognostication and prediction of recurrence risk, and antenatal testing. Classification and clinical assessment are complicated by the fact that a single phenotype is often caused by different genes, and that mutations in a gene may present with a variety of phenotypes (see Fig. 71-3).

Testing for neuropathies associated with inborn errors of metabolism is based on the clinical and neurophysiologic phenotype. Careful attention needs to be paid to other clinical findings that may guide diagnosis, such as cognitive deficits, vision or hearing loss, evidence of other organ dysfunction, and abnormalities on neuroimaging and biochemical investigations.

CLASSIFICATION OF CMT

CMT Type 1

Autosomal dominant demyelinating CMT—CMT type 1—is the most common form of CMT in most populations. Five genes for CMT1 are known (Table 71-2). Most patients present with the "classical" CMT phenotype in the first two decades of life, with a steppage gait, frequent falls, and development of pes cavus. Distal sensory loss is generally mild. There is marked slowing of motor conduction (<38 m/s), and sensory nerve action potentials (SNAPs) are generally lost. Nerve biopsy is

usually not required for diagnosis, but if performed shows a hypertrophic demyelinating neuropathy with onion bulb formation. The most common form, CMT1A, is caused by duplications in the peripheral myelin protein 22 gene on chromosome 17. Deletions in the same gene cause hereditary neuropathy with liability to pressure palsies (HNPP), which presents with recurrent mononeuropathies after minor compressive stresses. Other forms of CMT1 are very uncommon. Genes implicated in CMT type 1 can also cause Déjerine–Sottas syndrome, a severe demyelinating neuropathy that presents before the age of 2 years.

CMT Type 2

Axonal forms of CMT—CMT type 2—are relatively uncommon and can be difficult to distinguish from sporadic axonal neuropathies. CMT2 has been linked to at least 13 loci and 10 genes (Table 71-3). The most common form, CMT2A, is caused by mutations in the gene for a mitochondrial fusion protein, mitofusin 2 (*MFN2*). Mutations in *MFN2* can cause the classic CMT phenotype or can be associated with early-onset severe weakness, long-tract signs, and/or optic atrophy. Other forms of type 2 CMT may be associated with prominent sensory loss and a mutilating arthropathy, early involvement of the distal upper extremities, and pyramidal signs.

Other CMT Types

CMT4 defines a group of rare autosomal recessive demyelinating neuropathies that are generally seen in specific ethnic populations and associated with other physical abnormalities such as vocal cord paresis, glaucoma, and scoliosis. Nerve biopsy is generally required for diagnosis.

X-linked CMT (CMTX) is the second most common form of inherited neuropathy, affecting 10–15% of all CMT patients. Cardinal features of this disorder are absence of male-to-male transmission within kindreds, onset in the first two decades of life, and intermediate nerve conduction velocities (25–45 m/s) with evidence of a mixed axonal and demyelinating neuropathy. CMTX presents in adolescent or adult males with frequent falls, exercise intolerance, and cramping. Progression is associated with development of tremor, weakness, wasting, and sensory loss in the hands. By the fourth to sixth decade, most men have moderate or severe functional impairment with difficulty walking. Central nervous system (CNS) involvement is seen in a minority of individuals with CMTX. Carrier females are generally less severely affected.

CMT subtypes with clinical and neurophysiologic evidence of a pure motor neuropathy are designated **distal hereditary motor neuropathy** (dHMN). Sensory action potentials are reduced or absent in CMT, but always normal in dHMN. Distal HMN is associated with histopathologic evidence of axonal degeneration, and it is classified on the basis of age of onset, mode of inheritance, and clinical evolution.

The **hereditary sensory neuropathies** (HSNs) are a group of uncommon disorders associated with prominent sensory loss, skin ulcers, and arthropathy. Complications of these disorders include recurrent injuries, ulceration, osteomyelitis, and amputations.

Acquired Polyneuropathies

Ted M. Burns, Michelle Mauermann, and Jayashri Srinivasan

72

DIAGNOSTIC APPROACH

Clinical Vignette

A 51-year-old woman complained of acute onset of right hand weakness and pain for 2 weeks and acute onset of painful left foot drop for 3 days. She describes the pain as being "burning and aching" and associated with some prickling and "pins and needles" sensation. Over the past month she has also experienced low-grade fevers, fatigue, malaise, and an unexplained 15-pound weight loss. Her past medical history is only remarkable for adult-onset asthma, for which she uses an inhaler as needed. She is on no other medications. The family history is unremarkable. She does not smoke or drink alcohol. Review of systems is otherwise negative, including for any symptoms of autonomic nervous system dysfunction.

Her examination was noteworthy for marked weakness and sensory loss in the right ulnar nerve and left peroneal nerve distributions; there was also sensory loss over the lateral aspects of the left foot. Nerve conduction studies (NCS) and needle electromyography (EMG) confirmed moderate to severe right ulnar, left peroneal, and left sural mononeuropathies. NCS/EMG demonstrated relatively recent-onset, prominent axonal damage without any findings of prominent demyelination.

Laboratory testing was remarkable for a very elevated erythrocyte sedimentation rate of 82 mm/hour (nonspecific indicator of systemic inflammation). Hypereosinophilia was present on the complete blood count (CBC). A left sural nerve biopsy was performed confirming the clinical suspicion of vasculitic neuropathy. She was diagnosed with Churg–Strauss syndrome with vasculitic neuropathy and was started on high-dose corticosteroids. This led to gradual resolution of her symptoms; 18 months later, there were only minimal residual deficits in the involved peripheral nerves.

The evaluation for the etiology of a patient's polyneuropathy can be very challenging for many reasons, including the fact that there are more than 100 potential etiologies (Fig. 72-1). Ultimately the polyneuropathy is determined to be acquired (i.e., caused by some other disease or exposure) in one third of cases (Box 72-1), inherited in another one third of cases (see Chapter 71), and—in spite of appropriate testing—idiopathic in the remaining one third of cases. In order to focus on a smaller list of potential etiologies so that the evaluation can be simplified, we believe that it is best for the clinician to first characterize the polyneuropathy and the patient. We will present one method for characterizing neuropathy that is easy to remember, based on four simple clinical questions about the neuropathy and the patient: "What?" "Where?" "When?" and "What setting?"

"What?" refers to what nerve fiber modalities (motor, sensory, autonomic, or a combination) are involved? The identification of sensory nerve involvement, at a minimum, allows the clinician to exclude other neuromuscular diseases not associated with sensory dysfunction, such as disorders of anterior horn cells (e.g., amyotrophic lateral sclerosis), neuromuscular transmission (e.g., myasthenia gravis), or of muscle (myopathy). When sensory symptoms and signs are present, it is useful to characterize neuropathic sensory symptoms into "positive" or "negative" because acquired neuropathies are usually accompanied by positive neuropathic sensory symptoms and inherited neuropathies are usually not. Positive sensory symptoms may be painful (e.g., "burning," "freezing," or "throbbing") or painless (e.g., "tingling" or "swelling") (Box 72-2). Paresthesias and pain (positive neuropathic sensory symptoms) are common complaints for patients with diabetic, vasculitic, alcoholic, or uremic neuropathy and patients with Guillain–Barré syndrome (GBS) or chronic inflammatory demyelinating polyradiculoneuropathy (CIDP). In the clinical vignette presented above, the patient had prominent positive neuropathic sensory symptoms, strongly suggesting that the etiology of her neuropathy is acquired rather than inherited. Patients with neuropathy often also complain of exaggerated discomfort to painful sensory stimuli (hyperalgesia) and to nonpainful sensory stimuli (allodynia). Patient complaints indicative of negative neuropathic sensory symptoms include loss of sensation and imbalance (i.e., sensory ataxia). Most patients with neuropathy have some degree of motor nerve involvement that at times is overshadowed by the sensory complaints. Our patient had prominent motor nerve fiber involvement.

Identification of autonomic nerve involvement can be an important clue because only a small number of neuropathic processes affect both autonomic and somatic nerves (e.g., GBS, paraneoplastic neuropathy, diabetic neuropathy, amyloid neuropathy) (Box 72-3). Autonomic symptoms include lightheadedness, syncope, diarrhea, constipation, postprandial bloating, early satiety, urinary complaints, erectile dysfunction, abnormal or absent sweating, and dry mouth and eyes (Fig. 72-2). Our patient did not have discernible autonomic nervous system involvement.

"Where?" refers to the distribution of nerve damage. An important diagnostic watershed is the determination of whether the process is "length dependent" (e.g., distal) or not. Length-dependent neuropathies manifest first in the feet and are symmetric. Non–length-dependent neuropathies are not necessarily evident initially in the feet and may be asymmetric, focal, or multifocal. The etiology of length-dependent neuropathies is usually inherited, metabolic/toxic, or idiopathic whereas a neuropathy that is not length dependent is often caused by an immune-mediated or infectious process.

Our vignette patient clearly had a neuropathy that was not length-dependent (it was multifocal). Some examples of non–length-dependent neuropathies are polyradiculoneuropathies

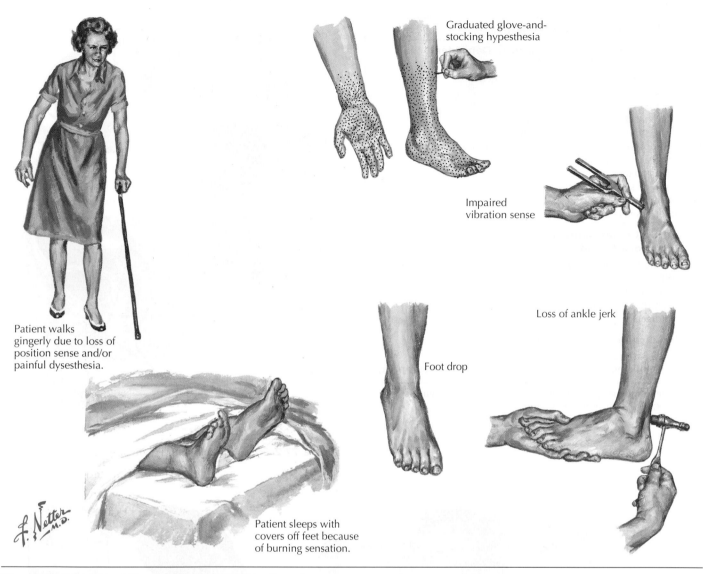

Graduated glove-and-stocking hypesthesia

Impaired vibration sense

Loss of ankle jerk

Foot drop

Patient walks gingerly due to loss of position sense and/or painful dysesthesia.

Patient sleeps with covers off feet because of burning sensation.

Figure 72-1 Peripheral Neuropathies: Clinical Manifestations.

Box 72-1 Neuropathies Associated with Systemic Diseases

Diabetes mellitus
Toxins
Critical illness polyneuropathy
Vasculitis
Amyloidosis
HIV
Lyme
Uremia
Paraneoplastic
Sarcoidosis
Mitochondrial disorders
Fabry disease

(e.g., GBS), plexopathies (often inflammatory), sensory ganglionopathy (e.g., paraneoplastic subacute sensory neuronopathy caused by small cell lung cancer), and multifocal mononeuropathies (e.g., mononeuritis multiplex caused by vasculitis). Our patient's presentation was of painful multifocal mononeuropathies, which is typical of mononeuritis multiplex caused by vasculitis.

"When?" refers to the temporal evolution of the neuropathy. Because of confusion over what is meant by "acute," "subacute," and "chronic," it is often best to describe symptom onset based on whether or not the neuropathic symptoms had a compelling, definite date of onset. A definite date of symptom onset almost always indicates an acute or subacute onset typical of an immune-mediated or infectious etiology. A less-exact date of onset suggests a gradual or insidious onset, indicative of inherited, idiopathic, or toxic/metabolic etiologies. The pace of progression following symptom onset is also an important consideration. Symptom onset and pace of progression often correlate in a predictable manner, owing largely to the underlying mechanism. Mononeuritis multiplex caused by systemic vasculitis, which is at the top of the differential diagnosis for our vignette patient, typically presents with a series of painful mononeuropathies of acute onset, occurring one after the other with the rapid development of significant morbidity. Our patient's description of acute-onset mononeuropathies is typical of mononeuritis multiplex.

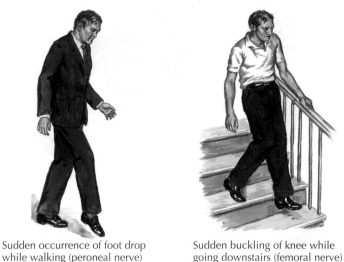
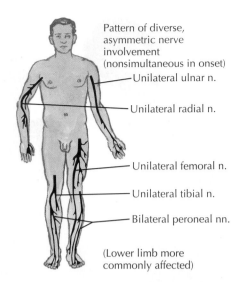

Sudden occurrence of foot drop while walking (peroneal nerve)

Sudden buckling of knee while going downstairs (femoral nerve)

Pattern of diverse, asymmetric nerve involvement (nonsimultaneous in onset)

Unilateral ulnar n.

Unilateral radial n.

Unilateral femoral n.

Unilateral tibial n.

Bilateral peroneal nn.

(Lower limb more commonly affected)

Polyarteritis nodosa with characteristic multisystem involvement

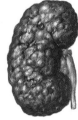
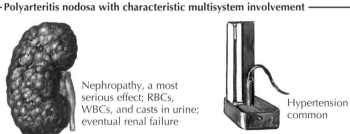
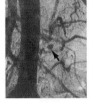
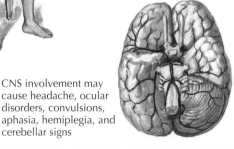
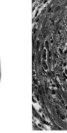
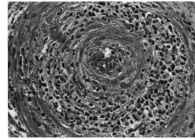

Myalgia and/or arthralgia often associated with abdominal problems, anorexia, fever, and weight loss

Nephropathy, a most serious effect; RBCs, WBCs, and casts in urine; eventual renal failure

Hypertension common

Angiogram showing microaneurysm of small mesenteric artery

CNS involvement may cause headache, ocular disorders, convulsions, aphasia, hemiplegia, and cerebellar signs

Inflammatory cell infiltration and fibrinoid necrosis of walls of small arteries lead to infarction in various organs or tissues

Figure 72-5 Mononeuritis Multiplex due to Systemic Vasculitis.

quickly—because undiagnosed and untreated systemic vasculitis may be fatal. See discussion on vasculitic neuropathies below.

Clinical Vignette

A 72-year-old man reported a 4-year history of numb feet characterized as a feeling of "cotton between the toes." Walking on bare feet became uncomfortable. The numbness ascended circumferentially to his ankles. He no longer trusted his balance to put on his pants without support. Difficulty wiggling the toes was the only indication of weakness. He had no symptoms in his hands or face, indications of dysautonomia, or systemic illness. His medications included a diuretic and a multivitamin. He had no toxic exposure or affected family members. The patient appeared well and had bilateral hammertoe deformities. Neurologic findings included an inability to spread his toes and intrinsic foot muscle atrophy. Muscle stretch reflexes were normal in the arms, diminished at the knees, and absent at the ankles. There was a distal maximal graded stocking distribution sensory loss to light touch, pinprick, temperature, vibration, and proprioception to mid calf bilaterally. He wobbled slightly on Romberg testing but did not fall.

EMG demonstrated a length-dependent, primarily axonal, sensorimotor polyneuropathy. An undefined hereditary sensory neuropathy could not be excluded, although his children were examined clinically and electrodiagnostically. Laboratory investigation did not demonstrate an etiologic mechanism. Nerve biopsy was not indicated.

The symmetric pattern of sensory and reflex loss and the subtle distal motor involvement supported the length-dependent

---

Box 72-4 Primary Demyelinating Polyneuropathies

Length-Dependent Polyneuropathy Pattern
Charcot–Marie–Tooth disease (types 1, 3, 4)
Anti-MAG syndrome
Metachromatic leukodystrophy
Globoid cell leukodystrophy

Polyradiculoneuropathy Pattern
Guillain–Barré syndrome
CIDP
Diabetes
POEMS syndrome

Multifocal Neuropathy Pattern
Multifocal motor neuropathy with conduction block
Multifocal CIDP (Lewis–Sumner syndrome, MADSAM)
Hereditary neuropathy with liability to pressure palsy

Anti-MAG, anti–myelin-associated glycoprotein; CIDP, chronic inflammatory demyelinating polyradiculoneuropathy; MADSAM, multifocal acquired demyelinating sensory and motor; POEMS, polyneuropathy, organomegaly, endocrinopathy, monoclonal gammopathy, and skin changes.

Box 72-5 Length-Dependent Polyneuropathies

Hereditary
Charcot–Marie–Tooth disease
Hereditary sensory neuropathy (HSN or HSAN)
Idiopathic
Amyloidosis
Mitochondrial disorders

Idiopathic
Cryptogenic sensory or sensorimotor polyneuropathy

Dysimmune/Inflammatory
Amyloidosis
Monoclonal gammopathy of unknown significance
Sjögren syndrome (LDPN most common phenotype, may associate with SN, trigeminal neuropathy)
Rheumatoid arthritis
Sarcoidosis (LDPN most common phenotype, may produce MM, cranial neuropathy, usually occurs in established disease)
Vasculitis (25–30% of neuropathy cases present as LDPN, may be presenting manifestation, MM more typical)

Infectious
HIV
Lyme disease

Malnutrition
B-vitamin deficiency (B_{12}, thiamine)

Metabolic
Critical illness polyneuropathy
Diabetes mellitus and impaired glucose tolerance
Gluten-sensitive enteropathy
Hypothyroidism
Uremia

Toxic
Alcohol abuse
Pyridoxine (B_6) toxicity (sensory neuronopathy mimicking LDPN)
Environmental or industrial exposure
  Arsenic
  Hexacarbons
  Lead
  Mercury
  Organophosphates
  Thallium
Prescription drugs
  Amphiphilic cationic drugs (amiodarone, chloroquine, perhexiline)
  Colchicine (neuromyopathy)
  Disulfiram
  Hydralazine
  Isoniazid
  Metronidazole
  Nitrofurantoin
  Nitrous oxide
  Nucleosides (ddC, ddI, d4T for AIDS)
  Paclitaxel
  Thalidomide
  Vincristine

CIDP, chronic inflammatory demyelinating polyradiculoneuropathy; CMT, Charcot–Marie–Tooth neuropathy; GBS, Guillain–Barré syndrome; HNPP, hereditary neuropathy with liability to pressure palsy; LDPN, length-dependent polyneuropathy; MM, mononeuritis multiplex; MMN, multifocal motor neuropathy; PNSS, positive neuropathic sensory symptoms; SN, sensory neuropathy.

---

nature of his neuropathy. Although his hammertoes were compatible with a hereditary neuropathy, positive sensory symptoms, his age, and the absence of affected family members made Charcot–Marie–Tooth disease (CMT) an unlikely consideration. Distal sensory symptoms could occur with myelopathies; however, the characteristic distribution of clinical findings and absence of urinary sphincter problems was consistent with a length-dependent polyneuropathy (LDPN). Annual follow-up revealed minimal progression of his neuropathy.

IDIOPATHIC LENGTH-DEPENDENT POLYNEUROPATHIES

Polyneuropathies are one of the most common neurologic disorders; the length-dependent pattern is the most prevalent. Although there are many recognized causes of polyneuropathy, specific mechanisms have not been identified in 30–40% of patients, and these patients are deemed to have idiopathic neuropathy (Box 72-5).

Peripheral nerve axons are fine-caliber distal portions of long individual cells, sometimes longer than 1 m. They depend on their cell bodies, within dorsal root ganglia or anterior horns, and their axonal transport mechanisms for nutrition and other factors for maintenance of homeostasis. Length-dependent patterns of dysfunction are thought to relate to impaired cell body metabolism or axonal transport within the nerves' most vulnerable components. As the neuropathy progresses, the fingers typically become symptomatic when lower extremity symptoms have ascended to approximately the mid-shin to knee level. Very rarely in advanced cases, the chin, nose, and midline trunk are involved.

Typical patients with primary sensory LDPN note tingling, numb, or burning sensations, often pronounced at rest, particularly at night. Occasionally, exercise exacerbates these unpleasant sensations. When weakness is present, foot and toe extensors

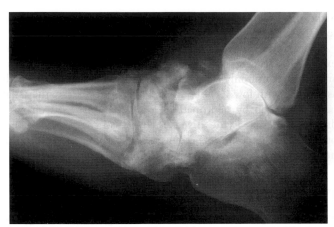

Lateral plain film of ankle and foot demonstrates severe proliferative degenerative changes that are typical of the multiple injuries sustained because of lack of sensation.

Figure 72-7 Neuropathic Foot (Charcot Neuropathy).

gangrene of the toes requiring surgery such as amputations (Fig. 72-7). Motor strength is usually preserved and electrodiagnostic studies will reveal a length-dependent sensory predominant axonal process. Treatment of this condition consists of improved control of diabetes and symptomatic treatment of neuropathic pain. Medications such as gabapentin, pregabalin, and tricyclic antidepressants are used for neuropathic pain.

Diabetic polyradiculoneuropathy (Bruns–Garland syndrome) is an asymmetric painful condition seen in patients with poor diabetic control. Lumbar involvement presents with severe pain in the legs; clinical examination will demonstrate significant asymmetric proximal greater than distal weakness of the lower extremities. Diabetic polyradiculoneuropathy can also involve the thoracic dermatomes, resulting in severe abdominal or thoracic pain. Nerve conduction studies will reveal findings suggestive of lumbar root, plexus, and peripheral nerve involvement. Nerve biopsies may reveal perivascular inflammatory infiltrates and findings of ischemic injury, suggesting that the pathogenesis may be immune mediated. Immune-modifying treatments such as IVIG or prednisone may be beneficial.

Diabetic autonomic neuropathies present with pupillary (Argyll Robertson pupil), sweat, gastrointestinal (gastroparesis, diarrhea), urologic (erectile dysfunction), and cardiovascular (orthostatic hypotension, bradycardia) dysfunction.

Cranial neuropathies such as pupil-sparing third nerve palsy or facial palsy may be associated with diabetes. The incidence of compressive neuropathies is also significantly higher in diabetic patients.

COBALAMIN DEFICIENCY

Cobalamin (vitamin B_{12}) deficiency frequently occurs in people older than age 60. The most common etiology is pernicious anemia, an autoimmune disease that leads to impaired absorption of cobalamin due to the absence of intrinsic factor in the setting of atrophic gastritis. Other causes include dietary avoidance (vegetarians), gastrectomy, gastric bypass surgery, and nitrous oxide abuse. The neuropathy associated with cobalamin deficiency can be similar to other toxic/metabolic etiologies in that there is distal numbness and positive neuropathic sensory symptoms. However, many patients have a non–length-dependent presentation. These patients often present with sensory symptoms beginning in the hands, or simultaneously in the hands and feet. Commonly there is no pain. The neuropathy might begin suddenly, similar to other acquired neuropathies, rather than with a gradual insidious onset. This may occur immediately after surgery requiring general anesthesia wherein nitrous oxide was used for induction. This agent will cause a precipitous sensory polyneuropathy when the patient has very low cobalamin stores, something that may have previously been recognizable. The neuropathy often coexists with a myelopathy, which serves as a clue to the diagnosis but can also make it difficult to differentiate symptoms that are primarily attributable to the neuropathy rather than the myelopathy.

It is important to diagnose cobalamin deficiency as it is a treatable neuropathy. In order to make the diagnosis, the serum B_{12} levels should be evaluated. If they are below normal range, replacement therapy should be initiated. In those patients with B_{12} levels in the low normal range (less than 300 pg/mL), it is important to check the serum homocysteine and methylmalonic acid levels as these will be elevated in cobalamin-deficient patients. Another important clue to cobalamin deficiency is elevation of the mean corpuscular volume (MCV). Electrophysiological studies demonstrate an axonal neuropathy, and somatosensory evoked potentials and magnetic resonance imaging (MRI) may aid in demonstrating a coexisting myelopathy with involvement of the posterior columns. Cobalamin deficiency should be treated with vitamin B_{12} replacement therapy. The route of therapy (intramuscular vs. oral) and duration of therapy depends on the underlying cause and severity of the deficiency.

GUILLAIN–BARRÉ SYNDROME

Clinical Vignette

A 47-year-old man reported a 10-day history of progressive distal and proximal weakness and paresthesias in his arms and legs. He did not report bowel or bladder dysfunction, dysarthria, dysphagia, or dyspnea. He remembered a mild and transient upper respiratory infection 2 weeks before onset of his neuropathic symptoms but otherwise had been well. His medical, family, and social history were unremarkable. He was not taking medications.

Vital signs were normal without orthostatic hypotension or tachycardia. Forced vital capacity and negative inspiratory force were normal. Neurologic examination demonstrated mild facial and symmetric primarily distal weakness in the lower and upper extremities. The patient was areflexic, and his toes were flexor to plantar stimulation. Vibration and joint position sensation were abnormal at the toes and ankles but normal at the fingers. Pinprick, temperature, and light touch sensation were normal, with no spinal cord "sensory level." The patient displayed mild dysmetria with heel-to-shin testing but performed well on finger-to-nose testing. His gait was characterized by weakness, with bilateral foot drop, and he was unsteady. The Romberg test was abnormal.

Cerebrospinal fluid (CSF) examination results demonstrated increased protein of 107 mg/dL and only 3 WBCs. EMG disclosed multifocal signs of demyelination. This clinical and laboratory set of findings was highly suggestive of GBS. The significant degree of weakness made him a good candidate for immunomodulatory therapy. Plasmapheresis (PE) was begun on the second hospital day, with IVIG held in reserve. His autonomic and respiratory statuses were monitored closely. Except for mild intermittent tachycardia, the patient remained free of dysautonomia or respiratory compromise. By day 9 of hospitalization, the patient was walking without assistance. He was transferred to a rehabilitation unit after completing the PE. At follow-up 4 weeks later, he was asymptomatic.

The patient's rapidly evolving polyneuropathy affected motor and sensory function in a non–length-dependent fashion. Presentation with generalized areflexia, concomitant with antecedent respiratory infection, was typical of GBS. Subsequent electrodiagnostic and CSF examination results confirmed this diagnosis.

Guillain–Barré syndrome is a classic acute autoimmune polyneuropathy (Fig. 72-8). Characteristically, it presents in a previously healthy person with the rapid onset of symmetric weakness, areflexia, and generally minimal sensory symptoms with the exception of severe pain in some individuals. Typical CSF findings are an albuminocytologic dissociation with increased protein and fewer than 5–10 WBCs. Additional findings include gait ataxia and cranial and autonomic nerve involvement. Although GBS is the most common cause of acute flaccid paralysis, a primary spinal cord lesion and rarely a poliomyelitis-like illness such as seen now with the West Nile virus, must always be considered early in the clinical course.

GBS, sometimes known as **acute inflammatory demyelinating polyradiculoneuropathy (AIDP)**, and **chronic inflammatory demyelinating polyradiculoneuropathy** (CIDP) are common acquired polyradiculopathies. Both are autoimmune processes that share the unusual feature of significant widespread peripheral—often including nerve root (Fig. 72-9) and sometimes cranial nerve—involvement. Consequently, these disorders are categorized as **polyradiculoneuropathies** rather than polyneuropathies.

The major clinical difference between GBS and CIDP is the temporal course. GBS is a monophasic illness of acute onset that usually reaches a nadir within 1–4 weeks and then gradually improves (see Fig. 72-8). CIDP has a slower onset and more prolonged course that is progressive, monophasic, or relapsing. Most cases of childhood or adult CIDP present within 6 months of symptom onset. Sometimes CIDP can present acutely, mimicking GBS, to be diagnosed correctly only later when a clinical relapse occurs.

The immune attack in GBS and CIDP is widespread and occurs proximally at the nerve roots and distally at the motor axon terminal. These two sites are theoretically more vulnerable because of their less complete blood–nerve barriers. Both cellular and humoral immune mechanisms seem to be involved. Lymphocytes and macrophages are the effector cells involved in damaging myelin and the adjacent axons (see Fig. 72-8). Motor, sensory, and autonomic nerves are affected. The weakness and sensory disturbances are due to nerve fiber action potential conduction block (secondary to demyelination) or conduction failure (due to axon damage).

The pathophysiology of GBS, and perhaps CIDP, relates to the immune system probably being first primed as it responds to foreign molecules, such as a virus or bacteria. Later, the immune system inappropriately attacks host tissue that shares homologous epitopes, for example, gangliosides found on the cell wall of certain bacteria and the peripheral nerve myelin of the host. This pathologic process has been termed molecular mimicry. In keeping with molecular mimicry, approximately two thirds of patients with GBS give a history of antecedent infection. Campylobacter jejuni and cytomegalovirus are the most frequent antecedent infections in GBS, usually as gastroenteritis or respiratory infection 1–4 weeks before the appearance of GBS symptoms. Antecedent infection is observed less commonly in CIDP.

The cardinal features of GBS and CIDP are predominantly symmetric motor symptoms with less consistent sensory symptoms affecting all limbs. Furthermore, the proximal involvement in GBS and CIDP, rather than the classic distal weakness of a polyneuropathy, aids the distinction of a polyradiculoneuropathy. Typically, in GBS and CIDP, motor symptoms overshadow sensory paresthesias such as "tingling" or "pins and needles." These symptoms are more pronounced distally in a stocking-glove distribution. Back pain is common in GBS, particularly in children, but is not found in CIDP. At times, pure motor or pure sensory variants of GBS or CIDP occur but remain recognizable because of the frequently associated prodrome; the acute, symmetric, and generalized pattern of weakness; the areflexia; and the supportive information gained by electrodiagnostic and CSF examinations.

Gait difficulty often occurs early on in patients with polyradiculoneuropathies. It may manifest as trouble climbing stairs, arising from chairs, unsteadiness, falls, or difficulty with arm use. Facial weakness occurs in more than half of patients with GBS but is much less common in CIDP. Ophthalmoplegia, dysarthria, and dysphagia may occur in both disorders, more frequently in GBS.

Neurologic examination demonstrates prominent proximal and distal weakness, rarely slightly asymmetric. More subtle proximal and distal strength should be sought by having the patient rise from a chair, step up on a step, kneel on one knee and stand, walk on the heels, and walk on the toes. Reduced or absent muscle stretch reflexes are important early clinical clues that the symptoms are likely from a peripheral nerve disorder. However, retention of reflexes may occur in early GBS and occasionally in CIDP. There is an associated mild distal sensory impairment in the feet.

Respiratory compromise occurs in 15–30% of patients with GBS. Endotracheal intubation for airway protection and mechanical ventilation for diaphragmatic weakness are necessary. Airway and respiratory compromise are rare in CIDP.

Pathogenesis

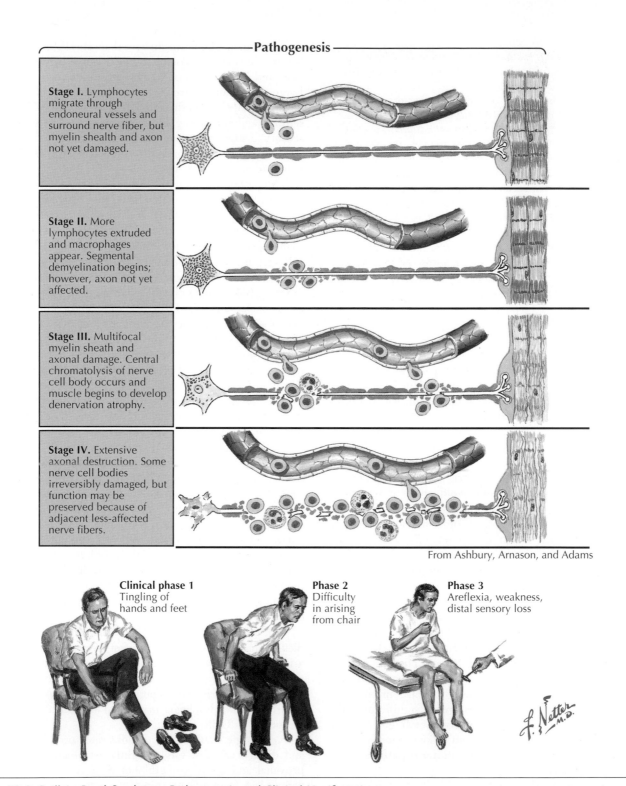

Stage I. Lymphocytes migrate through endoneural vessels and surround nerve fiber, but myelin sheath and axon not yet damaged.

Stage II. More lymphocytes extruded and macrophages appear. Segmental demyelination begins; however, axon not yet affected.

Stage III. Multifocal myelin sheath and axonal damage. Central chromatolysis of nerve cell body occurs and muscle begins to develop denervation atrophy.

Stage IV. Extensive axonal destruction. Some nerve cell bodies irreversibly damaged, but function may be preserved because of adjacent less-affected nerve fibers.

From Ashbury, Arnason, and Adams

Clinical phase 1
Tingling of hands and feet

Phase 2
Difficulty in arising from chair

Phase 3
Areflexia, weakness, distal sensory loss

Figure 72-8 Guillain–Barré Syndrome: Pathogenesis and Clinical Manifestations.

The autonomic nervous system is frequently involved in GBS, especially in severe cases. Dysautonomia in GBS commonly manifests as sinus tachycardia but may result in other cardiac arrhythmias or labile blood pressures that may be life threatening and warrant close observation. Urinary retention, adynamic ileus, and constipation sometimes occur. Overt dysautonomia in CIDP is rare.

DIFFERENTIAL DIAGNOSIS OF DEMYELINATING POLYNEUROPATHIES

Subjective sensory symptoms have differential diagnostic importance favoring GBS or CIDP over other motor unit disorders, including myopathies, neuromuscular transmission disorders, or

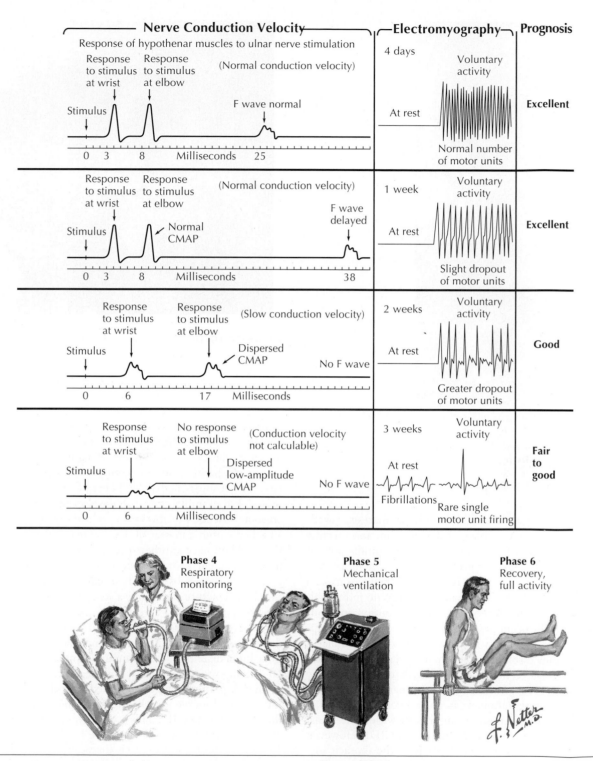

Figure 72-8 Guillain–Barré Syndrome: Electrophysiologic Findings and Clinical Manifestations.

motor neuron disorders. However, the possibility of acute spinal cord lesion or other fulminating forms of polyneuropathy should always be considered.

Because sensory symptoms also occur with **myelopathies**, the possibility of an acute or subacute myelopathy with evolving spinal cord compression that may necessitate emergent intervention must always be considered, especially early in the patient's clinical course. Important clues to the possibility of a myelopathy include the preservation or hyperactivity of muscle stretch reflexes, Babinski signs, a cord level on careful sensory testing and sphincter dysfunction. Patients presenting with a polyradiculoneuropathy do not have a spinal cord sensory level, and preservation of muscle stretch reflexes is unusual in GBS and CIDP, although such may occasionally occur for ≥48 hours.

Transverse myelitis (TM) is the most common acute spinal cord lesion leading to confusion in the differential diagnosis of

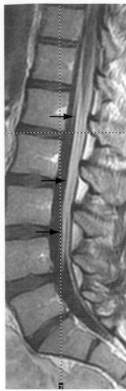

Sagittal T1 post-gadolinium-enhanced MRI demonstrating diffuse enhancement of cauda equina (arrows)

Figure 72-9 Guillain–Barré.

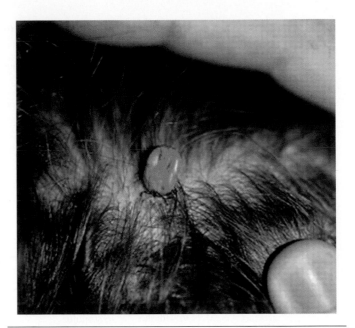

Figure 72-10 Tick Embedded in Scalp Causing Tick Paralysis. *(Courtesy Dr. Thomas Swift.)*

GBS. Criteria for diagnosis of TM include paraparesis, a well-defined sensory level, severe bladder dysfunction, and myelitic findings on MRI. Often motor and sensory symptoms present equally but motor findings may predominate. Sphincter control is lost in most patients with TM. It may be difficult to make a clinical differential between GBS and TM in some individuals without spinal cord MRI. Although urinary retention and constipation occasionally occur in GBS for the first day, these symptoms are very suggestive of a myelopathy, a conus medullaris, and/or cauda equina disorders. And when present in GBS, these symptoms are always very short-lived, usually clearing in a day or so. Thus, whenever sphincter difficulties persist in a patient with a GBS-like presentation, it is most likely that there is another pathophysiologic mechanism present within the spinal cord. Back pain is common in GBS but not in CIDP. However, when it has a radicular quality, particularly in the thoracic distribution, a thoracic **spinal mass lesion**, **dural AVM**, or TM must be considered.

The temporal course is of primary importance for **differentiating GBS and CIDP** from many other peripheral neuropathies. Patients with GBS and CIDP can usually give a specific date of symptom onset. This contrasts with many other acquired or inherited polyneuropathies wherein the onset is so insidious that the patient has no recall as to its precise timing.

Patients with **mononeuritis multiplex** (MNM) usually have an associated systemic or primary peripheral nervous system vasculitis. The precise temporal profile of the patient's clinical symptomatology, that is, stepwise and asymmetric, is the primary diagnostic clue, in direct contrast to CIDP, which has a symmetric evolution. Typically MNM patients have sudden acute mononeuropathies, often affecting 4–6 specific nerves, particularly the peroneal, median, and ulnar, within a 2- to 6-week time period. For example, they may develop an acute foot drop from an acute vasculitis to the vasa nervorum of the peroneal nerve, and then within a matter of days acute sensory or motor loss in the distribution of another specific peripheral nerve such as the median or ulnar with numbness in the specific fingers supplied by these nerves. Subsequently if many nerves become involved, the clinical picture can mimic a symmetric generalized polyneuropathy. An increased erythrocyte sedimentation rate, often in the range of 60–100 mm/hour and a peripheral nerve biopsy demonstrating vasculitis provide important diagnostic information. Immediate high-dose immunosuppressive therapy, such as 60–100 mg prednisone daily, is indicated.

In **tick paralysis**, an unidentified tick saliva toxin most likely interacts with nerve ion channels, producing an acute paralytic illness mimicking GBS. This is most common in girls and young women, in whom ticks can become hidden in their scalp hair. Examiners must always search for ticks in any patient with an acute flaccid paralysis. These are relatively large sized when engorged and easily recognized (Fig. 72-10) when one carefully examines the scalp. In North America, the recovery is rapid and complete after the tick is dislodged.

A number of **toxins**, including marine origin (red tide, ciguatoxin), metals (arsenic), solvents (hexacarbons), insecticides (organophosphates), and native plants such as Buckthorn, may produce acute generalized neuropathy. GBS may be the presenting sign of **HIV** before AIDS is definitively diagnosed. The findings of a disparate CSF examination with an inordinate pleocytosis are clues to search for CD4 cell count deficiencies and other clinical and laboratory signs of AIDS. **Paralytic polio** is preceded by a prodrome that includes back pain similar to GBS. Its multifocal and asymmetric pattern, the absence of sensory signs or symptoms, and CSF pleocytosis are distinguishing features. EMG demonstrates axon loss confined to motor nerves, consistent with anterior horn cell localization. **Diphtheria** is no longer of concern in industrialized nations, with the exception of parents who withhold immunization from their children. However, it still occurs in less fortunate economic settings. Acute intermittent and variegate **porphyria** may produce an acute generalized sensorimotor neuropathy mimicking GBS. Previous attacks, a family history of similar disorders, concomitant abdominal pain, and mental status changes are clinical clues that typify this rare biochemical disorder. An axonal character defined by EMG, rather than the typical demyelinating neuropathy of GBS, raises the possibility of porphyria.

Botulism and **myasthenia gravis** may produce an acute generalized weakness. Botulism is typically acute in onset and myasthenia is usually more indolent, although myasthenia gravis can have a relatively rapid presentation with cranial nerve and peripheral distribution weakness. Neither produces sensory system involvement. Both have a predilection for oculobulbar musculature. Botulism may also have prominent manifestations of cholinergic dysautonomia. EMG may be required for distinction from GBS. **Lambert–Eaton myasthenic syndrome (LEMS)** may mimic CIDP with a subacute onset of proximal weakness and areflexia. History of tobacco addiction and a dry mouth suggest LEMS (Chapter 74).

Severe **hypokalemia** and **hypophosphatemia** may produce weakness on an acute, generalized basis. Weakness severe enough to mimic GBS does not usually occur until potassium decreases to less than 2 mEq/mL and phosphate decreases to less than 1 mg/mL. Both typically occur in clinical contexts where severe hypokalemia or hypophosphatemia could be anticipated. **Hypokalemia** weakness is thought to be myopathic and is unassociated with sensory changes. **Hyperkalemia** with acute severe generalized weakness may also mimic GBS. Addison disease becomes an important diagnostic consideration. Barium carbonate poisoning, severe vomiting and diarrhea, and clay ingestions have also presented with similar clinical pictures. Sensory symptoms and signs in **hypophosphatemia** resemble GBS more closely than hypokalemic and hyperkalemic states.

AIDP AND CIDP VARIANTS

There are several recognized variants of GBS. There are acute axonal forms of GBS, which represents 5–10% of cases of GBS in North America but is more common in Japan and China. **Acute motor axonal neuropathy (AMAN)** tends to affect mostly children and large epidemics are seen in northern China during the summer. The onset of weakness is abrupt and is often preceded a few weeks by an upper respiratory or other infection. There are no sensory symptoms or signs. The CSF demonstrates albuminocytologic dissociation. The recovery usually begins within 3 weeks and is often complete. **Acute motor and sensory axonal neuropathy (AMSAN)** presents in adults and can affect any geographic location and occur during any season. There is involvement of sensory nerves and the course is often more protracted with severe residual disability. The most

recognized variant is **Miller Fisher syndrome (MFS)**. MFS usually follows an infection, such as *Campylobacter jejuni*. MFS presents with external ophthalmoplegia, ataxia, and areflexia, although all of these components need not be present. Facial weakness and dysarthria are particularly common in MFS. Many patients often have "overlapping GBS" with flaccid quadriparesis. Anti-GQ1b antibodies are present in approximately 95% of patients with acute MFS.

Chronic inflammatory demyelinating polyradiculoneuropathy associated with an IgG or IgA monoclonal gammopathy of undetermined significance usually presents clinically like CIDP, without a monoclonal protein, and treatment response is similar. However, an IgG-λ or IgA-λ (lambda) monoclonal gammopathy suggests the possibility of **POEMS syndrome** (polyneuropathy, organomegaly, endocrinopathy, monoclonal gammopathy, and skin changes, particularly hyperpigmentation). Often an osteosclerotic or osteolytic bony lesion can be identified by performing a "metastatic bone" standard radiograph survey. Focused beam radiation therapy to these tumors can dramatically improve all POEMS syndrome aspects.

In contrast, an acquired demyelinating polyneuropathy associated with an IgM monoclonal protein frequently presents with more predominant sensory symptoms and signs, including sensory ataxia. It is less responsive to standard CIDP treatments. Many patients with a demyelinating polyneuropathy with an IgM monoclonal protein have high titers of antibodies to myelin-associated glycoprotein. It is thought that the IgMs are directed at myelin-associated glycoprotein epitopes on peripheral nerve constituents, and thereby are possibly pathogenic. GBS is not associated with monoclonal gammopathies.

Although the confirmation of GBS or CIDP primarily rests on clinical features, **CSF analysis**, EMG (see Fig. 72-8), serum immunophoresis, and treatment response provide the best means to make a precise diagnosis. An increased level of CSF protein (>50 mg/dL) without pleocytosis (<10 cells/mm^3) is common in GBS and CIDP. CSF examination is often normal within the first week of GBS; however, approximately 90% of patients with CIDP and patients with late GBS have an increased level of CSF protein. Although 10–50 cells/mm^3 in the CSF may occur in GBS, more than 50 cells/mm^3 must arouse suspicion of an alternate diagnosis, including Lyme neuroborreliosis, HIV-associated polyradiculoneuropathy, poliomyelitis, or lymphomatous meningoradiculitis.

EMG provides a definitive means to assess the presence of a peripheral neuropathic process, ruling out other causes such as disorders of neuromuscular transmission or myopathy. EMG can demonstrate widespread involvement of spinal roots and peripheral nerves, usually defining the process as demyelinating, although well-recognized axonal variants exist with GBS as noted above. In GBS or CIDP, the motor and sensory conduction velocities are abnormally slow, with prolonged distal motor and F-wave latencies and often absent H reflexes. Nonuniform slowing, conduction block at sites not prone to entrapment, and abnormal temporal dispersion are commonly found in GBS and CIDP but not in most inherited demyelinating polyneuropathies. Conduction block is present when there are significant reductions in compound motor nerve action potential amplitude and area, with proximal versus distal stimulation. Temporal dispersion is characterized by abnormal prolongation of compound motor nerve action potential duration with proximal but not distal stimulation. Conduction velocities on routine nerve conduction studies may be normal when inflammatory lesions are more proximal, for example, in nerve roots or early in the disease course. Documentation of absent F waves, conduction block, temporal dispersion, or a combination of these is helpful for diagnosis of early GBS wherein more widespread slowing of conduction is not yet present. Another important feature of the electrodiagnostic studies can be the pattern of "sural sparing," which means there is a normal sural sensory response in the setting of abnormal median and sensory antidromic sensory responses; this may be seen in CIDP.

Usually, blood laboratory study results are unremarkable in GBS and CIDP. The most important exception is the occasional occurrence of a monoclonal protein in patients with CIDP; this usually represents a monoclonal gammopathy of undetermined significance. When this is a λ monoclonal antibody, it may signify a malignancy, such as osteosclerotic or osteolytic myeloma in POEMS as noted above, multiple myeloma, or Waldenström macroglobulinemia.

TREATMENT

Care of patients with GBS varies from watchful waiting to emergency intervention, but initially always in a hospital because of the potential for rapid respiratory compromise. Patients with mild GBS who are able to ambulate are often cared for without specific treatment. Those individuals who are unable to walk, who develop respiratory compromise, or who exhibit rapid progression require treatment with plasmapheresis (PE) or IVIG. Both treatments are effective, but only if given within 1–2 weeks of onset, when the autoimmune attack is still active. Concomitant or sequential use of these therapies usually has no value. IVIG is given as a 2.0 g/kg dosage over 2–5 days. PE is given as five plasma exchanges of 1 plasma volume each over 9–10 days. Oral steroids are not effective for GBS. Respiratory failure is common in GBS; one third of patients require mechanical ventilation. Early on in the course of GBS, negative inspiratory force and vital capacity must be monitored closely in all patients. Autonomic dysfunction is also seen frequently. Labile hypertension and arrhythmias occur frequently, often prompting observation and management in the intensive care unit.

Treatment of patients with CIDP having significant disability with oral corticosteroids, IVIG, and PE is useful. Predetermined neurologic end points, such as strength, gait, and reflexes, must be monitored closely. In CIDP, clinical improvement usually occurs within a few weeks. **Oral steroids**, usually prednisone, are also efficacious in CIDP. The initial dose is usually 40–60 mg/day, transitioned to every-other-day dosing, then tapered and discontinued. The potential acute and chronic risks must be considered when deciding on steroid treatment and its duration. PE is not used as frequently as oral steroids or IVIG for CIDP because it is more invasive and not any more efficacious. In addition, the response to PE may be more transient. Nonetheless, PE remains an option, especially for patients who do not respond to IVIG or steroids.

Most patients with GBS have a good prognosis, particularly those who primarily have the disorder limited to demyelination without significant axonal involvement where the course may be more prolonged. Most recover within a few months, although recovery is not always complete. A small percentage is left with some disability, and rarely, permanent disability primarily involving distal weakness in the feet. Occasional (approximately 1–2%) mortalities do occur in GBS. Most deaths are from preventable respiratory complications or autonomic derangement. Supportive care, including emotional and nutritional support, judicious pain management, and prophylaxis for common complications of hospitalized, immobile patients (deep venous thrombosis and decubitus ulcers) is important.

The long-term outcome varies for patients with CIDP who are treated with conventional therapy. Most return to normal strength although some require intermittent IVIG to maintain improvement. Unfortunately, a rare patient progresses despite aggressive immunotherapy.

SENSORY NEURONOPATHIES

Clinical Vignette

A 64-year-old lifelong smoker awakened with unexplained, poorly described pain in her left groin unrelated to position or movement. Within 2 weeks, pains developed in a multifocal distribution. Her feet, her hands, and the right posterior part of her scalp became numb. She experienced increasing difficulty maintaining balance and walking, particularly in the dark or with her eyes closed.

Examination revealed a chronically ill woman who initially seemed to give incomplete effort during manual muscle testing. This was corrected by having her directly visualize tested body parts. Muscle stretch reflexes were absent in the ankles and knees and diminished but present in the arms. Vibration, position, and, to a lesser extent, pain and temperature sensations were absent in the feet and variously diminished more proximally. Pinprick was less well perceived in the right posterior part of the scalp than in the left.

Within 2 months of onset, the patient could not open her mouth and reported blurred vision. Examination disclosed apparent trismus and a direction-changing nystagmus. EMG revealed absent sensory nerve action potentials in the lower extremities and reduced sensory nerve action potentials in the hands. Motor conduction and needle electrode examination results were normal.

An acute-onset sensory polyneuropathy developed in this patient. Her clinical profile suggested a non–length-dependent process typical of a dorsal root ganglion cell sensory neuronopathy. This rapid temporal evolution in a smoker was a particularly ominous sign suggestive of a **paraneoplastic sensory neuronopathy**. Her subsequent development of trismus and nystagmus suggested concomitant brainstem encephalitis, another paraneoplastic syndrome that occurs in patients with small cell lung cancer. Chest imaging and subsequent biopsy of an anterior mediastinal mass confirmed the suspected small cell lung cancer. Anti-Hu antibodies confirmed the paraneoplastic relation between the sensory neuronopathy and lung tumor.

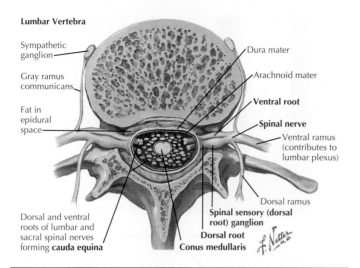

Lumbar Vertebra

Sympathetic ganglion

Gray ramus communicans

Fat in epidural space

Dura mater

Arachnoid mater

Ventral root

Spinal nerve

Ventral ramus (contributes to lumbar plexus)

Dorsal ramus

Spinal sensory (dorsal root) ganglion

Dorsal root

Conus medullaris

Dorsal and ventral roots of lumbar and sacral spinal nerves forming **cauda equina**

Figure 72-11 Spinal Nerve Origin: Sensory Components.

Box 72-6 Sensory Neuronopathy Pattern Dorsal Root Ganglion

Sjögren syndrome
Cancer
   Paraneoplastic
      Small cell lung
      Non-Hodgkin lymphoma
   Cisplatin toxicity
Other medications
   Pyridoxine
   Thalidomide
Idiopathic
Spinocerebellar ataxia

Box 72-7 Causes of Axonal Length-Dependent Sensory Polyneuropathy (LDPN)*

Idiopathic
Diabetes mellitus
Toxins
B-vitamin deficiency
Sjögren syndrome
Amyloidosis (primary systemic or hereditary)
HIV
Hereditary sensory neuropathies

*LDPN, length-dependent polyneuropathy.

Most patients with peripheral neuropathies present with slowly ingravescent sensory symptoms and signs typical of a **length-dependent polyneuropathy** (LDPN). Another, smaller population of sensory-impaired individuals has pathophysiology primarily affecting the sensory neuron cells within the dorsal root ganglion (in contrast to neuropathies, affecting the distal nerve axon) (Fig. 72-11). They are described as having a primary **sensory neuronopathy**. The acute onset is often typified by a painful, noxious clinical picture with a generalized distribution. The dorsal root ganglia (DRG) sensory peripheral nerve cell bodies are the primary target of the disease process in patients with sensory neuronopathies. This anatomic locale explains why these disorders present with a non–length-dependent clinical pattern. Disproportionate loss of position and other discriminatory modalities occur when large sensory fibers are affected. Severe sensory ataxia frequently presents. Distinguishing between sensory LDPN and sensory neuronopathy is important because their differential diagnoses vary considerably. Often, a clinically suspected diagnosis can be confirmed with EMG.

In **paraneoplastic sensory neuronopathy (PSN)**, it is proposed that similar molecular and antigenic components in DRG and small cell lung carcinoma cells set the stage for molecular mimicry. PSN typically has an acute to subacute painful presentation. It occurs in approximately 1% of patients with small cell lung cancer, rarely with other malignancies. The paraneoplastic syndrome may precede malignancy recognition by years. One or more additional paraneoplastic neurologic syndromes eventually develop in approximately 75% of these patients.

Sjögren syndrome is an immunologically mediated process associated with several neuropathy phenotypes that may evolve acutely or chronically. The classic sensory neuronopathy form is uncommon. It is clinically indistinguishable from other DRG lesions, particularly paraneoplastic sensory neuronopathy. Women are more commonly affected. Diagnostic findings include the sicca complex with dry eyes and mouth, antibodies directed against SSA and SSB, inflammatory involvement of salivary glands on lip biopsy, or a combination of these.

Sensory neuronopathy is a well-recognized dose-related and dose-limiting **toxicity of cisplatin and carboplatin**.

Pyridoxine in large doses (1–2 g daily) may cause irreversible sensory neuronopathy syndromes. Doses, as small as 200 mg/day, over extended periods may have similar toxic potential. **Vitamin B$_{12}$ deficiency** and **tabes dorsalis** have strong predispositions to affect the posterior columns. They present with sensory ataxia. Patients with B$_{12}$ deficiency frequently experience paresthesias, often initially in the hand in a non–length-dependent manner, but may also have generalized painful neuropathies. **Tabes dorsalis** is rarely seen today. This complication of tertiary syphilis is typified by its unusual clinical manifestations, including paroxysms of severely uncomfortable lightning pains and ataxia. Many sensory neuronopathy patients with ataxic neuropathies do not have definable pathophysiologic mechanisms, **idiopathic sensory ganglionopathy**. As with idiopathic or cryptogenic disease categories, this remains a diagnosis of exclusion. Often clinically indistinguishable from paraneoplastic sensory neuronopathy presenting with a sensory ataxia, these disorders may evolve acutely or chronically and occur predominantly in women.

EMG is the initial study because it provides a means to differentiate between LDPN and sensory neuronopathy. Almost all patients with LDPNs, even those without clinical weakness, have EMG evidence of motor involvement. These are recognized by motor nerve conduction study changes, needle electrode examination abnormalities, or both (Fig. 72-12). Patients with a primary DRG lesion, that is, sensory neuronopathy, have only sensory nerve conduction study abnormalities.

When sensory neuronopathies are confirmed, subsequent ancillary testing is limited to disorders known to cause such patterns (Box 72-6). The various causes of sensory LDPN may also require consideration (Box 72-7). Testing for serum anti-Hu

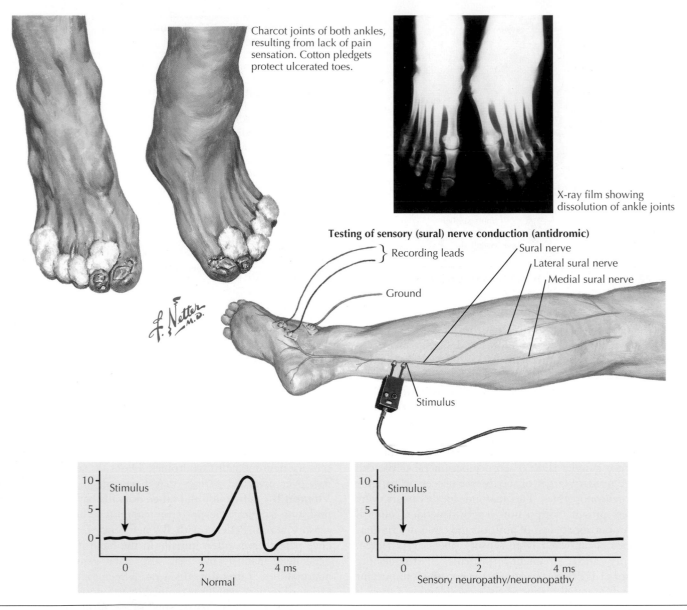

Charcot joints of both ankles, resulting from lack of pain sensation. Cotton pledgets protect ulcerated toes.

X-ray film showing dissolution of ankle joints

Testing of sensory (sural) nerve conduction (antidromic)

Recording leads

Sural nerve

Lateral sural nerve

Medial sural nerve

Ground

Stimulus

Stimulus — Normal

Stimulus — Sensory neuropathy/neuronopathy

Figure 72-12 Hereditary Sensory Neuropathy.

antibodies is indicated in sensory neuronopathy evaluation, particularly for patients with a smoking or asbestos-exposure history. They are sensitive and specific for paraneoplastic neurologic disorders, particularly those with occult malignancies such as small cell lung cancer. Chest CT is indicated because the neuropathy may precede malignancy recognition by several years. Patients with suspected Sjögren syndrome require serologic tests, particularly SSA and SSB antibodies. Other potentially beneficial studies include the Schirmer test of lacrimation and slit lamp examination of the conjunctiva after Rose-Bengal staining. Minor salivary gland (usually lip) biopsy is performed if the diagnosis remains unconfirmed with less invasive means. Vitamin B_{12} levels and a serologic test for syphilis are important for evaluation of patients with large-fiber sensory dysfunction.

When the vitamin B_{12} level is borderline, the more sensitive blood or urine tests for homocysteine, methylmalonic acid, or both are helpful. A nerve biopsy is usually not indicated in sensory neuronopathies.

TREATMENT AND PROGNOSIS

Symptomatic treatment for discomfort associated with sensory neuronopathy and other sensory predominant neuropathies is important. Potential neurotoxins require identification and subsequent elimination. An empiric approach may include carefully considering discontinuation of medication begun at illness inception. The degree of recovery depends on the nature, intensity, and duration of the exposure. Successful recovery may occur rapidly or be protracted, in keeping with known limitations of nerve regeneration. Patients with severe sensory ataxia may require canes, crutches, walkers, or wheelchairs as these allow safe, independent mobility.

Meticulous foot hygiene should be emphasized when patients have prominent loss of pain perception. This includes monitoring for unnoticed painless injuries with the predisposition to become easily infected. Pain is a prominent component and necessitates empathetic management and appropriate use of analgesics, including narcotics. In Sjögren syndrome, reports of successful responses to various immunomodulating therapies are gaining recognition. IVIG was effective in a patient who had been ill for 5 years before treatment. Paraneoplastic sensory neuropathies are generally resistant to therapies, including a variety of immunomodulating agents. This seems paradoxical to the excellent evidence supporting an underlying autoimmune mechanism. Specific treatment of the underlying neoplasm, when identified, may be successful, but seems to have little or no impact on the neuropathy. These patients usually have an inexorable downhill course. Prognosis varies depending on the underlying cause of the neuropathy and the extent of axonal damage before treatment initiation. Specific treatments for sensory neuropathies are lacking, disappointing most patients. Sometimes sensory neuronopathies are debilitating with loss of independence. Severe cases may prevent independent ambulation, even with gait aids.

ADDITIONAL RESOURCES

AAN practice parameter: Practice Parameter: Evaluation of distal symmetric polyneuropathy: Role of autonomic testing, nerve biopsy, and skin biopsy (an evidence-based review). Neurology 2009;72:1.

Barohn RJ. Approach to peripheral neuropathy and neuronopathy. Semin Neurol 1998;18:7-18.

Burns TM. Guillain-Barre Syndrome. Seminars in Neurology 2008;28:152-167.

Dispenzieri A. POEMS syndrome. Blood Reviews 2007;21:285-299.

Dispenzieri A, Kyle RA, Lacy MQ, Rajkumar SV, Therneau TM, Larson DR, Greipp PR, Witzig TE, Basu R, Suarez GA, Fonseca R, Lust JA, Gertz MA. POEMS syndrome: definitions and long-term outcome. Blood 2003: 101:2496-2506.

Dyck PJ, Dyck PJ, Grant IA, Fealy RD. Ten steps in characterizing and diagnosing patients with peripheral neuropathy. Neurology 1996;47(10-17).

England JD, Asbury AK. Peripheral neuropathy. Lancet 2004;363:2151-2161.

Mauermann ML, Burns TM. The evaluation of chronic axonal neuropathies. Seminars in Neurology 2008;28:133-151.

Pourmand R. Evaluating patients with suspected peripheral neuropathy: do the right thing, not everything. Muscle Nerve 2002;26:288-290.

Sabin TD. Classification of peripheral neuropathy: The long and the short of it. Muscle and Nerve 1986;9:711-719.

Saperstein DS. Chronic acquired demyelinating polyneuropathies. Seminars in Neurology 2008;28:168-184.

Saperstein DS, Wolfe GI, Granseth GS, et al. Challenges in the identification of cobalamin-deficiency polyneuropathy. Arch Neurol 2003;60:1296-1301.

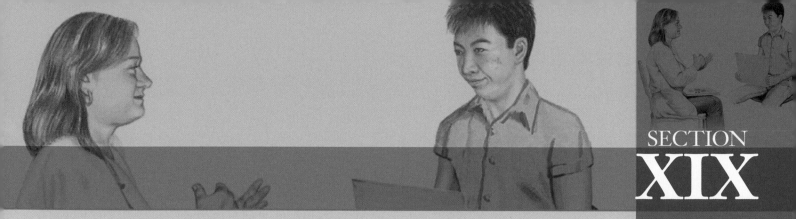

Neuromuscular Transmission Disorders

Myasthenia Gravis

73

Ted M. Burns and H. Royden Jones, Jr.

Clinical Vignette

A healthy 63-year-old man presented with a 6-week history of the gradual onset of asymmetric eyelid drooping and double vision. His ptosis and diplopia fluctuated in severity, being more noticeable later in the day. His wife noted that his speech sounded slurred near the end of the day or after he had been speaking uninterrupted for a few minutes. Neurologic examination revealed asymmetric, left worse than right, ptosis and dysconjugate eye movements in several directions of gaze with associated weakness of eye closure, neck flexion, and mild proximal limb weakness.

Nerve conduction studies and needle electromyography (EMG) demonstrated normal motor and sensory action potentials. Repetitive motor nerve stimulation testing demonstrated a 35% decrease in the ulnar compound muscle action potential (CMAP) amplitude between the first and fourth stimuli. Acetylcholine receptor (AChR) antibodies were present in significantly abnormal titers. Results of computed tomographic (CT) scanning of the mediastinum were unremarkable. Immunosuppressive and pyridostigmine bromide (Mestinon) treatments were initiated.

This vignette is typical of a myasthenia gravis (MG) patient with fatigable and fluctuating muscle weakness. MG almost always begins with ocular muscle weakness manifesting as ptosis, dysconjugate gaze, and eye closure weakness (Fig. 73-1). The symptoms of MG often spread to involve "bulbar" muscles, causing fatigable and fluctuating dysarthria, chewing weakness, and dysphagia. Respiratory, neck, and limb muscles can also become weak. An autoimmune basis for MG has been recognized since 1960. Overall, women are more commonly affected. Peaks of onset are seen in women in the second and third decades and for men in the fifth and sixth decades. The overall prevalence, estimated at 1 per 10,000, has increased over the past 40 years because of improved recognition, treatment, and survival.

ETIOLOGY AND PATHOGENESIS

The most common cause of acquired MG is the abnormal development of antibodies to immunogenic regions (epitopes) on or around the nicotinic AChR of the postsynaptic endplate region at the neuromuscular junction (NMJ) (Figs. 73-2 and 73-3). These AChR antibodies trigger immune-mediated degradation of the AChRs and their adjacent postsynaptic membrane. The loss of large numbers of functional AChRs decreases the number of muscle fibers that can depolarize during motor nerve terminal activation, resulting in a decreased generation of muscle fiber action potentials and subsequent muscle fiber contraction. Blocking of neuromuscular transmission causes clinical weakness when it affects large numbers of fibers.

The nicotinic AChR contains five subunits arranged radially around a transmembrane ion channel (Fig. 73-4). The antibodies generated in MG are usually directed against the alpha subunit of the AChR. These antibodies may bind at or near the acetylcholine-binding site, directly preventing acetylcholine binding, or may alter receptor function through other mechanisms, such as increased receptor degradation or complement-mediated receptor lysis.

CLINICAL PRESENTATION

Myasthenia gravis is typically classified as ocular, generalized, neonatal, congenital, or drug-induced. At presentation, weakness is confined to the ocular muscles in 80% of patients. Within 1–2 years, more generalized weakness develops in 85–90% of these individuals (see Fig. 73-1). In those few patients with primary ocular MG in whom bulbar or generalized weakness do not develop during the first 2 years, further progression to generalized MG is significantly less likely although it may occur as late as 8–10 years later (these patients are classified as having ocular MG).

Fatigability is one of the most important clinical characteristics seen in MG. Typically these patients describe worsening of their symptoms late in the day or during sustained exercise. Transient improvement occurs with rest, and symptoms often progress during the day. On examination, ocular fatigability (ptosis and/or diplopia) can be demonstrated on sustained upward or lateral gaze. Generalized weakness eventually occurs in 80% of all patients with acquired MG. Cardinal symptoms include fluctuating weakness, variably affecting the ocular, bulbar, and extremity musculature. Most patients initially demonstrate asymmetric diplopia and ptosis. Pupillary responses are always normal in contrast to some other disorders of neuromuscular transmission such as botulism.

Facial weakness manifests as weakness of eye and mouth closure. Occasionally bulbar symptoms such as chewing, and swallowing weakness (dysphagia) or slurred speech (dysarthria), are the presenting complaints. Characteristically MG patients with bulbar weakness have no problem when they begin to eat their meal, but increasing difficulties develop within the same sitting, particularly as they attempt to chew foods such as meats. Typically the speech becomes soft with a nasal breathy "twang" to the voice after a few minutes of uninterrupted speaking. Respiratory muscle involvement is potentially life threatening because of the risk of respiratory failure from hypoventilation. Neck extension weakness can lead to patients having difficulty holding up their heads. Increasing proximal muscle weakness results in problems with raising the arms overhead and/or with arising from chairs or climbing stairs.

Weakness may progress during weeks or months. Long-lasting spontaneous remission rarely occurs. Occasionally, after a brief period of modest symptoms, patients with new-onset MG may have a precipitous crisis-like presentation.

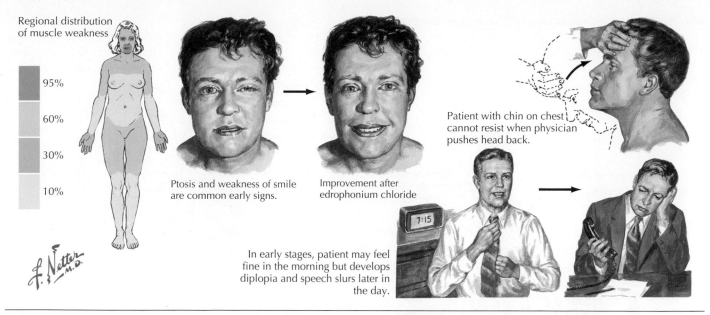

Figure 73-1 Myasthenia Gravis: Clinical Manifestations.

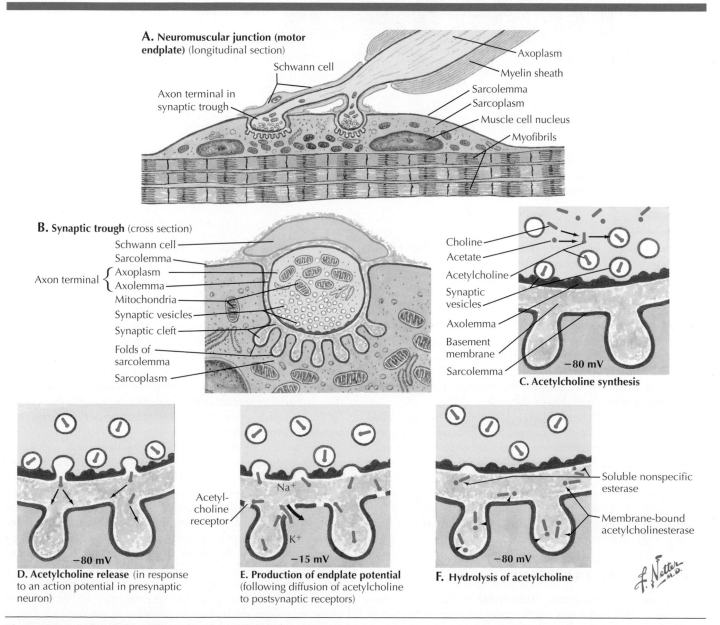

Figure 73-2 Somatic Neuromuscular Transmission.

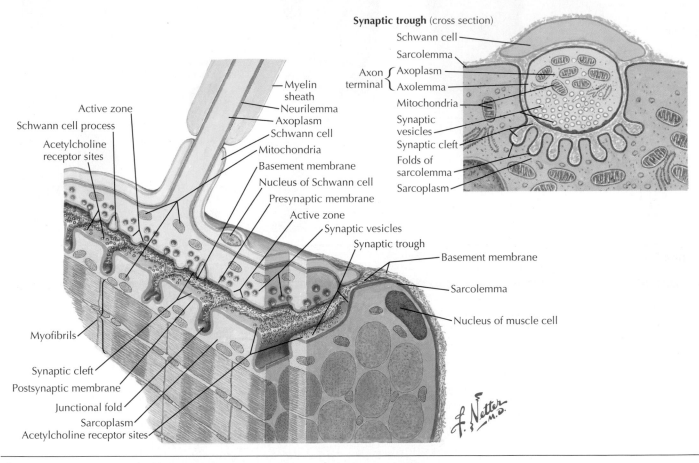

Synaptic trough (cross section)

Figure 73-3 Neuromuscular Transmission.

Exacerbations are often precipitated by hot weather (which affects the kinetics of the acetylcholinesterase enzyme system), intercurrent illness, menstruation, pregnancy, or concurrent thyrotoxicosis. Certain medications that affect NMJ function (e.g., antibiotics such as aminoglycosides) may exacerbate and even precipitate incipient MG. Myasthenic crises may cause respiratory failure, requiring assisted ventilation and treatment with plasmapheresis, intravenous immunoglobulin, and corticosteroids. For those patients already being treated with corticosteroids, a crisis is sometimes precipitated by injudicious discontinuation or rapid dosage decrease.

Women with MG have a 15–20% chance of having a child who is affected by transient weakness, poor suck, and respiratory depression related to transplacental transfer of anti-AChR antibodies, transient neonatal MG. Usually, the infant is affected for only a few months, and management with anticholinesterase medication, such as neostigmine, is sufficient. Transient neonatal myasthenia should be differentiated from the uncommon congenital myasthenia, which is a genetic condition arising from altered NMJ structure or function.

DIFFERENTIAL DIAGNOSIS

Myasthenia gravis presenting with ocular or bulbar weakness may mimic other diseases of the nervous system, although usually the evaluation to confirm the diagnosis of MG is

straightforward because of the characteristic presentation of MG, particularly the fluctuating and fatigable quality of pure motor manifestations that tend to develop in a "top down" sequence (i.e., first ocular, then bulbar). In patients with initial ocular and/or bulbar weakness, multiple sclerosis or brainstem tumor may sometimes be suspected, but fatigability and fluctuation of symptoms is usually atypical for both of these disorders; however, MS patients sometimes have a component of easy fatigue. Additionally multiple sclerosis and neurologic tumors usually involve multiple neurologic nonmotor systems, such as the cerebellar system, corticospinal tract (causing hyperreflexia, Babinski signs), optic nerve and tract, urinary system, and sensory nervous systems.

The sudden development of diplopia, dysarthria, and weakness may suggest a brainstem stroke. A third nerve palsy secondary to a posterior communicating artery aneurysm or diabetes mellitus can mimic ocular MG. Thyroid orbitopathy frequently leads to diplopia mimicking ocular MG. Rarely, multiple cranial neuropathies are the presenting sign of leptomeningeal inflammatory disorders, such as sarcoidosis, tuberculosis, or fungal infections. Similarly, metastatic cancer can invade the leptomeninges and very rarely mimic MG. A brain magnetic resonance image (MRI) is particularly useful for differentiating these conditions. When bulbar dysfunction is prominent and diplopia and ptosis are absent, the bulbar presentation of amyotrophic lateral sclerosis requires consideration. The Miller Fisher variant of

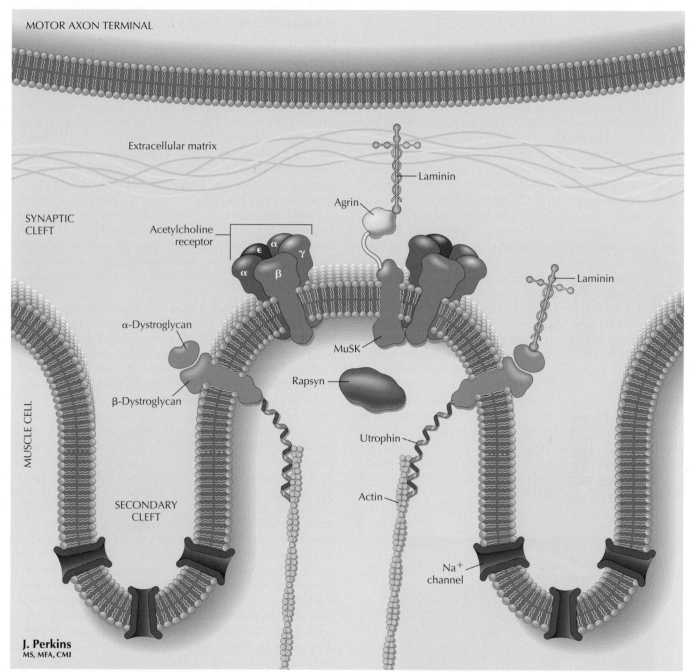

MOTOR AXON TERMINAL

Extracellular matrix

Laminin

Agrin

SYNAPTIC
CLEFT

Acetylcholine
receptor

ε α γ
α β

Laminin

α-Dystroglycan

MuSK

Rapsyn

β-Dystroglycan

MUSCLE CELL

Utrophin

Actin

SECONDARY
CLEFT

Na⁺
channel

J. Perkins
MS, MFA, CMI

Schematic representation of the normal neuromuscular junction, adult acetylcholine receptor in the postsynaptic muscle membrane and other important associated proteins.

Figure 73-4 Acetylcholine Receptor and Neuromuscular Junction.

Guillain–Barré syndrome presents with ocular muscle paresis, mimicking MG, but is usually associated with ataxia and areflexia and often abnormal pupillary responses. The Lambert–Eaton myasthenic syndrome occasionally involves the bulbar musculature, but peripheral weakness and systemic symptoms are more prominent. Rarely, polymyositis or muscular dystrophy may present with lower bulbar weakness but diplopia and ptosis are not usually seen; however, we have seen patients with this at Lahey. EMG is helpful in differentiating between myopathies, neuropathies, and disorders of neuromuscular transmission.

DIAGNOSTIC APPROACH

The patient's history and examination are the most important information directing one to a diagnosis of MG. Ancillary testing is necessary to confirm the diagnosis. Assays for antibodies to AChR are positive in approximately 85% of patients with generalized MG. Individuals with purely ocular MG have an approximately 50% incidence of positive AChR antibodies. Another 7% of patients with generalized MG have antibodies to muscle-specific tyrosine kinase (MuSK) (see Fig. 73-4). The remaining 8% of patients with generalized MG are classified as having "seronegative" generalized MG; that is, MG without a known accompanying autoantibody.

The electrodiagnostic NCS/EMG hallmark finding of MG is the presence of an electrodecremental response of the CMAP amplitude during slow (i.e., 2- or 3-Hz) repetitive motor nerve stimulation. In unaffected individuals, inherent functional reserve in neuromuscular transmission ("the safety factor") usually enables preservation of CMAP amplitude during repetitive stimulation. However, in MG, the loss of functional AChRs can result in a decrement of 10% or more between the first and fourth CMAP amplitudes on repeated stimulation. Repetitive stimulation of peripheral nerves is usually conducted on the ulnar and spinal accessory motor nerves, and sometimes the facial nerve. Single-fiber EMG, a more technically demanding test of NMJ function, records single muscle fiber discharges. In MG, the firing interval between individual muscle fibers of the same motor unit (i.e., jitter) is often increased, and there may be intermittent blocking of neuromuscular transmission. Single-fiber EMG has a sensitivity of more than 90% in ocular and generalized MG.

Computed tomographic or MR imaging of the mediastinum is an important diagnostic test in suspected MG. Ten to 15% of MG patients have thymomas; these may be benign (75–90%) or malignant thymic tumors (Fig. 73-5). Of those patients not having thymomas, 70% have thymic lymphoid follicular hyperplasia. Anti–striational muscle antibodies are present in 90% of patients with myasthenia and thymoma.

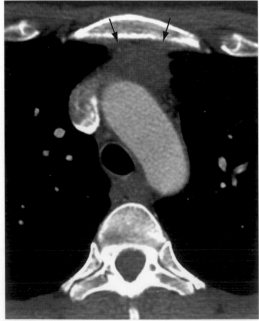

Axial CT scan of upper chest demonstrates a soft tissue mass anterior to the enhancing aorta (arrows).

Figure 73-5 Thymoma.

MANAGEMENT AND PROGNOSIS

Before the mid-1930s, there were no treatments for MG, and consequently the mortality rate for MG was approximately as high as 70%. The discovery and widespread use of anticholinesterase therapy (e.g., pyridostigmine) in the 1930s resulted in a dramatic reduction in mortality rate to approximately 30%. The anticholinesterase therapies work by decreasing the rate of breakdown of acetylcholine at the NMJ (Fig. 73-6). Pyridostigmine (e.g., Mestinon) is generally started at 30–60 mg orally every 6–8 hours. The dosage is titrated depending on the clinical response of the patient. Doses of more than 120 mg every 3–4 hours may cause cholinergic crisis, with paradoxically increased weakness (sometimes to a marked degree), increased salivation, abdominal cramping, diarrhea, and muscle fasciculations. Anticholinesterase therapy, however, does not treat the basic pathophysiologic process (i.e., autoimmunity), and thus, most patients with generalized MG require some form of immunosuppressive therapy.

Immunotherapy, often used in conjunction with pyridostigmine, has very substantially contributed to the reduction in MG mortality to less than 10%. Corticosteroids are the initial treatment of choice to induce remission of this autoimmune disorder. Oral prednisone is generally effective for achieving remission in MG. Some experts prefer to start patients on high-dose prednisone (e.g., 60 mg/day), whereas others prefer to start at lower doses and increase the dose until remission is achieved. The choice depends on the patient's clinical status. For those who are acutely ill and hospitalized with careful monitoring in an intensive care unit, one can safely begin with high doses of 40–60 mg prednisone daily. In contrast, for those who have mild MG and are being treated as outpatients, one needs to start slowly with 10–20 mg daily. This is gradually increased by 10 mg every 3–4 days. When corticosteroids were first tried in patients with MG, a paradoxical worsening occurred that was severe enough to dissuade the earlier investigators from recommending corticosteroids for this disorder. It was not for another quarter century, until the autoimmune nature of MG was documented, that it was recognized that smaller doses could be safely used in an outpatient setting. After MG patients have achieved remission for 1–2 months, usually at the level of 40–80 mg daily, the prednisone dose is gradually tapered. If these patients have been on a daily dosage schedule, for example, 60 mg at remission, they can be switched to alternate-day therapy, initially decreasing the off- or low-day dose by 10-mg decrements every 2–4 weeks.

The physician and patient must monitor for the many potential side effects of prednisone that commonly occur, especially at the higher doses used in MG. Some steroid therapy complications are significant, including aseptic necrosis of the femoral head, osteoporosis, and increased likelihood of infection, diabetes mellitus, cataracts, and serious psychomotor depression.

Azathioprine (Imuran) and mycophenolate mofetil (CellCept) are other options for long-term immunotherapy in MG. These serve as steroid-sparing agents but have a significant latency for therapeutic efficacy. They cannot be substituted for corticosteroids per se but rather are introduced so that eventually steroids can be gradually decreased while long-term immunosuppression is maintained with these agents. The usual dosage

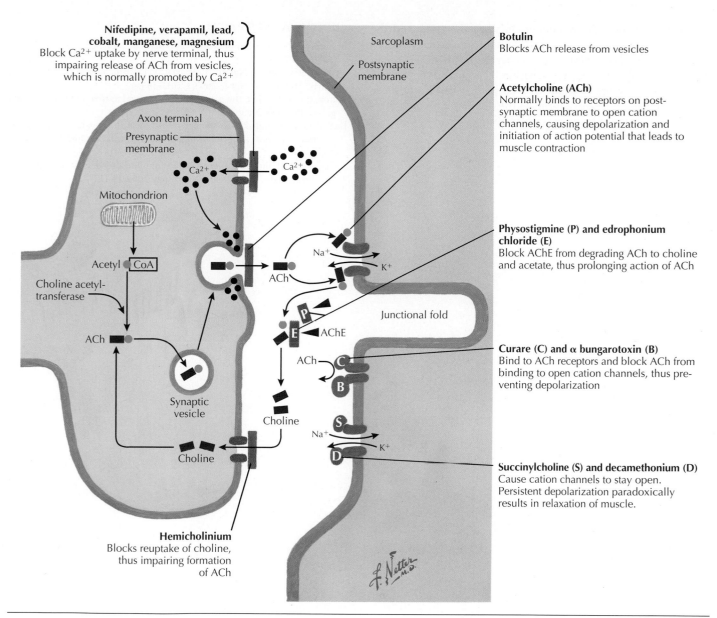

Figure 73-6 Pharmacology of Neuromuscular Transmission.

for azathioprine is 100–150 mg/day. Mycophenolate mofetil is typically prescribed at 1000–1500 mg twice a day. Both azathioprine and mycophenolate mofetil have potential side effects that must be discussed with the patient. Intravenous immunoglobulin is an important therapeutic option for short-term symptomatic control in the acutely ill patient. The usual total dosage is 2.0 g/kg divided over 2–5 days. Plasma exchange removes acetylcholine receptor (or MuSK) antibodies from the blood and produces rapid but transient clinical improvement. Plasmapheresis is particularly useful during myasthenic crises or steroid-related exacerbations, in preparation for thymectomy and other surgical procedures, and occasionally as maintenance therapy in patients refractory to other therapies.

Thymectomy is recommended treatment for AChR antibody–positive patients younger than 60 years with generalized MG. However, thymectomy may not be as beneficial in patients who are MuSK antibody–positive and seronegative patients.

Approximately 10–15% of patients with MG have an associated thymoma. Up to 25% of these thymomas are malignant. Both the benign and malignant entities are associated with a significant elevation of the anti–skeletal muscle antibody levels. All patients with a thymoma, regardless of their age, must undergo a thymectomy.

Respiratory failure (i.e., "myasthenic crisis"), secondary to diaphragmatic muscle weakness, is the most serious potential complication with MG. Pulmonary function should be carefully monitored in newly diagnosed patients and those experiencing disease relapses. The advent of positive-pressure and volume-controlled ventilation in 1965 was an important breakthrough in the management of MG, resulting in a substantial lowering of the mortality rate of patients with MG.

Long-term outcome in MG has improved markedly. In previous decades, up to 25% of patients died of respiratory failure within 3 years after diagnosis. However, with the widespread availability of multiple immunomodulatory therapies and the improved treatment of respiratory failure, more than 90% of patients, even those with severe generalized myasthenia, can achieve a symptom-free status within 1 year. A few patients continue to be more resistant to treatment, particularly those with the antibody-negative forms of the disease, for which therapeutic concepts are being reevaluated.

ADDITIONAL RESOURCES

Briemberg HR. Neuromuscular diseases in pregnancy. Seminars Neurology 2007;27:460-466.

Grob D, Brunner N, Namba T, Pagala M. Lifetime course of myasthenia gravis. Muscle and Nerve 2008;37:141-149.

Hilton-Jones D. When the patient fails to respond to treatment: myasthenia gravis. Practical Neurol 2007;7:405-411.

Luchanok U, Kaminski HJ. Ocular myasthenia: diagnostic and treatment recommendations and the evidence base. Current Opinions Neurol 2008;21:8-15.

Mahadeva B, Phillips LH, Juel VC. Autoimmune disorders of neuromuscular transmission. Seminars in Neurology 2008;28:212-227.

Other Neuromuscular Transmission Disorders

74

Ted M. Burns and H. Royden Jones, Jr.

Clinical Vignette

A 58-year-old woman presented with a 3-month history of progressive fatigue and lower extremity weakness, especially noticeable when she was walking up and down stairs or arising from a chair. Lately she had noted mildly slurred speech, transient double vision with eyelid droop, and dry mouth. Her past medical history was unremarkable. She had a 60-pack-year history of cigarette smoking. Examination was remarkable for mild weakness of orbicularis oculi, neck flexor, deltoid, triceps, and hip flexor and hip extensor muscles bilaterally. She had difficulty arising from a chair. Muscle stretch reflexes were absent on routine testing but elicitable after 10 seconds of isometric exercise.

Serum creatine kinase and acetylcholine (ACh) receptor antibody study results were normal. Nerve conduction studies (NCS) demonstrated low compound muscle action potentials (CMAPs) on most motor nerve conduction studies. A 15% decrement of CMAP amplitude was observed with 3-Hz repetitive motor nerve stimulation of the ulnar nerve. After 10 seconds of exercise, the ulnar CMAP amplitude facilitated approximately 300%, which is typical of a presynaptic neuromuscular transmission disorder. She was diagnosed with Lambert–Eaton myasthenic syndrome (LEMS). Serum voltage-gated P/Q calcium channel (VGCC) antibodies were later found to be elevated, consistent with LEMS.

A chest radiograph showed a right hilar mass; its biopsy revealed small cell lung cancer (SCLC). The patient received chemotherapy, as well as 3,4-diaminopyridine for symptomatic treatment of LEMS, resulting in some modest improvement in strength. She died 16 months later from complications of SCLC.

LAMBERT–EATON MYASTHENIC SYNDROME

Although rare, LEMS is the most frequently occurring presynaptic neuromuscular transmission disorder in adults. In approximately 50% of cases, LEMS is associated with cancer, especially SCLC. When LEMS is not associated with cancer, a primary autoimmune etiology is suspected. The paraneoplastic and nonparaneoplastic forms of LEMS share an autoimmune pathophysiologic mechanism. VGCC antibodies are detected in more than 90% of patients with either paraneoplastic or nonparaneoplastic LEMS. Antibodies to SOX1 have been identified in the majority of paraneoplastic LEMS patients but are not found in patients with nonparaneoplastic LEMS, and thus may prove valuable in evaluating for the presence or absence of cancer in a patient with LEMS. LEMS associated with lung cancer usually presents in past or present smokers, and clinical manifestations of LEMS often begin months to years before diagnosis of the malignancy. Therefore, a timely LEMS diagnosis may expedite the lung cancer diagnosis and influence treatment and prognosis. LEMS unassociated with cancer usually occurs in younger nonsmokers, especially women.

The vignette in this chapter illustrates cardinal LEMS symptoms and signs: proximal extremity weakness, reduced or absent muscle stretch reflexes, and complaints of fatigue and dry mouth, with milder symptoms of ocular and oropharyngeal weakness. Because of the patient's history of cigarette smoking, paraneoplastic LEMS was the prime consideration. The muscle stretch reflexes demonstrated improvement after 10 seconds of exercise, indicative of a presynaptic neuromuscular junction transmission disorder, and this corresponded to the NCS of postexercise facilitation of the CMAP amplitude.

LEMS often provides an early diagnosis of SCLC because the immune response producing LEMS is believed to begin early in tumor evolution. However, by the time LEMS was diagnosed in the preceding vignette, the SCLC had metastasized and prognosis was poor.

ETIOLOGY AND PATHOPHYSIOLOGY

Under normal conditions, neuronal depolarization opens VGCCs on the presynaptic axon terminal membrane, resulting in calcium influx within the nerve terminal. Intracellular calcium binds to calmodulin and mobilizes acetylcholine (ACh) vesicles that are released into the synaptic cleft (Fig. 74-1). The VGCCs are the primary site of immunopathology in LEMS. Divalent IgG autoantibodies cross-link the calcium channels, disrupting their function, resulting in inadequate release of presynaptic ACh vesicles from motor and autonomic cholinergic nerve terminals. The release of fewer ACh quanta at the neuromuscular junction decreases the probability of reaching the "all or none" depolarization threshold of a muscle fiber and thus the likelihood of the muscle fiber action potential (MFAP) generation. It is this drop out of a significant number of MFAP generation that results in low CMAPs on routine NCS.

The VGCCs expressed on SCLC cells and other neoplasms provide the presumed antigenic stimulus for antibody production to VGCC in the paraneoplastic form of LEMS. The precise antigenic stimulus in the nonparaneoplastic varieties of LEMS remains to be identified. Muscle weakness, fatigue, and autonomic symptoms result because the VGCC antibodies reduce the ACh release at motor and autonomic nerve terminals, impairing synaptic transmission.

CLINICAL PRESENTATION

The clinical presentation is similar in primary autoimmune and secondary paraneoplastic LEMS. Fatigue is a prominent and early symptom in LEMS patients. Patients with LEMS also

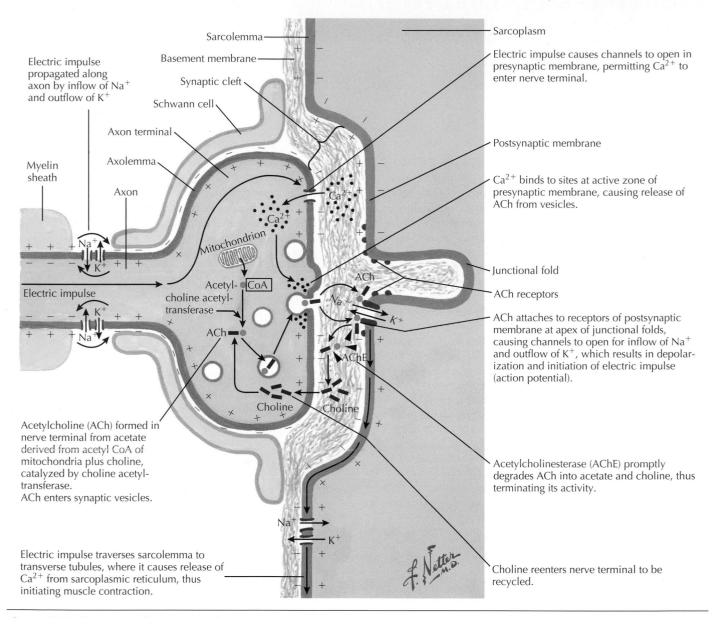

Sarcolemma

Basement membrane

Synaptic cleft

Schwann cell

Axon terminal

Axolemma

Myelin sheath

Axon

Electric impulse propagated along axon by inflow of Na$^+$ and outflow of K$^+$

Electric impulse

Acetyl-choline acetyltransferase

CoA

Mitochondrion

Ca^{2+}

Ca^{2+}

ACh

Choline

Choline

Na$^+$

ACh

Na$^+$

K$^+$

AChE

Acetylcholine (ACh) formed in nerve terminal from acetate derived from acetyl CoA of mitochondria plus choline, catalyzed by choline acetyltransferase.
ACh enters synaptic vesicles.

Na$^+$

K$^+$

Electric impulse traverses sarcolemma to transverse tubules, where it causes release of Ca^{2+} from sarcoplasmic reticulum, thus initiating muscle contraction.

Sarcoplasm

Electric impulse causes channels to open in presynaptic membrane, permitting Ca^{2+} to enter nerve terminal.

Postsynaptic membrane

Ca^{2+} binds to sites at active zone of presynaptic membrane, causing release of ACh from vesicles.

Junctional fold

ACh receptors

ACh attaches to receptors of postsynaptic membrane at apex of junctional folds, causing channels to open for inflow of Na$^+$ and outflow of K$^+$, which results in depolarization and initiation of electric impulse (action potential).

Acetylcholinesterase (AChE) promptly degrades ACh into acetate and choline, thus terminating its activity.

Choline reenters nerve terminal to be recycled.

Figure 74-1 Physiology of Neuromuscular Junction.

complain of proximal weakness, especially lower extremity weakness, sometimes mimicking a myopathy. The complaints of fatigue and proximal weakness often may seem disproportionate to the objective examination findings. When patients with suspected LEMS do not have objective detectable weakness, it may be better appreciated by watching individuals rise from a chair or climb stairs (Fig. 74-2). Muscle stretch reflexes are typically reduced or absent and this finding can be an important clue to the diagnosis. Postexercise potentiation of depressed or absent muscle stretch reflexes and of muscle strength is often demonstrable and signifies a presynaptic neuromuscular junction transmission disorder.

Oculopharyngeal weakness in the form of diplopia, ptosis, dysphagia, and dysarthria is frequently reported but is usually relatively mild. Autonomic symptoms, including dry mouth or erectile dysfunction in men, should prompt clinicians to consider LEMS. In fact, it is unlikely—although not

impossible—for a patient with LEMS to be without symptoms of dry mouth. Patients with LEMS also sometimes complain of vague sensory symptoms, such as tingling and numbness.

DIAGNOSTIC APPROACH

Appropriate NCS testing is crucial in the diagnosis of LEMS (Fig. 74-3). Most patients with LEMS have low-amplitude CMAPs on routine nerve conduction studies. The identification of low baseline CMAP amplitudes should prompt postexercise facilitation testing. This is performed by having the patient isometrically contract the muscle from which the CMAP is being recorded (e.g., abductor digiti quinti minimi) for 10 seconds followed by nerve stimulation and measurement of the CMAP. In patients without LEMS (or another presynaptic neuromuscular junction transmission disorder), there will be no change or only modest increase (<100%) in the size of the CMAP

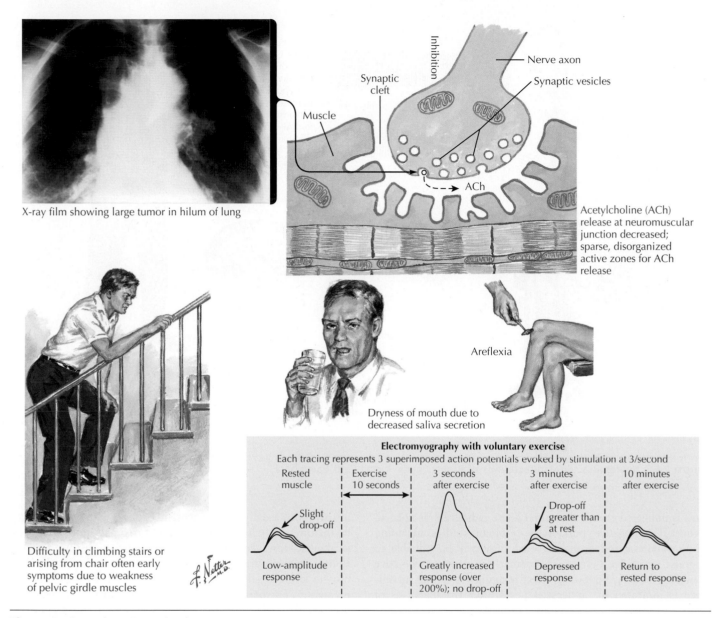

X-ray film showing large tumor in hilum of lung

Acetylcholine (ACh) release at neuromuscular junction decreased; sparse, disorganized active zones for ACh release

Dryness of mouth due to decreased saliva secretion

Areflexia

Difficulty in climbing stairs or arising from chair often early symptoms due to weakness of pelvic girdle muscles

Electromyography with voluntary exercise

Each tracing represents 3 superimposed action potentials evoked by stimulation at 3/second

Rested muscle	Exercise 10 seconds	3 seconds after exercise	3 minutes after exercise	10 minutes after exercise
Slight drop-off			Drop-off greater than at rest	
Low-amplitude response		Greatly increased response (over 200%); no drop-off	Depressed response	Return to rested response

Figure 74-2 Lambert–Eaton Syndrome.

amplitude. The differentiation between a presynaptic and a postsynaptic neuromuscular junction transmission disorder is that brief (10–15 seconds) voluntary exercise, or rarely, if necessary, high-frequency (20–50 Hz) repetitive motor nerve stimulation, leads to marked (>100%) facilitation of the baseline CMAP in patients with LEMS (presynaptic) but not those with myasthenia gravis (MG) (postsynaptic). In addition to testing for postexercise facilitation, slow (e.g., 2- or 3-Hz) repetitive motor nerve stimulation demonstrating decrement of CMAP amplitude of more than 10% can further support the diagnosis of a neuromuscular transmission disorder. Many electromyography (EMG) laboratories routinely combine the slow repetitive motor nerve testing with the 10-second exercise testing in order to search simultaneously for both the postexercise facilitation (of the first CMAP following brief exercise) and the decrement (of the subsequent CMAPs during slow repetitive nerve studies) seen in postsynaptic disorders.

Serum VGCC antibody testing is also very helpful in diagnosing LEMS. Abnormally high titers of VGCC antibodies are found in approximately 90% of patients with LEMS. High titers of VGCC are also found in 20–40% of patients with SCLC who do not have LEMS. Therefore, a positive VGCC antibody test result does not necessarily diagnose LEMS; the typical clinical and EMG findings are needed to support the diagnosis.

Approximately 50–70% of patients with LEMS have an associated cancer (usually SCLC); therefore, a search for malignancy must be initiated in each patient diagnosed with LEMS. Antibodies to SOX1 have recently been identified in the majority of patients with paraneoplastic LEMS but not in patients with LEMS unassociated with cancer, and thus serological testing for SOX1 may become a valuable aid in searching for cancer in patients who present with LEMS. Imaging for cancer (e.g., chest computed tomographic [CT] scan, chest magnetic resonance imaging scan, and positron emission tomographic [PET]

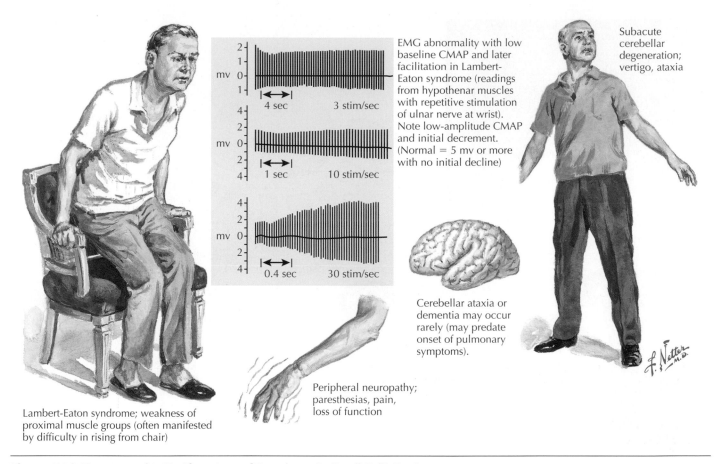

EMG abnormality with low baseline CMAP and later facilitation in Lambert-Eaton syndrome (readings from hypothenar muscles with repetitive stimulation of ulnar nerve at wrist). Note low-amplitude CMAP and initial decrement. (Normal = 5 mv or more with no initial decline)

Subacute cerebellar degeneration; vertigo, ataxia

Cerebellar ataxia or dementia may occur rarely (may predate onset of pulmonary symptoms).

Peripheral neuropathy; paresthesias, pain, loss of function

Lambert-Eaton syndrome; weakness of proximal muscle groups (often manifested by difficulty in rising from chair)

Figure 74-3 Neuromuscular Manifestations of Bronchogenic (Small Cell) Carcinoma.

scan) is indicated even if the initial chest radiograph is normal. If the CT is negative, pulmonary cytologic studies, including sputum analysis and bronchial washings, may be valuable to diagnose occult lung tumors, particularly in patients who have a smoking history. Follow-up chest imaging for cancer surveillance is indicated for at least 4 years after the diagnosis of LEMS, in patients with a smoking history.

DIFFERENTIAL DIAGNOSIS

The combination of symptoms of weakness and dry mouth sometimes mimics the hyperventilation syndrome, hysteria, malingering, or depression. These conditions should be in the differential early in the evaluation but an appropriate history-taking and examination, combined with appropriate NCS/EMG testing, should allow the physician to easily distinguish a psychological etiology from a neurologic cause. The neurologic disorders that most often mimic LEMS are MG, myopathy, and a chronic polyneuropathy. Unlike LEMS, MG typically has a preponderance of ocular or bulbar symptoms—diplopia, ptosis, dysarthria, and dysphagia—early in its course, whereas in LEMS, oculobulbar symptoms are less commonly the presenting symptoms and usually remain mild. Prominent autonomic symptoms, such as dry mouth and erectile dysfunction, are characteristic of patients with LEMS but are often overlooked by patients and/or clinicians. Other rare presynaptic neuromuscular transmission disorders (e.g., botulism and magnesium

intoxication) usually present acutely. Patients with inflammatory myopathies also have predominant proximal limb and neck weakness. However, these patients do not demonstrate facilitation of strength immediately after testing of each muscle. The muscle stretch reflexes are usually preserved in patients with myopathy. Furthermore, patients with myopathy typically do not complain of autonomic and sensory symptoms; serum CK is usually elevated, which would be unexpected in LEMS. Chronic inflammatory demyelinating polyradiculoneuropathy (CIDP), with its insidious onset of proximal weakness and areflexia, also enters the LEMS differential diagnosis. Nerve conduction studies in CIDP demonstrate features of acquired demyelination (e.g., slowed conduction velocities, conduction block, temporal dispersion), findings never seen in LEMS. Moreover, patients with CIDP usually have prominent sensory nerve symptoms and signs, whereas in LEMS sensory symptoms are typically mild.

TREATMENT AND PROGNOSIS

Chemotherapy, radiation therapy, and surgery are the primary treatment modalities for LEMS-associated lung cancer. Cancer treatment often leads to symptomatic improvement in LEMS, presumably by removing the antigenic stimulus and thus downgrading the immune response. Symptomatic treatment of LEMS aims to improve neuromuscular transmission. The anticholinesterase medication pyridostigmine (Mestinon) can improve neuromuscular transmission by inhibiting breakdown of Ach at the neuromuscular junction. In contrast to MG, pyridostigmine alone is not very effective for LEMS but it is often worth trying because it is a relatively benign treatment option. Common and dose-limiting side effects are abdominal cramps and diarrhea.

3,4-Diaminopyridine (3,4-DAP) promotes ACh release from the presynaptic portion of the neuromuscular junction by prolonging the VGCC open time. It is available for use primarily in Europe but in the United States requires local institutional review board approval and a concomitant submission to the FDA for compassionate use. Caution is advised because central nervous system irritability, manifested by seizures, is a major adverse effect. Anticholinesterases, such as pyridostigmine, potentiate the effects of 3,4-DAP and thus may be particularly beneficial when combined with 3,4-DAP.

Immunomodulation therapy is also sometimes used to inhibit the immune system's response directed at the neuromuscular junction. Unfortunately, for LEMS patients with cancer, immunomodulation may also inhibit the response of the host's immune system to the cancer, potentially worsening the cancer. Corticosteroids (e.g., prednisone), intravenous immunoglobulin, and plasmapheresis are some of the immunotherapies that may be beneficial to LEMS patients with profound weakness. These treatments are more commonly prescribed to nonparaneoplastic LEMS patients.

Several medications may exacerbate LEMS symptoms and should be used cautiously in LEMS; these include cardiac drugs, that is, adrenergic and calcium channel–blocking agents, and antiarrhythmic agents, such as procainamide and quinidine. Aminoglycoside antibiotics, magnesium citrate cathartics, quinine, and lithium may also worsen the neuromuscular transmission defect, increasing weakness. Anesthesiologists must be aware of the diagnosis of LEMS in their patient and use medications that do not prolong postoperative respiratory depression. On rare occasions, postanesthesia respiratory failure is the initial manifestation of LEMS.

Prognosis depends on whether LEMS is associated with malignancy and on the stage of malignancy. Most patients with LEMS and SCLC have a median survival of a few years. However, early detection improves prognosis, and consequently it is important to diagnose LEMS quickly and to search aggressively for cancer. In contrast, the prognosis in patients with primary autoimmune LEMS without SCLC is good; some patients live for more than 20 years after diagnosis. These patients with nonparaneoplastic LEMS often respond positively to immunomodulation and symptomatic therapy.

Clinical Vignette

A 4-month-old boy was brought to the emergency room by his parents because of a 2-day history of decreased activity and constipation. He was born at 39 weeks' gestation; development prior to admission was normal. On admission to the hospital, he appeared lethargic and dyspneic. His respiratory rate was 32 per minute and heart rate was 156 beats per minute. His oxygen saturation was 89% on room air and 100% on oxygen administered nasally.

Examination was remarkable for bilateral ptosis, sluggishly reactive pupils of 4 mm diameter, and bilateral facial weakness. He demonstrated minimal spontaneous movement. He was hypotonic and hyporeflexic. Baseline laboratory studies were unremarkable. NCS/EMG demonstrated an abnormality in neuromuscular transmission with modest posttetanic facilitation with rapid repetitive motor nerve stimulation of the ulnar nerve. Infantile botulism was suspected. He was treated with meticulous supportive care and intravenous human botulism immune globulin. Stool cultures later confirmed the diagnosis of Clostridium botulinum (type E) intoxication.

BOTULISM

Botulism is a rare, naturally occurring disease that is caused by release of toxin from *C. botulinum*. The toxins of *C. botulinum* exert their action on the presynaptic neuromuscular junction by blocking the release of ACh. Infantile botulism is more common than adult botulism. Early recognition of infantile and adult botulism can lead to expedited treatment.

ETIOLOGY AND PATHOPHYSIOLOGY

Botulism is caused by the toxin from *C. botulinum*, which is found ubiquitously in soil and water sediments. There are seven distinct toxins, designated by letters A–G, produced by *C. botulinum*, but human cases of botulism are caused only by toxin types A, B, E, and rarely F. Under normal conditions in the human intestine, any ingested spores of *C. botulinum* are excreted without germination or toxin production, and thus cause no harm. It is only rarely, more so in infants, that *C. botulinum* colonizes and produces enough toxin in the intestine to produce botulism.

Infant botulism is the most common form of botulism, with approximately 100 cases reported in the United States each year. Colonization of *C. botulinum* is believed to occur in some infants because the normal gut flora has not yet been entirely established and thus is unable to prevent the colonization of *C. botulinum*. The colonization of *C. botulinum* allows for elaboration of the toxins and development of infant botulism.

Food-borne botulism is caused by the ingestion of food contaminated with *C. botulinum*. Home-canned foods are a common source of intoxication. There are approximately 20 cases per year of foodborne botulism in the United States. Wound botulism is another form of botulism that occurs almost exclusively among injection drug users. Other less common forms of botulism are adult intestinal toxemia botulism, inhalation botulism, and iatrogenic botulism.

CLINICAL PRESENTATION, DIAGNOSTIC APPROACH, AND DIFFERENTIAL DIAGNOSIS

The presentation of botulism is distinctive with symmetrical cranial motor nerve palsies followed by descending flaccid paralysis, including the respiratory muscles. Extraocular muscle weakness (cranial nerves 3, 4, and 6) causes diplopia. Bilateral ptosis is common. Pupillary response is often impaired, resulting in blurry vision. Facial and oropharyngeal weakness, causing dysphagia and dysarthria, are prominent. Limb and axial weakness often develop; diaphragmatic and accessory breathing muscle weakness can cause respiratory compromise. Muscle stretch reflexes are lost. Autonomic nervous system dysfunction, including dry mouth, constipation, and postural hypotension, also occur. Cognition and the sensory system are unaffected.

The differential diagnosis includes MG, Guillain–Barré syndrome (GBS), LEMS, stroke syndromes, and tick paralysis. The very rapid progression of relatively symmetric cranial motor neuropathies followed by axial and limb weakness and dysautonomias (pupillary abnormalities, dry mouth, and constipation) are atypical for MG. On NCS/EMG testing, the presence of, or absence of, significant postexercise or posttetanic facilitation also helps to differentiate a presynaptic from postsynaptic neuromuscular junction transmission disorder. Furthermore, infants are unlikely to develop autoimmune MG and adults are unlikely to develop botulism, so age of onset is an important consideration. Demonstration of *C. botulinum* in a patient's stool sample or in cultures of a wound strongly favors botulism, whereas antibodies in serum for the acetylcholine receptor support a diagnosis of MG. GBS, particularly the Miller Fisher variant of GBS, can mimic botulism. Age of onset can again be helpful as GBS is uncommon in infants. Cerebrospinal fluid (CSF) protein is elevated in most cases of GBS, including most cases of Miller Fisher syndrome, whereas CSF protein is normal in botulism. NCS/EMG is often very helpful in detecting evidence of demyelination in GBS and the characteristic electrodiagnostic features of a presynaptic disorder of neuromuscular transmission in botulism (as discussed above in the LEMS section). Tick paralysis can essentially be excluded by a meticulous skin examination, including the scalp; in cases of North American tick paralysis, tick removal leads to a rapid recovery. However in Australia, the inciting tick's toxin has an effect sometimes lasting a few months.

TREATMENT AND PROGNOSIS

Meticulous supportive care is the mainstay of treatment, with most patients requiring treatment in the intensive care setting.

About half of infants with botulism will require intubation and mechanical ventilation. Infants who require ventilator support will do so for a median of 11 weeks. The vast majority will require nasogastric tube feeding for a median of 3 weeks. Antitoxin therapy can arrest progression of weakness and decrease the duration of paralysis, and requires consideration, especially if given within the first 24 hours of symptom onset. Human botulism intravenous immunoglobulin is approved by the United States Food and Drug Administration for the treatment of infant botulism. Almost all patients will recover completely without residual deficits, but this occurs slowly over weeks to months because the toxin binding to the nerve terminal is noncompetitive and irreversible, necessitating nerve terminal regeneration for recovery.

ADDITIONAL RESOURCES

Burns TM, Russell JA, Lachance DH, Jones HR. Oculobulbar involvement is typical with Lambert-Eaton Myasthenic Syndrome. Ann Neurol 2003;53:270-273.

Gutmann L, Phillips LH, Gutmann L. Trends in the association of Lambert-Eaton myasthenic syndrome with carcinoma. Neurology 1992;42:848-850.

Lambert EH, Eaton LM, Rooke ED. Defect of neuromuscular conduction associated with malignant neoplasms. Am J Physiol 1956;187:612-613.

Lambert EH, Rooke ED. Myasthenic state and lung cancer. In: Brain WR, Norris FH, editors. The Remote Effects of Cancer on the Nervous System. New York, NY: Grune and Stratton; 1965. p. 67-80.

Lennon VA, Kryzer TJ, Griesmann GE, et al. Calcium-channel antibodies in the Lambert-Eaton syndrome and other paraneoplastic syndromes. N Engl J Med 1995;332:1467-1474.

McEvoy KM, Windebank AJ, Daube JR, Low PA. 3,4-Diaminopyridine in the treatment of Lambert-Eaton myasthenic syndrome. N Engl J Med 1989;321:1567-1571.

O'Neil JH, Murray NMF, Newsom-Davis J. The Lambert Eaton myasthenic syndrome: a review of 50 cases. Brain 1988;111:577-596.

Sabater L, Titulaer M, Saiz A, Verschuuren J, Güre AO, Graus F. SOX1 antibodies are markers of paraneoplastic Lambert-Eaton myasthenic syndrome. Neurology 2008;70:924-928.

Sanders DB. Lambert-Eaton myasthenic syndrome: clinical diagnosis, immune-mediated mechanisms, and update on therapies. Ann Neurol 1995;37(suppl 1):S63-S73.

Sobel J. Botulism. Clinical Infectious Diseases 2005;41:1167-1173.

Tim RW, Sanders DB. Repetitive nerve stimulation studies in the Lambert-Eaton myasthenic syndrome. Muscle Nerve 1994;17:995-1001.

Tseng-Ong L, Mitchell WG. Infant botulism: 20 years' experience at a single institution. J Child Neurol 2007;22:1333-1337.

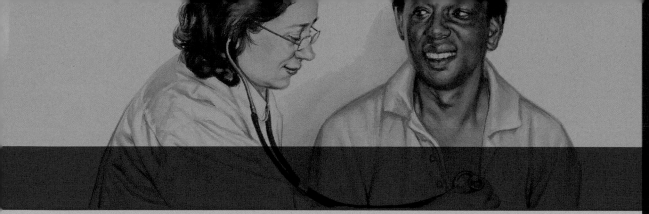

Myopathies

Hereditary Myopathies

Jayashri Srinivasan, Miruna Segarceanu, Doreen Ho, and H. Royden Jones, Jr.

75

Hereditary muscle disorders are usually generalized muscle disorders that are progressive and are variously categorized as channelopathies, metabolic and mitochondrial myopathies, muscular dystrophies, and congenital myopathies (Table 75-1).

CHANNELOPATHIES

There are a few inherited skeletal muscle disorders that typically have an acute onset mimicking an acquired myopathy; this is especially so when there is no known family history. These disorders are primarily the various channelopathies or inborn errors of metabolism affecting either glycogen or lipid metabolism.

PERIODIC PARALYSIS AND CONGENITAL MYOTONIC DISORDERS

Clinical Vignette

A 52-year-old physician presented with increasing nonfluctuating weakness characterized by problems climbing stairs and more recently arising from low seats. In early adolescence, he had first experienced recurrent episodes of postexercise relatively severe proximal extremity weakness that interfered with his walking, especially stepping up and getting out of chairs as well as problems lifting his arms overhead and using his hands. At his worst, as an adolescent, he could not stand or raise his hands and arms over his head. He never had symptoms that implicated any cranial nerve or respiratory muscle dysfunction. Between these intermittent episodes of weakness he was totally asymptomatic, his clinical neuromuscular examination was normal, and he could play singles tennis.

These periods of exercise-induced weakness typically were precipitated by brief periods of rest. Most events resolved within 30–120 minutes; however, on rare occasions his weakness might last a few days. Acetazolamide, a carbonic anhydrase inhibitor, 250 mg three times daily, significantly diminished the frequency of these attacks and allowed him to play tennis regularly. As he reached middle age, this physician began to note more chronic symptomatology on a daily basis. This did not respond to various pharmacologic interventions. By this time, one of his two sons and a daughter were beginning to experience similar periodic spells of weakness.

Occasionally he also noted some hand stiffness as well as inability to open his eyelids immediately after squinting. This suggested a myotonic component, something that was later confirmed by electromyography (EMG). Myotonia is a nonspecific finding occurring with hyperkalemic periodic

paralysis (HyperKPP), as well as various other channelopathies presenting with myotonic syndromes. DNA testing confirmed the diagnosis of a sodium channelopathy that typified the HyperKPP in this patient as well as his children.

Comment: This patient is a classic example of individuals having periodic paralysis; symptoms typically begin in mid-childhood. Although the use of a carbonic anhydrase inhibitor initially protected him from frequent attacks of weakness, as he reached his fifth and sixth decades he developed a fixed proximal weakness that limits his activities of daily living (ADL).

The various genetically determined hyperkalemic or hypokalemic channelopathies are phenotypically similar disorders related to abnormal ion passage within the muscle membrane ion channels. Their clinical picture is stereotypical as illustrated by the above vignette. It is often difficult to document the occurrence of the transient hyperkalemia or hypokalemia as it is unusual to evaluate the patient during an episode per se where the abnormal values typically occur. On the rare occasion when a persistent hyperkalemia is demonstrated, and there is no genetic component, adrenal insufficiency (Addison disease) must be considered in the differential diagnosis.

Variable mutations within genes encoding muscle membrane ion channels are responsible for the different forms of periodic paralyses as well as other myotonic disorders (Table 75-2). Most of these patients have an autosomal dominant inheritance. During the episodic paralyses, the skeletal muscle membrane excitability transiently disappears. The degree of weakness may vary from one family member to another; boys and men are more often significantly affected.

Hyperkalemic periodic paralysis (HyperKPP) and paramyotonia are *sodium* channel disorders, whereas hypokalemic periodic paralysis (HypoKPP) is due to voltage-gated *calcium* channel dysfunction. The congenital myotonias are *chloride* channel disorders inherited in either a dominant (Thomsen disease) or recessive (Becker disease) fashion.

CLINICAL PRESENTATION

Although most instances of weakness related to periodic paralysis have a symmetric distribution, occasionally a patient may have a focal or asymmetric distribution of weakness. The latter occurs when a few specific muscles are overutilized; for example, we had a jeweler who developed symptoms confined to his dominant hand, obviously the side that he primarily used most of his working day. The hypokalemic patient may also have paralytic events precipitated by rest after exercise, as well as occurring subsequent to either a significant carbohydrate intake, or ethanol ingestion and sometimes cold weather. Bulbar and

Table 75-1 Hereditary Myopathies

Myopathy	Type	Locus	Gene Product
Dystrophies			
Myotonic			
Classic distal	1[†]	AD 19q13	Myotonin protein kinase
Proximal (PROMM)	2[†]	AD 3q21	ZNF9 (zinc finger protein)
Limb-girdle	1A	AD 5q22–34	Myotilin
	1B	AD 1q11–21	Lamin A/C
	1C	AD 3p25	Caveolin-3
	1D	AD 6q23	FDC-CDM
	1E	AD 7	?
	1F	AD 7q32.1–32.27q32.1–32.2	?
	1G	4q21	?
	2A	AR 15q15	Calpain-3
	2B[‡]	AR 2p13	Dysferlin
	2C[‡]	AR 13q12	γ-Sarcoglycan+
	2D[‡]	AR 17q12	α-Sarcoglycan+ (adhalin)
	2E[‡]	AR 4q12	β-Sarcoglycan+
	2F[‡]	AR 5q33	δ-Sarcoglycan+
	2G	AR 17q11	Telethonin
	2H	AR 9q31–33	E3 ubiquitin ligase
	2I	AR 19q13.3	Fukutin-related protein
	2J	AR 2q31	Titin
	2K	AR 9q34.1	POMT1
	2L	AR 9q31	Fukutin
Dystrophinopathies			
	Duchenne	XR Xp21	Dystrophin
	Becker		
Facioscapulo-humeral	‡	AD 4q35	?
Scapuloperoneal		AD 12	?
Emery-Dreifuss	1[‡]	X Xq28	Emerin
	2	AD 1q11–q21	Lamin A/C, nesprin-1 and -2
Oculopharyngeal	‡	AD 14q11.2–q13	Poly (A) binding protein 2
Bethlem		AD 21q22, 2q37	Collagen type VI Subunit α1 or α2
		AD 2q37	Collagen type VI Subunit α3
Congenital muscular dystrophy			
	Classic CMD[‡]	AR 6q22–23	Laminin-α2 chain of merosin
	α7 Integrin CMD	AR 12q13	Integrin α7
	Fukuyama	AR 9q31–33	Fukutin
	Walker-Warburg	AR ?	?
	Muscle-eye-brain	AR 1p32–34	O-mannose β-1,2-N-acetylglucosaminyl transferase
	Rigid spine	AR 1p35–36	Selenoprotein N1
Congenital myopathies			
	Central core	AD 19q13.1	Ryanodine receptor
	Nemaline	AD 1q21–23	α-Tropomyosin
	Nemaline	AR 2q21.2–22	Nebulin
	Nemaline	AR 1q42	α-Actin
	Nemaline	AD 9p13	β-Tropomyosin
	Nemaline	AR 19q13	Troponin T
	Centronuclear	AR?	?
	Myotubular	X Xq28	Myotubularin
	Myotubular	AR?	?
	CFTD	?	?
	Myofibrillar	AD 11q22	α,β-Crystallin
	Myofibrillar	AD 2q35	Desmin
	Myofibrillar	AR?	?

Continued

Table 75-1 Hereditary Myopathies—cont'd

Myopathy	Type	Locus	Gene Product
Metabolic Glycogen storage			
	II–Acid maltase deficiency§	AR 17q21–23	α1,4-Glucosidase
	III–Debrancher deficiency§	AR 1p21	Amylo-1,6-glucosidase
	IV–Branching enzyme deficiency§	AR 3	Branching amylo-1,4-1,6-transglucosidase
	V–Myophosphorylase deficiency		
	VII–Phosphofructokinase		
Lipid storage	Carnitine deficiency	AR/AD	

AD, autosomal dominant; AR, autosomal recessive; CFTD, congenital fiber–type disproportion; CMD, congenital muscular dystrophy; nesprin, nuclear envelope spectrin repeat proteins; PROMM, proximal myotonic myopathy; X, X linked.
†DNA mutational analysis commercially available.
‡Immunostain commercially available.
§Biochemical analysis available.

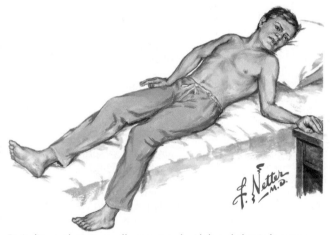

Periodic paralysis is usually associated with hypokalemia but may also occur with hyperkalemia or normokalemia. Hyperthyroidism may also be associated with hypokalemic periodic paralysis. Although extremity weakness is often profound, the respiratory and cranial nerve innervated muscles are spared.

Figure 75-1 Periodic Paralysis.

respiratory muscles are not affected. However, by midlife the periodic events usually cease and some individuals may develop a fixed weakness as illustrated in the above vignette.

Paramyotonia congenita is an even more uncommon hyperkalemic disorder often associated with periodic paralysis. Similar to myotonia congenita, cold weather exacerbates muscle stiffness in paramyotonia. In contrast to myotonia congenita, where rest promotes weakness, exercise exacerbates the stiffness in paramyotonia congenita patients.

Myotonia congenita, a *chloride* channelopathy, is especially aggravated by immobility and ameliorated by exercise and warming; here the myotonia per se is easily elicited on examination. Fixed weakness is not usually present in dominant myotonia congenita. A rather unique characteristic of Thomsen disease variant is the pseudo-hypertrophy of the skeletal muscles providing the patient with a rather pseudo-herculean habitus (Fig. 75-2). It may be so profound that athletic coaches

enthusiastically encourage these individuals to participate in sports activities. Unfortunately, some of these individuals may develop a mild progressive weakness. Transient episodes of true weakness precipitated by sudden movements after rest that are relieved by exercise are characteristic of myotonia congenita. Interesting examples include a baseball player who cannot run after hitting the ball or a subway rider who wishes to get off when the train stops but is frozen in place or falls when he arises to leave the train.

DIFFERENTIAL DIAGNOSIS

Myasthenia gravis (MG) classically has a remitting relapsing course predominantly confined to ocular as well as bulbar muscles and to a lesser extent proximal extremity musculature. MG is typified by fluctuating, rarely acute weakness with a very definitive diurnal variation (see Chapter 73).

Patients with *fatigue and nonorganic weakness* often report periods of episodic muscle pain. These symptoms per se are not components of the various channelopathies or MG. Furthermore, these individuals do not have any family history of neuromuscular disease, as do the various channelopathies. The patient with *functional weakness* frequently has a "consistent inconsistency" or "giveway component" to their weakness. One must take care as on occasion the Lambert–Eaton myasthenic syndrome (LEMS) is confused with this type clinical picture because of its posttetanic potentiation that mimics the giveway of the nonorganic seen in the nonorganically ill individual.

Addison disease requires urgent consideration during the evaluation of any acute, generally weak patient presenting with hyperkalemia. Because thyrotoxicosis has a symptomatic link to periodic paralysis, such patients, particularly young Asian men, must also be screened for clinical signs and laboratory findings of thyroid dysfunction.

DIAGNOSTIC APPROACH

The clinical history is the best means to diagnose a channelopathy. This may be relatively simple in patients with a positive family history examined while symptomatic and documented to

Table 75-2 Channelopathies Affecting Skeletal Muscle

	Age at Onset	Duration of Episodes	Weakness	Myotonia	Precipitants	Alleviating Factors	Gene Mutation/ Inheritance and Cation
Hyperkalemic periodic paralysis	Infancy–early childhood	Minutes–hours	Episodic, possibly permanent later in life	Possibly (between episodes of weakness) EMG (+)	Potassium loading, cold, fasting, rest, after exercise	Carbohydrate loading, exercise	CN4A 17q23: AD Sodium channel
Paramyotonia congenita	Infancy	Minutes	Very uncommon	Present EMG (+)	Repeated exercise, cold, fasting	Warming	SCN4A 17q23: AD Sodium channel
Sodium channel myotonia	Childhood–adolescence	Variable	Very uncommon	Present (often painful)	Rest after exercise, potassium loading, fasting	—	SCN4A 17q23: AD Sodium channel
Hypokalemic periodic paralysis	Puberty	Hours–days	Episodic, possibly permanent later in life	Absent	Cold, rest after exercise, carbohydrate loading	Potassium loading, exercise	CACNLA3, SCN4A 17q23: AD Calcium channel
Myotonia congenita	Infancy–early childhood	Minutes	Uncommon	Present EMG (+)	Exercise after rest, cold	Repeated exercise	CLC-1 7q: AD (Thomsen), AR (Becker) Chloride channel
Anderson-Tawil syndrome	Childhood–adolescence	Variable	Episodic, can have cardiac arrythmias and distinctive skeletal abnormalities	No	Usually hypokalemia but can be normo or hyperkalemic during attacks	—	KCJN2 (ATS1) encoding for Kir2.1

AD, autosomal dominant; AR, autosomal recessive.

have an abnormal serum potassium level or found to have demonstrable myotonia on EMG. In sporadic cases, diagnosis may prove elusive, especially when clinical examination results are normal and provocative testing does not demonstrate any biochemical or neurophysiologic abnormalities.

Whether the underlying channelopathy leads to hyperkalemia or hypokalemia, the serum potassium is normal between attacks. The clinician rarely has the opportunity to obtain a serum specimen during an event per se. However, during episodes of hyperkalemic periodic paralysis the serum potassium is elevated. It is between events that the cold-induced and EMG-defined myotonia occurs. Similarly, the hypokalemic periodic paralysis patient has low serum potassium findings, also confined to the precise time of paralysis.

Measurement of the serum potassium level is indicated in any patient observed during spontaneous episodes of weakness or, if recurrent, an attack of periodic paralysis.

Currently, the availability of a few DNA studies has greatly enhanced the specificity of the diagnostic evaluation of a patient with a question of periodic paralysis. These include DNA testing for the skeletal muscle *sodium* channel as seen in *HyperKPP* and the skeletal muscle *calcium* channel specific for *HypoKPP*.

The previously used provocative studies, such as carbohydrate loading to make one hypokalemic, are no longer of much value today.

Nerve conduction studies sometimes demonstrate decreased compound motor action potential amplitudes in the rare instance one has the opportunity to examine a patient during an episode of periodic paralysis; otherwise, these are normal. In the EMG laboratory, having the potential periodic paralysis patient exercise for prolonged periods may lead to progressive diminution in compound motor action potential amplitudes. Much more rarely, when evaluating a patient during individual episodes of periodic paralysis, needle EMG will demonstrate that affected muscles are electrically inactive as they are fully depolarized. Myotonic discharges occur on EMG in the *sodium* channelopathy HyperKPP, as well as the chloride channelopathies. This electrophysiologic finding is particularly useful in the differential diagnosis of hyperkalemic and paramyotonic varieties from the nonmyotonic hypokalemic variety. Clinical myotonia is often not evident in HyperKPP although it may be so in paramyotonia when exposed to the cold.

Provocative testing, such as carbohydrate loading, is occasionally required in patients with clinical histories highly

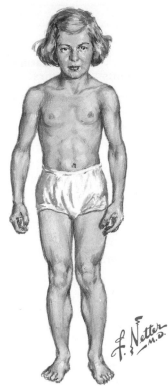

Myotonia and muscular overdevelopment.
Disease affects both males and females.

Figure 75-2 Myotonia Congenita (Thomsen Disease).

suggestive of periodic paralysis and in whom DNA testing is negative. This allows for documentation of abnormal serum potassium levels during episodes of weakness. A controlled clinical setting with appropriate monitoring equipment and facilities for emergent care must be available before initiating this testing. Serum creatine kinase levels are usually normal or minimally increased in the periodic paralyses and myotonic disorders.

Muscle biopsy is normal early in the course of periodic paralyses. However, after patients develop persistent weakness, biopsy may demonstrate vacuolar myopathy with tubular aggregates. Biopsy is rarely necessary for diagnosis.

TREATMENT AND PROGNOSIS

The treatment of choice for a patient having an acute attack of periodic paralysis is by correction of abnormal potassium levels. Severe hyperkalemia necessitates emergency treatment with intravenous (IV) glucose and insulin. Inhaled β-adrenergic agents or ingestion of carbohydrates is fine for less severe episodes. With any patient experiencing his or her first episode of hyperkalemia-associated paralysis, Addison disease is always a diagnostic possibility; therefore, the administration of IV corticosteroids is indicated after a serum cortisol level is obtained. IV potassium or in the milder case oral supplementation is the best means to care for the patient with a hypokalemic episode. These are prevented by avoiding dietary carbohydrate loads.

Maintenance therapy with the carbonic anhydrase inhibitor (CAI) acetazolamide is usually indicated to prevent attacks. Paradoxically, this is equally effective in patients with

hyperkalemic or hypokalemic periodic paralysis. Dichlorphenamide, another CAI, is currently under study; previously it had become a mainstay therapy that seemed to be better than acetazolamide; however, the manufacturer withdrew it from production. It is hoped that this will soon return to the neurologist's pharmacologic armamentarium. When treatment of myotonia per se is required, therapy with mexiletine or other membrane stabilizers is usually effective.

Generally, a diminution in frequency and severity of periodic paralysis attacks occurs in middle age. However, in some patients with periodic paralysis, as in the initial vignette of this chapter, permanent proximal weakness develops with increasing age. This is only minimally responsive to carbonic anhydrase inhibitors and awaits a better therapy.

GLYCOGEN AND LIPID STORAGE DISORDERS

Clinical Vignette

A 16-year-old boy presented with severe muscle pain and very dark urine subsequent to outrunning police officers who were concerned about his teenage prank. Because of his persistently dark urine he was taken to his family physician. An evaluation for liver disease was commenced after he was noted to have aspartate aminotransferase (AST) levels that were extraordinarily elevated. Paradoxically all other liver function tests (LFTs) were normal. His liver biopsy demonstrated "excess" glycogen but was otherwise unremarkable, and the serum creatine kinase (CK) level was found to be 50 times normal. Myoglobin was demonstrated in his urine. The patient was admitted to the hospital and treated with vigorous IV hydration. His symptoms resolved within several days.

The forearm exercise test (FET) failed to demonstrate the normally expected postexercise increase in lactate but did have significant and normal elevations of the venous ammonia levels. The latter demonstrated that the patient had successfully stressed his muscle metabolism. The combination of no change in lactate and appropriate rise in ammonia levels was classic for the presence of a glycogen storage disease. Subsarcolemmal blebs seen on a periodic acid-Schiff–stained muscle biopsy specimen were consistent with glycogen excess. Biochemical analysis demonstrated decreased levels of myophosphorylase, confirming the diagnosis of McArdle disease.

Comment: This is a classic example of muscle phosphorylase deficiency (Fig. 75-3) with onset in adolescence when individuals for the first time have the muscle power to allow them to stress their metabolic system to the point of actual muscle necrosis and subsequent myoglobinuria, the feature that most commonly brings them to medical attention.

Glycogen storage disorders (GSDs) are very uncommon clinical entities. The classic picture is one of exercise-induced painful muscle cramps, associated with myoglobinuria. The concomitant laboratory documentation of profound elevated serum CK levels and myoglobinuria strongly implicates either

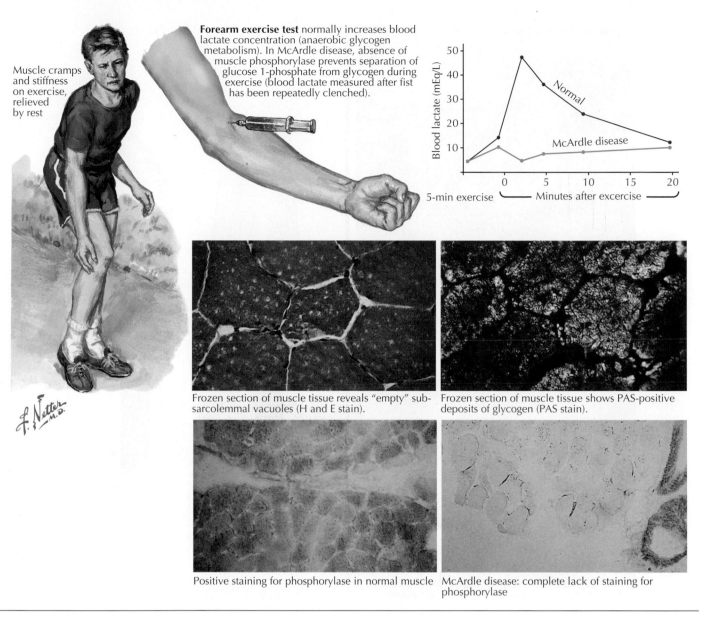

Forearm exercise test normally increases blood lactate concentration (anaerobic glycogen metabolism). In McArdle disease, absence of muscle phosphorylase prevents separation of glucose 1-phosphate from glycogen during exercise (blood lactate measured after fist has been repeatedly clenched).

Muscle cramps and stiffness on exercise, relieved by rest

Frozen section of muscle tissue reveals "empty" sub-sarcolemmal vacuoles (H and E stain).

Frozen section of muscle tissue shows PAS-positive deposits of glycogen (PAS stain).

Positive staining for phosphorylase in normal muscle

McArdle disease: complete lack of staining for phosphorylase

Figure 75-3 McArdle Disease.

a carbohydrate or lipid enzymatic deficiency of inborn metabolism (Fig. 75-4; Table 75-3). Very rarely prolonged use of one extremity, in isolation, will uncover the presence of a previously unsuspected glycogen storage disease (GSD). Muscle phosphorylase deficiency, an inborn error of glycogen metabolism, is the most common of these GSD myopathies.

PATHOPHYSIOLOGY

Skeletal muscle function is extremely energy dependent. Normal muscle metabolism requires the presence of both circulating glucose and free fatty acids (Figs. 75-5 and 75-6). At rest, muscles use fatty acids for basal metabolic demands. When one first begins to vigorously exercise, usually within the first 10 minutes, the glycolysis of glycogen, already stored within muscle tissues, is the primary energy source as its breakdown produces glucose but for a relatively short time period. However, when

the vigorous exercise is prolonged past these first few minutes, the body shifts to anaerobic glycolysis. This is manifested clinically by the *second wind phenomenon*. Here lipid stores, in the form of free fatty acids, are mobilized as the primary source of energy. Effective glycolysis is blocked in the various muscle glycogenoses. This essentially deprives muscle of the initial need for glucose, and consequently an accumulation of under-utilized glycogen occurs within muscle. In essence, that is, these muscles are inappropriately stressed by what for most healthy persons is no more than strenuous exercise.

GENETICS

Muscle phosphorylase deficiency usually has a dominant inheritance pattern. In contrast, the much more rare phosphoglycerate kinase deficiency is usually X-linked. The remaining other glycogenoses, as well as the various disorders of lipid

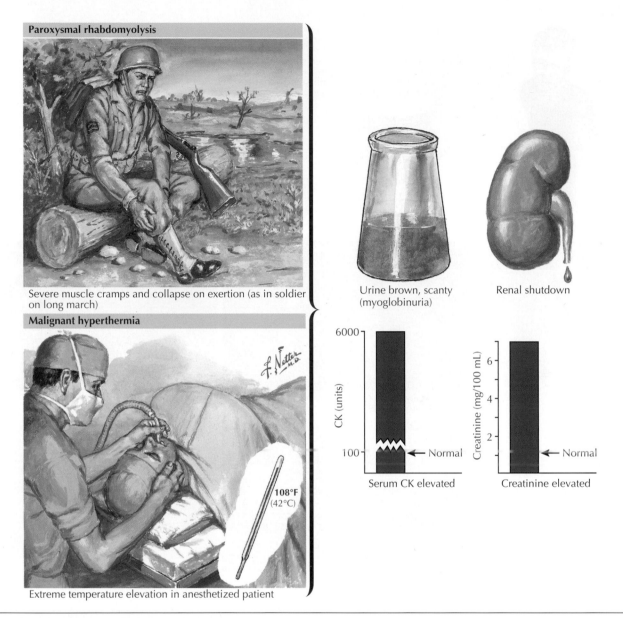

Paroxysmal rhabdomyolysis

Severe muscle cramps and collapse on exertion (as in soldier on long march)

Malignant hyperthermia

Extreme temperature elevation in anesthetized patient

108°F (42°C)

Urine brown, scanty (myoglobinuria)

Renal shutdown

6000

CK (units)

100 — Normal

Serum CK elevated

Creatinine (mg/100 mL)

— Normal

Creatinine elevated

Figure 75-4 Myoglobinuric Syndromes.

Table 75-3 Myopathies Presenting with Exercise Intolerance

Glycogenoses	Respiratory Chain Defects	Lipid Metabolism Disorders
Myophosphorylase deficiency (McArdle disease)—Type V	Complex 1 deficiency	Carnitine deficiency
Phosphofructokinase deficiency (Tauri disease)—Type VII	Coenzyme Q$_{10}$ deficiency	Carnitine palmitoyltransferase deficiency
Phosphorylase B kinase deficiency—Type VIII	Complex III deficiency	Very long chain, long chain, medium chain, or short chain acyl CoA dehydrogenase deficiency
Phosphoglycerate kinase deficiency—Type IX	Complex IV deficiency	3-Hydroxy Acyl-CoA dehydrogenase deficiency protein deficiency
Phosphoglycerate mutase deficiency—Type X	Complex V deficiency	Glutaric aciduria type II (electron-transferring flavoprotein and CoQ oxidoreductase deficiencies)
Lactate dehydrogenase deficiency—Type XI	Combination of I to V	Neutral lipid storage disease with myopathy; neutral lipid storage disease with ichthyosis
Beta enolase deficiency—Type XII		

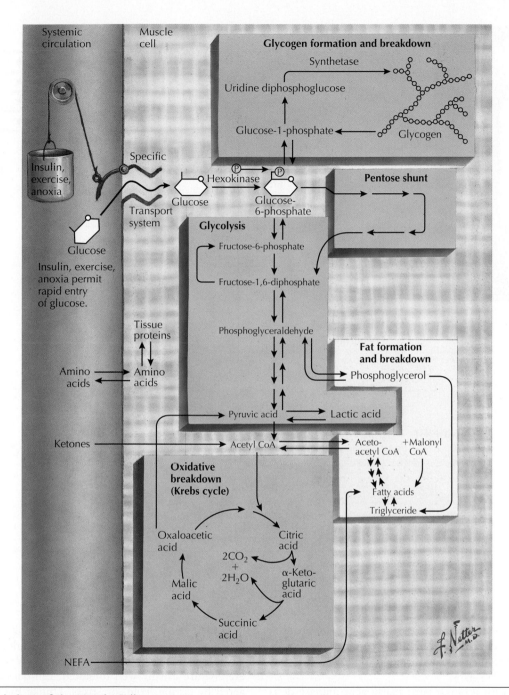

Figure 75-5 Metabolism of the Muscle Cell.

metabolism, the respiratory chain defects, and muscle adenylate deaminase deficiency are usually recessively inherited. As based on the specific enzyme deficiency, there are 12 different types (I-XII) of GSDs. Type V, McArdle disease, is the most common, presenting with classic exercise-induced painful symptomatology (see Fig. 75-3). Similar phenotypes occur with types VII, IX, X, and XI GSDs.

CLINICAL PRESENTATION

Severe painful muscle cramping and stiffness occurring after exertion are the hallmark of an enzymatic deficiency

glycogen or lipid storage disorder. There may be a characteristic second-wind phenomenon, where brief periods of rest at the onset of myalgia alleviate symptoms and enable prolonged exercise. Symptomatic relief may come with rest (see Fig. 75-4). Recurrent myoglobinuria is common, and permanent weakness may develop in older patients. Patients with myalgias and exercise intolerance, with or without hyperCKemia, are commonly evaluated by neuromuscular specialists. The exercise-induced symptomatology with the subsequent myalgia (in contrast to joint or soft tissues), muscle stiffness, and myoglobinuria provide the primary diagnostic criteria for investigating the possibility of a metabolic myopathy. Although specific defects

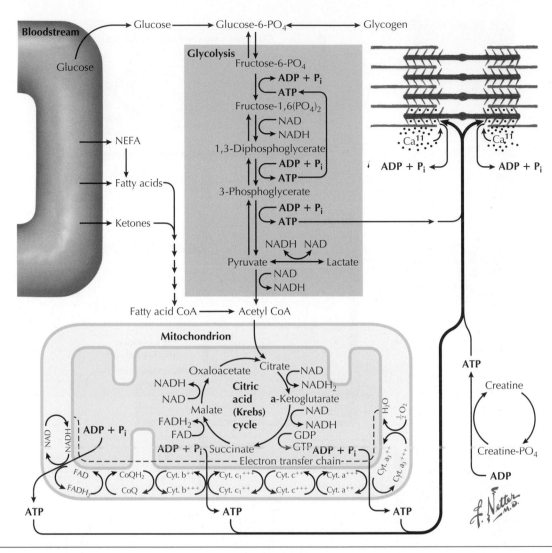

Figure 75-6 Regeneration of ATP for Source of Energy in Muscle Contraction.

of muscle energy metabolism, as described in this chapter, are sometimes precisely defined, more commonly and very frustratingly, specific enzymatic defects cannot be identified in this setting.

A few patients with a GSD, particularly acid maltase deficiency in the adult, present with fixed, often progressive weakness. These individuals have no typical history of episodic symptomatology.

Muscle adenylate deaminase deficiency is a controversial "disorder" because it is not clear that this is a discrete biochemical disorder. These patients also experience exertional muscle cramping, stiffness, weakness, and pain. However, in contradistinction to a GSD they do not demonstrate an appropriate increase in serum ammonia levels after forearm exercise, but do have the normal increase in serum lactate, indicating normal glycogen metabolism. Myoglobinuria is rare in muscle adenylate deaminase deficiency, which may represent a disorder of defective purine metabolism.

Carnitine palmitoyltransferase II deficiency is the most common disorder of lipid metabolism. Dynamic symptoms include myalgia without muscle cramping. Most commonly, young men present with recurrent myoglobinuria after prolonged but not necessarily strenuous exercise. Brief periods of exercise are usually well tolerated. Episodes also may be triggered by fasting, cold, or stress. Unlike the glycogenoses, no second-wind phenomenon is seen, fixed weakness does not develop, and serum CK values may normalize between episodes.

Mitochondrial myopathies need to be considered in the setting of ptosis and ophthalmoparesis. These are the clinical signatures of these very uncommon disorders; however, these clinical findings are not present in every phenotype. These myopathies are defined by alterations in mitochondrial structure and function; there is a rather marked clinical heterogeneity. Furthermore, the involvement of other end organs, particularly those with high energy requirements such as the kidneys, liver, and brain, is typically found in patients with a mitochondrial myopathy. However, on occasion these rare myopathies occur in a solitary fashion mimicking the glycogen and lipid storage disorders.

DIAGNOSTIC APPROACH

Precise diagnosis of a GSD requires biochemical findings manifested by an abnormal FET. Baseline measurement of plasma lactate, pyruvate, and ammonia are obtained. The patients then vigorously exercise their hand for 1–2 minutes (see Fig. 75-6). Subsequently serial lactate and ammonia determinations are made immediately after exercise and 1, 3, 6, and 10 minutes thereafter. Normally there is a fivefold rise in serum lactate and a tenfold rise in the serum ammonia level. *Glycogen metabolism storage disorders* are suspected where there is failure to achieve the normal increase of serum lactate. *Muscle adenylate deaminase deficiency* is defined by a lack of the expected increase in plasma ammonia after exercise and the normal increase in serum lactate. The test sensitivity is dependent on patient effort. Permanent weakness or rhabdomyolysis, leading to renal impairment, either one precipitated by the ischemic testing format has been rarely reported. Therefore we no longer include an induced ischemic component to this study.

Muscle tissue histochemical analysis is also important. Here one obtains a muscle biopsy and then utilizes specific stains looking for the presence, or absence, of the enzyme muscle phosphorylase. When this is not abnormal, then other GSDs, or even more rarely, inborn errors in muscle lipid metabolism must also be assessed. Genetic testing for CPT2 is available, so biopsy can be avoided if clinical suspicion is high.

IDIOPATHIC HYPERCKEMIA

It is normal to find a moderate postexercise hyperCKemia increase in healthy individuals. Typically, this CK elevation is less than five times the upper limit of normal after a moderately vigorous exercise, whether skiing or playing an intense game of singles tennis or participating in various types of football, basketball, or rugby, for example. These elevated CK levels return to normal standards within 3–8 days postexercise.

Evaluation of patients who have nonspecific symptoms or who are serendipitously found to have increased CK is often frustrating in the absence of clinically demonstrated weakness or specific EMG abnormalities. The yield of muscle biopsy in search of glycogen or lipid storage changes is relatively low, even with extensive histochemical staining and DNA tests. Abnormalities found on routine analysis of muscle biopsy specimens do not accurately predict abnormalities on biochemical testing. Some metabolic myopathies are skeletal muscle specific. Here one needs to specifically study the involved muscles. Other metabolic disorders of muscle are more systemically distributed and can be detected on enzymatic testing of fibroblasts or leukocytes.

Respiratory chain mitochondrial disorders are characterized by marked increases in baseline serum lactate or pyruvate, as well as demonstration of metabolic acidosis and dicarboxylic or aminoaciduria.

EMG generally does not provide a useful diagnostic medium as it is usually normal in these various energy metabolic defects. The one exception is if one has the opportunity to perform the EMG while the patient is actually experiencing an active and often painful contracture, when there will be total electrical silence. This finding is unique to glycogen storage disorders. GSD type II, also known as acid maltase (alpha glucosidase) deficiency, is the one other exception where there are classic EMG findings of a very active myopathy mimicking polymyositis; the findings here are frequently most profound in the paraspinal musculature. Parenthetically, adult-onset acid maltase patients most commonly present with clinical findings similar to polymyositis. Overall the primary utility of EMG in this group of metabolic skeletal muscle disorders is to provide a means to exclude other motor unit processes before moving on to other studies.

Lymphocyte or cultured skin fibroblast analysis supersedes the need for muscle biopsy in certain metabolic myopathies. Testing is available for many glycogenoses and disorders of lipid metabolism. With the exception of complex IV deficiency, analysis for respiratory chain disorders is generally available only on a research basis.

MUSCLE BIOPSY

Abnormal accumulation of glycogen or lipid may be detected in a muscle biopsy specimen using periodic acid-Schiff or oil red O staining, respectively. Muscle phosphorylase, phosphofructokinase, and myoadenylate deaminase deficiency are the primary enzyme-specific stains available for metabolic myopathies. Lipid stains may be normal or show mild lipid accumulation in carnitine palmitoyltransferase II deficiency. Biochemical testing of muscle is available for some myopathies (Table 75-4).

The diagnosis of a mitochondrial myopathy is supported by finding ragged red fibers. These are detected by the modified Gomori trichrome and succinic dehydrogenase stains or by myofibers that do not stain with cytochrome-c oxidase. Mitochondrial mutational analysis is available for a limited number of mutations.

Table 75-4 Biochemical Analyses Available for Specific Metabolic Myopathies

Glycogen Storage	Lipid Storage	Mitochondrial	Purine
Acid maltase	Carnitine	NADH dehydrogenase	Myoadenylate deaminase
Neutral maltase	Carnitine palmitoyltransferase	NADH cytochrome-c reductase	Adenylate kinase
Phosphofructokinase		Succinate dehydrogenase	
Phosphorylase		Succinate cytochrome-c reductase	
Phosphorylase β kinase		Cytochrome-c oxidase	
Phosphoglycerate kinase		Citrate synthase?	
Phosphoglycerate mutase		Fumarase	

TREATMENT AND PROGNOSIS

One crucial caveat is that patients with hyperCKemia, regardless of cause, have an increased risk for development of malignant hyperthermia (see Fig. 75-4, bottom). This is a potentially life-threatening anesthesia-induced complication of certain fluorinated hydrocarbon inhalation agents such as halothane. Thus, we suggest that any patient with hyperCKemia wear a MedicAlert bracelet at all times to alert the anesthesiologist to the potential for this life-threatening disorder.

Most patients with metabolic myopathies learn to adapt to limited exercise tolerance. No specific treatments are available for most of these conditions. Isolated reports attribute clinical benefit in the glycogenoses to aerobic training, high-protein diets, and creatine supplementation. However, none are proven reliable therapies. Patients with carnitine palmitoyltransferase II deficiency often can prevent attacks by increasing dietary carbohydrate intake before prolonged exercise or during febrile illness.

Myoglobinuria is always a major concern as it is a major risk for acute renal failure because there is deposition of myoglobin within renal tubules potentially leading to renal shutdown. This is a significant problem with the various muscle metabolism glycogenoses and lipid storage disorders. As much as 50% of patients with recurrent myoglobinuria experience episodes of acute renal insufficiency. Patients who are at risk for myoglobinuria are advised to seek prompt medical attention if such occurs. Treatment includes forced diuresis and alkalinization. A complete recovery is expected if the episodes are appropriately managed.

Metabolic myopathies are generally nonprogressive disorders, although fixed weakness develops with increasing age in some patients who have a glycogenosis. This is particularly the case with acid maltase deficiency. Once this disorder presents in middle age, there is early potential for significant respiratory compromise. In a few patients with the very rare carnitine palmitoyltransferase II deficiency, respiratory muscle involvement also occurs. This may require ventilatory support during episodes of severe weakness. Generally, these episodes are reversible with appropriate supportive care.

MUSCULAR DYSTROPHIES

These are genetically determined myopathies distinguished from congenital myopathies by their generally progressive clinical course and characteristic dystrophic histology profile, that is, myofiber degeneration, regeneration, and fibrosis and fatty replacement (Fig. 75-7, bottom panel). The milder dystrophies, for example, oculopharyngeal muscular dystrophy, may lack some of these classic histologic features.

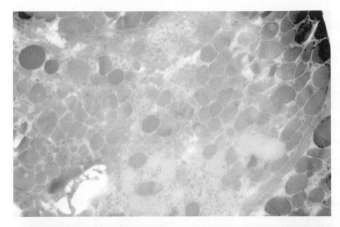
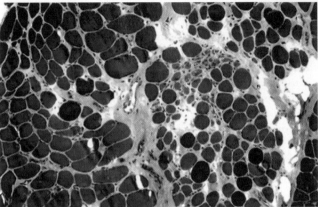

Muscle biopsy specimens showing necrotic muscle fibers being removed by groups of small, round phagocytic cells (**top,** trichrome stain) and replaced by fibrous and fatty tissue (**bottom,** H and E stain).

Figure 75-7 Duchenne Muscular Dystrophy: Muscle Biopsy Specimens.

Clinical Vignette

A 42-year-old man presented with weakness that developed gradually over 5 years. He noticed reduced strength in his lower extremities; he had difficulty climbing stairs, had reduced handgrip, and occasionally tripped when he walked. He had had cataract surgery at the age of 32. His father had developed walking problems in his fifties and had apparently died suddenly in his early sixties, probably due to an arrhythmia. On questioning, he admitted to dysphagia.

On examination, he had bilateral ptosis, temporalis wasting, mild proximal weakness and bilateral foot drop. Reflexes were reduced throughout. Sensory examination was normal. Forced handgrip revealed slow relaxation (clinical myotonia). Electrodiagnostic studies revealed normal nerve conduction studies. EMG showed evidence of myotonic discharges with small myopathic units in all muscles tested. Genetic testing revealed 1200 CTG repeats on chromosome 19q13 for the myotonin protein kinase (DMPK).

Myotonic muscular dystrophies are the most common adult forms of muscular dystrophy. They are genotypically heterogeneous.

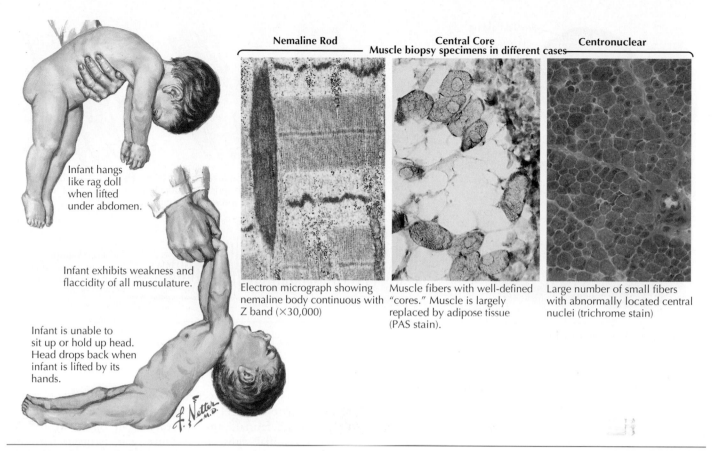

Nemaline Rod

Central Core

Muscle biopsy specimens in different cases

Centronuclear

Infant hangs like rag doll when lifted under abdomen.

Infant exhibits weakness and flaccidity of all musculature.

Infant is unable to sit up or hold up head. Head drops back when infant is lifted by its hands.

Electron micrograph showing nemaline body continuous with Z band (×30,000)

Muscle fibers with well-defined "cores." Muscle is largely replaced by adipose tissue (PAS stain).

Large number of small fibers with abnormally located central nuclei (trichrome stain)

Figure 75-8 Congenital Myopathies: Floppy Infant.

MYOTONIC MUSCULAR DYSTROPHY, TYPE 1 (DM1)

The classic autosomal dominant form usually presents in early adulthood but may be recognized from the neonatal period presenting as a floppy infant similar to some of the congenital myopathies and congenital dystrophies (Fig. 75-8). This condition presents with distal weakness that progresses to involve proximal muscles. Myotonia is delayed skeletal muscle relaxation and is best demonstrated with a forceful handgrip or by thenar muscle eminence percussion. Temporalis, masseter, and sternocleidomastoid wasting, frontal balding, and ptosis contribute to the characteristic myotonic facies (Fig. 75-9). Facial, pharynx, tongue, and neck muscles are also weak. Limb weakness predominantly affects distal extensor muscle groups and then progresses proximally.

Various systemic problems occur concomitantly with myotonic muscular dystrophy, Type 1 (DM1): impaired gastrointestinal dysmotility, alveolar hypoventilation, cardiac conduction defects, and cardiomyopathy. The last three often shorten life expectancy. Neurobehavioral manifestations include hypersomnolence, apathy, depression, personality disorders, and cognitive impairment. Premature posterior subcapsular cataracts are common and may sometimes provide the essential clue leading to the initial diagnosis of DM1. Testicular atrophy and impotence occur in men. Pregnant women have a high rate of fetal loss.

Laboratory investigations demonstrate that the CK may be mildly elevated. Nerve conduction studies are normal. Needle EMG predominantly demonstrates myotonic potentials. Muscle biopsy is characterized by an increase in internal nuclei, atrophy, pyknotic clumps, and ring fibers. Genetic testing for the myotonin protein kinase (DMPK) will reveal >37 CTG repeats on chromosome 19q13.2. Greater repeat lengths are associated with more severe disease. Amplification of repeat size occurs in newborn babies of mothers with DM1 resulting in congenital dystrophy.

PROXIMAL MYOTONIC MYOPATHY (DM2)

Proximal myotonic myopathy (PROMM) DM2 is another autosomal dominant myotonic disorder that presents in adults or, rarely, in children. Patients present with myotonia, myalgia, and proximal weakness. Weakness begins in the legs and is slowly progressive. Patients may describe episodic fluctuation in their weakness and may experience severe muscle pain. Ptosis, facial weakness, and weakness of the respiratory muscles are uncommon in DM2. Associated systemic abnormalities include cataracts, cardiac arrhythmias, and testicular atrophy. The proximal weakness and absence of signature features make DM2 a more difficult clinical diagnosis than DM1.

Serum CK may be mildly increased. EMG demonstrates myotonia, which often provides an important diagnostic clue when evaluating patients with typical clinical pictures of proximal myopathies. Genetic studies for zinc finger protein 9 on chromosome 3 will reveal >177 base pairs CCTG expansion.

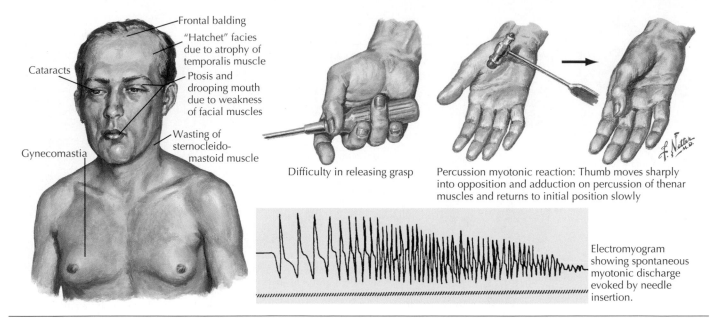

Frontal balding

"Hatchet" facies due to atrophy of temporalis muscle

Cataracts

Ptosis and drooping mouth due to weakness of facial muscles

Gynecomastia

Wasting of sternocleido-mastoid muscle

Difficulty in releasing grasp

Percussion myotonic reaction: Thumb moves sharply into opposition and adduction on percussion of thenar muscles and returns to initial position slowly

Electromyogram showing spontaneous myotonic discharge evoked by needle insertion.

Figure 75-9 Myotonic Dystrophy.

LIMB-GIRDLE MUSCULAR DYSTROPHIES

Limb-girdle muscular dystrophies (LGMDs) are a genetically heterogeneous group of disorders wherein the precise classification is rendered more complicated by the frequency of variable phenotypes resulting from mutations of the same gene. It is difficult to distinguish clinically the various subtypes of LGMD, although patterns of weakness or other clinical features may suggest various genotypes. Classification of LGMDs is by number (1 for dominant inheritance, 2 for recessive) and letter (usually in the order of discovery of the chromosomal locus) (see Table 75-1).

Weakness in these individuals typically has a symmetric limb-girdle pattern, usually affecting the proximal leg muscles before the shoulder girdle. There is relative sparing of facial, oculomotor, pharyngeal, and neck muscles. Onset is usually before the age of 20 years, although LGMD is frequently unrecognized until early middle life, and women and men are affected as frequently. Systemic involvement is uncommon. CK increases range from normal to 20 times normal. Genetic testing is available for some of the LGMD.

DYSTROPHINOPATHIES

These dystrophinopathies are the most common muscular dystrophies occurring during childhood and in some adults. Dystrophin is a subsarcolemmal protein present in skeletal and cardiac muscle. Dystrophin along with the sarcolemmal proteins forms the dystrophin-sarcoglycan complex (Fig. 75-10).

Duchenne Muscular Dystrophy

Duchenne muscular dystrophy (DMD) is a primarily X-linked recessive dystrophinopathy; however, in a third of patients this occurs sporadically, presenting in early childhood with proximal weakness and difficulty walking (Fig. 75-11). Untreated patients,

usually boys, become wheelchair dependent by midadolescence. Calf hypertrophy, heel cord shortening, and blunted intellect help to differentiate this disorder from other myopathies. Common initial signs are a clumsy gait, frequent falls, and proximal lower extremity weakness. Children cannot rise from a squatting position on the floor and use their hands to push off on their legs (Fig. 75-12). Most patients are wheelchair bound by 12 years of age.

An associated cardiomyopathy is common and can cause arrhythmias or congestive heart failure. Respiratory failure due to neuromuscular weakness may be exacerbated by the development of kyphoscoliosis and contractures. Most patients die of respiratory or cardiac complications in the second or third decade of life unless they choose long-term mechanical ventilation. Smooth muscle involvement may occur, manifesting as an ileus or gastric atony.

Female carriers often have asymptomatic hyperCKemia but very rarely do present with symptomatic myopathies as adults.

CK levels are significantly elevated to approximately 30–50 times normal. Serum molecular genetic testing for mutations in the dystrophin gene is the first step in children in whom a dystrophinopathy is suspected. This is positive in approximately two thirds of these boys. When DNA analysis is negative, a muscle biopsy is indicated for dystrophin immunostaining, immunoblotting, or Western blot analysis. Immunostaining demonstrates that most fibers are devoid of dystrophin in DMD. Electrodiagnostic studies and muscle biopsy, once the mainstays of diagnosis, are no longer necessary in most cases. Needle EMG demonstrates myopathic-appearing motor units as well as profuse fibrillation potentials.

Becker Muscular Dystrophy

Becker muscular dystrophy (BMD) is another X-linked dystrophinopathy that is allelic to DMD. This usually presents with a

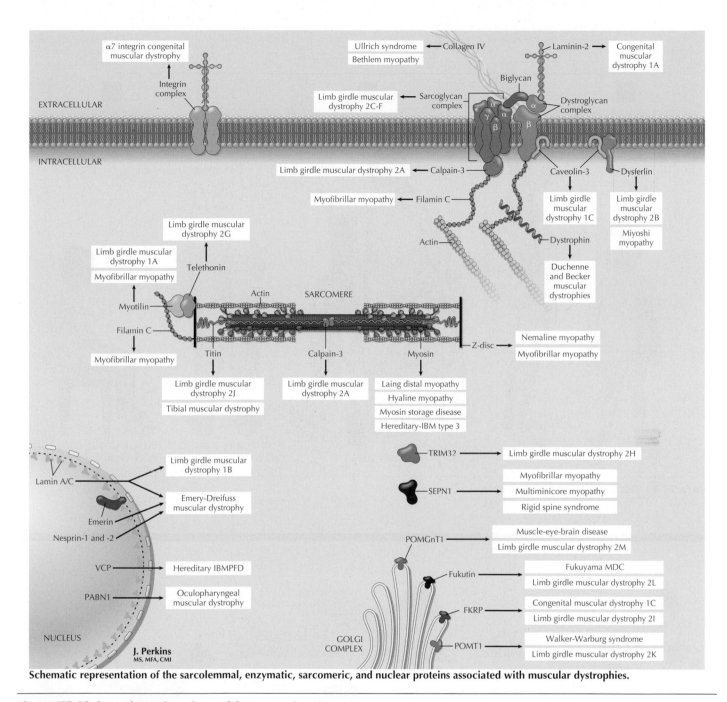

Schematic representation of the sarcolemmal, enzymatic, sarcomeric, and nuclear proteins associated with muscular dystrophies.

Figure 75-10 Sarcoglycan Complex and Sarcomere Proteins.

milder phenotype. Patients present with difficulty walking in the late first or early second decade of life. BMD is sometimes manifest by exertional myalgias, cardiomyopathy, or asymptomatic increased serum CK levels. Increased CK may not occur early on; some patients have normal values in childhood and increased serum CK levels develop later in their 20s. Life expectancy is still reduced but usually significantly longer than in DMD. Diagnosis is similar to that of DMD. Mutations that result in in-frame mutations are more likely to present with the BMD phenotype.

In both BMD and the rare female carrier, muscle biopsy demonstrates a mix of dystrophin staining and nonstaining fibers. Both immunoblotting and immunostaining results for dystrophin in muscle biopsies are quantitatively and qualitatively abnormal in BMD.

Treatment of Dystrophinopathies

No specific treatment is available to treat these disorders. Long-term corticosteroid therapy in ambulatory patients may help somewhat to ameliorate the course of DMD. Corticosteroid is often associated with significant side effects and patients will need to be monitored for weight gain, stunted growth, osteoporosis, and mood changes. Aggressive treatment of heart failure

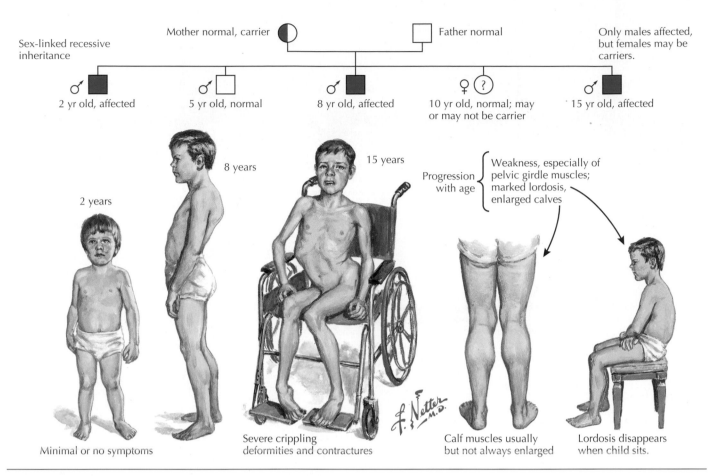

Sex-linked recessive inheritance

Mother normal, carrier ◐ — □ Father normal

Only males affected, but females may be carriers.

♂ ■ 2 yr old, affected

♂ □ 5 yr old, normal

♂ ■ 8 yr old, affected

♀ (?) 10 yr old, normal; may or may not be carrier

♂ ■ 15 yr old, affected

2 years

8 years

15 years

Progression with age { Weakness, especially of pelvic girdle muscles; marked lordosis, enlarged calves

Minimal or no symptoms

Severe crippling deformities and contractures

Calf muscles usually but not always enlarged

Lordosis disappears when child sits.

Figure 75-11 Duchenne Muscular Dystrophy.

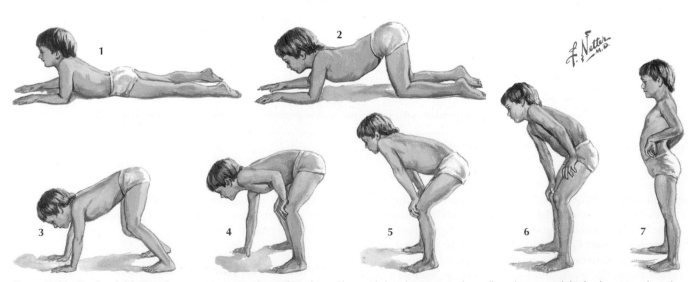

1   2   3   4   5   6   7

Characteristically, the child arises from prone position by pushing himself up with hands successively on floor, knees, and thighs, because of weakness in gluteal and spine muscles. He stands in lordic posture.

Figure 75-12 Duchenne Muscular Dystrophy: Gowers maneuver.

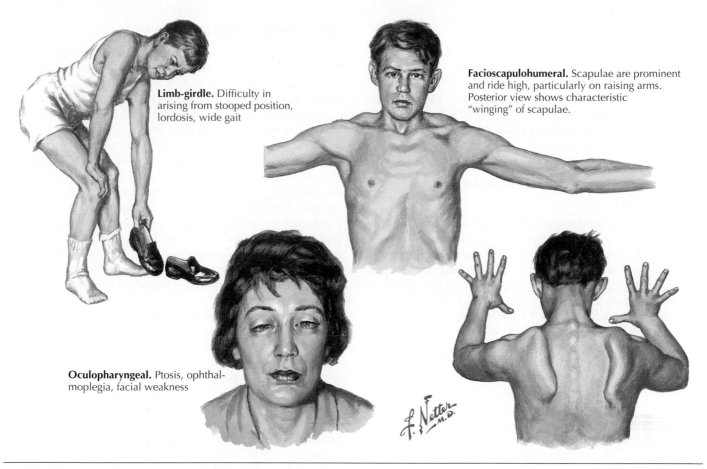

Limb-girdle. Difficulty in arising from stooped position, lordosis, wide gait

Facioscapulohumeral. Scapulae are prominent and ride high, particularly on raising arms. Posterior view shows characteristic "winging" of scapulae.

Oculopharyngeal. Ptosis, ophthalmoplegia, facial weakness

Figure 75-13 Other Types of Muscular Dystrophy.

and consideration for cardiac transplant in patients is also recommended; this is especially important in patients with BMD presenting with cardiomyopathy. Supportive treatment including physical, occupational, speech, and respiratory therapy are important aspects in the care of these patients.

FACIOSCAPULOHUMERAL MUSCULAR DYSTROPHY

Facioscapulohumeral (FSH) muscular dystrophy is a dominantly inherited disorder with variable penetrance. Patients may present with facial weakness and scapular winging in the second to fifth decade of life (Fig. 75-13). Atrophy and weakness of biceps and triceps muscles typically occur; paradoxically, there is relative sparing of deltoid and forearm strength. Ankle dorsiflexors are usually first affected in the lower extremity. An asymmetric pattern of weakness is a common feature. Abdominal muscle weakness and a Beevor sign (caudal or rostral movement of the umbilicus with head flexion) may be present. Variations in phenotype include the rare absence of any demonstrable facial weakness. An infantile form presents with a rapidly progressive course leading to wheelchair dependency by the age of 10 years.

Electrodiagnostic studies demonstrate myopathic findings. Genetic testing (a D4Z4 repeat contraction on chromosome 4q35) reveals mutations on the 4q35 chromosomal region. More

recently a subset of patients with FSHD who do not have this contraction has been observed.

SCAPULOPERONEAL SYNDROMES

These various disorders need consideration in the differential diagnosis of FSH. The genetic pattern in scapuloperoneal syndromes may be autosomal dominant or recessive, sometimes X-linked, or even sporadic. Usually, these children present with arm weakness before a foot drop is recognized. Most patients have normal longevity with relatively mild disability.

EMERY–DREIFUSS MUSCULAR DYSTROPHY

This is inherited in either an X-linked or autosomal dominant manner. Distinctive features include a humeroperoneal (elbow flexion and extension, foot dorsiflexion) pattern of weakness and contractures (especially of the Achilles tendons, elbows, and posterior cervical muscles). Most patients present with contractures causing difficulty extending the elbows and dorsiflexing the ankles.

Cardiac conduction defects are common causes of stroke and life-threatening arrhythmias, and sometimes the clinically presenting feature of this disorder. Genetic tests will reveal mutations in the EMD gene on chromosome Xq28 (X-linked form) or in the LMNA gene on chromosome 1q11-23 (autosomal dominant form).

BETHLEM MYOPATHY

This is an autosomal disorder similar to Emery–Dreifuss muscular dystrophy with early childhood onset. It is an indolent myopathy also having prominent elbow flexion contractures but without cardiac complications.

OCULOPHARYNGEAL MUSCULAR DYSTROPHY

This autosomal dominant myopathy is particularly prevalent in North America among individuals of French Canadian ancestry. Most patients present in mid- to late adulthood with ptosis and dysphagia. Mild proximal weakness and ophthalmoparesis may develop. Genetic testing for the presence of a GCG repeat in the PABN1 gene on chromosome 14q11.1 if positive will confirm the diagnosis (see Fig. 75-13, bottom right panel).

MYOFIBRILLAR (DESMIN) MYOPATHY

Genetically and phenotypically, this disorder is characterized by desmin or other protein accumulation within the muscle. Electron microscopy (EM) findings demonstrate the presence of myofibrillar disruption, probably due to Z-disk disruption. The clinical phenotype is varied. Diagnosis is made by the presence of the characteristic histologic features. It can present at any age with proximal or distal weakness. Surveillance for associated cardiomyopathy, ventilatory insufficiency, or both is required. Mutations have been identified in myotilin, ZASP, filamin-C, desmin, selenoprotein n, alphabeta crystallin, and bag-3. Pattern of inheritance is variable.

CONGENITAL MUSCULAR DYSTROPHIES

These are a heterogeneous group of recessively inherited neonatal disorders commonly confused with congenital myopathies, particularly when infants are hypotonic, often presenting as floppy babies. Children with congenital muscular dystrophy often have joint contractures or arthrogryposis. Some forms are associated with associated brain or ocular abnormalities. These clinical features coupled with increased CK values and dystrophic muscle histology distinguish congenital muscular dystrophies from congenital myopathies and other infantile neuromuscular disorders.

DISTAL MYOPATHIES OR MUSCULAR DYSTROPHIES

The distal myopathies are rare and present with progressive, distal weakness and may be sporadic or inherited. The distal myopathies are classified based on the inheritance, pattern of weakness, and histopathologic findings (Table 75-5). It is important to remember that other myopathies can present with a distal pattern of weakness, for example, DM1, EDMD, FSHD, scapuloperoneal, nemaline myopathy, and centronuclear myopathy due to dynamin-2 mutation.

CONGENITAL MYOPATHIES

These disorders are usually evident at birth or in infancy. They may be severe but often tend to be only minimally progressive if the child survives infancy. Affected children are often limited in their physical capacities, but many live to adulthood. These myopathies are typically named for key histologic features, for example, nemaline (threadlike) rods.

The most common congenital myopathies are centronuclear (myotubular) myopathy, central core disease, and nemaline myopathy (see Fig. 75-8, bottom panel). These are well-defined clinically and genetically heterogeneous disorders. Concomitant congenital skeletal changes such as high arched palates and kyphoscoliosis are commonplace and are suggestive of these genetically determined disorders. Although the presentation is usually that of a floppy infant, some individuals are mildly affected and may not present until early to midadulthood. Babies surviving infancy tend to have minimal progression and reasonable life expectancy.

Centronuclear myopathy, previously called myotubular myopathy, is a disorder associated with characteristic muscle biopsy findings of central nuclei. It is seen as an X-linked recessive neonatal disorder frequently causing death from respiratory insufficiency in infancy, or rarely presents indolently in childhood or early adulthood. Ptosis and ophthalmoparesis help distinguish this from other congenital myopathies. Muscle biopsy demonstrates nuclei in the center of the fiber, sometimes forming longitudinal chains. Mutations in myotubularin or dynamin are linked to this condition.

Central core myopathy presents in infancy or childhood with generalized weakness. Muscle biopsies demonstrate cores that appear in type 1 fibers and are seen on NADH stains as nonstaining regions. Z-band streaming and myofibrillar disruption may result in the formation of cores. This condition is associated with an increased risk for malignant hyperthermia; this is particularly seen on exposure to volatile anesthetics or depolarizing neuromuscular blockers.

Nemaline myopathy can present at any age from infancy to adulthood and is phenotypically and genetically heterogeneous. Affected children have delayed motor milestones, but those surviving past infancy eventually achieve some degree of functional independence. On muscle biopsy there is type 1 predominance, with the presence of nemaline rods in the subsarcolemmal region best seen on Gomori trichrome stain. EM is useful to confirm the presence of the rods. The rods are thought to represent disrupted Z-disk structure.

The diagnosis of congenital myopathies is usually confirmed with routine histochemical staining of muscle in concert with the appropriate phenotype. A few metabolic myopathies can be diagnosed by histochemical staining, but many require biochemical analysis of the muscle biopsy specimen or other tissue.

HEREDITARY INCLUSION BODY MYOPATHY

The hereditary inclusion body myopathies (IBMs) are difficult to classify. They manifest in the second or third decades of life and are histologically identical to sporadic IBMs but without inflammation. Two forms are allelic to distal myopathies. Their

Table 75-5 The Distal Myopathies

	Initial Muscle				Chromosome		
	Age at Onset	Group Involved	Serum CK	Muscle Biopsy	Inheritance	Linkage	Gene
Nonaka (hIBM type 1)	Early adulthood	AC legs	N or sl ↑	Rimmed vacuoles	AR	9p1–q1	GNE
Miyoshi	Early adulthood	PC legs	↑ × 10–150	Myopathic changes, occasional inflammation	AR	2p13	Dysferlin
Laing	Childhood to adulthood	AC legs, neck flexors	↑ × 1–3	Myopathic changes	AD	14q11	
Myofibrillar myopathy (desmin)	Childhood to adulthood	Hands or AC legs	N or sl ↑	Myopathic changes with vacuoles or cytoplasmic inclusions	AD, sporadic, ? AR, ? X-linked	2q35, 11q21–23, 12q, 10q22.3	Various genes
Welander	Late adulthood	Finger and wrist extensors	N or sl ↑	Myopathic changes, vacuoles	AD	2p13	
Udd	Late adulthood	AC legs but can be highly variable	N or ↑ CK	Dystrophic, can have rimmed vacuoles	AD/AR		2q31 mutation in gene for titin
Markesbury-Griggs	Late adulthood	AC legs	N or ↑ CK	Myofibrillar myopathy and rimmed vacuoles	AD		ZASP (Z-band alternatively spliced PDZ motif-containing protein)
Distal myopathy with vocal cord and pharyngeal weakness	Late adulthood	AC legs, finger extensors, late vocal cord and pharyngeal weakness	N or ↑ × 3–6	Vacuolar myopathy	AD	5q31 [*]	

AC, anterior compartment; AD, autosomal dominant; AR, autosomal recessive; CK, creatine kinase; N, normal; PC, posterior compartment; sl, slight; ↑, increased.
*Previously thought localized to 5q31 but now thought of as linked to MATR3 gene on X chromosome.

genetic bases relate to mutations in the gene encoding the enzyme complex UDP-N-acetylglucosamine-2-epimerase-N-acetylmannosamine kinase (GNE), which catalyzes the rate-limiting step in sialic acid production. An autosomal dominant form of hereditary IBM associated with frontotemporal dementia and Paget disease of the bone has been linked to mutations in the gene encoding for valsolin containing protein (VCP). Another form presents with congenital arthrogryposis and has been linked to mutations in the MYH2 gene.

DIAGNOSTIC APPROACH TO GENETIC MYOPATHIES

The diagnostic testing required in patients with generalized chronic myopathies varies depending on clinical presentation (Table 75-6), as provided in guidelines for routinely and selectively ordered tests. Many diagnostic tools are available for evaluating a patient with an apparent myopathy. Extensive analyses of muscle should be undertaken only when warranted by a reasonable index of clinical suspicion.

TREATMENT

General goals for the management of chronic myopathies are largely supportive rather than disease specific and do not usually affect the natural disease course (Box 75-1).

Corticosteroids are often used in ambulatory patients with DMD or BMD. There is evidence suggesting that these drugs may delay wheelchair dependency by years in afflicted males. This benefit occurs despite the potential drawbacks of steroids in individuals who have not grown to full stature and who are prone to complications of immobility. Myoblast transfer in the dystrophinopathies and gene transfer in LGMD have been attempted without notable success. Carnitine supplementation in lipid-storage myopathies is effective in few patients, presumably those with primary rather than secondary causes of carnitine deficiency.

Symptomatic myotonia is uncommon in DM1 and DM2. Mexiletine is probably the most effective treatment but requires caution in light of the risk of aggravating possible cardiac conduction problems.

Table 75-6 Evaluation of a Patient with Suspected Muscle Disease*

Primary Studies	Studies That May Be Indicated in Some Patients
EMG CK	Muscle biopsy Potassium (serum) Aldolase Lactate (serum) Thyroid function tests, electrolytes Anti–acetylcholine receptor antibodies Nonischemic forearm exercise testing (lactate, ammonia) Nonischemic forearm exercise testing (venous O_2) Total eosinophil count Immunofixation (serum) DNA mutational analysis for dystrophinopathy DNA mutational analysis for FSH muscular dystrophy DNA mutational analysis for oculopharyngeal muscular dystrophy DNA mutational analysis for specific mitochondrial disorders DNA mutational analysis for myotonic muscular dystrophy types I and II Myositis-specific antibodies Forced vital capacity Electrocardiogram, echocardiogram Slit-lamp examination

*CK, creatine kinase; FSH, facioscapulohumeral.

Box 75-1 Management Goals in the Chronic Proximal/Generalized Myopathies

Maintenance of optimal, independent neuromuscular function for as long as possible, with particular attention to ambulation, via durable medical equipment and occupational therapy evaluation and intervention

Reduction in the risk of falls and injury through home modification, durable medical equipment, or physical therapy instruction

Patient comfort maintenance:

Prevention or correction of joint contractures, particularly spine deformities and kyphoscoliotic cardiopulmonary disease

Appropriate nutrition maintenance of (adequate calories in those with feeding difficulties; caloric restrictions in those with a propensity to obesity)

Genetic counseling where needed

Aspiration pneumonia prevention or prompt treatment (when appropriate)

Cardiac/Pulmonary support: Recognition and treatment of associated congestive heart failure, symptomatic cardiac conduction defects, and pulmonary hypertension

Malignant hyperthermia prevention: Patient should alert anesthesiologist prior to surgery of the potential for this life-threatening disorder

Identification of patient (or parental) goals in situations in which the severity of the illness may be anticipated to significantly shorten the patient's life expectancy (with provision of adequate counseling)

Cardiomyopathies, with or without cardiac conduction abnormalities, occur in several of these disorders. Serial electrocardiographic surveillance and echocardiographic screening are important if the natural disease history or the patient's symptoms raise the possibility of accompanying cardiac dysfunction. Cardiac transplantation is rarely considered in BMD or other myopathies wherein congestive heart failure is the dominant symptom.

PROGNOSIS

Despite the paucity of disease-specific therapies, accurate diagnosis remains important for prognostic and counseling purposes. Precise definition of inheritance patterns is particularly important in myopathic disorders wherein the activities of daily living and life expectancy are diminished, especially where prenatal testing may be available. Affected patients, and sometimes their families, need to be made aware of all implications of their diagnoses as tactfully and honestly as possible. The issues are even more compelling when dealing with an affected child. Many patients and their families have the misconception that all muscle diseases have a natural course similar to DMD. Those with more indolent disorders including certain congenital myopathies and milder forms of muscular dystrophy can often be reassured that the expected natural history is one of mild progression and normal life expectancy.

ADDITIONAL RESOURCES

Amato AA, Russell JA. Neuromuscular Disorders. New York: McGraw-Hill; 2008.

Jones HR. Case presentation and discussion. June 5, 1997. Case records of the Massachusetts General Hospital. N Engl J Med 1998;339:182-191.

Miller A. Muscle disease. In: American Academy of Neurology. Continuum. Philadelphia, Pa: Lippincott Williams & Wilkins; 2006. p. 12.No 3.

Moxley R. Channelopathies affecting skeletal muscle in childhood. In: Jones HR, De Vivo D, Darras, editors. Neuromuscular Disorders of Infancy, Childhood, and Adolescence. Philadelphia, Pa: Butterworth-Heinemann; 2003. p. 783-812.

Neuromuscular disease center—Washington University, St. Louis. www.neuro.wustl.edu/neuromuscular.

North K, Goebel HH. Congenital myopathies. In: Jones HR, De Vivo D, Darras BT, editors. Neuromuscular Disorders of Infancy, Childhood, and Adolescence. Philadelphia, Pa: Butterworth-Heinemann; 2003. p. 601-632.

North K, Jones K. Congenital muscular dystrophies. In: Jones HR, De Vivo D, Darras BT, editors. Neuromuscular Disorders of Infancy, Childhood, and Adolescence. Philadelphia, Pa: Butterworth-Heinemann; 2003. p. 633-648.

Olafsson E, Jones HR, Guay AT, et al. Myopathy of endogenous Cushing's syndrome: a review of the clinical and electromyographic features in eight patients. Muscle Nerve 1994;17:692-693.

Snyder R. Bioethical issues. In: Jones HR, De Vivo D, Darras, editors. Neuromuscular Disorders of Infancy, Childhood, and Adolescence. Philadelphia, Pa: Butterworth-Heinemann; 2003. p. 1279-1286.

Acquired Myopathies

76

Jayashri Srinivasan, Miruna Segarceanu, Doreen Ho, and H. Royden Jones, Jr.

Myopathies are disorders that adversely affect muscle function (Greek "myo" = muscle and "pathy" = suffering). Insights from molecular biology are changing the traditional classification of muscle disorders and opening new areas of investigation.

CLASSIFICATION

Current classifications of the myopathies remain suboptimal because of incomplete knowledge of the precise pathogenesis of many disorders and the complexity of genotypic–phenotypic correlations. Historic classifications begin by distinguishing between acquired and inherited myopathies. This chapter reviews the different categories of acquired myopathies.

Clinical Vignette

The patient is a 33-year-old woman who presents with a 6-month history of difficulty climbing stairs. Recently she noticed she could not climb the 10 steps from her basement. She has also developed problems picking up jars from shelves of tall cabinets as well as inability to keep her hands over her head to brush her hair. Her ability to swallow has been fine and she has not experienced any shortness of breath. Her examination was significant for bilateral weakness of her hip flexors (iliopsoas), deltoids, biceps, and triceps. Muscle stretch reflexes were diminished but present. Sensory examination was normal.

Serum creatine kinase (CK) was increased to 1200 IU/L (six times normal). Electromyography (EMG) demonstrated normal nerve conduction studies. However, needle examination was abnormal, with large numbers of short-duration, low-amplitude, polyphasic motor unit potentials associated with scattered fibrillation potentials and complex repetitive discharges.

Comment: This patient's presentation is typical for a myopathic process with the clinical picture of evolving proximal weakness, elevated serum CK, and abnormal EMG.

The common nongenetically determined myopathies are classified into those having a primary inflammatory process, an underlying endocrinopathy, a toxic pathophysiology, or an underlying associated systemic disorder. Much less commonly, a few infectious agents, such as trichinosis, may lead to a primary myopathy. Myopathies typically present with symmetric symptoms and signs of muscle weakness affecting the proximal limbs and paraspinal musculature (Fig. 76-1). Asymmetric, distal, generalized, or regional patterns of weakness also occur in certain distinct myopathies such as inclusion body myositis (IBM). Less commonly, ventilatory muscles or cardiac muscles are primarily affected. Myopathies occasionally present with periodic weakness, exercise-induced muscle pain, or stiffness.

Muscle weakness is a common defining feature of a variety of peripheral motor unit disorders. Myopathies are included in the same differential diagnosis as neuromuscular transmission disorders, motor neuron disease, as well as rare demyelinating polyneuropathies. Muscle stretch reflexes are generally normal, and sensation is usually unaffected in primary myopathies. The presence of certain distinguishing clinical features may help in the diagnosis of a myopathy. These include the pattern of weakness (e.g., presence of ptosis, ophthalmoparesis, ventilatory muscle weakness, scapular winging, and head drop) or other clinical features (e.g., contractures, skeletal dysmorphisms, calf hypertrophy, myotonia, cardiac involvement, or subtle to marked dermatologic changes). Another very important diagnostic determinant is an assessment of the clinical temporal profile (e.g., the rate of progression), any history of a relapsing (periodic) weakness, diurnal variation, and symptoms that occur only with exertion. Other important factors include genetic predisposition, medication and toxin exposure, and other organ system involvement.

DIAGNOSTIC APPROACH

Patients who present with symptoms of myalgia and muscle weakness with a normal muscle strength examination and with normal or mildly elevated serum creatine kinase (CK) levels are common in clinical practice. Such patients are diagnostically and therapeutically challenging. Definable myopathic disorders are uncommon in patients who present with muscle pain, fatigue, or exercise intolerance in the absence of objective clinical, laboratory, or electrophysiologic abnormalities.

LABORATORY EVALUATION

The serum CK is characteristically increased in many myopathies; this may vary from a 2- to 50-fold increase, although in most myopathies CKs are usually in the 500–5000 IU/mL range (Fig. 76-2). When this enzyme is abnormally elevated, its serum levels do not closely parallel disease severity or activity. Serum aldolase levels are also frequently elevated in myopathies; its increase generally parallels the increase in CK, although many clinical neuromuscular specialists do not routinely order an aldolase level. However on occasion it may be elevated with a normal CK as illustrated in the Cushing syndrome vignette reported later in this chapter.

An increased CK level is a nonspecific finding vis-à-vis the diagnosis of myopathies. Other motor unit disorders (such as motor neuron disease, amyotrophic lateral sclerosis, or spinal muscular atrophy) and systemic processes (particularly myxedema) are commonly associated with increased CK of two to

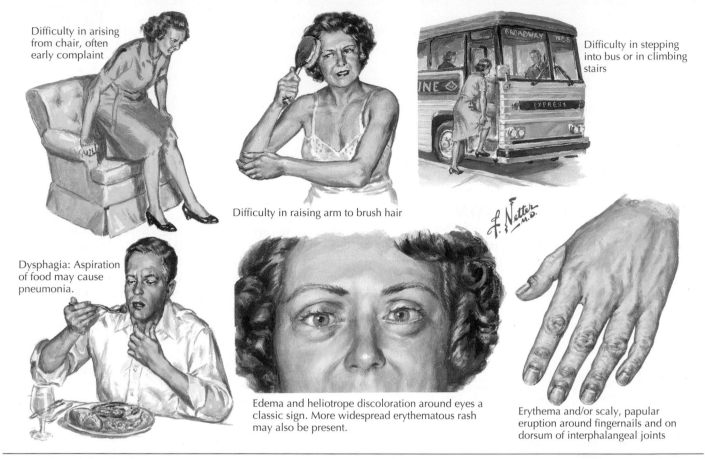

Difficulty in arising from chair, often early complaint

Difficulty in raising arm to brush hair

Difficulty in stepping into bus or in climbing stairs

Dysphagia: Aspiration of food may cause pneumonia.

Edema and heliotrope discoloration around eyes a classic sign. More widespread erythematous rash may also be present.

Erythema and/or scaly, papular eruption around fingernails and on dorsum of interphalangeal joints

Figure 76-1 Polymyositis and Dermatomyositis.

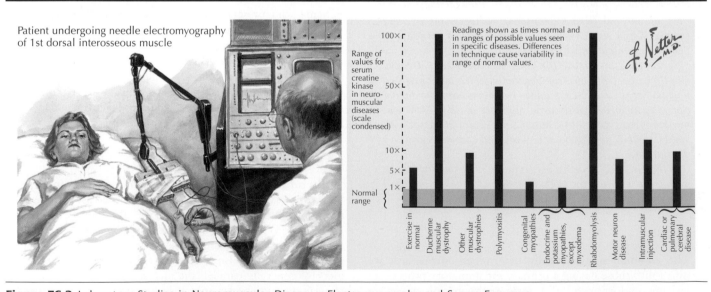

Patient undergoing needle electromyography of 1st dorsal interosseous muscle

Range of values for serum creatine kinase in neuro- muscular diseases (scale condensed)

Readings shown as times normal and in ranges of possible values seen in specific diseases. Differences in technique cause variability in range of normal values.

Normal range

Exercise in normal
Duchenne muscular dystrophy
Other muscular dystrophies
Polymyositis
Congenital myopathies
Endocrine and potassium myopathies, except myxedema
Rhabdomyolysis
Motor neuron disease
Intramuscular injection
Cardiac or pulmonary cerebral disease

Figure 76-2 Laboratory Studies in Neuromuscular Diseases: Electromyography and Serum Enzymes.

five times normal levels. Conversely, the serum CK can be normal in certain patients with DM and IBM.

Patients with persistently increased CK levels sometimes associated with muscle pain but without clinically demonstrable weakness, family history, or exposure to potentially myotoxic substances are classified as having *hyperCKemia*. Despite

thorough clinical and laboratory examination, it is often difficult to assign a specific pathophysiologic mechanism to this finding. HyperCKemia is often an elusive clinical challenge. However, it is important to emphasize that although no diagnosis per se is defined, the finding of hyperCKemia deserves serious consideration. Such individuals are at an increased risk of developing malignant hyperthermia (MH) if they require surgery under general anesthesia. Certain induction agents, particularly the halogenated ones, namely halothane, are particularly prone to inducing this life-threatening complication in patients with hyperCKemia. Therefore, we suggest that our hyperCKemia patients wear a *MedAlert* bracelet to always call the attention of anesthesiologists to this finding and thus potentially prevent an episode of MH (Fig. 76-3).

Serum aspartate and alanine aminotransferases (AST and ALT) are frequently elevated in many myopathies as these enzymes are released by diseased muscle. Rarely some patients with clinically unsuspected myopathies undergo unnecessary evaluation for liver disease when AST and ALT elevations are found and the CK has not been checked. Other liver function studies (e.g., gamma glutamyl transpeptidase and prothrombin time) are normal, providing another clue to the probability of a primary skeletal muscle rather than a hepatic disorder.

Routine biochemistry and hematologic laboratory tests are usually normal in patients with myopathy. Serum potassium levels should be checked to exclude Addison disease with hyperkalemia. Various muscle disorders characterized by episodic periodic paralysis may sometimes have either hypokalemia or hyperkalemia if they are tested during the overt period of paralysis. However, these patients most often have normal potassium values if tested between episodes of weakness. Serum markers of inflammation such as the erythrocyte sedimentation rate (ESR) and C-reactive protein (CRP) may be elevated in some acute myopathies. Thyroid function evaluation (serum TSH levels) must be considered in all patients presenting with an acute or chronic myopathy. Both hypothyroidism and rarely hyperthyroidism may present with primary muscle involvement. Appropriate endocrine evaluation is necessary in myopathic patients when a more obvious diagnosis is not apparent. These also include pituitary adrenal disorders such as Cushing syndrome or Addison disease, and very rarely hyperparathyroidism. In certain ethnic groups, for example, Chinese and Hispanics, thyrotoxicosis may be associated with hypokalemia and a proximal myopathy resembling periodic paralysis.

The serum *myositis-specific and myositis-associated antibodies* are other testing parameters that are useful in the evaluation of some patients with a myopathy. However, as these are present in fewer than half of all patients with polymyositis and dermatomyositis, routine serologic testing for these antibodies is of limited use. The presence of *anti-Jo-1 (antibody to histidyl t-RNA synthetase)* antibodies suggests potential end organ comorbidity, for example, interstitial lung disease (Fig. 76-4).

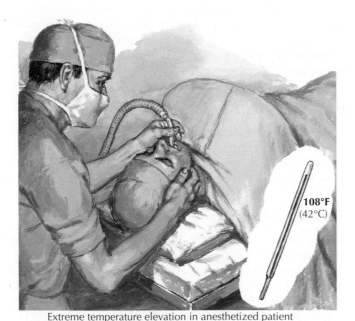

108°F
(42°C)

Extreme temperature elevation in anesthetized patient

Figure 76-3 Malignant Hyperthermia.

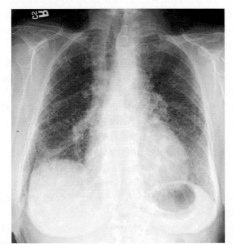

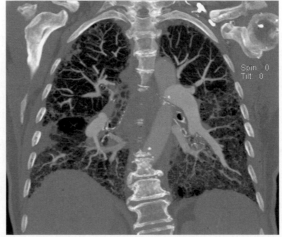

A. PA chest film shows extensive pulmonary fibrosis with typical honeycomb pattern.

B. Coronal reconstruction of chest from CTA shows extensive interstitial thickening, cystic changes, and honeycombing bilaterally with cystic changes involving more the upper than lower lungs. Confluent pleural thickening is seen laterally on the right.

Figure 76-4 Severe pulmonary fibrosis.

Signal recognition particle antibodies are most often associated with necrotizing myopathies and may suggest a poor treatment response.

Sometimes polymyositis is associated with an underlying connective tissue disorder. In those patients, serologic markers for the underlying disease may be positive. These include antinuclear antibody (ANA), and/or rheumatoid factor. On occasion, the presence of these antibodies can aid in the diagnosis of the occasional patient for whom the history is not definitive. This is especially so when there is diagnostic confusion between the possibility of an acquired inflammatory myopathy and a genetically determined dystrophy. When polymyositis and, less commonly, dermatomyositis is associated with other collagen-vascular diseases, the combination is referred to as an overlap syndrome. Systemic lupus erythematosus (SLE), systemic sclerosis, rheumatoid arthritis, and Sjögren syndrome may have weakness as a component of their myriad symptoms and signs. In these cases, muscular weakness exceeds what arthritis alone can account for. They are characterized by elevated titers of *anti–U1/U2-ribonucleoprotein antibodies, PM-Scl antibodies or SSA* antibodies in scleroderma, Sjögren syndrome, SLE, or mixed connective tissue disease. Dermatomyositis is rarely associated with other collagen-vascular diseases, with the exception of scleroderma.

Paraneoplastic antibody evaluation may occasionally be helpful in the differential diagnosis of proximal weakness. This is particularly so in patients with Lambert–Eaton myasthenic syndrome (LEMS) who often present with symptoms emulating a myopathy. These individuals have elevated levels of *voltage-gated calcium channel antibodies*. This finding, in addition to the classic EMG nerve conduction studies typically seen in LEMS, is very specific for this diagnosis. In addition, anti-Hu antibodies may be positive in patients with myopathy associated with small cell lung cancer.

Immunofixation to look for the presence of serum monoclonal protein is necessary in certain instances if either amyloid myopathy or sporadic late-onset nemaline myopathy (SLONM) is in the differential diagnosis. Approximately 20% of patients with IBM also have a MGUS. Appropriate endocrine evaluation is necessary in myopathic patients when a more obvious diagnosis is not apparent.

Vitamin D levels are also important. Rarely hypovitaminosis D may present with a myopathy. Similarly, patients with primary or secondary osteomalacia may present with proximal weakness. Elevated serum calcium and alkaline phosphatase values may point toward these underrecognized disorders.

ELECTROMYOGRAPHY

EMG evaluation of patients with suspected myopathies is important (Fig. 76-5, and see Fig. 76-2). Results of routine nerve conduction studies are normal in myopathies, with the exception of diminished compound muscle action potential amplitudes in more severe disorders. The primary EMG abnormalities in the myopathies are classically found at the time of the needle examination. Classic findings of a myopathy include the presence of abnormally low amplitude, short duration, and polyphasic motor unit potentials (MUPs). It is typical for these patients to have both an early recruitment and increased numbers of MUPs early on in the muscle activation for a given effort. Destruction of myofibrils or muscle membrane results in abnormal insertional activity, particularly fibrillation potentials and complex repetitive discharges. Inflammatory myopathies, several dystrophies, and various myotonic muscle disorders may be distinguished by the presence of myotonic potentials on needle EMG.

Concomitantly, EMG helps to exclude disorders that affect other anatomic sites within the peripheral motor unit, particularly those with symmetric proximal weakness mimicking a myopathy. These include motor neuron disorders, such as amyotrophic lateral sclerosis, spinal muscular atrophy type 3, chronic inflammatory demyelinating polyneuropathies, neuromuscular transmission disorders (particularly Lambert–Eaton myasthenic syndrome), and myasthenia gravis. Results of EMG are often normal in the various endocrine, mitochondrial, and congenital myopathies.

IMAGING STUDIES

Magnetic resonance imaging (MRI) of muscles in addition to EMG to look for signal change abnormalities is useful in patients with inflammatory myopathies as it may help in the selection of a diseased muscle that can be a potential biopsy site.

MUSCLE BIOPSY

Muscle biopsy is the definitive diagnostic tool for many myopathies (Fig. 76-6). The selection of the biopsy site is important; muscles that are unaffected, that are severely affected (are at end stage), or have been recently subjected to EMG evaluation should be avoided. Muscles commonly biopsied include the vastus lateralis, deltoid, and biceps brachii. The gastrocnemius muscle is often avoided due to the possibility of incidentally discovered neurogenic atrophy. The upper lumbosacral muscles, thoracic paraspinal muscles, such as the multifidus, and much less commonly the cervical paraspinal muscles provide an alternative site for biopsy. On reflection one recognizes that these muscles are indeed the most proximal ones and thus more prone to show early changes of an active myopathic process.

The muscle biopsy specimen per se is divided into separate aliquots for formalin fixation, paraffin embedding, and immediate freezing. The formalin-fixed piece is stained with hematoxylin and eosin (H and E) because this permits a rapid means for initial evaluation. This is especially useful for identifying inflammatory myopathies where such a diagnosis offers the potential for successful therapeutic intervention. Frozen specimens are best for other stains, including nicotinamide adenosine dinucleotide dehydrogenase (NADH), modified Gomori trichrome, adenosine triphosphatase, and lipid and glycogen stains (Fig. 76-7 and see Fig. 76-5).

Muscle biopsy specimens are also subjected to biochemical analysis, mutational analysis, and electron microscopy, when these techniques are indicated. Inherited myopathies, such as the various muscular dystrophies, are evaluated by immunohistochemical stains, immunoblotting; testing is available for calpain, caveolin, dysferlin, the dystroglycans, dystrophin, laminin-2 (formerly merosin), and the sarcoglycans.

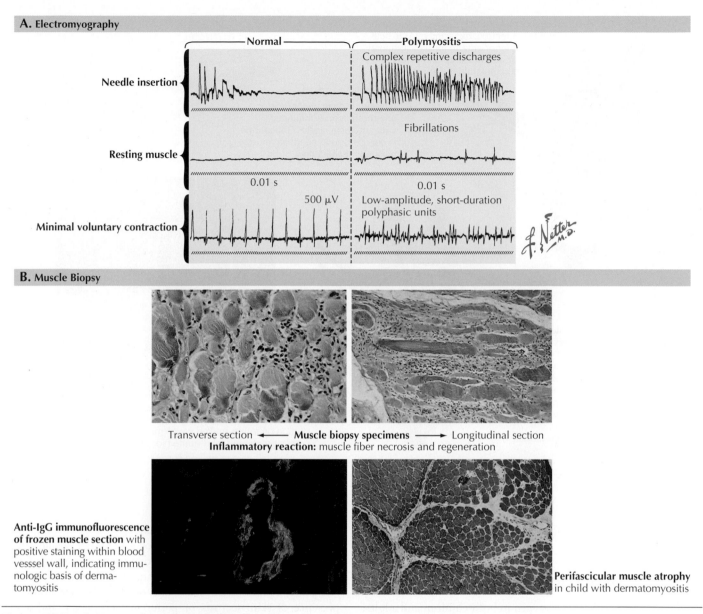

A. Electromyography

Normal — Polymyositis

Needle insertion

Complex repetitive discharges

Resting muscle

Fibrillations

0.01 s   0.01 s

500 μV   Low-amplitude, short-duration polyphasic units

Minimal voluntary contraction

B. Muscle Biopsy

Transverse section ◄── **Muscle biopsy specimens** ──► Longitudinal section
Inflammatory reaction: muscle fiber necrosis and regeneration

Anti-IgG immunofluorescence of frozen muscle section with positive staining within blood vesssel wall, indicating immunologic basis of dermatomyositis

Perifascicular muscle atrophy in child with dermatomyositis

Figure 76-5 Polymyositis/Dermatomyositis.

SPECIFIC INFLAMMATORY MYOPATHIC DISORDERS

There are three primary inflammatory disorders: polymyositis, dermatomyositis, and inclusion body myositis. Necrotizing myopathies are usually not considered to be inflammatory myopathies although there is some evidence that they may respond to immune-modifying treatment.

POLYMYOSITIS

This inflammatory myopathy is seen mainly in adults and presents subacutely usually over a period of several weeks to a few months. Clinically an important means for distinguishing polymyositis (PM) from dermatomyositis (DM) is the absence of skin involvement in PM. However, DM may also rarely present without skin involvement (sine dermatitis). Various criteria have

been proposed to make a definitive diagnosis of PM. Usually PM patients present with symmetric proximal weakness, involving the upper and lower extremities. Mild dysphagia, myalgia, and systemic symptoms, such as polyarthritis, may accompany the weakness. Rarely patients may present with either a clinically isolated head drop, or respiratory muscle weakness. Acid maltase deficiency, glycogen storage disease type II, needs to be considered in those individuals presenting primarily with pulmonary manifestations.

EMG is often abnormal and may show characteristic findings, myopathic motor units, and increased insertional activity, with fibrillation potentials and complex repetitive discharges. Laboratory studies reveal an elevated CK level. Muscle biopsy demonstrates perimysial and endomysial inflammatory infiltrate with CD8+ T cells invading nonnecrotic muscle fibers (see Fig. 76-5). Interstitial lung disease can be seen in 10–20% of patients with PM and may be associated with positive anti-Jo1 antibody. Cardiac involvement (cardiomyopathy and congestive heart

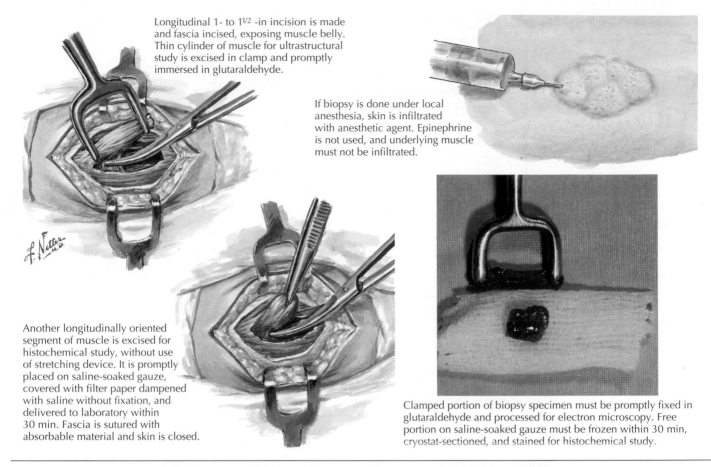

Longitudinal 1- to 1½-in incision is made and fascia incised, exposing muscle belly. Thin cylinder of muscle for ultrastructural study is excised in clamp and promptly immersed in glutaraldehyde.

If biopsy is done under local anesthesia, skin is infiltrated with anesthetic agent. Epinephrine is not used, and underlying muscle must not be infiltrated.

Another longitudinally oriented segment of muscle is excised for histochemical study, without use of stretching device. It is promptly placed on saline-soaked gauze, covered with filter paper dampened with saline without fixation, and delivered to laboratory within 30 min. Fascia is sutured with absorbable material and skin is closed.

Clamped portion of biopsy specimen must be promptly fixed in glutaraldehyde and processed for electron microscopy. Free portion on saline-soaked gauze must be frozen within 30 min, cryostat-sectioned, and stained for histochemical study.

Figure 76-6 Muscle Biopsy: Technique.

failure) is common, although the incidence of these associated conditions is unknown.

DERMATOMYOSITIS

Dermatomyositis (DM) is also seen in both children and adults. Proximal weakness develops insidiously over weeks. The characteristic rash may accompany or precede the myopathy (see Fig. 76-1). The rash is present over the exposed areas of the face, neck, and arms. Other dermatologic manifestations include heliotrope rash over the eyelids and erythematous rash over the knuckles, known as Gottron papules (Fig. 76-1, bottom). Nail bed examination will often demonstrate capillary telangiectasia. Occasional DM patients never develop this classic rash; here the differential diagnosis from PM is made on the classic pathologic findings of perifascicular atrophies in the muscle biopsy. In contrast, some patients present with the classic DM rash but paradoxically have no signs of a clinical myopathy (*amyopathic DM*). Other systemic manifestations include calcinosis, dysphagia, cardiomyopathy, and interstitial lung disease (ILD) (see Fig. 76-4). As in PM, ILD may be associated with positive anti-Jo 1 antibodies in some patients.

Dermatomyositis in adults may be associated with underlying malignancy. The cumulative incidence rate of malignancy varied from 20% at 1-year post DM diagnosis to approximately 30% five years after the diagnosis of DM. Adult patient should undergo evaluation for a possible underlying malignancy. The intensity of diagnostic evaluation for a potential occult cancer is determined individually. Factors that point to a higher likelihood of a paraneoplastic relationship include age at diagnosis >52 years, a rapid onset of skin and/or muscular symptoms, the presence of skin necrosis or periungual erythema, and a low baseline level of complement factor C4. This association with malignancy is not seen in juvenile DM and rarely if ever in polymyositis. A general physical examination, a thorough review of systems, a chest radiograph or computed tomography (CT), a mammogram (in women), a complete blood count (CBC), urinalysis, and stool guaiac, colonoscopy, Pap smears in women, and CT scan of abdomen and pelvis are considered a reasonable screening protocol.

Laboratory tests typically demonstrate the elevated CK. ANA and anti-Jo1 may be elevated. MRI usually shows inflammation in affected muscles. EMG will reveal characteristic myopathic changes in established disease. The characteristic histopathology in DM is perifascicular atrophy although this may not be seen in early disease (see Fig. 76-5). Inflammation is not prominent; when present it is seen in the perimysial and perivascular regions.

The pathogenesis of DM is thought to be a microangiopathy. A membrane attack complex (MAC) can be demonstrated on capillaries. Electron microscopy (EM) may reveal tubuloreticular inclusions in endothelial cells.

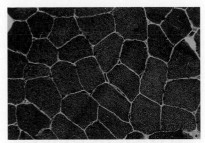

Cryostat section of normal adult muscle stained with hematoxylin and eosin. Muscle fibers are uniform in size and stain pink with eosin; their sarcolemmal nuclei are peripherally located and stain blue with hematoxylin.

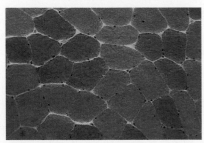

Cryostat section of normal adult muscle treated with modified Gomori trichrome stain, which stains muscle fibers greenish blue and sarcolemmal nuclei dark red.

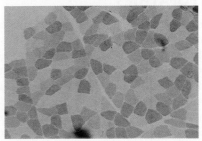

Cryostat section of normal muscle from adult male (ATPase stain, pH 4.6). Type II fibers, which contain low amounts of acid-stable ATPase, are subtyped into IIA (lightest) and IIB (intermediate) fibers. Type I (darkest) fibers contain largest amount of acid-stable ATPase. Each of these 3 fiber types amounts to about 1/3 of total number.

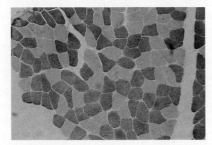

Cryostat section of normal muscle from adult male (ATPase stain, pH 9.4), showing typical checkerboard pattern with about twice as many type II fibers, which are high in alkali-stable ATPase and hence stain darkly.

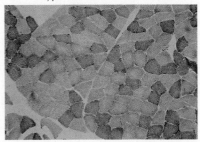

Cryostat section of normal adult muscle stained with NADH, an oxidative enzyme that reacts with mitochondria, sarcoplasmic reticulum, and T tubules. Type I fibers stain more darkly.

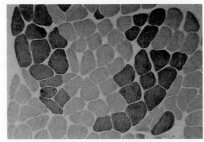

Cryostat section of reinnervated skeletal muscle stained with ATPase (pH 9.4), showing grouping of 2 fiber types: type I (lighter), type II (darker). Compare with normal section stained with ATPase (pH 9.4) above.

Figure 76-7 Sections from Muscle Biopsy Specimens.

TREATMENT OF POLYMYOSITIS AND DERMATOMYOSITIS

Muscle disorders are best managed by considering disease-specific therapies, genetic counseling, and various forms of supportive care. Unfortunately, few specific pharmacologic therapies are currently available for the myopathies. Directed therapies are anticipated for a number of genetic disorders but are not yet available.

Specific Pharmacologic Therapies

Polymyositis, dermatomyositis, and idiopathic, inflammatory, and granulomatous myopathies are often somewhat responsive to immunomodulation treatments. Prednisone is the gold standard, although its efficacy has never been confirmed in a well-designed prospective study; typically, prednisone equivalents of 1–1.5 mg/kg/day are started. In order to diminish the severity of the corticosteroid side effects, alternate-day dosing and appropriate dose tapers must be considered as soon as symptoms are adequately controlled. Sequential CK measurements may be useful in following disease activity, and a rise in CK may herald a clinical relapse while on treatment. Previous tuberculosis exposure should be excluded before initiation of steroid treatment. Vitamin D and calcium are regularly supplemented in patients on prednisone, particularly in women. Bone densitometry is indicated for patients at risk of osteopenia. Serum glucose and potassium levels need to be monitored at regular intervals and treated or supplemented when needed.

Other immunomodulation therapies including intravenous immunoglobulin (IVIG), plasma exchange, azathioprine, methotrexate, mycophenolate mofetil, and monoclonal antibody against CD20-positive lymphocytes, known as rituximab, are available.

INCLUSION BODY MYOSITIS

Clinical Vignette

A 74-year-old woman complained of progressive difficulty walking dating back the past 5 years. Recently she found it especially difficult to negotiate her stairs at home. She also reported several falls in the past 6 months, all of them due to "knee buckling and legs giving out." Lately she had noted difficulty using her hands, especially when she needed to grip things firmly.

Neurologic examination revealed significant weakness of the finger flexors bilaterally; quadriceps weakness was also present—this was severe on the left and mild on the right. There was also mild weakness of the right wrist, ankle dorsiflexors, and neck flexors. Ankle jerks were diminished; the remainder of muscle stretch reflexes and sensory examination results were normal.

Serum CK was increased to 900 IU/L. Nerve conduction studies were normal. EMG revealed a mixed myopathic–neuropathic pattern of motor units with increased insertional activity and fibrillation potentials. Muscle biopsy of the left quadriceps demonstrated endomysial inflammation and atrophic and hypertrophic fibers. Rimmed vacuoles were identified with a modified Gomori trichrome stain. Electron microscopy revealed tubofilament inclusion bodies in affected fibers.

Inclusion body myositis is the most common inflammatory myopathy occurring in patients older than age 50. It is often an insidiously progressive condition often presenting after years of subtle symptoms. Men are more commonly affected. IBM is frequently characterized by the finding of an asymmetric weakness that typically affects the finger and wrist flexors in the upper extremities as well as quadriceps and tibialis anterior in the lower extremities. Dysphagia may also occur. An associated sensory neuropathy may occur in IBM patients. Usually there is no involvement of the other systems. Unlike that in PM or DM, there is no associated interstitial lung disease, myocarditis, or malignancy.

Laboratory tests reveal an elevated CK (usually three to six times normal). EMG will usually reveal myopathic findings although occasionally the clinical and EMG findings may be misinterpreted as being consistent with amyotrophic lateral sclerosis. However, the mixture of myopathic as well as neurogenic changes often provides a clue to the primary pathophysiology. Muscle biopsy demonstrates endomysial inflammation and the characteristic rimmed vacuoles, which may stain positive for amyloid, although sampling error may occur and the absence of rimmed vacuoles does not exclude the possibility of IBM. Intranuclear and intracytoplasmic tubulofilament inclusions are demonstrated by electron microscopy.

The precise pathogenesis of IBM is unknown. Muscle biopsy demonstrates a definite inflammatory component. However, despite therapeutic trials of a number of various immunosuppressive pharmacologic agents, none of the traditional immunomodulation therapies are beneficial.

The general prognosis for an IBM patient is of a slowly ingravescent course with various limitations, particularly due to finger flexor weakness, that impairs fine manipulations such as buttoning clothes, handwriting, and putting keys into locks. However, the overall affect on these patients is such that there is not an increased mortality rate; their major hazard relates to the potential for aspiration secondary to upper pharyngeal muscle involvement.

OTHER ACQUIRED MYOPATHIES

TOXIC MYOPATHIES

Many pharmacologic agents may cause myopathies as rare adverse effects of their use (Box 76-1). The almost ubiquitously utilized HMG–CoA reductase inhibitor (statin) class of lipid-lowering agents may cause a necrotizing myopathy in a small percentage of these patients. Muscle biopsies in severely affected patients demonstrate necrosis and mitochondrial changes.

More commonly, a slightly larger percentage develops an asymptomatic hyperCKemia. This is thought to be related to subclinical muscle inflammation. On other occasions, some patients taking statins present with myalgias, and/or proximal weakness. Very rarely a rhabdomyolysis may develop in this setting. The risk for muscle toxicity increases in patients simultaneously exposed to multiple potentially myotoxic drugs. Fibric acid derivatives and niacin also occasionally demonstrate myotoxic properties.

Chloroquine may cause an amphiphilic neuromyopathy. These patients classically demonstrate both a peripheral neuropathy and a myopathy. This combination is very typical for chloroquine per se and the physician always needs to inquire about the possibility of the patient utilizing this medication. The serum CK level is often modestly increased in this setting. Muscle biopsy characteristically reveals an autophagic vacuolation, with markedly increased staining for acid phosphatase.

Chronic administration of steroids, typically at doses higher than 30 g/day, can also cause a myopathy. Steroid myopathy can present acutely or subacutely, classically with preferential involvement of the proximal lower extremities. Bulbar and distal muscles, sensation, and reflexes are typically spared.

Box 76-1 Toxic Myopathies	
Alcohol	Leuprolide
Aminocaproic acid	Lithium
Amiodarone	l-Tryptophan
Chloroquine/ hydroxychloroquine	Neuromuscular blocking agents
Cholesterol-lowering agents	Omeprazole
Cimetidine	Penicillamine
Colchicine	Procainamide
Corticosteroids	Propofol
Cyclosporine	Rifampin
Emetine	Tacrolimus
Illicit drugs (intramuscular injections)	Toluene (inhalation)
	Vincristine
Ipecac	Vitamin E
Labetalol	Zidovudine
Lamotrigine	

Importantly, CK is normal. Nerve conduction and needle EMG are typically normal, and muscle biopsy may demonstrate atrophy of type II (especially IIB) fibers, lipid droplets within type I fibers, and rarely abnormal mitochondria on electron microscopy.

Amiodarone is an antiarrhythmic drug that causes a neuromyopathy similar to that produced by chloroquine. It can also cause myopathy indirectly, by inducing hypothyroidism.

Colchicine may also cause either a myopathy or neuropathy, which may be related to colchicine-induced alteration of microtubular function. CK is usually increased, and muscle biopsies demonstrate autophagic vacuoles. Symptoms improve with drug discontinuation.

Immunosuppressive agents including cyclosporine and Tacrolimus may cause generalized myalgias and proximal muscle weakness within months after starting therapy. The pathogenic basis for this effect is still unknown; there is some suggestion that cyclosporine myotoxicity may have a pathogenesis similar to that of statins. There is a further increased risk of developing a myopathy when patients take both cyclosporine and statins.

Labetalol is an antihypertensive drug that has been associated with rare reports of necrotizing myopathy. Symptoms improve after discontinuation of the drug.

Propofol is a relatively newer anesthetic agent increasingly used in sedating ventilated patients. There have been reports of rhabdomyolysis and myoglobinuria described in children, but not in adults. Vincristine, a chemotherapeutic agent, acts by disrupting the polymerization of tubulin into microtubules. It is classically associated with a severe sensorimotor axonal neuropathy, but occasionally it can also cause proximal muscle weakness accompanied by myalgias.

Zidovudine (AZT), a primary therapy for HIV infection, can induce a myopathy related to mitochondrial dysfunction. The myopathies caused by zidovudine and by HIV infection are clinically indistinguishable. CK values are usually increased. EMG does not distinguish between toxic AZT and HIV myopathies. Muscle biopsies demonstrate endomysial inflammation. Prominent ragged red fibers suggest AZT-induced mitochondrial abnormalities. AZT myopathies usually improve on drug cessation.

CRITICAL ILLNESS MYOPATHY

Critical illness myopathy (CIM) is also referred to as acute quadriplegic myopathy or myopathy associated with thick filament (myosin) loss. It is probably the most common cause of generalized weakness identified for patients having a prolonged stay in the ICU. CIM is commonly seen in patients treated with high doses of corticosteroids or neuromuscular blocking drugs. Often these patients were initially septic and developed multiorgan failure. It may be associated with a sensorimotor axonal polyneuropathy (critical illness neuropathy).

The weakness in these patients develops over several days. It is often not recognized until there is an attempt to wean the patient from their ventilator. Clinical examination reveals a profound, occasionally asymmetric, weakness, with reduced muscle stretch reflexes, but a normal sensory examination. Serum CK is increased in less than half of these patients. Muscle biopsies may demonstrate muscle fiber necrosis, atrophy of type 1 and 2 fibers, and patchy loss of uptake with adenosine triphosphatase stains; the latter correlates with electron microscopic demonstration of thick filament (myosin) loss. The pathogenesis of this entity is not known.

HYPOKALEMIC MYOPATHIES

Hypokalemia is a rare metabolic cause of an acute myopathy (Fig. 76-8). The presentation may mimic Guillain–Barré syndrome. ICU observation is recommended because of potential serious cardiac arrhythmias that the severe hypokalemia may induce. The differential diagnosis includes various potassium-losing diuretics and corticosteroids and other medications (e.g.,

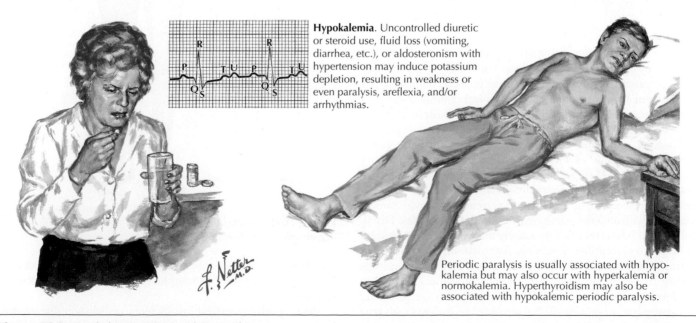

Hypokalemia. Uncontrolled diuretic or steroid use, fluid loss (vomiting, diarrhea, etc.), or aldosteronism with hypertension may induce potassium depletion, resulting in weakness or even paralysis, areflexia, and/or arrhythmias.

Periodic paralysis is usually associated with hypokalemia but may also occur with hyperkalemia or normokalemia. Hyperthyroidism may also be associated with hypokalemic periodic paralysis.

Figure 76-8 Hypokalemia Associated Myopathy.

laxatives, lithium, or amphotericin). Chronic alcoholism, rarely hyperaldosteronism or a villous adenoma of the colon, and very excessive intakes of licorice, are other important causes of hypokalemia-induced weakness.

ENDOCRINE MYOPATHIES

Clinical Vignette

A 41-year-old woman had typical myopathic symptoms. Her husband noted that her emotions were more labile. Neurologic examination demonstrated moderate proximal weakness. Serum CK was normal but the aldolase was mildly elevated. When she returned for her EMG, the neurologist noted generalized bruising that resembled that of patients taking corticosteroids, although neither was she taking same nor were there any apparent other common stigmata of Cushing syndrome. The patient's EMG demonstrated myopathic motor unit potentials with fibrillation potentials.

Because of her obvious classic dermatologic stigmata, Cushing syndrome was considered in the differential of this slowly evolving myopathy. Serum cortisol and particularly urinary free cortisol levels as well as 24-hour 17-OH corticosteroids were increased. An endocrinologist also found historical evidence of easy bruising, and recent-onset hypertension; this exam demonstrated very mild increase in facial hair, slight mooning of her facies, but no abdominal striae or shoulder hump. Elevated ACTH levels led to the diagnosis of a corticotrophin-producing pituitary tumor.

Comment: This patient's clinical picture was suggestive of a proximal myopathy and the easy bruising on examination led to the suspicion of Cushing syndrome. Clinically the typical features of Cushing syndrome were quite subtle. Her EMG findings were surprising because most endocrine myopathies, including corticosteroid-induced myopathies, are not associated with myopathic MUPs or abnormal insertional activity. Despite such, laboratory tests confirmed the diagnosis of Cushing disease.

Disorders of the adrenal, thyroid, parathyroid, and pituitary glands can result in subacute or, less commonly, acute myopathies. Interestingly, muscle involvement in such conditions may be apparent before patients develop typical clinical findings of their primary endocrinopathy. This is well illustrated by the prior vignette.

Cushing syndrome due to hyperadrenocorticism is either primary, iatrogenic, or rarely secondary to excessive pituitary secretion of ACTH (Fig. 76-9). This is one of the more common causes of an endocrine myopathy. Patients with Cushing syndrome, irrespective of etiology, experience proximal muscle weakness with atrophy usually starting in the hip girdles. Distal, bulbar, and ocular muscles are usually unaffected. Women seem to be more susceptible than men. Alternate-day corticosteroid dosing schedules and enriched protein diets may reduce susceptibility to iatrogenic induced Cushing syndrome. The serum CK level is usually normal. EMG is normal in iatrogenic steroid myopathy but is occasionally "myopathic" in patients with true Cushing syndrome. Muscle biopsy demonstrates a nonspecific

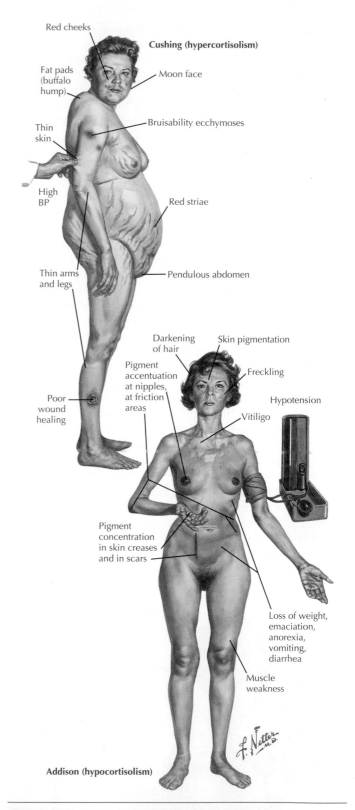

Figure 76-9 Cushing (hypercortisolism) and Addison (hypocortisolism) Syndrome.

type II muscle fiber atrophy. The pathogenesis of the myopathy is poorly understood but may be related to increased protein catabolism.

Primary adrenocortical insufficiency or Addison disease may be associated with a myopathy. Addison disease is characterized

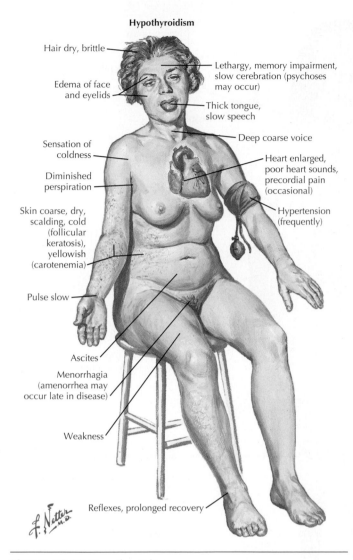

Hypothyroidism

Hair dry, brittle

Edema of face and eyelids

Lethargy, memory impairment, slow cerebration (psychoses may occur)

Thick tongue, slow speech

Deep coarse voice

Sensation of coldness

Heart enlarged, poor heart sounds, precordial pain (occasional)

Diminished perspiration

Hypertension (frequently)

Skin coarse, dry, scalding, cold (follicular keratosis), yellowish (carotenemia)

Pulse slow

Ascites

Menorrhagia (amenorrhea may occur late in disease)

Weakness

Reflexes, prolonged recovery

Figure 76-10 Hypothyroidism.

by weight loss, bronzing of the skin, hypotension, and hyperkalemia (see Fig. 76-9). Muscle weakness may be an early symptom of this disease and may be due to the associated hyperkalemia.

Thyroid dysfunction is another important consideration in the differential diagnosis of adult-onset myopathies. Hypothyroidism-associated myopathy is characterized by proximal weakness, fatigue, slowed movements and reflexes, stiffness, myalgia, and muscle cramps (Fig. 76-10). An elevated CK, sometimes up to 10 times normal, is a common finding in hypothyroid patients.

Hyperthyroidism-induced myopathy may also present with weakness, and the incidence of weakness in patients with thyrotoxicosis is high (up to 82%). Patients with thyrotoxicosis tend to have proximal muscle weakness and fatigue as prominent complaints (Fig. 76-11). Serum enzyme levels including CPK and AST tend to be normal.

In addition to typical myopathic features, hyperthyroid patients have brisk muscle stretch reflexes, thyroid eye disease with proptosis, and impairment of extraocular muscle function. Furthermore, myasthenia gravis occurs in approximately 5%

of thyrotoxic patients. Asian males with hyperthyroidism also have a propensity to hypokalemic periodic paralysis. Serum CK and routine electrodiagnostic study results are usually normal.

Hyperparathyroidism may be associated with a painful myopathy. This most likely relates to an interchange with vitamin D metabolism and resultant osteomalacia.

OSTEOMALACIA, HYPOVITAMIN D MYOPATHY

Lack of vitamin D can lead to decreased calcium and phosphorus absorption and secondary hyperparathyroidism with eventual osteomalacia. This is associated with an unusual but very treatable myopathy with associated bone pain, loss of appendicular height, and kyphoscoliosis.

Although usually considered in chronic renal failure, osteomalacic myopathy may also occur in patients receiving long-term treatment with phenytoin or with various malabsorptive syndromes. Individuals taking statins are more prone to developing symptomatic myositis secondary to hypovitaminosis D. Supplementation of same may totally relieve the symptoms of a painful myopathy while continuing to utilize the statin medication. An unusual setting for development of hypovitaminosis D and osteomalacia occurs in societies where women traditionally are almost totally veiled whenever outside of their homes. Serum vitamin D levels may be very low while CK and electrodiagnostic studies are normal. Muscle biopsy, if performed, demonstrates type II fiber atrophy. Vitamin D and calcium supplementation can lead to excellent improvement.

GRANULOMATOUS MYOPATHIES

Although patients with sarcoidosis often have granulomas in muscle tissue, most commonly these patients have no clinical evidence of a myopathy. However, when these are symptomatic, focal pain, atrophy, or generalized proximal weakness may be seen. Diagnosis usually requires involvement of other end organs typically involved by sarcoidosis, particularly the liver or lungs. Nonspecific inflammatory granulomatous myopathies are rare, although they may be seen with underlying myasthenia gravis and thymoma. Ocular and bulbar symptoms attributable to myasthenia may accompany proximal weakness.

EOSINOPHILIC MYOPATHY

This myopathy is usually present as a component of the hypereosinophilic syndrome. The pattern of weakness is indistinguishable from that of the inflammatory myopathies. Systemic features of hypereosinophilic syndrome involve the heart, lungs, skin, kidneys, and gastrointestinal tract.

INFECTIOUS MYOPATHIES

Human immunodeficiency virus (HIV) infection may produce a primary inflammatory myopathy with subacute or chronic proximal weakness and myalgia. Typically seen in patients with CD4 counts of less than 200/mm³, HIV myopathy may be difficult to distinguish from polymyositis.

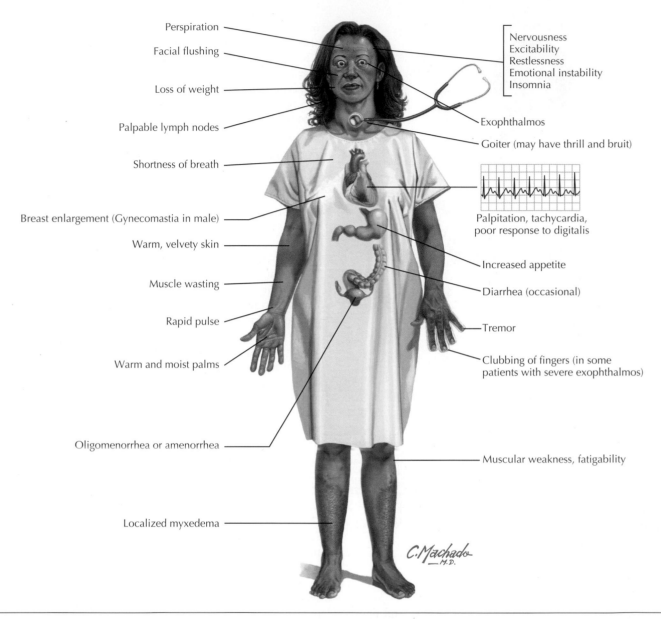

Perspiration

Facial flushing

Loss of weight

Palpable lymph nodes

Shortness of breath

Breast enlargement (Gynecomastia in male)

Warm, velvety skin

Muscle wasting

Rapid pulse

Warm and moist palms

Oligomenorrhea or amenorrhea

Localized myxedema

Nervousness
Excitability
Restlessness
Emotional instability
Insomnia

Exophthalmos

Goiter (may have thrill and bruit)

Palpitation, tachycardia, poor response to digitalis

Increased appetite

Diarrhea (occasional)

Tremor

Clubbing of fingers (in some patients with severe exophthalmos)

Muscular weakness, fatigability

Figure 76-11 Hyperthyroidism (Graves Disease).

Nonspecific viral syndromes, particularly in relation to the enteric and influenza viruses, often cause significant myalgia in their prodromal phases. An acute relatively specific viral myositis occasionally occurs in children. It presents with prominent calf pain and toe walking. The CK level is usually increased; EMG may demonstrate myopathic changes, and muscle biopsy reveals scattered necrotic and regenerating fibers. The course is self-limiting. Rarely, there may be severe muscle rhabdomyolysis with significant increase of CK, myoglobinuria, and consequent metabolic derangement.

Trichinosis, typically caused by the ingestion of inadequately cooked pork, is the most common parasitic infection of muscle. Some patients have a prodrome of nausea, vomiting, and periorbital edema within days after exposure. Strikingly severe myalgia, weakness, fever, and sometimes encephalopathy then develop. Occasionally, trichinosis causes a chronic myopathy. Typically there is an associated eosinophilic leukocytosis. The serum CK level may be increased. Muscle biopsy sometimes demonstrates organisms and eosinophilic infiltration.

Pyomyositis is a rare primary bacterial infection characterized by a focal myopathy. This is primarily seen in the tropics. It is more common in immunodeficient individuals. A variety of gram-positive and -negative organisms have been associated with this. Muscle pain, tenderness, and fever are prominent. Neutrophilic leukocytosis and bacteremia also occur. CT and MRI of muscle may demonstrate muscle abscesses.

PARANEOPLASTIC NECROTIZING MYOPATHY

Paraneoplastic necrotizing myopathies are rare and are typically associated with lung, gastrointestinal, or adenocarcinoma. They typically present with gradually progressive proximal weakness with or without myalgias. The serum CK level is often increased.

Necrotic muscle fibers with "pipestem" arterioles and capillaries with perivascular inflammation are notable histologic findings.

TREATMENT OF MYOPATHIES

Toxic myopathies and critical illness myopathy most commonly resolve within weeks to months of withdrawal of the offending agent. In this instance treatment is supportive, and most patients fully recover muscle strength.

The myotoxicity of cholesterol-lowering agents creates a common and vexing clinical problem. In some patients, CK increases and myalgia persist long after cholesterol-lowering agents are withdrawn. The basis for this phenomenon is unknown. However, recent evidence suggests that some people with statin myopathy are vitamin D deficient. Replacement of same while maintaining statin therapy leads to complete recovery in most of these individuals.

Endocrine myopathies are responsive to treatment of hormonal excess or deficiency. Corticosteroid-induced endocrine myopathies usually respond to cessation of steroid therapy or treatment of primary pituitary or adrenal lesions. Some infectious myopathies, such as trichinosis, may respond to antimicrobial agents, corticosteroids, or both. Treatment of pyomyositis consists of appropriate antibiotics and surgical drainage of abscesses.

SUPPORTIVE THERAPIES

The goal of all treatments is maximization of patient function. Most patients with significant myopathies benefit from the involvement of a physiatrist early in the course of their illness. Rehabilitation specialists are best able to decide what form of support aids, including braces, canes, crutches, walkers, wheelchairs, lift chairs, stair lifts, elevators, bed rails, and lifting devices, are best suited for the individual patient. Lift chairs are beneficial to ambulatory patients with proximal weakness that precludes them from independently rising from a chair. Elevators and stair lifts are valuable when accessing more than one floor. Newer lift systems allow patient transfers with the help of a single individual. Crutches are of limited value for patients with myopathy because of concomitant arm weakness.

PROGNOSIS

Control rather than immediate cure is often the most realistic initial management goal. DM and PM eventually stabilize or achieve a good to excellent remission, but drug therapy may be required for months or years. Patients with IBM usually have a normal lifespan but some require a wheelchair within 10–15 years after diagnosis. Patients with endocrine, metabolic, infectious, toxic, and vitamin D deficiency myopathies that are usually amenable to treatment generally have an excellent prognosis. The prognosis of paraneoplastic necrotizing myopathies is dependent on that of the underlying malignancy.

ADDITIONAL RESOURCES

Ahmed W, Khan N, Glueck CJ, et al. Low serum 25 (OH) vitamin D levels (<32 ng/mL) are associated with reversible myositis-myalgia in statin-treated patients. Transl Res 2009 Jan;153(1):11-16.

Amato AA, Barohn RJ. Inclusion body myositis: old and new concepts. J Neurol Neurosurg Psychiatry 2009;80:1186-1193.

Amato AA, Russell JA. Neuromuscular Disorders. New York: McGraw-Hill; 2008.

Davies NP, Hanna MG. The skeletal muscle channelopathies: distinct entities and overlapping syndromes. Curr Opin Neurol 2003;16:559-568.

DiMauro S, Lamperti C. Muscle glycogenoses. Muscle Nerve 2001;24: 984-999.

Engel AG. Metabolic and endocrine myopathies. In: Walton NJ, editor. Disorders of voluntary muscle. 5th ed. Edinburgh: Churchill-Livingstone; 1988.

Engel AG, Banker BQ, editors. Myology. New York: McGraw-Hill; 1986.

Fardet L, Dupuy A, Gain M, et al. Factors associated with underlying malignancy in a retrospective cohort of 121 patients with dermatomyositis. Medicine (Baltimore) 2009 Mar;88(2):91-97.

Felice KJ, Schneebaum AB, Jones HR. McArdle's disease with late onset symptoms. J Neurol Neurosurg Psychiatry 1992;55:407-408.

Ferrante MA, Wilbourn AJ. Myopathies. In: Levin KH, Luders HO, editors. Comprehensive Clinical Neurophysiology. Philadelphia, Pa: WB Saunders; 2000. p. 268-281.

Griggs RC, Engel WK, Resnick JS. Acetazolamide treatment of periodic paralysis. Ann Int Med 1970;73:39-48.

Griggs RC, Mendell JR, Miller RG. Evaluation and Treatment of Myopathy. Philadelphia, Pa: FA Davis Co; 1995.

Haller RG, Knochel JP. Metabolic myopathies. In: Johnson RT, Griffin JW, editors. Current Therapy in Neurologic Disease. St. Louis, Mo: Mosby-Year Book; 1993. p. 397-402.

Jones, HR, Darras, B, De Vivo DC. Neuromuscular disorders of infancy, childhood, and adolescence: a clinician's approach. Elsevier Health Sciences 2002.

Katirji B, Al-Jaberi MM. Creatine kinase revisited. J Clin Neuromusc Dis 2001;2:158-163.

McManis PG, Lambert EH, Daube JR. The exercise test in periodic paralysis. Muscle Nerve 1986;8:704-710.

Miller A. Muscle disease. In: American Academy of Neurology. Continuum. Philadelphia, Pa: Lippincott Williams & Wilkins; 2006. p. 12:No 3.

Moxley RT III. Channelopathies affecting skeletal muscle in childhood: myotonic disorders including myotonic dystrophy and periodic paralysis. In: Jones HR, De Vivo DC, Darras BT, editors. Neuromuscular Disorders of Infancy, Childhood, and Adolescence. Philadelphia, Pa: Butterworth-Heinemann; 2003. p. 1017-1035.

Muthukrishnan J, Jha S, Modi KD, et al. Symptomatic primary hyperparathyroidism: a retrospective analysis of fifty one cases from a single centre. J Assoc Physicians India 2008 Jul;56:503-507.

Al-Said YA, Al-Rached HS, Al-Qahtani HA, et al. Severe proximal myopathy with remarkable recovery after vitamin D treatment. Can J Neurol Sci 2009 May;36(3):336-339.

Simmons A, Peterlin BL, Boyer PJ, et al. Muscle biopsy in the evaluation of patients with modestly elevated creatine kinase levels. Muscle Nerve 2003;27:242-244.

Tonin P, Lewis P, Servidei S, et al. Metabolic causes of myoglobinuria. Ann Neurol 1990;27:181-185.

Warren JD, Blumberg PC, Thompson PD. Rhabdomyolysis. Muscle Nerve 2002;25:332-347.

Index

Page numbers followed by *f* indicate figures; *t*, tables; *b*, boxes.